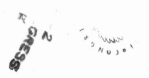

D1466012

DUNCAN E. REID, M.D.

Kate Macy Ladd Professor of Obstetrics and Gynecology,
Harvard Medical School; Chief of Staff,
Boston Hospital for Women

KENNETH J. RYAN, M.D.

Professor of Reproductive Biology,
Chairman, Department of Obstetrics and Gynecology
University of California, San Diego
La Jolla, California

KURT BENIRSCHKE, M.D.

Professor of Reproductive Biology and Pathology
Department of Obstetrics and Gynecology
University of California, San Diego
La Jolla, California

PRINCIPLES AND MANAGEMENT OF HUMAN REPRODUCTION

W. B. SAUNDERS COMPANY — Philadelphia · London · Toronto

W. B. Saunders Company: West Washington Square
Philadelphia, Pa. 19105

12 Dyott Street
London, WC1A 1DB

833 Oxford Street
Toronto 18, Ontario

Principles and Management of Human Reproduction   ISBN 0-7216-7532-8

Print No.:   9   8   7   6   5   4   3   2

*This book is dedicated
to those who
work toward achievement of
the initial right of man
to be born without handicap
and the privilege of woman
to bear without injury*

Preface

In keeping with concepts put forth in Reid's *Textbook of Obstetrics* (Saunders, 1962), its transformation into *Principles and Management of Human Reproduction* has occurred in a setting of burgeoning knowledge in this field, stimulated to a large extent by societal concern about the quantity and quality of human life.

Advances have occurred in our understanding of many aspects of reproductive processes which have altered the approach to the care of patients. As a consequence of endocrine and reproduction research, one can measure steroid and protein hormones with precision in minute amounts of blood throughout the cycle and pregnancy. Human follicle-stimulating and luteinizing hormones are available for induction of ovulation, and the isolation and structural identity of hypothalamic releasing hormones have been achieved. Details of the dynamics of the feto-placental unit during human pregnancy are more completely defined.

Genetic assessment of the fetus in utero, of the newborn, and of prospective parents has contributed materially to a rational approach in management of and counseling in hereditary diseases, including mental retardation and congenital defects. Monitoring of the fetus in utero by electronic and chemical means assures a more adequate surveillance of the infant's health prior to birth, even to the point of predicting respiratory competence in the newborn period. Treatment and prevention of the hitherto disastrous consequences of diseases such as choriocarcinoma and Rh isoimmunization are dramatic examples of progress made in recent years.

Principles and Management of Human Reproduction has been divided into sections covering: endocrine and neuroendocrine control, physiology, pathology, clinical obstetrics, neonatology, and public health aspects of reproduction.

This arrangement was designed to aid readers of varying backgrounds and interest, the "student of medicine," whether he be in medical school, internship-residency training, or the clinical practice of obstetrics and gynecology.

It is the hope that principles have been emphasized, controversy identified, and the minutiae of a specialty avoided. Thus, it has been the authors' objective to relate the process of human reproduction to the general framework of medicine and biology. Emphasis has been placed on the interaction of medical and surgical diseases in pregnancy and on the disciplines fundamental to the understanding of reproductive processes. The concern here has been to see obstetrics and the physiology of human reproduction in a meaningful relationship. Furthermore, the ultimate aim of medical science is the prevention of disease, and the first step must be related to life at its inception.

DUNCAN E. REID

KENNETH J. RYAN

KURT BENIRSCHKE

Acknowledgments

As stated in the Preface, if obstetrics and related areas of gynecology are to be soundly practiced and patients optimally served, it is imperative that the more basic aspects of human reproduction be emphasized. To attain this objective, two former associates and authorities in reproductive biology, Drs. Kenneth J. Ryan and Kurt Benirschke, kindly accepted my request to assume joint authorship.

In Part I Dr. Ryan presents a unified concept of endocrinology, particularly as it relates to the development and growth of the new individual and the overall process of reproduction. Dr. Benirschke is responsible for much of Parts II and III, particularly genetics, immunology, the biology of multiple pregnancy, and the role of infection in the outcome of the fetus and newborn.

I am indebted to Drs. Fred H. Allen, Jr., and Irving Umansky for the chapter on Erythroblastosis Fetalis. Also, Dr. Jerold F. Lucey contributed immeasurably to the chapters on the evaluation and examination of, and conditions and diseases in, the newborn. Each has brought to his writing the background of a rich clinical experience.

The remarks on psychiatric states most often encountered in women in the childbearing age reflect my long-time association with Dr. Mandel E. Cohen.

The manuscript has been under the supervision of Miss Ruth E. Brown. We are deeply grateful for her infinite patience and efforts and her meticulous concern for each chapter.

Finally, the assistance and patience of the W. B. Saunders Company was again in evidence. The authors are especially obligated to Miss Elizabeth Taylor, and the expert advice and help of Mr. John L. Dusseau is again deeply appreciated.

DUNCAN E. REID, M.D.

Contents

PART I

The Endocrine and Neuroendocrine Control of Reproduction

"Endocrines are nature's gift to man and beast, without them he can neither grow nor reproduce. They are the architects of love and marriage, the paramount basis of every social order."[*] These "endocrines" do not work alone, however; they depend upon a complex nervous system–endocrine interplay that regulates the fundamental processes of reproduction and homeostasis.

As animal life evolved from unicellular to multicellular organisms, from aquatic to terrestrial forms, from asexual to sexual reproduction, from monoecious (hermaphrodites) to dioecius (separate sexes) individuals, the endocrine glands and their neurologic control mechanisms continually developed and adapted to the needs imposed by these changes in life style and means of replication. Endocrine and neurologic processes have been the facilitating bases for the evolution of reproduction, and it is supposedly not the hormones themselves that have evolved and varied so much as the diverse roles that they play in different species. Hence one finds the same hor-

mones—estrogens, progestins, oxytocins—in a broad spectrum of animal life (fish, birds, reptiles, and mammals) but the hormonal function in any given animal seems to depend upon an evolutionary need.

EVOLUTION OF REPRODUCTION

The general forms of evolutionary reproductive processes from those in simple animal life to the eutherian mammals and man include:

1. *Reduction of the number of ova shed for fertilization at any given time, from the extremes of millions in fish to one in the human.* This reduction in number of ova released to one a month in man created a requirement for careful control of ovulatory timing and the need for a high success rate for fertilization and fetal development via internal fertilization and viviparity, all subject to evolving neuroendocrine control.

2. *Internal fertilization.* This means of fertilization is characteristic of all land forms of animal life (as well as of some fish) and was accomplished by changes in socialization and the cues for sexual receptivity,

---

[*]Greep, R. O.: The Presidential Address of the Endocrine Society. Endocrinology: orphan and Cinderella science. Endocrinology, 79:823, 1966.

such as the estrus phenomenon, which are under endocrine direction.

3. *Retention of the embryo and fetus within the mother and birth of live young by ovoviviparity or viviparity.* This process is seen not only in mammals but also in insects, cartilaginous and bony fish, amphibia, and reptiles. Viviparity, at least in man and most mammals, imposed the requirement for development of immune tolerance by the mother for the infant maintained within her. Requirements were also generated for physical accommodation of the conceptus, for life support by exchange of nutrients and wastes, and finally for a mechanism of parturition, all of which are largely endocrine-regulated.

4. *Development of new organs for exchange in the form of extraembryonic membranes and placenta.* These organs fulfill the needs imposed by viviparity as already noted.

5. *Acquisition by the placenta of endocrine function and provision for postpartum nutrition by lactation.* Placental endocrine function seems to be an accommodation to a lengthening of the gestational period and insures hormonal support of pregnancy for prolonged periods. Postpartum lactation and maternal behavior provide a degree of nutritional and physical security for the newborn that is especially critical for terrestrial animals with a limited number of offspring.

REPRODUCTIVE ENDOCRINOLOGY IN MAN

The status of reproduction in man at this point in evolution consists of: monthly ovulation of a single ovum, internal fertilization, a long gestational period, viviparity, a hormonally active placenta, parturition through a pelvic girdle modified by the erect posture, and postpartum lactation. This is a far cry from the simplest forms of replication, division of a single cell in a unicellular organism, or the release of eggs by fish with external fertilization. Reduced to its fundamentals, however, reproduction in man and other mammals represents no more than a continuum of hereditary information passed on from one generation to the next by the germ cells. The entire body may be viewed as merely a repository, conveyer, and incubator for the gametes which are sequestered in the gonads await-

ing release, fertilization, and development. This continuous and cyclic process is thus fundamentally simple in the concept of a germ cell continuum but extremely complex in the organizational control of the body in accomplishing the task.

For reproduction in all higher forms of animal life certain hormones such as estrogens and progestins are essential. A large part of the working of reproductive endocrinology depends on how and where such hormones are produced and how they influence gestation. To provide these hormones in proper association with gamete development and fertilization requires a highly complex interplay between the central nervous system, the hypothalamus, the gonadotropin-secreting adenohypophysis, the steroid- and gamete-producing gonads, and the reproductive tract. After implantation there is an interaction between the developing fetus, the placenta, and the maternal organism that supersedes much of the endocrine mechanism of the nonpregnant state. In the chapters that follow, the discussion of the reproductive process will be developed by consideration of: the hormones, the endocrine glands that produce them, and finally the integrative mechanisms that control the various aspects of the reproductive cycle.

HORMONES OF REPRODUCTION

The most proximate circulating effector substances now known for control and maintenance of gestation are hormones, of which six should be singled out for consideration in detail: estrogens, progesterone, human chorionic gonadotropin, human chorionic somato-mammotropin (placental lactogen), oxytocin, and pituitary prolactin. These six hormones figure extensively in the literature of obstetrics and reproduction because of their central role in various aspects of the pregnant state.

In addition to estrogens and progestins, the androgens and the pituitary gonadotropins are involved in the reproductive cycles of both male and female, and hormonal substances such as relaxin and catecholamines and the more recently discovered prostaglandins have as yet poorly understood roles in human reproduction.

The other major hormonal substances, namely growth hormone, insulin, adrenal corticoids, and thyroxin, generally contribute homeostatic support for the pregnant state, which is essential but somewhat peripheral to the direct endocrine control of gestation. These latter hormones are essential for good health in general and for replication as just one of the normal bodily functions. Their absence can be immediately life-threatening to the human whether pregnant or not. On the other hand, absence of sex hormones and gonadotropins is not immediately life-threatening but their presence is more fundamentally essential for reproduction to take place.

These various substances will be discussed under the general classifications of steroid (Chapter 1) and protein or polypeptide hormones (Chapter 2) with emphasis on those most directly involved in the reproductive processes.

Chapter 1

Steroid Hormones and Prostaglandins

UNIFIED CONCEPT OF STEROID BIOSYNTHESIS AND METABOLISM

Steroids are a class of hormones with a common basic chemical structure related to the cholesterol backbone (Fig. 1).[3] These steroids have certain group characteristics in regard to biosynthesis and metabolism which simplify consideration of their biologic behavior. These characteristics may be catalogued as broad generalizations which follow:

1. Steroids are ultimately derived from the simple two-carbon substance acetate via

CHOLESTANE
C_{27}

PREGNANE
C_{21}

ANDROSTANE
C_{19}

ESTRANE
C_{18}

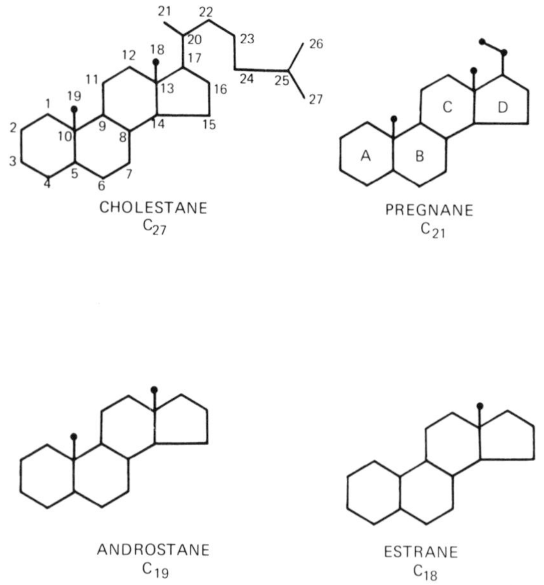

Figure 1. Common steroid skeleton. The intersections and apices of lines in these figures represent a carbon atom numbered as in the cholestane molecule. The four rings are designated according to letters as illustrated in the pregnane structure.

Active hormones and sterols occurring in nature have corresponding basic carbon structures—cholesterol (C-27), progesterone (C-21), testosterone (C-19), and estradiol (C-18)—but differ from the illustration in terms of ring and side-chain carbon substituents and unsaturated bonds in the A or B rings.

cholesterol (or a cholesterol-like intermediate) and pregnenolone. The steroids can be synthesized de novo from acetate by any of the major steroid-producing endocrine organs: ovary, testis, or adrenal (Fig. 2). These pathways are similar for any of these endocrine tissues, and each of these organs can make any type of steroid hormone.[4] The adrenal can synthesize not only corticoids but progestins, androgens, and estrogens as well; the testis can synthesize androgens, progestins, estrogens, and corticoids, as can the ovary. Although the adrenal usually produces corticoids and adrenal androgens, the testis usually produces androgens, and the ovary usually produces estrogens and progestins, the potential for "aberrant steroid production" becomes manifest in disease states or after malignant change. Examples are estrogens from the adrenal in certain tumors, estrogens and androgens from the adrenal in the adrenogenital syndrome, and androgens from the ovary in polycystic ovary disease. These types of deviant steroid secretion become less mysterious when one realizes that in most endocrine tissues progestins are converted to androgens and androgens to estrogens in the usual course of events. The disease states can be associated with blocks or defects in the enzymatic steps that are most characteristic for a particular endocrine gland, or with acceleration of a minor pathway. Recognition of this is clinically important since such abnormalities are usually associated with defects in reproduction (Table 1).

2. Not only the pathways for steroid hormone formation but also the location and types of enzymes involved are remarkably similar for each of these endocrine tissues. Only the control mechanisms, tropic hormones, and histology vary. As a conse-

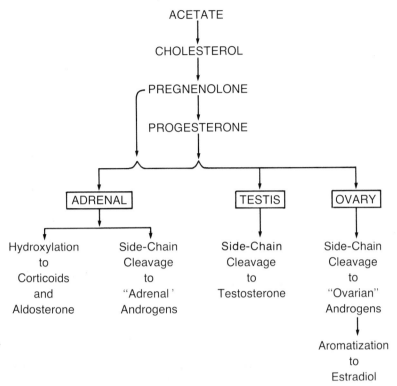

Figure 2. Unified concept of steroid formation.

TABLE 1. COMMON FEATURES OF STEROID-PRODUCING ENDOCRINE TISSUES

Steps in Steroid Biosynthesis	Adrenal		Testis		Ovary		Placenta	
	Normal Activity	Disease Defect	Normal Activity	Disease Defect	Normal Activity	Disease Defect	Normal Activity	Disease Defect
Acetate to cholesterol	+++		+++		+++		+	
Cholesterol to pregnenolone	+++		+++		+++		++++	
Pregnenolone to progesterone	+++	↓ Adreno-genital syndrome	+++		+++		++++	
Hydroxylation to corticoids and aldosterone	++++	Tumor Cushing's ↑ disease ↓ Adreno-genital syndrome	±	Rare in ↑ tumors	−	Rare in ↑ tumors	−	
Side-chain cleavage to androgens	+++	↑ Adreno-genital syndrome	++++		++	↑ Poly-cystic disease	−	
Aromatization to estrogens	±	↑ Tumors ↑ Adreno-genital syndrome	++	↑ Tumors	+++	↓ Poly-cystic disease	++++	↓ Sulfatase deficiency

Of special note: (1) The capacity of all tissues to convert acetate to cholesterol, but the relative deficiency of activity of the placenta. (2) The capacity of all tissues to convert cholesterol to pregnenolone and thence to progesterone. (3) Increased androgen production via side-chain cleavage in adrenogenital syndrome and polycystic ovary disease and absence of such production in the placenta. (4) Aromatization of androgens to estrogens in essentially all tissues, but in the case of the placenta the androgen substrate is delivered via the blood stream as a conjugate which must be cleaved prior to further metabolism.

TABLE 2.   PREHORMONES IN ENDOCRINOLOGY

Prehormones	*Active Hormone Product*
Pregnenolone sulfate	Progesterone
Dehydroepiandrosterone sulfate	Estradiol
Androstenedione	Estrone; testosterone
16-Hydroxydehydroepiandrosterone sulfate	Estriol

quence, the pathways for each of the hormones to be listed are equally applicable to any of the steroid-producing endocrine tissues.

3. Steroids can also be synthesized from intermediate blood-borne precursors such as cholesterol, pregnenolone, testosterone, androstenedione, or dehydroepiandrosterone by "incomplete" endocrine organs, such as the liver or placenta, that form steroids from acetate poorly or not at all. Some of these intermediate precursors such as dehydroepiandrosterone or androstenedione have little direct hormonal action themselves but can in this manner be converted to potent hormones, i.e., estradiol or testosterone.[1] These precursors have thus been designated as "prehormones" (Table 2).

4. Metabolism of steroids following secretion occurs in many tissues of the body but the liver's central location, abundant blood flow, and repertory of enzymes allow it to play the major role. In general, steroids are metabolized and usually made less biologically active by reduction of double bonds; cleavage of side chains; addition, reduction, or oxidation of hydroxyl groups (Fig. 3); and conjugation with the acidic moieties sulfate or glucuronate.[2] Note that with prehormones in the blood, the liver or other tissues could convert a steroid into either a more or a less biologically active substance. The factors that regulate this balance in steroid metabolism are as yet not fully understood, but clearly important. In the male, for instance, too much estrogen can be produced by peripheral conversion of androstenedione to estrone, rather than its usual conversion and excretion by way of the androgen metabolites, 17-ketosteroids.

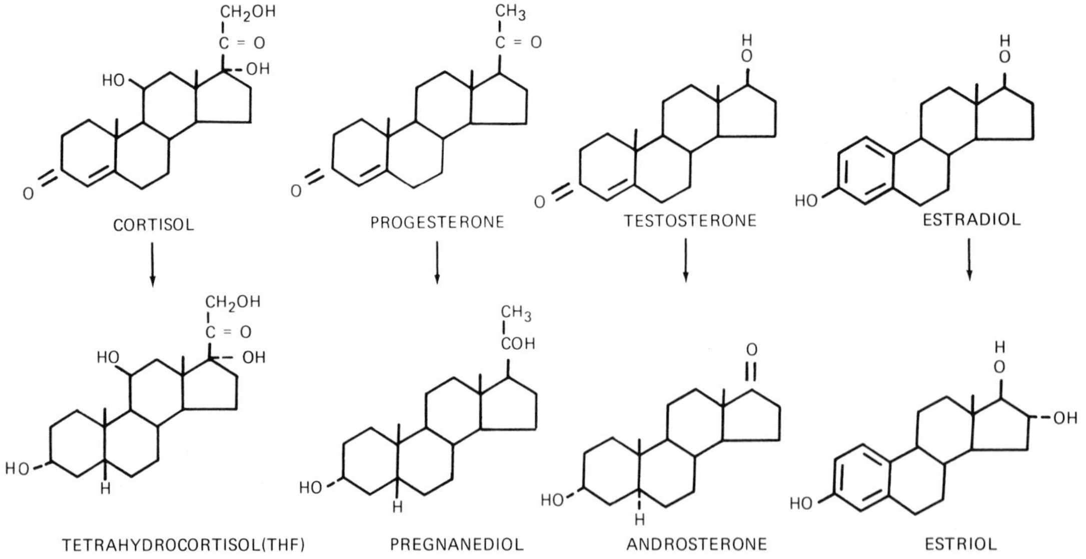

Figure 3. Examples of common steps in steroid catabolism. 1. Ring A double-bond reduction in all steroids except estrogens. 2. Reduction of the ketonic oxygen at position C-3. 3. Opportunity for stereoisomerism at positions C-3 (hydroxyl in α position on THF, androsterone, and pregnanediol), C-5 (hydrogen in β position in THF and pregnanediol and α position in androsterone), C-20, C-16, and any other asymmetric carbon substitution. 4. Steroid hydroxylation (at C-16 in estriol) possible at essentially any carbon position, but most frequent at positions C-2, C-6, C-16, and C-17.

BIBLIOGRAPHY

1. Baird, D., Horton, R., Longcope, C., and Tait, J. F.: Steroid prehormones. Perspect. Biol. Med., 11: 384, 1968.
2. Dorfman, R. F., and Ungar, F.: Metabolism of Steroid Hormones. Academic Press, New York, 1965.
3. Fieser, L. F., and Fieser, M.: Steroids. Reinhold Publishing Corp., New York, 1959.
4. Ryan, K. J.: Synthesis of hormones in the ovary. In Grady, H., ed.: The Ovary. Williams and Wilkins, Baltimore, 1963.

ESTROGENS

Estrogens may be defined as hormones that produce characteristic biologic effects such as cornification of the vaginal mucosa, growth of the uterus, estrus behavior in animals, and development of a proliferative endometrium in a gonadectomized subject.[7] More simply stated, estrogens are the hormones of femininity and as such are the major determinants of the development and functional maintenance of the female secondary sex characteristics, the breasts, the feminine body type, and metabolism. It should be stressed that estrogen effects are ultimately the result of the degree of responsiveness of the end-organ to the estrogen and also of a complex interplay of this hormone with any other steroids present, such as androgens or progestins.

Men and women have both estrogens and androgens circulating in their blood at the same time and yet masculinity in the male and femininity in the female are usually readily apparent. It is not the absolute amount of estrogen available that determines its effect but the relative amount of competing androgen present that can interfere with estrogen expression. For example, in the syndrome of testicular feminization the relative amounts of hormone present are appropriate but the tissues do not respond normally to androgens and a genotypic male resembles a phenotypic female.[5]

These variables (end-organ response and the presence of other hormones) are undoubtedly the determinants of the wide spectrum of bodily habitus, breast development, hair growth, and reproductive activity observed in different women. Although the word estrogen is derived from its capacity to induce sexual receptivity, estrus behavior or heat in animals, human sexuality is so steeped in overlying social custom and culture that no consistent direct effects of estrogen on sexual behavior in the human have been verified. (It is interesting that only the androgens when used in large doses, as for palliation of breast cancer, have resulted in increased libido in the human female.)

CHEMISTRY

The first natural estrogens to be described were estradiol, estrone, and estriol, which bear the metabolic relationships indicated in Figure 4. Estradiol is the most active or parent compound, and is secreted by the

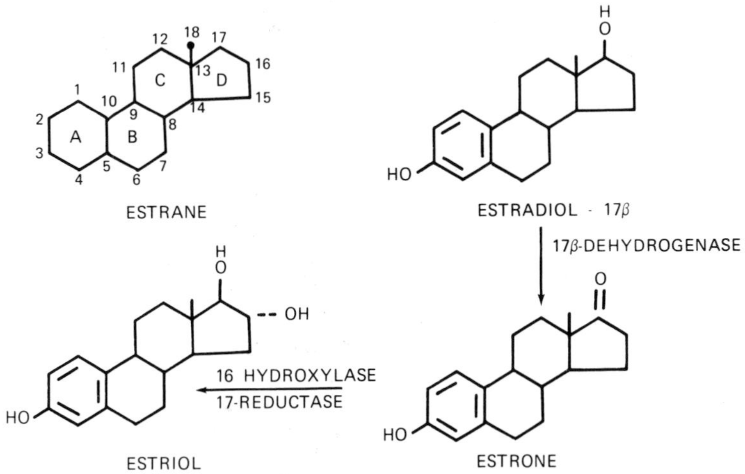

Figure 4. Major natural estrogens.

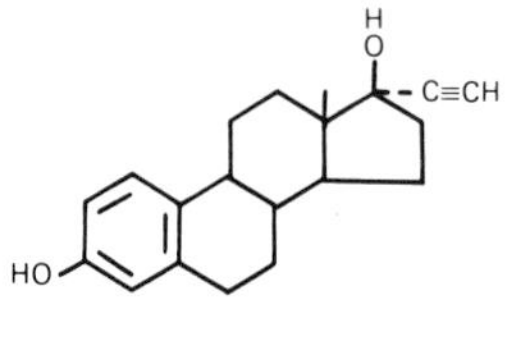

Figure 5. Common synthetic estrogens.

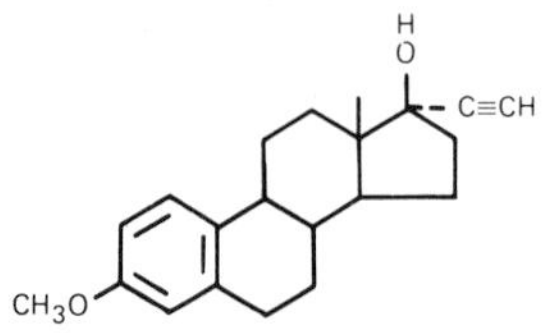

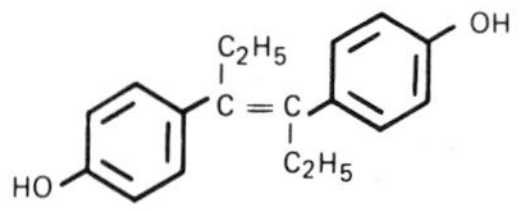

ovary and placenta. The estrogens are cyclopentanoperhydrophenanthrene derivatives similar to all steroid hormones but are typified by their 18 carbons, aromatic A ring, and the associated phenolic hydroxyl group at carbon position 3 (Fig. 4). There are no estrogens now known that do not contain an aromatic ring. Most of the natural estrogens have limited value in therapy because of their rapid metabolism and the need for parenteral administration. The chief pharmacologic estrogenic agents now employed in medicine are synthetic compounds and modified natural hormones that are effective when given orally (Fig. 5). The biologic effects of these substances are all quite similar in spite of their widely differing structures and metabolism.

BIOSYNTHESIS

The formation of estrogens can occur de novo from acetate in the ovary,[13] testis, or adrenal, and the pathway utilized can most simply be presented in diagrammatic form (Fig. 6). While complex at first encounter, the pathway can be simplified by division into three component steps: (1) acetate conversion to cholesterol, and cholesterol conversion to pregnenolone and thence to progesterone (Fig. 7); (2) the hydroxylation at C-17 and cleavage of the pregnenolone or progesterone side chains to form androgens (Fig. 8); and finally (3) the aromatization of the androgens to form estrogens (Fig. 9).[8] The pathway was elaborated by showing that each of the steps did, in fact, take place in these tissues, that acetate

could be converted to each of the intermediates (Table 3), and that the amounts of estrogen formed increased when the precursor tested was closer to the end of the biosynthetic chain (Table 4).[10, 13-16, 19-21]

Of note are the precursor roles of progesterone and testosterone. These are active hormones when released into the blood stream but may serve as intermediates in the tissue. As mentioned earlier, acceleration or blockage at these steps could result in secretion of an aberrant hormone. In addition, as outlined in Figures 6 and 8, there are parallel alternate routes to the estrogens via for example: (1) progesterone, 17-hydroxyprogesterone, and androstenedione to estrone; or (2) pregnenolone, 17-hydroxypregnenolone, dehydroepiandrosterone, and androstenedione to estrone. These alternate pathways may be important in controlling the types and amounts of intermediates involved.

In addition to the de-novo estrogen pathway from acetate in conventional endocrine tissues, estrogens can be formed from blood-borne precursors[3, 4] in either the liver or placenta. In pregnancy the major source of estrogens appears to be the placental pathway: (1) from dehydroepiandrosterone sulfate to dehydroepiandrosterone, androstenedione, and finally to estrone (Fig. 10); or (2) from 16-hydroxydehydroepiandrosterone sulfate to 16-hydroxydehydroepiandrosterone, 16-hydroxyandrostenedione, 16-hydroxyestrone, and on to estriol (Fig. 11). While the placenta cannot synthesize steroids from acetate very effectively (see Table 1) and therefore cannot synthesize dehydroepiandrosterone, it can utilize this

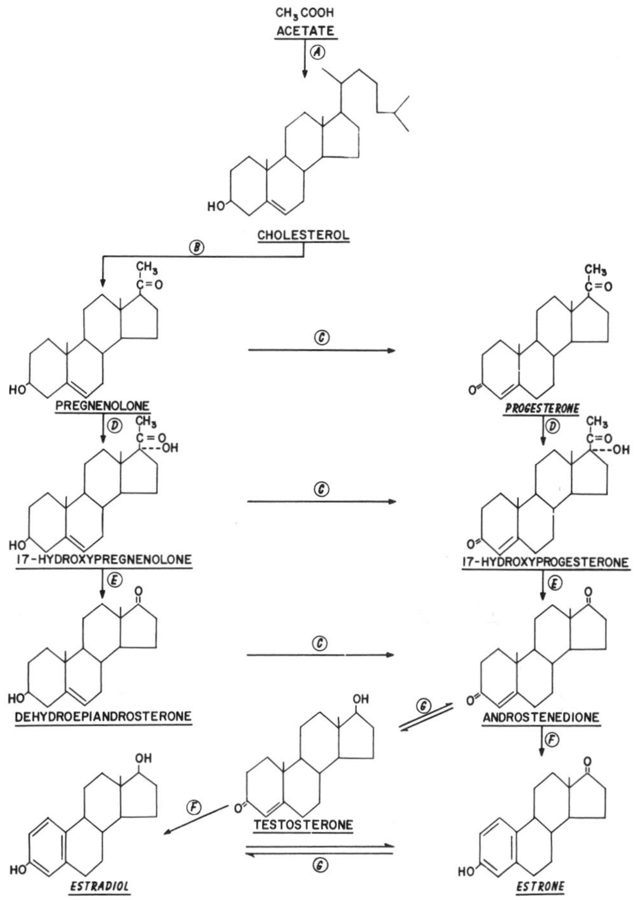

Figure 6. Pathway for estrogen biosynthesis from acetate. (From Smith, O. W., and Ryan, K. J.: Amer. J. Obstet. Gynec., 84:141, 1962.)

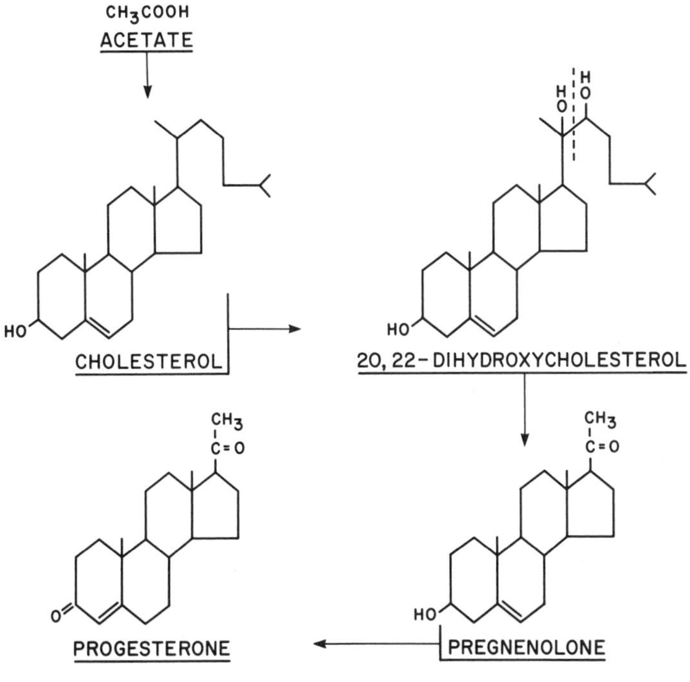

Figure 7. Pathway for progesterone synthesis from acetate. (From Ryan, K. J., in Marcus, C. C., and Marcus, S. L., eds.: Advances in Obstetrics and Gynecology. Williams and Wilkins, Baltimore, 1966.)

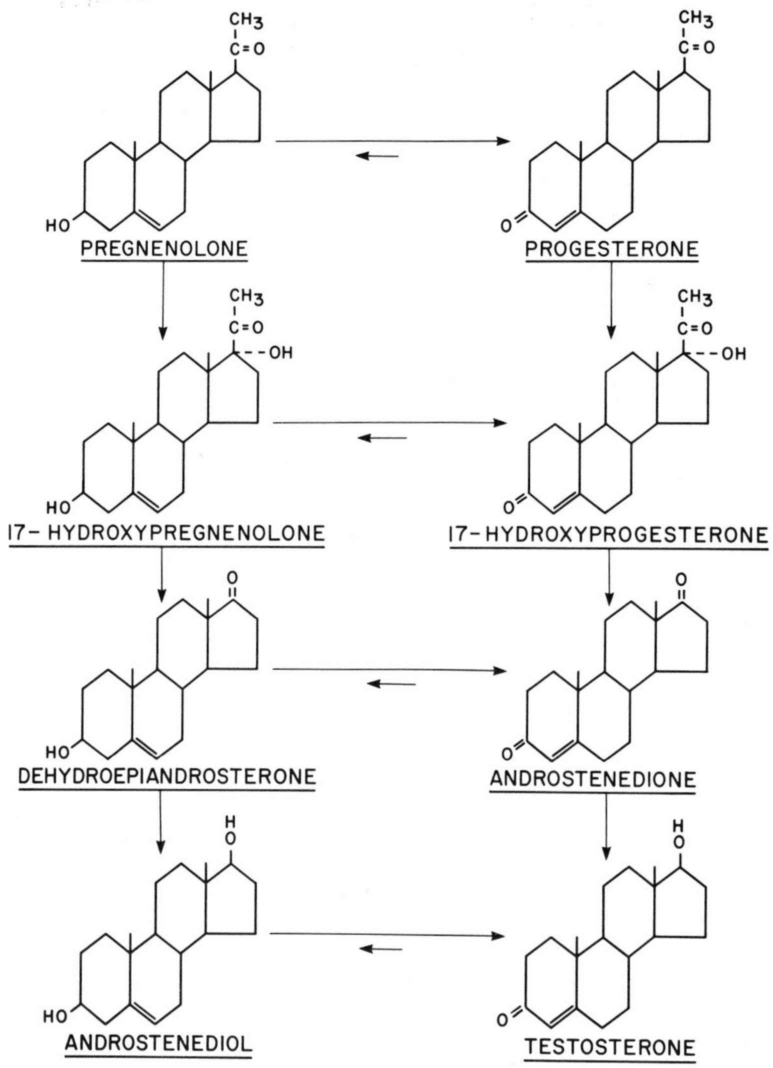

PREGNENOLONE   PROGESTERONE

17-HYDROXYPREGNENOLONE   17-HYDROXYPROGESTERONE

DEHYDROEPIANDROSTERONE   ANDROSTENEDIONE

ANDROSTENEDIOL   TESTOSTERONE

Figure 8. Androgen formation from pregnenolone and progesterone. (From Ryan, K. J., Marcus, C. C., and Marcus, S. L., eds.: Advances in Obstetrics and Gynecology. Williams and Wilkins, Baltimore, 1966.)

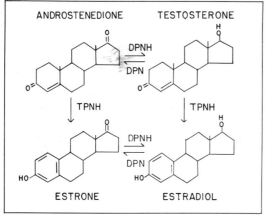

Figure 9. Aromatization of androgens to form estrogens. (From Ryan, K. J., in Popjak, G., ed.: Biosynthesis of Lipids. Proceedings of the Fifth International Congress of Biochemistry, Vol. 7. Pergamon Press, New York, 1963.)

TABLE 3. **SPECTRUM OF RADIOACTIVE STEROIDS DERIVED FROM ACETATE-C^{14} BY HUMAN OVARIAN FOLLICULAR TISSUE IN VITRO**[*]

Steroid Formed	Amount (cpm)
Cholesterol	758,765
Progesterone	545
17-Hydroxyprogesterone	2,950
Androstenedione	10,463
Pregnenolone	5,600
17-Hydroxypregnenolone	1,380
Dehydroepiandrosterone	10,200
Estrone	26,300
Estradiol	35,400

[*]From Ryan, K. J., and Smith, O. W.: J. Biol. Chem., 236:2207, 1961.

TABLE 4. INCREASING YIELD OF ESTROGEN
FORMATION IN THE OVARY FROM
PRECURSORS CLOSEST TO END OF THE
BIOSYNTHETIC PATHWAY

Precursor	Per Cent Yield of Estrogens
Acetate	0.03
Cholesterol	0.09
Progesterone	5.6
Androstenedione	15.3

°From Ryan, K. J., in Marcus, C. C., and Marcus, S. L., eds.: Advances in Obstetrics and Gynecology. Copyright 1966, The Williams & Wilkins Co., Baltimore Md. 21202, U.S.A., p. 340.

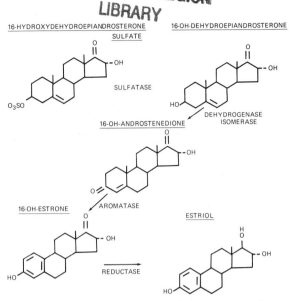

Figure 11. Pathway for estriol formation in the placenta.

sulfurylated compound, which is synthesized in and secreted from the maternal and fetal adrenals. This substance or its 16-hydroxylated derivative reaches the placenta by way of the circulation and undergoes the steps outlined in Figures 10 and 11. The fetal contribution of precursors appears to be the major one since estrogen levels are low in pregnancy if the fetus has no adrenal or dies in utero (see p. 118). In such cases maternal urinary and plasma estriols are low.

METABOLISM

Estrogens are metabolized largely by hydroxylation of the molecule at carbon 2, 6, 7, 14, 15, 16, or 18, as well as by oxidation or reduction of the oxygenated functions at several of these positions.[6] Thus estradiol, the parent hormone, can be converted to estrone and estrone to the estriols (see Fig. 4). Estriols can exist in any one of four possible epimeric forms and can be further modified into metabolites with combinations of hydroxyl and ketone functions at carbons 16 and 17 (α-ketols) (Fig. 12). Methyl ether formation can also occur with C-2-hydroxylated estrogens. By and large, most of the metabolites have much less biologic activity than estradiol. The metabolites are further altered by conjugation as the sulfate or glucuronate and when in the blood stream are bound to proteins as well. The conjugated metabolites are ultimately excreted via the urine. There is no evidence that the aromatic A ring is reduced, so that natural estrogens and their metabolites can be recognized and identified by the presence of this structural characteristic.

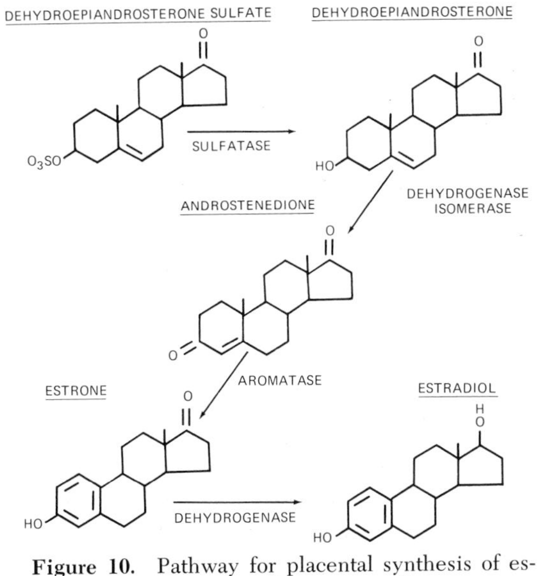

PRODUCTION AND EXCRETION

Estrogen levels in blood and urine are low during infancy and childhood but generally rise gradually until the onset of cyclic ovarian function at menarche when adult values are reached. In the adult female, blood levels of estradiol and excretion of urinary metabolites vary during the cycle, being highest at ovulation and in the luteal phase (Fig. 13). Total production of estra-

Figure 10. Pathway for placental synthesis of estradiol from dehydroepiandrosterone sulfate.

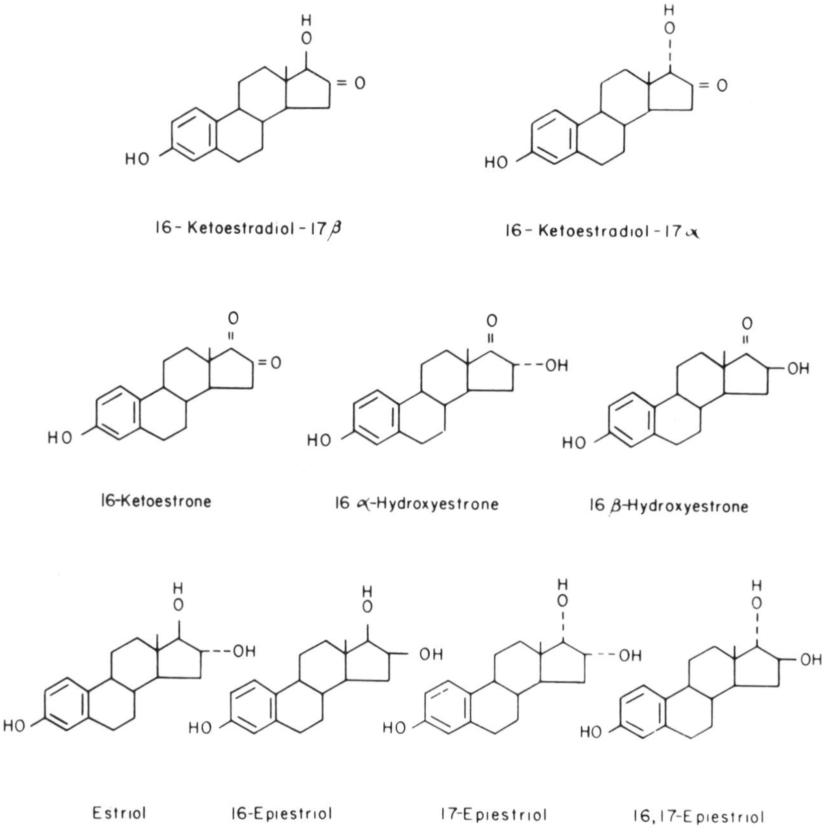

Figure 12. The many possible epimeric estriols and ketols isolated from in vivo and in vitro studies. (From Ryan, K. J., in Behrman, S. J., and Kistner, R. W., eds.: Progress in Infertility. Little, Brown and Co., Boston, 1968.)

diol is 250 to 500 mcg./24 hours and the blood level of free estradiol is 0.05 mcg./ 100 ml. at the highest point in the cycle.[1] Urinary excretion of metabolites similarly varies from a low of 20 mcg./24 hours early in the cycle to 80 mcg./24 hours at the peak.[8]

Males and most postmenopausal women have blood and urine values below those seen in the early part of the cycle; usually the blood level of estradiol is 0.003 mcg./ 100 ml. and total estrogens in urine equal 10 mcg./24 hours.

Estrogens can also be found in bile, in which they are excreted and reabsorbed through the bowel wall. Little estrogen is excreted via the feces in man, in contrast to many animal species.

During pregnancy estrogens in blood and urine rise progressively to levels of 20 mcg./ 100 ml. in blood and 40 mg./24 hours in urine (see p. 118). The bulk of urinary estrogen in pregnancy is estriol. Estrogens are also found in amniotic fluid and in the fetal blood stream at concentrations higher than in the mother.

BIOLOGIC EFFECTS AND PHARMACOLOGIC USES

The biologic effects of the estrogens can be divided into two general categories: those concerned with reproductive functions[7] and those responsible for metabolic effects.[17] Although it is not certain that these effects can arbitrarily be separated in the whole bodily economy, they are presented in this manner for the sake of clarity.

EFFECTS ON SECONDARY SEX STRUCTURES

By the very nature of the endocrine control of pregnancy, human embryos (male or female) never develop in the absence of maternal and placental estrogens and hence we cannot be certain what role these hormones play in embryologic development of the Müllerian system; it has been assumed that estrogens do not play a determining part in the differentiation of second-

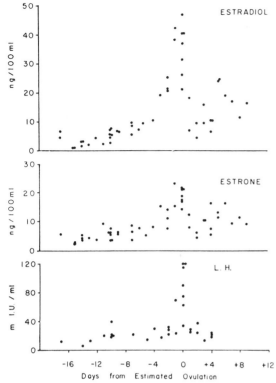

ESTRADIOL

ESTRONE

L. H.

Days from Estimated Ovulation

Figure 13. Concentration of luteinizing hormone (LH), unconjugated estrone, and estradiol-17β in peripheral plasma of women during the menstrual cycle (n=51). Day 0 in the graph is the day of estimated ovulation. (From Baird, D. T., and Guevara, A.: J. Clin. Endocr., 29:149, 1969.)

ary sex structures, in contrast to the need for specific factors in male differentiation. In addition, the fetus metabolizes and conjugates estrogens extensively to forms which may have limited biologic activity.

After birth and during the period of childhood small amounts of estrogens are produced but the secondary sex organs remain in an infantile state until the time of puberty. In the absence of ovaries the secondary sex structures remain undeveloped during adult life, and in the case of ovarian failure at the climacteric the reproductive organs that were developed atrophy. In this respect estrogens are essential for the development and maintenance of an adult female reproductive system. The effects upon these structures are the following.

Vagina

Under the effects of estrogens the vaginal mucosa develops from a thin columnar layer to a multi-layered structure, with cornification and shedding of the superficial cells. This is the basis for the bioassay

of estrogens in animals (Allen-Doisy test) and humans (cornification count). The degree of cornification and the type of cells present are reflections of estrogen presence and dosage. Estrogens can change an infantile vaginal pattern to an adult one or an atrophic vaginal pattern of old age into that seen in the active reproductive years. (See Vaginal Cycle, p. 99).

Cervix

Estrogens cause the cervix to grow in size and vascularity, to develop mucous glands, and to secrete cervical mucus which has a chemical content and physical behavior characteristic of estrogen stimulation. The ferning and spinbarkeit (elasticity) of the cervical secretions are typical of this estrogen effect. (See Cervical Cycle, p. 99).

Uterus

Estrogens cause endometrial gland and blood vessel proliferation and are necessary for the baseline maintenance of the endometrial cells and the preliminary modification of the cells for superimposed progesterone effects. (See Menstrual Cycle, p. 97.)

The myometrium hypertrophies in response to estrogens, and its electrical and contractile activities are modulated in some as yet incompletely understood way, so that myometrial irritability is altered.

Fallopian Tubes

The fallopian tubes develop both their mucosal lining and musculature under the influence of estrogen and the contractability, secretion, and function of the tubes are dependent on these steroid hormones. (See Oviductal Cycle, p. 99.)

Ovaries

The effects of estrogens on the ovaries are complex and not fully understood, but at present one can state that they appear to increase the response of the ovarian follicle to pituitary gonadotropin stimulation at the local level.[18] When amounts of estrogen so small that they have no systemic effects are implanted in one ovary, the ovary so treated responds with greater follicular proliferation than the untreated contralateral gonad. Estrogens also appear to have local effects on the function of the corpus luteum but these are not yet completely defined. Thus, this is one example of a hormone having an effect on its gland of origin such that it stimulates growth of the cells that produce the hormone. In animals estrogens can also moderate the ovarian atrophy caused by hypophysectomy.

Breasts

Estrogens are responsible for growth and development of the nipple, areola, and breast duct but total breast integrity depends on other ovarian, adrenal, thyroid, and pituitary hormones as well. The response of breast tissue to estrogen stimulation is a good example of variable endorgan response since cosmetic production of increased breast development is unpredictable when estrogens are used pharmacologically for this purpose in otherwise normal women. When estrogens have been used in males for palliation of prostatic carcinoma, many of the aforementioned effects upon the breast have been apparent, and in agonadal women estrogens can be used to develop adult tissue from an infantile form. (See Mammary Gland and Lactation, p. 127.)

Hair Growth

Estrogens are perhaps needed for pubic and axillary hair growth but this effect depends to a large extent on an interplay with the effects of androgenic ovarian and adrenal steroids.

Endocrine Glands

PITUITARY. Estrogens have varying effects on pituitary structure and function depending on dosage. It is believed that their locus of action is the hypothalamus, which secondarily controls pituitary activity. In small dosage estrogens may stimulate gonadotropin *release*; although this is reasonably well documented in animals, it is by no means definitely established in man. In larger dosage, estrogens are among the most effective inhibitors of gonadotropin production and release and form a part of most preparations compounded for contraceptive purposes (see p. 62).

The vasomotor symptoms of the climacteric can be relieved by estrogens but at a dosage level below that required to significantly lower the elevated gonadotropin levels. The site of action and chain of events for relief of menopausal vasomotor symptoms are not understood.

After castration pituitary structure changes and certain castration cells become apparent. This can be prevented with estrogen replacement.

THYROID. Estrogens cause an increase of thyroid-binding globulin in the blood and result in an elevated protein-bound iodine (PBI) level. In pregnancy, there is a tendency for the thyroid to enlarge but whether this is due to an effect of estrogen is not known (see p. 124).

ADRENAL. Estrogens have profound effects on adrenal steroid formation and metabolism and also on adrenal structure in animals and humans. Under the influence of estrogens, the level of transcortin, or cortisol-binding globulin, is increased, the half-life of adrenal steroids in blood is lengthened, and adrenal hormone metabolism is decreased. Evidence of these changes is striking during pregnancy (see p. 125).

EFFECTS ON METABOLISM

Estrogens have profound effects on many metabolic processes not directly related to reproduction.[17]

Electrolytes

The resorption of sodium and water by the renal tubule is increased by estrogens, with resultant production of edema and circulatory compromise when persons with heart disease or cirrhosis are given estrogens therapeutically. Whether the edema of pregnancy or the premenstrual syndrome is based in part on this estrogen effect is not certain. The mechanism of the estrogen effect is unknown but it has recently been postulated that estrogens actually cause sodium excretion by counteracting the effect of aldosterone, as is the case with progesterone. As a consequence, the level of aldosterone rises and the net effect is one of salt retention.

Calcium, Bone Dynamics, and Epiphyseal Closure

Estrogens are one of the determinants of bone integrity and calcium balance. After castration or menopause, osteoporosis and a negative calcium balance can be ameliorated by estrogen administration. This forms one of the bases for postmenopausal replacement therapy. Estrogens influence epiphyseal closure and can cause premature limitation of bone growth by their presence prior to attainment of adult stature. They have been used therapeutically to prevent inordinate height in young girls.[2]

Lipoproteins, Cholesterol-Phospholipid Ratios, and Coronary Atherosclerosis

It is well known that women in their reproductive years are less prone to coronary disease than are men of comparable age, but this difference tends to disappear 15 years after the menopause in association with prolonged absence of ovarian function.

The lipoproteins and cholesterol-phospholipid ratios are characteristically different in men and women and these sex-linked differences can be manipulated by withdrawal of male or female hormones and/or institution of estrogen or androgen administration. On the basis that these cholesterol and lipoprotein dynamics may be related to atherosclerosis, estrogens have been given to male survivors of coronary occlusions and prophylactically to postmenopausal women. The scientific validity of this practice is still under scrutiny.

Carbohydrate Metabolism

Studies in animals and humans have shown that estrogens have effects on carbohydrate metabolism, but the response is not well defined and may be dose-related.

In some instances the diabetic state seemed to be aggravated cyclically at menses and ameliorated by estrogens; in other instances the reverse observations, with hyperglycemia and aggravation of diabetes in response to estrogens, have been noted. Estrogens have an effect on serum growth hormone levels and hence might influence carbohydrate metabolism directly or indirectly. Diabetogenic effects of contraceptive drugs have been reported, with elevation of serum insulin, but the contributions of estrogen as opposed to progestin in these effects have not yet been completely resolved. Mestranol alone can, however, alter carbohydrate tolerance (see Insulin, p. 125).

Anabolic Action

Estrogens can cause increases in serum copper and ceruloplasmin levels and in nitrogen retention. Effects on iron dynamics and hemoglobin synthesis are not completely defined but there is a characteristic sex-linked difference in erythrocyte and hemoglobin level—it is lower in women than in men.

Skin and Blood Vessels

Skin pigmentation, especially of scars and the areolar areas of the breast, can be increased by estrogens but the pathway for this effect is not known.

Angiomata or "spiders" of pregnancy and cirrhosis are attributed to estrogens but again the precise mechanism for this effect is unknown. On the other hand, the changes in blood vessels of the genital tract appear to be a relatively more predictable and specific effect of these hormones.

OVERALL EFFECTS IN PREGNANCY

From the foregoing list of biologic effects of estrogens, and from what will follow on estrogen control of the menstrual cycle (p. 105), it is clear that these hormones are necessary for fertilization and implantation and may be important for ovulation. Once the pregnancy is established it is difficult to select out the specific continuing role of the estrogens in view of the contributions of the many other hormones and bodily changes. In some animals in which the placenta does not produce estrogens and the ovary is needed for the maintenance of pregnancy, both estrogen and progesterone must be replaced if the pregnancy is to continue after ovarian ablation. In other animals progesterone but not estrogens must be replaced after ovarian removal for pregnancy to be maintained. It is possible that estrogen is made in the placenta in these latter species or that estrogen is not always essential once pregnancy is established. In the human, in which estrogen and progesterone are produced in the placenta and neither the ovaries nor replacement therapy with estrogen or progesterone is needed after oophorectomy, it is not possible to test whether estrogens really play an essential role throughout pregnancy, although the bias of history and scientific custom is in favor of such an indispensable requirement for these hormones.

In any case, many of the breast changes; skin pigmentation; uterine growth, accommodation, and smooth muscle activity; anabolic tendencies; pituitary quiescence; changes in thyroid and adrenal function; electrolyte and water retention; altered carbohydrate metabolism; and vascular and connective tissue changes of pregnancy are believed to be due in part to estrogenic effects. The contributory role of the other hormones in pregnancy will be considered in subsequent sections.

BIBLIOGRAPHY

1. Baird, D. T., and Guevara, A.: Concentration of unconjugated estrone and estradiol in peripheral plasma in nonpregnant women throughout the menstrual cycle, castrate and postmenopausal women and in men. J. Clin. Endocr., 29:149, 1969.
2. Frasier, S. D., and Smith, F. G., Jr.: Effect of estrogens on mature height in tall girls: a controlled study. J. Clin. Endocr., 28:416, 1968.
3. Longcope, C., Kato, T., and Horton, R.: Conversion of blood androgens to estrogens in normal adult men and women. J. Clin. Invest., 48:2919, 1969.
4. MacDonald, P. C., Rombaut, R. P., and Siiteri, P. K.: Plasma precursors of estrogen. I. Extent of conversion of plasma Δ^4-androstenedione to estrone in normal males and nonpregnant normal, castrate and adrenalectomized females. J. Clin. Endocr., 27:1103, 1967.
5. Morris, J. M., and Mahesh, V. B.: Further observations on the syndrome, "testicular feminization." Amer. J. Obstet. Gynec., 87:731, 1963.
6. O'Donnell, V. J., and Preedy, J. R. K.: The oestrogens. In Gray, C. H., and Bacharach, A. L., eds.: Hormones in Blood, Vol. 2. Academic Press, New York, 1967, pp. 109–186.
7. Papanicolaou, G. N., Traut, H. F., and Marchetti, A. H.: The Epithelia of Women's Reproductive Organs. Commonwealth Fund, New York, 1948.
8. Ryan, K. J.: Biological aromatization of steroids. J. Biol. Chem., 234:268, 1959.

9. Ryan, K. J.: Metabolism of C-16 oxygenated steroids by human placenta: The formation of estriol. J. Biol. Chem., 234:2006, 1959.
10. Ryan, K. J.: Biogenesis of estrogens. In Popjak, E., ed.: Biosynthesis of Lipids. Proceedings of the Fifth International Congress of Biochemistry, Vol. 7. Pergamon Press, New York, 1963, p. 381.
11. Ryan, K. J.: Steroid metabolism in the human ovary. In Marcus, C. C., and Marcus, S. L., eds.: Advances in Obstetrics and Gynecology. Williams and Wilkins, Baltimore, 1966, p. 340.
12. Ryan, K. J.: Biosynthesis end metabolism of ovarian steroids. In Behrman, S. J., and Kistner, R. W., eds.: Progress in Infertility. Little, Brown and Co., Boston, 1968, p. 275.
13. Ryan, K. J., and Smith, O. W.: Biogenesis of estrogens by the human ovary. I. Conversion of acetate-1-C^{14} to estrone and estradiol. J. Biol. Chem., 236:705, 1961.
14. Ryan, K. J., and Smith, O. W.: Biogenesis of estrogens by the human ovary. II. Conversion of progesterone-4-C^{14} to estrone and estradiol. J. Biol. Chem., 236:710, 1961.
15. Ryan, K. J., and Smith, O. W.: Biogenesis of estrogens by the human ovary. III. Conversion of cholesterol-4-C^{14} to estrone. J. Biol. Chem., 236:2204, 1961.
16. Ryan, K. J., and Smith, O. W.: Biogenesis of estrogens by the human ovary. IV. Formation of neutral steroid intermediates. J. Biol. Chem., 236:2207, 1961.
17. Salhanick, H. A., Kipnis, D. M., and Vande Wiele, R. L.: Metabolic Effects of Gonadal Hormones and Contraceptive Steroids. Plenum Press, New York, 1969.
18. Smith, B. D., and Bradbury, J. T.: Ovarian response to gonadotrophins after pretreatment with diethylstilbestrol. Amer. J. Physiol., 204:1023, 1963.
19. Smith, O. W., and Ryan, K. J.: Biogenesis of estrogens by the human ovary. The conversion of androstenedione-4-C^{14} to estrone and estradiol in high yield. Endocrinology, 69:869, 1961.
20. Smith, O. W., and Ryan, K. J.: Biogenesis of estrogens by the human ovary. Formation of neutral steroid intermediates from progesterone-14-C^{14}, androstenedione-4-C^{14} and cholesterol-4-C^{14}. Endocrinology, 69:970, 1961.
21. Smith, O. W., and Ryan, K. J.: Estrogen in the human ovary. Amer. J. Obstet. Gynec., 84:141, 1962.

PROGESTERONE

Progesterone is *the* hormone of pregnancy and more specifically *the* hormone of mammalian viviparity. Biologically it is effective upon tissues that have previously been primed with estrogens and adds upon the foundation of estrogen effects a superstructure of uterine endometrial and myometrial changes that allow and sustain implantation and uterine muscle "quiescence." These two primary effects, the secretory "progestational" endometrium and the progesterone-dominated muscle activity, are major aspects of the endocrine roots of human pregnancy.[2] To be sure, the details of endocrine control of myometrial activity are far from established, but at the heart of the matter will almost certainly be a progesterone effect.

Progesterone or a progestational substance is therefore a hormone that will produce characteristic effects in an estrogen-primed endometrium *or* will maintain pregnancy in an animal deprived of progestins, as by removal of the corpus luteum of pregnancy. These characteristics form the bases for several biologic assays. It should be emphasized that many synthetic so-called progestins do not have both properties, being able to stimulate the endometrium but not being capable of maintaining pregnancy in oophorectomized animals.

Establishment of a relationship between the corpus luteum, the maintenance of pregnancy in rabbits, and the production of a secretory endometrium provided an experimental system for the search for the chemical mediator. Subsequently, in the early 1930s Corner and Allen isolated progesterone from corpora lutea and the chemist Butenandt described its structural formula. Thus, progesterone was established as a major hormone of the corpus luteum and pregnancy. When it was discovered that in some species the corpus luteum was not necessary for the maintenance of pregnancy, the explanation was not a lack of need for this hormone, but the fact that the placenta could also produce it.

CHEMISTRY

Progesterone is a steroid hormone of the pregnane series; it and the more recently discovered dihydroprogesterones represent the only known natural progestational agents. Structural formulas are illustrated in Figure 14. Progesterone is a C-21 compound. Testosterone when suitably modified has progestational activity and the 19-nor derivative of testosterone forms the root compound for many of the oral progestational agents (Fig. 15). The progesterone molecule suitably modified also provides the basis for active synthetic progestational agents (Fig. 16).[13]

BIOSYNTHESIS

Progesterone can be produced by the adrenal gland, testis, and ovarian follicle but its major sources for secretion into the blood stream are the corpus luteum and placenta. In the ovary, progesterone can be synthesized from acetate or cholesterol via the steps illustrated in Figure 7. The cholesterol side chain is hydroxylated at carbons 20 and 22, and cleavage of the side chain between these two carbons produces pregnenolone and an isocaproic aldehyde or acid residue. Pregnenolone is converted to progesterone by a facile enzymatic system that changes the 3β hydroxyl group to a ketone and shifts the double bond from C-5 to C-4. Similar steps occur in the human placenta but the formation of cholesterol from acetate is limited in the placenta, and

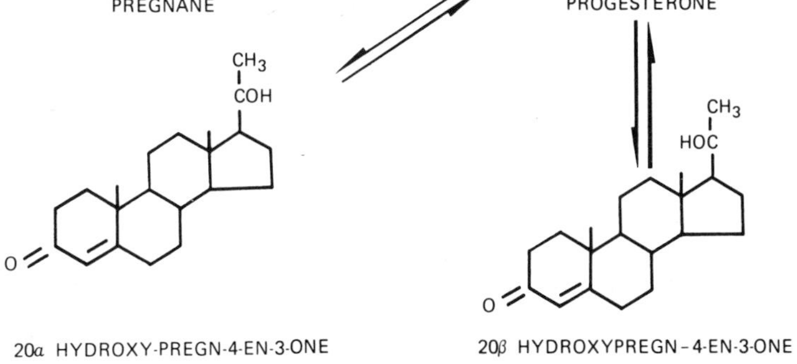

Figure 14. Naturally occurring progestins.

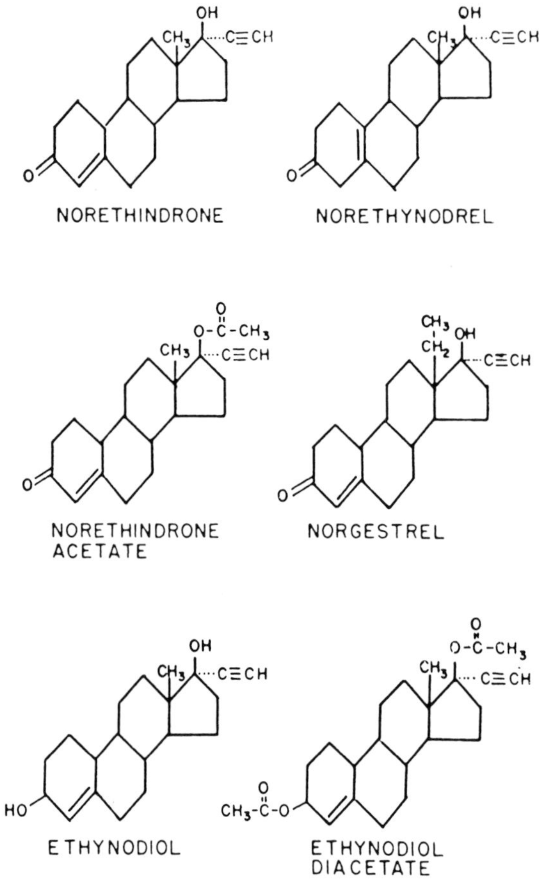

Figure 15. Structural formulas of progestins related to 19-nortestosterone. (From Sanders, F. J.: Fed. Proc., 29:1211, 1970.)

PRODUCTION AND EXCRETION

Progesterone secretion varies of course with the stage of the ovarian cycle and hence blood levels and excretion of urinary metabolites fluctuate depending upon the presence of a corpus luteum. During the follicular phase of the cycle prior to ovulation pregnanediol in the urine is 1 mg./24 hours and the blood levels of progesterone are barely detectable, at amounts below 0.001 mcg. per milliliter. After ovulation and corpus luteum formation, peak progesterone blood levels are 0.02 mcg. per milliliter (Fig. 18),[4] and urinary pregnanediol rises to 2 to 5 mg./24 hours. The production rate of progesterone is approximately 2.6 mg./24 hours in the follicular phase of the cycle and 22 mg./24 hours after corpora lutea secretion.[9]

During pregnancy, the production rate rises to 300 mg./24 hours at term and blood levels are over 0.120 mcg. per milliliter. Pregnanediol excretion reaches levels of 40 mg./24 hours in the last trimester (see p. 118).[3]

PHARMACOLOGIC USES

Although a complete review of the uses of progesterone and synthetic progestins in blood-borne cholesterol or pregnenolone provides the more immediate precursors for progesterone rather than de novo synthesis from acetate (see p. 116).

METABOLISM

Progesterone can be readily converted by the liver to saturated pregnane derivatives which are conjugated with glucuronic acid and excreted in the urine. A well known metabolite is pregnanediol (5β-pregnane-3α,20α-diol) which constitutes approximately 20 per cent of the metabolic disposition of progesterone. Other metabolites are epimers of pregnanediol with various combinations of the possible isomeric substitutes at carbons 3, 5, and 20 (Fig. 17).[14]

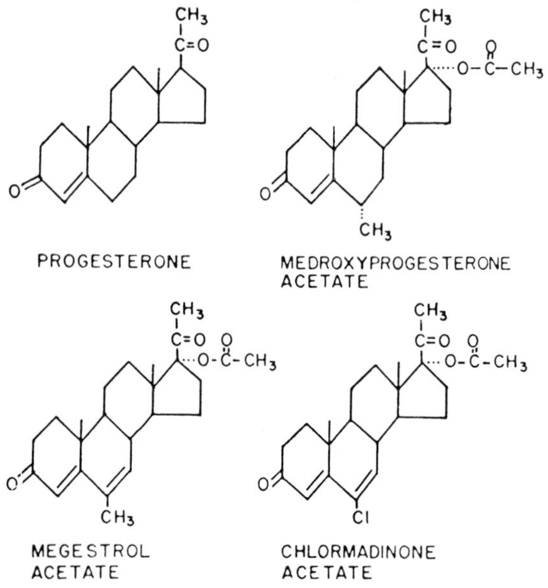

Figure 16. Structural formulas of various progestins related to progesterone. (From Sanders, F. J.: Fed. Proc., 29:1211, 1970.)

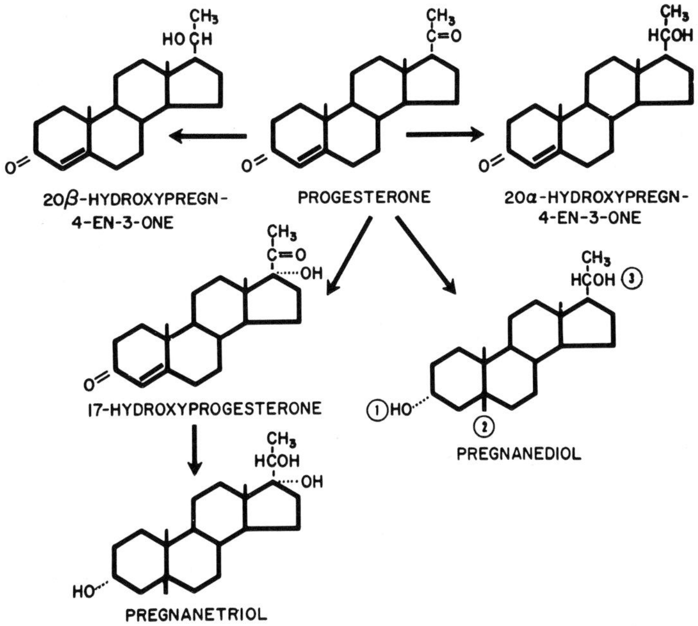

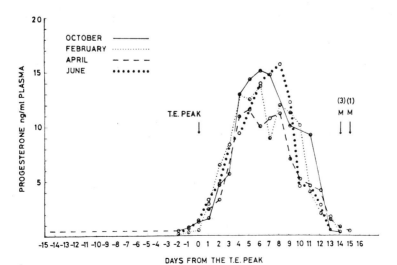

Figure 17. Metabolism of progesterone. Epimeric forms of pregnanediol are possible by alteration of the substituent at positions labeled 1, 2, and 3 (carbon positions 3, 5, and 20 of the steroid numbering system). (From Ryan, K. J., in Marcus, C. C., and Marcus, S. L., eds.: Advances in Obstetrics and Gynecology. Williams and Wilkins, Baltimore, 1966.)

clinical medicine cannot be given in this presentation, several important examples are presented.

Progesterone itself is relatively inactive when given by mouth and consequently has been replaced to a considerable extent in clinical usage by a wide variety of orally effective synthetic compounds (Figs. 15 and 16). The important aspect of this transition in the types of pharmacologic agents used is that not all of the synthetic compounds have a spectrum of activity identical with that of progesterone.[12] Care must be exercised in selecting the compound with the effects desired and avoiding those with undesirable effects such as virilization and other androgenic properties.

Control of Abnormal Endometrial Bleeding

The effect of progesterone on the estrogen-primed endometrium makes it an ideal agent for controlling estrogen withdrawal and breakthrough bleeding that typify anovulatory dysfunctional uterine bleeding. This constitutes one major gynecologic use based on physiologic properties. Most of the synthetic agents are also highly effective.

Figure 18. Plasma progesterone during the luteal phase of the menstrual cycle. T. E. peak, timing of ovulation by basal body temperature elevation; M., menses. (From Johansson, E. D. B.: Acta Endocr., 61:592, 1969.)

Contraception

Synthetic progestins are the basic constituent of contraceptive medications. They act as a synergist with an estrogen in hypothalamic inhibition of gonadotropin production and release, and they produce a more predictable type of endometrial bleeding response than that obtained with estrogen alone.[13] Progestins may also contribute to contraception by affecting cervical, endometrial, or ovarian factors.

Threatened Abortion, High-Risk Pregnancy, Endometriosis, and Endometrial Carcinoma

Since progesterone has been shown to have a quieting effect on the myometrium, its therapeutic and prophylactic use in threatened and habitual abortion has been extensive. It should be pointed out that many of the synthetic progestins suggested for this use cannot maintain pregnancy in oophorectomized animals in which progesterone itself is effective. Double-blind studies and those utilizing urinary pregnanediol excretion as a guide to case selection have failed to reveal a beneficial effect of progesterone. This failure may be masked by the fact that many abortions are not due primarily to progesterone deficiency. Progestins have also been used in diabetic pregnancies but the benefits of such therapy have not been conclusively established. In any case, the use of replacement estrogens and progestins in pregnancy is at present an empiric exercise that awaits definitive evaluation. Similarly, progestins have not been of practical use in delaying the onset of labor or stopping premature labor when it occurs. Progesterone is effective in delaying labor in animals and its lack of effect in the human may be related to the dynamics of its metabolism and to failure to achieve a sufficient local level at the myometrial site. There is some evidence that locally administered progesterone can diminish uterine activity but this is not sufficient for clinical application.

Synthetic progestins have been administered in high dosage continuously to produce decidualization and gland atrophy in cases in which ectopic endometrium causes symptoms in the entity known as endometriosis. Such a course of therapy has been called a pseudopregnancy.

Progestins in very high dosage have also been effective in causing regression of the metastases of carcinoma of the endometrium as a palliative form of treatment.[5, 6]

BIOLOGIC EFFECTS

Progesterone, like the estrogens, has biologic effects upon both the reproductive system and the general bodily economy. Unlike the estrogens, which have primary growth-initiating effects on the reproductive tract, progesterone normally exerts its effects secondarily on an estrogen-primed substrate.

Lining of Reproductive Tract

VAGINA. Progesterone alters an estrogen-primed human vaginal epithelium, causing desquamation of superficial cell layers, decrease in the thickness of the lining, and infiltration with leukocytes. The desquamated cells are less acidophilic and more folded. These changes can be used as a crude correlation with the relative amounts of estrogens and progestins in the body, for diagnosing ovulation, and, according to some cytologists, for predicting the outcome of threatened or habitual abortion in early pregnancy. (See Vaginal Cycle, p. 99.)

CERVIX. The epithelium of the endocervix, having been stimulated by estrogens, is altered by progesterone, which causes flattening of the cells and changes in the amount, viscosity, and ferning ability of the cervical mucus. These changes in cervical mucus are also used as a guide to determine the presence of progesterone. (See Cervical Cycle, p. 99.)

ENDOMETRIUM. The proliferative type of endometrial lining produced by estrogens is converted into a secretory endometrium by progesterone. The changes in the glands include evidence of secretion, tortuosity, and glycogen deposition. The stromal cells are altered in shape and size and the end-effect is the so-called decidual cell.[10] These effects are dependent upon the proper ratio and timing of estrogen and progesterone action and result in a proper implantation bed should conception occur. The blood vessels are also altered in the direction of increased tortuosity, coiling, and growth. Failure of implantation to occur, with withdrawal of progesterone and estrogen, results in endometrial regression and typical menstrual bleeding which is much more predictable in timing, completeness, and character than the type of bleeding following estrogen priming alone. (See p. 99.)

FALLOPIAN TUBES. The columnar cells of the fallopian tube are flattened and their secretion is affected by progesterone action on the estrogen-prepared lining.

Myometrium and Smooth Muscle

Progesterone has a characteristic ability to decrease the amplitude and interval of contractibility of smooth muscle. It is this action upon myometrium which is believed partially responsible for the ability of the uterus to retain a growing fetus without expulsion prior to term.[2] Estrogen generally has an opposite effect but may be synergistic with progesterone. The exact relationship of the hormonal action to the molecular events of muscle contractibility are unknown and there is some controversy about the relative roles played by estrogens, progesterone, oxytocin, catecholamines, and nerve pathways in the maintenance of pregnancy and the initiation of labor.

Attempts to relate the onset of labor to changes in progesterone or estrogen concentration have thus far not been enlightening since blood levels vary from species to species and no consistent pattern can be observed.

Progesterone has similar effects on the smooth muscle of the fallopian tubes and ureters.

Breasts

Progesterone causes development of acini and lobules of the estrogen-primed breast and prepares it for lactation, which depends on many other hormones working in concert.

Central Nervous System

Progesterone in high dosage may be an anesthetic agent. In physiologic amounts, it is responsible for the thermogenic shift that occurs in midcycle after the corpus luteum is formed.[1] It is believed that the action of progesterone is at the level of the hypothalamus. During pregnancy, with gradually increasing levels of progesterone, the basal body temperature elevation is maintained and then gradually declines

in the face of continued presence of progesterone. Progesterone also affects gonadotropin synthesis and release from the pituitary by action on hypothalamic centers. This appears to be dose-related, and involves inhibition of luteinizing hormone release and stimulation of lactogenic hormone release although the details are not yet established. Progesterone itself is a relatively poor inhibitor of pituitary function on a weight basis but is synergistic with estrogens in this regard. Synthetic progestins are much more active than progesterone in their effects on pituitary function.

Renal Function and Metabolism

Progesterone has been demonstrated by Landau[3, 7, 8] to have catabolic effects in causing nitrogen excretion and to cause water and electrolyte loss by its ability to antagonize the effects of aldosterone at the renal tubule. Subsequent to the renal effect of progesterone, compensatory secretion of aldosterone is believed to occur so that the net effect may appear to be water retention. The relationship of these progesterone actions to premenstrual edema and the tendency to water retention in pregnancy has not been clarified as yet.

ORIGIN IN HUMAN PREGNANCY

Progesterone is essential for pregnancy in all higher forms of animal life and as described earlier is produced by the corpus luteum and placenta.[3, 11] The evidence for this is as follows:

1. The corpus luteum source of progesterone has been established by: (a) isolation from the tissue; (b) isolation from ovarian vein blood in higher concentration than in the periphery; (c) perfusion studies of ovaries containing corpora lutea and in-vitro enzymatic studies which demonstrate the capacity to synthesize the hormone.

The ability to maintain pregnancy after removal of the corpus luteum, with essentially unchanged levels of progesterone in the blood or pregnanediol in the urine, suggests that the corpus luteum function is not critical after six to seven weeks, when the placental function is well established. In many pregnancies, the corpus luteum actually regresses before term, as demonstrated at laparotomy for cesarean section. On the other hand, progesterone can be isolated from some corpora lutea at term, and although they are not essential, some corpora lutea may function throughout pregnancy.

2. The evidence for progesterone formation by the human placenta includes: (a) its presence in blood and placental tissue in increasing amounts as pregnancy progresses, with increased excretion of metabolites in urine, all of which decline after delivery of the placenta; (b) its presence in pregnancy in the absence of pituitary, ovaries and adrenals; (c) the higher level of progesterone in effluent blood leaving the placenta than in maternal or fetal blood; (d) the presence of enzymatic systems in the placenta which can synthesize progesterone; (e) the presence of progesterone after fetal demise until the placenta is delivered, and the continued presence of progesterone in abdominal pregnancy when the infant has been delivered and the placenta left in situ (see Placenta, p. 95, and Maternal-Placental Unit, p. 116).

BIBLIOGRAPHY

1. Buxton, C. L., and Atkinson, W. B.: Hormonal factors involved in the regulation of basal body temperature during the menstrual cycle and pregnancy. J. Clin. Endocr., 8:544, 1948.
2. Corner, G. W., and Csapo, A.: Action of the ovarian hormones on uterine muscle. Brit. Med. J., 1:687, 1953.
3. Ehrlich, E. N., Laves, M., Lugibihl, K., and Landau, R. L.: Progesterone-aldosterone interrelationships in pregnancy. J. Lab. Clin. Med., 59: 588, 1962.
4. Diczfalusy, E., and Troen, P.: Endocrine functions of the human placenta. Vitamins Hormones, 19: 229, 1961.
5. Johansson, E. D. B.: Progesterone levels in peripheral plasma during the luteal phase of the normal human menstrual cycle measured by a rapid competitive protein binding technique. Acta Endocr., 61:592, 1969.
6. Kennedy, B. J.: Progestogens in the treatment of carcinoma of the endometrium. Surg. Gynec. Obstet., 127:103, 1968.
7. Kistner, R. W., Griffiths, C. T., and Craig, J. M.: Use of progestational agents in the management of endometrial cancer. Cancer, 18:1563, 1965.
8. Landau, R. L., Bergenstal, D. M., Lugibihl, K., and Kascht, M. E.: The metabolic effects of progesterone in man. J. Clin. Endocr., 15:1194, 1955.
9. Landau, R. L., and Lugibihl, K.: Inhibition of the sodium-retaining influence of aldosterone by progesterone. J. Clin. Endocr., 18:1237, 1958.
10. Little, B., Tait, J. F., Tait, S. A. S., and Erlenmeyer, F.: The metabolic clearance rate of progesterone in males and ovariectomized females. J. Clin. Invest., 45:901, 1966.
11. Long, O., and Bradbury, J. T.: Induction and maintenance of decidual changes with progesterone and estrogen. J. Clin. Endocr., 11:134, 1951.
12. Ryan, K. J.: Hormones of the placenta. Amer. J. Obstet. Gynec., 84:1695, 1962.
13. Salhanick, H. A., Kipnis, D. M., and Vande Wiele, R. L.: Metabolic Effects of Gonadal Hormones and Contraceptive Steroids. Plenum Press, New York, 1969.
14. Sanders, F. J.: Endocrine properties and mechanism of action of oral contraceptives. Fed. Proc., 29:1211, 1970.
15. Van Der Molen, H. J., and Aakvaag, A.: Progesterone. In Gray, C. H., and Bacharach, A. L., eds.: Hormones in Blood, Vol. 2. Academic Press, New York, 1967, p. 221.

ANDROGENS

Androgens are the hormones of masculinity and as such are concerned with the development and maintenance of the sexual apparatus, bodily habitus, special metabolic characteristics, psyche, and libido of the male.[6, 14] In spite of this, androgens are present in both sexes, and in the pregnant female. Their ultimate physiologic effects depend, as with the estrogens, on the endocrine milieu and the conditioned and inherent sensitivity of target tissues.

HISTORY AND CHEMISTRY

Although an endocrine role for the testes was clearly established by reimplantation of the extirpated gonads into capons by Berthold in the mid 19th century, it was almost another hundred years before the male hormone was finally identified.

In 1931, Butenandt first isolated from urinary extracts a crystalline androgenic substance, androsterone, which was later shown to be a urinary metabolite of the primary testicular hormone. Another steroid, androstene-olone (dehydroepiandrosterone), was also found in urine and later shown to be a precursor of the testicular hormone. It was only with preparation of extracts of endocrine tissue in the mid 1930s that a much more potent and primary product of the testes was identified as the testosterone we now know as the male hormone.

Androstenedione, a weak androgen and

testosterone precursor, was first produced chemically and only later identified as a natural product of endocrine tissue. Dihydrotestosterone, another natural hormone, was also known to the chemist by synthesis before its isolation from tissue was accomplished. The relationships of these hormones are demonstrated in Figure 19.

The androgens are steroid hormones with 19 carbons and differ from the C_{21} progesterone and corticoids by the absence of a side chain and from the C_{18} estrogens by the presence of the methyl group, which is attached to carbon 10. The basic carbon ring structure is, of course, the same as for cho-

lesterol and the other steroids except for these differences. The A ring of testosterone, like that of progesterone and the corticoids, and unlike that of the aromatic estrogens, has a double bond at carbon 4 and a 3-keto group which provides absorption of ultraviolet light at 240 mμ. Unlike all other active hormonal steroids, the reduced-ring A compounds androsterone and dihydrotestosterone are potent compounds. Reduction of the A ring of other $\triangle^4$-3-ketones like progesterone or corticoids renders them inactive.

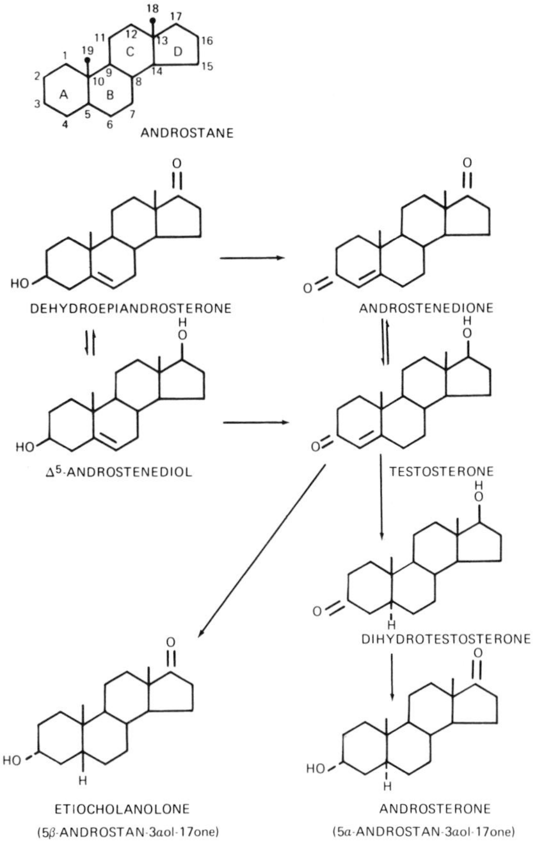

BIOSYNTHESIS

The androgens can be formed from the C-21 compounds pregnenolone or progesterone by 17-hydroxylation and side-chain cleavage in the testis, ovary, and adrenal.[7] The interstitial cells of the testes, the follicle, stroma, and corpus luteum of the ovary, and the zona fasciculata and reticularis of the adrenal are the locales of androgen hormone synthesis. The pathway for synthesis is illustrated in Figure 8. Testosterone is largely a testicular secretory product although small amounts of testosterone can also be released by the ovary and adrenal. In certain tumors or hyperplasia of the adrenal and in ovarian tumors and polycystic disease, marked secretion of testosterone may result in female hirsutism.

Ordinarily in the female, the adrenal and ovary both secrete androstenedione in the ratio of 2:1 *for their relative production* and since this is a weak androgen there are few masculinizing effects. In the same disease states in which the ovary or adrenal secretes excess testosterone, both androstenedione and dehydroepiandrosterone may also be secreted in excess.[3, 4, 16] Both androstenedione and dehydroepiandrosterone can be converted peripherally (as in the liver) to testosterone, and thus elevated levels of testosterone in the female can be the result of either excess secretion, as such, or peripheral transformation from weak androgens. In any case, androstenedione is a normal constituent of the female blood stream, in levels higher than in the male. The role of this hormone in female physiology is unknown.

Dehydroepiandrosterone as the sulfate ester is a normal secretory product of the

Figure 19. Examples of androgen biosynthesis and metabolism.

1. Testosterone can be derived from Δ^5-androstenediol without involving androstenedione.
2. Dihydrotostosterone and androsterone are both metabolites and active androgens.
3. Any of the androgens illustrated can give rise to the 17-ketosteroids, androsterone, and etiocholanolone.
4. Other metabolites that are stereoisomers of etiocholanolone and androsterone at positions C-3 and C-5 are possible as well as metabolites with ketonic functions at both C-3 and C-17.

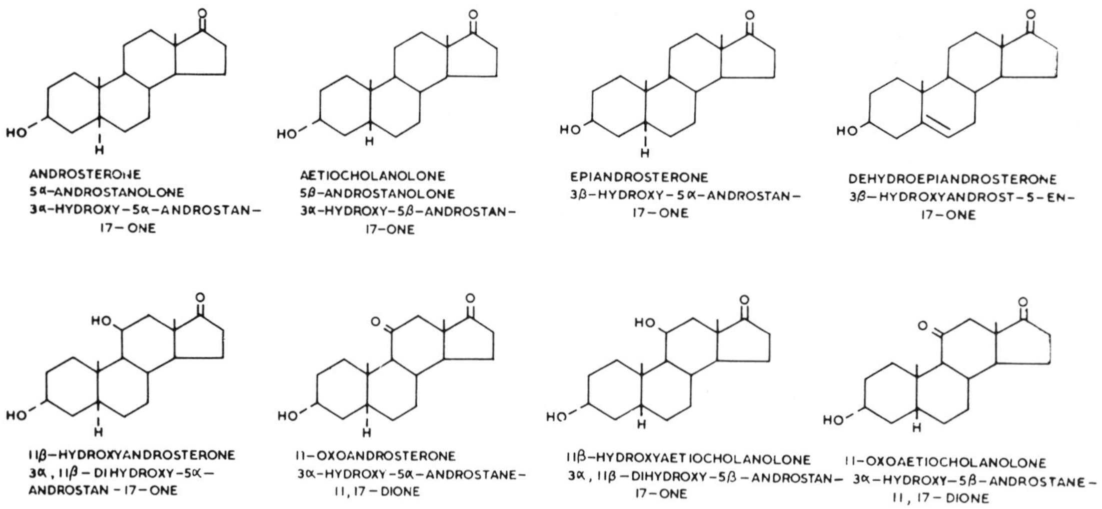

ANDROSTERONE
5α-ANDROSTANOLONE
3α-HYDROXY-5α-ANDROSTAN-17-ONE

AETIOCHOLANOLONE
5β-ANDROSTANOLONE
3α-HYDROXY-5β-ANDROSTAN-17-ONE

EPIANDROSTERONE
3β-HYDROXY-5α-ANDROSTAN-17-ONE

DEHYDROEPIANDROSTERONE
3β-HYDROXYANDROST-5-EN-17-ONE

11β-HYDROXYANDROSTERONE
3α, 11β-DIHYDROXY-5α-ANDROSTAN-17-ONE

11-OXOANDROSTERONE
3α-HYDROXY-5α-ANDROSTANE-11, 17-DIONE

11β-HYDROXYAETIOCHOLANOLONE
3α, 11β-DIHYDROXY-5β-ANDROSTAN-17-ONE

11-OXOAETIOCHOLANOLONE
3α-HYDROXY-5β-ANDROSTANE-11, 17-DIONE

Figure 20. Structural formulas of 17-ketosteroids. Those in the upper row are derived from both the gonads and adrenals, and those in the lower row exclusively from the adrenal glands. (From Loraine, J. A., and Bell, E. T.: Hormone Assays and Their Clinical Application, ed. 2. Williams and Wilkins, Baltimore, 1966.)

adrenal in both male and female. It is present in the blood stream of both sexes in high concentration and aside from its precursor role for placental estrogens in pregnancy its function is unknown (see Feto-Placental Unit, p. 117). It may play a role in puberty and development of pubic and axillary hair growth. Dehydroepiandrosterone can also be synthesized in testis and ovary.

In addition, the adrenal secretes 11-oxygenated C-19 steroids such as adrenosterone and these may contribute to total androgenic effects (Fig. 20).

METABOLISM

Testosterone, androstenedione, and dehydroepiandrosterone are excreted in the urine as conjugated 17-ketosteroids or as steroid alcohols with reduced ring structures. The levels of 17-ketosteroids in the urine of a female are an indicator largely of adrenal function except when ovarian hyperactivity exists. In the male, two thirds of the 17-ketosteroids are of adrenal origin and one third are of testicular origin. The various androgenic metabolites are illustrated in Figure 20.

The male metabolizes testosterone at a much greater rate than the female. If women are given testosterone over a long period, the turnover of the steroid will increase, since metabolic clearance is related to the blood level of the hormone. This difference in metabolism does not pertain to androstenedione. As noted in Table 5, the metabolism of testosterone is two times greater in the male than in the female, a difference that is obliterated in hirsute women who have elevated blood testosterone levels. Of the testosterone in the blood of normal women, 49 per cent is formed by peripheral conversion from androstenedione (see prehormones, p. 6).[1, 8, 15, 18]

The protein that binds testosterone is increased by estrogens and both the binding protein and blood levels of testosterone and androstenedione are above normal during pregnancy. Levels of androgens in fetal blood are also elevated although there is no significant difference between male and female fetuses in this respect. Although the blood testosterone in pregnant women is elevated, its binding to the increased amounts of protein reduces the androgenic potential and virilization does not occur.[2, 5, 12, 13, 18]

SECRETION AND PRODUCTION RATES AND CHANGES IN PREGNANCY

In the male, the production rate of testosterone is 7 mg./24 hours and the blood levels average 0.6 mcg./100 ml. Blood production rates and concentration of testosterone in the female are 0.35 mg. per day and 0.04 mcg./100 ml, respectively. Androstenedione is produced at a rate of 1.4 to 3.0 mg./24 hours and 3.0 to 4.0 mg./24 hours in male and female, respectively.[9, 11, 15, 17] It is of interest that during development

TABLE 5. ANDROGEN DYNAMICS IN THE HUMAN MALE AND FEMALE

	Androgen	MCR° (L./day)	Blood Level (mcg./100 ml.)	PR† (mg./day)
Adult male	Testosterone	1179–1288	0.768	5.78–7.08
	Androstenedione	2210	0.03–0.17	1.4–3.0
Adult female	Testosterone	545–675	0.042	0.29–0.35
	Androstenedione	2070	0.05–0.185	3.3–3.7
Hirsute female	Testosterone	1067	0.06–0.09	1.7
	Androstenedione	2300	0.28	6.0
Pregnant female	Testosterone		0.140	
	Androstenedione		0.420	
Newborn cord blood	Testosterone		0.056	
	Androstenedione		0.10	

°MCR—Metabolic clearance rate.
†PR—Production rate.

the ratio of the weak androgen androstenedione to testosterone, a strong androgen, gradually declines as puberty approaches in the male. The blood level of androstenedione seems to be relatively constant throughout the menstrual cycle, whereas blood levels of androgens rise during pregnancy[2] and urinary androgens may vary with the cycle,[10] with higher values in the luteal phase.

BIOLOGIC EFFECTS AND PHARMACOLOGIC USES

Testosterone has primary effects in providing a positive nitrogen balance as well as in stimulating the male secondary sex organs, lowering the voice, and affecting hair distribution and libido.[6, 14] Attempts have been made to dissociate the anabolic from the masculinizing effects, with incomplete success. Most anabolic steroids have masculinizing activity as well. Testosterone can antagonize estrogen effects on the uterus and vagina and has slight progestational properties. There are very few clinical uses for androgens in female endocrinology, although they have been used to control uterine bleeding, modulate estrogen effects, and prevent breast engorment post partum. Use in uterine bleeding has largely been discarded. In the male, testosterone and various synthetic derivatives are used largely for replacement therapy. An interesting clinical entity, testicular

feminization, demonstrates the principle of end-organ refractoriness to testosterone.

Androgens have effects on the developing hypothalamus in experimental animals and, as indicated on page 61, can influence the pattern of gonadotropin secretion in later life. Whether this is applicable to primates and the human is unknown but it could be important in the genesis of diseases such as polycystic ovaries.

MECHANISM OF ACTION

Studies of androgen effects on tissues in the presence of metabolic inhibitors suggest that the mechanism of action of these hormones is via specific stimulation of new protein and enzyme synthesis by augmented replication of messenger RNA. Recent work has also suggested that dihydrotestosterone is the primary hormone at the tissue level since testosterone is readily converted to this active metabolite in the target organ. Further elucidation of the mechanism of action and the active hormone at the site of action is anticipated.

SUMMARY

Although androgens are clearly the hormone of the male, where their function in development and the maintenance of the sexual apparatus is clearly evident, these hormones are also present in the female, where their role is largely unknown. Not only the testis, but also the ovary and adrenal can synthesize androgens and in disease states can secrete amounts sufficient to cause masculinization in the female. Androgen blood levels rise during pregnancy but this is probably masked by the high quantities of estrogens present and by increased protein binding. Clinical use of androgens is largely confined to replacement therapy in the male. Attempts are constantly being made to separate the anabolic effect of androgens from their masculinizing properties to produce an anabolic steroid for use in debilitating diseases, but as yet none has been completely successful.

BIBLIOGRAPHY

1. Abraham, G. E., Lobotsky, J., and Lloyd, C. W.: Metabolism of testosterone and androstenedione in normal and ovariectomized women. J. Clin. Invest., 48:696, 1969.
2. August, G. P., Tkachuk, M., and Grumbach, M. M.: Plasma testosterone-binding affinity and testosterone in umbilical cord plasma, late pregnancy, prepubertal children, and adults. J. Clin. Endocr., 29:891, 1969.
3. Bardin, C. W., Hembree, W. C., and Lipsett, M. B.: Suppression of testosterone and androstenedione production rates with dexamethasone in women with idiopathic hirsutism and polycystic ovaries. J. Clin. Endocr., 28:1300, 1968.
4. Bardin, C. W., and Lipsett, M. B.: Testosterone and androstenedione blood production rates in normal women and women with idiopathic hirsutism or polycystic ovaries. J. Clin. Invest., 46:891, 1967.
5. Bird, C. E., Green, R. N., and Clark, A. F.: Effect of the administration of estrogen on the disappearance of ³H-testosterone in the plasma of human subjects. J. Clin. Endocr., 29:123, 1969.
6. Dorfman, R. I., and Shipley, R. A.: Androgens; Biochemistry, Physiology and Clinical Significance. Wiley, New York, 1956.
7. Eberlein, W. R., Winter, J., and Rosenfield, R. L.: The androgens. In Gray, C. H., and Bacharach, A. L., eds.: Academic Press, New York, 1967, p. 187.
8. Horton, R., Shinsako, J., and Forsham, P. H.: Testosterone production and metabolic clearance rates with volumes of distribution in normal adult men and women. Acta Endocr., 48:446, 1965.
9. Kirschner, M. A., and Coffman, G. D.: Measurement of plasma testosterone and △⁴-androstenedione using electron capture gas-liquid chromatography. J. Clin. Endocr., 28:1347, 1968.
10. Longhino, N., Tajić, M., Vedris, M., Janković, D., and Drobnjak, P.: Urinary excretion of androstenedione, testosterone, epitestosterone and dehydroepiandrosterone during the normal menstrual cycle. Acta Endocr., 59:644, 1968.
11. Mayes, D., and Nugent, C. A.: Determination of plasma testosterone by the use of competitive protein binding. J. Clin. Endocr., 28:1169, 1968.
12. Mizuno, M., Lobotsky, J., Lloyd, C. W., Kobayashi, T., and Murasawa, Y.: Plasma androstenedione and testerone during pregnancy and in the newborn. J. Clin. Endocr., 28:1133, 1968.
13. Pearlman, W. H., Crepy, O., and Murphy, M.: Testosterone-binding levels in the serum of women during the normal menstrual cycle, pregnancy, and the post-partum period. J. Clin. Endocr., 27:1012, 1967.
14. Pincus, G.: The physiology of ovarian and testis hormones. In Pincus, G., and Thimann, K. V., eds.: The Hormones, Vol. 3. Academic Press, New York, 1955.
15. Southren, A. L., Gordon, G. G., and Tochimoto, S.: Further study of factors affecting the metabolic clearance rate of testosterone in man. J. Clin. Endocr., 28:1105, 1968.
16. Southren, A. L., Gordon, G. G., Tochimoto, S., Olivo, J., Sherman, D. H., and Pinzon, G.: Testosterone and androstenedione metabolism in the polycystic ovary syndrome: studies of the percentage binding of testosterone in plasma. J. Clin. Endocr., 29:1356, 1969.
17. Southren, A. L., Gordon, G. G., Tochimoto, S., Pinson, G., Lane, D. R., and Stypulkowski, W.: Mean plasma concentration, metabolic clearance and basal plasma production rates of testosterone in normal young men and women using a constant infusion procedure: effect of time of day and plasma concentration on the metabolic clearance rate of testosterone. J. Clin. Endocr., 27:686, 1967.
18. Vermeulen, A., Verdonck, L., Van der Straeten, M., and Orie, N.: Capacity of the testosterone-binding globulin in human plasma and influence of specific binding of testosterone on its metabolic clearance rate. J. Clin. Endocr., 29:1470, 1969.

PROSTAGLANDINS

Prostaglandins are lipid substances originally isolated from seminal fluid in 1930; they have since been detected in many tissues including the central nervous system, amniotic fluid, endometrium, decidua, and umbilical cord. There are six primary prostaglandins, each containing 20 carbons and a cyclopentane ring with minor differences in substituents and unsaturation (Fig. 21). Prostaglandins PGE_1, PGE_2, and PGF_2 have been studied in relation to effects on the myometrium, induction of labor, and abortion as well as influences upon corpus luteum function.[4, 10] Although there are differences in the response of the uterus to the several types of prostaglandins studied, labor has been induced in late pregnancy with PGF_2 and PGE_2 and ther-

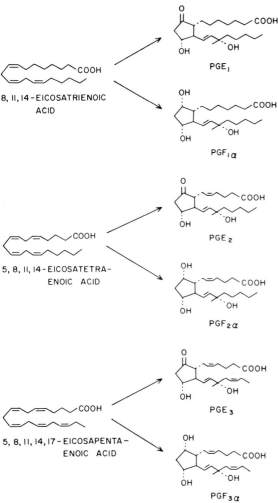

8, 11, 14 - EICOSATRIENOIC ACID

PGE₁

PGF₁α

5, 8, 11, 14 - EICOSATETRA-ENOIC ACID

PGE₂

PGF₂α

5, 8, 11, 14, 17 - EICOSAPENTA-ENOIC ACID

PGE₃

PGF₃α

Figure 21. The primary prostaglandins and the three primary precursors. (From Speroff, L., and Ramwell, P. W.: Amer. J. Obstet. Gynec., 107:1111, 1970.)

apeutic abortion has been accomplished in the first and second trimester after intravenous infusion of PGF_2.[1, 2, 3, 5, 6, 7]

Amniotic fluid of patients in spontaneous labor has been demonstrated to contain PGE_1 and PGF_2 but that of patients not in labor has been found to have small or no detectable amounts of these substances; these findings suggest a relationship of these agents with labor.

Prostaglandin F_2 has been reported to cause corpus luteum regression in both the sheep and the rhesus monkey when administered in vivo, an effect presumed to be related to effects upon blood flow.[8, 9]

Thus far the data on the biologic properties of prostaglandins have been meager but as knowledge of their action on the reproductive system has become available in the last few years, interest and study have proliferated rapidly. It is still too early to predict the ultimate role of prostaglandins in normal reproductive physiology or their possible function as pharmacologic agents.

BIBLIOGRAPHY

1. Beazley, J. M., Dewhurst, C. J., and Gillespie, A.: The induction of labour with prostaglandin E_2. J. Obstet. Gynaec. Brit. Comm., 77:193, 1970.
2. Bygdeman, M., Kwon, S. U., Mukherjee, T., Roth-Brandel, U., and Wiqvist, N.: The effect of the prostaglandin F compounds on the contractility of the pregnant human uterus. Amer. J. Obstet. Gynec., 106:567, 1970.
3. Embrey, M. P.: The effect of prostaglandins on the human pregnant uterus. J. Obstet. Gynaec. Brit. Comm., 76:783, 1969.
4. Horton, E. W.: Hypotheses on physiological roles of prostaglandins. Physiol. Rev., 49:122, 1969.
5. Karim, S. M. M., and Filshie, G. M.: Therapeutic abortion using prostaglandin $F_{2×}$. Lancet, 1:157, 1970.
6. Karim, S. M. M., Hillier, K., Trussell, R. R., Patel, R. C., and Tamusange, S.: Induction of labour with prostaglandin E_2. J. Obstet. Gynaec. Brit. Comm., 77:200, 1970.
7. Karim, S. M. M., Trussell, R. R., Hillier, K., and Patel, R. C.: Induction of labour with prostaglandin $F_{2α}$. Obstet. Gynaec. Brit. Comm., 76:769, 1969.
8. Kirton, K. T., Pharriss, B. B., and Forbes, A. D.: Luteolytic effects of prostaglandin $F_{2α}$ in primates. Proc. Soc. Exp. Biol. Med., 133:314, 1970.
9. McCracken, J. A., Glew, M. E., and Scaramuzzi, R. J.: Corpus luteum regression induced by prostaglandin $F_{2α}$. J. Clin. Endocr., 30:544, 1970.
10. Speroff, L., and Ramwell, P. W.: Prostaglandins in reproductive physiology. Amer. J. Obstet. Gynec., 107:1111, 1970.

Chapter 2

Protein Hormones

Progress in our understanding of placental, pituitary, and other protein hormones has been markedly enhanced: (1) by isolation, purification, structural identification, and, in some instances, actual synthesis of these complex substances;[1, 3] (2) by preparation of species-specific human material in purity and quantity suitable for clinical use, as in the cases of pituitary gonadotropins and growth hormone; and (3) by development of highly sensitive and specific assay methods which can be used for repeated determinations in small samples of blood to measure dynamic hormonal changes in the ovulatory cycle, in childhood, in stress, and during pregnancy.[2, 4–6] The assay technique most widely used is a radioimmunoassay method in which the amount of binding of a radioactively labeled (^{131}I) standard protein hormone to a specific antigen is altered by the concentration of the unknown plasma hormone to be measured. Thus the sensitivity of radioactive tracer measurement has been coupled with the specificity of an immunologic antigen-antibody reaction. With this procedure growth hormone, insulin, pituitary gonadotropins, and placental hormones have all been quantitated during various phases of the reproductive cycle.

Several aspects of the physiology of the protein hormones bear emphasis. Unlike the steroids, which are essentially structurally identical in all the animals in which they occur, the protein hormones isolated from various species vary in their physical-chemical characteristics and amino acid composition. As a consequence, it is not surprising that these proteins are recognized as foreign substances in cross-species administration and that antibodies are formed which interfere with clinical use but can be used for assay. In addition, a species specificity exists which results in many of these animal protein hormones being inactive when tested for certain effects in man, as in the case with growth hormone and gonadotropins. A summary of these protein hormones is presented in Table 1. The hypophyseotropic hormones (hypothalamic releasing and inhibiting factors) will be considered with Hypothalamus (p. 58).

BIBLIOGRAPHY

1. Friesen, H., and Astwood, E. B.: Hormones of the anterior pituitary body. N. Eng. J. Med., 272: 1272, 1328, 1965.
2. Jaffe, R. B., and Midgley, A. R., Jr.: Current status of human gonadotropin radioimmunoassay. Obstet. Gynec. Survey, 24:200, 1969.
3. Li, C. H.: Current concepts on the chemical biology of pituitary hormones. Perspect. Biol. Med., 11: 498, 1968.
4. Midgley, A. R.: Radioimmunoassay for human follicle-stimulating hormone. J. Clin. Endocr., 27:295, 1967.
5. Midgley, A. R., Jr.: Radioimmunoassay: a method for human chorionic gonadotropin and human luteinizing hormone. Endocrinology, 79:10, 1966.
6. Wide, L., Roos, P., and Gemzell, C.: Immunological determination of human pituitary luteinizing hormone (LH). Acta Endocr., 37:445, 1961.

HUMAN CHORIONIC GONADOTROPIN (HCG)

Human chorionic gonadotropin (HCG) is a glycoprotein hormone produced by the placenta during human pregnancy. Secretion occurs predominantly into the maternal rather than the fetal circulation and large quantities of the hormone can ultimately be recovered from maternal urine, the first demonstrable levels being present as early as 10 days after conception.[54] Assay of HCG in maternal urine has been utilized for more than 25 years as a test for pregnancy that is especially helpful in the period before maternal and fetal physical changes can provide confirmation. The functions of HCG have not been completely established but it is likely that a major role for this hor-

TABLE 1. PROTEIN HORMONES

Tissue Source	Hormone	Major Biological Properties	Structure	Molecular Weight	Comment
Placenta	Human chorionic gonadotropin (HCG)	Luteinizing, luteotropic	Glycoprotein	30,000	Cross-reacts immunologically with human pituitary LH
	Human chorionic somatomammotropin (Placental lactogen, HPL)	Lactogenic, metabolic, growth-promoting, diabetogenic	Protein	38,000 (2 chains of 20,000)	Cross-reacts immunologically with human pituitary growth hormone
	Human chorionic thyrotropin	Thyroid-stimulating		–	Cross-reacts immunologically with *bovine* TSH
Anterior pituitary	Follicle-stimulating hormone (FSH)	Follicle growth, synergism with LH for steroid production, spermatogenesis	Glycoprotein	29,000	
	Luteinizing hormone (LH)	Steroid production, ovulation hormone	Glycoprotein	26,000	Cross-reacts immunologically with HCG
	Growth hormone, somatotropin	Skeletal and visceral growth, metabolic effects	Protein	21,500	Cross-reacts immunologically with HPL Has some LTH activity
	Adrenocorticotropin (ACTH)	Control of adrenal growth and secretion	Polypeptide	4,500	Has been synthesized in laboratory
	Prolactin Luteotropin (LTH)	Mammotropic, lactogenic, luteotropic	Protein	25,000	Not yet isolated as a distinct hormone in human
	Thyrotropin (TSH)	Thyroid stimulation	Glycoprotein	26,000-30,000	
	Melanocyte-stimulating hormone (MSH)	Melanocyte stimulation	Polypeptide	2,734	Has amino acid sequence in common with portion of ACTH
Neurohypophysis	Oxytocin	Uterine stimulation, milk letdown	Polypeptide	1,007	Octapeptide synthesized in laboratory
	Vasopressin	Antiduretic	Polypeptide	1,084	Octapeptide synthesized in laboratory

mone is as a luteotropin. HCG can stimulate and prolong the otherwise transient existence of the corpus luteum, thereby assuring a continued supply of ovarian progesterone until the placenta can itself secrete this steroid which is essential for the maintenance of pregnancy. This transition from an ovarian to a placental progesterone source occurs at about six to eight weeks of gestation. Other functions for HCG which have been postulated but not confirmed include tropic actions on the placenta itself and on the fetal adrenals and gonads.

CHEMISTRY

Several detailed physical-chemical studies have been carried out on extensively purified HCG with potencies of 12,000 to 18,000 international units per milligram of hormone.[4, 5, 8, 21, 23, 43, 47, 52] Since HCG is not available as a pure or homogeneous preparation, all measurements of this hormone are compared to an international standard and reported for biologic assay and immunoassay in terms of international units.[6] The molecular weight has been variously assigned as 27,000 to 59,000 with the spread probably due to the fact that the molecule can exist as a dimer of two polypeptide chains of the 27,000 molecular weight size.

The polypeptide portion accounts for 66 per cent of the molecular weight and amino acid analysis reveals remarkably high values for proline, cystine, and serine, with no free SH groups. The carbohydrate content of the molecule represents 33 per cent of its weight, with 11 residues of N-acetylglucosamine, 9 of mannose and galactose, 8 of sialic acid, 3 of N-acetylgalactosamine, and 1 of fucose per glycopeptide chain of 27,000.[4, 5] The molecule is unique in its high content of sialic acid, and the varying potencies and heterogeneity of isolated preparations have been attributed to alterations in the sialic acid content during purification. It is suggested that each peptide chain has attached to it two large multiple-branched heteropolysaccharide units and three short oligosaccharide chains.[5] The function of the carbohydrate portion of the molecule is unknown but it is essential for biologic activity since enzymatic removal of sialic acid abolishes the hormone's biologic properties.[7] Antigenicity of the molecule is, however, not altered under these conditions.[40]

HCG shares with pituitary luteinizing hormone (LH) an immunologic cross-reactivity,[33, 57] and review of their amino acid and carbohydrate compositions reveals similarities including comparable molecular weights, but HCG does differ in having more total carbohydrates and specifically much more sialic acid.

BIOLOGIC EFFECTS

Chorionic gonadotropin has biologic properties similar but not identical to those of pituitary LH.[15, 18] In common with LH it causes luteinization of ovarian follicular and interstitial cells, induces ovulation of follicles primed by follicle-stimulating hormone (FSH) and LH, causes stimulation of the interstitial cells of the testis, enhances progesterone production by the isolated corpus luteum in vitro, and stimulates testosterone synthesis by the testis. These properties may be demonstrated not only in the human but also in various test animals that provide a basis for biologic assays to be described later.

The molecular basis for the mechanism of action of HCG has not yet been established but has been a matter of intense investigation. Increased steroid hormone synthesis is a major consequence of HCG action on the gonads. It has been variously postulated that this effect is produced by one or more of the following mechanisms: increased acetate-to-cholesterol conversion; increased cholesterol 20α-hydroxylation; provision of an accessible pool of preformed steroid precursor such as cholesterol esters; or provision of increased amounts of cofactors to augment the biosynthetic reactions required in progesterone, androgen, and estrogen formation.

In addition, HCG increases enzyme activities in ovarian cells and increases blood flow to the organ. Some activities of HCG are abolished by inhibitors of RNA and protein synthesis; this suggests a locus of action in the direction of new enzyme or protein formation. Some of the actions of HCG and LH can be mimicked by cyclic-AMP, which also increases luteal progesterone production in association with increased RNA and protein synthesis.[31] Furthermore, LH and presumably HCG can increase the concentration of cyclic-AMP in the corpus luteum by activating the enzyme adenyl cyclase. In this respect, cyclic-AMP has been considered an intracellular messenger for LH and HCG. At this point the molecular action of HCG or LH is still a matter of conjecture.

HCG has the unique property, not shared to the same extent by LH, of extending the functional life of the corpus luteum beyond its usual duration in the ovarian cycle of primates (the differences between LH and HCG with respect to luteotropic properties may depend on the fact that HCG is less rapidly cleared from the blood and less rapidly metabolized than the pituitary hormone by a factor of 10). Human placental lactogen (HPL) is also luteotropic but its role relative to HCG is unknown. These properties of HCG and perhaps HPL are believed to be of importance in the endocrine control of early pregnancy in maintaining an ovarian source of steroid hormones until the placental endocrine activity supervenes. This role for HCG has been challenged but the data available are sufficiently suggestive to maintain this hypothesis as the most attractive one for HCG function in early human pregnancy. In the human, the onset of menstruation as a result of corpus luteum failure has been delayed 13 to 19 days by exogenous HCG; progesterone metabolites in the urine have been maintained and histologic changes in the corpora lutea suggestive of pregnancy have been observed in endometrium and ovary.[12, 13, 44] Similar prolongation of the cycle length and histologic changes in the corpora lutea were observed after HCG administration to monkeys.[25] HCG does appear to have significant inherent FSH activity, with a ratio of 500:1 of HCG to FSH potencies, that is apparent only at high dosage of HCG.[1] Although there have been reports that an FSH-like activity is present in pregnancy urine, the significance of these reports has not yet been established with respect to whether it is a separate hormone or part of the spectrum of HCG activities.[42]

HCG is present throughout pregnancy including the later months when its presumed role in corpus luteum maintenance is no longer required. No function for HCG during this period has been assigned but the suggestion has been offered that it may have a regulatory effect on placental steroid production or fetal endocrine tissues. Some effects of HCG upon placental steroid production have been reported on the basis of perfusion studies in which formation of estrogens or estrogen metabolites was augmented.[4] HCG may also have stimulatory effects upon the fetal adrenals and gonads in utero.[28, 29]

THE PLACENTA AS A SITE OF HCG FORMATION

Studies in the early 1900s demonstrated the presence of gonadotropic principles in placental extracts but the gross nature of HCG production in pregnancy was established by Aschheim and Zondek between 1927 and 1929. They demonstrated its presence in human pregnancy blood and urine and devised their classic test for its assay in immature mice. Although they originally believed that HCG was of pituitary origin, further studies by many investigators established HCG as a placental secretory product unique to the human and to trophoblastic tissue, although material similar to it has been described in several other primates.[24, 50, 51]

Evidence for the placental origin of HCG includes the following:[18] (1) it can be extracted directly from the placenta; (2) it is present in pregnancy urine and blood after implantation and disappears after delivery; (3) HCG is present in body fluids after fetal demise, when the cord is clamped experimentally, and when the placenta is left in situ in abdominal pregnancies, and its concentration in fetal blood is relatively low—all of these facts eliminating the fetus as a source of the hormone; (4) following hypophysectomy during pregnancy, HCG continues to be present—this fact eliminating the pituitary as a source; (5) HCG can be produced by placental tissue implanted into

the anterior chamber of the eye of experimental animals and by placental transplants in other animal sites; (6) HCG can be produced by placental tissue in culture and by placental perfusions in vitro; (7) immunofluorescent techniques localize HCG to the trophoblast and to the syncytial cell layer of the placenta; and (8) not only normal placental tissue, but trophoblast of diverse cellular types, including choriocarcinoma in either the male or female and hydatidiform mole, can produce HCG.

CELLULAR ORIGIN OF HCG

The cellular locus of HCG formation had been postulated to be the cytotrophoblastic layer of the placenta; this conclusion is based on positive histochemical staining for glycoprotein in that cell type and also on the correlation of the dynamics of morphologic cell changes and HCG excretion— i.e., the cytotrophoblastic cell is most apparent at the time of highest HCG titers in blood and urine. In addition, tissue culture production of HCG was believed due to a surviving cytotrophoblastic cell type in the culture. Immunofluorescent techniques have more recently localized the intracellular site of HCG to the syncytiotrophoblastic cell in both placenta and choriocarcinoma. Insofar as localization of the hormone cannot absolutely demonstrate site of synthesis, the cell of origin is still in question but the most likely site of production now appears to be the syncytiotrophoblast, which is ultimately derived from the cytotrophoblastic cell.[36, 37, 48, 49]

HCG ASSAY

Requirements for the assay of HCG in body fluids or tissues depend to a large extent on the nature of the clinical or research application of the data. Pregnancy tests require a simple yes or no answer and for these a qualitative assay of reasonable specificity and sensitivity is adequate. Measurements of HCG for describing the endocrine dynamics of reproduction or for following patients with malignant trophoblastic disease require quantitative assays of higher specificity and precision.[30] The general classes of HCG assay available are either of a biologic or of an immunologic type.

Bioassay

Biologic assays of HCG depend upon measurement of the response of the ovary or testis of experimental animals (rats, mice) to the gonadotropin. These tests include the primary response of increase in ovarian weight or hyperemia, or the secondary response of increase in size of secondary sex organs produced by the increased steroidogenesis in gonadotropin-stimulated gonads (Table 2). The latter tests include measurement of increases in weight of uterine, prostatic, or total male accessory reproductive organs. Expulsion of ova or sperm from amphibia is also utilized for HCG assay.[30]

Immunoassay

The capacity of HCG and other protein hormones to evoke a specific antibody response upon injection into animals has been utilized to prepare antisera for use in immunologic assay. For the assay to be specific, an antigen, in this case HCG, of highest purity must be available. Although the purest antigens now used are still not completely homogeneous on immuno-electrophoresis, they can be employed for practical purposes. Antisera to HCG cross-react with human pituitary LH and it is believed that the two molecules share common immunologic determinants. There are, however, methods of distinguishing between the two hormones so that the low maternal levels at implantation or the low values in cord blood can be identified specifically as HCG and not LH.[34, 54]

The three general types of immunologic assays used are: *hemagglutination-inhibition*, which depends on the ability of HCG to inhibit an agglutination reaction between HCG-coated red cells and HCG antisera; *complement-fixation tests*, which rely on the utilization of complement in antigen-antibody interaction; and *radioimmunoassay*, which depends upon competition of the HCG to be measured with radioactively labeled HCG for sites on the antibody.

Pregnancy Tests Based on HCG Assay

The pregnancy tests utilized can best be summarized in tabular form (Table 3). Several of these are now of only historical interest since the speed and convenience of the immunoassays are supplementing almost all others in practical use. The reliability of all such tests is comparable and all are suitable for routine clinical usage.[26, 30, 32, 45]

HCG LEVELS IN PLACENTA, URINE, AND SERUM

Quantitative measurements of HCG have relied predominantly on bioassay in the past, but radioimmunoassay is now becoming a major technique employed because of its sensitivity. Of the bioassay methods only the measurement of male rat accessory organs allows assay of HCG in untreated pregnancy sera.[30] It is also apparent that immunologic and biologic assays do not always measure the same substance since biologically inactive material may give an immunologic response. Even if the biologic

TABLE 2. BIOASSAY METHODS FOR HCG

Primary Effects Upon Gonads	Secondary Effects Upon Reproductive Tract
Rat ovarian weight	Rat uterine weight
Rat ovarian hyperemia	Rat vaginal smears
Expulsion of toad spermatozoa	Rat total or ventral prostate weight
	Seminal vesicle weight
	Total accessory reproductive organs

TABLE 3. PREGNANCY TESTS

Test	End-Point	Time Involved
Aschheim-Zondek	Hemorrhagic follicles and corpora lutea in immature mice	5 days
Friedman	Ovulation in rabbits	24–48 hours
Kupperman	Hyperemia in rat ovaries	2 hours
Hogben	Ovulation by the toad	24 hours
Galli Mainini	Expulsion of sperm from male amphibia	2 hours
Latex slide test	Immunologic agglutination of latex particle on a slide	2 minutes
Hemagglutination-inhibition	Inhibition of hemagglutination reaction	2 hours

potency is reduced experimentally by alteration in the carbohydrate portion of the molecule, immunoassay remains undisturbed since the carbohydrate is not involved in the antigenic structure of the molecule. As a consequence, curves of HCG excretion in urine during pregnancy vary according to the technique utilized.[2, 38, 39, 46]

Normal Pregnancy

HCG can be detected in pregnancy urine some 9 to 16 days[27, 54] post conception (Fig. 1, 2). It rises progressively to reach a characteristic peak between days 50 to 70 and then declines to a more or less constant level until term (Fig. 3). A similar pattern is observed for the concentration of HCG in the placenta.[17] The values in urine at the peak by bioassay are 20,000 to 100,000 I.U. HCG per day and later in pregnancy the values range between 4000 and 11,000 I.U. There is almost a parallelism between values in serum and urine, there being an equivalent unitage per liter of serum and urinary excretion per 24 hours.[30] HCG values of 0.252 I.U. per milliliter and 0.388 I.U. per milliliter have been reported for cord arterial and venous plasma, respectively.[9]

The values obtained by immunoassay in the early stages of pregnancy have usu-

ally been lower than those reported for bioassay and the characteristic first trimester peak is less marked. As the immuno-

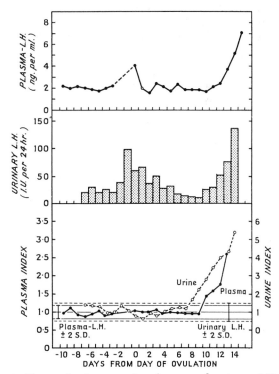

Figure 1. Increase in plasma and urinary LH (HCG) signaling placental production of hormone within 10 to 12 days after ovulation. (From Wide, L.: Lancet, 2:863, 1969.)

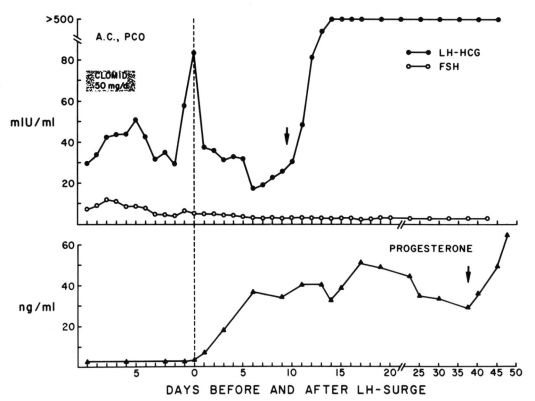

Figure 2. Serum FSH (○—○), LH-HCG (●—●) (upper curves), and progesterone (lower curve) during a Clomid-induced ovulatory cycle and during the early period of ensuing pregnancy. Arrow in upper curve indicates rise of HCG within 10 days of ovulation. Arrow in lower curve indicates shift from corpus luteum to placental progesterone production. Note low FSH throughout. (From Yen, S. S. C., Vela, P., and Ryan, K. J.: J. Clin. Endocr., 31–7, 1970.)

assay methods have been refined and made more specific, the immunologic and bio-assay data have become comparable (Fig. 4)[46] but quantitative differences still persist.[2, 11] There is no diurnal variation for HCG levels in serum and values in multiple pregnancies appear to be higher. Higher HCG levels in serum have been reported in association with female fetuses compared to males.[10] The difference was statistically highly significant and suggests a possible fetal relationship to HCG production or metabolism. The disappearance curve of HCG in plasma has two components and the complete disappearance of HCG after delivery takes several days. HCG half-life averages 8 hours (Figs. 5 and 6). The metabolic clearance rate of HCG is similar for men and nonpregnant women. The renal clearance of HCG reported in the literature varies between 0.38 and 0.95 ml. per minute. Clearance values did not vary during pregnancy

in normal, mildly pre-eclamptic, hypertensive, or diabetic patients. In severe pre-eclampsia the clearance declined. Because of the relatively constant renal clearance during pregnancy, it is assumed that variations in serum and urine levels are determined by alterations in production or inactivation rather than in excretion. The percentage of secreted HCG that finally reaches the urine in measurable form has been estimated at 20 per cent. It is therefore impossible at this time to calculate actual production rates for HCG but the range would be some 16 to 30 mg. per day at the peak level in the first trimester and about 1.4 mg. per day at term.[35, 41, 56]

Hydatidiform Mole and Choriocarcinoma

Patients with hydatidiform moles tend to have higher urine and serum-HCG levels

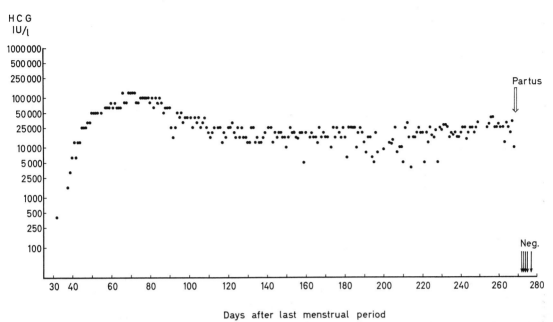

Figure 3. Immunologic activity in 222 morning urines from one woman with a normal pregnancy. (From Wide, L.: Acta Endocr., 41:[Suppl. 70]1, 1962.)

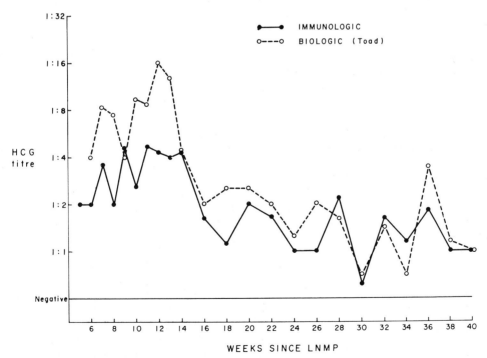

Figure 4. Calculated immunologic and biologic levels of HCG excretion throughout pregnancy for one of five normal subjects. (From Taymor, M. L., Goss, D. A., and Tamada, T.: Fertil. Steril., 17:613, 1966.)

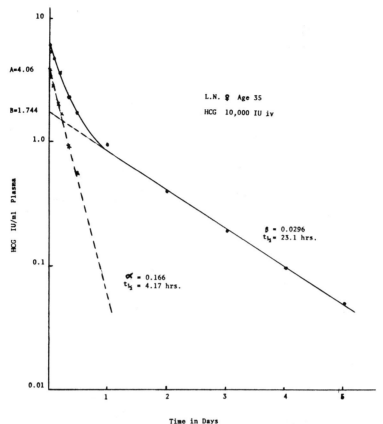

Figure 5. Semilogarithmic plot of plasma concentration after intravenous administration of 10,000 I.U. of HCG, indicating its half-life in plasma. (From Rizkallah, T., Gurpide, E., and Vande Wiele, R. L.: J. Clin. Endocr., 29:92, 1969.)

than women with normal pregnancies, with average values over 300,000 I.U. per liter of urine. With evacuation of the mole the HCG titer is markedly reduced in one month and HCG is absent after three months in 91 per cent of cases (Fig. 7). In complicated cases or those with retention of tissue, values remain elevated. Patients with choriocarcinoma also secrete large quantities of HCG and their response to chemotherapy or surgery can be followed by serial quantitative assays (Fig. 8).[16, 17, 19, 20, 38, 55]

Abnormal Pregnancy

ABORTION. Studies during early pregnancy suggest that the levels of HCG may be abnormally low in paients with threatened or habitual abortion. Reported experience is variable, however, and a definite relationship between pregnancy outcome and HCG levels is difficult to establish, although recent immunologic assays demonstrate a correlation. Levels of HCG in ectopic pregnancy appear to be below normal even at first examination.

PRE-ECLAMPSIA AND DIABETES. It has been reported that in severe pre-eclampsia, with or without diabetes, HCG levels are apt to be elevated, but the significance and utility of these findings are yet to be discovered. Results of HCG assay in pregnancy with hyperemesis or Rh incompatibility have been variable depending on the assay utilized and the degree of the

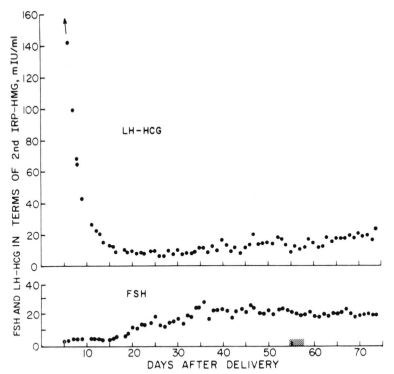

Figure 6. Decline in HCG concentration after delivery of the placenta and rise of FSH as cyclic ovarian function resumes. (From Jaffe, R. B., Lee, P. A., and Midgley, A. R., Jr.: J. Clin. Endocr., 29:1281, 1969.)

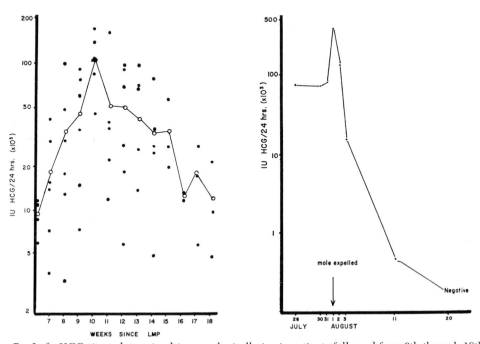

Figure 7. Left, HCG titers determined immunologically in six patients followed from 6th through 18th week since last menstrual period. Mean titer is depicted by line joining open circles. Titers of HCG (I.U. per 24 hr.) are graphed on a log scale. Right, HCG titers determined immunologically in patient with a benign (Group I) mole. (From Goss, D. A., and Taymor, M. L.: Fertil. Steril., 16:151, 1965.)

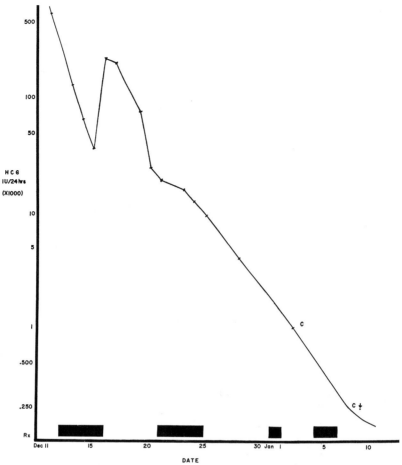

Figure 8. HCG titers determined immunologically in patient with metastatic choriocarcinoma. Periods of treatment with actinomycin D (8 μg./kg.) are depicted by solid bars. Titers of HCG (I.U. per 24 hr.) are graphed on log scale. (From Goss, D. A., and Taymor, M. L.: Fertil. Steril., 16:151, 1965.)

disorder. Such assays have not thus far been of clinical importance in the management or understanding of the processes studied.

SUMMARY

HCG is a protein hormone produced by the placenta in human pregnancy with chemical and biologic properties similar to those of pituitary LH. It has in addition a characteristic ability to extend the life of the corpus luteum of the cycle. This is believed to be a major function of HCG in the transition from ovarian to placental endocrine control of primate pregnancy. HCG is detectable in serum and urine in very early pregnancy and can be measured by biologic and immunologic means. The excretion pattern characteristically has a first trimester peak which roughly coincides in time with the transition from ovarian to placental endocrine activity. The presence of the hormone in urine has traditionally been used as a diagnostic pregnancy test. In hydatidiform mole and choriocarcinoma the hormone levels are higher and do not have the characteristic patterns of normal pregnancy; this allows diagnosis and evaluation of response to treatment by serial assays of the hormone. Measurement of HCG has not yet proved widely applicable in the management of other complications of pregnancy such as threatened abortion, but with the newer immunologic assays, hormone measurement may be of clinical assistance. The biologic function of the hormone in later pregnancy is unknown, and its mechanism of action at any time also remains to be determined.

BIBLIOGRAPHY

1. Albert, A.: Follicle-stimulating activity of human chorionic gonadotropin. J. Clin. Endocr., 29:1504, 1969.
2. Baechler, C., Bell, E. T., Borth, R., Brody, S., Carlstrom, G., Kerr, M. G., and Menzi, A.: Comparison of two immunochemical and three biological methods for the assay of human chorionic gonadotrophin in serum. Acta Endocr., 61:117, 1969.
3. Bagshawe, K. D., Wilde, C. E., and Orr, A. H.: Radioimmunoassay for human chorionic gonadotrophin and luteinising hormone. Lancet, 1:1118, 1966.
4. Bahl, O. P.: Human chorionic gonadotropin. I. Purification and physicochemical properties. J. Biol. Chem., 244:567, 1969.
5. Bahl, O. P.: Human chorionic gonadotropin. II. Nature of the carbohydrate units. J. Biol. Chem., 244:575, 1969.
6. Bangham, D. R., and Grab, B.: The second international standard for chorionic gonadotropin. Bull. WHO, 31:111, 1964.
7. Barr, W. A., and Collee, J. G.: Differences in the biological and immunological activities of human chorionic gonadotrophin after the removal of sialic acid by enzymic hydrolysis. J. Endocr., 38:395, 1967.
8. Bell, J. J., Canfield, R. E., and Sciarra, J. J.: Purification and characterization of human chorionic gonadotropin. Endocrinology, 84:298, 1969.
9. Berle, P., and Schultze-Mosgau, H.: Choriales Gonadotropin im Plasma der Arteria und Vena Umbilicalis. Acta Endocr., 58:339, 1968.
10. Brody, S., and Carlstrom, G.: Human chorionic gonadotropin pattern in serum and its relation to the sex of the fetus. J. Clin. Endocr., 25:792, 1965.
11. Brody, S., and Carlstrom, G.: Human chorionic gonadotropin in abnormal pregnancy. Serum and urinary findings using various immunoassay techniques. Acta Obstet. Gynec. Scand., 44:32, 1965.
12. Brown, W. E., and Bradbury, J. T.: A study of the physiologic action of human chorionic hormone; the production of pseudopregnancy in women by chorionic hormone. Amer. J. Obstet. Gynec. 53:749, 1947.
13. Browne, J. S. L., and Venning, E. H.: The effect of intramuscular injection of gonadotropic substances on the corpus luteum phase of the human menstrual cycle. Amer. J. Physiol., 123:26, 1938.
14. Cedard, L., Varangot, J., and Yannotti, S.: Biosynthèse et metabolisme des oestrogènes dans le placenta humain perfusé d'incube in vitro. II. Variation des réactions enzymatiques en fonction de l'âge de la grossesse. Europ. J. Steroids, 1:287, 1966.
15. Deanesly, R.: The endocrinology of pregnancy and foetal life; production of gonadotrophic and luteotrophic hormones in pregnancy. In Parkes, A. S., ed.: Marshall's Physiology of Reproduction, Vol. III. Little, Brown and Co., Boston, 1966, pp. 950–964.
16. Delfs, E.: Quantitative chorionic gonadotropin, prognostic value in hydatidiform mole and chorionepithelioma. Obstet. Gynec., 9:1, 1957.
17. Diczfalusy, E., Nilsson, L., and Westman, A.: Chorionic gonadotrophin in hydatidiform moles. Acta Endocr., 28:137, 1958.
18. Diczfalusy, E., and Troen, P.: Endocrine functions of the human placenta, human chorionic gonadotropin. Vitamins Hormones, 19:233, 1961.
19. Fox, F. J., and Tow, W. S. H.: Immunologically determined chorionic gonadotrophin titers in Singapore women with hydatidiform mole, choriocarcinoma, and normal intrauterine pregnancy. Amer. J. Obstet. Gynec., 95:239, 1966.
20. Goss, D. A., and Taymor, M. L.: A rapid immunologic method for the semiquantitative determination of human chorionic gonadotropin in urine. Fertil. Steril., 16:151, 1965.
21. Got, R., and Bourillon, R.: Critères de pureté de la gonadotropine choriale humaine. Bull. Soc. Chim. Biol., 42:31, 1960.
22. Got, R., Bourillon, R., and Michon, J.: Les constituants glucidiques de la gonadotropine choriale humaine. Bull Soc. Chim. Biol., 42:41, 1960.
23. Goverde, B. C., Veenkamp, F. J. N., and Homan, J. D.: Studies on human chorionic gonadotrophin. II. Chemical composition and its relation to biological activity. Acta Endocr., 59:105, 1968.
24. Hampton, J. K., Jr., Levy, B. M., and Sweet, P. M.: Chorionic gonadotropin excretion during pregnancy in the marmoset, Callithrix jacchus. Endocrinology, 85:171, 1969.
25. Hisaw, F. L.: The placental gonadotrophin and luteal function in monkeys (Macaca mulatta). Yale J. Biol. Med., 17:119, 1944.
26. Hobson, B. M.: Pregnancy diagnosis using the pregnosticon haemagglutination inhibition test. J. Obstet. Gynaec. Brit. Comm., 75:718, 1968.
27. Jaffe, R. B., Lee, P. A., and Midgley, A. R., Jr.: Serum gonadotropins before, at the inception of, and following human pregnancy. J. Clin. Endocr., 29:1281, 1969.
28. Lauritzen, C., and Lehmann, W.-D.: Levels of chorionic gonadotrophin in the newborn infant and their relationship to adrenal dehydroepiandrosterone. J. Endocr., 39:173, 1967.
29. Lauritzen, C., Shackleton, C. H. L., and Mitchell, F. L.: The effect of exogenous human chorionic gonadotrophin on steroid excretion in the newborn. Acta Endocr., 61:83, 1969.
30. Loraine, J. A., and Bell, E. T.: Hormone Assays and Their Clinical Application, ed. 2. Williams and Wilkins, Baltimore, 1966, pp. 83–113.
31. Marsh, J. M.: The stimulatory effect of luteinizing hormone on adenyl cyclase in the bovine corpus luteum. J. Biol. Chem., 245:1596, 1970.
32. Mayo, R. W., and Thompson, R. B.: Comparison of pregnancy tests. Obstet. Gynec., 25:699, 1965.
33. Midgley, A. R., Jr.: Radioimmunoassay: a method for human chorionic gonadotropin and human luteinizing hormone. Endocrinology, 79:10, 1966.
34. Midgley, A. R., Jr., Fong, I. F., and Jaffe, R. B.: Gel filtration radioimmunoassay to distinguish human chorionic gonadotrophin from luteinizing hormone. Nature, 213:733, 1967.
35. Midgley, A. R., Jr., and Jaffe, R. B.: Regulation of human gonadotropins. II. Disappearance of human chorionic gonadotropin following delivery. J. Clin. Endocr., 28:1712, 1968.
36. Midgley, A. R., Jr., and Pierce, G. B.: Immunohistochemical localization of human chorionic gonadotrophin. J. Exp. Med., 115:289, 1962.

37. Midgley, A. R., Jr., Pierce, G. B., Jr., Deneau, G. A., and Gosling, J. R. G.: Morphogenesis of syncytiotrophoblast *in vivo*: an autoradiographic demonstration. Science, 141:349, 1963.
38. Mishell, D. R., Jr., and Davajan, V.: Quantitative immunologic assay of human chorionic gonadotropin in normal and abnormal pregnancies. Amer. J. Obstet. Gynec., 96:231, 1966.
39. Mishell, D. R., Jr., Wide, L., and Gemsell, C. A.: Immunologic determination of human chorionic gonadotropin in serum. J. Clin. Endocr., 23:125, 1963.
40. Mori, K. F.: Antigenic structure of human gonadotropins: importance of protein moiety to the antigenic structure of human chorionic gonadotropins. Endocrinology, 86:97, 1970.
41. Rizkallah, T., Gurpide, E., and Vande Wiele, R. L.: Metabolism of HCG in man. J. Clin. Endocr., 29:92, 1969.
42. Robyn, C., Pertrusz, P., and Diczfalusy, E.: Follicle stimulating hormone-like activity in human chorionic gonadotrophin preparations. Acta Endocr., 60:137, 1969.
43. Schuurs, A. H. W. M., de Jager, E., and Homan, J. D. H.: Studies on human chorionic gonadotrophin. III. Immunochemical characterisation. Acta Endocr., 59:120, 1968.
44. Segaloff, A., Sternberg, W. H., and Gaskill, C. J.: Effects of luteotropic doses of chorionic gonadotropin in women. J. Clin. Endocr., 11:936, 1951.
45. Tamada, T., Taymor, M. L., and Stark, J.: A rapid immunologic method for the semiquantitative determination of low concentrations of human chorionic gonadotropin in urine. Amer. J. Obstet. Gynec., 95:249, 1966.
46. Taymor, M. L., Goss, D. A., and Tamada, T.: Immunologic and biologic titers of human chorionic gonadotropin throughout normal pregnancy. Fertil. Steril., 17:613, 1966.
47. Taymor, M. L., Todd, R., and Blatt, W. F.: Preparation of human chorionic gonadotrophin of high specific activity. J. Endocr., 36:417, 1966.
48. Thiede, H. A., and Choate, J. W.: Chorionic gonadotropin localization in the human placenta by immunofluorescent staining. II. Demonstration of HCG in the trophoblast and amnion epithelium of immature and mature placentas. Obstet. Gynec., 22:433, 1963.
49. Thiede, H. A., Choate, J. W., and Bindschadler, D. D.: Chorionic gonadotropin localization in the human placenta by immunofluorescent staining. I. Production and characterization of anti-human chorionic gonadotropin. Obstet. Gynec., 22:310, 1963.
50. Tullner, W. W.: Urinary chorionic gonadotropin excretion in the monkey (Macaca mulatta)—early phase. Endocrinology, 82:874, 1968.
51. Tullner, W. W., and Gray, C. W.: Chorionic gonadotropin excretion during pregnancy in a gorilla. Proc. Soc. Exp. Biol. Med., 128:954, 1968.
52. van Hell, H., Matthijsen, R., and Homan, J. D. H.: Studies on human chorionic gonadotrophin. I. Purification and some physicochemical properties. Acta Endocr., 59:89, 1968.
53. Wide, L.: An immunological method for the assay of human chorionic gonadotrophin. Acta Endocr., 41:(Suppl. 70)1, 1962.
54. Wide, L.: Early diagnosis of pregnancy. Lancet, 2:863, 1969.
55. Wide, L., and Hobson, B.: Immunological and biological activity of human chorionic gonadotrophin in urine and serum of pregnant women and women with a hydatidiform mole. Acta Endocr., 54:105, 1967.
56. Wide, L., Johannisson, E., Tillinger, K.-G., and Diczfalusy, E.: Metabolic clearance of human chorionic gonadotrophin administered to non pregnant women. Acta Endocr., 59:579, 1968.
57. Wilde, C. E., Orr, A. H., and Bagshawe, K. D.: A sensitive radioimmunoassay for human chorionic gonadotrophin and luteinizing hormone. J. Endocr., 37:23, 1967.

HUMAN PLACENTAL LACTOGEN (HPL; CHORIONIC SOMATO-MAMMOTROPIN)

The isolation in 1962 of a distinct new placental protein hormone culminated more than 30 years of scattered observations on the isolation of lactogenic and growth hormone-like principles from the human placenta.[21] Although it has been variously called human placental lactogen (HPL), chorionic "growth hormone-prolactin," and human purified placental protein, this hormone has now been established as a single substance with lactogenic, luteotropic, and growth hormone-like activities which is produced by trophoblastic tissue and may account for some of the heretofore unexplained metabolic alterations of pregnancy.[6–8, 13, 15, 23] The designation chorionic somato-mammotropin has now been suggested.

CHEMISTRY

Although further purification and characterization of HPL is still in progress, several reports have been published indicating a molecular weight of 30,000 to 38,000 with an amino acid composition remarkably similar to that of human pituitary growth hormone.[5, 6, 34, 42] Analysis suggests also that HPL is a dimer of two polypeptide chains of equivalent weight of 19,000 held together by hydrogen bonding without interchain disulfide links. There is no evidence for significant amounts of lipid or carbohydrate in the molecule.

Immunodiffusion studies by many investigators have revealed a reaction of partial identity with human growth hormone and this observation, originally made by Josimovich and MacLaren, facilitated its identification and purification.[12, 21] Degradation of purified HPL and comparison with human growth hormone reveal marked similarities in amino acid composition and tryptic peptides which provide a structural basis for the common biologic and immunologic characteristics of the two hormones.[5, 34]

BIOLOGIC EFFECTS

For convenience, the biologic properties of HPL will be reviewed under three headings: lactogenic, luteotropic, and growth hormone-like effects. It should be clearly indicated, however, that the full spectrum of activity and the metabolic significance of this hormone in human pregnancy are not yet established. In contrast to HCG, placental lactogen was isolated first by immunologic rather than biologic assays and it is only now, after its chemical and immunologic identities have been established, that widespread testing of its biologic function has begun.

Prolactin Activity

HPL produces a response in the pigeon crop sac assay at 10 to 50 per cent of the activity of National Institutes of Health sheep prolactin and also stimulates milk production after intramammary injection into pseudopregnant rabbits.[20, 21] Casein synthesis and histologic development in organ culture are both stimulated by HPL in a manner indistinguishable from that of ovine pituitary prolactin.[40, 41] Whatever role HPL may play in mammary development during pregnancy, it is no longer present in the maternal organism at the time of lactation since it is cleared from the body in one day after delivery.[24, 25]

Luteotropic Activity

HPL has luteotropic properties similar to those of sheep prolactin in terms of the response of hypophysectomized rats to a decidomata-producing stimulus and its ability to delay estrus in cycling rats.[19] These properties are shared by such related substances as prolactin and growth hormone. Whether HPL is luteotropic in the human has not been established, but

Josimovich has postulated that it might be synergistic with HCG in the maintenance of the corpus luteum of early pregnancy.[17]

Growth Hormone-Like Activity

In the original report of its isolation, Josimovich and MacLaren indicated that HPL had little or no growth-promoting activity as measured by assay of tibial plate growth in the hypophysectomized rat, but in later work the ability of HPL to synergistically potentiate the effect of human growth hormone (HGH) in the same assay was established.[16, 18] HPL also enhances the insulin resistance induced by HGH. The synergistic effects of HPL did not occur with bovine growth hormone. Other investigators have reported growth hormone-like activity of HPL in the rat tibial epiphysis assay and in its effects upon the incorporation of radioactive sulfate into costal cartilage, but at a lower level of potency than growth hormone.[15]

HPL will stimulate the incorporation of glucose into fat in experimental animals at a dose 100 times that required of growth hormone and will also cause lipolysis from isolated fat cells.[11, 43] Body weight gain by hypophysectomized rats was found to be proportional to the HPL injected, and HPL stimulated protein synthesis in skeletal muscle in a manner analogous to growth hormone. In addition, HPL causes elevation in free fatty acids of fasting animals and deposition of glycogen in myocardial and skeletal muscle in hypophysectomized animals.[1] In the human, it has been reported that HPL induces a rise in free fatty acids[14] and alters glucose metabolism in hypopituitary subjects. In normal subjects, there is an impairment of glucose tolerance after a 12-hour infusion of HPL.[2]

The administration of up to 200 mg. of HPL per day did not induce nitrogen retention in an adult or a juvenile hypopituitary patient in one study, while in another evaluation of the hormone at a higher dose level, both nitrogen and potassium retention were obtained, with direct evidence of growth-promoting activity. The somatotropic activity of HPL is thus not clearly defined as yet, but it appears certain that it is a substance with the capacity to potentiate pituitary growth hormone action and also has many of the metabolic potentials of the pituitary hormone but at a higher dose level.[32] In direct contrast to growth hormone, however, the levels of HPL in plasma are not altered by either hypoglycemia or hyperglycemia, but like growth hormone HPL is a significant physiologic antagonist of insulin and may be a "diabetogenic" factor in pregnancy.[22, 26, 27, 29] It has been established that pituitary growth hormone levels are not elevated during pregnancy[45] and hence any increased somatotropic activity present may well be due to the synergistic or direct action of HPL.

THE PLACENTA AS A SITE OF HPL FORMATION

Evidence for the placental origin of HPL includes the following: (1) it is present in high concentration in placental tissue from three and a half weeks' gestation to term, and in urine and serum in increasing concentrations as pregnancy advances, and disappears after delivery in one day; (2) it is present in the serum and placenta of a hypophysectomized pregnant patient and is not detected in maternal or fetal pituitary; (3) it is present in higher concentration in retroplacental and ovarian vein blood than in the periphery and is not present in decidua; (4) it is present in hydatidiform moles and choriocarcinoma in males; (5) its concentration in the fetus is low and it is present in the trophoblast of a blighted ovum; (6) it can be produced in vitro by tissue culture of placenta;[9, 38, 39] (7) it has been localized to syncytiotrophoblast by immunofluorescent technique.[33]

HPL MEASUREMENT IN SERUM AND URINE

Since HPL was first detected and identified by immunologic means, sensitive and specific assays were readily available for measurement during pregnancy.[3, 13, 24, 28, 36, 44] Early work was confused by the immunologic cross-reaction of pituitary growth hormone with HPL but this problem was largely overcome by preparation of purified antigens and by recognition of the fact that HPL is present in serum at many times the concentration of growth hormone. The earlier erroneous reports on elevations of growth hormone in pregnancy were due to the immunologic cross-reactivity. The half-life of HPL in plasma is about 20 minutes; this explains its rapid disappearance after delivery. It has been calculated that the placenta secretes from 1 to 2 grams a day at term.[25] There is no diurnal variation in blood levels and no change due to physical activity. Levels in serum are detectable early in pregnancy and rise progressively to 2 to 10 mcg. per milliliter at term (Fig. 9), with disappearance from plasma by four hours post partum. The levels in umbilical cord blood are just barely measurable and equal at least 1/300 of the maternal levels.[24] The actual values reported for HPL in blood are currently being downgraded as the assay methods become more refined. In any case, the levels are many times higher than those of growth hormone in the latter months of pregnancy.

Relatively small amounts of HPL reach

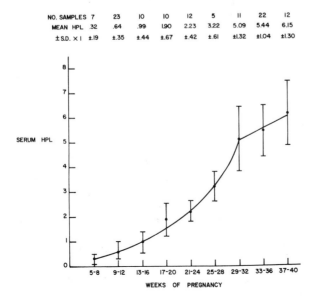

NO. SAMPLES	7	23	10	10	12	5	11	22	12
MEAN HPL	.32	.64	.99	1.90	2.23	3.22	5.09	5.44	6.15
±S.D. × I	±.19	±.35	±.44	±.67	±.42	±.61	±1.32	±1.04	±1.30

Figure 9. Average levels of serum HPL (± 1 standard deviation) throughout normal pregnancy (HPL is shown in micrograms per milliliter). (From Saxena, B. N., Emerson, K., Jr., and Selenkow, H. A.: New Eng. J. Med., 281:225, 1969.)

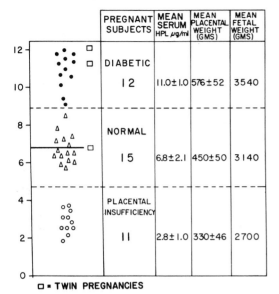

	PREGNANT SUBJECTS	MEAN SERUM HPL μg/ml	MEAN PLACENTAL WEIGHT (GMS)	MEAN FETAL WEIGHT (GMS)
DIABETIC	12	11.0±1.0	576±52	3540
NORMAL	15	6.8±2.1	450±50	3140
PLACENTAL INSUFFICIENCY	11	2.8±1.0	330±46	2700

□ = TWIN PREGNANCIES

Figure 10. Serum HPL levels in the third trimester (more than 32 weeks), showing the relation between HPL and placental and fetal weights. The placentas were weighed after removal of the cord and fetal membranes according to the method of Benirschke and Driscoll. (From Saxena, B. N., Emerson, K., Jr., and Selenkow, H. A.: New Eng. J. Med., 281:225, 1969.)

As shown in Figure 11, levels of HPL tend to be low and do not rise normally in cases of placental insufficiency. It is possible that this assay, coupled with other tests of fetal or placental function such as estriol excretion (see p. 118), may be of assistance in determining the management of high-risk pregnancies.

the urine unchanged, with values of 100 mcg. per day at 56 days' gestation and 105 mcg. per day at 265 days' gestation. There is a correlation between HPL levels in blood and placental and fetal weight (Fig. 10).[30] Values tend to be high in diabetic pregnancies.

There has been no widespread clinical use of HPL measurement as yet although it has been proposed as an assay for placental function[10, 30, 35, 37] in abnormal pregnancy and with trophoblastic disease.

SUMMARY

HPL is a protein hormone produced by the human placenta with immunologic, chemical, and biologic properties similar to those of pituitary growth hormone. In addition, it has lactogenic and luteotropic activities similar to those of prolactin. In the human, pituitary growth hormone and prolactin have overlapping activities and the question of a distinct pituitary prolactin hormone has not been completely resolved by isolation. HPL is present in early pregnancy and rises progressively in placenta, serum, and urine. Its range of biologic activity has been the basis for suggestions that it is an important metabolic hormone of pregnancy affecting breast development and carbohydrate and fat metabolism, and perhaps acting as a synergist with HCG to maintain corpus luteum function. The most significant potential of HPL to affect pregnancy lies in its capacity to antagonize insulin action and thus contribute to the "diabetogenic" nature of the pregnant state.

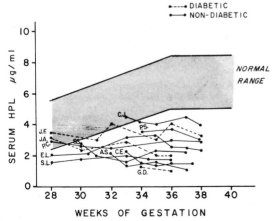

- - - - DIABETIC
——— NON-DIABETIC

NORMAL RANGE

Figure 11. Serum HPL levels in chronic placental insufficiency. (From Saxena, B. N., Emerson, K., Jr., and Selenkow, H. A.: New Eng. J. Med., 281:225, 1969.)

BIBLIOGRAPHY

1. Beas, F., Salinas, A., and Pak, N.: Action of "chorionic growth hormone-prolactin" on growth and carcass composition of hypophysectomized rat. Proc. Soc. Exp. Biol. Med., 131:1171, 1969.
2. Beck, P., and Daughaday, W. H.: Human placental lactogen: studies of its acute metabolic effects and disposition in normal man. J. Clin. Invest., 46:103, 1966.
3. Beck, P., Parker, M. L., and Daughaday, W. H.: Radioimmunologic measurement of human placental lactogen in plasma by a double antibody method during normal and diabetic pregnancies. J. Clin. Endocr., 25:1457, 1965.
4. Catt, K. J., Moffat, B., and Niall, H. D.: Human growth hormone and placental lactogen; structural similarity. Science, 157:321, 1967.
5. Catt, K. J., Moffat, B., Niall, H. D., and Preston, B. N.: Purification and physiochemical properties of human placental lactogen. Biochem. J., 102:27c, 1967.
6. Florini, J. R., Tonelli, G., Breuer, C. B., Coppola, J., Ringler, I., and Bell, P. H.: Characterization and biological effects of purified placental protein (human). Endocrinology, 79:692, 1966.

7. Friesen, H.: Further purification and characterization of a placental protein with immunological similarity to human growth hormone. Nature, 208:1214, 1965.

8. Friesen, H.: Purification of a placental factor with immunological and chemical similarity to human growth hormone. Endocrinology, 76:369, 1965.

9. Friesen, H. G.: Biosynthesis of placental proteins and placental lactogen. Endocrinology, 83:744, 1968.

10. Genazzani, A. R., Aubert, M. L., Casoli, M., Fioretti, P., and Felber, J.-P.: Use of human-placental-lactogen radioimmunoassay to predict outcome in cases of threatened abortion. Lancet, 2:1385, 1969.

11. Genazzani, A. R., Benuzzi-Badoni, M., and Felber, J. P.: Human chorionic somato-mammotropine (HCSM): lipolytic action of a pure preparation on isolated fat cells. Metabolism, 18:593, 1969.

12. Greenwood, F. C., Hunter, W. M., and Klopper, A.: Assay of human growth hormone in pregnancy at parturition and in lactation. Brit. Med. J., 1:22, 1964.

13. Grumbach, M. M., and Kaplan, S. L.: On the placental origin and purification of chorionic "Growth Hormone-Prolactin" and its immunoassay in pregnancy. Trans. N.Y. Acad. Sci., 27:161, 1964.

14. Grumbach, M. M., Kaplan, S. L., Abrams, C. L., Bell, J. J., and Conte, F. A.: Plasma free fatty acid response to the administration of chorionic "growth hormone-prolactin." J. Endocr., 26:478, 1966.

15. Grumbach, M. M., Kaplan, S. L., Sciarra, J. J., and Burr, I. M.: Chorionic growth hormone-prolactin (CGP): Secretion, disposition, biologic activity in man, and postulated function as the "growth hormone" of the second half of pregnancy. Ann. N.Y. Acad. Sci., 148:501, 1968.

16. Josimovich, J. B.: Potentiation of somatotrophic and diabetogenic effects of growth hormone by human placental lactogen (HPL). Endocrinology, 78:707, 1966.

17. Josimovich, J. B.: Maintenance of pseudopregnancy in the rat by synergism between human placental lactogen and chorionic gonadotrophin. Endocrinology, 83:530, 1968.

18. Josimovich, J. B., and Atwood, B. L.: Human placental lactogen (HPL), a trophoblastic hormone synergizing with chorionic gonadotrophin and potentiating the anabolic effects of pituitary growth hormone. Amer. J. Obstet. Gynec., 88:867, 1964.

19. Josimovich, J. B., Atwood, B. L., and Goss, D. A.: Luteotrophic, immunologic and electrophoretic properties of human placental lactogen. Endocrinology, 73:410, 1963.

20. Josimovich, J. B., and Brande, B. L.: Chemical properties and biological effects of human placental lactogen (HPL). Trans. N.Y. Acad. Sci., 27:161, 1964.

21. Josimovich, J. B., and MacLaren, J. A.: Presence in the human placental and term serum of a highly lactogenic substance immunologically related to pituitary growth hormone. Endocrinology, 71:209, 1962.

22. Kalkhoff, R., Schalch, D. S., Walker, J. L., Beck, P., Kipnis, D. M., and Daughaday, W. H.: Diabetogenic factors associated with pregnancy. Trans. Ass. Amer. Physicians, 77:270, 1964.

23. Kaplan, S. L., and Grumbach, M. M.: Studies of a human and simian placental hormone with growth hormone-like and prolactin-like activities. J. Clin. Endocr., 24:80, 1964.

24. Kaplan, S. L., and Grumbach, M. M.: Serum chorionic "growth hormone-prolactin" and serum pituitary growth hormone in mother and fetus at term. J. Clin. Endocr., 25:1370, 1965.

25. Kaplan, S. L., Gurpide, E., Sciarra, J. J., and Grumbach, M. M.: Metabolic clearance rate and production rate of chorionic growth hormone-prolactin in late pregnancy. J. Clin. Endocr., 28:1450, 1968.

26. Martin, J. M., and Friesen, H.: Effect of human placental lactogen on the isolated islets of Langerhans *in vitro*. Endocrinology, 84:619, 1969.

27. Riggi, S. J., Boshart, C. R., Bell, P. H., and Ringler, I.: Some effects of purified placental protein (human) on lipid and carbohydrate metabolism. Endocrinology, 79:709, 1966.

28. Samaan, N., Yen, S. C. C., Friesen, H., and Pearson, O. H.: Serum placental lactogen levels during pregnancy and in trophoblastic disease. J. Clin. Endocr., 26:1303, 1966.

29. Samaan, N., Yen, S. C. C., Gonzalez, D., and Pearson, O. H.: Metabolic effects of placental lactogen (HPL) in man. J. Clin. Endocr., 28:485, 1968.

30. Saxena, B. N., Emerson, K., Jr., and Selenkow, H. A.: Serum placental lactogen (HPL) levels as an index of placental function. New Eng. J. Med., 281:225, 1969.

31. Saxena, B. N., Refetoff, S., Emerson, K., Jr., and Selenkow, H. A.: A rapid radioimmunoassay for human placental lactogen. Amer. J. Obstet. Gynec., 101:874, 1968.

32. Schultz, R. B., and Blizzard, R. M.: A comparison of human placental lactogen (HPL) and human growth hormone (HGH) in hypopituitary patients. J. Clin. Endocr., 26:921, 1966.

33. Sciarra, J. J., Kaplan, S. L., and Grumbach, M. M.: Localization of anti-human growth hormone serum within the human placenta: evidence for a human chorionic 'growth hormone-prolactin'. Nature, 199:1005, 1963.

34. Sherwood, L. M.: Similarities in the chemical structure of human placental lactogen and pituitary growth hormone. Proc. Nat. Acad. Sci., 58:2307, 1967.

35. Spellacy, W. N., Carlson, K. L., and Birk, S. A.: Human placental lactogen levels as a variable of placental weight and infant weight. Amer. J. Obstet. Gynec., 95:118, 1966.

36. Spellacy, W. N., Carlson, K. L., and Birk, S. A.: Dynamics of human placental lactogen. Amer. J. Obstet. Gynec., 96:1164, 1966.

37. Spellacy, W. N., Cohen, W. D., and Carlson, K. L.: Human placental lactogen levels as a measure of placental function. Amer. J. Obstet. Gynec., 97:560, 1967.

38. Suwa, S., and Friesen, H.: Biosynthesis of human placental proteins and human placental lactogen (HPL) *in vitro*. I. Identification of ³H-labeled HPL. Endocrinology, 85:1028, 1969.

39. Suwa, S., and Friesen, H.: Biosynthesis of human placental proteins and human placental lactogen (HPL) *in vitro*. II. Dynamic studies of normal term placentas. Endocrinology, 85:1037, 1969.

40. Turkington, R. W.: Induction of milk protein synthesis by placental lactogen and prolactin *in vitro*. Endocrinology, 82:575, 1968.
41. Turkington, R. W., and Topper, Y. J.: Stimulation of casein synthesis and histological development of mammary gland by human placental lactogen *in vitro*. Endocrinology, 79:175, 1966.
42. Turtle, J. R., Beck, P., and Daughaday, W. H.: Purification of human placental lactogen. Endocrinology, 79:187, 1966.

43. Turtle, J. R., and Kipnis, D. M.: The lipolytic action of human placental lactogen on isolated fat cell. Biochim. Biophys. Acta, 144:583, 1967.
44. Yen, S. S. C., Pearson, O. H., and Rankin, J. S.: Radioimmunoassay of serum chorionic gonadotropin and placental lactogen in trophoblastic disease. Obstet. Gynec., 32:86, 1968.
45. Yen, S. S. C., Pearson, O. H., Stratman, S.: Growth hormone levels in maternal and cord blood. J. Clin. Endocr., 25:655, 1965.

FOLLICLE-STIMULATING HORMONE AND LUTEINIZING HORMONE

FOLLICLE-STIMULATING HORMONE (FSH)

Follicle-stimulating hormone (FSH) is a glycoprotein hormone of pituitary origin that stimulates ovarian follicle growth in the female and testicular seminiferous tubule growth and spermatogenesis in the male.

ISOLATION AND CHEMISTRY

FSH has been isolated from extracts of animal pituitaries, from human pituitaries obtained at autopsy, and from human menopausal urine, where it is present in large quantities. The human material has been sufficiently purified for analysis of amino acid composition and carbohydrate content. The molecular weight has been variously estimated at 30,000 to 41,000 and the carbohydrates, which constitute 25 per cent of the weight of the hormone, include sialic acid, mannose, galactose, and glucosamine.[2, 18-20] The carbohydrate portion of the hormone is essential for activity since enzymes that remove the sialic acid also abolish the biologic effects.[16] In addition it is believed that a D-galactopyranosyl unit is important for antigenicity.

BIOLOGIC EFFECTS

In the female, follicle growth proceeds to a definite but minimal level in the absence of pituitary hormones, and FSH stimulates the follicle to enlarge by proliferation of granulosa cells, increase of follicular fluid, and orientation of theca cells concentrically around the follicle (see Ovary, p. 72). Hormone production is, however, minimal to absent and ovulation will not occur unless luteinizing hormone (LH) is also present.[7] Appropriate amounts of FSH and LH can induce normal follicle development and ovulation in the absence of the pituitary.[1, 3, 5, 9, 14, 21, 22]

In the male, seminiferous tubule development and spermatogenesis do not occur in the absence of FSH and the atrophy of the testes that follows hypophysectomy can be overcome by administration of FSH. As with ovarian follicular development, the accompanying action of LH (or interstitial cell-stimulating hormone) is necessary to produce complete testicular function by stimulating testosterone production from the Leydig, or interstitial, cells. Testosterone is necessary for normal testicular function.[6, 10, 13, 15]

CONTROL OF EXCRETION

FSH is produced and secreted in response to a FSH-releasing hormone which travels to the pituitary via the hypophyseal portal system from the hypothalamus. The hypothalamic centers that control FSH release are in turn influenced by humoral factors such as steroid hormones or by neurologic impulses from higher brain centers as described in the sections in Chapter 3 on the hypothalamus and adenohypophysis. In the absence of estrogens (or androgens), FSH-releasing factor is unchecked and FSH is secreted in large quantities; hence the rise of FSH levels in blood and urine after castration or menopause. These elevated levels can be reduced by exogenous administration of estrogens (or androgens). If the pituitary is grafted away from the hypothalamus, it loses its capacity to secrete FSH because of lack of FSH-releasing hormone from the hypothalamus.

DYNAMICS AND LEVELS IN BODY FLUIDS

During childhood blood levels of FSH rise slowly from less than 5 milli-I.U. per milliliter at age eight to 10 milli-I.U. per milliliter, approaching the adult range, by age 14. The factor that initiates the rise at puberty is not known (Fig. 12). During adult life the levels are relatively constant at 10 to 15 milli-I.U. per milliliter in the male. In the female the values are similar but they fluctuate during the cycle, with a midcycle peak (Fig. 13), and blood and urine levels increase several fold at menopause or following castration. From ages 9 to 13 and in adulthood females have higher FSH levels than males.

FSH is cleared from the body slowly and has a metabolic clearance rate half that of LH (Fig. 14). After menopause, FSH production increases some 15-fold but metabolism is essentially unaltered (Table 4),[4] so that blood levels reach high values. FSH levels are low throughout pregnancy,[8, 17] reflecting pituitary inactivity.

ASSAY METHODS

Biologic activity of FSH can be assayed by its capacity to cause augmentation of ovarian weight when administered to rats or mice in the presence of sufficient chorionic gonadotropin. More recently FSH

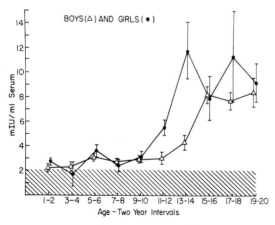

| GIRLS | 16 | 6 | 9 | 8 | 15 | 24 | 18 | 7 | 4 | 8 |
| BOYS | 21 | 17 | 28 | 24 | 29 | 21 | 20 | 18 | 14 | 7 |

Figure 12. Serum concentrations of FSH in boys and girls aged 1 through 20 analyzed at two-year intervals. The shaded area is below the mean minimal detectable dose. Brackets indicate standard errors. (From Lee, P. A., Midgley, A. R., Jr., and Jaffe, R. J.: J. Clin. Endocr., 31:248, 1970.)

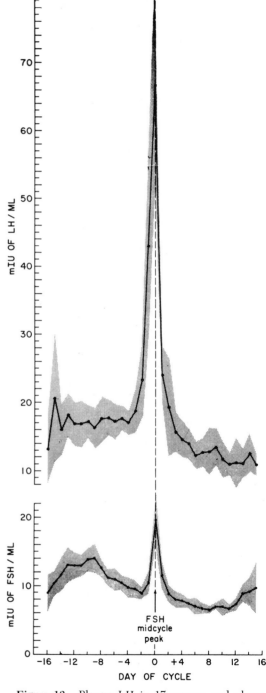

Figure 13. Plasma LH in 17 women and plasma FSH in 21 women: mean ±2 s.e. All cycles are centered on the FSH midcycle peaks. (From Cargille, C. M., Ross, G. T., and Yoshimi, T.: J. Clin. Endocr., 29:12, 1969.)

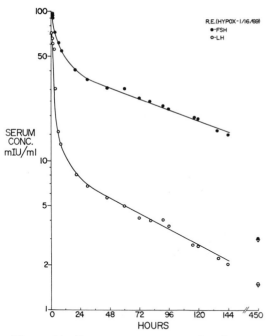

R.E.(HYPOX-1/16/69)
●-FSH
○-LH

Figure 14. Disappearance curves of endogenous serum FSH and LH following hypophysectomy. Note much slower rate for FSH and compare the curves of both with that for HCG shown in Figure 5. (From Yen, S. S. C., Llerena, L. A., Pearson, O. H., and Littell, A. S.: J. Clin. Endocr., 30:325, 1970.)

in blood has been measured by the development of antibodies to the purified hormone. The radioimmunoassay method utilizes the antibody to measure the competitive binding of the unknown titer of hormone against a standard amount of radioactively labeled FSH.

LUTEINIZING HORMONE

Luteinizing hormone (LH) is a glycoprotein of pituitary origin that in association with FSH causes morphologic changes (luteinization) in theca and granulosa cells of the ovarian follicle which are accompanied by ovarian hormone secretion. LH also causes rupture (ovulation) of the fully developed follicle and in the male causes development of Leydig cells, testicular growth, and testosterone secretion. The designation interstitial cell-stimulating hormone (ICSH) has been used synonymously with LH.

ISOLATION AND CHEMISTRY

Like FSH, LH has been isolated from animal pituitaries, human autopsy pituitary tissue, and postmenopausal urine. The human material, a glycoprotein, has been characterized as to amino acid and carbohydrate content and assigned a molecular weight of approximately 26,000.[2, 18] LH has one third less sialic acid and hexosamine than FSH and is less susceptible to inactivation by neuraminidase. It cross-reacts immunologically with HCG.

BIOLOGIC EFFECTS

In the female, LH (in the presence of FSH) causes steroid secretion by the follicle and ultimately morphologic changes described as luteinization of the granulosa and theca cells. A suitably prepared follicle will respond to a rapid elevation of blood LH (LH surge) by ovulating, by way of a mechanism that is as yet unknown (see Ovarian Follicle, p. 74).[9, 22] The corpus luteum which forms after ovulation responds to LH by increased hormone secretion. The interstitial and stromal cells of the ovary also secrete increased amounts of hormones upon exposure to LH.

Current theories for LH action invoke: (1) its capacity to make steroid precursors (such as cholesterol) more readily available; or (2) its capacity to stimulate new protein synthesis of the enzymes necessary for augmented hormone secretion.

In the male LH (or ICSH) will overcome Leydig cell atrophy after hypophysectomy

TABLE 4. PRODUCTION AND METABOLISM OF PITUITARY GONADOTROPINS

| | FSH | | LH | |
	MCR* (ml./min.)	PR† (mU/min.)	MCR (ml./min.)	PR (mU/min.)
Premenopausal	14.2	146	24.4	734
Postmenopausal	12.6	2141	25.6	2400

*MCR—metabolic clearance rate.
†PR—production rate.

and will maintain testosterone production. The mechanism involved is believed to be similar to that of its effects on the corpus luteum.

CONTROL OF EXCRETION

Like FSH, LH is produced and secreted in the pituitary in response to a releasing factor (LH-releasing factor) reaching the appropriate pituitary cells via the hypophyseal portal system. If the pituitary is transplanted away from the hypothalamus it loses its capacity to synthesize and release LH.

Discharge of LH-releasing factor from the hypothalamic neurons is regulated by the feedback effects of steroid hormones such as estrogens or progestins on the hypothalamus and other brain structures. In addition, neural impulses that ultimately affect gonadotropin levels funnel to the hypothalamus from other areas of the brain as a consequence of alterations in the external or internal environment. Hence such factors as light or emotional state may influence reproductive function. One unique aspect of LH release in the female is the ovulatory surge, a timed repetitive discharge of LH that results in follicle rupture and ovulation. It is postulated that there may be different hypothalamic centers controlling tonic and cyclic or ovulation-inducing release of LH.

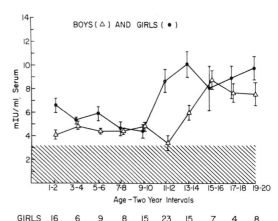

Figure 15. Serum concentrations of LH in boys and girls aged 1 through 20 analyzed at two-year intervals. The total number of boys and girls in each category is indicated. The shaded area is below the mean minimal detectable dose. Brackets indicate standard errors. (From Lee, P. A., Midgley, A. R., Jr., and Jaffe, R. J.: J. Clin. Endocr., 31:248, 1970.)

contraceptive pills. After castration or menopause, the LH levels rise many fold owing to the lack of gonadal hormone effects on the hypothalamus. These high levels can be reduced with exogenous estrogens.

LH is cleared from the body faster than FSH (Fig. 14) and much more rapidly than HCG (p. 34). The production rate is increased three- to five-fold in the menopausal years but, as with FSH, metabolism is unchanged and blood levels rise (see Table 4).

DYNAMICS AND LEVELS IN BODY FLUIDS

LH levels are low in childhood and gradually rise until puberty, when they rise rather sharply to approach adult levels (Fig. 15). The pattern of secretion in the adult male and female is naturally different, the male having a more or less tonic or constant level at 5 to 10 milli-I.U. per milliliter, and the female having a cyclic pattern with a classic midcycle surge to levels of 80 milli-I.U. per milliliter just before ovulation (Fig. 13). From ages 8 through 15, levels in females are higher than in males. The midcycle release of LH can be inhibited by administration of steroid hormones; this is the basis of action of the

ASSAY METHODS

Biologic function of LH can be determined by its capacity to cause depletion of ascorbic acid from suitably prepared rat ovaries or by measurement of its effect on the prostate or seminal vesicles of hypophysectomized immature male rats. The LH effect on the male accessory sex organs is dependent upon stimulation of testicular testosterone production. LH has been isolated in a form pure enough for use as an antigen for antibody formation and the development of immunologic methods, including radioimmunoassay, and, as noted on page 32, the antibody so produced will cross-react with HCG.

BIBLIOGRAPHY

1. Abrams, C. A. L., Grumbach, M. M., Dyrenfurth, I., and Vande Wiele, R. L.: Ovarian stimulation with human menopausal and chorionic gonadotropins in prepubertal hypophysectomized female. J. Clin. Endocr., 27:467, 1967.
2. Butt, W. R.: The Chemistry of the Gonadotrophins. Charles C Thomas, Springfield, Ill., 1967.
3. Buxton, C. L., Kase, N., and van Orden, D.: The effect of human FSH and HCG on the anovulatory ovary. Amer. J. Obstet. Gynec., 87:773, 1963.
4. Coble, Y. D., Kohler, P. O., Cargille, C. M., and Ross, G. T.: Production rates and metabolic clearance rates of human follicle stimulatory hormone in premenopausal and postmenopausal women. J. Clin. Invest., 48:359, 1969.
5. Crooke, A. C., Butt, W. R., Carrington, S. P., Morris, R., Palmer, R. F., and Edwards, R. L.: Pregnancy in women with secondary amenorrhoea treated with human gonadotrophins. Lancet, 1:184, 1964.
6. Danezis, J. M., and Batrinos, M. L.: The effect of human postmenopausal gonadotropins on infertile men with severe oligospermia. Fertil. Steril., 18:788, 1967.
7. Eshkol, A., and Lunenfeld, B.: Purification and separation of follicle stimulating hormone (FSH) and luteinizing hormone (LH) from human menopausal gonadotrophin (HMG). III. Effects of a biologically apparently pure FSH preparation on ovaries and uteri of intact, immature mice. Acta Endocr., 54:91, 1967.
8. Faiman, C., Ryan, R. J., Zwirek, S. J., and Rubin, M. E.: Serum FSH and HCG during human pregnancy and puerperium. J. Clin. Endocr., 28:1323, 1968.
9. Gemzell, C.: Human pituitary gonadotropins in the treatment of sterility. Fertil. Steril., 17:149, 1966.
10. Gemzell, C., and Kiessler, B.: Restoration of human spermatogenesis by menopausal gonadotrophins. Lancet, 1:1196, 1964.
11. Kohler, P. O., Ross, G. T., and Odell, W. D.: Metabolic clearance rate and production rates of human luteinizing hormone in pre- and postmenopausal women. J. Clin. Invest., 47:38, 1968.
12. Lee, P. A., Midgley, A. R., Jr., and Jaffe, R. B.: Regulation of human gonadotropins. VI. Serum follicle stimulating and luteinizing hormone determinations in children. J. Clin. Endocr., 31:248, 1970.
13. Lunenfeld, B., Mor, A., and Mani, M.: Treatment of male infertility. I. Human gonadotropins. Fertil. Steril., 18:581, 1967.
14. Marshall, J. R., Jacobson, A., and Hammond, C. B.: Dose response relationships of ovulation induction with human menopausal gonadotropin. J. Clin. Endocr., 29:106, 1969.
15. Martin, F. I. R.: The stimulation and prolonged maintenance of spermatogenesis by human pituitary gonadotrophins in a patient with hypogonadotrophic hypogonadism. J. Endocr., 38:431, 1967.
16. Mori, K. F.: Antigenic structure of human gonadotropins: contribution of carbohydrate moiety to the antigenic structure of pituitary follicle-stimulating hormone. Endocrinology, 85:330, 1969.
17. Parlow, A. F., Daane, T. A., and Dignam, W. J.: On the concentration of radioimmunoassayable FSH circulating in blood throughout human pregnancy. J. Clin. Endocr., 31:213, 1970.
18. Reichert, L. E., Jr., Kathan, R. H., and Ryan, R. J.: Studies on the composition and properties of immunochemical grade human pituitary follicle stimulating hormone (FSH): Comparison with luteinizing hormone (LH). Endocrinology, 82:109, 1968.
19. Roos, P.: Human follicle-stimulating hormone. Acta Endocr., 59(Suppl. 131):3, 1968.
20. Saxena, B. B., and Rathnam, P.: Purification of follicle-stimulating hormone from human pituitary glands. J. Biol. Chem., 242:3769, 1967.
21. Taymor, M. L., Sturgis, S. H., Goldstein, D. P., and Lieberman, B.: Induction of ovulation with human postmenopausal gonadotropin. III. Effect of varying dosage schedules on estrogen and pregnanediol excretion levels. Fertil. Steril., 18:181, 1967.
22. Vande Wiele, R. L., and Turksoy, R. N.: The use of human menopausal and chorionic gonadotropins in patients with infertility due to ovulatory failure. Amer. J. Obstet. Gynec., 93:632, 1965.
23. Yen, S. S. C., Llerena, L. A., Pearson, O. H., and Littell, A. S.: Disappearance rates of endogenous follicle-stimulating hormone in serum following surgical hypophysectomy in man. J. Clin. Endocr., 30:325, 1970.
24. Yen, S. S. C., and Vicic, W. J.: Serum follicle-stimulating hormone levels in puberty. Amer. J. Obstet. Gynec., 106:134, 1970.
25. Yen, S. S. C., Vicic, W. J., and Kearchner, D. V.: Gonadotropin levels in puberty. I. Serum luteinizing hormone. J. Clin. Endocr., 29:382, 1969.

LUTEOTROPIN AND PROLACTIN

LUTEOTROPIN

The term luteotropin is used to refer to a protein hormone that can activate and maintain the corpus luteum when it is formed from the recently ovulated follicle. The concept of such a function has been derived from the study of the laboratory rat and mouse and uncritically applied to man and other mammals, where its pertinence must be questioned since in the latter group of animals there is less evidence that corpora lutea of the cycle require this tropic substance to survive.

In the rat and mouse (but not in man or most mammals) the corpus luteum that forms after ovulation is relatively inactive. Ovulation occurs every four or five days and the corpora lutea regress rapidly, producing little progesterone. The relatively inactive corpus luteum of the rat or mouse cycle is converted into a progesterone-producing, active organelle that lasts for 12 days when a pituitary hormone called luteotropin is released as a result of nervous stimuli associated with mating or cervical irritation. This luteotropin is believed to be identical with prolactin (see below), which is the pituitary hormone required for milk production. The corpus luteum formed after ovulation in man, on the other hand, is usually fully active and does not require (as far as is known) external stimuli such as mating to maintain its function. There is as yet no evidence that gonadotropins other than FSH and LH are required for ovulation in man, or that once the corpus luteum is formed another luteotropin is required to maintain it for its usual life span and function during the cycle. The best evidence for this is that in women who lack pituitary function because of hypophysectomy or tumor, ovulation can be induced with exogenous FSH and LH and the corpus luteum produced thereby is similar to that formed normally. There is thus no evidence for the necessity of a separate luteotropin in the human cycle, although a continuous lower level of LH must be maintained.

Since human pituitary LH can stimulate progesterone production in the corpus luteum, luteotropic properties have been ascribed to it and, as noted before, the corpus luteum once formed still requires its presence.

In addition, HCG can prolong the life and steroid-secreting function of the corpus luteum of the cycle (see Human Chorionic Gonadotropin) and in this sense HCG is also considered luteotropic, but of course it is not operative in the nonpregnant state.

For the present, the concept of a separate luteotropin as a gonadotropic principle can be applied to only a limited number of mammals. Even the possibility of such a process in man is complicated by the fact that prolactin, which is identical with luteotropin in animals (see below), has not as yet been isolated from human pituitaries and the luteotropic hormone derived from animals is not active in man. A critique of the possible role of luteotropin in mammalian species has been prepared by Rothchild.[2] What is known about the chemistry and physiology of animal luteotropin-prolactin will be considered in the following section.

PROLACTIN

A pituitary protein hormone that has been demonstrated to be primarily responsible for mammary growth and lactation has been variously designated prolactin, mammotropin, lactogenic hormone, and, as already indicated, luteotropin because of its action on the corpus luteum of certain animals.[1]

ISOLATION AND CHEMISTRY

Prolactin has been isolated in relatively pure form from sheep, bovine, pig, and rat pituitaries but not as yet from a human source. The molecular weight of the sheep hormone is approximaely 25,000 and the amino acid composition has been determined. In contrast to FSH and LH, the molecule contains no carbohydrate moieties.

All protein fractions obtained from human pituitaries that have prolactin activity also have significant growth hormone properties and the two biologic actions have not been completely dissociated. Hence the possible coexistence of the two hormonal properties in one molecule has been postulated. There are, however, experimental and clinical situations in which there are disparities between the two hormonal actions. In tissue culture of human fetal pituitaries and in certain patients with pituitary tumors, the lactogenic factor predominates, giving rise to speculation that separate prolactin and growth hormones will ultimately be described for the human (see p. 132).

BIOLOGIC EFFECTS

In the pigeon, prolactin stimulates the growth of the crop sacs, bilateral esophageal pouches used for providing nutrition to the young by regurgitation of desquamated epithelium from the crop sac wall. Prolactin induces proliferation of the epithelial lining of the crop and also increases production of a caseous fluid called "crop milk." The analogy to mammalian lactation and the capacity of a mammalian lactogenic hormone to induce these changes are striking.

Prolactin induces milk formation in mammalian species when the breasts are suitably prepared by prior stimulation with estrogen, progesterone, and adrenal steroids. Growth hormone, insulin, and thyroid hormone are also necessary for normal lactation to occur. The effects of prolactin on milk production can be demonstrated by local injection into the mammary ducts, which results in further lobuloalveolar growth as well as the activation of milk formation.

The necessity for practically all other hormones to participate in the preparation for lactation provides difficulties in demonstrating the action of prolactin and has resulted in some confusion about its fundamental role.

Apparently prolactin and growth hormone can induce breast growth in animals in the absence of estrogen and progestins, while the latter steroid hormones may have no effect on breast tissue in the absence of the pituitary in certain experimental situations. There is, for instance, a pituitary tumor occurring in rats which will induce lobuloalveolar breast growth in adrenalectomized, orchidectomized rats. Prolactin is therefore considered the hormone primarily concerned with both breast growth and milk production. Prolactin can induce lobuloalveolar development and casein synthesis in mammary tissue grown in organ culture. Prolactin also has certain central nervous system effects which are responsible for nest-building activities and maternal behavior.

CONTROL OF EXCRETION

In contrast to most other pituitary hormones, prolactin production and release is under tonic inhibition by the hypothalamus via the action of a prolactin-inhibiting hormone. If the pituitary is removed from the hypothalamus, prolactin production and release increases, while that of other pituitary hormones diminishes whether the pituitary is simply transplanted to a distant site, the pituitary stalk is cut, or the excised pituitary is maintained in organ culture. The effects of prolactin-inhibiting hormone can be demonstrated in such organ culture, where it decreases prolactin production in vitro.

Estrogen in low dosage will facilitate prolactin release, as will many pharmacologic agents such as reserpine and ataractic drugs.

It is believed that high dosage of estrogens or progestins or both will inhibit prolactin release; hence the absence of lactation until parturition is accomplished. Suckling, of course, stimulates prolactin release and is a major physiologic process for continued lactation. Prolactin control will be considered further in the section on lactation (Chapter 4).

DYNAMICS AND LEVELS IN BODY FLUIDS

In view of the lack of certain knowledge of the presence and identity of pituitary prolactin as a separate human hormone, past measurements in human blood and urine have limited meaning. The recent identification of the placental lactogen (see Human Placental Lactogen) has cast doubt on the older studies using bioassay during pregnancy since they may have been measuring the placental hormone.

In nonpregnant patients with galactorrhea there is no change in growth hormone levels as measured by radioimmunoassay; hence the possible role of growth hormone as the lactogenic agent cannot be demonstrated and the search for a separate human prolactin continues. In addition, growth hormone is not elevated in postpartum lactation or galactorrhea. Growth hormone is not present in ateliotic dwarfs who have normal postpartum milk production (see p. 132).

ASSAY METHODS

Prolactin can be measured by its capacity to stimulate crop sac growth in pigeons and this provides the basis for the most useful bioassay method. Other measurements have been based on its capacity to induce mammary growth, and to prolong the rat estrus cycle because of its luteotropic properties (see Luteotropin).

Immunologic assays have been developed for animal prolactin but this method cannot be applied to human material until a human prolactin is identified.

BIBLIOGRAPHY

1. Forsyth, I. A.: Prolactin and placental lactogens. In Gray, C. H., and Bacharach, A. L., eds.: Hormones in Blood. Vol. 1. Academic Press, New York, 1967, p. 233.
2. Rothchild, I.: The nature of the luteotrophic process. J. Reprod. Fertil., Suppl. 1, p. 49, 1966.

SOMATOTROPIN (GROWTH HORMONE)

Somatotropin, or growth hormone, is a major secretory product of the adenohypophysis that directly controls growth and metabolic processes of the body. These somatotropin effects on normal development and homeostasis are subtle, however, and it is only at the extremes of its range of influence that the biologic potential of this hormone is dramatically revealed. In excess, somatotropin causes marked bone and soft tissue overgrowth: gigantism before epiphyseal fusion, and acromegaly thereafter. Absence of somatotropin may result in dwarfism in the developing child or metabolic derangements in the adult. As a consequence, there has been an intense interest in any possible role that growth hormone might play in both normal and abnormal fetal development and the profound physiologic changes occurring in the pregnant woman.

ISOLATION AND CHEMISTRY

Somatotropins have been isolated in relatively pure form as protein hormones from the pituitaries of many species including man, and their physical and chemical properties have been described.[1] The amino acid sequence for human pituitary growth hormone has been mapped, revealing a single-chain structure of 188 amino acids with a molecular weight of 21,500. Systematic study of somatotropins from different animal sources has indicated widely varying molecular weights, immunochemical identity, and biologic effectiveness in cross-species administration. Refinement of purification procedures, along with partial degradation of animal material, now suggests that there may be a biologically active core that is common to the hormone from most species and that there is a potential for more immunologic and biologic cross-reactivity than was at first appreciated.

Since only human or primate growth hormone is effective in man, it is fortunate that somatotropin resists autolysis in autopsy material and up to 10 per cent of the dry weight of the gland can be isolated as active hormone. The pituitary content of somatotropin does not appear to vary significantly with age.

PLASMA LEVELS AND CONTROL AND DYNAMICS

Plasma growth hormone levels vary considerably depending upon activity and metabolic state so that random sampling provides limited information. In the adult at rest after overnight fasting, levels are in the range of 1 to 2 millimicrograms per milliliter. Deviations from this baseline state are produced by insulin and hypoglycemia, exercise, fasting, and amino acid infusion. The increase of plasma levels from any of these stimuli may range from 10 to 50 millimicrograms. Estrogens augment the response to such stimuli and the growth hormone rise after exercise, for instance, is greater in women than in men.

The fetus and the newborn child have growth hormone levels in the acromegalic range, averaging 50 to 60 millimicrograms per milliliter. Values in children during the growing years are lower, similar to those found in the adult, although the growth hormone response to metabolic stimuli is more exaggerated in the newborn child than in later years. Since the half-life of somatotropin in blood is 40 minutes or less, changes in blood levels are rapid and must be correlated with metabolic state to have any meaning.

BIOLOGIC EFFECTS

It has been postulated that growth hormone regulates the metabolic activity of the body by responding to changes in energy-producing material in the blood. The growth hormone effects are summarized in Table 5.

TABLE 5. BIOLOGIC EFFECTS OF SOMATOTROPIN

Site of Action	Metabolic Effect of Somatotropin
Protein	1. Increased tissue uptake of amino acids 2. Drop in plasma amino acids 3. Increase in carcass protein 4. Increase RNA synthesis
Skeleton	1. Proliferation of epiphyseal cartilage 2. Increased connective tissue synthesis
Fat	1. Mobilization of fat depots to liver 2. Ketogenesis 3. Rise in plasma nonesterized fatty acids
Carbohydrate	1. Modulation of insulin effects 2. Decrease of glucose tolerance and glucose utilization

Although levels of somatotropin are high in fetal and newborn blood, it is believed that the hormone plays little role in growth and development until six months or more post partum. In anencephalic fetuses, somatic development may be normal and the pituitary dwarf does not start deviating from the growth curve until some six months to two years of life. In childhood and adult life the metabolic needs for growth and homeostasis are apparently met by growth hormone influences on protein, carbohydrate, and fatty acid metabolism.

CHANGES IN PREGNANCY

Growth hormone levels are unchanged in maternal serum during pregnancy.[2] On the other hand, the response to hypoglycemic and amino acid stimuli are blunted; this effect can also be created in nonpregnant women by administration of progestational agents.[3] In addition, the presence of chorionic somato-mammotropin (HPL) provides a growth hormone-like substance in great excess which can potentiate the effects of the pituitary growth hormone as well as exercise its own biologic effects. The result may be the basis for the "diabetogenic" effects of pregnancy, with decreased glucose tolerance and elevated levels of free fatty acids in serum.

BIBLIOGRAPHY

1. Li, C. H.: Current concepts on the chemical biology of pituitary hormones. Perspect. Biol. Med., 11: 498, 1968.
2. Yen, S. S. C., Samaan, N., and Pearson, O. H.: Growth hormone levels in pregnancy. J. Clin. Endocr., 27:1341, 1967.
3. Yen, S. S. C., Vela, P., and Tsai, C. C.: Impairment of growth hormone secretion in response to hypoglycemia during early and late pregnancy. J. Clin. Endocr., 31:29, 1970.

OXYTOCIN

Oxytocin is a neurohypophyseal peptide hormone that is present in practically all vertebrates and has the property in mammals of stimulating both uterine contractibility and milk ejection or letdown.[1] Dale first described the ability of posterior pituitary extracts to cause uterine contractions in 1906 and soon thereafter the milk-ejecting effects of this extract were reported.[3, 7] The possible role of oxytocin in the initiation or facilitation of human labor and its clinical application to obstetric management warrant a detailed review of its chemical and physiologic properties.

STRUCTURE

Originally oxytocin and the other neurohypophyseal hormone, vasopressin, were considered to be one large protein molecule having two hormonal actions. It is now known that in the natural state both hormones are bound to a large protein of molecular weight 30,000 called neurophysin. If neurophysin with both hormones attached is dialyzed, the hormonal activities remain with the large protein. If the molecule is subjected to electrodialysis or treatment with acid, however, the smaller hormones are released and can easily be separated.[8]

The structure of oxytocin was elaborated by du Vigneaud and his collaborators and by Tuppy and Michl and finally synthesized by du Vigneaud in 1953.[4] The hormone is a cyclic octapeptide with a five-membered ring held together by sulfhydryl bonds with a chain of three amino acids attached (Fig. 16). It is alkali-unstable and loses activity

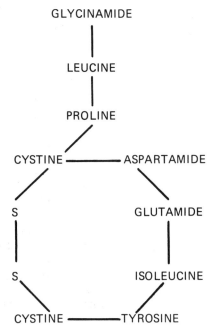

Figure 16. Structural formula for oxytocin.

if the disulfide bridge is disrupted. Many analogues have been synthesized by substitution of different amino acids into the molecule. This usually results in diminished activity or in a compound that can actually inhibit the action of the natural hormone. Removal of the amino acid chain or alteration of the exact size of the ring structure diminishes activity, but if the free amino group of cysteine in the 1-position is removed, this desamino compound provokes greater myometrial response than oxytocin.

BIOSYNTHESIS AND SECRETION

Oxytocin is believed to be synthesized in the neurons of the paraventricular or supraoptic nuclei, or both, of the hypothalamus. The hormone, packaged in dense neurosecretory granules, travels down the axons along the neurohypophyseal tract to their terminus in the neurohypophysis where they are released in response to stimuli reaching the hypothalamus.[2, 8] Stimulation of the cervix or uterus by distention can result in oxytocin release by a "positive feedback" system called the Ferguson reflex.[5] The stimulation of suckling will also cause oxytocin release, and both mechanisms for oxytocin secretion can function

without evoking vasopressin responses.[6] Various anesthetics, drugs, and alcohol can inhibit neurohypophyseal secretion, and the effect of alcohol has been used clinically in attempts to inhibit premature labor.

The pathways for the neurologic tracts involved in either suckling or genital stimulation of oxytocin release have not been well defined. Lesions deep in the lateral funiculi of the spinal cord interfered with lactation in experimental animals and stimulation of specific areas of the brain stem or forebrain could result in milk ejection. The final path for all afferents appears to be the cells of the paraventricular and supraoptic nuclei.

Emotional disturbances causing inhibition of the milk-ejecting reflex have been observed in animals and women, suggesting a central control for oxytocin release. In addition, progesterone can inhibit the hypothalamic centers for hormone release and it is probable that humoral feedback mechanisms exist for regulation of neurohypophyseal function.

METABOLISM

There exist in many tissues and in the blood aminopeptidases that can disrupt the ring structure of oxytocin. As a consequence the half-life of the hormone in the human blood stream is about 3 minutes. The placenta contains peptidases that will destroy both oxytocin and vasopressin and in pregnancy the level of aminopeptidases in the blood is elevated. It has been suggested but certainly not as yet adequately justified that the high levels of oxytocin peptidases prevent premature effects of oxytocin on the uterus and that perhaps a decrease in these inactivating enzymes finally allows sufficient oxytocin to reach the myometrium to trigger labor.

BIOLOGIC EFFECTS

Uterus

Oxytocin stimulates the myometrial cell, resulting in increased rate and intensity of contraction.[1] The hormone ordinarily lowers the membrane potential of smooth muscle but the effects produced depend on the physiologic state of the animal. Immature or ovariectomized animals that are estrogen-deficient have uteri that are unresponsive to oxytocin. Estrogens sensitize the myometrium to oxytocin and lower the threshold stimulus; progesterone tends to counteract the estrogen effects and raises the threshold for oxytocin action. Surprisingly, vasopressin is more active in stimulating the nonpregnant uterus than is oxytocin. As pregnancy progresses, the sensitivity of the myometrium to oxytocin increases such that the threshold dose changes from 100 mU. per minute in early pregnancy to 1 mU. per minute at 32 weeks' gestation. In the isolated state the muscle can also be made unresponsive to oxytocin by washing it free of calcium or other cations.

Mammary Gland

Oxytocin stimulates contraction of the myoepithelial cells of the breast; this causes milk to be expressed through the lactiferous ducts into sinuses and the main mammary ducts. Many mammalian species cannot lactate without this milk-ejecting effect of oxytocin. The exquisite sensitivity of the breast to oxytocin is increased as pregnancy advances.

Blood Pressure and Renal Function

The biologic effects of oxytocin overlap with those of vasopressin. The synthetic oxytocin molecule can cause antidiuresis and even water intoxication if too much hormone is given with excess hypotonic fluid during induction of labor. Rarely oxytocin may produce hypotension or hypertension when administered in excess dose in clinical situations.

ASSAY AND BLOOD LEVELS

The most sensitive and specific assay for oxytocin is based on its ability to cause milk ejection and thereby increase mammary intraductal pressure, which can be measured in various laboratory animals. The response of the uterus to oxytocin stimulation is a less reliable measure of the hormone owing to difficulties in standardizing the assay and to the possible presence of other substances which can affect myometrial activity. Attempts are now being made to measure oxytocin during pregnancy and labor, but results are still meager and not sufficiently reliable to depend upon at this time. Estimates for levels during late labor are of the order of 5 to 20 μU. per milliliter.

CLINICAL USE

The induction of labor was first demonstrated in animals with crude posterior pituitary extracts in 1926, and was subsequently applied to the clinical management of patients as more highly purified materials became available (see Induction of Labor, p. 652). For this purpose, the pure synthetic material can now be utilized and administration carried out with a constant-flow infusion pump for adequate control. As stated earlier, the most striking aspect of the uterine response to oxytocin is the exquisite sensitivity when the patient is "ready" for labor.

BIBLIOGRAPHY

1. Caldeyro-Barcia, R., and Heller, H., eds.: Oxytocin. Pergamon Press, New York, 1961.
2. Cross, B. A.: Neural control of oxytocin secretion. In Martin, L., and Ganong, W. F., eds.: Neuroendocrinology. Academic Press, New York, 1966, p. 217.
3. Dale, H. H.: On some physiological actions of Ergot. J. Physiol., 34:163, 1906.
4. du Vigneaud, V., et al.: The synthesis of an octapeptide amide with hormonal activity of oxytocin. J. Amer. Chem. Soc., 75:4879, 1953.
5. Ferguson, J. K. W.: A study of the mobility of the intact uterus at term. Surg. Gynec. Obstet., 73: 73:359, 1941.
6. Fox, C. A., and Knaggs, G. S.: Milk-ejection activity (oxytocin) in peripheral venous blood in man during lactation and in association with coitus. J. Endocr., 45:145, 1969.
7. Ott, J., and Scott, J. C.: The action of infundibulin upon the mammary secretion. Proc. Soc. Exp. Biol. Med., 8:48, 1910.
8. Sawyer, W. H.: Vertebrate neurohypophysial principles. Endocrinology, 75:981, 1964.

RELAXIN

Relaxin was initially described in the late 1920s as a corpus luteum hormone that could cause relaxation of the pelvic ligaments of the guinea pig.[5, 6] Although discovered at approximately the same time and from the same tissue as progesterone, relaxin has had a much more ambiguous chemical and physiologic identity than progesterone or any other hormone associated with reproduction. At the present time the assignment of any role for relaxin in human reproduction would be tenuous at best. It is, however, appropriate to discuss this substance in view of its use in clinical medicine, which is controversial and has been discontinued, and its possible role in the evolution of adaptive mechanisms in pregnancy.

ISOLATION AND CHEMISTRY

Relaxin can be isolated from corpora lutea, placenta, or uterus depending on the species. The sow corpus luteum and the placenta of the rabbit are especially rich sources of the material, and it has also been isolated from the human placenta.[1] Relaxin activity can be extracted with aqueous solvents and is sensitive to proteolytic enzymes. It has been concluded that it is a polypeptide of roughly 10,000 molecular weight. Amino acid analyses have been performed although a completely homogeneous preparation has not yet been described.[2, 3]

BIOLOGIC EFFECTS

The major physiologic effects of relaxin are three in number—pelvic adaptation, uterine contractibility, and cervical ripening or dilatation—and are best described separately.[1, 4, 5, 7]

Pelvic Adaptation

Burrowing mammals and other species with a narrow pelvic outlet have evolved mechanisms to allow parturition of young through a birth canal that would otherwise be too small. These adaptive mechanisms include either bone or cartilage resorption, leaving the pelvis open, as in the pocket gopher, or relaxation of pelvic ligaments,

as in the mouse or guinea pig. In some species bone resorption is brought about by estrogen alone and the pelvis of male and female differ on this hormonal basis. In other species estrogen alone can cause relaxation of the pelvic ligaments but this is augmented by the more rapid specific additive effects of relaxin. Progesterone appears to stimulate relaxin secretion in some species but antagonizes relaxin effects in the mouse, so that there are species differences. In some animals pelvic adaptation appears to be independent of hormonal effects. The relaxin effects appear to be due to alteration of the ground substance with breakdown of collagen fibers and change in water content.

The confusion about relaxin has been due to the facts that it must have an estrogen-primed substrate to work on, estrogens have effects in the absence of relaxin, progesterone has variable effects, and wide species differences exist. This spectrum of action, coupled with inability to isolate a pure substance, has created a credibility gap as to physiologic role and identity, if not in the guinea pig then certainly in the human where a specific action has never been consistently demonstrated or clearly accepted.

Uterine Contractibility

Relaxin preparations have been demonstrated to inhibit myometrial activity both in vivo and in vitro. On this basis it was once marketed as an agent to prevent premature labor in human pregnancy. The relaxin inhibition can be demonstrated only in certain species, and only in an estrogen-primed animal, and it does not appear to affect oxytocin action on the uterus. The clinical effectiveness of relaxin in premature human labor has never been established.

Cervical Dilatation

Like the relaxation of the pelvic ligaments, changes occur in the uterine cervix during pregnancy which, close to term, have been characterized as effacement and softening. Relaxin is believed to cause depolymerization of connective tissue and an increase in water content of the cervix similar to the changes in the pelvic ligaments. The effects in different species have been variable and the use of relaxin to soften the cervix and hasten delivery in human pregnancy, although controversial, has been largely discredited.

DYNAMICS AND CONTROL

Relaxin increases in the tissues and blood of animals during gestation and a gradual rise in blood relaxin has been reported for the rabbit, cow, and human.[7] The increase in relaxin in the rabbit persists in the absence of the ovaries if the pregnancy is maintained with progesterone. Progesterone can elicit elevations in blood relaxin in ovariectomized animals treated with estrogen and progesterone but not in hysterectomized animals. The uterus is therefore also considered a source of the hormone.

SUMMARY

While it seems likely that there is, in fact, a hormonal substance, relaxin, which can cause softening of pelvic ligaments of certain mammals in a more or less specific fashion, assignment of a role to this hormone in human reproduction must be deferred. With so many aspects of pelvic adaptation, labor, and cervical ripening remaining undefined, a possible physiologic function for this or other as yet unidentified agents must, however, be considered. For the present, relaxin can best be regarded as an adaptive mechanism for pelvic relaxation in certain mammals whose birth canal has a narrow outlet. Relaxation of pelvic ligaments occurs also in the human. Cervical softening and ripening certainly are antecedents of human labor, and relaxin is present in the human placenta and blood, but more study is needed to establish cause-and-effect relationships.

BIBLIOGRAPHY

1. Deanesly, R.: The endocrinology of pregnancy and foetal life: Relaxin—a hormone of pregnancy. In Parkes, A. S., ed.: Marshall's Physiology of Reproduction, Vol. III. Little, Brown and Co., Boston, 1966, p. 994.
2. Frieden, E. H., and Hisaw, F. L.: The biochemistry of relaxin. Recent Progr. Hormone Res., 8:333, 1953.
3. Griss, G., Peck, J., Engelhorn, R., and Tuppy, H.: The isolation and purification of an ovarian polypeptide with uterine-relaxing activity. Biochem. Biophys. Acta, 140:45, 1967.
4. Hall, K.: An evaluation of the roles of estrogen, progesterone and relaxin in producing relaxation of the symphysis pubis of the ovariectomized mouse, using the technique of metachromatic staining with toluidine blue. J. Endocr., 13:384, 1956.
5. Hall, K.: Relaxin. J. Reprod. Fertil., 1:368, 1960.
6. Hisaw, F. L., and Zarrow, M. X.: The physiology of relaxin. Vitamins Hormones, 8:15 1950.
7. Zarrow, M. X., Holmstrom, E. G., and Salhanick, H. A.: The concentration of relaxin in the blood serum and other tissues of women during pregnancy. J. Clin. Endocr., 15:22, 1955.

Chapter 3

Endocrine Organs of Reproduction

The endocrine glands involved in reproduction represent a diverse array of tissues with highly specialized functions that are dependent upon interlocking control mechanisms. As a group, these organs are critically influenced by one another for their integrated control of reproductive cycles as well as for their own anatomic and secretory integrity. Furthermore changes in the patterns of endocrine gland activity during the life cycle of an individual are based upon these interdependent relationships. Physiologic stages of life such as puberty, adult reproductive function, and menopause are all outward clinical expressions of these changes and are covered in Chapter 4, Integrative Functions in Reproduction. The endocrine glands are considered under the subdivisions of: the central nervous system–pituitary group, which produce protein and peptide hormones; the steroid-producing glands, comprising the gonads and adrenal; and the placenta, which secretes both types of hormones.

HYPOTHALAMUS AND PINEAL

HYPOTHALAMUS

STRUCTURE AND FUNCTION

The hypothalamus is a primitive portion of the brain ordinarily associated with control of fundamental homeostatic, vegetative, and reproductive functions such as water balance, appetite regulation, sexual and gonadal activity, emotional behavior, temperature control, and sleep.[6] Our basic concern with hypothalamic function at this point is related to its control over the adenohypophysis and neurohypophysis, which is reflected in regulation of sexual and reproductive processes.[8]

Anatomically the hypothalamus is part of the forebrain and diencephalon. Its boundaries are ill defined and extend fore and aft from just anterior to the optic chiasma to the mammillary bodies in the floor and wall of the third ventricle, which divides it in half. The thalamus lies above; below, the base of the hypothalamus narrows into an infundibulum or pituitary stalk extending into the neurohypophysis, or posterior pituitary, which is derived from the floor of the third ventricle. The adenohypophysis, or anterior lobe of the pituitary, is in apposition to the neural lobe and pituitary stalk and is derived from the roof of the buccal cavity from which it is detached in embryonic development. Thus the two lobes of the pituitary are of diverse origin and, as might be expected, function differently.[25]

The hypothalamus contains some 16 groups or nuclei of neuronal cells with nerve fibers coming to them from olfactory centers, the thalamus, and the cortex, and with fibers going out from them to the thalamus, midbrain, brain stem, and hypophysis. Certain unique features of the hypothalamus related to endocrinology and reproduction bear emphasis. The hypothalamic cells can produce hormones which travel down the axons by axoplasmic flow into the neurohypophysis to be released into the blood stream as the neurohypophyseal secretory products vasopressin and oxytocin.[4] In addition, the hypothalamic neurons can produce hormones which are released into vascular channels flowing to the adenohypophysis and thereby regulate the synthesis and release of anterior pituitary hormones (Fig. 1).[14] These vascular channels are designated the hypophyseal portal circulation. Blood directed downward from the hypothalamus to the anterior pituitary constitutes the principal hypophyseal blood supply.

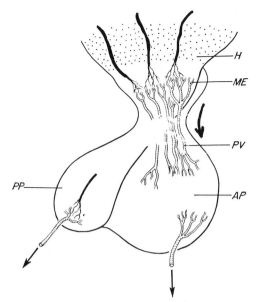

Figure 1. Midline sagittal section through the base of the hypothalamus and pituitary gland to show the structures concerned in the regulation of anterior pituitary activity. Nerve fibers from the hypothalamus enter the median eminence of the tuber cinereum to end on the primary plexus of the hypophyseal portal vessels. It is postulated that releasing factors pass from these nerve terminals into the portal vessels and are carried to the anterior pituitary gland to regulate its secretory activity. This is probably a mechanism similar to that obtaining in the posterior pituitary gland, where peptides are discharged from nerve endings into the general circulation. (From Fawcett, C. P., Reed, M., Charlton, H. M., and Harris, G. W.: Biochem. J., 106:229, 1968.)

In a real sense the pituitary has little independent hormonal action. Of the seven protein hormones produced in the adenohypophysis and the two hormones released from the neurohypophysis, only one, prolactin, is synthesized and released more effectively by the pituitary when it is removed from the hypothalamus and maintained as a transplant or in organ culture. All other hormonal function of the pituitary appears to be dependent upon close hypothalamic regulation.[26] With its extensive afferent nervous system pathways and its unique relation to the pituitary, the hypothalamus is truly the center of neuroendocrine integration (Fig. 2).[24]

Hypothalamic Hormones

Aside from oxytocin and vasopressin which are, in fact, produced in the hypothalamus and transported to and released

from the neurohypophysis, there are some seven to nine hormones or factors produced in the hypothalamus which apparently direct adenohypophyseal hormone production and release either by stimulation, inhibition, or both. Although most of these factors have not been isolated in pure form

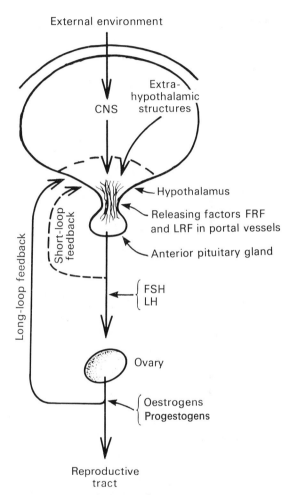

Figure 2. The central nervous-pituitary-ovarian axis. Ovarian function is regulated by the blood concentration of anterior pituitary gonadotropic hormones (follicle-stimulating hormone. FSH: luteinizing hormone, LH). The secretion of FSH and LH is in turn dependent on the transportation of releasing factors (follicle-stimulating hormone releasing factor, FRF; luteinizing hormone releasing factor, LRF) from hypothalamic nerve terminals to the anterior pituitary gland by the hypophyseal portal vessels. The hypothalamus itself appears to act as a major integrative center. It appears to have some autonomous function in maintaining anterior pituitary activity. This in turn is modulated by (1) neural inputs from extrahypothalamic brain structures (such as the amygdaloid nuclei), some of which mediate environmental influences, and (2) hormonal feedback through the long-loop (solid line), and possibly (and therefore denoted by an interrupted line) short-loop, systems. (From Harris, G. W., and Naftolin, F.: Brit. Med. Bull., 26:3, 1970.)

there is sufficient evidence for their existence and specificity to warrant discussion at this time.[14] The other hypothalamic hormones, oxytocin and vasopressin, will be considered under the neurohypophysis.

These hypothalamic factors have been designated hypophyseotropic hormones and their existence has been postulated on the basis of: the unique anatomic relationship between the hypothalamus and pituitary, with the portal circulatory system; the results of stalk section and pituitary transplantation experiments; and the stimulatory and inhibitory effects on pituitary function produced by chemical and physical manipulation of hypothalamic nuclei. Extracts of the hypothalamus from animals and humans have been isolated and purified which in vivo and in vitro can influence pituitary function.[14] In certain experimental states after hypothalamic lesions or following castration or hypophysectomy, the quantity of active principles in these extracts may be altered. At one point oxytocin and vasopressin were considered to be the releasing factors since they can cause ACTH release from the pituitary. More potent and specific substances have subsequently been discovered. In each instance the hypophyseotropic hormones have been isolated essentially free of one another and of other known hormonal substances.

Studies and attempts at characterization of the following hypophyseotropic hormones are currently in progress.

CORTICOTROPIN-RELEASING FACTOR (CRF). Hypothalamic extracts from rat, sheep, and cow material have been prepared which are active in releasing ACTH both in vivo and in vitro. Similar activity has been isolated from pituitary stalk blood. The activity of the extracts cannot be accounted for by their content of vasopressin or oxytocin.[14]

LUTEINIZING HORMONE-RELEASING FACTOR (LRF). Extracts of the stalk–median eminence region of the hypothalamus yielded the richest source of a heat-stable substance sensitive to proteolytic enzymes which caused release of luteinizing hormone. LRF was also found in peripheral blood. If LH release was inhibited by prior administration of estrogens, LRF still caused LH secretion.[5, 13, 15]

Porcine LRF was administered intravenously to a total of eight men and women with and without prior hypothalamic suppression by steroid hormone administration. In each case there was an increase in LH and FSH in the blood stream within half an hour.[11, 21] The question of contamination of the LRF with FSH-releasing factor or a nonspecific gonadotropin response could not be resolved, but it is clear that the porcine hypothalamic hormone is active in man. A control injection of vasopressin produced no significant rise in either LH or FSH.

FOLLICLE-STIMULATING HORMONE–RELEASING FACTOR (FSHRF). A substance extracted from the stalk–median eminence region was separated from LRF and could cause FSH release even when FSH was otherwise inhibited by prior administration of estrogen or a hypothalamic lesion.[9, 10]

PROLACTIN-INHIBITING FACTOR (PIF). As previously mentioned in the discussion of prolactin, the secretion of this hormone is under tonic inhibition which is removed when the pituitary is separated from the hypothalamus. Hypothalamic extracts will inhibit the release of prolactin from the transplanted pituitary in vivo and in vitro, although PIF is not as yet purified to the extent of LRF or FSHRF.

GROWTH HORMONE-RELEASING FACTOR (GHRF). Extracts from the hypothalamus can be prepared which cause release of growth hormone both in vivo and in vitro with pituitary incubation. This factor appears to be distinct from other releasing factors.

THYROTROPIN-RELEASING FACTOR (TRF). This factor has now been characterized chemically and synthesized, and its structure is that of a tripeptide of glutamic acid, histidine, and proline (Fig. 3).[1, 2, 16, 23]

Other possible hypothalamic hormones include growth hormone-inhibiting factor (GIF), and melanocyte-stimulating hormone–releasing (MRF) and inhibiting factors (MIF).[14] These are much less well characterized.

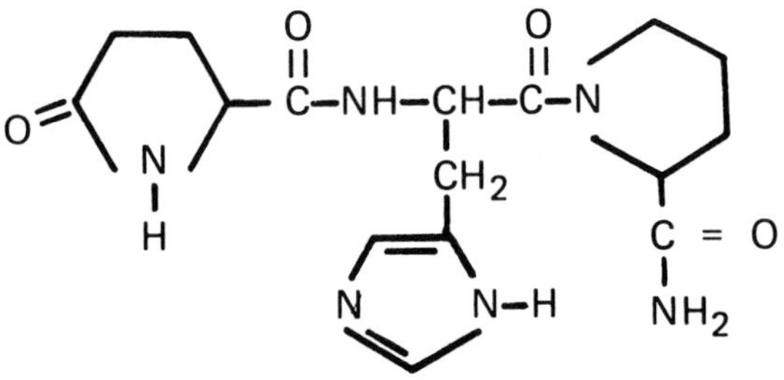

Figure 3. Thyrotropin releasing factor: 2-pyrrolidone-5-carboxyl-histidyl-proline-amide; L-(pyro) glu-L-his-L-pro(NH$_2$).

The simple structure of TRF and the fact that LRF is active in man have led to the belief that there will not be significant species variations of structure or function in these various hypothalamic hormones.[22]

LIFE CYCLE AND CONTROL OF FUNCTION

It is the central position of the hypothalamus in practically all aspects of neuroendocrine control that makes understanding of its function so critical for the student of reproductive biology.[3, 5] There are two different fundamental rhythms of the hypothalamopituitary system for the male and female of most mammalian species. In the male there is a more or less baseline tonic discharge of FSH and LH during active reproductive periods which may be seasonal, as in certain domestic and wild animals, or continuous, as in the human. This maintains the gonads and spermatogenesis. In the female there is a baseline discharge of FSH and LH for ovarian maintenance, but in addition there is the distinguishing feature of a cyclic surge type of discharge of LH which causes ovulation at regular intervals during active reproductive periods, which are continuous in the adult human until menopause.

From animal studies, it has been learned that the hypothalamus is influenced by testosterone in intrauterine life or the early neonatal period to create the male pattern. This can be demonstrated experimentally in certain animals either by removing the source of androgen by castration of the newborn male or by administration of testosterone to the female in the neonatal period. In the latter case the female animal at maturity will be anovulatory and the hypothalamic control of pituitary function will be similar to that of the male. That this is hypothalamic and not pituitary control can further be demonstrated by pituitary transplants to test animals, in which case the pituitary action is directed by the hypothalamic control of the recipient. A pituitary from a normal female animal behaves as a male gland when transplanted next to the hypothalamus of a male recipient. It is postulated that this type of hypothalamic programming could be the basis of certain naturally occurring anovulatory states in the human.[3, 5]

In addition, during otherwise normal reproductive life, the reproductive cycle is controlled by neurologic, endocrine, homeostatic, or pharmacologic cues which funnel through the hypothalamus and thence via the hypothalamohypophyseal portal system direct pituitary and ultimately all endocrine and reproductive function. Hypothalamic and pituitary function begin in utero during development.[7, 12, 20] The onset of puberty is believed to be associated with the maturation of the hypothalamic centers and, in a sense, with a change in the threshold of hypothalamic nuclei to internal and external stimuli which can trigger their function. The pituitary of an immature animal transplanted to a mature recipient will function in a normal adult fashion. How hypothalamic maturity is achieved is at present a complete mystery.

For each type of hypothalamic function it has been possible to map out anatomic areas which appear to be related to a specific endocrine role. This type of mapping has been based on the effects of localized lesions or local applications of stimulatory or inhibitory substances. There is considerable overlap of these areas, and it has not as yet been possible to assign function as discretely as one would hope. It has further been suggested that the neurons responsible for a given releasing or inhibiting factor have more or less direct access to a cluster of the pituitary cells they affect via the hypophyseal portal system.

Hypothalamic control can be influenced by a wide variety of mechanisms, and a few examples are given here.

Negative Feedback System

It has been demonstrated quite extensively that there is a reciprocal relationship between the level of blood-borne hormones of the adrenal, thyroid, and gonads and the blood levels of the pituitary tropic hormone for the target endocrine glands (Fig. 4). For instance, the amount of cortisol secretion is proportional to the level of ACTH reaching the gland per unit time, and the secretion of ACTH is in turn modulated by the cortisol level reaching the appropriate center in the central nervous system. Classic examples are observed after adrenalectomy, thyroidectomy, or gonadectomy, when the levels of ACTH, TSH, or FSH and LH rise (Fig. 5).[17] Conversely, the levels of the tropic hormones can be reduced by

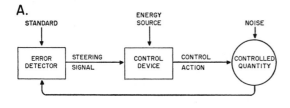

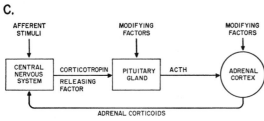

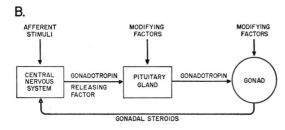

Figure 4. Comparison of concepts of feedback systems in physics and neuroendocrinology. A, Feedback system as of a thermostat controlling a furnace. B, Analogous hormonal feedback system controlling gonadal functions. C, Corresponding control system of the adrenal cortex. (From Scharrer, E., and Scharrer, B.: Neuroendocrinology, Columbia University Press, New York, 1963.)

Other Hormonal Feedback Mechanisms

In addition to the relatively gross negative feedback mechanism, there are other less well understood effects on hypothalamic and pituitary functions. These include the capacity of low levels of estrogens or progestins to trigger gonadotropin release, while higher levels are inhibitory (Fig. 6). Hormones may also have effects on other portions of the brain and only secondarily affect the hypothalamus. An internal feedback mechanism has also been suggested in which the level of ACTH influences the hypothalamic CRF and thereby helps control its own secretion, along with cortisol. In the case of PIF, progesterone can inhibit its release or action so that prolactin is secreted in what is a positive feedback system.

External and Internal Stimuli

Although it has not been possible as yet to specifically implicate the hypothalamus in the chain of events by which external stimuli affect reproductive function, it is highly likely that the hypophyseotropic hormones are involved as intermediates. The duration, intensity, and even the wavelength of light can influence reproductive cycles (see Pineal). Constant light can result in anovulation in rats, and alteration

administration of the appropriate exogenous hormone of the target gland, as in the case of depressing elevated gonadotropin levels with estrogens after menopause or castration. The original concept was that the target gland hormone exerted its inhibitory effect directly upon the pituitary, but the hypothalamus is now looked upon as the center for these inhibitory influences in most cases. The thyroid-TSH interplay is an exception; the pituitary itself can also be autonomously responsive to thyroid hormone levels. With corticosteroids, estrogens, and progestins, the hypothalamus appears to be the main receptor area influencing the pituitary release of hormones via the hypophyseotropic hormones. In any case this is a simplistic push-pull mechanism that cannot explain all of the varied and fine control exerted in regulating hormone levels in response to cyclic reproductive function or homeostatic need.

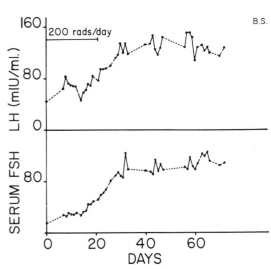

Figure 5. Effect of ovarian irradiation on serum gonadotropins. Irradiation was initiated on day 0. An example of release from feedback inhibition. (From Ostergard, D. R., Parlow, A. F., and Townsend, D. E.: J. Clin. Endocr., 31:43, 1970.)

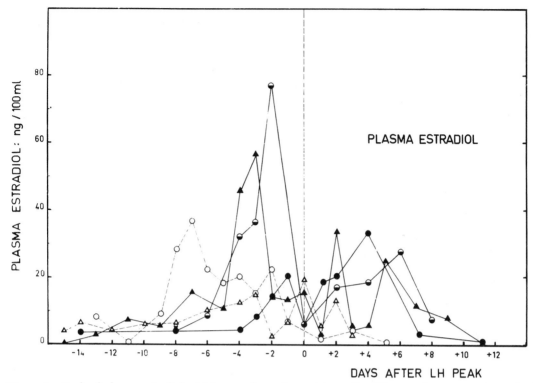

Figure 6. Peak of plasma estradiol which precedes and may trigger the LH surge that creates the midcycle peak of gonadotropins. (From Dufau, M. L., Dulmanis, A., Catt, K. J., and Hudson, B.: J. Clin. Endocr., 30:351, 1970.)

in light can affect reproductive function in seasonally breeding animals. Olfactory stimuli may affect the course of pregnancy in mice so that the presence of a new male will cause interruption of gestation. This does not occur if the male is castrated or if the female is made anosmatic. Other external factors such as visual cues or abnormal auditory stimuli may affect ovulation or courtship behavior. In reflex ovulators, such as the cat or rabbit, ovulation occurs only upon mating and the mechanism appears to involve reflex pathways from the cervix to the hypothalamus as well as higher brain centers. Under certain circumstances, suckling at the breast and cervical stimulation can also stimulate hypothalamic release of prolactin and oxytocin. Finally, many pharmacologic agents such as reserpine or chlorpromazine affect ovulation and gonadotropin secretion.

With such a wealth of experimental data as a background, it is not unreasonable to propose that many instances of unexplained anovulation seen in the human will ultimately be demonstrated to be the result of specific disruption of the neuroendocrine pathways involving the hypothalamus.

PINEAL

The mammalian pineal is believed to be a neuroendocrine gland with regulatory effects upon reproductive function, including control of the onset of puberty.[18, 19] Uncertainty about the physiologic role of the pineal stems from comparative studies in lower vertebrates where this organ serves as a photosensory receptor containing cells similar to those of the retina. It is the so-called third eye of lower animals.

Since a direct photosensory function has been lost in mammals, the pineal would have been considered a completely vestigial organ, except for the fact that precocious puberty in children has been associated with destruction of the gland by malignancy. Recent biochemical and physiologic studies indicate that the mammalian pineal can in fact be influenced by light via neurologic pathways from the ganglion cells of the retina. In addition, the pineal produces a hormone, melatonin, which has effects upon gonadal activity.

The pineal is a 4 by 8 mm. ovoid structure situated in the midline of the brain at the posterior superior apex of the third ventricle. It is derived from an evagination of the diencephalon during development. Histologically the pineal has nerve endings in direct approximation to secretory cells, suggesting a neuroendocrine function. The neural connections between the eyes and the pineal are believed to follow a pathway via the inferior accessory optic tract to the superior cervical ganglion and thence via postganglionic sympathetic fibers to the gland at the apex of the third ventricle.

CONTROL OF FUNCTION

In periods of total darkness, the pineal is most active, whereas prolonged light causes inhibition of function. Continuous illumination causes decrease in weight of the gland and in the size of cells, reduces lipid stores, and prevents synthesis of large amounts of melatonin, a pineal hormone. Darkness has a reverse effect on glandular structure and function.

PINEAL HORMONES

Melatonin was first isolated from the pineal glands of beef cattle by Lerner and was shown to have the property of lightening the skin color of amphibians by reversing the darkening effect of melanocyte-stimulating hormone. It has been demonstrated that the pineal can also secrete norepinephrine and serotonin but that it is completely unique in its capacity to synthesize melatonin (Fig. 7).

In mammals melatonin has biologic effects that are quite distinct from the skin pigmentation effects originally described in amphibians. This methoxyindole compound generally inhibits endocrine function. Exogenous melatonin administered to experimental animals causes decrease in ovarian weight, delays puberty in immature animals, and causes reduction in size of the accessory sex organs of male rats. Pinealectomy has a reverse effect and studies of pineal ablation and treatment with melatonin provide evidence that there may be other hormones produced by the pineal. The inhibitory effects of melatonin on gonadal function are believed to be mediated indirectly by the hypothalamus.

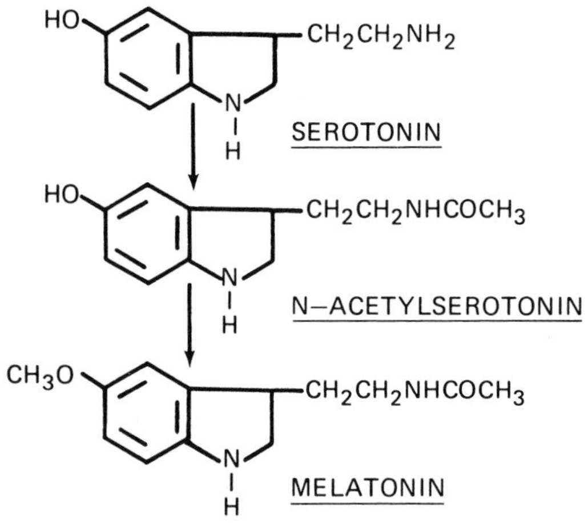

Figure 7. Biosynthetic steps in the synthesis of melatonin by the pineal.

PHYSIOLOGY OF THE PINEAL

Possible roles in mammalian reproduction have been assigned to the pineal on the basis of studies involving removal of the gland, replacement of pineal extracts or melatonin to pinealectomized animals, and evaluation of the effects of prolonged light and dark periods on both the pineal gland itself and reproductive endocrine activity.

In general, the pineal is most active in animals that are blinded or kept in total darkness. Under these circumstances, melatonin production is high and there is an inhibition of gonadal activity, presumably by an effect upon the hypothalamus and gonadotropin release since pinealectomy causes an increase in adenohypophyseal content of gonadotropins. Direct effects of melatonin on the median eminence and reticular formation have also been described.

The effects of blinding or darkness are obliterated if the pineal is removed. Prolonged exposure to light, on the other hand, inhibits pineal function and results in increased gonadal activity, exemplified by such situations as continuous estrus in rats. Pinealectomy in some animals also results in increased thyroid function, suggesting effects not only on reproduction but upon endocrine activity in general.

Although there are many unanswered questions regarding the pineal, it is reasonably certain that this gland plays an important role in endocrinology and may be a major mediator for the effects of environmental cues, such as light periods, upon reproductive functions.

BIBLIOGRAPHY

1. Bowers, C. Y., Schally, A. V., Enzmann, F., Boler, J., and Folkers, K.: Porcine thyrotropin releasing hormone is (Pyro) Glu–His–Pro (NH$_2$). Endocrinology, 86:1143, 1970.
2. Burgus, R., Dunn, T. F., Desiderio, D., Ward, D. N., Vale, W., and Guillemin, R.: Characterization of ovine hypothalamic hypophysiotropic TSH-releasing factor. Nature, 226:321, 1970.
3. Davidson, J. M.: Control of gonadotropin secretion in the male. In Martini, L., and Ganong, W. F., eds.: Neuroendocrinology. Academic Press, New York, 1966, pp. 565–599.
4. Everett, J. W.: Neuroendorcine aspects of mammalian reproduction. Ann. Rev. Physiol., 31:383, 1969.
5. Flerko, B.: Control of gonadotropin secretion in the female. In Martini, L., and Ganong, W. F., eds.: Neuroendocrinology. Academic Press, New York, 1966, pp. 613–654.
6. Ganong, W. F.: Neuroendorcine integrating mechanisms. In Martini, L., and Ganong, W. F., eds.: Neuroendocrinology. Academic Press, New York, 1966, pp. 1–11.
7. Gitlin, D., and Biasucci, A.: Ontogenesis of immunoreactive growth hormone, follicle-stimulating hormone, thyroid-stimulating hormone, luteinizing hormone, chorionic prolactin and chorionic gonadotropin and the human conceptus. J. Clin. Endocr., 29:926, 1969.
8. Harris, G. W., and Naftolin, F.: The hypothalamus and control of ovulation. Brit. Med. Bull., 26:3, 1970.
9. Igarashi, M., and McCann, S. M.: A hypothalamic follicle stimulating hormone-releasing factor. Endocrinology, 74:446, 1964.
10. Igarashi, M., Yokota, N., Ehara, Y., Mayuzumi, R., Hirano, T., Matsumoto, S., and Yamasaki, M.: Clinical effects with partially purified beef hypothalamic FSH-releasing factor. Amer. J. Obstet. Gynec., 100:867, 1968.
11. Kastin, A. J., Schally, A. V., Gual, C., Midgley, A. R., Jr., Bowers, C. Y., and Diaz-Infante, A., Jr.: Stimulation of LH release in men and women by LH-releasing hormone purified from porcine hypothalami. J. Clin. Endocr., 29:1046, 1969.
12. Levina, S. E.: Endocrine features in develop-
ment of human hypothalamus, hypophysis, and placenta. Gen. Comp. Endocr., 11:151, 1968.
13. McCann, S. M., Dhariwol, P. S., and Porter, J. C.: Regulation of the adenohypophysis. Ann. Rev. Physiol., 30:589, 1968.
14. McCann, S. M., and Porter, J. C.: Hypothalamic pituitary stimulating and inhibiting hormones. Physiol. Rev., 49:240, 1969.
15. Mittler, J. C., Arimura, A., and Schally, A. V.: Release and synthesis of luteinizing hormone and follicle-stimulating hormone in pituitary cultures in response to hypothalamic preparations. Proc. Soc. Exp. Biol. Med., 133:1321, 1970.
16. Nair, R. M. B., Barrett, J. F., Bowers, C. Y., and Schally, A. V.: Structure of porcine thyrotropine releasing hormone. Biochemistry, 9:1103, 1970.
17. Ostergard, D. R., Parlow, A. F., and Townsend, D. E.: Acute effect of castration on serum FSH and LH in the adult woman. J. Clin. Endocr., 31:43, 1970.
18. Relkin, R.: The pineal gland. New Eng. J. Med., 274:944, 1966.
19. Reiter, R. J., and Fraschini, F.: Endocrine aspects of the mammalian pineal gland: a review. Neuroendocrinology, 5:219, 1969.
20. Rice, B. F., Ponthier, R., Jr., and Sternberg, W.: Luteinizing hormone and growth hormone activity of the human fetal pituitary. J. Clin. Endocr., 28:1071, 1968.
21. Root, A. W., Smith, G. P., Dhariwal, A. P. S., and McCann, S. M.: Ovine hypothalamic extract has luteinizing hormone releasing activity in man. Nature, 221:570, 1969.
22. Schally, A. V., Arimura, A., Bowers, C. Y. Wakabayashi, I., Kastin, A. J., Redding, T. W., Mittler, J. C., Nair, R. M. G., Pizzolato, P., and Segal, A. J.: Purification of hypothalamic releasing hormones of human origin. J. Clin. Endocr., 31:291, 1970.
23. Schally, A. V., Redding, T. W., Bowers, C. Y., and Barrett, J. F.: Isolation and properties of porcine thyrotropin-releasing hormone. J. Biol. Chem., 244:4077, 1969.
24. Scharrer, E., and Scharrer, B.: Neuroendocrinology. Columbia University Press, New York, 1963.
25. Scheiber, V.: The Hypothalamo-hypophysial System. Publishing House of the Czechoslovak Academy of Sciences, Prague, 1963.
26. Szentagothai, J., Flerko, B., Mess, B., and Halasz, B.: Hypothalamic control of the anterior pituitary. Akademiai Kiado, Publishing House of the Hungarian Academy of Sciences, Budapest, 1962.

ADENOHYPOPHYSIS

The adenohypophysis, pars distalis, or anterior pituitary, as it is variously called, was once thought to be the "conductor of the endocrine orchestra." Its function now seems more closely analogous to that of the concert master who follows the cues of the hypothalamic maestro. The anterior pituitary produces protein hormones that regulate the growth, anatomic maintenance, and secretory function of other endocrine glands as well as influencing body growth, metabolism, and lactation. The gland is not autonomous as once thought but is regulated by hypophyseotropic hormones reaching it via the hypophyseal portal system from the hypothalamus.

STRUCTURE

The adenohypophysis is derived from the primitive oropharynx. An evagination,

Rathke's pouch, becomes separated from the oral cavity during embryonic development and ultimately lies in apposition to the neural lobe of the pituitary and the pituitary stalk encased in a fossa, the sella turcica, of the sphenoid bone. The pituitary gland is 10 by 15 by 6 mm. in size and weighs half a gram, of which three fourths is adenohypophysis. The major blood supply is from the hypophyseal portal system along the pituitary stalk, and if the stalk is severed infarction of the gland occurs. This vascular system is also susceptible to thrombosis in periods of shock that results in the occasional pituitary failure (Sheehan's syndrome) seen after hemorrhage during pregnancy. The nerve supply is limited and serves mainly vasomotor functions. It was, in fact, the lack of secreto-motor nerve fibers that provided a clue for the importance of the hypophyseal portal chemotransmitter system.

The cytology of the adenohypophysis is complex and it is believed that each of the many hormones produced has a unique cell type of origin.[1, 3, 4, 6, 8-10, 13] The cells have been characterized according to size, staining characteristics, and granule content. The assignment of the origin of a hormone to a particular cell type has, for instance, been based upon association of secretory products with specific tumor cells. In acromegaly, excess growth hormone production is associated with an adenoma composed of acidophilic cells. In Cushing's syndrome, in which ACTH is the hormone secreted in excess, or in myxedema, in which there is excess TSH, there is an abundance of distinct cell types to which is attributed the role of hormone producer. Attempts have been made to localize hormones to their cells of origin by immunofluorescent techniques and by immuno-enzyme histochemistry.[1, 6, 8] In pregnancy and in lactation there is an abundance of special cells associated with each physiologic state.[3] Disagreement and some confusion exists because of the purely subjective and descriptive nature of assignment of hormones to cells and the variability in different animal species. In addition, the cells vary in granule content and staining depending on their physiologic state and the stains used (Table 1).

ADENOHYPOPHYSEAL HORMONES

The hormones of the anterior pituitary have been described in more detail in Chapter 2, Protein Hormones. One important characteristic of pituitary hormones is their apparent species specificity, so that only human or primate growth hormone and gonadotropins are fully active in man. Fortunately, these hormones are resistant to autolysis and can be isolated from pituitary glands removed at human autopsy, and thus made available for clinical use. A summary of the hormones, their activities, and the major control mechanisms is given in Table 2.[5]

TABLE 1.   PITUITARY HORMONES AND ADENOHYPOPHYSEAL CELL TYPES

Hormone	Cell Type	Cell Stain	Associated Tumors or Physiologic State
Somatotropin	Alpha, Somatrotroph	Acidophil	Acromegaly Gigantism
Thyrotropin (Thyroid-stimulating hormone)	Theta, Thyrotroph	Cyanophil	Myxedema
Corticotropin (Adrenocortico-tropic hormone)	Gamma, Corticotroph	Neutrophil, Basophil	Cushing's disease
Follicle-stimulating hormone and interstitial cell-stimulating hormone (LH)	Delta, Gonadotroph	Cyanophil	Castration
Prolactin	Epsilon-eta, Lactotroph	Acidophil	Pregnancy Lactation
Melanocyte-stimulating hormone	Zeta, Melanotroph	Basophil	

TABLE 2. PITUITARY HORMONES AND PHYSIOLOGICAL EFFECTS

Hormone	Physiologic Effect	Control Mechanisms
Growth hormone (STH)	Causes protein synthesis Causes mobilization of fat (NEFA) Causes growth of epiphyseal cartilage Antagonizes insulin action	1. Insulin causes increase in blood level 2. Lowered blood sugar causes increase 3. Amino acids cause increase
Corticotropin	Stimulates adrenal growth and cortisol secretion	1. Stress increases 2. Lowered cortisol increases 3. Elevated cortisol decreases
FSH	Causes follicle growth Causes spermatogenesis	Estrogen decreases
LH (ICSH)	1. Causes follicle growth and stimulates estrogen synthesis 2. Causes ovulation 3. Stimulates Leydig cells and testosterone synthesis	1. Estrogen and progesterone in low dose may trigger ovulatory surge 2. High steroid levels cause decrease
Thyrotropin (TSH)	Stimulates thyroid growth and hormone synthesis	1. Low thyroxin causes increase 2. High thyroxin causes decrease
Prolactin	1. Initiates milk secretion, causes mammary growth 2. Maintains corpus luteum in certain species	1. Suckling causes release 2. Cervical stimulation causes release
Melanocyte-stimulating hormone	Stimulates melanocytes and skin pigmentation	Absence of cortisol in Addison's disease causes elevation

LIFE CYCLE AND CONTROL OF SECRETION

The pituitary is active from early in intrauterine life, when evidence of ACTH, growth hormone, and TSH secretion is apparent. If the pituitary is absent in the fetus with anencephaly, the adrenal may not develop. In addition, growth hormone in fetal blood can be measured and its levels are higher than in maternal blood. This growth hormone is absent if the fetus is anencephalic. There is good evidence that these proteins do not cross the placenta from the mother and that the pituitary hormones measured in fetal blood are of fetal origin. All during childhood there is evidence for baseline secretion of gonadotropins, and the levels rise gradually and then change abruptly at the time of sexual maturation (see FSH and LH, p. 45). At menopause, elevated gonadotropin levels are the rule into quite advanced age.

It has been reported that growth hormone, luteotropin, FSH, LH, TSH, MSH, oxytocin, and vasopressin can be detected by bioassay in human fetal pituitaries. With more specific immunoassays, FSH, TSH, LH, and growth hormone were detected after incubating fetal pituitary cells in vitro with radioactive precursors. Hormones could be detected by nine weeks' gestational age, well within the period of cellular differentiation of the fetal pituitary (see Hypothalamus, p. 61).

Control of the adenohypophysis is predominantly by way of the hypophyseal portal system involving hypophyseotropic hormones released from the hypothalamus on cue from neurologic and endocrine stimuli. The range of hypothalamic controls have been reviewed previously. In addition, it has been further suggested that the various nuclei or centers of the hypothalamus are specific for a given releasing or inhibitory factor and that these hormones drain more or less directly to clusters of pituitary cells that are responsive to their action.

ALTERATIONS IN PREGNANCY

The pituitary increases grossly in size during pregnancy such that there is a di-

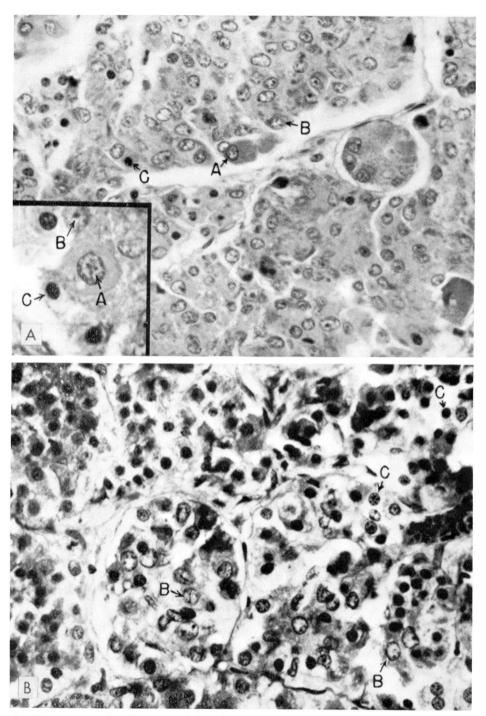

Figure 8. Photomicrographs of sections of the anterior hypophysis. A, The anterior hypophysis of a patient eight and a half months pregnant. × 300. Acidophil cells (A) and modified chromophobe cell, or "pregnancy cell" (B). Within the remainder of the gland are cells with pyknotic or darker-staining nuclei (C), which may be permanent components of the anterior lobe which are temporarily inactive or represent a stage of exhaustion of the pregnancy cell. The insert shows these different types of cells at higher magnification. B, The anterior hypophysis of a patient dying 19 hours post partum. × 300. The separation of the cells may be an indication of a certain amount of edema and fragility of the gland or it may be a fixation artifact. Regression of all cells is evident. Modified chromophobe (B) and inactive cells (C) are readily observed, but normal acidophil cells are not distinguishable. (Courtesy of Dr. Donald G. McKay.)

rect relationship of weight with increased parity and with the female sex. In addition, there is an increase in the number of a large chromophobe cell referred to as a "pregnancy cell."[9, 10, 13] Lobules of the gland contain clusters of these cells, which are characterized by large vesicular nuclei with clumped chromatin, a relatively indistinct cell membrane, and pale cytoplasm. Scattered among these cells are a few larger acidophilic cells with distinct cell membranes. Both types of cells are shown in more detail in the insert in Figure 8. In addition, there are cells with pyknotic, darkly stained nuclei, scanty vacuolated cytoplasm, and indistinct cell membranes. The function, if any, of these cells during pregnancy is not clear, but it is noteworthy that they are seen in fairly large numbers, and they are predominant in the involuting gland post partum (Fig. 8).

It has been suggested that the pituitary may increase in size and cause pressure on the optic chiasm sufficient to result in some loss of bitemporal visual acuity. It is unlikely that any such pressure effect is due to a normal physiologic change, and if visual disturbances should develop in pregnancy, they should be regarded as abnormal.

It has been demonstrated in the monkey that the pituitary is not necessary for the maintenance or successful termination of pregnancy.[11, 12] Moreover, one patient with metastatic breast cancer, who had undergone a complete hypophysectomy (later proved at autopsy) in the 26th week of pregnancy, was subsequently followed. Although she required supportive therapy in the form of cortisone, thyroid, and Pitressin, this patient was successfully delivered at the 36th week of pregnancy after a relatively uneventful labor. The newborn was normal in every respect, and is now thriving. This case and others in the literature indicate that pregnancy, together with fetal growth, may proceed independent of the maternal pituitary.[7]

Functionally, there is no evidence for increased growth hormone secretion in pregnancy and blood levels do not change. Levels of pituitary gonadotropins are low in human pregnancy (Fig. 9)[2] and the pituitary can be removed without a change in the production of placental hormones that maintain pregnancy.[7] Both the thyroid and adrenal appear to have increased activity during pregnancy. There is some tendency toward thyroid enlargement, but the elevation in thyroid hormone in blood is due largely to increased protein binding. The increase in blood cortisol in pregnancy is also due largely to increased protein bind-

Figure 9. Low levels of FSH throughout pregnancy, documenting lack of pituitary function. See also Figures 2 and 6 in Chapter 2. (From Faiman, C., Ryan, R. J., Zwirek, S. J., and Rubin, M. E.: J. Clin. Endocr., 28:1323, 1968.)

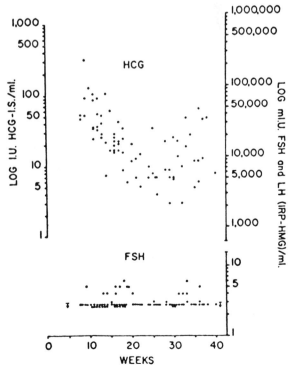

ing, with a much smaller increase in free cortisol. There is little specific information on alterations in pituitary activity relative to ACTH during gestation but serum TSH levels do rise. A placental TSH has, however, now been described and its function is unknown. Finally, pituitary prolactin appears to be released after parturition, as evidenced by analogies with animal studies which are described in the section on lactation (p. 132).

BIBLIOGRAPHY

1. Bain, J., and Ezrin, C.: Immunofluorescent localization of the LH cell of the human adenohypophysis. J. Clin. Endocr., 30:181, 1970.
2. Faiman, C., Ryan, R. J., Zwirek, S. J., and Rubin, M. E.: Serum FSH and HCG during human pregnancy and puerperium. J. Clin. Endocr., 28:1323, 1968.
3. Goluboff, L. G., and Ezrin, C.: Effect of pregnancy on the somatotroph and the prolactin cell of the human adenohypophysis. J. Clin. Endocr., 29:1533, 1969.
4. Halmi, N. S., and McCormick, W. F.: The delta cell of the human hypophysis in childhood. J. Clin. Endocr., 29:1036, 1969.
5. Harris, G. W., and Donovan, B. T.: The Pituitary Gland, Vols. 1, 2, 3. University of California Press, Berkeley, 1966.
6. Kawarai, Y., and Nakane, P. K.: Localization of tissue antigens on the ultrathin sections with peroxidase-labeled antibody method. J. Histochem. Cytochem., 18:161, 1970.
7. Little, B., Smith, O. W., Jessiman, A. G., Selenkow, H. A., Van't Hoff, W., Eglin, J. M., and Moore, F. D.: Hypophysectomy during pregnancy in a patient with cancer of the breast; case report with hormone studies. J. Clin. Endocr., 18:425, 1958.
8. Nakane, P. K.: Classifications of anterior pituitary cell types with immunoenzyme histochemistry. J. Histochem. Cytochem., 18:9, 1970.
9. Pearse, A. G. E.: Cytological and cytochemical investigations on the foetal and adult hypophysis in various physiological and pathological states. J. Path. Bact., 65:355, 1953.
10. Severinghaus, A. E.: The cytology of the pituitary gland. In The Pituitary Gland; an Investigation of the Most Recent Advances. Williams and Wilkins, Baltimore, 1938.
11. Smith, P. E.: Non-essentiality of hypophysis for maintenance of pregnancy in rhesus monkeys. Anat. Rec., 94:497, 1946.
12. Smith, P. E.: Continuation of pregnancy in rhesus monkeys (Macaca mulatta) following hypophysectomy. Endocrinology, 55:655, 1954.
13. Somers, S. C.: Pituitary cell relations to body states. Lab. Invest., 8:588, 1959.

NEUROHYPOPHYSIS

The neurohypophysis is the site of storage and release of two hormones important in reproduction and homeostasis, oxytocin and vasopressin.[1-3] Oxytocin stimulates milk letdown and uterine contractibility, while vasopressin is an antidiuretic and pressor substance.

STRUCTURE

The neurohypophysis, which is not an endocrine gland in its own right, comprises the posterior (or neural) lobe of the pituitary, the infundibulum, and the median eminence. Actually, the functional unit responsible for production, storage, and secretion of the hormones consists of the neurons and axons originating in the hypothalamic supraoptic and paraventricular nuclei which extend into the neurohypophysis.

NEUROHYPOPHYSEAL HORMONES

The hormones oxytocin and vasopressin are octapeptides that were synthesized in the laboratory by du Vigneaud, an accomplishment recognized by a Nobel prize in chemistry in 1955. The hormones are stored in association with a large protein molecule of molecular weight 30,000 called neurophysin which is found to contain varying proportions of oxytocin and vasopressin but can exist with predominantly one or the other hormone. This neurosecretory material can be visualized under the microscope as granules in the cell and its axons. These granules apparently are transported by "axoplasmic flow" from the cell to the axon terminals in the neurohypophysis where they are stored for release when triggered by appropriate stimuli to the hypothalamus. It has been demonstrated in certain species that the supraoptic neurons are the origin of vasopressin and the paraventricular neurons the origin of oxytocin.

Evidence for the neurosecretory process is based on the observations that the hormonal activity can be extracted from the supraoptic and paraventricular nuclei. In addition, the neurosecretory granules move down the axons and disappear distal to any lesion of the tract. If hormone release is stimulated, the granules decrease markedly.

Oxytocin and vasopressin are octapeptides with a five-membered amino acid ring held together with a sulfhydryl bond and with a tail of three amino acids (Fig. 10). Oxytocin has been found in the pituitaries of practically all mammalian species in which it has been sought. Surprisingly, vasopressin (see Fig. 10) and oxytocin have identical physical structures except for two different amino acids at positions 3 and 8 in the molecule. It should not be surprising that the pure compounds have overlapping biologic effects. While vasopressin has an activity of 300 units per milligram in vasopressor activity, oxytocin has an activity of 9 units. The antidiuretic activities of the two molecules bear a similar relationship. Conversely, with uterine activity and milk ejection, oxytocin has an activity of about 400 units per milligram, while vasopressin has activities of 9 units and 50 units per milligram, respectively, in the two test systems.

All neurohypophyseal peptides require the intact disulfide bond for activity but various substitutions and alterations in the molecule modify activity even to the point of exceeding the potency of natural hormones.

While vasopressin of most species has an arginine at position 8, the vasopressin of the domestic pig and hippopotamus has a lysine at this site and the two are designated arginine and lysine vasopressin, respectively (Fig. 10).

In nonmammalian vertebrates, an analogue of these mammalian hormones has been characterized as arginine vasotocin, which can be isolated from chickens and amphibians. The relationships of structure,

biologic activity, and animal distribution have been of interest from a comparative point of view. Obviously, these structurally similar molecules have been adapted to the changing needs for control of water balance, reproduction, and lactation imposed by evolutionary trends.

CONTROL OF SECRETION

The control of neurohypophyseal secretion is via neurologic or humoral stimuli upon the hypothalamic nuclei. The activities of these nuclei have been demonstrated by the deficiencies produced by lesions involving the hypothalamus, and by the activities evoked by electrical stimulation of ascending pathways, midbrain, or hypothalamus. There are also osmoreceptors, probably in the hypothalamus, that respond to infusions of hypertonic solutions. The major stimuli for vasopressin release include water deprivation, plasma hyperosmolarity, and changes in blood volume and pressure. The major stimuli for oxytocin release are suckling and distention of the lower reproductive tract and uterus in response to coitus or parturition.

The two neurohypophyseal hormones are stimulated separately and it is possible to evoke oxytocin release to suckling, as evidenced by milk ejection, without a concomitant antidiuresis. Similarly, antidiuresis from vasopressin release can be stimulated without evidence of oxytocin secretion.

Various anesthetics and drugs as well as alcohol can inhibit neurohypophyseal secretion.

Oxytocin

$$CyS\text{-}Tyr\text{-}Ileu\text{-}Glu(NH_2)\text{-}Asp(NH_2)\text{-}CyS\text{-}Pro\text{-}Leu\text{-}Gly(NH_2)$$
$$1 \quad 2 \quad 3 \quad\quad 4 \quad\quad\quad 5 \quad\quad 6 \quad 7 \quad 8 \quad\quad 9$$

Arginine vasopressin

$$CyS\text{-}Tyr\text{-}Phe\text{-}Glu(NH_2)\text{-}Asp(NH_2)\text{-}CyS\text{-}Pro\text{-}Arg\text{-}Gly(NH_2)$$

Lysine vasopressin

$$CyS\text{-}Tyr\text{-}Phe\text{-}Glu(NH_2)\text{-}Asp(NH_2)\text{-}CyS\text{-}Pro\text{-}Lys\text{-}Gly(NH_2)$$

Arginine vasotocin

$$CyS\text{-}Tyr\text{-}Ileu\text{-}Glu(NH_2)\ Asp(NH_2)\text{-}CyS\text{-}Pro\ Arg\ Gly(NH_2)$$

Figure 10. Formulas of neurohypophyseal hormones (see text). (From Sawyer, W. H.: Pharmacol. Rev., 13:225, 1961.)

ALTERATION IN PREGNANCY

Although toxemia with its attendant water retention and hypertension was at one time linked to possible excess of the antidiuretic principle, vasopressin, there is little specific information on changes of function of the neurohypophysis in pregnancy in relation to either oxytocin or vasopressin. In any case, labor and delivery are generally uncomplicated in patients with diabetes insipidus, and there is still controversy about whether there is a role for oxytocin in either the initiation of labor, the facilitation of delivery, or both.

BIBLIOGRAPHY

1. Bern, H. A., and Knowles, F. G. W.: Neurosecretion. In Martini, L., and Ganong, W. F., eds.: Neuroendocrinology, Vol. 1. Academic Press, New York, 1966, p. 187.

2. Sawyer, W. H.: Neurohypophysial hormones. Pharmacol. Rev., 13:225, 1961.

3. Sawyer, W. H., and Mills, E.: Control of vasopressin secretion. In Martini, L., and Ganong, W. F., eds.: Neuroendocrinology, Vol. 1. Academic Press, New York, 1966, p. 139.

OVARY

The ovaries are paired, almond-shaped organs attached to the posterior leaf of the broad ligament by the mesovarium lying posterior and lateral to the uterus and inferior to the fallopian tubes. In this position the ovary can serve its dual function as a site of ovum development and release and as an endocrine gland.[4, 15] The two processes are interdependent and coordinated in the periodic cycles characteristic of adult ovarian function.

At maturity each ovary averages 3.5 cm. in length, 2 cm. in width, and 1 cm. in thickness, and in addition to the support of the mesovarium, the ovary is slung between the uterus and lateral pelvic wall by two ligaments running within the leaves of the broad ligament. The ovarian ligament connects one pole of the ovary to the uterus just below the insertion of the oviduct while a suspensory ligament containing ovarian vessels and nerves connects the opposite pole of the ovary to the lateral pelvic wall. The surface of the ovary facing the lateral pelvic wall lies in a fossa ovarica, a depression bounded by the external iliac and obturator vessels. The gross appearance of the surface of the ovary varies with age and function. In childhood, the ovary is smooth, white, and glistening, with the occasional nodularity produced by follicle cysts. This generally persists into adult life with the addition of the hemorrhagic orange-yellow discolorations produced by ruptured follicles and corpora lutea. When ova and follicles are depleted in later life, the ovary becomes smaller, pale, scarred, and corrugated by the functional activity of prior years.

OVARIAN DEVELOPMENT

Our knowledge of gonadal embryogenesis is largely descriptive, and considerable controversy has existed over the years regarding the origin of specific cell types. The general consensus is that the germ cells that give rise to ova and sperm are separated during the early cleavage stages and can just be identified in the yolk sac epithelium at about four weeks. At this time, they are large ameboid cells that stain intensely for alkaline phosphatase. The epithelial cells overlying the mesonephric bodies give rise to the cortex of the gonads and ultimately the granulosa and Sertoli cells of the ovary and testis, respectively, while the underlying mesenchyme contributes to the medulla of the gonad from which are derived the testicular tubular system and interstitial cells and the ovarian stroma that supplies theca cells of the follicle. With a common developmental heritage, it is not surprising that ovarian stroma and testicular interstitial cells share common steroidogenic potentials with one another and with the adrenal tissue that is derived in close proximity from the same embryonic mesonephric ridge.

The ovary develops from this epithelium and underlying mesenchymal tissue of the urogenital ridge under the influence of primary germ cells which migrate to this area from the primitive hindgut. The movement of such cells has actually been documented by time-lapse photography. The primary germ cells are set aside in very early development in keeping with the concept of germ-plasm continuum, and if their migration from the hindgut to the genital ridge is interrupted, definitive gonads do not form and significant endocrine function never develops. The primary ovarian germ cells divide extensively into oogonia, which are enveloped by a single layer of cortical granulosa cells forming the primitive follicles, which are, in turn, surrounded by mesenchymal stroma. Near the time of birth the oogonia are transformed into primary oocytes, which develop further only in relation to follicular maturation and ovulation.

At 20 weeks of intrauterine life ova number in the millions but subsequent degeneration leaves only some 750,000 potential primary oocytes at birth (Fig. 11). There is a constant atresia during development and adult reproductive life so that the numbers of oocytes continually decline

A

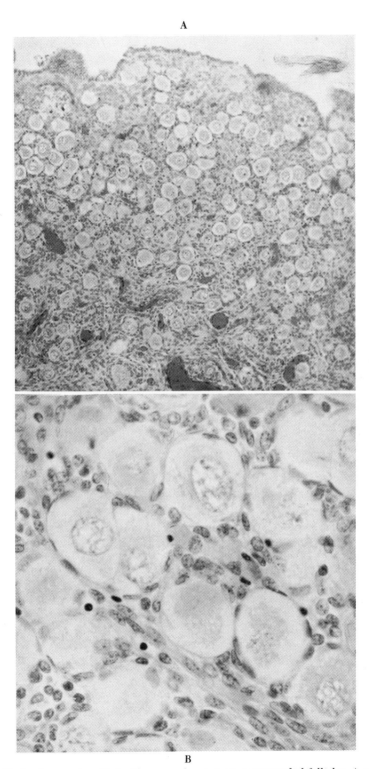

B

Figure 11. Photomicrographs of infantile ovary showing many primordial follicles. A, × 50; B, × 400.

until the supply is essentially completely exhausted at the time of menopause. Of these thousands of potential ova only some 500 are ovulated and would be available for fertilization; the rest are destroyed by as yet unexplained mechanisms and selection in the process of atresia.

From the newborn period to puberty, the ovary is functionally quiescent, producing little in the way of hormones. At the same time, however, the ovary undergoes structural changes with follicle development, occasional cyst formation, and continued atresia or loss of oocytes.

In the adolescent period, the ovaries come under the stimulatory effects of pituitary gonadotropins and an ovarian cycle develops with periodic ovum release and hormonal activity. The initiating event for puberty is believed to be maturation of the hypothalamus and its stimulation of cyclic pituitary hormonal activity.

At maturity, the ovary is a uniquely dynamic organ with cyclic changes in structure and function that persist all during adult reproductive life. The structural sequence of follicular development, ovulation, and corpus luteum formation is accompanied by a functional sequence of hormonal secretion patterns that are responsible for preparing the reproductive tract for conception and implantation. During pregnancy, the ovary is more or less quiescent again because of the intervention of the endocrine mechanisms associated with the placenta and conceptus. Exhaustion of oocytes at the climacteric converts the ovary into a structurally less active organ, with variable endocrine function.

Consideration of the ovary therefore must be in relationship to its longitudinal changes with age (ovarian life cycle, Table 3) and, during the active reproductive period, in relationship to the dynamic structural and functional changes of the cycle. The ovary contains at various times in the cycle discrete structural and functional units: the follicle, the corpus luteum, the stroma, and the hilum. Each will be considered in turn.

OVARIAN FOLLICLE

Follicular Structure and Ovulation

The most primitive follicles consist of a single oocyte surrounded by a layer one cell deep of flattened granulosa cells lying within the cortex close to the surface of the ovary. As the oocyte increases in size, the surrounding granulosa cells grow and divide, developing a concentric ring several layers thick which is, in turn, enveloped by circles of specialized stromal cells, the theca interna, and an outer layer of less differentiated stromal cells, the theca externa. In essence, the follicle consists of ovum, granulosa cells, and theca interna and externa layers from within outward and represents a primary structural and functional unit for reproduction and endocrine activity. The granulosa and thecal layers

TABLE 3. OVARIAN LIFE CYCLE*

Age	Status of Ova	Ovarian Structures Present	Hormonal Activity
Fetal	Plentiful	Stroma and follicles	Minimal
Childhood	Plentiful	Stroma and follicles	Minimal estrogens
Adolescence, puberty	Declining	1. Stroma and follicles 2. Start of ovulation and corpora lutea 3. Anovulation common	Estrogens and progesterone
Adult, reproductive	Declining	Follicle, corpora, and stroma	1. Estrogens in follicular phase 2. Estrogens and progesterone in luteal phase
Perimenopausal	Markedly declining	1. Stroma and follicles 2. Corpora lutea in ovulatory cycles 3. Anovulation common	1. Estrogens in anovulatory cycles 2. Estrogens and progesterone with ovulation
Menopause	Absent	Stroma	Androgens from stroma; occasionally estrogens

*From Ryan, K. J.: Int. J. Gynec. Obstet., 8:608, 1970. The Williams & Wilkins Co., Baltimore, Md. 21202, U.S.A.

are separated by a fine membrana propria, and only the thecal layer is invested with capillaries, there being no direct blood supply to the granulosa. With increased growth, the follicle is positioned deeper in the ovary. The ovum can be observed to have a thin surrounding vitelline or true cell membrane and a thicker clear homogeneous membrane, the zona pellucida, to which is attached a single layer of granulosa cells called the corona radiata. The corona remains with the ovum after ovulation but must be dispersed before fertilization can take place (Fig. 12).

The ovum grows to a size of 0.140 mm., and the follicle increases in diameter up to 10 mm. The increase in follicular size is accomplished by the development of a fluid-filled cavity or antrum in addition to granulosa cell proliferation. As the fluid cavity enlarges, the ovum is displaced eccentrically, surrounded by a mound or tuft of granulosa cells, the cumulus, with which it is discharged at the time of follicular rupture. The remainder of the follicle wall surrounding the fluid is covered by several layers of granulosa cells (Fig. 12). At full maturity the follicle bulges above the surface of the ovary, and the point of rupture thins into an area known as the stigma, the site from which the ovum discharges. Actual rupture is probably caused by increased distensibility and local enzymatic destruction of the follicular wall. Although other mechanisms have been favored, there is insufficient information as yet to assign a cause-and-effect priority. Study of follicular fluid reveals that it contains the high-molecular-weight mucopolysaccharides hyaluronic acid and chondroitin sulfate, and that these depolymerize prior to ovulation. Recent consideration of the mechanics of ovulation provides a basis for reconciling the distensibility and necrobiosis theories and suggests that both may be involved.

Follicle Atresia

Since usually only one follicle ruptures each month in the human, many developing follicles obviously reach a halfway point toward full maturation and then regress without release of an ovum. These follicles, after reaching a certain size, can be seen to lose the ovum by cytolysis. The granulosa cells degenerate, the follicular fluid is resorbed, the follicle wall collapses, the surrounding theca cells undergo degeneration, and the entire follicle is ultimately replaced by a hyaline scar. This represents the fate of most developing follicles and proceeds unremittingly during the entire ovarian life span until the supply of follicles is exhausted.

Follicular Control

The follicle can develop to the antrum stage and undergo atresia in the absence of any tropic control, but for full follicular development and ovulation to occur the ovary must be stimulated by a combination of pituitary follicle-stimulating hormone and luteinizing hormone for some 9 to 14 days. Neither hormone alone is effective.

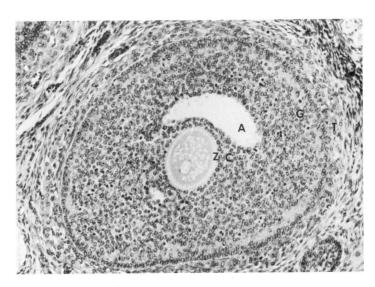

Figure 12. Ovarian follicle. *Z*, Zona pellucida surrounding ovum; *C*, Cumulus of granulosa cells; *A*, Beginning antrum and follicular fluid; *G*, granulosa cells; *T*, thecal cells.

After full follicular development, ovulation is triggered one day after stimulation by a surge of LH. This course of events can be documented by correlating FSH and LH blood levels with follicular development and rupture or by producing these ovarian changes in patients without pituitary function by appropriate exogenous administration of these hormones. The response of the ovarian follicles to gonadotropins is itself augmented by estrogens, and since follicle growth is associated with estrogen production, the process involves a positive self-priming or snowballing phenomenon.

Puberty and Follicle Growth

This cyclic development of ovarian follicles and ovulation commences at the time of puberty, presumably when maturation of the hypothalamic control centers occurs. It should be remembered that the pituitary tropic hormones FSH and LH are released under the influence of hypothalamic hypophyseotropic hormones which are, in turn, governed by internal and external environmental influences including steroid hormones. The ovary can ordinarily respond to gonadotropins long before it is called upon to do so and gonadotropin can be produced and released by the pituitary even in childhood. The series of events that triggers the onset of cyclic ovarian function is at present completely unknown.

Follicle Function: Maturation of Ova and Steroidogenesis

During follicle maturation the ova increase in size and are presumably supplied with nutritional stores and developmental information by the surrounding granulosa or nurse cells. It is also possible that cortical field information that imparts polarity and specific cytoplasmic distribution to the ovum is supplied during this period. It should be remembered that the nuclear genetic information of the fertilized egg can be expressed and is controlled only in a cell properly programmed for development. In addition, expulsion of the first polar body and completion of meiosis occurs at the time of ovulation.

The endocrine function of the follicle has been determined by: (1) correlating urinary or blood steroid production with the timing of follicular development; (2) measuring steroids in follicular fluid in various stages of the cycle in health and in disease states; (3) studying the enzymes of the whole follicle and of individual cells that are concerned with steroidogenesis; (4) re-creation of the natural chain of events by artificial administration of gonadotropins and use of all of the foregoing together. By these methods it has been established that the follicle is a major source of estrogen, which it can synthesize de novo from acetate, that the follicle can also synthesize progestins and androgens, which it uses as estrogen precursors, and that the follicular secretory products are estradiol-17β, androstenedione, 17-hydroxyprogesterone, dehydroepiandrosterone, and progesterone, in order of relative biologic importance and effective amounts.

Urinary Steroids During Follicular Development

Measurement of estrogens in urine during follicular development during the normal cycle or after FSH and LH administration indicates a gradual elevation of estrogen metabolites. In the urine a peak occurs near the time of ovulation, with average levels of total estrogens (estriol, estrone, estradiol) starting at 20 mcg./24 hours at the start of the cycle and rising to 80 mcg./24 hours at the time of ovulation. Estrogen levels are low in childhood prior to cyclic follicular function and decline at menopause after such function disappears. If the follicles are overstimulated by gonadotropins, the amounts of estrogen increase, reaching near-pregnancy levels. Since androgens are derived principally from the adrenal, ovarian contributions to urinary 17-ketosteroids are usually overshadowed except in disease states.

Blood Steroids During Follicle Development

Measurements of estrogen in peripheral blood reveal a pattern similar to urinary excretion with elevations of estrogens from the start of the cycle to the point of ovulation. Since there is a lag in excretion, the blood estrogen peak anticipates the urinary one by about a day.

Steroids measured in effluent blood from the ovary containing the ripe follicle have excess progesterone, 17-hydroxyprogesterone, androstenedione, dehydroepiandrosterone, and estradiol-17β compared to the

TABLE 4. PLASMA STEROIDS IN A 34-YEAR-OLD PATIENT, GRAVIDA 3, PARA 3,
DATED 12 DAYS POSTMENSTRUAL[*]

Steroid	Peripheral Plasma (μg./100 ml.)	Ovarian Plasma	
		Right (μg./100 ml.)	Left[†] (μg./100 ml.)
Progesterone	0.149	0.393	1.550
17α-Hydroxyprogesterone	<2.000	<2.000	4.437
20α-Hydroxy-4-pregnene-3-one	0.276	0.040	0.108
20β-Hydroxy-4-pregnene-3-one	0.011	0.015	0.024
Androstenedione	0.683	8.520	8.852
Testosterone	0.083	0.190	0.242
Dehydroepiandrosterone	1.861	3.956	4.236
Estrone	0.038	0.071	0.172
Estradiol	0.125	0.359	1.760

[*]From Mikhail, G.: Clin. Obstet. Gynec., 10:29, 1967.
[†]Ovary containing the ripe follicle.

other ovary or the periphery, although both ovarian effluents exceed the peripheral levels (Table 4).

Steroids in Follicular Fluid

All of the steroids thus far described in urine and blood have been isolated from the follicular fluid.

Enzymatic Capacity of Follicle Wall and Isolated Granulosa and Theca Cells

On the basis of histochemical staining and the correlations of steroid production with anatomic changes, various enzymatic capacities have been assigned to the individual cell types that comprise the follicle wall. This has now been tested directly in several species, including man. The ripe ovarian follicle can readily synthesize estrogen from acetate in accord with the pathway shown in Figure 6 in Chapter 1, and as one approaches the end-product the rate of precursor conversion increases, giving credence to the biosynthetic scheme illustrated. Both the granulosa and the theca cell when isolated free of each other can synthesize estrogens in a similar manner but with quantitative differences. The granulosa cell piles up progesterone and 17-hydroxyprogesterone, while the theca cell converts most intermediates into the estrogens. The two cells seem to work synergistically in producing more hormone than either alone. This has given rise to a two-cell theory for estrogen formation which has been substantiated by separation and recombination studies in vitro (Tables 5 and 6).

TABLE 5. PERCENTAGE YIELD OF STEROIDS PRODUCED BY GRANULOSA
AND THECA CELLS IN VITRO FROM ACETATE-1-^{14}C

Steroid[†]	Yield (%)		
	Granulosa	Theca	Combined Granulosa and Theca
Progesterone	0.10	0.001	0.032
Androstenedione	0.002	0.001	0.003
Estrone	0.002	0.004	0.02
Estradiol	—	0.004	0.016

[*]From Ryan, K. J.: Int. J. Gynec. Obstet., 8:608, 1970. The Williams & Wilkins Co., Baltimore, Md. 21202, U.S.A.
[†]Note that the major steroid isolated from granulosa was progesterone and from theca, estradiol. The combined cells synthesized four times the amount of estrogen as did the theca alone.

TABLE 6. STEROIDS FORMED BY HUMAN GRANULOSA AND THECA CELLS IN VITRO

	Product	
Precursor	Granulosa	Theca
Pregnenolone	Progesterone	Progesterone
	17-Hydroxyprogesterone	17-Hydroxyprogesterone
		Androstenedione
		Estrone
		Estradiol
Progesterone	17-Hydroxyprogesterone	17-Hydroxyprogesterone
		Androstenedione
		Estrone
		Estradiol

°From Ryan, K. J., in Behrman, S. J., and Kistner, R. W., eds.: Progress in Infertility. Little, Brown and Co., Boston, 1968, p. 275.

CORPUS LUTEUM

Structure

The corpus luteum, or yellow body, derives its name from the carotene pigment it contains, and its structure is formed from the collapsed ovulated follicle. The follicle is initially filled with blood. The remaining granulosa cells of the follicle proliferate to become luteinized or larger polyhedral cells with a granular cytoplasm. Some fluid is secreted into the ruptured follicle and along with the blood forms a coagulum. There is ingrowth of theca cells, which also become luteinized, and this is accompanied by blood vessel invasion (Fig. 13). The membrana propria as a discrete entity dividing granulosa and theca disappears and the cells are somewhat intermixed. The fully developed corpus luteum is reconstituted to a size similar to that of the preovulatory follicle from which it was derived and consists mainly of convoluted groupings of cells with a central thin coagulum.[3] The unique feature of the corpus luteum of the cycle is its limited life span. After an average life of 10 to 14 days the luteal cells undergo fatty degeneration. The cells gradually disappear and the debris is removed by phagocytosis. There is an increase in connective tissue, disappearance of blood vessels, and decrease in overall size to form a corpus albicans, which ultimately blends into the ovarian stroma. The factors controlling the degeneration of corpora lutea are incompletely understood.

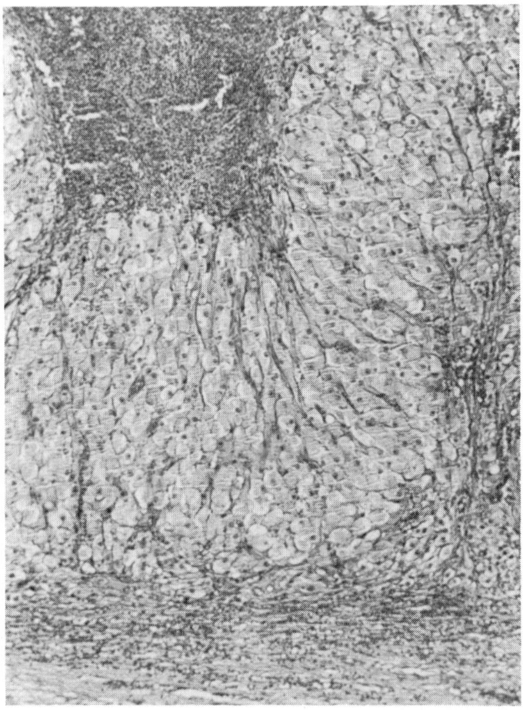

Corpus Luteum of Pregnancy

If pregnancy intervenes and implantation takes place, the corpus luteum does not regress but enlarges two- to three-fold and remains functional for another 8 to 10 weeks (Fig. 14), after which time it may slowly disappear or remain throughout the duration of pregnancy with a diminished secretory role, ending finally as a corpus albicans. During pregnancy the granulosa and theca cells contain lipid deposits and a fine granular cytoplasm.[2, 5, 6, 8, 9, 14]

Figure 13. Corpus luteum soon after ovualation.

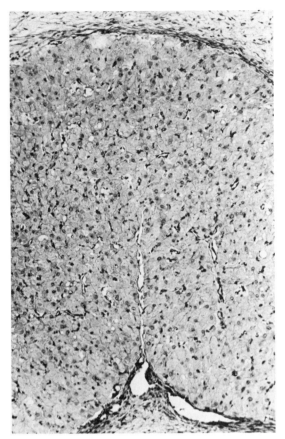

Figure 14. Corpus luteum at eight weeks of pregnancy.

maintained indefinitely; this suggests the intervention of other factors in its degeneration. The uterus has no effect on luteal function in man, in contast to other species.[1]

Corpus Luteum Function: Progesterone Formation

By utilizing the same criteria as for studies with the follicle, hormone secretion by the corpus luteum can be documented by correlation of its life span with blood and urinary hormone and metabolite levels, extraction of hormones from the isolated luteal tissue, assay of effluent ovarian blood, and in-vitro enzyme assays.

Urinary Steroids in the Luteal Phase

Following ovulation, the urinary level of pregnanediol, a progesterone metabolite, rises, and this increase persists for the duration of the cycle, dropping just before menstruation. The levels range from 1 mg./24 hours during follicular growth to 4 to 6 mg./24 hours after ovulation. Levels of total estrogens increase to values comparable to the ones obtained with the peak follicular activity.

Control of Corpus Luteum Growth and Function

The functional corpus luteum forms spontaneously after ovulation in the human and other animals and does not require the luteotropic hormone necessary for maintaining luteal function in the rat. Rat luteotropin is released by cervical stimuli or coitus, and in the absence of such a special tropic hormone the corpus luteum does not persist in this species. In the human, even with no pituitary function, stimulation with FSH and HCG is followed by ovulation and a normal luteal phase. HCG, however, has a long-life and if human pituitary LH is used to induce ovulation, the corpus luteum does not persist for its normal time unless it is supplied with small amounts of LH. Luteinizing hormone may therefore be a luteotropic principle in man and other animals. Either LH or HCG will stimulate corpus luteum synthesis of hormones in vivo and in vitro. Although the life of the corpus luteum can be extended by HCG it cannot be

Blood Steroids During Corpus Luteum Function

Immediately after ovulation, blood progesterone increases from barely detectable levels to a peak of 12 to 16 millimicrograms per milliliter and drops again just before menstruation. Assays of ovarian vein blood from the side bearing the corpus luteum reveal elevated levels of progesterone, 17α-hydroxyprogesterone, 20α-hydroxy-4-pregnene-3-one, and estradiol, and the values are higher than those for blood from either the contralateral ovary or the periphery (Table 7).

Steroids in Luteal Tissue

All of the steroids isolated from ovarian vein blood have also been obtained by extraction of isolated luteal tissue, including progesterone, 20α-hydroxypregn-4-en-3-one, 17-hydroxyprogesterone, androstenedione, estradiol, and estrone.

TABLE 7. PLASMA STEROIDS IN A 28-YEAR-OLD PATIENT, GRAVIDA 3, PARA 3,
DATED 3–4 DAYS POSTOVULATORY

| | | Ovarian Plasma | |
Steroid	Peripheral Plasma (ug./100 ml.)	Left (μg./100 ml.)	Right† (μg./100 ml.)
Progesterone	2.130	2.570	47.100
17α-Hydroxyprogesterone	<2.000	<2.000	4.050
20α-Hydroxy-4-pregnene-3-one	0.314	0.500	1.390
Androstenedione	0.533	1.710	1.760
Dehydroepiandrosterone	1.638	2.080	1.680
Esterone	0.039	0.080	0.065
Estradiol	0.058	0.193	0.418

°From Mikhail, G.: Clin. Obstet. Gynec., 10:29, 1967.
†Ovary with the corpus luteum.

Enzymatic Capacity of Luteal Tissue

Unfortunately, one cannot readily separate granulosa from theca cells in the corpus luteum, and studies of enzymatic capacity do not distinguish which cell type is contributing to hormone production. In any case, luteal tissue can carry out all of the steroid synthetic reactions from acetate through cholesterol to progesterone. Progesterone (as in the follicle) can be converted to androgens and estrogen. The corpus luteum favors progesterone formation, however, and the Δ^5 compounds, pregnenolone and dehydroepiandrosterone, which figure prominently in estrogen biosynthesis in the follicle, seem to be less involved in luteal tissue (Table 8). Hence, in the follicle pregnenolone seems to be a favored precursor of estrogen via 17-hydroxypregnenolone and dehydroepiandrosterone, while in the corpus luteum progesterone accumulates and appears to be the preferred source of estrogen via 17-hydroxyprogesterone and androstenedione (see p. 8).

OVARIAN STROMA

The ovarian stroma consists of densely packed spindle-shaped cells in the cortex and a more loosely arranged connective tissue in the medullary and hilar regions. These stromal cells give rise to the theca interna and externa, and occasionally contain nests of luteinized or interstitial cells in a condition termed hyperthecosis. In the

TABLE 8. PER CENT DISTRIBUTION OF STEROIDS FORMED IN THE HUMAN FOLLICLE,
CORPORA LUTEA, AND STROMA FROM ACETATE°

Follicle		Corpora Lutea		Stroma†	
Steroid	Per Cent Formed Compared to Estradiol	Steroid	Per Cent Formed Compared to Progesterone	Steroid	Per Cent Formed Compared to Androstenedione
Estradiol	100	Progesterone	100	Androstenedione	100
Estrone	74	17-Hydroxyprogesterone	26	Dehydroepiandrosterone	19
Androstenedione	30	Androstenedione	12	17-Hydroxyprogesterone	18
Dehydroepiandrosterone	29	Estradiol	10	Testosterone	10
Pregnenolone	16	20α-Hydroxypregn-4-	3	Progesterone	—
17-Hydroxyprogesterone	8.3	en-3-one		Estradiol	—
17-Hydroxypregnenolone	3.9				
Progesterone	1.5				

°From Ryan, K. J., in Behrman, S. J., and Kistner, R. W., eds.: Progress in Infertility. Little, Brown and Co., Boston, 1968, p. 275.
†Follicular phase of the cycle.

absence of recognizable follicles or corpora lutea, the remaining stroma is capable of synthesizing hormones from acetate and the predominant product appears to be androgenic steroids, although estrogens can also be produced (Table 8). This tissue is responsive in vitro to gonadotropic stimulation, with increased hormone production. It is likely that in periods of anovulation or after menopause the stroma can contribute to the secretory function of the ovary.

HILAR CELLS

The hilus appears to be continuous with the stroma of the medullary region but is distinguished as the portal for major blood vessels and nerves into the ovary. Hilar or Leydig cells, a counterpart of the testicular cell type, can usually be found in the ovary and are present occasionally in nests in the form of a Leydig cell tumor. These cells are polyhedral with an eosinophilic cytoplasm that contains the crystalloids of Reinke, by which criterion their identity can be established. Studies of the hilar region of the ovary indicate a potential for steroid production similar to that of the stroma.

SUMMARY OF OVARIAN FUNCTION AND STRUCTURE IN RELATION TO AGE AND CONTROL MECHANISMS

From the foregoing, it can be appreciated that the ovary is a dynamic, heterogeneous tissue, and that its functional potential varies with the structural organelles available for hormone synthesis and ovum development at any given period during life.[10]

During fetal development, infancy, and childhood, the ovary can respond to stimulation and occasionally does so by cyst formation, even in the fetus in utero in response to the gonadotropic hormones of pregnancy. Many ova and follicles undergo atresia throughout prepubertal life, and even ovarian follicle cysts may be present, but no significant endocrine activity is evident until close to the age of menarche. At the onset of ovarian endocrine function, varied periods of anovulation between ovulatory cycles are sufficiently common to be considered a variant of normalcy. In such periods of anovulation only estrogens of follicular origin are present and the absence of corpora lutea and its progestational hormone is manifested in irregular menses.

After the ovarian cyclicity is established, many follicles continue to undergo atresia for every one ovulated. The ovary secretes predominantly estrogen during the follicular phase, and after ovulation, estrogen and progesterone from the corpus luteum (Table 9).[11, 12]

At the time of menopause, anovulation becomes more common and irregular menses are frequent owing to the absence of corpora lutea and progesterone formation. After the follicles are depleted only the stroma remains for hormonal secretion, which might be androgenic or estrogenic in nature.

Since the ovarian follicle and stroma can both secrete androgens normally, it is not surprising that in certain anovulatory conditions, such as polycystic ovary disease, excess androgen may be of ovarian origin. In such instances, inhibition of adrenal function with persistence of elevated androgen levels can assist in implicating the ovary.

TABLE 9. BLOOD LEVELS AND PRODUCTION RATES OF OVARIAN STEROIDS*

Hormone	*Blood Levels (μg. 100 ml.)*		*Production Rate*
	Follicular	Luteal	
Estradiol	0.02	0.01	200–500 μg./day
Androstenedione	0.130	0.145	3.4 mg./day
Progesterone	0.132	1.06	4 mg./day follicular phase
			30 mg./day luteal phase

*From Ryan, K. J., in Behrman, S. J., and Kistner, R. W., eds.: Progress in Infertility. Little, Brown and Co., Boston, 1968, p. 275.

BIBLIOGRAPHY

1. Beling, C. G., Marcus, S. L., and Markham, S. M.: Functional activity of the corpus luteum following hysterectomy. J. Clin. Endocr., 30:30, 1970.
2. Crisp, T. M., Dessouky, D. A., and Denys, F. R.: The fine structure of the human corpus luteum of early pregnancy and during the progestational phase of the menstrual cycle. Amer. J. Anat., 126:37, 1969.
3. Gillim, S. W., Christensen, A. K., and McLennan, C. E.: Fine structure of the human menstrual corpus luteum at its stage of maximum secretory activity. Amer. J. Anat., 126:409, 1969.
4. Grady, H., ed.: The Ovary. Williams and Wilkins, Baltimore, 1963.
5. Green, J. A., Garcilazo, J. A., and Maqueo, M.: Ultrastructure of the human ovary. I. The luteal cell at term. Amer. J. Obstet. Gynec., 99:855, 1967.
6. Guraya, S. S.: Histochemical study of human corpus luteum at term. Amer. J. Obstet. Gynec., 102:219, 1968.
7. Mikhail, G.: Sex steroids in blood. Clin. Obstet. Gynec., 10:29, 1967.
8. Nelson, W. W., and Greene, R. R.: The human ovary in pregnancy. Int. Abstr. Surg., 97:1, 1953.
9. Nelson, W. W., and Greene, R. R.: Histology of the human ovary during pregnancy. Amer. J. Obstet. Gynec., 76:66, 1958.
10. Richardson, G. S.: Ovarian physiology. New England Journal of Medicine Medical Progress Series, Little, Brown and Co., Boston, 1967.
11. Ryan, K. J.: Steroid metabolism in the human ovary. In Marcus, C. C., and Marcus, S. L., eds.: Advances in Obstetrics and Gynecology. Williams and Wilkins, Baltimore, 1966, p. 340.
12. Ryan, K. J.: Biosynthesis and metabolism of ovarian steroids. In Behrman, S. J., and Kistner, R. W., eds.: Progress in Infertility. Little, Brown and Co., Boston, 1968, p. 275.
13. Ryan, K. J.: Ovarian function and gynecologic endocrinopathies. Int. J. Gynec. Obstet., 8:608, 1970.
14. White, R. F., Hertig, A. T., Rock, J., and Adams, E.: Histological and histochemical observations on corpus luteum of human pregnancy with specific reference to corpora lutea associated with early normal and abnormal ova. Contrib. Embryol., 34:55, 1951.
15. Zuckerman, S., ed.: The Ovary, Vols. 1, 2. Academic Press, New York, 1962.

TESTIS

The testes are ovoid organs occupying a scrotal sac in most mammals. They share with the ovaries a dual function of endocrine and gametogenic activity.[1] Up to five weeks of fetal development the gonads of both sexes are morphologically indistinguishable, consisting of an outer cortex and inner medulla, which give rise in large part to the ovary and testis, respectively. The primitive germ cells migrate from the yolk sac to the gonadal ridge in a like manner for both sexes, and it is the chromosomal make-up of these cells that determines the specific gonadal development. In the testes, the sex cords condense to form seminiferous tubules and a tunica albuginea forms a fibrous layer separating the cords and the developing testes from the overlying epithelium. The mesenchyma separates the tubules and gives rise to the interstitial cells. This development differs from that in the ovary, in which a tunica does not form and the coelonic epithelium is not separated from the gonad at an early stage. The testes differ from the ovaries also in their movement from the abdominal cavity through the inguinal canal to the scrotum by the eighth month of gestation. The testes contribute testosterone or other androgens during development[2, 3] which influence the maintenance and formation of the wolffian system from the mesonephric ducts while also causing regression of the female müllerian system. In the normal course of events, the müllerian system forms in the absence of the gonad or in the presence of the ovary, so that the formation of the female reproductive tract is considered not to be dependent on hormones, at least not on those from the developing gonads. The role of maternal estrogen is, of course, unknown.

The wolffian system gives rise to the epididymal duct, vas deferens, seminal vesicles, and bladder tissue, while the müllerian system develops into the tubes and uterus. In the female, remnants of the wolffian system may persist and give rise to Gartner duct tumors in later life. The potential capacity of the testes to secrete hormones which might influence ductal development has been established. The interstitial cells are hypertrophied during fetal life and contain enzymes capable of forming testosterone.[2, 3]

In animal studies, removal of the testes can result in feminization of the duct system and external female genitalia. Masculinization of the female can be achieved even in the presence of the ovary by the administration of androgens. Sex reversal of the gonad itself is possible in amphibians and birds with steroid hormones but has not been achieved in mammals by this means. In a natural example of sex reversal, in cows the female of a pair of male-female twins has ovaries that have been transformed into immature testes, presumably by transfer of cells or possibly hormones from the male partner. Cross-placental circulation and passage of cells between the twins have been described. The female in such an instance is called a freemartin.

TESTICULAR HORMONES AND FUNCTION

The testes in adult life secrete predominantly testosterone, but other steroids can also be produced and released into the blood stream. These other hormones include estrogens, dehydroepiandrosterone, androstenedione, and occasionally C-21 steroids such as pregnenolone or progesterone. The possible role of testicular hormones other than testosterone is unknown. The potential for secretion of these other steroids becomes manifest in certain disease states, such as testicular feminization, or in testicular tumors.

Major hormone production of the testes is via the interstitial cells, the counterpart of the ovarian theca and stroma. It has been postulated that the Sertoli cells are analogous to the ovarian granulosa cells and produce testicular estrogens but this has not yet been established. The capacity of the testes to produce estrogens is prodigious in some species such as the horse, where the stallion testis represents the richest tissue source, male or female, of the hormone.

The role of the testis in reproduction is obviously two-fold; it acts as a source for the sperm, continually replenished by spermatogenesis, and also provides the male hormone necessary for maintenance of the reproductive tract and of interest in and capacity to reproduce.

CONTROL OF FUNCTION

The interstitial cells of the testis are active morphologically and functionally in intrauterine life and in the neonatal period, presumably as a result of gonadotropin stimulation from chorionic gonadotropin. After the newborn period, the interstitial cells regress and hormonal production is held in abeyance until puberty when it resumes. The triggering mechanism for male puberty is as much a mystery as that for the female but is believed to be associated with "maturation" of the central nervous system and hypothalamic centers that control gonadotropin release.

Follicle-stimulating hormone in the presence of adequate testosterone stimulates spermatogenesis, as shown by studies in hypophysectomized animals and men. Luteinizing hormone, or interstitial cell-stimulating hormone as it is also called, is tropic for interstitial or Leydig cell structure and testosterone secretion. Androgens can feed back to modulate gonadotropin release, and gonadotropin levels rise after castration, as in the female. Whether the estrogen produced by the testis also serves a physiologic function by influencing hypothalamic releasing factors is unknown.

BIBLIOGRAPHY

1. Albert, A.: The mammalian testis. In Young, W. C., ed.: Sex and Internal Secretion, ed. 3. Williams and Wilkins, Baltimore, 1961.
2. Huhtaniemi, I., Ikonen, M., and Vihko, R.: Presence of testosterone and other neutral steroids in human fetal testes. Biochem. Biophys. Res. Commun., 38:715, 1970.
3. Serra, G. B., Perez-Palacios, G., and Jaffe, R. B.: De novo testosterone biosynthesis in the human fetal testis. J. Clin. Endocr., 30:128, 1970.

ADRENAL

The adrenal cortical glands are paired organs formed in embryonic life from the same mesonephric ridge as the gonads, and they share with the gonads a common derivation from mesenchymal tissue for their steroid hormone-secreting cells. Chromaffin cells from the neural crest grow into the cortical tissue in early development and give rise to the medulla, which comes to lie in the center of the adrenal glands and produces predominantly catecholamines rather than the adrenal steroids of the cortex. One striking aspect of adrenal cortical physiology is its role during intrauterine life in providing hormonal precursors which when metabolized by the placenta result in the markedly elevated estrogen levels of human pregnancy.[5] Like the testis with its action in embryonic male duct formation, the adrenal apparently also has a functional role to play during intrauterine life, but in both sexes (see Feto-Placental Unit, p. 117).

ADRENAL HORMONES AND FUNCTION

In the adult, the adrenal cortex and medulla provide hormones which are involved in the control of fundamental metabolic processes, but it is the cortical hormones that are indispensable to life[2, 3] The adrenal cortex can produce more than 30 different steroids but the major hormones include cortisol and corticosterone as glucocorticoids, aldosterone as a mineralocorticoid, and dehydroepiandrosterone sulfate and androstenedione as adrenal androgens (Fig. 15). As with the testes and ovary, the capacity of the adrenals to produce other steroids becomes manifest in disease processes, including hyperplasia and tumors. The hormones produced by the adrenal cortex vary according to the age and functional state of the individual. In fetal life, the major hormone is dehydroepiandrosterone sulfate, and corticoid and aldosterone production is limited until the newborn period.[1, 5] During infancy and childhood, corticoids are produced in amounts proportional to body surface but significant amounts of adrenal androgens are not formed again until puberty or the

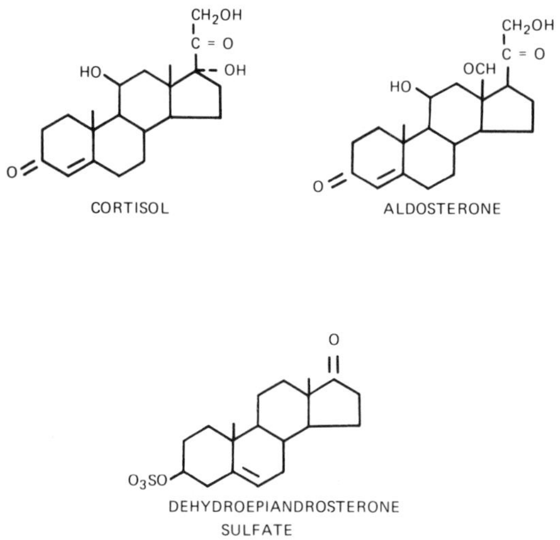

time of adrenarche, when dehydroepiandrosterone sulfate production again becomes a major factor. Whether this is the cause or the result of puberty is at present unknown. In older age, corticoid production continues but that of adrenal androgens may decline, providing an imbalance of catabolic versus anabolic hormones. Some believe that the osteoporosis or bone changes seen in old age may be due to this alteration in adrenal hormone secretion.

Adrenal Zonation and Cell Types Associated with Specific Steroid Production

During fetal life, the definitive cortex occupies a peripheral location surrounding a much larger mass of vacuolated cells arranged in cords that represent the fetal or provisional cortex (Figs. 16 and 17).[4] These cells are presumably the source of major adrenal hormone production in fetal life, producing largely dehydroepiandrosterone sulfate. The fetal cortex regresses toward the end of gestation and during the newborn period, with the resultant decrease in adrenal weight and change in function. As the fetal zone degenerates, the adult outer cortex begins to differentiate into three layers, a process that takes up to several years. Accompanying the structural change is the shift from dehydroepiandrosterone production to that of cortisol. In later childhood and adult life, the cortex has three zones of cortical cells; from the surface inward these are an outer zona glomerulosa, which produces aldosterone and to a lesser extent the glucocorticoids, a larger zona fasciculata consisting of cell columns, and a zona reticularis with a loose network of cells. The reticularis is in apposition to the medulla in a rather irregular fashion with columns of cortical cells protruding into the chromaffin tissue.[3] The fasciculata supposedly contributes to cortisol production, and it has been suggested that adrenal androgens may be produced in the reticularis, although the evidence is incomplete. The isolated adrenal medulla may also produce adrenal corticoids when tested in vitro but the complete exclusion of cortical cells would be difficult in such a study.

Although the provisional or fetal adrenal cortex is considered unique to the human, the fetal adrenals of many animal species

Figure 15.   Structural formulas of the major adrenal secretory products.

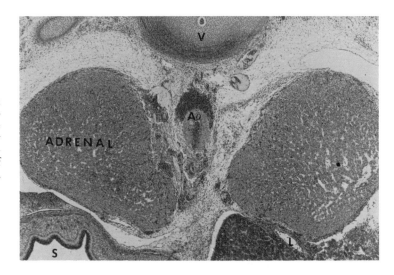

Figure 16. Cross-section through a 2 cm. human embryo (eight weeks) demonstrating large adrenal glands, almost entirely fetal zones with a small rim of cortex. Medulla growing into left of aorta (*A.*). *V*, Vertebral body; *L*, liver; *S*, stomach. H. & E. × 30.

are quite large during intrauterine life and may serve a similar function.

CONTROL OF FUNCTION

Pituitary release of corticotropin is critical for adrenal development since the adrenals will not form and function normally if the fetus has been hypophysectomized (as tested in animals) or is born without a pituitary (as in anencephaly in man) (Fig. 18). Whether there is another tropic hormone to control the production of the dehydroepiandrosterone sulfate so typical of fetal function is unknown but chorionic gonadotropin has been suggested as a possibility. When given to the newborn, chorionic gondotropin can stimulate increased dehydroepiandrosterone production. All through life the adrenal cortex is dependent upon ACTH, and in its absence the glands atrophy and lose their secretory function. The exception to this complete control of steroid secretion by ACTH is the production of aldosterone, which occurs largely, if

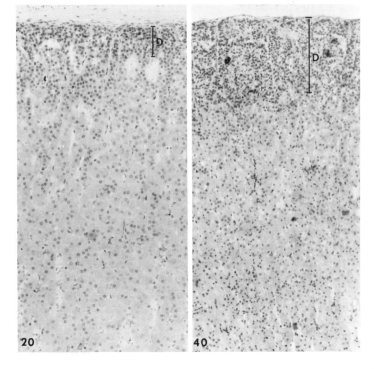

Figure 17. Fetal adrenal at 20 (left) and 40 (right) weeks at same magnification showing increase in definitive cortex (*D*) with increasing age. H. & E. × 25.

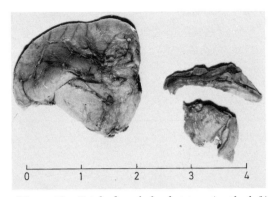

Figure 18. Fetal adrenal gland at term (on the left) compared with both organs removed from an anencephalic newborn (right); top right is a cross-section to show absence of fetal zone. (From Benirschke, K.: Verzleichende Endokrinologie der Fotalzeit. In Sympos. Deutsch. Ges. Endokr., Vol. 16, Springer-Verlag, Berlin, 1970.)

not exclusively, in the glomerulosa zone of the cortex, and is uniquely stimulated by angiotensin in response to electrolyte shifts and blood volume changes rather than by ACTH (see Renin-Angiotensin System, p. 126). The initial concept of adrenal cortical control was a simple negative feedback, with blood levels of cortisol influencing the hypothalamus and pituitary in a reciprocal fashion, causing production of more ACTH with low levels of cortisol and less ACTH with elevated levels. If corticoids are administered exogenously, ACTH release is depressed and the adrenals may atrophy and become less functional. There are certain disease states in which cortisol production is low because of adrenal enzyme defects and ACTH is released in greater amounts, as in the adrenogenital syndrome. The increased ACTH aggravates the condition by causing adrenal hyperplasia and release of the "wrong" steroids, such as adrenal androgens, in great excess. Exogenous administration of cortisol to control ACTH release can restore balance for the patient.

ACTH release is governed by a hypothalamic corticotropin-releasing factor and many of the stimuli that regulate adrenal function via ACTH release do so by effects upon the central nervous system. These stimuli may be nonspecific and include such stressful situations as extreme exercise, burns, surgery, hemorrhage, and psychic trauma. The stress probably evokes ACTH release in these instances by way of nervous pathways to the hypothalamus. There is a diurnal variation of adrenal secretion such that blood cortisol levels are elevated in the morning and reduced in the evening. In Cushing's disease, the diurnal variation is obliterated, and there is a tendency toward this in pregnancy and in states of adrenal hyperactivity. The morning elevation of adrenal secretion is anticipated by a rise in ACTH release in the morning. Shift in the day-night work cycle does not rapidly alter the diurnal variation but changes in latitude do seem to affect the pattern.

ADRENOCORTICAL FUNCTION IN PREGNANCY

Measurement of the secretion products of the maternal adrenal in blood and urine indicates increased function during pregnancy. Free and bound cortisol are both increased during pregnancy, even in evening samples, with a blunting of the diurnal changes. Estrogens can cause elevation in the blood levels of a cortisol-binding globulin called transcortin. This increase of transcortin occurs in pregnancy also, and the increase in blood cortisol of the pregnant state is undoubtedly due in large part to binding by transcortin, with presumably slower metabolism and release of the hormone. The elevation of levels of free cortisol in pregnancy is considered a reflection of increased adrenal activity although such a rise could be due to diminished excretion or catabolism as well. The half-life of cortisol and its metabolites in blood is extended during pregnancy, indicating some change in disposition of the hormone. Reflecting the blood changes, urinary metabolites of adrenal steroids also increase to values about twice the nonpregnancy levels. The adrenal response of corticoid excretion to ACTH is diminished, however, in the third trimester of pregnancy. The urinary 17-ketosteroids, as a measure of adrenal androgen production, are increased during pregnancy although blood levels of dehydroepiandrosterone sulfate are not uniformly different than in the nonpregnant state. This rise of urinary metabolites is, however, used as another basis for assuming increased adrenal function.

Aldosterone is increased in the pregnant state even in the face of an expanding sodium load. Two factors may be related to this increased secretion. Progesterone can antagonize aldosterone effects on the renal tubule and may cause a compensatory rise in aldosterone release. In addition, the renin-angiotensin system, which affects aldosterone production, is also more active during pregnancy. The net result is a doubling of urinary aldosterone conjugates by the end of gestation (see p. 126). Corticoids readily pass to the fetus from the mother and the relative lack of adrenal glucocorticoid production by the fetal adrenal noted earlier is not of physiologic significance until birth, when a transient low level of production by the newborn can be documented.

In spite of the functional changes in hormone secretion, the maternal adrenal does not appear to undergo the morphologic changes of hypertrophy noted in other animal species during pregnancy. Autopsy material taken from pregnant human subjects revealed no consistent histologic alterations.

For many years, it was assumed that the placenta had the potential to secrete adrenal hormones since there was evidence that some pregnant patients with Addison's disease required less replacement therapy. Actual study of placental tissue reveals little, if any, capacity to synthesize adrenal steroids. Patients with prior surgical adrenalectomy require full adrenocortical replacement when pregnant and thus any significant role for the placenta in adrenal steroid formation cannot be substantiated.

In view of the hyperfunctional state of the adrenal during pregnancy, measured in terms of aldosterone, cortisol, and androgens, many questions have been raised regarding possible adverse metabolic effects. In fact, few adverse effects are observed, but the tendency toward toxemia and the diabetogenic effects of pregnancy have been related to increased adrenal function without, as yet, adequate justification.

Of historical interest and practical significance is the fact that in devising the clinical use of corticoids in the treatment of rheumatoid arthritis, Hench used as a clue the improvement or regression of this disease during pregnancy. This was assumed to be due to the elevated levels of corticoids present during gestation. The levels of corticoids present in pregnancy are actually seldom high enough to be relied on for clinical efficacy in states in which cortisol administration is indicated. For treatment of hemolytic anemia and thrombocytopenia, for instance, the usual nonpregnancy dosage of adrenal hormones is necessary even in the pregnant woman.

BIBLIOGRAPHY

1. Dufau, M. L., and Villee, D. B.: Aldosterone biosynthesis by human fetal adrenal *in vitro*. Biochim. Biophys. Acta, 176:637, 1969.
2. Eisenstein, A. B., ed.: The Adrenal Cortex. Little, Brown and Co., Boston, 1967.
3. Forsham, P. H., and Melmon, K.: The adrenal cortex. In Williams, R. H., ed.: Textbook of Endocrinology. W. B. Saunders Co., Philadelphia, 1968, p. 287.
4. Johannisson, E.: The foetal adrenal cortex in the human. Acta Endocr., 58(Suppl. 130):1, 1968.
5. Villee, D. B.: Development of endocrine function in the human placenta and fetus. New Eng. J. Med. 281:473, 533, 1968.

THE PLACENTA

The placenta is a multi-functional organ that assumes the characteristics of: (1) *the liver*, with glycogen synthesis and energy production; (2) *the lung*, with oxygen-carbon dioxide exchange; (3) *the kidney*, with fluid and electrolyte clearance; (4) *the gastrointestinal tract*, with nutrient and waste product transfer; (5) *the pituitary*, in protein tropic and somato-mammotropin secretion; (6) *the ovary*, in estrogen and progesterone secretion; and probably many other as yet unknown functions. Fundamentally all of these activities can be classified into three broad groups that permitted viviparity to evolve: metabolism, transfer, and endocrine secretion.

PLACENTAL METABOLISM

The placenta has diverse metabolic properties that not only allow active transport and steroid and protein biosynthesis to occur, but in addition may serve as an early source of nutrients and energy for the developing embryo and fetus. In early pregnancy the placenta synthesizes glycogen and consumes oxygen at a higher rate than later in the gestational period. The declining capacity to synthesize glycogen in later pregnancy has been correlated temporally with the development by the fetal liver of this function. The placenta also synthesizes cholesterol from acetate, has an active glycolytic cycle, synthesizes fatty acids, has a pentose phosphate pathway and a tricarboxylic acid cycle, and develops energy via oxidative phosphorylation and electron transfer. Many of these functions are undoubtedly critical for the major placental roles of exchange and hormone production.

PLACENTAL TRANSFER

Transfer has many determinants, of which three may be singled out to help define the character of the process: (1) transfer mechanisms; (2) anatomic relationships of the tissues across which transfer occurs; and (3) the nature of the substances transported. Each is considered in turn.

TRANSFER MECHANISMS

Simple diffusion is a process of movement of substances across a membrane from an area of high concentration to one of lower concentration; it ceases when equilibrium is reached. This can be expressed quantitatively with Fick's law, in which the rate of diffusion is directly proportional to the concentration difference on the two sides of the membrane, directly proportional to the surface area of the membrane, and inversely proportional to the thickness of the membrane. A diffusion constant factor would include: molecular weight and shape, ionization, and solubility of the substance transferred. (See formula below.)

Many small-molecular-weight substances including electrolytes and drugs seem to pass across the placenta by simple diffusion.

Facilitated diffusion, like simple diffusion, is a process that is dependent upon a concentration gradient but, in addition, involves a carrier or selective sieve mechanism that permits more rapid and specific transfer. Transport of glucose and other substances may be by this mechanism. It has been theorized that appropriate fit of the shape of the molecule to the membrane "pore" may explain why one stereoisomer of a given compound passes more readily than another.

Active transport involves transfer against a gradient; it has a transport mechanism that can be saturated, that has specificity that can be inhibited by competition of another substance transported by the same mechanism, and that is noncompetitively inhibited by interference with metabolism of the cell. It has not yet been possible to verify which substances are transported across the human placenta by active transport since many of the criteria cannot be assayed by the methods available. The substances that are concentrated in the fetal blood against a lower maternal concentration may be transported actively from mother to fetus.

Pinocytosis involves active engulfment of droplets and particles by invaginations of the placental villi and movement of the particle across the cell to the the fetal blood stream. This may be important with large molecules such as proteins involved in the immune mechanism.

Breaks between cells in the villus may occasionally allow whole cells such as red blood cells to move from child to mother. Such breaks account for the occasions when fetal hemoglobin can be measured in the mother's blood as well as provide the genesis of Rh isoimmunization.

The transport mechanisms can be summarized as: simple diffusion based upon Fick's law, facilitated diffusion, which is faster than predictions based on concentration gradient; and active transport, which is an energy-requiring metabolic process.[9]

PLACENTAL STRUCTURE IN RELATION TO TRANSPORT

The extraembryonic membranes include the yolk sac, amnion, chorion, and allantois. The yolk sac is the most primitive form of transfer membrane and is utilized in lower animals to transport yolk material to the embryo. While the yolk sac is vestigial in man, it is still present and has been suggested as a possible route for transfer of proteins although its role is still controversial. The allantois usually merges with the chorion in forming the definitive pla-

Rate of diffusion =

$$\frac{\text{Diffusion constant} \times \text{Membrane area (Concentration of substance in mother} - \text{Concentration of substance in fetus}}{\text{Membrane thickness}}$$

centa, which, depending on its thickness, becomes the villous or labyrinthine structure through which most transfer occurs. The amnion surrounds the fluid-filled cavity enclosing the embryo and may itself provide passage of water and electrolytes without involving the placenta. The definitive placenta varies among animals in terms of its shape, the area in apposition to the maternal uterine wall, and the number of cell layers interspersed between the maternal and fetal blood streams. Grosser has classified placentas as *epitheliochorial* when between the maternal blood and the fetal chorion there are three layers — maternal blood vessel (endothelium), connective tissue, and uterine epithelium; as *syndesmochorial* when the uterine epithelium is lost; as *endotheliochorial* when the maternal blood vessel is in apposition to the chorion; and as *hemochorial* when the chorion is bathed in maternal blood, as in man (Table 10).

Perhaps to make up for differences in the number of layers between the chorion and maternal blood stream, the shape and area of placentas vary. The epitheliochorial placentas are usually membranous in type, lying in apposition to essentially the whole surface of the uterine lining. The syndesmochorial placentas are often small and disc-shaped (cotyledonary), whereas endotheliochorial placentas are zonary, having a bandlike shape. The hemochorial placenta of man is disc-shaped and fairly large, occupying a goodly portion of the uterine wall.

Since in the Fick law for diffusion the area and thickness of the membrane are critical factors for rate of transfer, consideration of placental structure is essential to an understanding of the dynamics of the process (Fig. 19).

Correlations have been made between the transfer rate of sodium per unit weight of placenta and the type of placentation; the epitheliochorial has the lowest rate and the hemochorial the highest (Fig. 19). Perhaps more important than the number of layers involved are the physical and chemical properties of the membranes and the surface area for exhange. As pregnancy progresses in the human, the placental villi become less cellular and thinner, vascularity increases, and the surface area of the whole placenta is greater. Accompanying this is a many-fold rise in the rate of sodium transfer with gestational age.

TRANSFER OF SPECIFIC SUBSTANCES

Gas Exchange

Oxygen is delivered to the fetus from the mother and carbon dioxide is exchanged by a simple diffusion mechanism influenced by the concentration gradients, thickness of the placenta, and placental area.[1] In addition, factors such as gas-carrying capacity of the maternal and fetal blood and the type of blood flow may be important. Partial pressure of the gas is proportional to concentration and is therefore used in studies instead of concentration since pressure is the driving force for gas diffusion.

The partial pressures of oxygen in fetal umbilical blood vessels are 15 mm. Hg O_2 and 28 mm. Hg O_2 in the artery and vein, respectively. The pCO_2 levels in umbilical blood are 55 mm. Hg and 40 mm. Hg in artery and vein. On the maternal side, the

TABLE 10. TISSUES SEPARATING THE MATERNAL AND FETAL BLOOD[*]

Morphological Type	Maternal Tissue			Fetal Tissue			Typical Examples
	Endothelium	Connective Tissue	Epithelium	Chorion	Connective Tissue	Endothelium	
Epitheliochorial	+	+	+	+	+	+	Pig, horse
Syndesmochorial	+	+	−	+	+	+	Sheep, cow
Endotheliochorial	+	−	−	+	+	+	Dog, cat
Hemochorial				+	+	+	Primates, bats, lower rodents, man, monkey
Hemoendothelial						+	Higher rodents

[*]From Barcroft, J.: Researches on Prenatal Life. Charles C Thomas, Springfield, Ill., 1948.

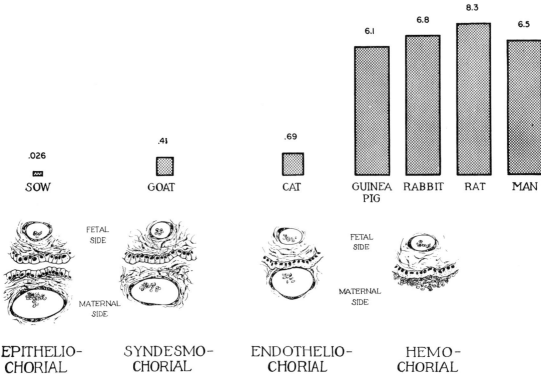

Figure 19. Variations observed in different types of placentas in the transfer rate of sodium per unit weight of placenta at the nine-tenths gestational age of the pregnancy, in accordance with Grosser's classification. The values for sodium are given in milligrams, while the relative magnitudes of transfer are denoted by the shaded rectangles. (From Flexner, L. B., et al.: Amer. J. Obstet. Gynec., 55:469, 1948.)

uterine artery partial pressures are 95 mm. Hg O_2 and 33 mm. Hg CO_2. The partial pressures in maternal uterine vein are 33 mm. Hg O_2 and 46 mm. HgCO_2. The values do not take into account shunts and other factors which would obscure true exchange values in the placenta (Table 11). These gradients do, however, reflect oxygen transfer to the fetus and carbon dioxide transfer to the mother.[1]

Factors related to oxygen- and carbon dioxide-carrying capacity of blood include blood pH, hemoglobin concentration, and hemoglobin affinity for oxygen. These factors tend to influence the rate and extent of gas exchange in addition to the actual process of membrane transfer, but their relative contributions are still controversial.

The fetal hemoglobin concentration is higher than that of the adult, and fetal red cells have a higher affinity for oxygen than adult red cells. A lower pH tends to cause oxygen release from hemoglobin and facilitates oxygen transfer to cells (Bohr effect). In operation, it is believed that the carbon dioxide and fixed acids reaching the maternal blood from the fetus increase oxygen release from the mother's blood. The release of oxygen favors a greater capacity of the blood for carbon dioxide (Haldane effect) and would allow the mother to take up more carbon dioxide. The loss of acid from the fetal side increases the fetal hemoglobin capacity for oxygen, in addition to the greater inherent affinity of fetal hemoglobin for this gas at a given pH. All of these factors would tend to favor proper gas exchange.

The dynamics of blood flow also influence gas exchange but are critical only when

TABLE 11. PARTIAL PRESSURES (MM. HG) OF O_2 AND CO_2 IN MOTHER AND FETUS

	Maternal Artery	Umbilical Vein	Umbilical Artery	Maternal Vein
pO_2	95	28	15	33
pCO_2	33	40	55	46

diffusion capacity is high. The flow of the maternal blood is at cross-current to villous capillary flow, and efficiency in gas exchange is intermediate between counter-current flow systems and concurrent flow systems, which favor equilibrium with maternal arterial gas tension and maternal venous gas tension, respectively. The diffusing capacity of the placenta can be increased by opening of more villous capillaries, a mechanism believed operative in adjustments to maternal blood with reduced amounts of oxygen at high altitudes. Changes in the rate of blood flow can also increase oxygen exchange.

Transfer of Nutrients and Waste Products

During very early development, the fetal cell mass presumably exchanges materials in the same way as any other cell of the maternal organism. However, as the embryo's growth separates it from direct access to exchange, the development of a fetal circulation to the placenta, which is bathed in maternal blood, provides the route for nutrient and waste product transfer.[2] Placental transfer has been studied in many animal species, but to a much lesser extent in the human. It is moreover not possible to predict except in the grossest manner whether our knowledge derived from animal studies is applicable to man. Other problems in understanding transfer are due to the limitation of the methods available for study. The techniques employed include following the movement of radioactive tracers from mother to fetus or fetus to mother and measurement of the concentration of substances in fetal and maternal blood. Such factors as binding of substances and metabolism in the fetus or placenta make careful evaluation of the data obtained necessary.

As the embryo and fetus grow, body size and composition change, and there are as yet no accurate methods for establishing minimal requirements for nutrients. It is assumed that there is, however, a safety factor such that excesses are usually present. The genesis of fetal malnutrition is understood only in the grossest terms of poor uterine blood perfusion and placental fibrosis or infarction.

Proteins are synthesized in the fetus from amino acids which are concentrated in the fetal blood stream against a gradient (Table

TABLE 12. TOTAL α-AMINO NITROGEN (NH_2-N) OF HUMAN MATERNAL AND FETAL PLASMA[*]

Fetal NH_2-N (mg./100 ml.)	Maternal NH_2-N (mg./100 ml.)	Ratio: $\dfrac{Fetal\ NH_2\text{-}N}{Maternal\ NH_2\text{-}N}$
6.70	2.23	3.00
5.19	3.16	1.64
3.94	2.40	1.63
5.03	3.10	1.62
4.32	2.78	1.55
4.69	3.37	1.39
4.30	3.31	1.30
4.42	3.70	1.23
4.62		
2.94	2.85	1.03

[*]From Crumpler, H. R., Dent, C. E., and Lindan, O.: Biochem. J., 47:223, 1950.

12). The natural amino acids are selectively transferred faster than the unnatural stereo-isomers and the mechanism can be saturated. Whole proteins such as globulins and even albumin may be transferred but usually in small amounts.

Carbohydrates are provided for the fetus in the form of glucose, which is derived both from the maternal blood stream and from breakdown of placental glycogen early in pregnancy, but only from maternal blood glucose later in pregnancy. The chief energy source for fetal metabolism is from glucose, which is transferred selectively at a rate different from fructose. The placenta can also convert glucose to fructose but the extent varies among animal species. The glucose level in the fetus ranges from 40 to 120 mg./100 ml. but is always lower than the maternal concentration. Administration of intravenous glucose to the mother results in its transfer to the fetus with increase to levels less than maternal values.

Lipids are transferred to the fetus poorly and by and large are catabolized by the placenta for resynthesis in fetal tissues (Table 13). Acetate crosses the placenta readily but cholesterol, fatty acids, and phospholipids are transferred slowly. Lipids are not extensively catabolized by the fetus.

Water is transferred readily to the developing fetus in increasing amounts as pregnancy progresses and, although there is exchange with the amniotic fluid, the bulk transport is across the placenta. In normal pregnancy the amniotic fluid is replaced at a half-time of 95 minutes. This time is longer in polyhydramnios and shorter in oligohydramnios. The rate of water ex-

TABLE 13. PLASMA LIPIDS AT BIRTH, COMPARED WITH THOSE OF ADULTS DETERMINED BY THE SAME METHOD[*]

	Cord Blood at Term (mg./100 ml. Oxalated Plasma)	Adult (mg./100 ml. Oxalated Plasma)[†]
Total lipids	198 ± 80	589 ± 87
Total fatty acids	140 ± 57	353 ± 56
Neutral fat	90 ± 50	154 ± 42
Phospholipid	61 ± 32	196 ± 23
Cholesterol – total	34 ± 15	162 ± 32
Cholesterol – combined (or ester)	20 ± 12	115 ± 27
Cholesterol – free	14 ± 7	47 ± 7
Cholesterol – % combined	59%	71%

[*]From Boyd, E. M.: Amer. J. Dis. Child., 52:1319, 1936.

[†]Concentrations somewhat lower than those of maternal plasma at term.

change is equivalent both to and from the infant.

Electrolytes are exchanged at a rate independent of water movement. Sodium transfer increases as pregnancy progresses, presumably because of thinning and increased vascularity of the placenta. The blood levels are equivalent in mother and fetus.

Minerals such as calcium, inorganic phosphorus, and iron are concentrated in the fetus against a gradient and move unidirectionally from the maternal side. Fortunately, radioactive metabolites such as plutonium-239, radium-226, and strontium-90 pass the placenta with difficulty. Iodides, however, pass the placenta and radioisotopes can be concentrated in the fetal thyroid.

Vitamins pass the placenta well and are present in higher concentration in the fetus if they are water-soluble (riboflavin, thiamine, vitamin B_{12}, and vitamin C). Fat-soluble vitamins (A and E) pass less readily and their levels are lower in fetal than maternal blood. Apparently, vitamin A is transferred as carotene and transformed into vitamin A by the fetus.

Waste products such as urea and uric acid are equivalent in maternal and fetal blood, passing the placenta by simple diffusion. Bilirubin is cleared by the placenta, and in spite of the inability of the fetus to conjugate this substance, high

levels, if they do occur in the fetus, make their appearance only after birth.

Transfer of Hormones

Steroid hormones pass through the placenta in both directions and free compounds rather than conjugates are preferentially exchanged. Most steroids are conjugated as sulfates in higher concentration in fetal than maternal blood and the placenta cleaves these conjugates during passage to the mother. Adrenal hormones, progestins, androgens, and estrogens are all exchanged in this manner.

Thyroid hormone as thyroxin is slowly transferred from mother to infant and high dosages must be administered to the mother to achieve significant transport. Tri-iodothyronine is more readily transferred.

Protein hormones such as gonadotropin, growth hormone, and insulin are poorly transferred. An anencephalic infant has low blood growth hormone levels, whereas normal infants have levels higher than the mother. Chorionic gonadotropin and placental lactogen are present at much lower levels in the fetus compared to the mother.

Transfer of Antibodies and Infectious Agents[4]

Some passive immunity is conferred upon the fetus by transplacental transfer of antibodies from the mother. Maternal immunity to measles, hepatitis, poliomyelitis, herpes, and diphtheria is positively related to the prevention or modification of illness in her newborn because of passive transfer of antibodies. The type of antibody transferred is selective, and only smaller protein molecules of the $gamma_2$-globulin size with a sedimentation pattern of 7S (Svedberg units) are passed to any extent.

There are natural experiments demonstrating that mothers that have no gamma globulins (agammaglobulinemia) give birth to infants who lack these proteins but develop them one to two months after delivery.

On the other hand, if the mother is normal but the infant has agammaglobulinemia, the child is born with gamma globulin transferred from the mother but these levels decline after delivery since the child cannot produce the proteins by itself.

The site of transfer of these proteins is the placenta in the human and many animals, but in the rabbit transfer through the yolk sac has been demonstrated. In some species, such as the pig, antibodies are not transferred at all.

The antibodies evoked by a given antigen have been shown to be heterogeneous in size and shape, ranging from 7S to 19S in sedimentation constants and varying in molecular weight. Isoantibodies that develop in the mother as anti-A, anti-B, or anti-Rh against the fetal blood group substances are examples of this heterogeneity. Only the smaller molecules are transferred; this explains why anti-Rh factors demonstrable in saline (19S) are not transferred to the fetus, whereas anti-Rh factors demonstrable in albumin (7S) are found in the offspring. This also explains why mothers of blood group O pass more antibodies to the fetus than mothers of blood group A or B.

Certain autoantibodies developing in the mother are also transferred to the fetus, including platelet antibodies in thrombocytopenic purpura, lupus factor, and antithyroid antibodies. These are usually rapidly cleared by the newborn but transient toxic signs may be present and occasionally the birth of a cretin has resulted.

Viruses associated with variola, varicella, measles, encephalitis, poliomyelitis, and rubella and coxsackie virus may pass through the placenta and cause prenatal infection, and, as in the case of rubella, congenital anomalies can result. Bacteria and protozoa such as Toxoplasma and the tubercle bacillus infect the placenta by creating lesions and then gain access to the fetal blood stream. Malaria and syphilis are transmitted in utero by this mechanism.

Transfer of Drugs

The passage of drugs from the maternal to the fetal blood is of practical clinical significance since such agents could have a bearing on the development of congenital malformation in the first trimester, on alterations of metabolism or physiologic status at any time in pregnancy, and on fetal function in the newborn period.[7, 9] While the vast majority of agents taken by pregnant women do not have deleterious effects on the fetus, certain notable exceptions have been demonstrated. Phocomelia from the sedative thalidomide if taken by the mother in the first trimester, fetal goiter from iodides or propylthiouracil, and severe congenital defects from folic acid antagonists all indicate the need for extreme caution in the use and timing of pharmacologic agents given to pregnant women. Caution dictates that drugs not be used unless essential, that they be particularly avoided during embryonic development and organogenesis up to the first 12 weeks of gestation, and that new agents be thoroughly tested before being marketed.

The placenta is considered to offer a cellular membrane for transfer that favors free passage by diffusion of lipoidal, poorly ionized, small-molecular-weight substances. Most pharmacologic agents used in clinical practice will cross the placenta. Tetracyclines used for combating maternal infections may discolor developing teeth and alter fetal long bone growth. The potential for toxicity of streptomycin can be realized in utero. Sulfonamide drugs may pass the placenta and alter bilirubin metabolism such that a risk of kernicterus is increased. Extensive study has been carried out in the transfer to the fetus of analgesics, sedatives, tranquilizers, and anesthetic agents given during labor and delivery. Aside from the muscle relaxants, such as succinylcholine and curare, which are transferred poorly, most of the agents used for conduct of labor will readily cross the placenta. Barbiturates, ether, chloroform, cyclopropane, meperidine, morphine, nitrous oxide, trichloroethylene, belladonna derivatives, and chlorpromazine have all been measured in cord blood at delivery after administration to the mother. Respiratory depression of the newborn may be the consequence depending upon dose and timing in relationship to delivery.

PLACENTAL SYNTHESIS OF HORMONES

The concept of the placenta as an endocrine organ has evolved over the years by the accumulation of clinical and experimental observations derived from many sources.[3] In 1905 Halban suggested a hormonal role for the placenta on the basis of changes in the mother that coincided with the term of pregnancy and did not seem explicable by other maternal or fetal endocrine activity. Extracts of placental tissue could evoke endocrine changes in animals similar to those produced by gonadotropins or estrogenic hormones, and the endocrine changes of pregnancy were observed in pregnant patients after oophorectomy or hypophysectomy, or with absence of the fetus, as in cases of hydatidiform mole. In more recent times, the hormones have been isolated and identified from placental tissue and the enzymatic steps for biosynthesis have been described in isolated systems.[3, 8] In the case of the steroid hormones, the concentration of steroid hormones in the blood leaving the placenta has been shown to be higher than that in the returning blood stream, and with protein hormones, de novo synthesis in tissue culture has been described.

Certain technical problems have always hampered the direct approach to a study of placental endocrine function. The placenta cannot be removed and replaced with an extract as in classic endocrine research since the pregnancy depends upon both transfer and hormonal activities and the two functions cannot be dissociated without destroying the fetus. The large quantity of blood pooled in the placental vessels always required that this be considered in preparing extracts to ensure that the hormone measured was not predominantly in blood rather than tissue. The problem of storage in the tissue rather than synthesis had to be considered as well. It was also learned that the placenta does not synthesize steroid hormones de novo as do other endocrine organs but instead utilizes blood-borne precursors from the mother and fetus. Finally, species variation in the endocrine control of pregnancy was recognized in the differing endocrine capacities of placental tissue from animals other than man, so that care is required in translating the laboratory result to the clinical situation.

Within the limitations imposed by critical review, the major hormones of the human placenta have been identified as: chorionic gonadotropin, chorionic somato-mammotropin (placental lactogen), estrogens (estradiol, estrone, estriol), and progesterone. A chorionic thyrotropin has recently been characterized[6] and relaxin has also been isolated from placental tissue. The evidence for many other hormones attributed to the placenta in the past has not withstood careful scrutiny and further experimental work will be necessary to assign any additional endocrine activity to this tissue.

The individual placental hormones and their relationships to endocrine regulation of pregnancy are covered in Chapters 1, 2, and 4. Selected aspects of placental endocrine function are discussed in the section that follows.

Placental Protein Hormones

Review articles on placental endocrine function as recently as 1961 and 1962 did not include chorionic somato-mammotropin or thyrotropin as definite hormones since evidence for their formation was not then available.[3, 8] In a similar manner, the clinical and circumstantial evidence for placental production of melanocyte-stimulating hormone, corticotropin, oxytocin, vasopressin, relaxin, and other as yet unspecified hormones may ultimately be corroborated with modern analytic techniques. For the present, chorionic gonadotropin, somato-mammotropin, and thyrotropin are the only well documented protein hormone products of the placenta, but one must be aware that the final word on the subject has not yet been written.

Chorionic gonadotropin is a glycoprotein with luteinizing, interstitial cell-stimulating, and luteotropic properties. The hormone has been demonstrated in blood and urine of the pregnant woman as well as in the placenta in high concentration. The most direct evidence for its synthesis by the placenta is based upon production by isolated cells in tissue culture. The hormone is produced in hypophysectomized pregnant women and by trophoblastic tissue in the absence of a fetus. It is believed to be important in the maintenance of the corpus luteum and is, of course, the basis for pregnancy tests (see Human Chorionic Gonadotropin, p. 28).

Chorionic somato-mammotropin is a protein hormone with growth-promoting, lactogenic, and some luteotropic properties. It has also been known as placental lactogen. It was first identified by immunologic techniques and noted to have partial cross-reactivity with pituitary growth hormone. The evidence for placental production has been already cited and significant synthesis of this hormone by the placental enzymes in isolated systems has been accomplished. The many changes in carbohydrate and lipid metabolism that occur in pregnancy have been attributed to this hormone (see Human Placental Lactogen, p. 40).

Chorionic thyrotropin has been identified in placental tissue and interestingly has immunologic cross-reactivity with bovine pituitary thyrotropin. Its function in pregnancy has not yet been determined.[6]

Placental Steroid Hormones

Estradiol, estrone, and estriol have been isolated in higher concentration in uterine vein blood than in uterine artery or peripheral blood, indicating secretion of these three hormones by the placenta. Placental microsomes contain the enzymes for converting blood-borne dehydroepiandrosterone sulfate to free dehydroepiandrosterone and thence to androstenedione. The androstenedione is readily aromatized to estrone by enzymes in the same subcellular compartment.

Similarly, testosterone may be formed and aromatized to estradiol. A comparable series of enzymatic steps converts 16α-hydroxydehydroepiandrosterone sulfate to free 16-hydroxylated androgens which are aromatized to estriol. The important aspects of placental production of estrogens are that the precursors arise from the fetus and its adrenals. In the absence of a conceptus (hydatidiform mole), when the fetus is dead, when the fetus has no adrenal (anencephaly), or when the placenta cannot cleave the sulfate because of an enzyme defect, estrogen production by the placenta and estrogen excretion in maternal urine is low. Since estriol is quantitatively the major metabolite, it is this hormone which is usually measured in urine. Estriol levels may be low if the mother's adrenals are absent but this is less consistent than the association between fetal deficiency and low estriol levels (see p. 118).

The placenta can also metabolize estrogens; various epimeric forms of estriol, α-ketols, and 2- and 6-hydroxylated steroids are the products.

The placenta does not have the enzymes necessary for formation of androgens from other steroids and hence cannot synthesize estrogens without a formed precursor. Nor can the placenta insert the 16-hydroxy group to form estriol directly from estrone or estradiol.

Progesterone has been isolated in higher concentrations in placental effluent blood than in the blood returning to this tissue, indicating active secretion. In contrast to effects on estrogen production, death of the fetus or anencephaly interferes less with progesterone levels. Blood cholesterol has been demonstrated to be a precursor of progesterone, and the enzymes for cholesterol conversion to pregnenolone and pregnenolone to progesterone have been characterized in placental tissues.

The placenta can also metabolize progesterone to 20α-dihydroprogesterone and 6-hydroxyprogesterone but more extensive catabolism occurs in other fetal or maternal tissues (see Fig. 17, p. 119).

There is little convincing evidence that the placenta can form adrenal hormones and for the moment estrogens and progesterone are the only steroids formed in placental tissue, but the placenta has many other enzymatic functions related to its endocrine and transfer activities.[5]

BIBLIOGRAPHY

1. Bartels, H., Moll, W., and Metcalfe, J.: Physiology of gas exchange in the human placenta. Amer. J. Obstet. Gynec., 84:1715, 1962.
2. Dancis, J.: The placenta in fetal nutrition and excretion. Amer. J. Obstet. Gynec., 84:1749, 1962.
3. Diczfalusy, E., and Troen, P.: Endocrine functions of the placenta. Vitamins Hormones, 19:229, 1961.
4. Freda, V. J.: Placental transfer of antibodies in man. Amer. J. Obstet. Gynec., 84:1756, 1962.
5. Hagerman, D.: Enzymology of the placenta. *In* Klopper, A., and Diczfalusy, E., eds.: Foetus and Placenta. Blackwell Scientific Publications, Oxford, 1969, p. 413.
6. Hennen, G., Pierce, J. G., and Freychet, P.: Human chorionic thyrotropin: further characterization and study of its secretion during pregnancy. J. Clin. Endocr., 29:581, 1969.
7. Moya, F., and Thorndike, V.: Passage of drugs across the placenta. Amer. J. Obstet. Gynec., 84:1778, 1962.
8. Ryan, K. J.: Hormones of the placenta. Symposium on the placenta. Amer. J. Obstet. Gynec., 84:1695, 1962.
9. Schanker, L. S.: Passage of drugs across body membranes. Pharmacol. Rev., 14:501, 1962.
10. Schultz, R. L.: Placental transport: A review. Obstet. Gynec. Survey, 25:979, 1970.
11. Sternberg, J.: Placental transfer: Modern methods of study. Amer. J. Obstet. Gynec., 84:1731, 1962.

Chapter 4

Integrative Functions in Reproduction

Reproduction in higher forms of animal life is characterized by integration of neurologic and endocrine activities. Complex and finely regulated systems provide the means for fertilization, gestation, birth, infant nutrition, and ultimately puberty, adult reproductive behavior, and the menopause. These integrated functions include: (1) *reproductive cycles* regulated by the neuroendocrine reflex typified by the human female menstrual cycle; (2) *pregnancy-specific reproductive endocrinology* involving maternal, fetal, and placental hormonal interaction, and the endocrine control of gestation length and labor; and (3) postpartum support of the newborn in the form of *lactation*.

The preceding sections covering the hormones and the glands that produce them provide the background for consideration of what is to follow.

CYCLIC CHANGES IN HORMONAL SECRETION AND REPRODUCTIVE TRACT MORPHOLOGY

The reproductive cycle is an integration of central nervous system–pituitary, ovarian, and reproductive tract rhythms that are constantly interacting.[17] The pattern of gonadotropin release in the normal cycle is not maintained unless ovaries are present that can respond with appropriate hormone secretion and feedback. In lower animals, more than in man, the ovarian cycle, especially the luteal phase, is affected by alterations in the reproductive tract that are produced by the ovarian hormones, and a cervical stimulus, such as coitus, can also affect central nervous system–pituitary function. The cycle, therefore, may be looked upon as a self-sustaining feedback system (Fig. 1). Removal or derangement of any component is apt to disrupt the cycle. The question of what provides order and in a sense starts the cyclic process is more or less at the state of "which came first, the chicken or the egg?" The ovary cannot secrete hormones properly unless it has cyclic gonadotropic stimulation, and gonadotropins are not released in an appropriate pattern unless there is ovarian steroid feedback. An understanding of the process complete enough to answer the questions has not yet been achieved, but the contributions of the individual components are reviewed here.

HYPOTHALAMIC-PITUITARY HORMONE CYCLE

The inherent rhythm of the hypothalamus which is established in fetal or neonatal life has already been described (p. 61). Presumably, there is a rhythmic secretion of releasing factors to the anterior pituitary during the cycle but actual changes in the hypophyseotropic hormones have not yet been measured. The cyclic variations of the pituitary gonadotropins FSH and LH have now been measured in blood during normal menstrual cycles and are typified by a midcycle surge of both FSH and LH one day prior to ovulation (Fig. 2).[2, 9, 10, 13–17, 21, 2] The pattern of gonadotropin release is dependent upon feedback effects of ovarian steroids on the hypothalamus.

OVARIAN HORMONE CYCLE

Estrogens are secreted throughout the cycle from ovarian follicles and from the

96

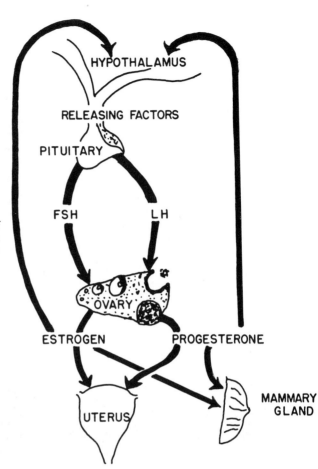

Figure 1. Diagrammatic representation of interplay of sex hormones and gonadotropins in a normally cycling woman. (From Drill, V. A.: Fed. Proc., 29:1209, 1970.)

corpus luteum during the luteal phase. The levels rise from day 1 of the cycle to reach a peak just prior to the gonadotropin surge and estrogens may, in fact, trigger this sudden release of FSH and LH.[1, 3–6, 8, 17] The estrogen levels decline precipitously with or just prior to ovulation and reach another peak in the midluteal phase.

Progesterone is present at low levels in the blood prior to ovulation and is secreted early in the cycle by both the ovary and the adrenal in amounts too small to produce recognizable end-organ effects. Soon after ovulation and corpus luteum formation progesterone levels rise some 10-fold, reach a peak in the midluteal phase, and decline just before menstruation (Fig. 3).

CYCLIC ENDOMETRIAL CHANGE AND MENSTRUATION

The endometrium is the "mucous" membrane lining the body of the uterus and is characterized by its specific growth responsiveness to estrogen and progesterone stimulation. With the variation in the relative and absolute amounts of the two ovarian hormones during the cycle the endometrium develops and wanes in timed sequence, menstruation occurring when hormonal support is withdrawn. The endometrium consists of three layers with differing histologic appearance and function. The basal layer is closest to the endometrium, responds poorly to hormones, is not sloughed at the time of menses, and provides the regeneration potential at the start of the cycle. A bipartite "functional" layer resting on the basalis consists of a midposition "spongiosum" and a superficial "compact" layer, which participate in the growth, differentiation, and regression of the cycle.

The blood supply of the endometrium is derived from two types of arterioles which branch off from the radiate artery of the myometrium. There is a short straight branch that supplies the basal layer of endo-

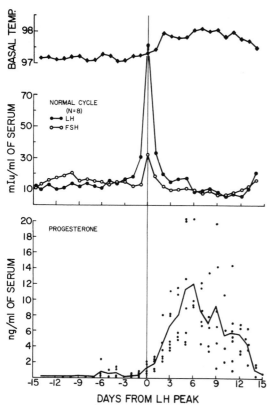

Figure 2. FSH, LH, and progesterone in serum during the menstrual cycle. (From Yen, S. S. C., Rankin, J., and Littell, A. S.: J.A.M.A., 211:1513, 1970.)

phase accompanying corpus luteum function and progesterone and estrogen secretion. Ovulation divides the modal cycle into two equal halves, consisting of the menstrual-proliferative phase and the secretory phase.

Proliferative Phase

The proliferative phase commences approximately five days after the start of menstruation and is under estrogen stimulation. The endometrium is thin, the surface epithelium is cuboidal, glands are straight, and the stroma is compact. Over the next eight or nine days there is an increase in mitotic activity in the glands, the nuclei appear pseudostratified, some loosening of the metrium which undergoes little change during the cycle, and the tortuous spiral arterioles which supply the functional layers and grow and regress with the endometrial changes of the zona spongiosa and compacta. Vasoconstriction and hemorrhage from the spiral arterioles are the prelude and genesis of menstrual bleeding. The spiral arteries are probably under hormonal control and each new cycle requires regrowth of the vessels.

The temporal relationships of gross and histologic endometrial change to ovarian hormone secretion during the cycle have been determined by: direct observation of primate endometrial implants into the anterior chamber of the eye of experimental animals, review of histologic sections of timed endometrial biopsies, and correlation of ovarian and endometrial histology when removed at surgery.[11] The cycle is divided into three phases, the *menstrual phase* during active bleeding, followed by the *proliferative phase* during follicular growth and estrogen secretion, and the *secretory*

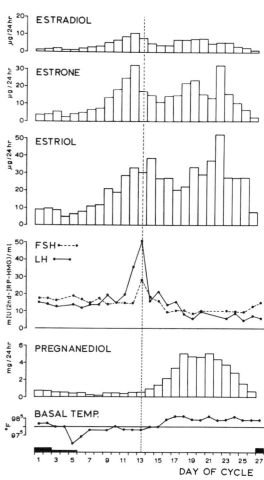

Figure 3. Ovarian hormone cycle. Pattern of daily 24 hour urinary estrogen and pregnanediol excretion and serum LH and FSH concentration in a normally menstruating subject. (From Gobelsmann, U., Midgley, A. R., Jr., and Jaffe, R. B.: J. Clin. Endocr., 29:1222, 1969.)

stroma occurs, stromal cell mitosis appears, and there is a general thickening of the endometrial layers (Fig. 4). Toward the end of the proliferative phase the glands become elongated and start coiling.

Secretory Phase

The secretory phase commences around the time of ovulation. It is due to progesterone secretion and is noted by early basal vacuolization in the glandular cells with displacement of the nuclei toward the gland lumen (Fig. 5). This is followed by secretion of glycogen into the gland lumen with movement of nuclei back to the base of the cell again (Fig. 6). The glands become saw-toothed and serrated in appearance, stromal edema is marked, and the stromal cells hypertrophy with increased cytoplasm typical of a decidual reaction. The spiral arterioles become prominent and at this point the three functional zones are most clearly demarcated into the basalis, spongiosa, and compacta.

Menstrual Phase

The menstrual phase merges into the late secretory phase (Fig. 7), with degeneration of the upper layers of endometrial cells, infiltration of white blood cells, congestion of the blood vessels with small hematomas, and finally desquamation and bleeding. The compacta and spongiosa layers are more or less completely lost and the regeneration starts from the glands that remain.

THE VAGINAL CYCLE

The vagina has a multi-layered epithelial covering consisting of a basal germinal cell row lying upon the basement membrane, with three additional zones of cells from within outward that are desquamated cyclically under hormonal influence (Fig. 8). The innermost layer next to the germinal cells consists of parabasal cells with thick rounded cytoplasm and a centrally placed vesicular nucleus. The next more superficial cell type is the precornified squamous cell, which is thin and platelike and has a rounded vesicular nucleus. The most superficial cells are the cornified squamous cells with the small pyknotic nucleus. The cells that are desquamated into the vaginal fluid

are evaluated by several methods: the karyopyknotic index, which is determined by the percentage of squamous cells with a pyknotic nucleus; the cornification count or index, reflecting cytoplasmic acidophilia of the squamous cells; and the maturation index, which reflects the percentage of parabasal, intermediate (precornified), and superficial (cornified) cells.

Estrogens cause thickening of the vaginal epithelial cell layer and an increase in the cornified cells. This is seen in the proliferative phase of the cycle. Progesterone following estrogen stimulation results in more precornified cells, clumping of the desquamated cells, and a background of leukocytes and cellular debris. This pattern is seen in the secretory phase of the cycle.

THE CERVICAL CYCLE

The endocervix is covered by a mucous gland-laden epithelium that merges into the squamous epithelial layer on the vaginal portion of the cervix externally and meets the endometrium at the inner os (Fig. 9). The endocervical epithelium is responsive to hormonal stimulation but the histologic changes in the cycle are not as dramatic or as well documented as those of the endometrium.[12] The cervical mucus does, however, change dramatically in the course of the cycle. Under estrogen stimulation the flow increases and the mucus becomes clear and less viscous. On a glass slide the mucus dries in a fernlike arborization because of its electrolyte content, which is typical of an estrogen effect. The mucus has a stringy tendency and can be stretched without breaking, a phenomenon known as spinbarkeit. In the secretory phase of the cycle under the influence of progesterone, the electrolyte content and physical-chemical characteristics of the mucus change, and "ferning" and spinbarkeit are no longer observed.

OVIDUCTAL CYCLE

The epithelium of the fallopian tubes varies with the cycle under the influence of hormones.[12] In the menstrual period, the epithelium is low, but under estrogen influence in the proliferative phase, the ciliated and secretory cells are taller. After

(Text continued on page 105.)

A

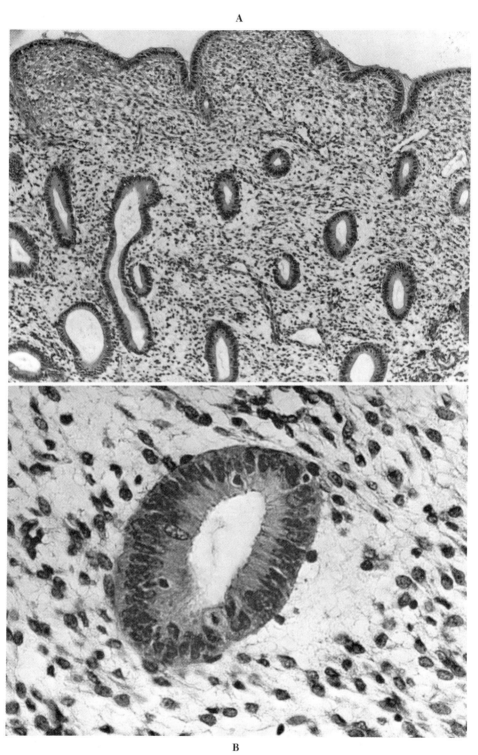

B

Figure 4. Photomicrographs of endometrium, beginning of late proliferative phase. A, × 150; B, × 400. (From Noyes, R. W., Hertig, A. T., and Rock, J.: Fertil. Steril., 1:3, 1950.)

A

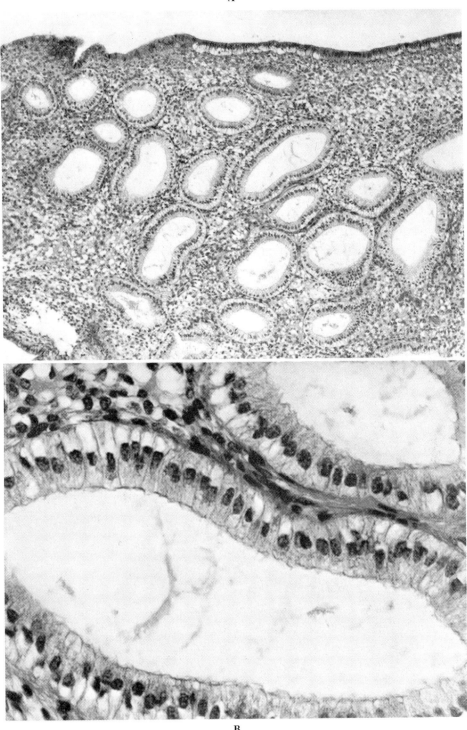

B

Figure 5. Photomicrographs of endometrium, early secretory phase. A, × 150; B, × 400. (Courtesy of Dr. Arthur T. Hertig.)

A

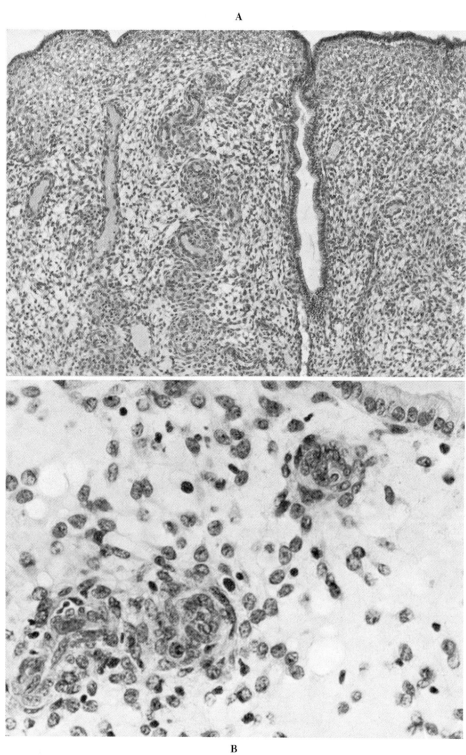

B

Figure 6.   Photomicrographs of endometrium, end of early secretory and beginning of late secretory phase (23 to 24 days). A, × 150; B, × 400. Prominent spiral vessel surrounded by predecidual change of the stroma. Edema of the latter is noteworthy. (From Noyes, R. W., Hertig, A. T., and Rock, J.: Fertil. Steril., 1:3, 1950.)

A

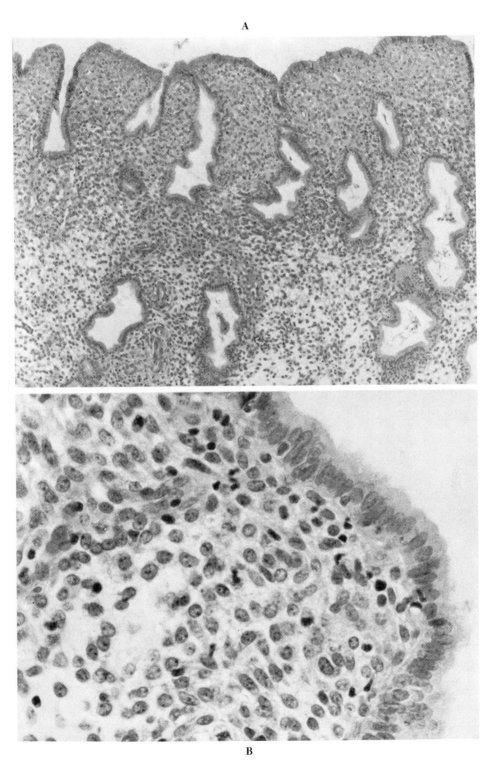

B

Figure 7. Photomicrographs of endometrium, late secretory phase (25 to 26 days — eleventh postovulatory day), showing loss of stromal edema. A, × 150; B, × 400. (From Noyes, R. W., Hertig, A. T., and Rock, J.: Fertil. Steril., 1:3, 1950.)

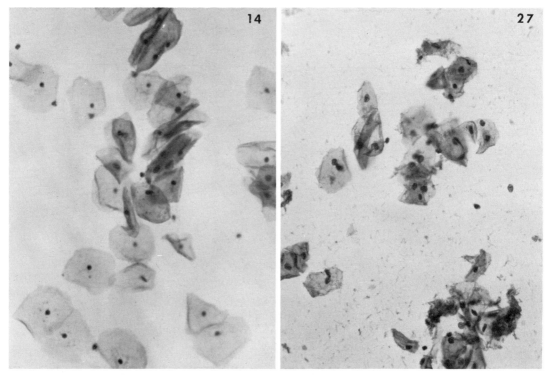

Figure 8.   Desquamated vaginal cells at day 14 and 27 of the cycle.

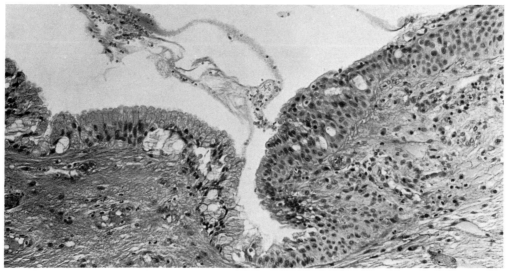

Figure 9.   Squamocolumnar junction of the cervix.

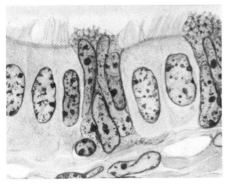

Figure 10. Epithelium of human fallopian tube prior to ovulation, showing the two principal cell types, ciliated cells and the so-called "secretory" cells. The secretory cells are the more highly basophilic. Eosin and methylene blue stain. × 2000. (Courtesy of Dr. Don Fawcett.)

ovulation, in the late secretory phase the secretory cells of the tube are prominent and glycogen content increases (Figs. 10 and 11).

THE MENSTRUAL CYCLE

The menstrual cycle is a repetitive phenomenon occurring in nonpregnant women during reproductive life that involves a patterned sequence of structural and functional changes in the reproductive system. The most apparent manifestation of a menstrual cycle is, of course, the monthly discharge of blood and endometrial debris from the uterine cavity, but many other, less overt changes are also taking place within the body. The cycle is thus a more complex physiologic process than the

simple monthly bleeding would indicate. The menstrual period is in reality determined by hypothalamic mechanisms which regulate pituitary gonadotropin secretion which, in turn, controls ovarian hormone release. The ovarian steroids, estradiol and progesterone, are the prime mediators of the cyclic changes that take place in the whole body, and especially stimulation of the endometrial development required for implantation. In the absence of an intervening pregnancy, the decrease of hormone secretion that occurs when the corpus luteum regresses initiates the degeneration of the uterine lining and supporting blood vessels which manifests itself as menstrual flow. Other cyclic events influenced by the hormones involve the neurologic system, metabolic processes, breasts, vagina, and cervix. (See Endometrial, Vaginal, Cervical, and Oviductal Cycles.)

It is obvious that the menstrual type of cycle is not fundamental for reproduction in the animal kingdom at large since its occurrence is restricted to the human and certain other primate species. While endometrial development is necessary for a fit implantation site in all viviparous animals, regression of that endometrium can take several forms, menstruation being just one example, based upon the peculiar cyclic uterine vascular development and regression that occurs in the human. Most mammals have endometrial regression in a less obvious manner.

The essential ingredients of the female reproductive cycle in all viviparous mammals including man are: (1) ovarian follicular development for ovulation and hormone secretion; (2) preparation of the reproductive tract for mating, conception, and implantation; and (3) recycling of all events should pregnancy not occur.

In most animals, the visual and behavioral clues of the cycle develop just before ovulation when the animal assumes mating behavior (heat or estrus). In species other than man, there may be slight vaginal bleeding at estrus, in addition to swelling of the external genitalia and submission to mating just before rupture of the follicle. These external events are largely unknown in the human, where the ovulatory period is more difficult to time directly (see Determinants of a Menstrual Cycle). The estrus cycle of animals is comparable to the menstrual cycle of man except for the timing and pat-

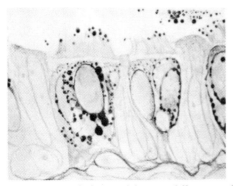

Figure 11. Epithelium of human fallopian tube, stained for glycogen. Coarse aggregates of glycogen are found principally in the ciliated cells and in the lumen of the tube. Glycogen is also found in the nonciliated cells at certain phases of the cycle. Periodic acid–Schiff reaction. × 2000. (Courtesy of Dr. Don Fawcett.)

tern of bleeding and behavioral activity. Cyclic patterns among animals also differ in regard to the ovulatory act itself. While most animals, including man, ovulate spontaneously in cyclic fashion at times specific for their species, the rabbit and cat, for example, ovulate reflexly in response to the coital stimulus and otherwise do not release an egg. Within these variations in cyclicity, the essential elements for reproduction are met by the same basic events of ovulation and preparation of the body for procreation.

BREEDING SEASONS AND FACTORS THAT AFFECT THE CYCLE

Reproductive cycles may occur in the human throughout the year, under wide extremes of environmental conditions, but many animals are fertile and exhibit estrus periods only at certain seasons and only under "favorable" life situations. The factors that regulate the occurrence of these fertile periods include: light-dark intervals, temperature, humidity, availability of food and water, and surroundings. Many wild animals will not breed in captivity, transporting animals from the northern to the southern hemisphere may reverse the reproductive season, and alterations of light exposure can change the timing of sexual activity. In man, it has been observed that ovulation and the menstrual cycle may be interfered with under conditions of stress and emotional trauma. Anovulation and amenorrhea may be associated with going off to summer camp or college and may also occur in relationship to mental illness such as anorexia nervosa. If light is supplied continuously to laboratory animals they may cease cycling and not ovulate. In mice, a pregnancy will be resorbed if the odor of a strange male is perceived, and this can be prevented by making the female anosmatic. The pathways for these environmental cues to the reproductive tract are via sight, hearing, smell, and exteroreceptor nerves to the central nervous system and hypothalamus, including perhaps the pineal (p. 63). The hypothalamus is also sensitive to alterations in internal metabolic derangements. It is thus understandable how emotional factors, disease, environmental changes, and metabolic alterations may interrupt the menstrual pattern by interfering with the neuroendocrine reflex even

if the detailed mechanisms cannot always be defined. As with animals, the human female may individually vary in her susceptibility to these disruptive stimuli.

AGE, REPRODUCTIVE FUNCTION, AND THE MENSTRUAL CYCLE

The female life span can be divided into periods that are a reflection of development, attainment, maintenance, and ultimate loss of reproductive function. These are in order: infancy and childhood, adolescence, adulthood, and climacteric and the postmenopausal years. The transition times of puberty and the climacteric are marked by the initiation (menarche) and cessation (menopause), respectively, of the menses. So many events in a woman's life are related to her menstrual activity that it is small wonder that the cycle has assumed a mystique over and above its procreative implications.

Infancy and Childhood

This period in the female's life is one of general somatic growth and development in a more or less physiologically asexual manner. Levels of gonadal hormones are low and roughly equivalent in the two sexes. The reproductive tract remains in the infantile state until toward the end of this period when levels of pituitary gonadotropins begin to rise slowly and both LH and FSH can be measured in increasing amounts in the blood stream; this is followed by elevations in the gonadal steroids typical of the two sexes: testosterone in boys, estradiol in girls. Vaginal bleeding may rarely occur during this period and, in the absence of the rare true precocious puberty, usually represents either a foreign body in the vagina, infection, or malignancy.

Adolescence and Puberty

Adolescence is a transition period between childhood and adulthood and represents: a rapid change in body size, composition, and shape, and maturation of the gonads, the reproductive tract, and secondary sexual characteristics. The individual loses the childhood body configuration and assumes the proportions of an adult. The growth spurt starts about the eighth year and the peak rate may be reached between the ages of 9½ and 14½ years. There is deposition of fat in positions characteristic of the female on the shoulders and hips. The breasts start to develop (thelarche) from ages 8 to 13, at about the same time as the growth of pubic hair, with axillary hair following some two years later. Menarche, or the beginning of menses, occurs between the age of 10 and 14, with the extremes of normalcy placed at 8 and 18 years. Variations in timing of all these events are quite common but the sequence is more predictable. The external genitalia develop adult characteristics with changes in the vulva, lengthening of the vagina, and alteration of the proportions of the uterus. The relatively long cervix and small fundus of the child is altered by more rapid growth of the body of the uterus so that proportions of the uterus are changed. The cyclic changes in vaginal cells, cervical secretions, and endometrium begin as a result of production of estrogen from the ovary. The initiating events of adolescence and menarche are unknown. It is believed that the ovaries can respond to gonadotropin stimulation long before they are called upon to do so. The current theory is that hypothalamic maturation is the triggering event, with subsequent stimulation of pituitary release of FSH and LH. The responses of the gonads and to a certain extent of the adrenals (adrenarche) result in the production of steroid hormones which stimulate the growth and development observed. That the brain or hypothalamus is the triggering mechanism has been shown in animals, where an infantile pituitary grafted into an adult hypophyseal fossa commences adult function immediately. The factors responsible for the maturation of the hypothalamus at the time of puberty are, however, unknown. Precocious puberty is rare and may occur in relation to hypothalamic, pineal, or cerebral tumors or infection. Premature development of the reproductive tract, breasts, and skeletal system may accompany hormone-producing tumors of the adrenals or gonads, or be present with hypothyroidism. This, of course, does not represent true precocious puberty, with which it might be confused. Many behavioral and emotional problems are associated with adolescence, including adjustment to adulthood and the interactions with parental authority and the opposite sex. It has not been possible to completely dissociate the influence of cultural effects from those produced by the altered physiologic state and the role of hormones. It is likely that the "trauma" of initiation into adulthood is an interaction of many of these factors.

Adult Life

The onset of menses signals the start of reproductive life. Menstrual cycles commence at ages 10 to 14 (8 to 18) and cease in the fourth or early fifth decade of life. There are indications that over the past 100 years the onset of menses has tended to occur at earlier ages, while the cessation of flow at menopause seems to be occurring later in life, so that the potential reproductive period is lengthened. Adult life is usually timed from the period when adolescent growth and development has been achieved and the menstrual cycle has entered a more or less regular pattern. At the menarche, as in the premenopausal years, missed periods and irregularity are typical. This is often associated with failure to ovulate regularly, with subsequent abnormalities in steroid hormone production and the bleeding pattern (see below).

The cycle length is judged from the first day of bleeding until the start of another menses, with an average interval of 24 to 32 days and a mode of 28 days. The length of bleeding averages from three to five days, with wide variation in duration and amount. The blood loss measures between 50 and 150 ml., with the largest amount lost in the first two days of flow.

It should be clearly understood that a menstrual cycle refers to endometrial development and regression (see Endometrial Cycle) in association with ovulation and consequent estrogen-progesterone synergism and withdrawal. In the absence of ovulation there is little or no progesterone since a corpus luteum is not formed, and the endometrium develops and regresses under the influence of estrogen alone. The withdrawal bleeding is not a true menstrual type and is characterized by more variability in interval, duration, and amount. Anovulatory bleeding is one of the most common causes of menstrual irregularities, and occurs most frequently at the beginning and end of the reproductive period.

DETERMINANTS OF A MENSTRUAL CYCLE. It is of importance to have determinants of a menstrual cycle in evaluating patients for problems of infertility and menstrual irregularity. The hallmark of a "normal" cycle is the occurrence of ovulation and formation of a corpus luteum, and most determinants are based upon indirect evidence for the release of an egg and corpus luteum production of progesterone.

A cycle is more apt to be normal if the interval is regular and the bleeding follows a normal pattern of duration and amount. Normal cycles are usually associated with symptoms of some breast tenderness, menstrual cramps, premenstrual tension, and even fluid accumulation. These are all variables and crude signs that progesterone and a corpus luteum have been present. More meaningful signs of progesterone formation are, in order of complexity and ease of determination: change in basal body temperature, variation in cervical mucus and vaginal epithelium, secretory (progesterone) changes in the endometrium, as determined by biopsy, elevation in urinary pregnanediol, and finally elevation of blood progesterone. The only absolute sign of ovulation is, of course, visualization of the egg or an ensuing pregnancy. Occasionally a corpus luteum can be identified at laparotomy or culdoscopy when the procedure is otherwise indicated. Some women have pain in the middle of their cycle ("mittelschmerz"), believed to be associated with release of the egg, and this too has been used as a crude indication of ovulation. It can be seen that man, unlike the animal with an estrus cycle, has had to develop techniques of his own for determining the ovulatory period.

The so-called average 28-day cycle can be divided into two phases based upon ovarian activity and uterine response. In the first 14 days the follicles are developing, estrogen production is increasing, and a "proliferative" or "estrogenic" response occurs in the endometrium. The second 14 days is ushered in by ovulation, with progesterone production and a "secretory" or "progestational" response of the endometrium. The most constant portion of the cycle regardless of total length is the postovulatory period, which is determined by the rather fixed limits of corpus luteum survival. In a menstrual cycle that is shorter than average, say of only 25 days, the proliferative period prior to ovulation may last only 11 days, while in a longer menstrual period of 40 days the preovulatory interval might be 26 days.

Menopause, Climacteric, and Postmenopausal Years

Cessation of menses for at least one year due to exhaustion of ovarian hormonal activity is designated the natural menopause, while loss of ovarian function due to surgical removal in the reproductive years, before natural ovarian senescence normally occurs, is considered a surgical menopause. The natural menopause usually starts in the latter half of the fourth decade or early fifth decade of life. Rarely a true natural menopause may occur at an age as early as the 30's but such an event requires substantiation to rule out disease processes that may cause anovulation and amenorrhea. Since the gonadotropin levels rise when ovarian endocrine function declines, measurement of a high urinary gonadotropin level will confirm that the pituitary is functioning and ovarian exhaustion is at fault.

Even though menstruation stops, the ovary may continue to secrete modest amounts of hormone for several years and there may be an occasional ovum or follicle remaining, Prior to the menopause, anovulation and irregular, estrogen-type withdrawal bleeding is common and a variant of normalcy.

While the menopause refers to the cessation of menstrual bleeding, the transition period of life from reproductive to postmenopausal years is called the climacteric and encompasses all of the physiologic and emotional changes that transpire. Symptoms at this time include hot flashes, sweating or vasomotor instability, nervousness, irritability, and depression. While hormonal replacement will ordinarily correct the symptoms of "hot flashes" or "flushes," not all of the problems are amenable to such therapy. The reaction to the changing pattern of life at the climacteric is often determined by the individual's prior adjustment and is highly variable.

The human is unique in having a long period of life when there is no reproductive function. Although fertility and efficiency in procreation decline with age in most animals, only the human has evolved a prolonged period of ovarian senescence.

During this time a true deficiency state of gonadal hormones may develop but usually takes up to 15 years to manifest itself in greater liability to heart disease and osteoporosis. This is the basis for use of estrogens in the postmenopausal years.

After menopause the ovarian stroma and the adrenals are capable of direct secretion of estrogens or secretion of androgens which can be peripherally converted to estrogens. Hence, there is considerable variability among individuals as to the extent of the deficiency.

Endometrial bleeding in the postmenopausal years is always considered abnormal and may be associated with: (1) no obvious cause and an atrophic endometrium on curettage; (2) effects of exogenous estrogens; (3) stimulation of the endometrium by a functioning ovarian tumor; and (4) endometrial cancer. Diagnostic curettage to rule out malignancy is required in the management of postmenopausal bleeding.

BIBLIOGRAPHY

1. Burger, H. G., Catt, K. J., and Brown, J. B.: Relationship between plasma luteinizing hormone and urinary estrogen excretion during the menstrual cycle. J. Clin. Endocr., 28:1508, 1968.
2. Cargille, C. M., Ross, G. T., and Yoshimi, T.: Daily variations in plasma follicle stimulating hormone, luteinizing hormone and progesterone in the normal menstrual cycle. J. Clin. Endocr., 29:12, 1969.
3. Corker, C. S., Naftolin, F., and Exley, D.: Interrelationship between plasma luteinizing hormone and oestradiol in the human menstrual cycle. Nature 222:1063, 1969.
4. Dufau, M. L., Dulmanis, A., Catt, K. J., and Hudson, B.: Measurement of plasma estradiol-17β by competitive binding assay employing pregnancy plasma. J. Clin. Endocr., 30:351, 1970.
5. Ferin, M., Tempone, A., Zimmering, P. E., and Vande Wiele, R. L.: Effect of antibodies to 17β-estradiol and progesterone on the estrous cycle of the rat. Endocrinology, 85:1070, 1969.
6. Ferin, M., Zimmering, P. E., and Vande Wiele, R. L.: Effects of antibodies to estradiol-17β on PMS-induced ovulation in immature rats. Endocrinology, 84:893, 1969.
7. Gobelsmann, U., Midgley, A. R., Jr., and Jaffe, R. B.: Regulation of human gonadotropins. VII. Daily individual urinary estrogens, pregnanediol and serum luteinizing and follicle stimulat-

ing hormones during the menstrual cycle. J. Clin. Endocr., 29:1222, 1969.
8. Kobayashi, F., Hara, K., and Miyake, T.: Further studies on the causal relationship between the secretion of estrogen and the release of luteinizing hormone in the rat. Endocr. Jap., 16:501, 1969.
9. Midgley, A. R., Jr., and Jaffe, R. B.: Regulation of human gonadotropins. IV. Correlation of serum concentrations of follicle stimulating and luteinizing hormones during the menstrual cycle. J. Clin. Endocr., 28:1699, 1968.
10. Neill, J. D., Johansson, E. D. B., Datta, J. K., and Knobil, E.: Relationship between the plasma levels of luteinizing hormone and progesterone during the normal menstrual cycle. J. Clin. Endocr., 27:1167, 1967.
11. Noyes, R. W., Hertig, A. T., and Rock, J.: Dating the endometrial biopsy. Fertil. Steril., 1:3, 1950.
12. Papanicolaou, G. N., Traut, H. F., and Marchetti, A. H.: The Epithelia of Women's Reproductive Organs. Commonwealth Fund, New York, 1948.
13. Saxena, B. B., Demura, H., Gandy, H. M., and Peterson, R. E.: Radioimmunoassay of human follicle stimulating and luteinizing hormones in plasma. J. Clin. Endocr., 28:519, 1968.
14. Stevens, V. C.: Comparison of FSH and LH patterns in plasma, urine and urinary extracts during the menstrual cycle. J. Clin. Endocr., 29:904, 1969.
15. Taymor, M. L., Aono, T., and Pheteplace, C.: Follicle-stimulating hormone and luteinizing hormone in serum during the menstrual cycle determined by radioimmunoassay. Acta Endocr., 59:298, 1968.
16. Taymor, M. L., Lieberman, B., and Rizkallah, T. H.: FSH excretion during the normal menstrual cycle. Fertil. Steril., 20:267, 1969.
17. Vande Wiele, R. L., et al.: Mechanisms regulating the menstrual cycle in women. Recent Progr. in Hormone Res., 26:63, 1970.
18. Yen, S. S. C., Llerena, O., Little, B., and Pearson, O. H.: Disappearance rates of endogenous luteinizing hormone and chorionic gonadotropin in man. J. Clin. Endocr., 28:1763, 1968.
19. Yen, S. S. C., Rankin, J., and Littell, A. S.: Hormonal relationships in the menstrual cycle. J.A.M.A., 211:1513, 1970.
20. Yoshimi, T., Strott, C. A., Marshall, J. R., and Lipsett, M. B.: Corpus luteum function in early pregnancy. J. Clin. Endocr., 29:225, 1969.
21. Yussman, M. A., and Taymor, M. L.: Serum levels of follicle stimulating hormone and luteinizing hormone and of plasma progesterone related to ovulation by corpus luteum biopsy. J. Clin. Endocr., 30:396, 1970.
22. Yussman, M. A., Taymor, M. L., Miyata, J., and Pheteplace, C.: Serum levels of follicle-stimulating hormone, luteinizing hormone, and plasma progestins correlated with human ovulation. Fertil. Steril., 21:119, 1970.

ENDOCRINOLOGY OF HUMAN PREGNANCY

Reproduction in man is a complex, endocrine-regulated process that for convenience can be considered under three general types of hormonal control systems (Table 1).

1. *Preimplantation endocrine systems* control the reproductive cycles in male and female and are required over and above the metabolic-homeostatic endocrine actions essential for normal health. Preimplantation hormonal function is required for gametogenesis, courtship, ovulation, coital activities, conception, and implantation. This is typified by cyclic pituitary gonadotropin release and ovarian estrogen-progesterone secretion in the female. Details of such endocrine activity have been covered in the sections on cyclic changes in hormones and reproductive tract (p. 96) and on the menstrual cycle (p. 105). These will not be reviewed further.

It should, however, be realized that the steroid hormones have several general metabolic actions as well as their reproductive ones, so that these classifications cannot be considered exclusive.

If fertilization or development were external to the maternal body, the reproductive endocrine cycles would be sufficient for control of the procreative process. The evolution of viviparity and a prolonged intrauterine gestation period created the requirement for the pregnancy-specific hormonal mechanisms to be considered next.

2. *Postimplantation endocrine systems* are *pregnancy-specific*. These activities control the integrity and duration of pregnancy once implantation has been established; the usual endocrine function of the ovarian cycle (menstrual cycle) would be expected to wane if a pregnancy had not

TABLE 1.   ENDOCRINOLOGY OF PREGNANCY

Type of Endocrine Control	Hormone	Endocrine Gland	Nonpregnant Activity	Activities and Requirements in Pregnancy
Preimplantation reproductive endocrine system	FSH	Pituitary	Cyclic pattern and midcycle surge	Quiescent
	LH	Pituitary	Cyclic pattern and midcycle surge	Probably quiescent—measurement interfered with by HCG
	Estrogens	Ovary	Cyclic pattern	Ovarian estrogen quiescent
	Progesterone	Corpus luteum of cycle	Cyclic pattern	Active through first 8-10 weeks of gestation via corpus luteum of pregnancy for both estrogen and progesterone
Pregnancy-specific, postimplantation reproductive endocrine system	HCG	Placenta	Absent except with choriocarcinoma	Maintains corpus luteum of pregnancy
	Estrogens	Corpus luteum of pregnancy and placenta	Absent except for ovarian cycle	Required in pregnancy
	Progesterone	Corpus luteum of pregnancy and placenta	Absent except for ovarian cycle	Required in pregnancy
	Chorionic somato-mammotropin	Placenta	Absent except with choriocarcinoma	Metabolic effects in pregnancy
	Oxytocin	Neurohypophysis	Present but function unknown	Facilitation of labor and/or delivery
Metabolic-homeostatic	Somatotropin	Pituitary	Growth and metabolism	Not increased; altered levels in response to blood glucose change blunted; potentiated by chorionic somato-mammotropin
	Thyrotropin	Pituitary	Metabolism	TSH increased; PBI elevated; inorganic iodine decreased; thyroid work increased; thyroxin-binding globulin increased

(Table continues on opposite page.)

occurred. This type of pregnancy-specific control is typified by the HCG secretion of the placenta which converts the corpus luteum of the cycle into a more long-lived corpus luteum of pregnancy to continue production of estrogen and progesterone. Later, estrogen and progesterone are secreted (in man and other species) by the placenta itself. Also involved in pregnancy-specific hormonal activities are oxytocin with its role in normal labor, chorionic somato-mammotropin with its general metabolic effects, postpartum pituitary prolactin for lactation, and relaxin for as yet poorly defined roles, at least in the human. There are indications of other endocrine influences on pregnancy which must await further study. Although many factors and hormones are involved, the essence of endocrine activity during human pregnancy is the provision of appropriate amounts of estrogens and progesterone which are required for reproduction in all higher forms of animal life. The shifts in endocrine control mechanisms that accomplish this continued supply of steroid hormone will be considered in some detail in the sections which follow.

3. *Metabolic-homeostatic endocrine systems* are required in both the pregnant and the nonpregnant state, but are not specific as far as reproduction is concerned. They allow pregnancy to occur as just one of many bodily functions. This type of activity is illustrated by the action of thyroid, adrenal, and pancreatic hormones on the general metabolism of the individual, but the effects and needs of such hormones are significantly modified by gestation and for that reason will constitute a part of our consideration of the endocrinology of pregnancy.

TABLE 1.   ENDOCRINOLOGY OF PREGNANCY *(Continued)*

Type of Endocrine Control	Hormone	Endocrine Gland	Nonpregnant Activity	Activities and Requirements in Pregnancy
Metabolic-homeostatic	Thyroxin	Thyroid		Replacement required in deficiency state
	ACTH Cortisol	Pituitary Adrenal	Metabolism	No known change in ACTH; adrenal steroid production increased Metabolism of adrenal steroids decreased Cortisol-binding globulin increased Free cortisol elevated; replacement required in deficiency state
	Aldosterone	Adrenal	Water and electrolyte balance	Production increased in pregnancy; renin-angiotensin system function elevated
	Insulin	Pancreas	Carbohydrate and fat metabolism	Insulin action on glucose handling up in early pregnancy, decreased in late pregnancy; blood insulin increased in late pregnancy Replacement required in deficiency state
	Catecholamines	Adrenal medulla	Homeostatic	Effects and changes in pregnancy not established
	Parathormone	Parathyroid	Calcium and phosphorous metabolism	Increased activity with pregnancy and lactation
	Vasopressin	Neurohypophysis	Water metabolism	Replacement required in deficiency state
	Melanocyte-stimulating hormone	Pituitary	Pigmentation	Activity increased in pregnancy

PREGNANCY-SPECIFIC ENDOCRINE ACTIVITIES

Formation of the Corpus Luteum of Pregnancy

After ovulation, the corpus luteum of the cycle is formed from the ruptured follicle and secretes estrogen and progesterone for only a limited time unless its function is prolonged by the intervention of implantation. Implantation of a conceptus is believed to affect corpus luteum viability by two possible processes: (1) the implanted trophoblast secretes a luteotropin (chorionic gonadotropin in the human), which stimulates continued luteal function; (2) the trophoblast alters the metabolism of the uterus which would otherwise release substances that cause luteal regression. In many animal species, the uterus cyclically releases as yet unidentified factors (luteolysins) which inhibit the endocrine secretion and survival of the corpus luteum. Hence, if hysterectomy is performed in such an animal while a corpus luteum is present, the cycle is prolonged and the corpus luteum does not disappear as readily; the process is reversed by injection of uterine extracts. Implantation in such species causes an effect similar to hysterectomy.

It is not yet certain whether the "lytic" substance of the uterus is operative in man (p. 79) and other primates, so that the only mechanism for luteal survival reasonably well established for human pregnancy is the luteotropic effects of chorionic gonadotropin. Chorionic gonadotropin is detectable in human blood as early as nine days post conception and the levels continue to rise for an additional two-month period before declining and reaching a low plateau for the remainder of pregnancy. The corpus luteum maintains its function for 8 to 10 weeks of gestation and in spite of the continued presence of chorionic gonadotropin may ultimately regress, implicating factors other than the luteotropin in its survival. The pituitary is not essential for maintenance of the corpus luteum of pregnancy since ovulation has been induced in hypopituitary subjects by administration of exogenous gonadotropins, and subsequent pregnancies continue without additional pituitary hormone administration.

By monitoring blood levels of hormones in man it can be demonstrated that corpus luteum function declines at six to eight

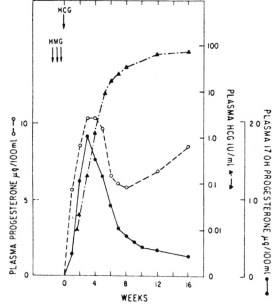

Figure 12. Mean plasma levels of progesterone, 17-hydroxyprogesterone and HCG which followed induction of ovulation with HMG-HCG. (From Yoshimi, T., Strott, C. A., Marshall, J. R., and Lipsett, M. B.: J. Clin. Endocr. 29:225, 1969.)

weeks of gestation, with a dip in the progesterone level followed by a secondary rise that is presumably due to secretion by the placenta. The metabolite 17-hydroxyprogesterone is secreted by the corpus luteum and not the placenta since its level in blood drops at six to eight weeks and does not rise as the progesterone level does (Fig. 12).

Comparative Studies of the Corpus Luteum Role in Pregnancy

OOPHORECTOMY-INTOLERANT MAMMALS. In many animal species pregnancy will terminate by abortion or resorption of the embryos if the ovaries or corpora lutea are removed at any time during the gestational period (Table 2). Pregnancy can be maintained in spite of corpora lutea removal in these animals if the correct relative and absolute amounts of estrogens and progestins are provided exogenously; this demonstrates the critical role of the corpus luteum in the provision of steroid hormones. These oophorectomy-intolerant mammals usually have a short gestational period, the corpus luteum remains structurally and functionally viable throughout pregnancy, and

TABLE 2.   OOPHORECTOMY-INTOLERANT MAMMALS[*]

Species	Gestation Length	Regression of Corpora	Placental Progesterone	Placental Estrogen	Placental Aromatization	Comments
			Class 1 — short gestation			
Opossum	12.5	No				No placental endocrine function
Hamster	16–19	No				
Mouse	20	No		No		Tolerates hypophysectomy-placental gonadotropin
Rat	21	No	No	No	No	Tolerates hypophysectomy-placental gonadotropin
Rabbit	30–32	No	No		No	Intolerant of hypophysectomy
Dog	58–63	Yes	No	No	No	Intolerant of hypophysectomy
			Class 2 — long gestation			
Sow	112–115	No	No	Yes	Yes	
Goat	151	No	No	Yes	Yes	Intolerant of hypophysectomy

[*]From Ryan, K. J., in Pecile, A., and Finzi, C., eds.: The Foeto-Placental Unit. Excerpta Medica Foundation, Amsterdam, 1969, pp. 120–131.

there is no evidence of significant placental hormone production. In some animals with a somewhat longer gestation period only progesterone needs to be replaced to maintain pregnancy after oophorectomy, suggesting that limited placental production of estrogen has developed. This placental activity can be verified experimentally.[40, 42]

OOPHORECTOMY-TOLERANT MAMMALS. In many animal species, including man, the course of natural pregnancy is not altered by oophorectomy or corpus luteum removal when it is performed at certain times during the gestation period (Table 3). This is due not to their lack of need for the corpora luteal steroids for pregnancy maintenance but rather to the fact that in these species the placenta has assumed the capacity to secrete estrogens and progesterone to replace the otherwise critical luteal function. These oophorectomy-tolerant mammals all require corpora luteal function in early pregnancy but lose dependence on this ovarian activity when the placental capacity to secrete steroids is sufficient to meet their needs. In the human, the ovaries have been removed from six weeks of gestation on without interference with pregnancy, while in some species oophorectomy is tolerated only in late gestation.

TABLE 3.   OOPHORECTOMY-TOLERANT MAMMALS[*]

Species	Gestation Length	Oophorectomy Time	Regression of Corpora	Placental Progesterone	Placental Estrogen	Placental Pregnenolone-Progesterone Conversion	Placental Aromatization	Coments
				Class 3 — short gestation				
Cat	63	49	Yes					Hypophysectomy intolerant
Guinea-pig	68	40	No	Yes			No	Tolerate hypox after 40 days
				Class 4 — long gestation				
Sheep	144	55	Yes	Yes	Yes	Yes	Yes	Tolerates hypox
Macaque	165	25		Yes	Yes	Yes	Yes	Tolerates hypox
Human	267	40	±	Yes	Yes	Yes	Yes	Tolerates hypox
Cow	280	207–230	No	Yes	Yes	Yes	Yes	
Horse	330	170–270	Yes	Yes	Yes	Yes	Yes	

[*]From Ryan, K. J., in Pecile, A., and Finzi, C., eds.: The Foeto-Placental Unit. Excerpta Medica Foundation, Amsterdam, 1969, pp. 120–131.

In almost all animals in the oophorectomy-tolerant category both estrogens and progesterone have been isolated from the placenta and the enzymatic activities for steroid production have been demonstrated by perfusion and in-vitro studies with the isolated tissue. Most of these mammals have a long gestational period during which the corpora lutea may actually regress prior to term. In some species such as the horse or elephant, succeeding crops of corpora lutea are utilized to maintain the supply of hormones until the placenta takes over, but in most animals the hormonal needs of prolonged gestation are met by placental endocrine function alone.

Compartmentalization of Endocrine Systems in Human Pregnancy

The major steroid hormones of human pregnancy, progesterone, estradiol, estriol, and their metabolites, are not simply the products of the usual type of endocrine gland synthesis, secretion into the blood stream, and peripheral metabolism.[51] There are three major compartments of relatively distinct endocrine activity—mother, placenta, and fetus—and two major tissue-blood exchange points—maternal-placental and feto-placental. Such a compartmentalization does not in reality represent a discontinuous isolation of the endocrine activity of mother, placenta, and child, but is rather the endocrinologist's device to separate out and study an otherwise unintelligible complexity of nature (Fig. 13).[40]

PLACENTAL COMPARTMENT. In respect to steroid hormone synthesis and secretion, the placenta is not a conventional endocrine organ. Although the placenta can synthesize cholesterol from small carbon fragments in a manner similar to other steroid-producing glands, it does not have the quantitative capacity to use this mechanism for the hormone production of human pregnancy. The placenta also lacks key enzymatic systems along the total biosynthetic pathway from cholesterol to estrogens. As outlined in the sections on the placenta and steroid hormones, this organ can readily transform cholesterol to progesterone and androgens to estrogens. From extensive clinical experience and clinical research studies, it is apparent that the cholesterol[22, 43] for progesterone synthesis is derived from the maternal blood stream and that the androgens for estrogen synthesis are derived predominantly from the maternal blood stream in early pregnancy and from the fetus in the later months of gestation.[9, 10, 18, 19, 34] The circulatory androgens are for the most part conjugated with sulfate, and the placenta has the enzymatic systems to cleave the complex and utilize the free androgen precursors in its steroid-producing machinery. A clinical case has been described in which the sulfatase was absent and estrogen production was low.[16] The placenta secretes its products in two

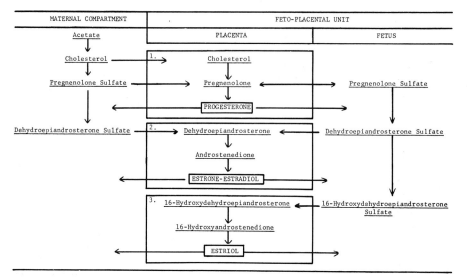

Figure 13. Major endocrine biosynthetic pathways in maternal and fetoplacental compartments. (From Ryan, K. J., in Pecile, A., and Finzi, C., eds.: The Foeto-placental Unit. Excerpta Medica Foundation, Amsterdam, 1969.)

directions, into both the maternal and fetal blood streams, and in addition transports steroid metabolites back and forth between mother and baby, although there is some quantitative and qualitative specificity to this function (Figs. 13, 14, and 15). Placental metabolism or degradation of steroids is quite limited compared to the activity in the maternal and fetal compartments.

MATERNAL COMPARTMENT. During pregnancy the usual reproductive endocrine functions of the maternal endocrine system are more or less quiescent. The pituitary gland is functionally inactive with respect to gonadotropins and the maternal ovaries are in a state of relative atrophy except for the occasional maintenance of the corpus luteum with limited activity. The other endocrine glands are to a certain extent "hyperactive" and there is evidence for increased thyroid and adrenal metabolism. The maternal adrenal continues to secrete dehydroepiandrosterone sulfate and this constitutes a major blood steroid. The maternal liver serves its usual function of extensive steroid metabolism and there is no evidence that metabolic clearance rates are altered. The major pathway for steroid excretion is via the urine.

FETAL COMPARTMENT. Fetal endocrine activity is quite different qualitatively from that in the adult. The distinctive features of hormonal metabolism in the developing individual in utero consist of: extensive conjugation of almost all steroids with sulfate, relatively high concentrations of steroids in the blood with levels often much higher than in the mother, the presence of a "fetal zone" in the adrenal which favors secretion of Δ^5 steroids like pregnenolone and dehydroepiandrosterone to the relative exclusion of the Δ^4 steroids like progesterone, androstenedione, and cortisol, and the capacity for extensive 16-hydroxylation of steroids. Some almost unique hydroxylations at positions 14 and 15 of the steroid molecule also occur in the fetus. The fetal liver can convert androgens to estrogens and is capable of 16-hydroxylation at a rate much greater than that of the adult organ.

There is still some controversy about how early the fetal adrenal develops the capacity to synthesize its steroids from acetate, and whether it relies on maternal precursors such as pregnenolone which cross the placenta for its building blocks.[47–49] In any

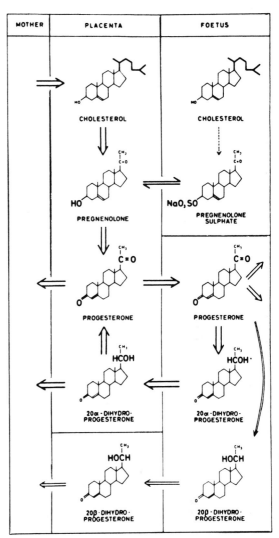

Figure 14. The metabolism of pregnenolone and progesterone in the human fetoplacental unit at mid-pregnancy. (From Diczfalusy, E., in Proceedings of the Second International Congress on Hormonal Steroids, Milan. Excerpta Medica International Congress Series, New York, 1966, p. 82.)

case, the placental secretion of pregnenolone, progesterone, androgens, and estrogens into the fetal blood stream provides a large hormonal substrate pool for metabolism within the fetus. The Δ^4 steroids, such as progesterone and androstenedione, which the fetus does not synthesize readily, are available by placental secretion for conversion to a myriad of end-products.

The fetal adrenal provides the bulk of the dehydroepiandrosterone sulfate precursor utilized by the placenta for its production of estradiol, and the fetal adrenal, with or without the aid of 16-hydroxylation by the liver, provides the 16-hydroxydehydroepi-

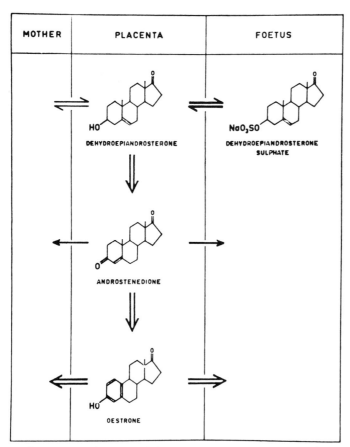

Figure 15. Simplified scheme of the metabolism of dehydroepiandrosterone sulfate in the human placenta in midterm. (From Diczfalusy, E., in Proceedings of the Second International Congress on Hormonal Steroids, Milan. Excerpta Medica International Congress Series, New York 1966, p. 82.)

androsterone for estriol formation (Fig. 16). After birth the precursors and their metabolites are still present in the neonate's blood[6, 13, 14, 36, 46] and urine but soon disappear as the remnants of fetal adrenal activity disappear.

The fetal testis is a remarkably large and functional organ with an ample supply of interstitial cells which disappear after birth, not to recur until puberty. The testis, like the adrenal, favors the secretion of $\triangle^5$ steroids. There is little evidence for significant ovarian hormonal activity in utero.

MATERNAL-PLACENTAL UNIT. As indicated by a classic experiment of Konrad Bloch in 1945, and more recently by studies of Hellig et al.,[22] the progesterone formed by the placenta is derived from maternal blood cholesterol. In-vitro enzymatic studies and placental perfusion have demonstrated limited capacity for de-novo acetate-to-cholesterol conversion by the placenta but facile transformation of cholesterol to pregnenolone and progesterone by this tissue.[43] Since maternal blood cholesterol is plentiful, the factors that might regulate progesterone synthesis are blood flow, transport into the cell, enzymatic capacity,

and enzyme mass rather than the availability of precursor.

The maternal blood stream also contains pregnenolone and pregnenolone sulfate[14] which could act as progesterone precursors upon reaching the placental cells, but their relative contribution is not known at this time.

The fetal blood stream could also provide pregnenolone sulfate and cholesterol for progesterone synthesis, but clinical studies demonstrate that even after intrauterine fetal demise, blood progesterone production remains elevated. The fetal contribution to this pathway seems to be limited in most cases.

The maternal blood stream also supplies dehydroepiandrosterone sulfate for possible placental conversion to estradiol and 16-hydroxydehydroepiandrosterone sulfate as an estriol building block, but both estradiol and estriol levels are low in the absence of a viable fetus or fetal adrenal, indicating a minor maternal contribution for most of pregnancy.[17, 20, 33, 34, 37, 39]

The estradiol and estriol secreted by the placenta into the maternal blood stream are extensively metabolized by the liver and

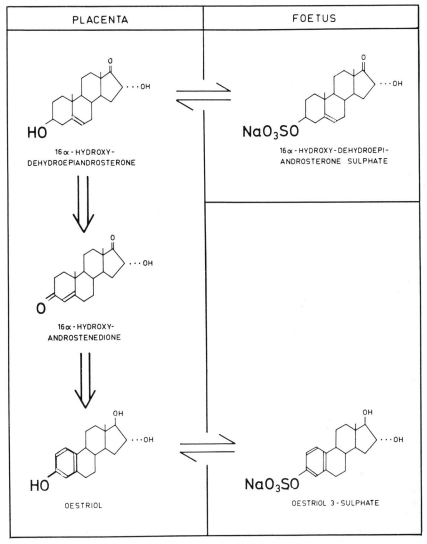

Figure 16. Principal pathway of estriol formation from 16α-hydroxy-dehydroepiandrosterone sulfate in the fetoplacental unit. (From Diczfalusy, E., and Marcuso, S., in Klopper, A., and Diczfalusy, E., eds.: Foetus and Placenta. Blackwell Scientific Publications, Oxford, 1969, p. 191.)

other tissues and excreted into the maternal urine as the 20 to 30 or so conversion products (Table 4) extractable from that source.[15, 23] Most of these excretion products are not biologically active.

The progesterone secreted by the placenta into the mother is also extensively metabolized for excretion as the stereoisomers of pregnanediol, the pregnanolones, and the pregnanediones.

There is as yet no evidence for a tropic control of placental function originating in the maternal organism.

FETO-PLACENTAL UNIT. Major clues for the existence of a feto-placental interaction (unit) were derived from the observations of Frandsen and Stakemann that mothers bearing anencephalic infants had low levels of estriol excretion[17–20] and the observations of Diczfalusy that the perfused fetus and placenta synthesized steroids that neither could alone.[9, 10] Clinical studies using radioactively labeled tracers in various experimental situations in patients with normal and abnormal pregnancies indicated that dehydroepiandrosterone sulfate derived from the fetus was the major precursor of placental estradiol and that 16-hydroxydehydroepiandrosterone sulfate was the major precursor of placental estriol (Figs. 15 and 16). These sulfurylated androgens have been isolated in high concentration from fetal blood[6, 13, 14, 36, 46] and the series of enzymatic steps was demonstrated in isolated placental enzyme systems[53, 54] long before their significance was estab-

TABLE 4. ESTROGENS IN HUMAN
PREGNANCY URINE[*]

Steroid	Amount mg./24 hr.
Estradiol	0.42–0.60
Estrone	1.2–1.4
Estriol	25–35
16 α Hydroxyestrone	0.6–1.6
16-Epi-estriol	0.35–0.80
16 β Hydroxyestrone	0.10–0.72
16-Oxo-17 β estradiol	0.2–1.10
16, 17-Epi-estriol	0.04–0.15
17-Epi-estriol	0.10–0.12
2-Methoxy-estrone	0.17–0.6
2-Methoxy-estriol	0.30
6 α Hydroxy-estrone	–
6-Hydroxyestriol	0.05–0.5
15 α Hydroxyesterone	–
15 α Hydroxyestradiol	–
15 α Hydroxyestriol	–
15 β Hydroxyesterone	–
15 β Hydroxyestradiol	–
18-Hydroxyesterone	–

[*]From Diczfalusy, E., and Marcuso, S., in Klopper, A., and Diczfalusy, E., eds.: Foetus and Placenta. Blackwell Scientific Publications, Oxford, 1969, p. 191.

lished.[40, 42, 43] This fetal precursor–placental product relationship for estrogen formation appears to be a major part of the feto-placental interaction. The estrogens produced along with other placental steroids such as progesterone and androstenedione are secreted into both the maternal and fetal blood stream. The fetus metabolizes the steroids it receives, conjugates them, and continually recirculates these metabolites with some placental transfer back to the mother for excretion (Fig. 17). Diczfalusy has reported in detail on the various aspects of fetal steroid metabolism.[9, 10] The amniotic fluid also contains large quantities of the steroids produced by the fetus and placenta.[1, 27, 44, 45]

Steroid Excretion in Human Pregnancy

The net result of maternal-placental and feto-placental interactions can be visualized in the maternal steroid blood levels and urinary excretion patterns as pregnancy progresses. These are illustrated in Figures 18, 19, and 20 and Table 4.

The rise in blood progesterone levels is relatively smooth as pregnancy advances except for the dip noted at the approximate crossover from a corpus luteum to a placental source of hormone (Figs. 12 and 20). The level of urinary pregnanediol (a progesterone metabolite), as determined by 24-hour collections, follows a relatively smooth curve, rising to a plateau in the later weeks of pregnancy (Fig. 19).

Total estrogen excretion in the urine and excretion of the individual metabolites follow a relatively smooth curve as the gestation period advances (Fig. 18). Although there are individual variations, estriol values can be roughly correlated with fetal weight. In addition to estrone, estradiol, and estriol, there are some 16 other estrogen metabolites excreted during pregnancy. Most of these compounds have no known biologic activity or function (Table 4).

Urinary 17-ketosteroids and pregnanetriols increase to lower overall levels than the pregnanediols or estrogens. The curves of HCG and HPL (Fig. 21) are included as a comparison with the pattern of steroid hormone excretion.

ESTRIOL AS A GUIDE OF FETAL WELL-BEING. Estrogen excretion in maternal urine increases some 1000-fold during pregnancy (see Fig. 18) and comprises largely estriol. As reviewed in the sections on estrogen synthesis and the feto-placental unit, estriol is synthesized by the placenta from precursors derived from the fetal adrenal and carried to it in the fetal blood stream. Once estriol is formed and secreted by the placenta its excretion in the maternal urine is dependent upon renal clearance and factors such as activity, posture, toxemia, and hypertension which can affect excretory function. Although the pathway for estriol formation and disposition is complex, the levels of estriol in urine, blood, or amniotic fluid can be used as a rough guide to fetal well-being[21, 35] provided that extraneous factors that affect the levels can be recognized. Serial values of maternal urinary estriol may be of prognostic value in determining an early delivery in a high-risk pregnancy (Fig. 22) when the amounts of estriol are clearly low and not rising normally. In practical experience this has been an adjunct to, rather than

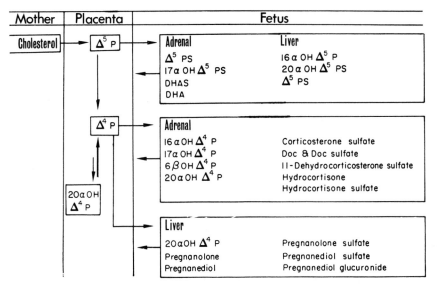

Figure 17. A scheme for the metabolism of pregnenolone and progesterone in the human placenta and fetus at mid-pregnancy. Δ^5 P = pregnenolone; Δ^5 PS = pregnenolone sulfate; 17α OH Δ^5 PS = 17α-hydroxypregnenolone sulfate; DHAS = dehydroisoandrosterone sulfate; DHA = dehydroisoandrosterone; 16α OH Δ^5 P = 16α-hydroxy-pregnenolone; 20α OH Δ^5 PS = 20α-dihydropregnenolone sulfate; 16α OH Δ^4 P = 16α-hydroxyprogesterone; 17α OH Δ^4 P = 17α-hydroxyprogesterone; 6β OH Δ^4 P = 6β-hydroxyprogesterone; 20α OH Δ^4 P = 20α-dihydro-progesterone; DOC = deoxycorticosterone. (From Younglai, E. V., and Solomon, S., in Klopper, A., and Diczfalusy, E., eds.: Foetus and Placenta. Blackwell Scientific Publications, Oxford, 1969, p. 249.)

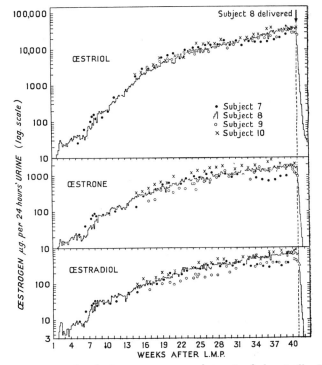

Figure 18. Urinary estrogen excretion during pregnancy, as determined chemically. (From Brown, J. B.: Lancet, 1:704, 1956.)

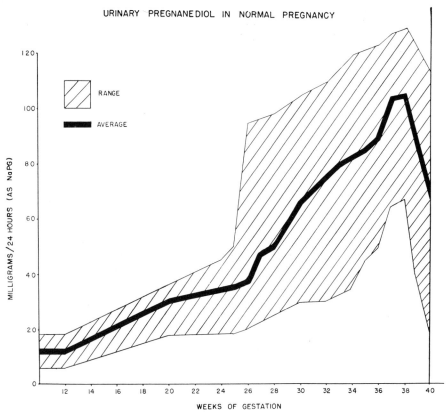

Figure 19.   Urinary pregnanediol calculated from the results of analyses for sodium pregnanediol glucuronide complex (NaPG). (Courtesy of Dr. O. W. Smith.)

a determinant of, clinical management. A similar use has been proposed for HPL excretion (p. 43) but this has been of somewhat less value than estriol excretion.

Since the estriol precursor is ultimately derived from the fetal adrenal, it is not surprising that exogenous corticoids given to the mother during pregnancy can cross the placenta and reduce adrenal hormone production, probably by feedback inhibition

of fetal ACTH. In any case, estriol excretion drops as a consequence of such adrenal steroid administration.[5, 52]

Fetal Endocrine Control of Gestational Length

The duration of pregnancy is fixed within remarkably narrow limits for every mam-

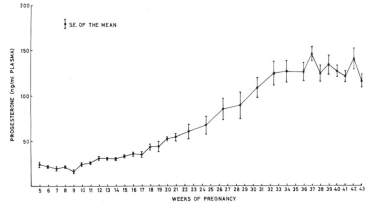

Figure 20.   Plasma progesterone levels during normal pregnancy. (From Johansson, E. D. B.: Acta Endocr., 61:607, 1969.)

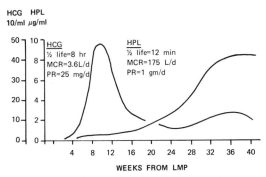

Figure 21. Serum levels of protein hormones throughout pregnancy. (Courtesy of Dr. S. S. C. Yen.)

born to survive. The mechanisms involved in controlling pregnancy length and in timing the onset of labor have been the object of considerable interest and controversy.[8]

Studies in animals have clearly indicated that when the fetus is removed from the uterus and the placenta is left in place, the placenta will be delivered at some future time, occasionally at full term. In clinical practice also, death of the fetus in utero (especially in the second trimester) does not always result in prompt delivery. These observations have been the basis for the impression that the fetus is not important in the timing of either gestational length or the onset of labor. Proposals for the mechanisms of pregnancy regulation and labor induction have invoked: placental progesterone effects on the myometrium,

malian species including man. How this is achieved is unknown, but evolution by natural selection has obviously favored those animals whose average length of gestation is neither too short (prematurity) nor too long (postmaturity) for their new-

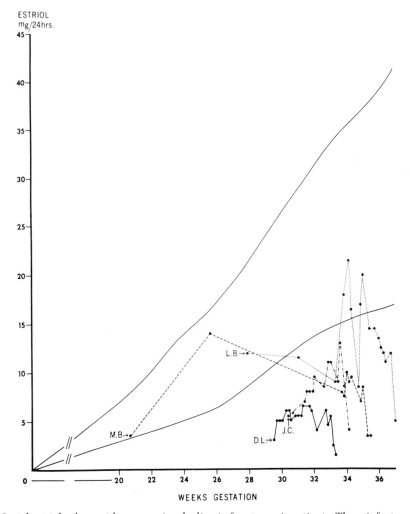

Figure 22. Serial estriol values with progressive decline in four toxemic patients. Three infants survived despite low birth weights. (From Magendantz, H. G., Klausner, D., Ryan, K. J., and Yen, S. S. C.: Obstet. Gynec., 32:610, 1968.)

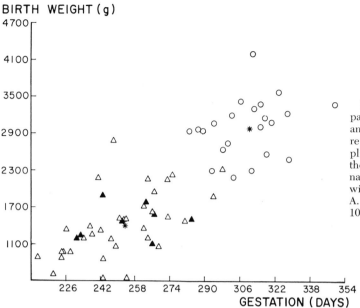

Figure 23. Gestational length in two patient populations of mothers bearing anencephalic offspring. The triangles represent those pregnancies with complications such as polyhydramnios, and the circles represent normal pregnancies. Anencephaly is often associated with prolonged gestation. (From Milic, A. B. M.: Amer. J. Obstet. Gynec., 104:134, 1969.)

neurohypophyseal oxytocin secretion, and pressure-volume relationships between the uterine contents and myometrial accommodation.[8] To this array of possibilities must be added fetal endocrine contributions to pregnancy length.

An endocrine mechanism in the prolonged pregnancies of Holstein-Friesian and Guernsey cows has been described. Recessive autosomal genetic constitutions of calf fetuses have been associated with fetal adrenal or pituitary malfunction and failure of the cow to deliver spontaneously.[24] These observations stimulated experimental study in sheep, where fetal pituitary destruction or fetal adrenalectomy caused prolonged pregnancy unless ACTH was infused into the hypophysectomized lamb in utero. Infusion of adrenal corticoids into the lamb but not into the ewe also caused prompt delivery whether the lamb was adrenalectomized or not.[3, 11, 12, 28-32] In the human, anencephaly of the fetus is associated with prolonged pregnancy unless hydramnios is present (Fig. 23). The possibility that a fetal adrenal secretory product contributes to pregnancy length must be considered.[2, 38, 50] The fetal adrenal secretes increasing quantities of cortisol as term approaches and cortisol can compete for protein binding sites with progesterone. The fetal adrenal also provides estrogen precursors for placental conversion to estrogens, as described in the sections of the biosynthesis of estrogens and the fetoplacental unit. As pregnancy progresses in the human, pregnanediol-estrogen ratios decline and estrogens may have a stimulatory effect on the myometrium.[26] It is not yet possible to establish the importance of either fetal corticoids or estrogen precursors in the control of pregnancy in man, but a role in domestic animals seems certain.

BIBLIOGRAPHY

1. Abramovich, D. R., and Wade, A. P.: Levels and significance of 17-oxosteroids and 17-hydroxycosteroids in amniotic fluid throughout pregnancy. J. Obstet. Gynaec. Brit. Comm., 76:893, 1969.
2. Anderson, A. B. M., Laurence, K. M., and Turnbull, A. C.: The relationship in anencephaly between the size of the adrenal cortex and the length of gestation. J. Obstet. Gynaec. Brit. Comm., 76: 196, 1969.
3. Bassett, J. M., and Thorburn, G. D.: Foetal plasma corticosteroids and the initiation of parturition in sheep. J. Endocr., 44:285, 1969.
4. Brown, J. B.: Urinary excretion of oestrogens during pregnancy, lactation, and the re-establishment of menstruation. Lancet, 1:704, 1956.
5. Brown, J. B., Beischer, N. A., and Smith, M. A.: Excretion of urinary oestrogens in pregnant patients treated with cortisone and its analogues. J. Obstet. Gynaec. Brit. Comm., 75:819, 1968.
6. Colas, A., Heinrichs, L. W., and Tatum, H. J.: Pettenkofer chromogens in the maternal and fetal circulations. Steroids, 3:417, 1964.
7. Coyle, M. G.: The urinary excretion of oestrogen in four cases of anencephaly and one case of

foetal death from cirrhosis of the liver. J. Endocr., 25:8, 1962.

8. Csapo, A. I., and Wood, C.: The endocrine control of the initiation of labour in the human. In James, V. H. T., ed.: Recent Advances in Endocrinology. Little, Brown and Co., Boston, 1968, p. 207.

9. Diczfalusy, E.: Steroid metabolism in pregnancy and in the foeto-placental unit. In Proceedings of the Second International Congress on Hormonal Steroids. Excerpta Medica International Congress Series, New York, 1966, p. 82.

10. Diczfalusy, E., and Marcuso, S.: Oestrogen metabolism in pregnancy. In Klopper, A., and Diczfalusy, E., eds.: Foetus and Placenta. Blackwell Scientific Publications, Oxford, 1969, p. 191.

11. Drost, M.: Bilateral adrenalectomy in the fetal lamb. Exp. Med. Surg., 26:61, 1968.

12. Drost, M., and Holm, L. W.: Prolonged gestation in ewes after foetal adrenalectomy. J. Endocr., 40:293, 1968.

13. Easterling, W. E., Jr., Simmer, H. H., Dignam, W. J., Frankland, M. V., and Naftolin, F.: Neutral C_{19}-steroids and steroid sulfates in human pregnancy. II. Dehydroepiandrosterone sulfate, 16 α-hydroxydehydroepiandrosterone, and 16 α-hydroxydehydroepiandrosterone sulfate in maternal and fetal blood of pregnancies with anencephalic and normal fetuses. Steroids, 8:157, 1966.

14. Eberlein, W. R.: Steroids and sterols in umbilical cord blood. J. Clin. Endocr., 25:1101, 1965.

15. Fishman, J., Brown, J. B., Hellman, L., Zumoff, B., and Gallagher, T. F.: Estrogen metabolism in normal and pregnant women. J. Biol. Chem., 237:1489, 1962.

16. France, J. T., and Liggins, G. C.: Placental sulfatase deficiency. J. Clin. Endocr., 29:138, 1969.

17. Frandsen, V. A.: The Excretion of Oestriol in Normal Human Pregnancy. Munksgaard, Copenhagen, 1963.

18. Frandsen, V. A.: The site of production of oestrogenic hormones in human pregnancy. Europ. Rev. Endocr., 1:227, 1965.

19. Frandsen, V. A., and Stakemann, G.: The site of production of oestrogenic hormones in human pregnancy. II. Experimental investigations on the role of the foetal adrenal. Acta Endocr., 43:184, 1963.

20. Frandsen, V. A., and Stakemann, G.: The site of production of oestrogenic hormones in human pregnancy. III. Further observations on the hormone excretion in pregnancy with anencephalic foetus. Acta Endocr., 47:265, 1964.

21. Greene, J. W., Jr., and Touchstone, J. C.: Urinary estriol as an index of placental function. Amer. J. Obstet. Gynec., 85:1, 1963.

22. Hellig, H., Gattereau, D., Lefebvre, Y., and Bolte, E.: Steroid production from plasma cholesterol. I. Conversion of plasma cholesterol to placental progesterone in humans. J. Clin. Endocr., 30:624, 1970.

23. Hobkirk, R., and Nilsen, M.: Observations on the occurrence of six estrogen fractions in human pregnancy urine. J. Clin. Endocr., 22:134, 1962.

24. Holm, L. W.: Prolonged pregnancy. Advances Vet. Sci., 11:159, 1967.

25. Johansson, E. D. B.: Plasma levels of progesterone in pregnancy measured by a rapid competitive protein binding technique. Acta Endocr., 61:607, 1969.

26. Klopper, A., and Billewicz, W.: Urinary excretion of oestriol and pregnanediol during normal pregnancy. J. Obstet. Gynaec. Brit. Comm., 70:1024, 1963.

27. Klopper, A., and Dennis, K. J.: The urinary excretion of oestriol after intra-amniotic injection of oestriol sulphate as a test of placental function. J. Obstet. Gynaec. Brit. Comm., 76:534, 1969.

28. Lanman, J. T., and Schaffer, A.: Gestational effects of fetal decapitation in sheep. Fertil. Steril., 19:598, 1968.

29. Liggins, G. C.: Premature parturition after infusion of corticotrophin or cortisol into foetal lambs. J. Endocr., 42:323, 1968.

30. Liggins, G. C.: Premature delivery of foetal lambs infused with glucocorticoids. J. Endocr., 45:515, 1969.

31. Liggins, G. C.: The foetal role in the initiation of parturition in the ewe. In Wolstenholme, G. E. W., and O'Connor, M., eds.: Ciba Foundation Symposium on Foetal Autonomy. J. and A. Churchill Ltd., London, 1969, p. 218.

32. Liggins, G. C., and Kennedy, P. C.: Effects of electrocoagulation of the foetal lamb hypophysis on growth and development. J. Endocr., 40:371, 1968.

33. MacDonald, P. C., and Siiteri, P. K.: Study of estrogen production in women with hydatidiform mole. J. Clin. Endocr., 24:685, 1964.

34. MacDonald, P. C., and Siiteri, P. K.: Origin of estrogen in women pregnant with an anencephalic fetus. J. Clin. Invest., 44:465, 1965.

35. Magendantz, H. G., Klausner, D., Ryan, K. J., and Yen, S. S. C.: Estriol determinations in the management of high-risk pregnancies. Obstet. Gynec., 32:610, 1968.

36. Magendantz, H. G., and Ryan, K. J.: Isolation of an estriol precursor, 16 α-hydroxydehydroepiandrosterone, from human umbilical sera. J. Clin. Endocr., 24:1155, 1964.

37. Michie, E. A.: Oestrogen levels in urine and amniotic fluid in pregnancy with live anencephalic foetus and the effect of intra-amniotic injection of sodium dehydroepiandrosterone sulphate on these levels. Acta Endocr., 51:535, 1966.

38. Milic, A. B., and Adamsons, K.: The relationship between anencephaly and prolonged pregnancy. J. Obstet. Gynaec. Brit. Comm., 76:102, 1969.

39. Nakayama, T., Arai, K., Yanaihara, T., Tabei, T., Satoh, K., and Nagatomi, K.: Oestrogen metabolism in anencephalus. Acta Endocr., 55:369, 1967.

40. Ryan, K. J.: Theoretical basis for endocrine control of gestation—a comparative approach. In Pecile, A., and Finzi, C., eds.: The Foeto-Placental Unit. Excerpta Medica Foundation, Amsterdam, 1969, pp. 120–131.

41. Ryan, K. J.: Endocrine control of gestational length. Amer. J. Obstet. Gynec., 109:299, 1971.

42. Ryan, K. J., and Ainsworth, L.: Comparative aspects of steroid hormones in reproduction. In Benirschke, K., ed.: Comparative Aspects of Reproductive Failure. Springer-Verlag, New York, 1967.

43. Ryan, K. J., Meigs, R., and Petro, Z.: The formation of progesterone by the human placenta. Amer. J. Obstet. Gynec., 96:676, 1966.

44. Schindler, A. E., and Ratanasopa, V.: Profile of steroids in amniotic fluid of normal and complicated pregnancies. Acta Endocr., 59:239, 1968.

45. Schindler, A. E., and Siiteri, P. K.: Isolation and quantitation of steroids from normal human amniotic fluid. J. Clin. Endocr., 28:1189, 1968.

46. Simmer, H. H., Dignam, W. J., Easterling, W. E., Jr., Frankland, M. V., and Naftolin, F.: Neutral C_{19}-steroids and steroid sulfates in human pregnancy. III. Dehydroepiandrosterone sulfate, 16 α-hydroxydehydroepiandrosterone, and 16 α-hydroxydehydroepiandrosterone sulfate in cord blood and blood of pregnant women with and without treatment with corticoids. Steroids, 8: 179, 1966.

47. Telegdy, G., Weeks, J. W., Archer, D. F., Wiqvist, N., and Diczfalusy, E.: Acetate and cholesterol metabolism in the human foeto-placental unit at midgestation; 3. Steroids synthesized and secreted by the foetus. Acta Endocr., 63:119, 1970.

48. Telegdy, G., Weeks, J. W., Lerner, U., Stakemann, G., and Diczfalusy, E.: Acetate and cholestrol metabolism in the human foeto-placental unit midgestation; 1. Synthesis of cholesterol. Acta Endocr., 63:91, 1970.

49. Telegdy, G., Weeks, J. W., Wiqvist, N., and Diczfalusy, E.: Acetate and cholesterol metabolism in the human foeto-placental unit at midgestation; 2. Steroids synthesized and secreted by the placenta. Acta Endocr., 63:105, 1970.

50. Trumbull, A. C., Anderson, A. B. M., and Wilson, G. R.: Maternal urinary oestrogen excretion as evidence of a foetal role in determining gestation at labour. Lancet, 2:627, 1967.

51. Villee, D. B.: Development of endocrine function in the human placenta and fetus. New Eng. J. Med., 281:473, 533, 1968.

52. Warren, J. C., and Cheatum, S. G.: Maternal urinary estrogen excretion: effect of adrenal suppression. J. Clin. Endocr., 27:433, 1967.

53. Wu, C. H., Flickinger, G. L., and Touchstone, J. C.: Conversion of dehydroepiandrosterone-7 α-^{3}H to oestrogens by corpus luteum, placenta, and placenta plus foetal viscera in early human pregnancy. Acta Endocr., 54:181, 1967.

54. Wu, C. H., Touchstone, J. C., and Flickinger, G. L.: Estrogen formation in vitro by fetoplacental tissues of midpregnancy. Amer. J. Obstet. Gynec., 102:862, 1968.

55. Yoshimi, T., Strott, C. A., Marshall, J. R., and Lipsett, M. B.: Corpus luteum function in early pregnancy. J. Clin. Endocr., 29:225, 1969.

56. Younglai, E. V., and Solomon, S.: Neutral steroids in human pregnancy: Isolation, formation and metabolism. In Klopper, A., and Diczfalusy, E., eds.: Foetus and Placenta. Blackwell Scientific Publications, Oxford, 1969, p. 249.

METABOLIC-HOMEOSTATIC ENDOCRINE SYSTEMS IN PREGNANCY

The total endocrine picture in reproduction is larger than the maternal-placental and feto-placental production of hormones just discussed. It also encompasses those metabolic and homeostatic processes that must adapt to the added load imposed by pregnancy. In general, the fetus and placenta do not compensate for most maternal endocrine deficiency states and, if anything, pregnancy increases the demands on the nonreproductive endocrine system. Thus, patients with surgical loss or hypoactivity of the pituitary, thyroid, pancreas, or adrenal before or during pregnancy must be given replacement hormones. The placenta has a prodigious capacity to synthesize various substances but not those ordinarily required for control of metabolism and homeostasis, and fetal hormones are not transferred in quantities sufficient to make up for absence of these in the mother.

Thyroid Function

For many years it was believed that pregnancy represented a state of mild "hyperthyroidism" with elevated oxygen consumption, fast pulse rate, increased protein-bound iodine, enlarged gland, and susceptibility to hypertension and toxemia. For the most part, these changes can be explained by factors other than net increase in active thyroid hormone secretion. The increased oxygen consumption is believed to represent the increased fetal and uterine requirements. As far as is now known, pituitary thyrotropin secretion is elevated in pregnancy but the role and contribution of the placental thyrotropin is unknown. Renal clearance of inorganic iodine is increased and the thyroid gland must clear twice as much blood to maintain the nonpregnancy level of iodine trapping.[1] The gland itself probably does increase in size but reliable objective documentation of this is difficult to obtain. In general, there is a clinical and historical impression that "goiter" is increased in the pregnant state. Histologically, there is a degree of hyperplasia and increased follicular size of the thyroid during pregnancy. Estrogens and pregnancy, probably because of estrogens, increase the circulating thyroid-binding globulin so that bound thyroid hormone (PBI) is increased in the blood stream but is not as available for metabolic action (Table 5). The in-vitro resin uptake test for radioactive thyroxin is evidence of this because, although the PBI is elevated in pregnancy, less of this material is available for transfer and

TABLE 5. COMPARISON OF THYROID FUNCTION IN MOTHER, NEWBORN, AND NONPREGNANT ADULT*

	PBI† (µg./100 ml.)	RT_3 (Fraction)	FT_4 (ng./100 ml.)	TBG (µg./100 ml.)	TSH (µU/ml.)
Maternal sera	6.96	0.68	1.84	54.2	7.17
Umbilical cord sera	7.08	0.913	2.19	37.3	11.8
Nonpregnant adult sera	4.0–8.0	0.8–1.2	1.4–2.5	16–24	0–5

*From Robin, N. I., Refetoff, S., Fang, V., and Selenkow, H. A.: J. Clin. Endocr., 29:1276, 1969.
†PBI – Protein-bound iodine; RT_3 – Triiodothyronine resin uptake; FT_4 – Free thyroxin; TBG – Thyroxin-binding globulin; TSH – Thyrotropin.

the competitive resin uptake is lowered.[13] In hyperthyroidism, with or without pregnancy, both the PBI and resin uptake are elevated. This provides a mechanism for distinguishing the elevated PBI of thyrotoxicosis and pregnancy. Thyroxin is only slowly transferred in either direction across the placenta. The mother bearing an athyrotic child must be given large doses in order to make some available to the fetus. Hypothyroid mothers do not receive sufficient thyroxin from the fetus to alter their blood thyroid levels and must receive exogenous hormones. Triiodothyronine is transferred across the placenta more readily than thyroxin.[6]

Adrenal Function

As with the thyroid, it was once thought that pregnancy caused adrenal hyperactivity, similar to Cushing's disease. It is now accepted, however, that this is partially but not a completely true picture of what is going on. The occasional regression of rheumatoid arthritis during pregnancy and the suspected associated hyperadrenal state were cited as clues which led to the clinical use of cortisone in treatment of the rheumatic diseases. There was some evidence that the placenta synthesized adrenal steroids and that addisonian patients improved in pregnancy. The altered carbohydrate metabolism, edema, and striae seen during both gestation and Cushing's syndrome were used as further evidence for increased adrenal function in pregnancy.

Recent evidence has clarified the situation somewhat. Corticotropin is not known to be increased in pregnancy and there is as yet no evidence that the placenta produces an adrenal tropic hormone. Patients with prior adrenal removal require cortisol replacement during pregnancy, and the

evidence for placental production of adrenal steroids does not withstand critical scrutiny.

Estrogens and pregnancy, because of estrogens, raise the cortisol-binding globulin, and as is the case with thyroxin, total blood corticoids are increased.[5, 14] Free active cortisol levels are higher than in the nonpregnant state and the diurnal variation is blunted so that there is a true state of hyperactivity, but at a lower level than originally anticipated.[10] The metabolism of the corticoids is altered and the half-life in blood is prolonged. Excretion of corticoid metabolites in the urine rises at a slow rate during pregnancy. The response of the adrenal to exogenous ACTH is, however, somewhat blunted during pregnancy.[4] The metabolic effects of the slightly increased free cortisol are yet to be clearly defined although this could contribute to the diabetogenic tendency seen in pregnancy.

Insulin

Carbohydrate and fat metabolism are markedly altered during pregnancy, and while all of the contributing factors are unknown, certain indications of possible mechanisms are now available. Chorionic somato-mammotropin has been shown to be diabetogenic and to counteract insulin effects in man. Free cortisol is increased and the response of growth hormone to hypoglycemia is impaired in late pregnancy as well. The oral glucose tolerance test is more apt to be abnormal during gestation than the intravenous test, but the roles of altered absorption and the different insulogenic effects of an oral versus an intravenous load have not been adequately explained.[11]

In any case, during early pregnancy, an intravenous glucose load is handled more efficiently than in late pregnancy, while the immunologically determined blood insulin levels rise as pregnancy advances.[15-17, 21] Later in pregnancy glucose handling is impaired. The poorer glucose clearance in the face of higher blood insulin levels is believed due to anti-insulin factors which might be based upon some of the mechanisms listed above. All of these effects would tend to make an existing diabetic state worse or might provoke glucose intolerance in someone with borderline pancreatic function. Similar effects are seen in patients after the administration of contraceptive steroids.[21]

Renin-Angiotensin System and Aldosterone

There is a complex homeostatic mechanism for the regulation of blood volume and water and electrolyte metabolism that is increased in activity during normal pregnancy.[12]

Conditions that reduce extracellular or blood volume cause increased release of renin from the juxtaglomerular cells of the kidney. Renin is an enzyme that acts on the blood-borne substrate angiotensinogen produced by the liver. The product is angiotensin I, a 10-amino acid polypeptide which is in turn converted by another enzyme to the active agent angiotensin II, an 8-amino acid peptide that specifically induces aldosterone secretion by the adrenal and also has a direct pressor effect on the vascular system. The sodium and water retention produced by aldosterone ultimately increases plasma volume and by a negative feedback mechanism reduces renin release and then adrenal production of aldosterone.

Estrogens have been reported to increase renin substrate and, to a lesser extent, blood levels of renin. The effect is more pronounced when sodium is restricted. During the third trimester of pregnancy, plasma renin activity is markedly elevated but returns to normal within six seeks post partum. No change in renin activity was observed for the first week after delivery, making it unlikely that the placenta or fetus is the source of renin during pregnancy. It is likely that at least some of the increased renin activity of the pregnant state is due to the high levels of estrogens.[2, 3, 7, 9] The increased renin activity is also believed responsible for the augmented production of aldosterone during gestation.[8, 18-20]

BIBLIOGRAPHY

1. Aboul-Khair, S. A., Crooks, J., Turnbull, A. C., and Hytten, F. E.: The physiological changes in thyroid function during pregnancy. Clin. Sci., 27:195, 1964.
2. Boonshaft, B., O'Connell, J. M. B., Jayes, J. M., and Schreiner, G. E.: Serum renin activity during normal pregnancy: effect of alterations of posture and sodium intake. J. Clin. Endocr., 28:1641, 1968.
3. Crane, M. B., and Harris, J. J.: Plasma renin activity and aldosterone excretion rate in normal subjects. I. Effect of ethinyl estradiol and medroxyprogesterone acetate. J. Clin. Endocr., 29:550, 1969.
4. Dickey, R. P., and Thompson, J. P.: Effect of ACTH and metyrapone on estriol, 17-hydroxycorticosteroid, 17-ketosteroid, pregnanediol and pregnanetriol excretion late in pregnancy. J. Clin. Endocr., 29:701, 1969.
5. Doe, R. P., Dickinson, P., Zinneman, H. H., and Seal, U.S.: Elevated nonprotein-bound cortisol (NPC) in pregnancy, during estrogen administration and in carcinoma of the prostate. J. Clin. Endocr., 29:757, 1969.
6. Dussault, J., Row, V. V., Lickrish, G., and Volpe, R.: Studies of serum triiodothyronine concentration in maternal and cord blood: Transfer of triiodothyronine across the human placenta. J. Clin. Endocr., 29:595, 1969.
7. Geelhoed, G. W., and Vander, A. J.: Plasma renin activities during pregnancy and parturition. J. Clin. Endocr., 28:412, 1968.
8. Jones, K. M., Lloyd-Jones, R., Riondel, A., Tait, J. F., Tait, S. A. S., Bulbrook, R. D., and Greenwood, F. C.: Aldosterone secretion and metabolism in normal men and women and in pregnancy. Acta Endocr., 30:321, 1959.
9. Menard, J., Malmejac, A., and Milliez, P.: Influence of diethylstilbestrol on the renin-angiotensin system of male rats. Endocrinology, 86:774, 1970.
10. O'Connell, M., and Welsh, G. W., 3rd: Unbound plasma cortisol in pregnant and Enovoid-E treated women as determined by ultrafiltration. J. Clin. Endocr., 29:563, 1969.
11. O'Sullivan, J. B., Snyder, P. J., Sporer, A. C., Dandrow, R. V., Jr., and Charles, D.: Intravenous glucose tolerance test and its modification by pregnancy. J. Clin. Endocr., 31:33, 1970.
12. Peart, W. S.: The renin-angiotensin system. Pharmacol. Rev., 17:143, 1965.
13. Robin, N. I., Refetoff, S., Fang, V., and Selenkow, H. A.: Parameters of thyroid function in maternal and cord serum at term pregnancy. J. Clin. Endocr., 29:1276, 1969.
14. Rosenthal, H. E., Slaunwhite, W. R., Jr., and Sandberg, A. A.: Transcortin: a corticosteroid-binding protein of plasma. X. Cortisol and progesterone interplay and unbound levels of these steroids in pregnancy. J. Clin. Endocr., 29:352, 1969.
15. Spellacy, W. N., and Goetz, F. C.: Plasma insulin in normal late pregnancy. New Eng. J. Med., 268:988, 1963.

16. Spellacy, W. N., Goetz, F. C., Greenberg, B. Z., and Ells, J.: Plasma insulin in normal "early" pregnancy. Obstet. Gynec., 25:862, 1965.

17. Spellacy, W. N., Goetz, F. C., Greenberg, B. Z., and Ells, J.: Plasma insulin in normal mid-pregnancy. Amer. J. Obstet. Gynec., 92:11, 1965.

18. Tait, J. F., and Little, G.: The metabolism of orally and intravenously administered labeled aldosterone in pregnant subjects. J. Clin. Invest., 47:2423, 1968.

19. Tait, J. F., Little, B., Tait, S. A. S., and Flood, C.: The mebabolic clearance rate of aldosterone in pregnant and nonpregnant subjects estimated by both single-injection and constant infusion methods. J. Clin. Invest., 41:2093, 1962.

20. Vande Wiele, R. L., Gurpide, E., Kelly, W. G., Laragh, J. H., and Lieberman, S.: The secretory rate of progesterone and aldosterone in abnormal late pregnancy. Acta Endocr., Suppl. 51, p. 159, 1960.

21. Yen, S. S. C., and Vela, P.: Effects of contraceptive steroids on carbohydrate metabolism. J. Clin. Endocr., 28:1564, 1968.

MAMMARY GLAND AND LACTATION

The mammary gland and lactation represent the only truly unique features of reproduction of the Mammalia and the major basis, of course, for designating them as a separate class of animals. In addition, the growth and function of the breasts involves the most exquisite integration of the nervous system and the reproductive and homeostatic hormones, a model of evolutionary adaptation.

MAMMARY GLAND DEVELOPMENT AND ANATOMY

In the embryo, a raised area of ectoderm appears on either side of the midline and is designated the mammary band. In the midline of this band, a ridge develops as the mammary crest and from this crest evolve the primitive mammary buds. These separate buds are epithelial nodules that give rise to the breast. The multiple nipples occasionally seen as accessory remnants in the human along the path of the mammary crest represent failure of normal involution to take place in all but the area that gives rise to the two definitive breasts. The mammary anlagen have been variously attributed to evolution from sweat glands, sebaceous glands, hair follicles, or de-novo development. The structure of the breast most closely approximates that of the sweat glands, but the mammae develop a capacity to respond to hormonal stimulation in a way that is different from the response of any of the possible homologues.[3, 6]

By the fifth month of fetal life, the ectodermal cells of the mammary bud proliferate and develop cords which give rise to the ducts of the adult gland. The underlying mesenchyne differentiates into zones from which the smooth muscle and connective tissue of the gland develop.

The nipple becomes prominent in the fifth and sixth months of fetal life but the mammary bud becomes depressed thereafter until term when it is pushed outward. Failure of the nipple to develop in this way may result in the various stages of inverted nipple seen in later life. From birth until puberty the breast in both males and females remains in a quiescent state until stimulated by the increased hormone levels typical of adolescence. There appears to be no innate difference between the breast tissue of the two sexes since even the male mammary gland can be made to grow (gynecomastia) and, rarely, secrete milk in response to appropriate hormonal and neurologic stimuli.

STRUCTURE OF ADULT MAMMARY GLAND

The human mammary glands are hemispheric organs lying on the pectoral muscles and deep fascia and occupying the space between the edge of the sternum and the ventral fold of the axilla from the level of the second rib to the sixth or seventh costal cartilage. Surmounting the breast just lateral and caudal to its center is the areola, a thin, pigmented, circular patch of skin from which the nipple protrudes surrounded by roughened elevations that represent sebaceous glands or glands of Montgomery.

The mammary gland parenchyma consists of a network of ducts branching out into a network of alveolar units. The alveoli are sacs made up of a layer of secretory cells surrounded by a covering of myoepithelial cells which can force milk into the duct system in response to oxytocin. A group of alveoli makes up a lobule, a group of which in turn makes up each of the 15 to 20 lobes of the breast. The intralobular ducts from alveoli lead to lactiferous ducts and thence to sinuses of which some 8 to 15 open on the surface of the nipple. The nipple is itself an erectile organ by virtue of both muscle contraction and vascular engorgement.[6, 8]

THE BREAST IN PREGNANCY

The breasts during the earlier weeks of pregnancy are firm and tender, and patients often complain of discomfort. Although the breasts usually continue to undergo some enlargement, they subsequently soften and the discomfort disappears. The glands of Montgomery often become prominent during pregnancy, and this is listed among the diagnostic signs of pregnancy. The areolar area tends to assume a greater degree of pigmentation. Shortly after the missed period, a slight amount of watery fluid may be expressed from the nipple, and in primiparous patients this is a useful sign in the diagnosis of pregnancy. In women who have recently borne children, however, especially those who have breast-fed their infants, secretion can be expressed from the nipple in the absence of pregnancy. As pregnancy advances, the fluid becomes whitish and thicker, and is known as colostrum.

During and after pregnancy the breast undergoes histologic changes which are quite characteristic for the three trimesters and for the periods of lactation and subinvolution. However, the various areas of the breast in pregnancy may respond differently to endocrine stimulation, with one lobule showing marked growth whereas an adjacent lobule may reveal little or no growth. During the first trimester the distal portions of the breast tubules reveal sprouting and epithelial proliferation with gland formation. The stroma of the lobules, which is composed of dense collagenous fibers, becomes displaced and compressed as the result of tubular growth. By the end of the 16th week the breast lobules are considerably enlarged. There is an increase in the number and the size of the glands with slight dilatation of the gland lumina which contain a small amount of secretion (Fig.

24A). The epithelial cells have a few vacuoles in the cytoplasm. During the middle trimester, the terminal ends of the tubules become dilated, and the cuboidal epithelium lining the glands acquires an increased fat content. In the last trimester, the epithelial cells lining the glands become flattened, and many of these cells have vacuoles in their cytoplasm. The glands are markedly dilated with inspissated acidophilic secretion (Fig. 24B). The connective tissue appears more cellular and the dense collagen bundles seen between the lobules in the earlier stages have largely disappeared.

The lactating breast reveals additional enlargement of the lobules. The secretion from the epithelial cells, which is now copious, distends the glands. The ducts leading to the tubules, which serve as a storehouse for the milk, likewise become distended. The connective tissue becomes markedly edematous in the intermediate postpartum period, during the time of breast engorgement (Fig. 25A). The cells of the gland, which now abut upon one another, show much vacuolated cytoplasm. At about the fourth or fifth postpartum day, the epithelial cells lining the acini contain many vacuoles consistent with established lactation (Fig. 25B). In the absence of breast feeding, involutional changes soon make their appearance, with the breast stroma again becoming prominent. The glands eventually collapse and the majority disappear. Phagocytosis and round cell infiltration are prominent features of these regressive changes. Late in the puerperium, or with reestablishment of the menses, the breast has returned morphologically to a nonpregnant state (Fig. 25C). Occasionally residual changes are observed, and in certain areas the lobules may retain their lactating appearance; this indicates that the gland may involute in a very irregular fashion.

HORMONAL CONTROL OF MAMMARY GROWTH AND LACTATION

The endocrine control of breast function is extremely complex and the details are still controversial.[3, 8] The techniques employed for studying the problem have

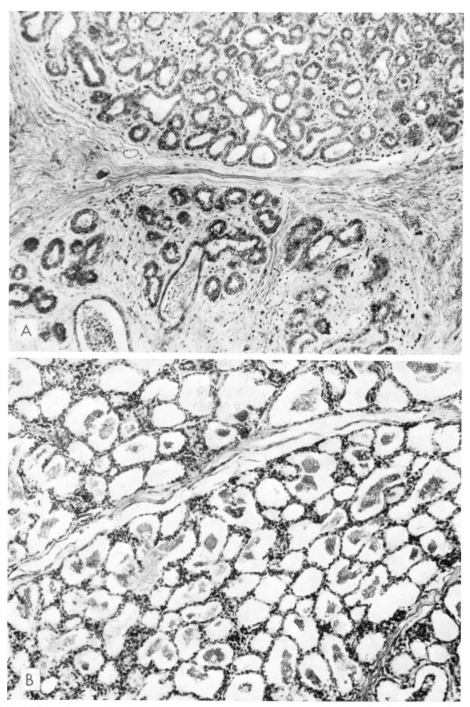

Figure 24. Photomicrographs of the breast during pregnancy. × 70. A, At 16 weeks, the few glands occupying the lower half of the photograph illustrate the fact that the breast may respond in an irregular fashion to the stimulus of pregnancy. A slight lymphocytic infiltration will be noted in this area. B, At about the thirtieth week of pregnancy, the heavy interlobular connective tissue is much less prominent. The glands of the lobule are dilated and filled with acidophilic material.

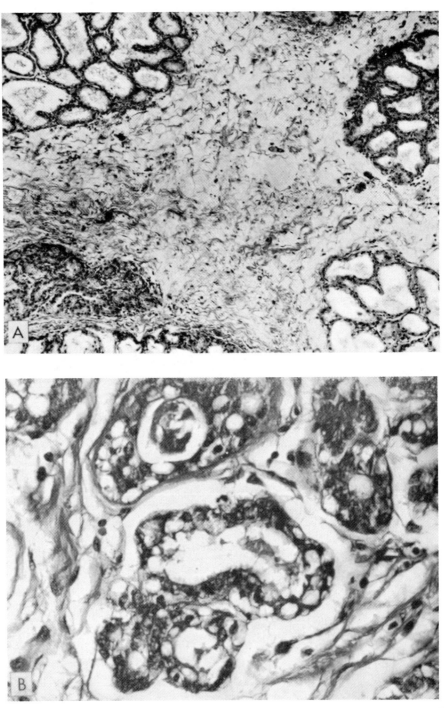

Figure 25.   Photomicrographs of the breast after delivery. A, At two days post partum. × 70. The gland lumina contain a granular precipitate and a few fatty macrophages. The period of engorgement is evident by the extreme degree of edema of the connective tissue. B, During lactation. × 400.

largely involved hormone replacement to animals after endocrine gland removal. Complete application to man is tenuous at best.

Estrogen can stimulate mammary duct growth in oophorectomized animals, and in high and prolonged dosage can stimulate some alveolar growth as well. Full alveolar development, however, requires the addition of the effects of progesterone to those already produced by prior estrogen. Thus, estrogen and progesterone appear to be synergistically and fundamentally involved in breast development. The effects of these two steroid hormones are observed in hypophysectomized animals but to a lesser extent than in animals with intact pituitary function. This pituitary deficiency can be overcome by the administration of prolactin or somatotropin or both in addition to the estrogen and progesterone. Complicating this picture is the fact that mammary growth can be induced in developed glands by prolactin and growth hormone in the absence of all steroid hormones. In essence, the total development of the breast is believed to involve both steroid and pituitary hormones. By studying pancreatectomized or hypophysectomized animals it can be demonstrated that, in order of decreasing need, insulin, cortisol, and thyroxin all contribute to normal mammary growth as well.

When a gland is fully developed, prolactin can induce milk secretion, even by local application into one of the main mammary ducts. Optimal milk secretion requires estrogen, progesterone, prolactin, somatotropin, insulin, cortisol, and to a lesser extent thyroxin. Once secretion is initiated, lactation can occur by movement of milk out of the alveoli and small ducts into the sinuses caused by the effect of oxytocin on the myoepithelial layer that surrounds the alveolar sac. In effect lactation therefore comprises two distinct processes, secretion of the milk into the alveoli and discharge of the milk via the milk-ejecting action of oxytocin. Once milk secretion is started by prolactin, the continued presence of prolactin is required but estrogen and progesterone can be dispensed with.

Thyroxin, cortisol, or insulin deficiency impairs milk production. The regulating action of the adrenal in electrolyte, carbohydrate, and protein metabolism makes its relationship to lactation obvious. Insulin is required for control of blood sugar levels

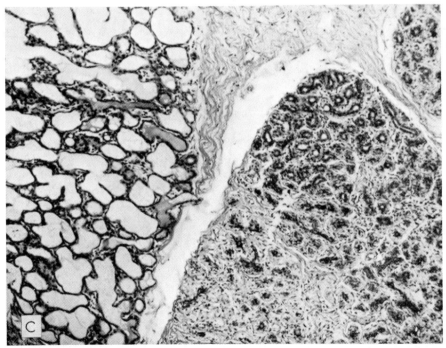

Figure 25. *Continued.* C, At six months post partum, and one month after cessation of nursing. × 70. The lobule on the left has retained the appearance of a lactating breast. The lobules on the right are decreased in size. The glands are narrowed and the cells are no longer vacuolated. The interlobular connective tissue has assumed its normal collagenous appearance.

and utilization. In diabetics the instability of blood sugar and changing insulin requirements, especially in the puerperium, may result in ineffective lactation. Parathormone can also be dispensed with if calcium and phosphorus blood levels are appropriately maintained.

In human pregnancy, a placental lactogen is present in large amounts until parturition and may play a role in breast development. The existence of a separate pituitary prolactin has not yet been established for the human and it has been postulated that somatotropin (which has lactogenic activity) may fill this role. On the other hand, blood levels of growth hormone are not elevated in normal lactating women post partum or during galactorrhea.[1, 14] Lactation can occur post partum in ateliotic dwarfs in the absence of plasma growth hormone as measured by radioimmunoassay,[14] and a decrease in growth hormone accompanies an increase in prolactin in tissue culture of both human and rhesus monkey adenohyophysis.[2, 9, 10] The only conclusion possible at present is that there is a distinct prolactin in the primate in spite of the failure thus far to isolate it.[5, 11] The possibility remains that it is very similar to human growth hormone chemically or that it represents a portion of the growth hormone molecule that is antigenically distinct.

Neurologic pathways, at least in certain animals, are not critical for lactation to occur since complete transplantation of the mammary gland has been carried out without a drop in milk production. In some animals oxytocin must be supplied after transplantation of the gland, presumably because of interruption of the reflex pathway for milk ejection.

CONTROL OF THE INITIATION OF LACTATION AT BIRTH

All of the hormonal components for lactation are present in the prenatal period but milk secretion does not begin until delivery has occurred. It is believed that the high levels of estrogen or progesterone inhibit prolactin release and perhaps prolactin action on the breast itself. At delivery, the sudden decrease in steroids would tend to remove all the inhibitory effects. Evidence for such a mechanism is based on the observation that administration of a high dose of estrogens in the first week post partum will usually prevent breast engorgement. It is

not known, however, whether this is due to prolactin inhibition.

Lactation will usually not occur in any pregnancy that terminates prior to the fourth or fifth month and hence a certain amount of the hormonal priming of pregnancy is required before the breast is prepared for lactation.

Suckling stimulates both continued prolactin secretion and oxytocin release and tends to maintain lactation in a form of positive feedback stimulation.

After delivery, the breast becomes greatly engorged and remains so for the first few days of the puerperium. During this prelactation period the breasts are often tender and uncomfortable. Engorgement, however, is not synonymous with milk production, for, although colostrum is more plentiful, little or no milk is evident during this period. Usually within four or five days after delivery, when the engorgement starts to subside, lactation is established. The breasts soften and, under the stimulus of suckling, become productive. The possibility of the excretion of drugs into milk, where they can gain access to the infant, should be borne in mind.[15]

LACTATION AMENORRHEA

Suckling and prolactin release tend to inhibit the production and secretion of FSH and LH and also the cyclic or ovulatory surge of LH responsible for ovulation. It is a prevalent belief, certainly among patients, that the phenomenon of lactation is associated with amenorrhea and, hence, that the lactating individual is temporarily infertile. Such is not the case, however, and although pregnancy is not common in lactating women who are amenorrheic, the reappearance of menstruation during lactation is not unusual, the approximate range varying enormously (between 40 and 75 per cent).[7] Of the women who conceived within a year after delivery, two thirds were lactating at the time, and one tenth of them never had a period prior to conceiving.[12] In addition, the cycle is more likely to reappear as the duration of feeding increases (Fig. 26). It is presumed that the stimulus of suckling inhibits the cycle and, hence, ovulation. As mentioned above, some 7 to 10 per cent of lactating women may conceive, but rarely in the absence of the menses. The patient should appreciate or be made aware of the fact that ovarian activity

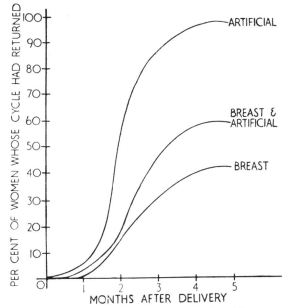

Figure 26. Return of menstruation after delivery, in relation to method of infant feeding. (From McKeown, T., and Gibson, J. R.: J. Obstet. Gynaec. Brit. Emp., 61:824, 1954.)

precedes uterine bleeding and conception can occur without prior menses. Why the menstrual cycle is suppressed must involve the influence of suckling on gonadotropin activity through the hypothalamic-pituitary axis.

Galactorrhea with amenorrhea may persist for long periods of time after breast feeding has been discontinued (Chiari-Frommel syndrome), may occur as a benign condition unassociated with pregnancy and postpartum lactation (Ahumada-del Castillo syndrome), or may occur in association with a pituitary tumor.[4, 13] Of note is the reciprocal relationship of the presence of prolactin production in the absence of gonadotropins which reflects the difference in normal control by the hypothalamus. Prolactin ordinarily is not secreted, owing to a hypothalamic inhibiting factor, and gonadotropins are ordinarily secreted in response to releasing factors. Tranquilizers of the phenothiazine type and other drugs can block hypothalamic control of the pituitary, causing galactorrhea and amenorrhea, in which case prolactin is released from its inhibition and gonadotropin secretion is inhibited. The etiology of the nonpregnancy type of galactorrhea is unknown. Aside from central nervous system tumors, the most frequent causal factor has been pharmacologic agents. In the benign cases,

there is a high rate of spontaneous remission.

BIBLIOGRAPHY

1. Benjamin, F., Casper, D. J., and Kalodny, H. H.: Immunoreactive human growth hormone in conditions associated with galactorrhea. Obstet. Gynec., 34:34, 1969.
2. Brauman, J., Brauman, H., and Pasteels, J.-L.: Immunoassay of growth hormone in cultures of human hypophysis by the method of complement fixation: comparison of the growth hormone secretion and the prolactin activity. Nature, 202:1116, 1964.
3. Cowie, A. T., and Folley, S. J.: The Mammary Gland and Lactation. In Young, W. C., ed.: Sex and Internal Secretions, Vol. 1, 3rd ed. Williams and Wilkins, Baltimore, 1961, p. 590.
4. Forbes, A. P., Henneman, P. H., Greswold, G. C., and Albright, F.: Syndrome characterized by galactorrhea, amenorrhea and low urinary FSH, comparison with acromegaly and normal lactation. J. Clin. Endocr., 14:265, 1954.
5. Goluboff, L. G., and Ezrin, C.: Effect of pregnancy on the somatotroph and the prolactin cell of the human adenohypophysis. J. Clin. Endocr., 29:1533, 1969.
6. Kon, S. K., and Cowie, A. T.: Milk: The Mammary Gland and Its Secretion. Academic Press, New York, 1961.
7. McKeown, T., and Gibson, J. R.: A note on menstruation and conception during lactation. J. Obstet. Gynec. Brit. Emp., 61:824, 1954.
8. Meites, J.: Control of mammary growth and lactation. In Martini, L., and Ganong, W. F., eds.: Neuroendocrinology, Vol. 1. Academic Press, New York, 1966, p. 669.
9. Nicoll, C. S., Parsons, J. A., Fiorindo, R. P., Nichols, C. W., Jr., and Sakuma, M.: Evidence of independent secretion of prolactin and growth hormone *in vitro* by adenohypophyses of rhesus monkeys. J. Clin. Endocr., 30:512, 1970.
10. Pasteels, J.-L., Brauman, H., and Brauman, J.: Etude comparée de la sécrétion d'hormone somatotrope par l'hypophyse humaine *in vitro* et de son activité lactogénique. C. R. Acad. Sci., 256:2031, 1963.
11. Peake, G. T., McKeel, D. W., Jarett, L., and Daughaday, W. H.: Ultrastructural, histologic and hormonal characterization of a prolactin-rich human pituitary tumor. J. Clin. Endocr., 29:1383, 1969.
12. Peckham, C. H.: On investigation of some effects of pregnancy noted six weeks after delivery. Bull. Johns Hopkins Hosp., 54:186, 1934.
13. Rankin, J. S., Goldpart, A. F., and Rakoff, A. E.: Galactorrhea-amenorrhea syndromes: postpartum galactorrhea-amenorrhea in the absence of intracranial neoplasm. Obstet. Gynec., 33:1, 1969.
14. Rimon, D. L., Holzman, G. B., Merinee, T. J., Rabinowitz, D., Barnes, A. C., Tyson, J. E. A., and McKusick, V. A.: Lactation in the absence of human growth hormone. J. Clin. Endocr., 28:1183, 1968.
15. Sapeika, N.: Excretion of drugs in human milk: a review. J. Obstet. Gynec. Brit. Emp., 54:426, 1947.

PART II

The Physiology
of Reproduction

Chapter 5

The Embryology and Anatomy of the Female Reproductive Tract

EMBRYOLOGY OF THE FEMALE REPRODUCTIVE TRACT

The anomalous embryonic development of the female reproductive system can lead to problems of intersexuality, infertility, pregnancy failure, or congenital neoplasms. On occasion, these aberrations can be traced to abnormalities in the embryonic urinary system and hindgut portion of the digestive system. In any consideration of the embryonic development of the female reproductive tract some reference must be made to the development of the latter two systems.

OVARY

The gonadal ridges are observed in embryos of five to six weeks' fertilization age (7 to 12 mm.), but the gonads remain sexually nondifferentiated until after the seventh week (17 to 20 mm.). During this interval of growth the gonadal ridge becomes covered by the splanchnic mesoderm overlying the urogenital ridge. In this location the mesoderm is modified to become the germinal epithelium, which will overlie

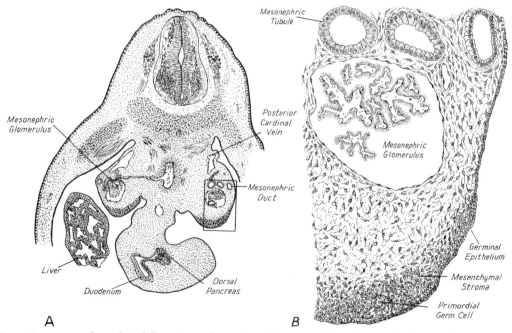

A   B

Figure 1. Section through indifferent gonad of 10 mm. human embryo. A, Drawing illustrating topography. ×30. B, Drawing of small area outlined by rectangle in A. ×200. (Figures 1 and 4 to 10 are used or modified by permission from Human Embryology, by B. M. Patten, 2nd ed., copyright 1953. Blakiston Division, McGraw-Hill Book Co., Inc.)

the tunica albuginea of the mature gonad (Fig. 1).

That the germ cells originate extra-gonadally is confirmed by human material, which shows that they are found among yolk sac endodermal cells or in the primitive hindgut. The original germ cells are probably set aside during early segmentation of the *germ disc* when it consists of five to eight cells. These cells migrate through the mesenchyme of the primitive mesentery (Fig. 2) and eventually lodge in the gonadal ridge, where they tend to arrange themselves near the surface close to the germinal epithelium (Fig. 3). At one time it was believed that the sex cells originate from germinal epithelium covering the gonad; if this were true, migration of the sex cells into the substance of the ovary would be restricted to the period of its early development because the tunica albuginea is well developed in 180 mm. embryos and separates the germinal epithelium from the ovarian mesenchyme.

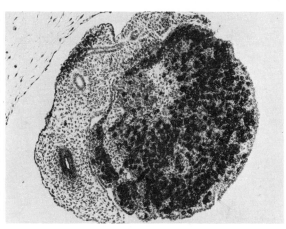

Figure 3. Right gonad of 35 mm. female embryo, containing many germ cells. ×90. (From McKay, D. G., Hertig, A. T., Adams, E. C., and Danziger, S., Anat. Rec., 117:201, 1953.)

In the male the sex cords, which are the primordia of the seminiferous tubules, appear much earlier than they do in the female (Fig. 4). Equally conspicuous are the interstitial cells. In the course of sex differentiation, the development of the internal and external sex organs in the male embryo is presumably under the influence of the rapidly growing interstitial cells. Earlier speculations regarding a further hormonal contribution by the fetal adrenals have not been supported by more recent investigations.

In the female embryo the gonadal tissue merely increases in mass during the period corresponding to that of rapid testicular development in the male. By the 17th to the 18th week (150 to 160 mm.), the embryonic ovary begins to differentiate; this process culminates in the formation of primary follicles. The mesenchyme near the hilus of the ovary becomes transformed into spindle-shaped stromal cells, and this process extends out through the medulla into the cortex. The stromal cells, which surround the primitive follicle, in turn enlarge to become theca cells. Prior to these stromal changes the pregranulosa cells of the sex cords arrange themselves about the primitive sex cell in a rosette pattern to form the anlage of the primary follicle, when they undergo transformation into cuboidal granulosa cells (Fig. 5).

Complete agreement is lacking with respect to the origin of the different types of cells composing the ovary. The rapidity with which the successive changes occur

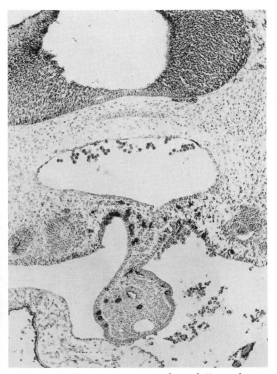

Figure 2. Transverse section through 5 mm. human embryo, showing spinal cord, aorta, urogenital ridges, and primitive gut. The primitive germ cells, outlined by the Seligman alkaline phosphatase technique, are present in the coelomic epithelium, connective tissue of the mesentery, and the developing gonadal folds. ×100. (From McKay, D. G., Hertig, A. T., Adams, E. C., and Danziger, S., Anat. Rec., 117:201, 1953.)

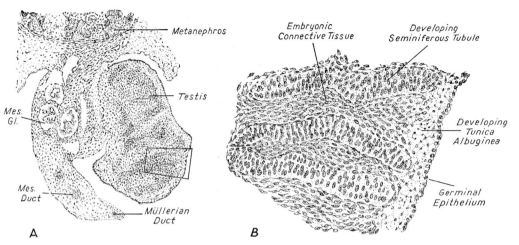

Figure 4. Drawing of cross-section through body of eight week (30 mm.) male embryo. A, Drawing illustrating topography. ×50. B, Small area of testis outlined in A. ×200. (From Patten.)

during embryonic development makes it difficult to identify the source of specific ovarian elements. The view has been presented that the sex cords originate from ovarian mesenchyme in situ, and these become modified to form epithelial granulosa cells. By histochemical methods, this theory has been confirmed. Also, it has been shown that this mesenchyme, derived from the medial side of the neighboring mesonephric ridge, gives rise to the covering epithelium of the gonad which no longer

need be referred to as "germinal" epithelium. Thus, the follicle with its sex cell has a dual origin: the theca or stromal cells from fetal connective tissue of the ovarian medulla, and the granulosa cells from the cortical mesenchyme. On the basis of their embryonic origin, the theca and granulosa cells in the female would be comparable to the interstitial (Leydig) and nourishing (Sertoli) cells in the male. It follows that the theca and interstitial cells are probably endocrinologically active, but the granulosa

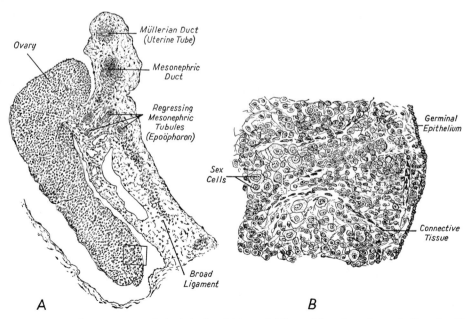

Figure 5. Drawing of cross-section through body of 11 week (65 mm.) female embryo. A, Drawing illustrating topography. ×30. B, Drawing of small area of ovary outlined by rectangle in A. ×200. (From Patten.)

and Sertoli cells are more likely endocrinologically inert. Whether granulosal lutein cells secrete progesterone or whether this function resides solely in the theca interna is debatable.

Ovarian Tumors

The genesis of certain ovarian tumors and their endocrine characteristics are related to the question of the origin of the various ovarian components. These rare ovarian tumors, some of which appear to attempt to recapitulate periods of gonadal development, may have a feminizing, a masculinizing, or no endocrine effect. Those that mimic the period of nondifferentiation are derived from germ cells; this type is known, in the female, as dysgerminoma and, in the male, as seminoma. These germ cell tumors may range from pure dysgerminoma without endocrine activity to a teratoma. Although there may be some infantilism of the uterus and external genitalia, such need not be the case provided one ovary is normal. Pregnancy, therefore, is not precluded. Most of these tumors come to light in the second or third decade of life, and are among the more common, albeit rare, tumors complicating pregnancy. The pure dysgerminoma is extremely radiosensitive and has a favorable prognosis, but unfortunately this is not true when other tissue elements are involved and the tumor is teratomatous in nature.

The feminizing endocrine tumors and their variants simulate histologically the period of differentiation of the granulosa and theca cells of the ovary. They are thought to originate either from superfluous granulosa tissue located mainly in the medullary portion of the ovary, in situ from the mesenchyme of the ovary, or from atretic follicles. They vary histologically and, depending on the predominance of the granulosal or of thecal tissue, are referred to as granulosa or theca cell tumors. Regardless of their appearance, these tumors are mainly estrogenic in their action, and the uterine endometrium is often proliferative and hyperplastic. A progestational effect apparently can occur, however, for a secretory endometrium is occasionally encountered. In the young, these tumors may lead to precocious puberty, followed by periods of amenorrhea, produced presumably by the effect of excessive amounts of estrogen with suppression of the gonadotropic activity of the pituitary. In the postmenopausal patient these tumors continue to stimulate the endometrium, resulting in uterine bleeding, and on occasion are associated with an endometrial cancer.

The masculinizing endocrine ovarian tumors arise either from nondifferentiated mesenchyme within the hilus of the ovary or from the deposition of adrenal rests within the ovary. Reference has been made to the dual mesenchymal origin of the stroma and the sex cords in the gonads of both sexes. A tumor that develops from this primitive bisexual mesenchyme is known as an arrhenoblastoma, and it more or less resembles the embryonic testis. Wolffian duct remnants, that is, the rete ovarii, are often contained within the hilar tissue. If a tubular structure predominates, there is little or no endocrine effect. However, in the majority of these tumors the interstitial, or Leydig, cells are abundant and are responsible for the masculinizing effect. The hilus of the ovary contains interstitial cells which may proliferate and become a tumor. This is a histologic and not a gross diagnosis. The clinical effects of such a tumor are similar to those of an arrhenoblastoma.

THE URINARY SYSTEM

The development of the urinary system in the female precedes, to a large extent, the formation of the reproductive tract. The

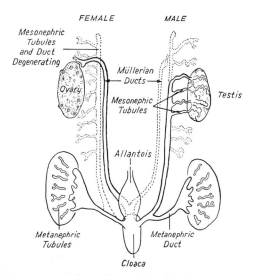

Figure 6. Relationship of the developing urinary system. (From Patten.)

mesonephros, or wolffian body, appears by the fourth week (5 mm.) as a derivative of the intermediate mesoderm. By the time the gonadal ridges have developed, the mesonephric duct has grown down to the urogenital sinus.

In the male, the mesonephric duct becomes connected to the seminiferous tubules of the newly formed testis by way of some of the mesonephric tubules and the rete (Fig. 6). Further, the mesonephric duct is the anlage of the epididymis, the vas deferens, and the ejaculatory duct. Thus, much of the mesonephric system is retained in the male, whereas in the female these structures regress.

Failure of the wolffian or mesonephric duct system to regress completely in the female may later give rise to occlusion cysts within the vestigial remnants (Fig. 7). The remnants within the mesosalpinx, should they accumulate fluid, may dissect laterally

between the tube and the upper pole of the ovary, such lesions being known as parovarian cysts. In-situ enlargement gives rise to broad-ligament cysts. Occasionally, these cysts develop in the lower generative tract lateral to the uterus and present as swellings along the lateral vaginal wall. In this area they are commonly referred to as Gartner's duct cysts. During pregnancy, such cysts have been known to enlarge to a size sufficient to obstruct labor. If necessary, fluid should be aspirated to allow for delivery; surgical removal is easily performed later, when the patient is not pregnant.

The metanephros, the precursor of the permanent kidney, arises partly as a bud of the mesonephric duct and in still greater part from portions of the intermediate mesoderm. The metanephric diverticulum first appears at the beginning of the fifth week on the posterior medial wall of the mesonephric duct near its junction with the

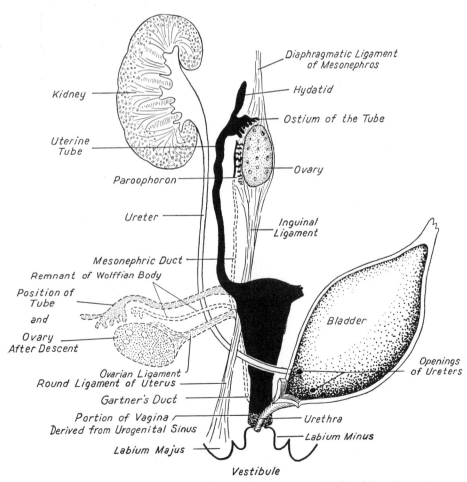

Figure 7. Development of the female reproductive tract. (Modified from Patten.)

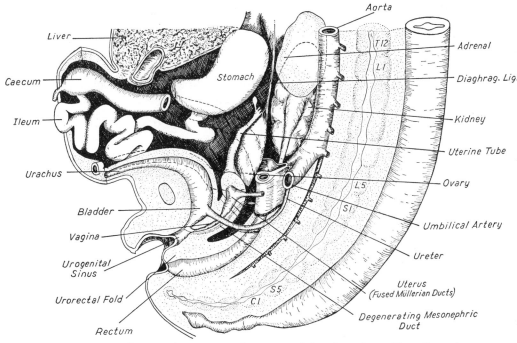

Figure 8.   The reproductive tract of a nine week female embryo. (From Patten.)

cloaca. The blind end of the diverticulum enlarges and grows dorsally and upward to form the ureter, renal pelvis, calices, and collecting tubules. The caudal portion of the metanephric diverticulum, near its origin from the mesonephric duct, becomes incorporated with the latter into the developing bladder and both attain independent openings. The openings of the metanephric diverticula persist as the ureteral orifices.

During growth and development, each metanephros undergoes changes in relative position, usually referred to as "ascent of the kidney" (Fig. 8). Initially, the metanephroi are situated caudal to the bifurcation of the umbilical arteries. They gradually move upward over the ridges formed by these vessels to lie on the dorsolateral body wall above the aortic bifurcation. Arising at the level of the fourth lumbar segment, the kidney is located at the 12th thoracic vertebra by the time of birth. Failure to ascend gives rise to the pelvic kidney which may cause obstructive labor.

CLOACA AND BLADDER

In embryos of the third or fourth week, the allantois has formed as an evagination of the hindgut. Soon after this, the genital tubercle appears, denoting the beginning of the formation of the external genitalia. The terminal portion of the hindgut becomes dilated to form the cloaca, which is separated from the external surface of the fetus by a thin double sheet of tissue, the cloacal membrane. During this time internal changes are taking place, with formation of the urorectal fold which divides the cloaca into a dorsal primitive rectum and a ventral urogenital sinus into which the mesonephric ducts open. Immediately after this division the cloacal membrane ruptures, and the urogenital sinus and rectum have individual openings (Fig. 8). Failure of the cloacal membrane to rupture results in atresia of the anal canal and an imperforate anus. The presence of this lesion should be immediately recognized by the obstetrician at the time of his initial physical examination of the newborn. Moreover, should this occur in the female, it is sometimes associated with a congenital rectovaginal fistula.

The midportion of the urogenital sinus dilates and becomes the urinary bladder, while the distal portion remains undilated and forms the urethra (Fig. 8). The upper portion of the bladder constricts to form the urachus, which is continuous with the allantoic stalk.

EXTERNAL GENITALIA

As in other portions of the reproductive system, there is a lag in differentiation of the external genitalia in the female, in contrast to that in the male. In the male embryo development of the external genitalia begins by the end of the sixth week, whereas in the female it is postponed until the end of the eighth week. Prior to the sixth week, the genital tubercle or eminence develops in the midventral line and cephalad to the cloaca. This structure contributes to the formation of the penis in the male and the clitoris in the female. On the cloacal surface of the tubercle appear the paired genital or urethral folds. Between these is the urethral groove, the floor of which, in the primitive state, is covered by the urethral membrane. This membrane soon ruptures, connecting the urethral groove with the urogenital sinus. During the eighth and ninth weeks (30 to 40 mm.), in the female, the cavernosa tissue forms and the genital tubercle assumes the shape of the glans of the clitoris. The genital folds in the male fuse to close the urethral groove and to include the penile urethra. Except in the region of the clitoris, where they regress, the genital folds persist in the female, but do not fuse, and later form the labia minora. The persistent urethral groove, therefore, becomes the vestibule of the vagina. The genital swellings that appear lateral to the tubercle and surround the urethral groove and folds are the primordia of the scrotum in the male and the labia majora in the female. In the female these genital swellings fuse only above the anal opening, to form the posterior labial commissure. The sex of the embryo can be determined at the end of the fifth week by careful dissection and measurement of the urethral groove, which at this stage is longer in the male than in the female embryo. Grossly, however, the sex of the embryo cannot be ascertained from the appearance of the external genitalia until about the third month.

PERINEAL MUSCLES

The perineal muscles are derived from the lower sacral myotomes. The primordia of these muscles surround the cloaca and, with the development of the vagina and anus, undergo modification to form sphincters about these structures. Fibers from the lateral margins of the muscles surrounding the anus give origin to the levator ani group. From the muscles about the newly formed vaginal orifice originate the ischiocavernosus and bulbocavernosus muscles (Fig. 9).

ACCESSORY SEX GLANDS

The accessory sex glands of the female arise from the urethra and urogenital sinus epithelium. The para-urethral ducts of Skene originate from the epithelium of the urethra. In the absence of closure of the genital folds below the clitoris, the ducts of Skene empty into the vestibule rather than into the urethra. The major vestibular glands (Bartholin's glands) arise from nearby epithelium of the vestibule. Skene's and Bartholin's glands are both subject to infection. In the former, Neisseria infection is the most likely, whereas a mixed infection can occur in Bartholin's glands.

THE REPRODUCTIVE TRACT

The müllerian duct system, which is the anlage of the oviducts, uterus, and upper part of the vagina, arises from an invagination of the coelomic epithelium. This process is usually observable by the fifth to sixth week (7 to 12 mm.), and by the end of the eighth week (30 mm.) the system extends from the cephalic portion of the mesonephros well into the pelvis in parallel arrangement with the wolffian duct system. The upper portion of the müllerian ducts lies lateral to the wolffian duct system but, at the lower border of the mesonephros, this relation becomes reversed. At the point where the müllerian ducts pass over the wolffian system they begin to fuse with each other to form the body of the uterus (Fig. 8). The portion above, which remains unfused, forms the oviducts; the fused distal portion forms the uterus, cervix, and major part of the vagina. To permit fusion, the müllerian ducts and the accompanying gonads migrate ventrally and toward the midline. The overlying peritoneum forms a mesentery-like structure, and with union of the müllerian ducts these leaves of peritoneum come to form the broad ligament of the uterus (Fig. 10). The müllerian ducts are joined by the ninth week (40 mm.), and at the 11th week (65 mm.) the

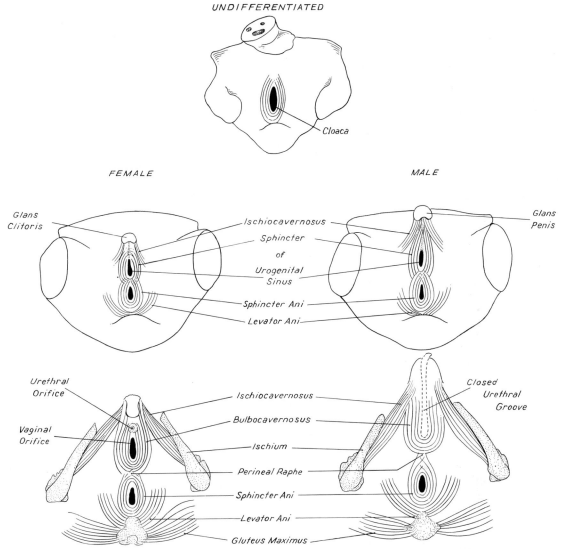

Figure 9.   Schematic diagrams showing developing perineal muscles in the two sexes. (Modified from Patten, after Papowski.)

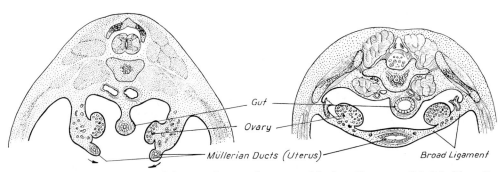

Figure 10.   Schematic cross-sectional diagram showing formation of the broad ligament. (Modified from Patten.)

septum separating the two ducts has disappeared, leaving a single uterine cavity. Demarcation between the vagina and uterus appears to be recognizable very early in embryonal development, for the cervix appears as a thickened area almost as soon as the müllerian ducts fuse with each other. Further demarcation is made possible later by the appearance of columnar epithelium lining the cervical and uterine canal, in contrast to the stratified epithelium that eventually covers the vagina and vaginal portion of the cervix.

With the formation of these structures of müllerian duct origin, the wolffian system undergoes regression and, by the 10th week (50 mm.), has lost its connection with the urogenital sinus. One portion of the wolffian system, the inguinal ligament of the mesonephros, is retained as a functioning structure. With descent of the ovary the upper part of this ligament becomes the ovarian ligament. The lower part becomes the round ligament of the uterus which, at its distal end, remains fixed in the labium majus (Fig. 7).

With fusion of the müllerian ducts, the primordium undergoes rapid growth caudally, to reach eventually the posterior wall of the urogenital sinus. The downward extension of the müllerian tissue results in a lengthening of the vaginal portion of the uterovaginal canal. The portion of the müllerian system that protrudes into the urogenital sinus is referred to as the müllerian tubercle. At the time that the müllerian tubercle reaches the urogenital sinus, the sinovaginal bulbs appear. These latter bodies are contributed by the urogenital sinus to the formation of the vagina. As the sinovaginal bulbs enlarge to encompass and fuse about the most distal müllerian tissue mass, the remnants of the wolffian bodies are displaced upward and at the same time the müllerian tubercle disappears. The lower part of the müllerian system, which is to become the vagina, continues to enlarge, and by the 15th week (120 mm.) the distal end of the uterovaginal canal has become temporarily occluded. During the 17th or 18th week (150 to 160 mm.) the cells in the center of this solid epithelial mass degen-

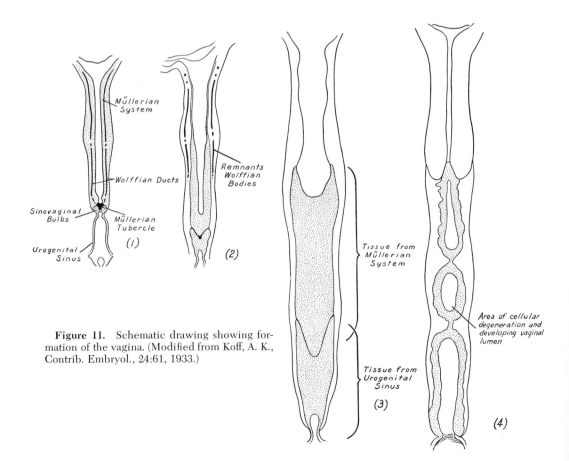

Figure 11. Schematic drawing showing formation of the vagina. (Modified from Koff, A. K., Contrib. Embryol., 24:61, 1933.)

erate, and the permanent vaginal lumen appears. The caudal end of the vagina opens into the vestibule through a newly formed aperture (Fig. 11). Circumscribing this opening is the hymen, derived from tissue at the junction of the urogenital sinus and vestibule.

In summary, the upper four fifths of the vagina is derived from the caudal portion of the müllerian system and the remainder arises as an epithelial outgrowth contributed by the urogenital sinus.

DEVELOPMENTAL ABNORMALITIES

The human uterus is in reality the product of growth and fusion of paired primordia, but the attainment of normal development depends on the regression of certain tissue as the result of this fusion (Fig. 12). The most common abnormality is the uterus subseptus unicollis, often referred to clinically as the arcuate uterus. This form arises as a result of incomplete fusion of the müllerian ducts with failure of decus-

sation of the muscle fibers and only partial regression of the intervening septum. During the later part of pregnancy, the arcuate uterus may be recognized on abdominal palpation by a broad flat form to the fundus with dimpling in the midline. Exaggeration of the abnormality gives rise to the bicornuate uterus, in which event the organ comprises two horns with a single cervix (unicollis). Complete failure of fusion of the müllerian ducts results in the production of a uterus didelphys, or double uterus. This condition is often associated with a duplication of the vagina. The other types of abnormality result mainly from failure of the medial wall of the fused müllerian ducts to regress. This partition may persist to produce a double uterus and septate cervix and vagina (Fig. 13). In addition, atresia may result in failure of the vagina to reestablish its lumen. Imperforation of the hymen, with failure to establish communication between the vagina and vestibule, may with the onset of the menses result in hematocolpos.

Because of the close approximation of the origin of their respective anlagen, it would

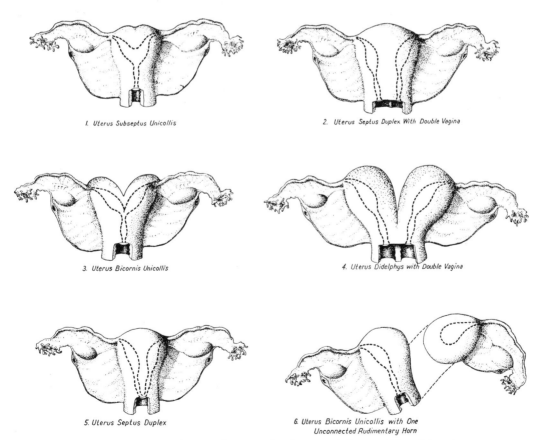

1. *Uterus Subseptus Unicollis*

2. *Uterus Septus Duplex With Double Vagina*

3. *Uterus Bicornis Unicollis*

4. *Uterus Didelphys with Double Vagina*

5. *Uterus Septus Duplex*

6. *Uterus Bicornis Unicollis with One Unconnected Rudimentary Horn*

Figure 12. Diagrams showing the major developmental abnormalities of the uterus.

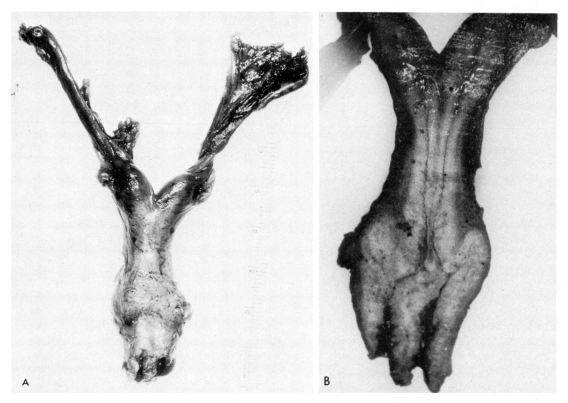

Figure 13. Reproductive tract from a newborn. A, Complete specimen, with tubal appendages and vagina. B, Midfrontal section through the same specimen, showing septation of the cervix and vagina.

be reasonable to suspect that abnormalities of the reproductive tract, the urinary tract, and the terminal portion of the large bowel and rectum might occur simultaneously. The rectum may open anywhere along the posterior wall of the vagina, even as high as its fusion with the cervix, and usually in the form of a fistulous opening. However, most congenital rectovaginal fistulas occur in the lower vagina.

The coexistence of anomalies of the urinary and reproductive tract has long been appreciated, and the extent of these abnormalities may range from the absence or displacement of one of the kidneys to stillbirth or neonatal death as a result of absence of both kidneys. Consequently, whenever anomalies of the female genital tract are detected, a search should always be made for urologic aberrations.

ANATOMY OF THE FEMALE REPRODUCTIVE TRACT

Knowledge of the surgical anatomy and obstetric landmarks of the bony and soft tissue structures of the female pelvis and reproductive tract is a prime requisite in the clinical management of pregnancy and of parturition, with its possible complications, and in the prevention of sequelae, particularly of a gynecologic nature. The concern here is with the overall anatomy of the female pelvis as it relates to reproduction.

BONY PELVIS

The bony pelvis is composed of the sacrum and the innominate bones. Each innominate bone consists of three parts: the ilium, the ischium, and the pubis. The junction of the ischium and ilium is indicated by the iliopectineal line. This line extends from the sacroiliac joint to the iliopectineal eminence anteriorly, and marks the division between the false and the true pelvis.

Within the surface of the ischium are two landmarks of particular obstetric importance: the ischial spines and ischial tuberosities. The pubis forms the anterior wall of the pelvis and, together with the lateral union of its superior ramus with the ischium, constitutes a portion of the superior boundary of the pelvis (Fig. 14). This point of fusion is marked by the iliopectineal eminence. The midline union of the superior and inferior rami of the two pubic bones constitutes the symphysis pubis.

Posteriorly the ilia join the sacrum at the sacroiliac synchondroses. Normally the sacrum is composed of five fused vertebral segments. An important feature of the first segment is the sacral promontory located on the anterior surface near its upper margin. Normally presenting a concave ventral surface, the sacrum ends at a level well below the inferior margin of the symphysis, and its lateral borders represent, functionally at least, an extension of the posterior border of the greater sacrosciatic notch. The sacrospinous ligament, extending from the lower portion of the sacrum to the ischial spine, constitutes the inferior border of the greater sacrosciatic notch.

To summarize, the anatomic landmarks of the bony pelvis and their relationships to each other have special interest in obstetrics for the following reasons: (1) The distance from the inferior border of the symphysis to the sacral promontory, i.e., the diagonal conjugate, is a determinant of the size of the pelvic inlet. (2) The curvature and location of the sacrum may influence the ability of the fetus to negotiate the birth canal. Normally the birth canal enlarges from inlet to outlet. (3) The ischial spines, literally absent in the subhuman primate, vary greatly in size in the human. They are extremely prominent in the male and all too often also in the female. Their presence can prevent advancement of the presenting part of the fetus in its passage through the midpelvis. An imaginary line between the spines (the intraspinous diameter) is highly important for obstetric purposes. It marks the division of the upper and lower pelves. Most important, when the normally flexed vertex descends to that line, it is assumed that clinically the biparietal diameter of the fetal vertex is passing or has passed the pelvic inlet, and the fetal head is now referred to as being "engaged." (4) The sacrosciatic ligament is a point of reference in the determination of the location of the ischial spines and in the estimation of the size of the sacrosciatic notch, which is a further index of the location and shape of the sacrum. A comparatively small notch suggests that the pelvis is convergent rather than normally divergent. (5) The size of the pubic arch and its contour, together with the distance between the ischial tuberosities, determine

Figure 14. Sagittal section of normal female pelvis.

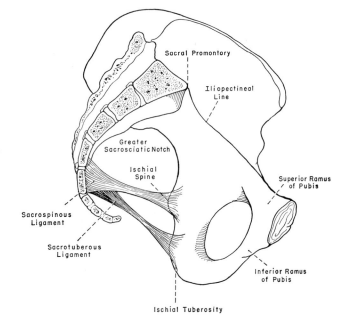

whether the pelvic outlet is ample to permit atraumatic birth, that is, to avoid disruption of the neighboring maternal tissues and harm to the fetus.

EXTERNAL GENITALIA

The external genitalia include the visible structures overlying the anterior compartment of the perineum and external to the deep layer of the superficial perineal fascia. Often included in the description of the external genitals are certain structures lying beneath the fascia, but these will be considered subsequently in the description of the deeper structure of the perineum.

The mons pubis, or mons veneris, is a fatty cushion that rests upon the symphysis pubis. Posterior to the mons is the vulva, consisting of the labia majora and minora, a portion of the clitoris, and the vestibule. The labia majora are rounded masses of tissue that form the lateral boundaries of the vestibule and are analogous to the scrotum in the male. Anteriorly the labia are continuous with the mons pubis, where they receive the insertions of the round ligaments. Posteriorly they merge in the midline anterior to the perineal body. In nulliparous women the labia majora are usually in close apposition, concealing the underlying parts, whereas after childbirth they become and remain separated (see Fig. 4 in Chapter 23). Their inner surface is covered by a moist mucous membrane; the integument of the outer convex surface is continuous with the adjacent skin. The connective tissue of the labia majora, beneath which lies a dense layer of fat, is permeated by an abundant plexus of blood vessels.

Medial to the labia majora are two triangular cutaneous folds, the labia minora, which correspond to the skin on the undersurface of the penis of the male. These folds enclose the vestibule and are much thinner and shorter than the labia majora. The labia minora converge anteriorly in the midline at the clitoris, and each terminates in two folds; the medial folds fuse to form the frenulum of the clitoris (Fig. 15). Posteriorly, the labia minora are connected below the vaginal orifice by a mucocutaneous fold of tissue, referred to as the fourchette, from which they merge into the substance of the labia majora. The labia minora consist of thin folds of tissue covered by stratified epi-

thelium with numerous papillae, and they contain many sebaceous follicles and some sweat glands. These folds are composed of connective tissue, a few nonstriated muscle fibers, many blood vessels, and abundant nerve endings.

The clitoris is a structure lying at the anterior region of the vulva. When the labia minora are separated, the parts of the clitoris visible are the glans, prepuce, frenulum, and a short portion of the body. Owing to the traction of the prepuce and frenulum, the glans or free end is directed inward toward the vaginal opening. The main body of the clitoris is beneath the deep layer of the superficial perineal fascia; this is considered in more detail in the description of the anatomy of the superficial compartment of the perineum.

The vestibule, or pudendal cleft, is bounded laterally by the labia minora, and opening into it are the urethra, the vaginal orifice, and on each side the ducts of Bartholin's glands. On either side of the urethral opening are the orifices of Skene's ducts, a set of periurethral glands.

The opening of the vagina varies in size, and its appearance is dependent upon the condition of the hymen and the perineal tissues. The hymen is a thin, membranous structure attached about the margin of the vaginal orifice. It presents marked differences in shape, most commonly being annular or crescentic in outline. In the virginal state the hymen has an aperture varying from pinpoint in size to one admitting one or two fingers. At the initial sexual intercourse the hymen tends to lacerate in several areas. It may fail to rupture, however, giving rise to difficult or painful intercourse, that is, dyspareunia. When the hymen is ruptured, its remnants are represented by nodular hymenal tags or carunculae myrtiformes. Conception may take place with the hymen intact, with the semen simply spilling, rather than being introduced, into the vagina.

PERINEUM

The perineum comprises the soft tissues included within the inferior pelvic plane. This diamond-shaped area is limited anteriorly by the symphysis pubis, laterally by the pubic arch and the gluteus maximus muscles, and posteriorly by the coccyx. The perineum may be divided into an *anterior*

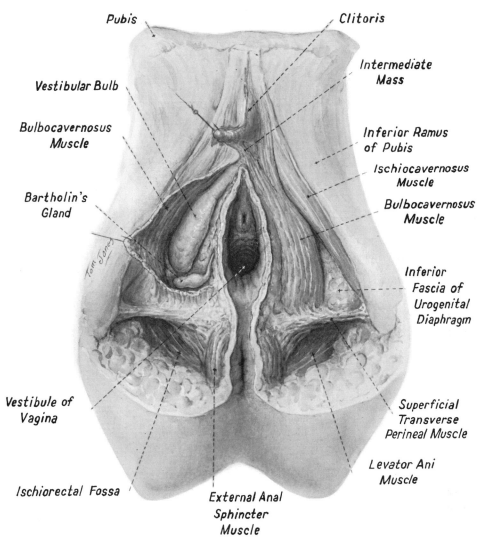

Figure 15. Anterior and posterior components of the female perineum. On the left side the bulbocavernosus muscle has been reflected to expose the bulb of the vestibule and the greater vestibular (Bartholin's) gland and duct. (Modified from Curtis, A. H., Anson, B. J., and Ashley, F. L., Surg., Gynec. Obstet., 74:708, 1942.)

and a *posterior* component, the division occurring along the course of the *superficial transverse perineal muscle.* Originating from the inner surface of the inferior ramus of the pubis and above the ischial tuberosity, this muscle inserts in the central point of the perineum anterior to the external anal sphincter (Fig. 15). The anterior component of the perineum can be further subdivided into a superficial and a deep compartment, the latter being better known as the urogenital diaphragm.

The superficial compartment is covered by the deep layer of the superficial perineal fascia, designated Colles' fascia, and is bounded above by the inferior fascia of the urogenital diaphragm (Figs. 15 and 16). As Colles' fascia overlies the anterior component of the perineum, it comes to envelop the superficial perineal muscle posteriorly and fuses with the inferior fascia of the urogenital diaphragm. Laterally, it becomes firmly attached to the pubic arch and ischial tuberosities. Consequently, the superficial compartment is enfolded except anteriorly, where Colles' fascia is continuous with the deep fascia of the abdomen (Scarpa's fascia). This has certain clinical implications, for an inflammatory condition or a hematoma occurring in this compartment may dissect

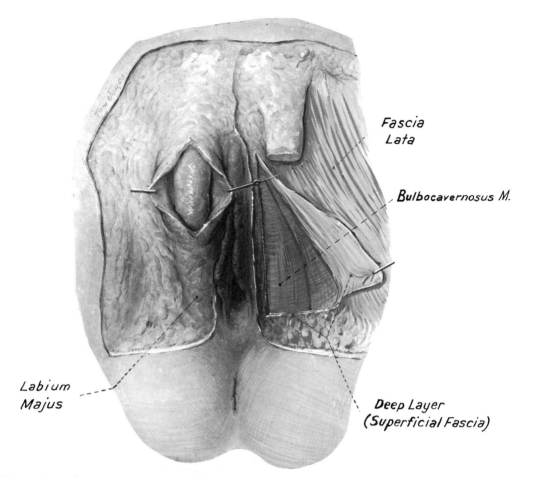

Fascia
Lata

Bulbocavernosus M.

Labium
Majus

Deep Layer
(Superficial Fascia)

Figure 16. Subcutaneous structures and layers of superficial fascia of the female perineum. On the left the superficial layer of the superficial fascia is exposed and in one area is excised longitudinally to reveal the round ligament. (Modified from Curtis, A. H., Anson, B. J., and Ashley, F. L., Surg., Gynec. Obstet., 74:708, 1942.)

anteriorly toward the pubis and, if extensive, over the lower abdominal wall. The process will not extend posteriorly beyond the superficial perineal muscle or the midpoint of the perineum. Contained between the two fascial planes of the superficial compartment are the perineal branches of the pudendal vessels and nerves, the superficial perineal muscles, Bartholin's glands, and the erectile tissues, with their investing musculature, comprising the clitoris (Figs. 15 and 17).

The clitoris is formed from two sources of erectile tissue; the body of the organ is derived from fusion of the corpora cavernosa, while the distal portion, or glans, is formed by the vestibular bulbs. The corpora cavernosa separate at the base of the clitoris and as crura are attached to the inner aspect of the upper portion of the rami of the pubis (Figs. 15 and 18). Overlying this

erectile tissue are the ischiocavernosus muscles. Contraction of these muscles retards venous return from the corpora cavernosa, allowing for erection, and at the same time draws the clitoris downward toward the vestibule, a function of some importance in sexual stimulation. The vestibular bulbs cover, in a caplike fashion, the fused ends of the corpora cavernosa to form the glans of the clitoris. These vestibular bulbs are covered by the bulbocavernosus muscles which insert posteriorly near the midpoint of the perineum. Contraction of these muscles has an effect on the clitoris similar to that of the ischiocavernosus muscles and, in addition, has a sphincterlike action about the vaginal orifice.

The deep compartment of the perineum is contained within the superior and inferior fascial layers of the urogenital diaphragm. As previously described, the inferior fascial layer of the urogenital diaphragm is continuous with the deep layer of the superficial fascia of the perineum. The superior fascia of the urogenital diaphragm joins the obturator fascia laterally, and in so doing bounds the floor of the anterior recesses of the ischiorectal fossae. Medially, this layer of fascia is in contact with the fascia over the inferior surface of the levator ani muscles, the main structures of the pelvic diaphragm. The superior and inferior fascial layers of the urogenital diaphragm fuse above the urethra anteriorly, forming the transverse ligament of the pelvis located beneath the symphysis pubis. Included between these layers of fascia of the urogenital diaphragm are the deep transverse perineal and the

sphincter muscles of the membranous urethra and the clitoral branches of the pudendal vessels and nerves.

The sphincter muscle arising from the upper portion of the pubic arch gives off constrictor fibers about the vagina and urethra, the fibers about the urethra being designated the external vesical sphincter. The deep perineal muscle, situated below the superficial perineal muscle, distributes its fibers posteriorly about the rectum and inserts in the midline between the rectum and the tip of the coccyx (Fig. 19).

The posterior component, containing the anal region, is bounded laterally by the ischial tuberosities and the sacrotuberous ligaments, and posteriorly by the coccyx. In

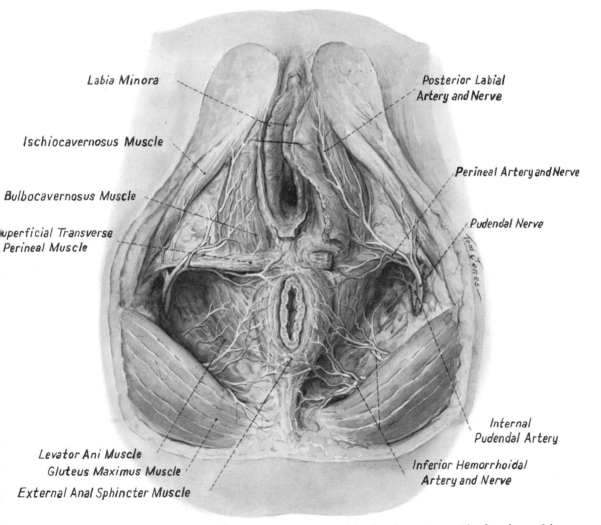

Figure 17. Superficial compartment of the anterior component of the female perineum. The deep layer of the superficial fascia has been removed, revealing the nerves and blood vessels supplying this region. (Modified from Anson, B. J., and Curtis, A. H., in Curtis, A. H., and Huffman, J. W.: Textbook of Gynecology, ed. 6. W. B. Saunders Co., Philadelphia, 1950.)

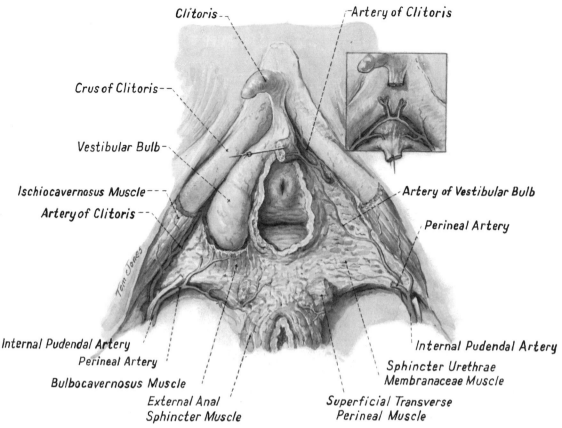

Figure 18. Arteries of the anterior component of the female perineum. The structures lying beneath the bulbocavernosus and ischiocavernosus muscles are exposed on the left. Insert: Subpubic anastomosis of the distal portion of the arteries of the clitoris. (Modified from Anson, B. J., and Curtis, A. H., in Curtis, A. H., and Huffman, J. W.: Textbook of Gynecology, ed. 6. W. B. Saunders Co., Philadelphia, 1950.)

contrast to the anterior component, this area is composed of only one compartment. In the lateral aspects of this anal triangle are the two ischiorectal fossae, the apices of which are anteriorly situated between the pelvic and urogenital diaphragms. These fossae extend inferiorly and diverge to a broad base along the gluteus maximus muscle. Here each is bounded medially by the rectum, laterally by the obturator fascia, and superiorly by the levator ani muscle. Infectious processes or hematomas developing in the area between the pelvic and urogenital diaphragms or in the posterior component of the perineum are contained within the ischiorectal fossae and tend to localize medial to the ischial tuberosity (Fig. 19).

The pelvic floor or diaphragm is composed of the different components of the levator ani muscles with their fascia, the group including the pubococcygeus and ilio-

coccygeus muscles. These structures separate the perineum from the pelvic cavity. The iliococcygeus muscle underlies the gluteus maximus muscle and is not obstetrically important. It takes origin from the tendinous arch of the obturator fascia, posterior to the pubococcygeus, and from the spine of the ischium. The muscle passes medialward to insert into the coccyx and the anococcygeal raphe. The pubococcygeus muscle originates from the posterior surface of the superior pubic ramus along the ventral aspect of the tendinous arch of the obturator fascia. Coursing downward and medialward, the muscle encircles the urethra, vagina, and anus, and merges into the central point of the perineum, fusing with the iliococcygeus muscle posteriorly. A median perineotomy or episiotomy, or a laceration extending from the vagina toward the rectum would involve the pubococcygeus muscle as well as the superficial perineal muscle and its fascial investment. In a mediolateral episiotomy the same structures are incised, in addition to the bulbocavernosus and deep transverse perineal muscles (Fig. 19).

In the areas where the bladder, vagina, and rectum pass through the pelvic floor or diaphragm, and the uterus enters the vagina, these viscera become surrounded with firm connective tissue, here known as the endopelvic fascia. This fascia, which is continuous with the fascia covering the inner or superior surface of the levator ani muscles, varies widely in its texture. This is exemplified by the portion that surrounds the cervix and the base of the bladder, which is considerably thicker and heavier than any of the other layers. From the anterior and lateral surfaces of the bladder, the endopelvic fascia is carried upward to cover the iliac vessels, behind which it encloses the ovarian vessels and contributes to the cervix to form the pillars of the bladder (pubovesicocervical fascia). The vagina and uterus are covered by a broad leaf of endopelvic fascia which sweeps up from the pelvic floor, forming a strong sheath at the junction of the cervix and vagina (uterovaginal fascia). Posteriorly, this layer continues to the sacrum to help form the uterosacral ligaments, and continues downward to the region of the rectovaginal septum as a loose

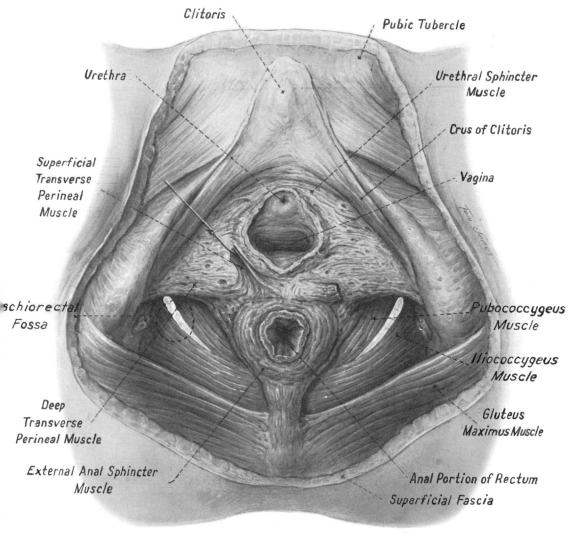

Figure 19. Deep compartment of the anterior component of the female perineum (urogenital diaphragm). The posterior component of the female perineum and a portion of the pelvic diaphragm or levator ani muscles may be observed. (Modified from Curtis, A. H., Anson, B. J., and Ashley, F. L., Surg., Gynec. Obstet., 74:708, 1942.)

fascial sheath about the rectum. Laterally, it is continuous with the fibrous tissue that makes up the round and cardinal ligaments. In the region of the cardinal ligaments the endopelvic fascia functions to hold the uterus, bladder, and vagina in proper relationship to each other (Fig. 20).

The importance of the endopelvic fascia (subject to confusing nomenclature) cannot be overemphasized, for it relates to nearly all surgical procedures involving the pelvis. It envelops all of the major pelvic structures —the rectum, the bladder, and, in the female, the vagina and uterus. Its two layers are in apposition, separated by loose areolar tissue. Dissection about the rectum, bladder, and vagina and uterus is facilitated if they remain between the layers of endopelvic fascia; this is the key to minimal bleeding. It is recognized that the endopelvic covering of one organ may become adherent to the layer covering an adjacent organ by infection or endometriosis. However, in the ab-

sence of disease, undue bleeding about the cervix or bladder at the time of hysterectomy or cesarean section indicates the endopelvic fascia has been penetrated through to the musculature of one of the pelvic structures. In the case of the peritoneum, it is impossible to free it from the endopelvic fascia, and no attempt should be made to dislodge it. The peritoneum will readily accompany the endopelvic fascia, as observed in an extraperitoneal cesarean section.

The injuries that may occur during labor and delivery frequently involve the supporting structures of the bladder, urethra, and rectum. Separation of the endopelvic fascia and pubococcygeus muscle causes the urethra and the internal bladder sphincter to drop away from their normal attachments. The resulting herniation of the urethra into the vagina is known as a *urethrocele*. The external sphincter of the membranous urethra may also be injured, but the internal urethral sphincter is of more importance in

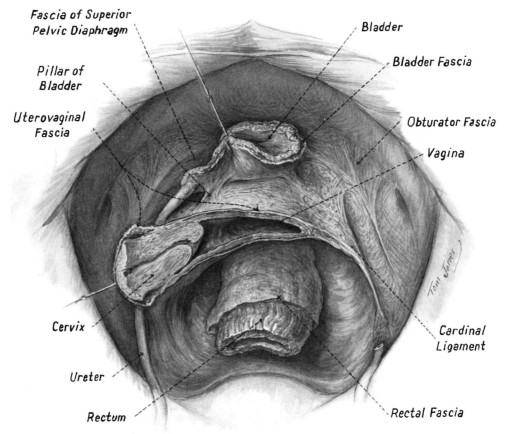

Figure 20. Investment of pelvic organs by endopelvic fascia. The cervix and upper two thirds of the vagina have been cut sagittally. The uterine collar of endopelvic fascia (uterovaginal fascia) is separated from the muscular wall of the cervix. (Modified from Curtis, A. H., Anson, B. J., and Beaton, L. E., Surg., Gynec. Obstet., 70:642, 1940.)

bladder control, and it is this structure that requires anatomic restoration in the cure of the condition known as urinary stress incontinence resulting from a urethrocele.

Disruption of the pubovesicocervical fascia and the pubococcygeus muscle may result in herniation of the bladder, or *cystocele*. When both urethra and bladder are involved, the condition is known as *urethrocystocele*. Incontinence is the symptom of urethrocele, and residual urine is the consequence of cystocele. Herniation of the rectum, or *rectocele* formation, is the result of damage to the middle third of the vagina and pelvic diaphragm. Minimal trauma may produce this lesion, because the vagina and rectum are so closely apposed, being separated by only a thin layer of endopelvic fascia. On rare occasions, in the presence of a congenitally deep rectovaginal pouch, a sliding herniation may develop in the posterior vaginal fornix which, because it may contain bowel and omentum, is known as an *enterocele*. Although regarded as being of congenital origin, the condition may be aggravated by parturition and may be identified for the first time in the puerperium. It should always be searched for at the time of vaginal hysterectomy and, if found, repaired.

Granted that tissue turgor, which differs among individuals, is a factor in the incidence of urinary stress incontinence, uterine prolapse, and other gynecologic consequences, these are usually the aftermath of labor and mode of delivery. To avoid these consequences, account must be taken of the shape and contour of the pelvic outlet. The pelvic arch places restrictions on the ability of the perineum to dilate in its entirety. Disruption of the posterior perineum can be prevented by a perineotomy performed at delivery. This in turn will protect the endopelvic fascia supporting the bladder from the pressure of the fetal occiput as it emerges from beneath the symphyseal region.

Thus, in the consideration of what is natural or what nature intended, one must acknowledge in the female human primate during parturition those anatomic characteristics of the pelvis that permit her the privilege of bipedal progression in the upright position. However, no woman should be subject to urinary stress incontinence or prolapse if she has received intelligent care during pregnancy, labor, and delivery.

VAGINA

The vagina is a musculomembranous canal surrounding the lower portion of the uterine cervix and extending to the vulva. Its upper third courses downward and backward, and its lower two thirds curves forward. Thus, it must be realized that when the female is in the supine position the vagina is directed almost precisely posteriorly. This fact has implications in avoiding discomfort on vaginal examination and in advising the patient with dyspareunia.

The vagina is related anteriorly to the fundus and base of the bladder and the urethra, from which it is separated by loose areolar tissue. Posteriorly, the upper portion of the vagina is separated from the rectum by a deep fold of peritoneum, which forms the cul-de-sac, or pouch, of Douglas. In the middle third of the vagina, the walls of the rectum and vagina are in close apposition to each other. Below this, the vagina and rectum again diverge to penetrate the pelvic floor, or diaphragm (Fig. 21).

The upper part of the vagina surrounding the cervix ends in a blind vault, or fornix. Projecting into this vault, the cervix subdivides this portion of the vagina into an anterior, a posterior, and two lateral fornices. The attachment of the vagina to the uterus is higher on the posterior than on the anterior surface, with the result that the posterior fornix is deeper than the anterior. The upper portion of the vagina is easily distensible, but the lower vagina, invested as it is by the musculature of the pelvic and urogenital diaphragms, distends or dilates less easily.

The muscles of the pelvic diaphragm, as they course toward their insertion, largely determine the shape of the vagina. There is an infolding of the vagina as the pubococcygeus portions of the levator ani muscles pass upward, giving the vagina an H configuration. The crossbar effect is produced by the collapse of the anterior and posterior walls, and the vertical arms are contributed by the columns of the pubococcygeus muscles. Contraction of the levator group of muscles decreases the size of the aperture of the vagina by drawing the lateral as well as the anterior and posterior walls together.

The vaginal wall is composed of three principal layers: an outer fibrous, a middle muscular, and an inner mucosal layer. The fibrous layer contains a nerve plexus and

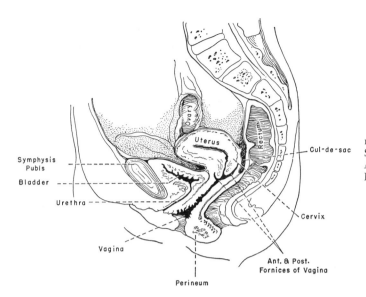

Figure 21. Sagittal section of the female reproductive tract. (Modified from Spalteholz, W.: Hand Atlas of Human Anatomy, ed. 7. J. B. Lippincott Co., Philadelphia, 1943.)

forms a dense sheath of connective tissue that serves to unite the vagina with surrounding structures. The muscular coat is composed of an outer layer of longitudinal and an inner layer of circular, smooth muscle fibers. The mucosa is a thick layer of stratified squamous epithelium, beneath which is a thin layer of connective tissue permeated by a network of blood vessels. Along the anterior and the posterior vaginal wall the mucosa form a longitudinal ridge from which numerous transverse ridges or rugae extend.

UTERUS AND CERVIX

The uterus occupies a position intermediate between the bladder and rectum. Its posterior wall is covered by peritoneum down to the cul-de-sac, whereas the anterior wall is covered only to the junction with the bladder (Fig. 21).

Flattened anteroposteriorly, the uterine cavity when opened laterally appears as an inverted cone with the cervix representing the apex (Fig. 22). The uterus can be divided both functionally and anatomically into the corpus and the cervix. The corpus comprises the main body of the uterus and contains certain subdivisions. The portion of the body superior to the insertion of the fallopian tubes is the fundus. In the inferior portion of the corpus and located just above the cervix is the isthmus, which measures a few millimeters in length. Softening of

this area, which can be detected on vaginal examination, is one of the early physical changes of the reproductive tract in pregnancy and is an invaluable sign in its diagnosis (Hegar's sign). In the course of pregnancy the isthmus becomes incorporated into the main body of the uterus and forms the major portion of the "lower uterine segment." The demarcation between the corpus and the isthmus is known as the "anatomic os." During pregnancy this demarcation is sometimes referred to as the "physiologic retraction ring," and it definitely marks the junction between the upper and lower uterine segments. In an occasional case of obstructed or prolonged labor, this area may become pathologically constricted. The inferior margin of the isthmus is the "histologic" or "internal os" of the cervix, which is further distinguished by the junction of the endometrial and endocervical mucosa.

The portion of the cervix above the attachment of the vagina, the portio supravaginalis, is in close relationship with the connective tissue beneath the bladder and the parametrial tissue within the broad ligament. The portion below the attachment of the vagina, the portio infravaginalis, projects into the vaginal fornices and at its tip presents an opening known as the "external os." In nulliparous women this is a small oval opening, whereas after childbirth it takes on the appearance of a transverse slit.

With the uterine corpus in an anterior position the cervix is located in the posterior fornix of the vagina. Certainly

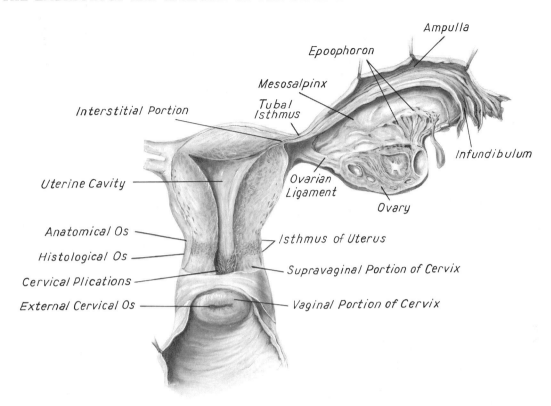

Figure 22. Longitudinal view of the female reproductive tract. (Modified from Spalteholtz, W.: Hand Atlas of Human Anatomy, ed. 7. J. B. Lippincott Co., Philadelphia, 1943.)

this is a favorable and perhaps in some instances a necessary position with respect to insemination. Frequently the cervix is located in the anterior fornix and behind the symphysis so that it is difficult on occasion to visualize it with a bivalve speculum. There are two reasons for the cervix to be in this position—either it is displaced forward by a mass in the cul-de-sac, in which case the corpus is likewise anterior, or by far more common, the uterus is in retroversion and the uterine corpus lies in the cul-de-sac. These distinctions must be kept in mind in a pelvic examination when the cervix is found in an anterior position.

The uterus is composed essentially of three decussating spiral systems of smooth muscle fasciculi, united by connective tissue. The arrangement of the muscle fibers may be traced to the müllerian ducts which, as they fuse, produce an interlacing pattern. The fibers of the outer layer are arranged predominantly in a longitudinal fashion, whereas the middle layer, which is much thicker, shows a circular arrangement. In addition, a very thin inner layer of longitudinal fibers in contact with the endometrium may be identified. The corpus and

isthmus are composed mostly of smooth muscle, but the ratio of fibrous tissue to muscle is much greater in the cervix.

The endometrium varies from 0.5 to 5.0 mm. in thickness, and consists of stroma and glands. Except for the gland openings, the outer surface of the endometrium is covered by a single layer of closely packed columnar cells. During pregnancy the stroma undergoes cellular alterations known as decidual change.

The cavity of the cervix, or endocervical canal, is lined by mucosa which forms a longitudinal ridge on the anterior and the posterior surface, from which secondary transverse ridges (cervical plications) circle the canal, giving it a herringbone appearance (Fig. 22). The mucosa is covered by narrow columnar epithelial cells. Beneath this layer and within the stroma are mucus-secreting racemose glands which open into the cervical canal. On occasion their openings become occluded to cause so-called nabothian cysts. The columnar epithelium lining the cervical canal merges with the squamous epithelium at the external os, the area being referred to clinically as the squamocolumnar junction.

LIGAMENTS

The uterus is suspended in position by a series of ligaments. From the lateral surfaces of the uterus to the fascia overlying the internal obturator and levator ani muscles are the broad ligaments, each consisting of a fold of peritoneum containing various structures. The superior and medial two thirds of each broad ligament contains the fallopian tube, while the lateral third forms the suspensory ligament of the ovary and serves to conduct the ovarian blood vessels (Fig. 23). The broad ligaments allow anteroposterior movements of the uterus but oppose lateral motion.

The round ligaments are fibromuscular cords, each of which arises from the lateral surface of the uterus below the insertion of the fallopian tube. Each runs in a forward, upward, and lateral direction, within the anterior leaf of the broad ligament, to the inguinal canal, through which it passes to terminate in the labium majus.

The function of maintaining the uterine corpus in anterior flexion, a state regarded as normal, is attributed to the round ligaments. Their ability to discharge this function is questioned by the finding that in some 40 per cent of nulliparous and adolescent females free of pelvic disease the uterus is found in retroversion, i.e., the reverse of what is regarded as normal. In women who have borne children, the incidence is probably higher. This suggests that there are perhaps other ligaments involved in maintaining the uterus in an anterior position.

During pregnancy obviously the round ligaments stretch. They appear as thumb-sized structures when pregnancy is near term. As might be anticipated, the stretching may cause discomfort and, on palpation of the ligaments, some degree of tenderness. The diagnosis of round ligament pain should be made only by exclusion. Mistakes have occurred when this easy diagnosis was invoked. Rather, repeated examination and

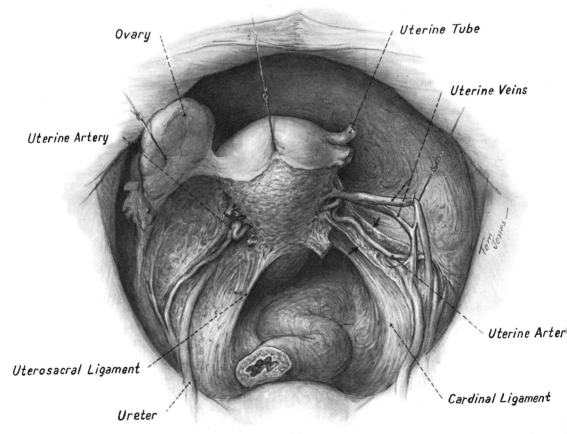

Figure 23. Subperitoneal structures within the broad ligament. The uterine tube, round ligament, and uterosacral ligaments have been removed on the right side. The arrows identify the cut margin of the parametrial tissues that invest the uterine artery. (Modified from Curtis, A. H., Anson, B. J., and Beaton, L. E., Surg., Gynec. Obstet. 70:642, 1940.)

a further search should be made to uncover a pathologic reason for the abdominal discomfort. Further, because the round ligaments stretch readily use of them alone in the infrequent and perhaps obsolete operation to correct a retroversion is of limited value. The retroversion is likely to reoccur postoperatively, perhaps within a matter of weeks or months.

The uterosacral ligaments originate from the posterior and upper portion of the cervix, pass laterally, and insert into the fascia covering the second and third sacral vertebrae. They act as stationary supports to the uterus, and tend to keep the cervix in the posterior fornix and oppose its displacement toward the symphysis (Fig. 23). This implies that in addition to surgical shortening of the round ligaments, the operation for correction or retroversion should include suturing the uterosacral ligaments together. This causes the cervix to be brought from an anterior position back into the posterior vaginal fornix and maintains it in that position.

The effectiveness of surgical approximation of the uterosacral ligaments is attested to by the results of the use of a suitable pessary to correct a retroversion. The same principle is involved, for, in the absence of pelvic disease, as the cervix is mechanically displaced posteriorly it is the rule rather than the exception for the corpus to move forward into an anterior position almost immediately or within a few days. Altering the position of the cervix and placing it in the posterior fornix changes the axis of the uterus and, abetted by intra-abdominal pressure, the corpus moves from the cul-de-sac to take up an anterior position. This simple procedure has both diagnostic and therapeutic value.

The cardinal ligaments are represented by the thickened inferior portion of the broad ligaments. They arise from the lateral walls of the cervix, where they may interdigitate with the originating uterosacral ligaments. The cardinal ligaments extend lateralward and insert into the fasciae of the internal obturator and levator ani muscles. The cardinal and uterosacral ligaments serve to immobilize the cervix and mark the most fixed portion of the uterus. Disruption of these ligaments leads to procidentia. In the operations devised to correct the prolapse and retain the uterus, these ligaments are sutured together in approximation to the anterior surface of the cervix following upward displacement of the bladder.

FALLOPIAN TUBES

The fallopian tubes (uterine tubes or oviducts) originate at the junction of the fundus with the main body of the uterus and extend to the region of the ovaries. Except for its distal portion, each tube is enclosed within the upper broad ligament. The portion of the broad ligament that invests the tube, known as the mesosalpinx (Fig. 22), contains nerves, blood vessels, and vestiges of the mesonephric duct system. As the tube courses lateralward along and ascends the pelvic wall, it curves about and envelops the upper pole of the ovary.

There are three subdivisions of the fallopian tube: the uterine or interstitial portion, included within the muscular wall of the uterus; the isthmus, which is the relatively straight portion immediately adjacent to the uterus; and the ampulla, the longest portion. A fourth division of the tube which may occasionally be considered for purposes of description is the infundibulum, the funnel-shaped lateral extremity of the tube (Fig. 22). The inner surface of the infundibulum is thrown into folds continuous with those of the ampulla, and these folds project outward, giving the extremity of the tube a fimbriated appearance. One fold, longer than the rest, remains attached to the mesosalpinx of the broad ligament and reaches toward the tubal pole of the ovary. This is the tubo-ovarian ligament, which is believed to aid in conducting the egg from the ruptured follicle into the lumen of the tube. The orifice of the fimbriated portion of the tube, communicating with the peritoneal cavity, is known as the abdominal ostium.

The musculature of the tube is arranged in two layers, an outer longitudinal layer and an inner circular layer. The mucosal lining of the tube is composed of a single layer of high columnar ciliated and unciliated epithelium resting on a thin basement membrane. During the menstrual cycle these cells undergo growth changes associated with increased secretory activity.

OVARIES

The ovaries are situated in the upper part of the pelvic cavity approximately at the origin of the external iliac veins and the brim of the pelvis, lateral to the uterus and behind the broad ligaments. Each is described as lying in a slight depression on the inner surface of the obturator muscle, known as the ovarian fossa, which occupies the area between the diverging external iliac and hypogastric vessels. The part of the ovary in contact with the ovarian fossa is referred to as the lateral surface, and that directed toward the uterus is the median surface. The extremes of the long axis of the ovary are designated the upper and lower or tubal and uterine poles, respectively.

The ovary is supported by a number of ligaments. The suspensory ligament of the ovary extends from its tubal or upper pole upward to the peritoneum of the pelvic wall. It represents the upper margin of the broad ligament which is not occupied by the fallopian tube and through which the ovarian vessels enter the broad ligament. The uterine or lower pole of the ovary is attached by the ovarian ligament to the lateral and posterior wall of the uterus below the insertion of the fallopian tube (Fig. 22). The position of the ovary within the pelvic cavity may vary normally. Retroversion of the uterus, growth of the uterus as in pregnancy, and variation in the length of the ligaments supporting the ovary, each may contribute to marked displacement. It is not uncommon for the otherwise normal ovary to prolapse into the cul-de-sac.

The ovary is composed of an outer zone, the cortex, and an inner portion, designated the medulla, through which the blood vessels and nerves enter. The cortex, which is covered with columnar epithelium, contains the ovarian follicles in various stages of development. These follicles are surrounded by stromal cells, some of which have endocrine function. The cortex varies in thickness and tends to become thinner with advancing years.

See Ovary, in Chapter 3.

BLOOD VESSELS

The blood supply to the organs of reproduction in the female is derived through the branches of the internal iliac and the ovarian arteries. These vessels pass through the loose areolar tissue beneath the pelvic peritoneum and the fascia overlying the muscles lining the lateral walls of the pelvis, and

approach the reproductive organs through the various supporting ligaments.

Originating from the common iliac artery inferior to its bifurcation, the internal iliac or hypogastric artery enters the true pelvis laterally at the point where the ureter dips over the brim of the pelvis. The artery continues along the wall of the pelvis on a level with the upper margin of the greater sciatic foramen, near which it divides into a posterior trunk and a small anterior trunk. For obstetric purposes the posterior trunk need not be considered.

The anterior trunk of the internal iliac or hypogastric artery gives origin to the middle hemorrhoidal artery and to the uterine, vaginal, and vesical arteries (Fig. 24), which are vessels of particular obstetric significance. The anterior branch is of major obstetric interest and importance, indeed, in any situation of uncontrolled bleeding in the pelvis. In critical obstetric situations, such as a uterine rupture with large broad ligament hematomas where the search for the disrupted uterine vessels is an exercise in futility, before the pelvis is explored, the hypogastric vessels should be identified and ligated. The peritoneum is incised lateral to the sacral promontory, and the incision is carried downward for several centimeters toward the posterior leaf of the broad ligament. The inner portion of the incised peritoneum together with the exposed ureter is retracted medially and the hypogastric arteries are identified near their origin and ligated (Fig. 24). A bilateral procedure will reduce the bleeding to manageable proportions and is truly lifesaving.

The uterine artery takes its origin near the ureter as the latter courses along the lateral wall of the pelvis. From the upper margin of the greater sacrosciatic notch, these two structures course downward and posteriorly in parallel arrangement until they reach the pelvic diaphragm. Entering the lower portion of the broad ligament, they then continue medially to approach the lateral margin of the uterus. Here the uterine artery passes above and superior to the ureter to enter the uterus at the junction of the cervix and corpus, where it divides into an ascending and a descending branch. The ureter turns downward and remains approximately 1.5 cm. away from and parallel to the cervix. Above the junction of the vagina and bladder, the ureter moves medially and

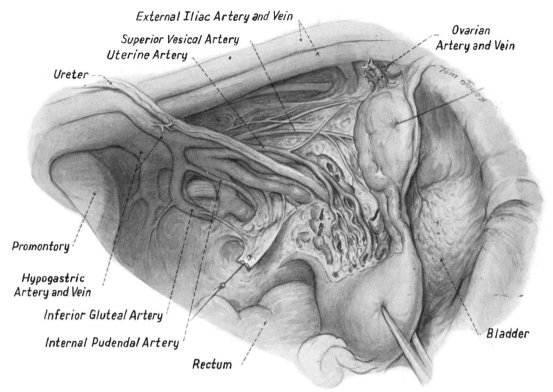

External Iliac Artery and Vein

Superior Vesical Artery

Uterine Artery

Ureter

Ovarian Artery and Vein

Promontory

Hypogastric Artery and Vein

Inferior Gluteal Artery

Internal Pudendal Artery

Rectum

Bladder

Figure 24. Anterior division of the hypogastric artery and veins of the posterior part of the left side of the pelvis. (Modified from Curtis, A. H., Anson, B. J., Ashley, F. L., and Jones, T., Surg., Gynec. Obstet., 75:421, 1942.)

enters the trigone of the bladder (Fig. 23).

The ascending or main branch of the uterine artery, which is noted for its spiral appearance, forms an extensive anastomosis with the ovarian artery and with the uterine artery of the opposite side. The corkscrew-like arrangement of the upper branch of the uterine artery allows the vessel to extend itself and accommodate to the growth of the uterus during pregnancy. The unspiraled descending branch forms an anastomosis with the vaginal artery, and with their increased size during pregnancy these pulsating vessels are easily palpated along the lateral side of the cervix at vaginal examination.

The vesical arteries, varying in number from one to six, are derived from the functional remnant of the umbilical artery. They originate near the beginning of the uterine artery, and pursue an anterior course along the lateral wall of the pelvis, curving medialward through the retroperitoneal space toward the bladder. Often these arteries sweep upward over the peritoneal surface of the anterior abdominal wall and anastomose with branches of the inferior epi-

gastric artery. When the abdomen is opened through a lower midline incision, arterial bleeding may be encountered from the peritoneal edge of the lower angle of the incision. This bleeding is from the terminal branches of the superior vesical arteries and denotes the proximity of the bladder.

The vaginal artery, which is the counterpart of the inferior vesical artery in the male, originates and pursues a course similar to that of the posterior branch of the vesical arteries. Near the cervicovaginal junction, the vessel passes around the cervix, anastomosing with its companion of the opposite side and the descending branch of the uterine artery. This artery is the source of the blood supply to the upper part of the vagina. If bleeding from the vaginal cuff is encountered at the time of complete abdominal hysterectomy in either the nonpregnant or the pregnant patient, it is derived from this vessel, as is also the bleeding from lacerations in the upper fornices of the vagina should such laceration occur during labor or delivery.

The obliterated umbilical arteries course from the lateral vesical margin to the dome of the bladder. At the midline where these vestigial vessels converge, the urachus or embryonal remnant of the allantois will be encountered as a ligament-like band of fibrous tissue. These structures must be incised in separating the prevesical or endopelvic fascia from the fundus of the bladder in the performance of extraperitoneal cesarean section. In rare cases of prolonged labor in which the lower uterine segment may become markedly elongated, the ureter may be displaced upward. In such circumstances the ureter may be encountered at the edge of the bladder slightly below the lateral reflection of the vesical peritoneum. This is the same area where the obliterated umbilical artery approaches the bladder. These structures can be differentiated on careful palpation, however, by demonstrating that the obliterated artery courses upward to the dome of the bladder, whereas the ureter passes downward to the region of the trigone.

The ovarian artery originates from the aorta distal to the renal artery, courses along the psoas muscles, and descends over the brim of the pelvis near the origin of the hypogastric artery. Here the ovarian artery passes above the ureter and gains entrance to the hilus of the ovary through the suspensory or infundibulopelvic ligament. Branches continue medially, forming an important surgical anastomosis with the ascending branch of the uterine artery.

The origin of the internal pudendal artery from the anterior trunk of the internal iliac artery is near the lumbosacral division of the sacral plexus. The vessel courses downward, leaving the pelvis through the greater sacrosciatic foramen to circle about the ischial spine. Penetrating the pelvic diaphragm, it emerges into the ischiorectal fossa. Before reaching the perineum the internal pudendal artery gives off one of its major branches, the inferior hemorrhoidal artery, which supplies the lateral and posterior portion of the external rectal sphincter. This vessel is injured only after the most unusual accident of delivery, involving lacerations about the anal sphincter or extension of a mediolateral episiotomy into the ischiorectal fossa. From the ischiorectal fossa and the lower margin of the urogenital diaphragm, the internal pudendal artery emerges to terminate in two branches, the perineal and clitoral arteries. Before dividing, the artery, with its accompanying vein, is in close

proximity to the pudendal nerve, a relation that is important in the performance of local block anesthesia of the perineum.

The perineal artery enters the superficial compartment of the perineum and, by branching vessels, supplies the surrounding structures, which include the ischiocavernosus, bulbocavernosus, and superficial perineal muscles. Penetrating the deep layer of the superficial perineal fascia (Colles' fascia) near the perineal body or central point of the perineum, the perineal artery anastomoses with its counterpart of the opposite side and the terminal branches of the inferior and middle hemorrhoidal arteries (Fig. 17). In an episiotomy, particularly of the midline type, the perineal artery commonly can be observed as a small spurting vessel beneath the cut edge of the deep layer of the superficial perineal fascia.

The clitoral branch of the internal pudendal artery enters the deep compartment of the anterior component of the perineum by penetrating the inferior fascia of the urogenital diaphragm. This artery supplies the membranous urethra and emerges again anteriorly into the superficial compartment of the perineum to terminate about the clitoris. Bleeding from lacerations occurring about the urethra and clitoris at delivery may be extensive, owing to the rich blood supply furnished by these terminal vessels (Fig. 18).

The veins of the generative tract have, in general, a pattern similar to that of the arteries, but certain differences can be noted in the extent of distribution. The blood from the vulva and perineum is collected by means of three independent venous channels. The external pudendal vein receives blood from the anterior portion of the pudendum and from the labia majora. The vessel then passes lateralward from beneath the mons to enter the fossa ovalis and empty into the greater saphenous vein of the femoral group. Venous drainage of this area of the vulva and particularly from the external portion of the clitoris may also be by way of the dorsal vein of the clitoris. This vessel pierces the upper margin of the transverse ligament of the pelvis to empty into the pudendal plexus situated about the vesical neck. From this plexus and the vesical plexus which lies along the margin of the bladder, the blood is collected and returned to the hypogastric or internal iliac vein by way of the vesical veins. The blood from the lower portion of the vulva and the structures within the different compartments of the perineum is returned through the internal pudendal veins to the hypogastric vein. The rich anastomoses between the veins of the vulva and perineum and the presence of many tributaries which empty into the systemic circulation at various points combine to make the treatment of varicosities rather unsatisfactory.

The major portion of venous blood from the uterus is drained by way of the uterine vein into the hypogastric vein, while the remainder drains through the ovarian or pampiniform plexus. On the right, these vessels empty into the caval circulation directly; on the left they empty by way of the renal vein. During pregnancy the veins surrounding the uterus, including those beneath the bladder, within the broad ligaments, and about the cervix and upper portion of the vagina, become greatly enlarged and engorged with blood. The veins in the broad ligaments appear medusa-like, and although they may be a centimeter or more in diameter during late pregnancy they regain their normal size soon after delivery.

The ability of these veins to expand to rather enormous proportions is seemingly important in the maintenance of a constant intrauterine venous pressure. With the enlarging uterus overlying the large pelvic veins, the amount of venous blood within them must be markedly altered when the pregnant patient changes position from the upright to the supine. These resultant fluctuations of venous pressure would be readily transferred to the uterine veins were it not for the ability of neighboring veins to compensate by this distention. Since the ovarian and uterine veins are devoid of valves, the only mechanism to maintain constant venous pressure within the uterus is the ability of the venous plexuses surrounding the uterus to expand and contract.

The middle hemorrhoidal vein connects with the superior and inferior branches and then passes outward on the surface of the levator ani muscles to empty into the hypogastric vein. Anorectal varicosities, or hemorrhoids, are very frequent during pregnancy and arise from the internal pudendal and hemorrhoidal vessels. The superior branch of the hemorrhoidal vessels, being a part of the portal system, lacks valves and is therefore particularly affected by the pressure from the growing uterus.

LYMPHATICS

The lymphatic drainage of the reproductive system occurs through two large groups of nodes. One group is situated below and distal to the inguinal ligament, which in turn communicates with the second group proximal to the ligament. The lymphatic vessels of the superficial and deep compartments of the perineum, including the anus, vulva, and lower third of the vagina, and those of the lower portions of the anterior abdominal wall drain into a large group of lymph nodes situated in the fossa ovalis. The efferent channels of these superficial inguinal and subinguinal nodes penetrate the deep fascia to connect with a deeper group of nodes. After receiving drainage from about the deeper structures of the clitoris, this deep subinguinal group of lymphatic channels joins with nodes lying above and lateral to the large pelvic vessels. The external and common iliac lymphatic chains also drain the bladder, after which they join with the aortic group. The cervical portion of the uterus and the upper two thirds of the vagina drain into the external and common iliac nodes directly or by way of the hypogastric group, while drainage from the uterine corpus and ovaries is into the aortic and ovarian lymphatics, respectively.

NERVES

The autonomic nerves that supply the reproductive system arise from T5 to T12 and from S2, S3, and S4. The sympathetic component with both motor and sensory fibers serves to innervate the body of the uterus and the adnexa, including the ovary. Sensory stimuli arising from the uterus are transmitted to the pelvic plexus or great cervicouterine ganglion of Lee-Frankenhäuser, located on the posterior uterine wall in close association with the uterosacral ligaments. The impulse travels upward over the inferior and middle hypogastric plexuses to the superior hypogastric plexus which is located below but close to the bifurcation of the aorta. From here it is carried over the aortic plexus to enter the cord at T11 and T12. By contrast, impulses from the fallopian tubes, the lateral portion of the broad ligaments, and the ovaries are transmitted over sympathetic fibers which accompany the ovarian vessels to enter the aortic plexus either directly or by way of the renal plexus. They likewise terminate at T11 and T12. That sensory impulses from the uterus course over the superior hypogastric plexus is deduced from study of patients who have had a presacral neurectomy for idiopathic dysmenorrhea. In patients who have undergone such surgery the first stage of labor is usually quite painless, and, in fact, they are unaware that they are in labor until the second stage is reached. Interruption of the hypogastric plexus by presacral neurectomy will not, however, abolish pain originating in the distal portions of the adnexa, for reasons cited above. Presumably, impulses arising in the lower uterine segment, cervix, and upper vagina pass through the pelvic plexus, from where they are carried over the parasympathetic component or pelvic nerve to enter the cord at S2, S3, and S4.

The sympathetic motor fibers leave the cord between T5 and T10, whereas the parasympathetic motor fibers originate from S2, S3, and S4. The motor control of the uterus has been the subject of much speculation. Earlier beliefs assigned to the sympathetic system the control of the circular muscle fibers of the uterus, particularly of the lower segment and cervix, and to the parasympathetic system the responsibility for the motor activity of the corpus. The present-day view, however, favors the belief that the sympathetic system is responsible for the neuromuscular activity of the upper uterine segment, while the lower uterine segment and cervix are under parasympathetic dominance. The fact that uterine contractions cease if the level of spinal anesthesia reaches T5 or T6 supports the contention that the motor control of the corpus is mediated by way of the sympathetic system.

Whatever nerve elements are present in the uterus apparently accompany the blood vessels as sympathetic nerve fibers. Nerve trunks enter the uterus along the branches of the uterine artery. In the inner portion of the uterine musculature branches of these trunks may be seen in association with the radial arteries. Nonmyelinated or vasomotor fibers and myelinated or sensory fibers have been seen in the basal layer of the endometrium, but sensory end-organs have not been demonstrated.

Although it is stated that the uterus may labor effectively without connections to the central nervous system, the statement can be taken with some reservation. This contention can be supported only when the lesion is above T5, which means the sensory loss is at or above the area of the nipple. Certainly spinal anesthesia that extends to this height will obliterate uterine contractions in the patient in labor. Reputedly patients with extensive thoracolumbar sympathectomies have productive labors; this procedure interrupts sympathetic trunks from T6 to L1 or L2 and spares the sacral parasympathetics. It is unlikely, however, that motor impulses passing over the latter nerves per se are concerned with uterine contractions.

The somatic innervation of the female reproductive tract involves the nerves which originate from L1 and L2 and from S2, S3, and S4. The group of nerves from the lumbar segments consists of the ilioinguinal, iliohypogastric, and genitocrural nerves. While branches of these converge over the mons, the ilioinguinal nerves continue down to supply the labia majora. The pudendal nerve, derived from the anterior rami of S2, S3, and S4, follows a course within the ischiorectal fossa similar to that of the internal pudendal artery. Classically, the nerve has been described as passing through the greater sacrosciatic notch and over the ischial spine to enter the lesser sacrosciatic notch and the pudendal canal. More recent anatomic study has shown that the pudendal nerve remains posterior to the ischial spine. The nerve emerges from the pudendal canal above the sacrotuberous ligament and, as it approaches the urogenital diaphragm, divides into two main terminal branches. The more superficial branch, the perineal nerve, accompanies the perineal artery and subdivides into labial nerves. The other branch, the clitoral nerve, passes with the clitoral artery into the deep compartment of the perineum and anteriorly occupies a more superficial location, to terminate over the anterior surface of the glans of the clitoris (Fig. 17). The inferior hemorrhoidal nerve supplying the anal region arises from the pudendal nerve just prior to this terminal division, or it may originate as a separate structure.

BIBLIOGRAPHY

Embryology

Benirschke, K.: Adrenals in anencephaly and hydrocephaly. Obstet. Gynec., 4:412, 1956.

Benirschke, K., and Bloch, E., and Hertig, A. T.: Concerning function of fetal zone of human adrenal gland. Endocrinology, 58:598, 1956.

Felix, W.: Development of the Urinogenital Organs; II. Development of Reproductive Glands and Their Ducts. In Keibel and Mall, eds.: Human Embryology, vol. 2. J. B. Lippincott Co., Philadelphia, 1912, p. 881.

Fischel, A.: Ueber die Entwicklung der Keimdrüsen des Menschen. (Origin of the sex cords.) Z. Ges. Ant., 92:34, 1930.

Gillman, J.: Development of gonads in man, with consideration of role of fetal endocrines and histogenesis of ovarian tumors. Contrib. Embryol., 32:81, 1948.

Jarcho, J.: Malformations of the uterus; review of subject including embryology, comparative anatomy, diagnosis and report of cases. Amer. J. Surg., 71:106, 1946.

Jones, H. W., and Jones, G. E. S.: Double uterus as etiological factor in repeated abortions. Amer. J. Obstet. Gynec., 65:325, 1953.

Koff, A. K.: Development of vagina in human fetus. Contrib. Embryol., 24:61, 1933.

Mansell, H., and Hertig, A. T.: Granulosa-theca cell tumors and endometrial carcinoma. Obstet Gynec., 6:385, 1955.

McKay, D. G., Hertig, A. T., and Hickey, W. F.: The histogenesis of granulosa and theca cell tumors of the human ovary. Obstet. Gynec., 1:125, 1953.

Meyer, R.: Pathology of some special ovarian tumors and their relation to sex characteristics. Amer. J. Obstet. Gynec., 22:697, 1931.

Novak, E.: Functioning tumors of ovary with special reference to pathology and histogenesis. J. Obstet. Gynaec. Brit. Emp., 55:725, 1948.

Pinkerton, J. H. M., McKay, D. G., Adams, E. C., and Hertig, A. T.: Development of the human ovary—a study using histochemical technics. Obstet Gynec., 18:152, 1961.

Spaulding, M. H.: Development of external genitalia in human embryo. Contrib. Embryol., 13:67, 1921.

Sternburg, W. H.: Morphology, androgenic function, hyperplasia, and tumors of human ovarian hilus cells. Amer. J. Path., 25:493, 1949.

Swift, C. H.: Origin and early history of primordial germ cells in the chick. Amer. J. Anat., 15:483, 1914.

Traut, H. F., and Butterworth, J. S.: Theca, granulosa, lutein cell tumors of human ovary and similar tumors of mouse's ovary. Amer. J. Obstet. Gynec., 34:987, 1937.

Wilson, K. M.: Correlation of external genitalia and sex glands in human embryo. Contrib. Embryol., 18:23, 1926.

Woolf, R. B., and Allen, W. M.: Concomitant malformations. Obstet. Gynec., 2:236, 1952.

Anatomy

Anson, B. J.: Atlas of Human Anatomy, ed. 2. W. B. Saunders Co., Philadelphia, 1963.

Burchell, R. C.: Internal iliac artery ligation: hemodynamics. Obstet. Gynec., 24:737, 1964.

Cleland, J. A. P.: Paravertebral anesthesia in obstetrics; experimental and clinical basis. Surg. Gynec. Obstet., 57:51, 1933.

Curtis, A. H., Anson, B. J., Ashley, F. L., and Jones, T.: Blood vessels of female pelvis in relation to gynecological surgery. Surg. Gynec. Obstet., 75:421, 1942.

Curtis, A. H., Anson, B. J., Ashley, F. L., and Jones, T.: Anatomy of the pelvic autonomic nerves in relation to gynecology. Surg. Gynec. Obstet., 75:743, 1942.

Hirsch, E. F., and Martin, M. E.: Distribution of nerves in adult human myometrium. Surg. Gynec. Obstet., 76:697, 1943.

Klink, E. W.: Perineal nerve block. Obstet. Gynec., 1:137, 1953.

Kuntz, A.: The Autonomic Nervous System. Lea & Febiger, Philadelphia, 1945.

Spalteholz, W.: Hand Atlas of Human Anatomy, ed. 7. J. B. Lippincott Co., Philadelphia, 1943.

Chapter 6

Gametogenesis and Fertilization

MITOSIS AND MEIOSIS

The somatic cells of man possess 46 chromosomes; 44 are autosomes and 2 are sex chromosomes. In the male the sex chromosomes are XY, and in the female they are XX. In the interphase state, i.e., when cells are not dividing and, usually, are productive of whatever their function (e.g., protein synthesis), the chromosomes are arranged in threadlike structures within the nucleus and cannot be individually recognized. They exist as pairs, one of each pair being derived from the paternal ancestor, and the other from the maternal ancestor.

The chromosomes may be visualized during *mitosis*, the process of cell division. Just prior to the time of division each chromosome duplicates an exact replica which remains attached to the master copy at the centromere until division. These structures subsequently condense, each thread now called a chromatid, and they may then be visualized. Their size and particular shapes allow the construction of karyotypes as shown in Figure 1 in Chapter 10. The spindle fibers of the mitotic spindle attach to the centromere and, at the time of division (anaphase), the chromatids of each chromosome separate one from another and are pulled by the spindle fibers into the respective daughter cells, whose nuclear membrane then reconstitutes. Thus, during mitosis each daughter cell receives the same chromosome complement as was present in the original cell prior to chromosome duplication. The latter process of DNA replication occupies a specific period in the cell cycle, the so-called S-phase (synthesis phase). The successive stages of mitosis are designated prophase, metaphase, anaphase, and telophase.

Gametogenesis, i.e., the formation of sperm and egg, employs an entirely different series of events that is termed *meiosis* (from the Greek verb "to lessen"). Meiosis is known to occur only in the germinal cells of the gonads and it comprises two cellular divisions, one following the other in close succession. The end-result of meiosis is that from a diploid (2n=46), or normal, precursor cell, four haploid (n=23) specialized elements arise. In the male these are four spermatozoa; in the female they are the large ovum plus three diminutive polar bodies.

Meiosis commences with a duplication of chromosomes (chromonemata) in the leptotene stage. In the subsequent zygotene stage the homologous elements pair, a process that must be envisaged in the following way: Inasmuch as two nearly identical elements of all chromosomes exist (except XY) they align and fuse in a zipper-like fashion, presumably because of their identical DNA structure. Pairing of homologues is essential for normal meiotic events to proceed and this phase is often called synapsis. This stage blends into pachynema at which time the "bivalents" shorten and develop focal and very characteristic thickened portions. It is this stage that allows, in ideal preparations, accurate description of chromosomes. The pachytene stage gives way to the diplonema at which time crossing-over may be observed. These crosses or chiasmata are sites of exchange between sister chromatids. Their number and location determine the shape of the bivalents and are relatively characteristic for individual species. It is from this crossing-over process that genetic variation arises in the forthcoming cell products. Thus, various pieces of chromosome material are exchanged between paternally derived and maternally derived homologous chromosomes. Subsequent to this event diakinesis with shortening of the bivalents occurs, the nuclear membrane disappears, a spindle apparatus forms, and metaphase I takes

166

place. The equatorial plate is formed and at anaphase I the chromosomes segregate into the two daughter cells of the first division which is complete in telophase I. It will be realized that the total amount of DNA per nucleus was doubled at the first stage and its original amount is reached again in the daughter cells of this first meiosis. Meiosis II commences very shortly after this event and is of very short duration. A spindle is formed, the nuclear membrane is dissolved, and at anaphase II the two attached chromatids are separated into daughter cells. Since no new synthetic period ensued, the results of meiosis II are two haploid (n=23) cells.

Abnormalities occur occasionally in mitosis and in meiosis. The most commonly observed is referred to as nondisjunction. By this term is meant that one (rarely more) element does not dissociate from the homologous partner and, failing to separate, is pulled into one daughter cell with its partner. In mitotic nondisjunction, the daughter cells will then contain 47 and 45 elements, respectively. Depending on the elements involved, such nondisjunction may be lethal to cellular function by the genetic imbalance it has caused. If it is not, the result is chromosomal "mosaicism," and should the event occur very early in embryonic life it leads to an individual composed of two or more types of cells. Most commonly such "mosaic" individuals are seen with the sex chromosomal anomalies.

Nondisjunction may also occur at meiosis I or II, and current evidence indicates that some environmental agencies may be critical. If the event occurs in meiosis I, then four unbalanced gametes result; if it happens in meiosis II only two abnormal gametes result, the genetic consequences being somewhat different. Fertilization of an abnormal gamete, say an ovum with n=24, by a normal spermatozoon (n=23) results in a trisomic individual. Various genetic evidence has been adduced to show that trisomics arise from disturbances in both meiosis I and II, occurring during oogenesis as well as during spermatogenesis. Second meiosis in the female usually follows sperm penetration and it has been shown in experimental animals that delayed fertilization interferes with normal meiotic events. Because trisomies occur more frequently with advancing maternal age, it has been suggested that the common denominator in their pathogenesis

may be delayed fertilization of an aging ovum, but direct observations are lacking as yet.

SPERMATOGENESIS

The germ cells are set aside early in embryologic development and multiply in the entodermal region. They are large cells, possessing much glycogen, alkaline phosphatase, and also ameboid motility. During the first six weeks of fetal development they migrate from the entodermal region via the mesentery to the gonadal ridge to which they are chemically attracted. Some also reach the circulation, as is the normal process in birds, and thence "home" to the gonad in a similar manner. Visual sexual differentiation in the human embryo begins at about 17 to 18 mm. length when cords are formed in the male, presumably because of the XY chromosome constitution of the gonadal stroma rather than because of the XY constitution of the migrating germ cells. The latter reach these cordlike structures and multiply within what are to become the seminiferous tubules among future Sertoli cells. After birth the population of germ cells (spermatogonia) is significantly reduced by an ill understood degenerative phase and the testis remains dormant until puberty. With the stimulation of the interstitial (Leydig) cells the spermatogonia once again become mitotically active and the highly complex process of spermatogenesis commences.

In the adult testis different types of spermatogonia can be identified by their tinctorial properties. They occur in groups and cytoplasmic bridges develop between many of them, presumably assuring synchronous meiotic process of clusters of germ cells. A distinct "wave" of meiosis, as is seen in many mammals to proceed along the seminiferous tubules, is not detected in man. Some spermatogonia continue to remain mitotic precursor cells while others proceed to develop into primary spermatocytes as they enter meiosis. Their nuclei become smaller and condensed as divisions proceed and the cytoplasm arranges itself to assume the tadpole-shaped structure in which the tail of the final spermatozoon develops.

The X and Y chromosomes of the spermatocyte cannot pair side by side, as is the case with all other chromosome pairs, because of their difference in size, structure, and gene content. The sex chromosomes are initially contained in what is referred to as the sex vesicle and pairing begins here in a highly characteristic end-to-end fashion. Although it is as yet uncertain, it is possible that minor segments of X and Y are exchanged here as is normal for other chromosomes at the site of chiasmata. From each primary spermatocyte two spermatozoa (spermatids) containing one X chromosome (n=23) and two spermatozoa containing one Y chromosome (n=23) develop. The entire time required for spermatogenesis from the appearance of earliest spermatocytes (meiosis) is estimated to be 64 days in man. After meiosis is completed the resultant haploid spermatids enter the complex process of spermiogenesis, i.e., maturation into a spermatozoon.

The Sertoli cells do not divide in adults but undergo significant cyclic changes correlated with the development of the germ cells. They are surrounded by germ cells; spermatocytes in turn are enveloped by cytoplasmic processes of the Sertoli cells. Presumably substances are passed from the latter into the spermatocytes, hence their description as nurse cells (Fig. 1). The entire process of spermatogenesis is regulated by pituitary gonadotropins. Follicle-stimulating hormone (FSH) is believed to exert a direct stimulating effect on the seminiferous tubules, while the interstitial cell-stimulating hormone (ICSH) aids spermatogenesis by causing the Leydig cells to secrete androgens. The androgenic hormones, in turn, not only assist in maintaining spermatogenesis but also are responsible for completion of the development of the male sex characteristics. In the normal male, pituitary gonadotropin may be detected in the urine prior to the somatic changes associated with puberty.

The appearance, within less than a year, of increased somatic growth and of pubic and axillary hair and the completion of development of the primary sex characteristics indicate the onset of puberty. These bodily changes usually occur between the ages of 12 and 14 years, but a wide range in these ages must be considered normal. Unless these changes occur before the age of 10 or after the age of 18, puberty need not be considered precocious or delayed. Beyond these limits deviations from normal sexual development in the male may be due to some of the same conditions that produce precocious menstruation or primary amenorrhea in the female.

Abnormal spermatogenesis, however, may occur in the absence of any demonstrable lesion. This suggests that an optimal pituitary-gonadal relationship is necessary for normal spermatogenesis to be completed. The presence of a high titer of urinary FSH in either the absence of testicular tissue or failure of function illustrates the reciprocal action between the pituitary and the testes. The correct proportion of

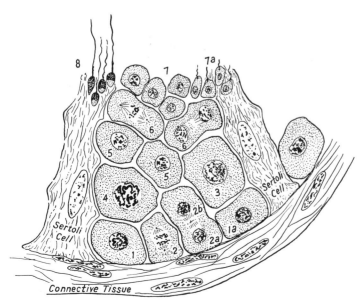

Figure 1. Semischematic view of segment of wall of active seminiferous tubule. (*1*) Spermatogonium divides (*2*) into two daughter cells (*2a* and *2b*), one of which (*2a*) remains peripherally located as a new spermatogonium (*1a*). The other daughter cell (*2b*) becomes a primary spermatocyte (*3*) and is moved closer to the lumen of the tubule. When fully grown (*4*) the primary spermatocyte divides and produces two secondary spermatocytes (*5, 5*). Each secondary spermatocyte divides (*6, 6*), producing spermatids (*7*). The spermatids become embedded in the tip of the Sertoli cells (*7a*), where they develop into spermatozoa (*8*) and, when mature, they are detached into the lumen of the tubule. (From Patten, B. M.: Human Embryology, 2nd ed. Blakiston Division, McGraw-Hill Book Co., Inc., New York, 1953.)

gonadotropic and gonadal hormones is believed to be as essential for optimal spermatogenesis as it is for ovulation in the female.

The maturing sperm eventually move out of the tubules and come to lodge within the epididymis, where they undergo final ripening. At this stage of their development the sperm cells are nonmotile and are rather sensitive to heat. They are protected from variations in temperature during their stay in the testis by the muscle of the scrotum, which will contract and relax in response to changes in environmental temperature. This muscular response serves to vary the thickness of the insulating scrotal wall. As spermatogenesis continues under the endocrine stimulation of the androgens, the older sperm are propelled into the vas deferens. Somewhere along the course of this structure they acquire both the power of motility and the ability to withstand the temperature within the body. The prostatic fluid has a glucose content two to three times that of blood plasma. This is undoubtedly essential as a source of supply of sufficient energy for the sperm not only to survive but to maintain a high state of motility.

Examination of specimens of semen from fertile males reveals a considerable variation in the metabolism, morphology, and physical activity of the spermatozoa. Although the metabolic rate of sperm from the same person is remarkably constant on repeated examination, there is a wide range in the metabolic rate of sperm from different men. This is only one example of the inherent difficulties encountered in attempts to establish what constitutes normal sperm behavior and to determine the relation of variations in morphology and motility to infertility. Nevertheless, there appear to be certain minimal requirements for a high fertility rate. The number of sperm contained in 1 ml. of normal seminal fluid is in the range of 60 million to 120 million. Microscopic examination of normal fresh human ejaculate (normally between 4 and 5 ml.) reveals that 80 per cent or more of the sperm are motile, and abnormal or immature forms do not exceed 10 to 15 per cent. It is believed that the presence of a larger proportion of these abnormal forms may contribute to male infertility, but this is apparently not a factor in the problem of repetitive abortion.

OOGENESIS

Primordial germ cells arrive in the fetal ovary in much the same way as in the male and rapid mitotic activity makes the embryonal ovary a large oblong structure composed of almost exclusively oogonia. From the gonadal stroma, cells differentiate which, initially, enclose groups of oogonia that are again connected one to another by cytoplasmic bridges. Cytoplasmic substances as large as mitochondria are known to be exchanged via these bridges, and groupwise proliferative events are assured by these connections. With advancing development the gonadal stromal elements come to surround individual oogonia which then separate the connections with other germ cells. These stromal cells assume cuboidal shape and ultimately develop into the granulosa layer of the follicle. Commonly at birth, and sometimes in mature ovaries, two or more oogonia are found to be enveloped by a single layer of granulosa cells.

After the sixth month of fetal development proliferative activity gradually ceases in the female germ cells and, contrary to the development in the testis, meiosis commences (Fig. 2). There is no further mitosis of germ cells and the newborn has a maximal complement of oogonia, usually estimated to be at least about 750,000. Their number decreases from then on by degenerative events and by follicular development. Counts indicate that between 6 and 15 years of age 439,000 are present; from 16 to 25 years there are 159,000; between 26 and 35 years there remain 59,000; and between 36 and 45 years there are 34,000. All have disappeared after menopause.

As the mitotic stages of germ cell maturation cease, meiosis commences; however, both stages occur side by side for some time. Leptotene stages of meiosis commence at approximately 13 weeks of gestation and proceed through zygonema and pachynema to the diplotene stage where all meiotic prophase is arrested for a prolonged period of time. The special stage of arrested prophase is usually referred to as the dictyate stage (dictyotene) but authors disagree whether this special stage can be recognized in man. In any event, it will be seen that chromosomes have already paired, the DNA has duplicated (i.e., the cell is tetraploid), and further development remains

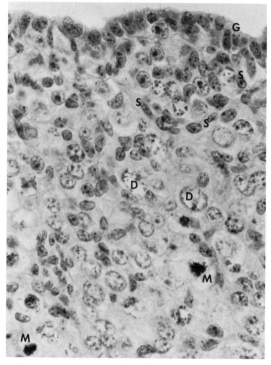

Figure 2. Ovary of 15 cm. crown-rump fetus, gestational age approximately 18 weeks. Oogonial mitoses (*M*) are still present but a majority of cells have entered meiotic prophase and are at the dictyate (*D*) stage. Their large nuclei are tetraploid at this stage which remains arrested until ovulation. Stromal cells (*S*) are sparse and begin to enclose groups of oogonia. The so-called germinal (*G*) epithelium is modified peritoneum and does not contribute to oogenesis. H & E × 700.

precluded by some unknown mechanism until the time of follicular development preparatory to ovulation. The cell in arrested meiotic prophase is referred to as the primary oocyte. Upon stimulation of the graafian follicle by gonadotropins meiosis is resumed and the first polar body is released, the secondary oocyte retaining the major portion of cytoplasm. Only a small amount of cytoplasm is given off with the first polar body. This division occurs immediately prior to ovulation, the second meiotic division occurring shortly after fertilization. In this second meiosis the second polar body is expelled and the original diploid chromosome content reduced to the haploid state (n = 23). Thus, when fertilization occurs with the haploid fertilizing spermatozoon the zygote attains the normal diploid number of man, 2n=46. It is possible that the first polar body also proceeds through a second meiotic division, but all three polar bodies, having virtually no cytoplasm, are destined to vanish. For a while they may be seen around the ovum,

within the zona pellucida (see Fig. 4).

Abnormalities occur in the process of female meiosis. If the second polar body is not eliminated a triploid cell (3n=67) may result. This is presumably the mechanism by which the frequent triploid abortuses arise. Nondisjunction of individual chromosomes may lead to trisomies, monosomies, and so forth, like the processes described earlier. It has been suggested that, in the absence of fertilization, abnormal circumstances may trigger on occasion further development of the secondary oocyte. Thus, it is envisaged that parthenogenetic development may lead to ovarian teratomata or dermoid cysts.

SEX DETERMINATION

The haploid ovum possesses 23 chromosomes, one of which is the X chromosome. Approximately half of the haploid spermatozoa contain a Y chromosome and half contain an X chromosome. Presumably only chance determines which of these two types fertilizes the ovum and thus an approximately equal number of 46 XY and 46 XX zygotes are formed. The fact that a slight male preponderance is found in neonates is offset by a greater loss of female zygotes in spontaneous abortion. Moreover, since zygotes with 45,XO chromosome constitution are not uncommon, particularly among aborted specimens, and because it is impossible to ascertain what the missing sex chromosome "should have been," it is not feasible to arrive at an accurate assessment of the sex ratio at conception.

For several weeks the fetal development proceeds along neuter lines. At approximately 17 to 18 mm. length it becomes possible to distinguish the testis because of its tubular structure. It is presumed that the Y chromosome in the XY stroma effects this structural change, since it is lacking in XO and XX embryos. Interstitial cell development is abundant early and the secretory products of these cells initiate internal and external masculinization. No evidence exists that the fetal ovary, on the other hand, plays an active role in shaping internal and external female sexual development. These structural changes may well occur because of the environment of female steroid hormones from the placenta.

An understanding of the mechanism of sex differentiation is important because of the relative frequency of abnormalities that occur. The earliest impetus for detailed studies came from the classic studies of Lillie and of Keller and Tandler. These investigators observed that when fraternal, heterosexual cattle twins have interplacental vascular connections, the male causes the female twin to develop into a sterile freemartin. In such animals the ovary is rudimentary, often having testis-like configuration, and the internal duct system is severely masculinized. The twins are also permanent blood chimeras. Hormonal factors were then postulated to effect the virilization of the female and extensive experiments by Jost and others have supported this concept. Still, the original mechanism by which a testis develops and the exact nature of hormonal factors are undetermined.

Although some continue to hold the opinion that sex differentiation of the duct system is also genetically determined, there is a large body of evidence to support the generally accepted view that the reproductive organs develop under endocrine influences. From earlier experiments in lower animals, fetal sexual dimorphism similar to that observed in the subhuman primate, as cited above, led to formulation of the dihormonic and monohormonic theories to explain the mode of sex differentiation of the duct system. The dihormonic theory stated that the primordia of the genital organs differentiated into a male or female reproductive system, depending on the predominance of androgens or estrogens present. The monohormonic theory proposed that differentiation of the duct system was due to the presence of sufficient amounts of androgens only. Under the terms of the monohormonic theory, male sexual development occurs only in the presence of physiologic amounts of male or testicular hormone, and female sexual development occurs in its absence. Considerable weight has been added to the monohormonic theory by castration experiments in rabbit fetuses. If the fetus is castrated on the 19th day, when the genital tract is still undifferentiated, sexual development of the duct system proceeds normally in the female fetus. Castration of the male fetus, on the other hand, results in the production of a female-like reproductive tract.

It is evident, experimentally, that sex differentiation of the duct system in the male is derived from its own gonad. In this regard, in the human, attention has been called to the fact that the interstitial or endocrine cells of the human fetal testes are especially prominent during the first half of gestation, suggesting that they may be endocrinologically active. Although these interstitial cells appear to regress later, their early prominence may indicate that they fulfill a necessary function during the crucial period of sex differentiation in the male. Rapid growth of the fetal adrenal occurs at the time when the interstitial cells of the testes are prominent. From studies already cited, there is little evidence to support the possibility that the fetal adrenal cortex affects the duct system of the male fetus.

ABNORMAL SEX DIFFERENTIATION

A wide variety of disorders exist in which abnormal internal or external sex differentiation takes place. These syndromes have found much clarification with our better understanding of steroid hormones and human cytogenetic disorders. They are authoritatively treated by Federman, and his work should be consulted for further details. Only the most common abnormalities will be mentioned here.

The external female genitalia are easily influenced by excessive androgen steroids during their development. Clitoral hypertrophy at birth should immediately lead to the suspicion of familial adrenal hyperplasia, the so-called adrenogenital syndrome. Because of an enzymatic deficiency in the homozygous abnormal infant, his adrenal is incapable of producing cortisol. Instead, a variety of precursors, some of them androgens, are secreted in large amounts that virilize the external genitalia. This cortisol deficiency must be promptly treated after birth, the clitoral hypertrophy being usually of a degree that does not require surgery. Maternal androgen (progestin) intake is also capable of causing a similar external masculinizing effect.

A variety of similar effects, or ambiguous external genitalia, are the result of simple or complex chromosomal anomalies. When confronted with such abnormalities it is usually wise to defer diagnosis and assignment of gender until competent chromosomal and endocrine studies have been undertaken. Of the chromosomal disorders the Turner syndrome, the Klinefelter syndrome, and true hermaphroditism are especially noteworthy.

Turner's syndrome, or ovarian agenesis, which is best described as gonadal dysgenesis, is often associated with a host of other anomalies. Most common among them are webbing of the neck and edema of the dorsum of the foot, which frequently can be recognized at birth. In this condition the external female genitalia are normal; the uterus and fallopian tubes are also normal, although small. Ovarian remnants—streak ovaries—are usually present but they lack germ cells. Therefore, ovulation and pregnancy do not occur in this syndrome. The condition is for some reason highly lethal in embryonic life, a majority of such zygotes appearing among the spontaneous abortuses. It is of interest to note that histologic study of such abortuses has shown a normal population of germ cells to be present. Presumably these die if the fetus develops to term for it is unusual to find oocytes at birth. Development of individuals with Turner's syndrome is retarded and most commonly these women are seen because of primary amenorrhea. Their nuclear chromatin pattern is negative, that is, the epithelial cells contain no sex chromatin (Barr bodies), and in most of the cases only 45 chromosomes are found, one X chromosome being present and the other missing. As indicated previously, such a deficiency could arise during meiosis by a process known as nondisjunction. Despite this anomaly, many patients with this syndrome lead reasonably normal lives but require estrogen substitution for the development of secondary sex characteristics.

Klinefelter's syndrome is important to the obstetrician, for some of his infertility patients may be married to individuals with this abnormality. Patients with this syndrome are sterile, with phenotypically normal external genitalia, underdeveloped testes (micro-orchidism), and frequently gynecomastia. Their buccal mucosal cells, however, are chromatin-positive. Their leukocytes often have drumsticks and most of these patients have 47 chromosomes, with an extra X chromosome (XXY). Three or four X chromosomes and additional Y chromosomes are occasionally found in this condition, with mental retardation a common additional finding.

True hermaphroditism is an uncommon condition in which the external genitalia may be normal or malformed. Often the condition is not recognized until later life when an ovary and testis or an ovotestis is found (Fig. 3), associated with a variety of changes in the duct systems. From the gross appearance of the gonad, it is difficult to predict whether the individual so afflicted will take on male or female characteristics at puberty. In an individual with ovotestes, the outcome will depend on the relative predominance of the testicular and ovarian hormones being secreted. Detailed chromosome studies have shown a majority of true hermaphrodites to have a 46,XX chromosome complement. Nevertheless, a substantial number of patients are composed of an admixture of cells. In fact many have a population of 46,XX admixed with 46,XY and are thus true chimeras. It is envisaged that either double fertilization, incorporation of a polar body, or fusion of two fraternal twin zygotes in early embryonic stages leads to this genotype.

Equally important is the realization that chromosomal numbers may be perfectly normal in certain types of genital maldevelopment. The most important in this group of genetic and hormonal disorders is the adrenogenital syndrome, leading to pseudohermaphroditism.

In recent years another condition has emerged which, unfortunately, is rarely properly diagnosed. This has led to much confusion and unhappiness in the rearing of children with so-called "**testicular feminization.**" These individuals are also called male pseudohermaphrodites, because phenotypically they appear as normal girls, yet their inguinal canals contain what look like testes. Often the diagnosis is made when a surgeon operates upon the labial inguinal hernias of apparently normal girls and finds their content to be testes. The buccal mucosal cells of individuals with this disorder have a negative chromatin pattern, and their chromosomes are apparently those of a normal male. The external genitalia are female; the vagina is short, and the uterus and tubes are absent. The testes are inguinal, labial, or intra-abdominal in location. Because growth is normal and menopausal symptoms ensue upon castration, early castration is ill advised, since substitution therapy then becomes necessary. On the other hand, there is evidence

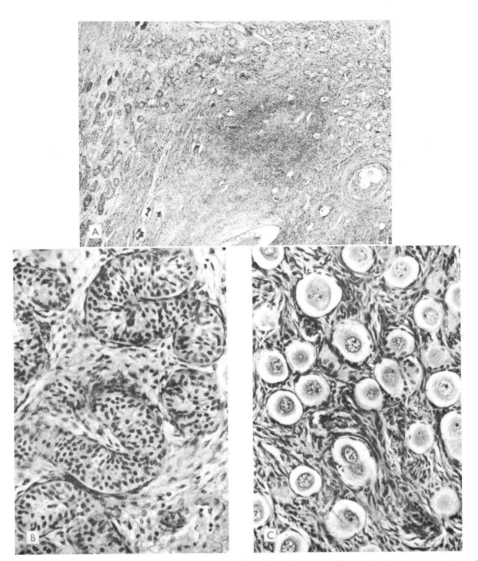

Figure 3. Photomicrographs of ovotestis in a hermaphrodite 2½ years of age. A, Low-power view, showing follicle formation in lower right-hand corner, and seminiferous tubules on the left. × 25. High-power views of (B) testicular and (C) ovarian elements. × 125. (Courtesy of Dr. Earl T. Engle.)

of an increased incidence of testicular tumors later in life, and orchiectomy should be considered around age 25. The androgen production by the testes is approximately normal, the reason for the feminine habitus being a hereditary deficiency of the end-organs (skin, breast, and so forth) to respond to these steroids.

INSEMINATION AND SPERM TRANSPORT

Normally about 500 million sperm, in some 4 to 6 ml. of ejaculate, are deposited in the posterior fornix of the vagina at copulation. With the uterine corpus in the normal anterior position, the external cervical os is directed into the posterior vaginal fornix, where it is bathed in the recently deposited semen. Despite the alkalinity of the seminal fluid, which is so essential in protecting the sperm from the acidity of the vaginal mucosa, there is a considerable sperm mortality immediately upon their deposition within the vagina. Sperm have been found in the vagina 48 to 72 hours after coitus, but within 4 to 6 hours the alkalinity of the semen is overcome by the acidity of the vaginal mucosa, and the sperm lose their reproductive potential.

One may ask why oligospermia need contribute to infertility when the number of spermatozoa deposited is usually so great. The answer is more apparent when it is realized that normally only a few thousand of these sperm have the ability to complete the journey into the distal portion of the uterine tube. Although the sperm concentration of semen may be fairly constant, the volume of fluid is decreased with frequent ejaculations. Therefore, under such circumstances, the relative decrease in the number of sperm available is sufficient on occasion to account for the existing infertility. Furthermore, adequate amounts of seminal fluid are desirable in overcoming the acidity of the vagina. Lack of a normal amount of ejaculate indicates that periods of sexual rest in the male may be helpful in the treatment of the infertile couple.

The original discovery of prostaglandins in the seminal fluid and the recent demonstration of the efficacy of some prostaglandins in initiating labor have raised important questions (Chapter 1). It has been shown that prostaglandins placed on tampons that are inserted into the vagina are capable of inducing uterine contractions and abortion. Although it has often been suggested that intercourse during pregnancy may be instrumental in causing labor, these claims have not been universally accepted and are vigorously denied by some.

After their deposition in the posterior fornix of the vagina, the motile spermatozoa journey upward through the cervical canal. Normally the cervix does not present a barrier to their passage. Their failure to pass through the cervix, however, may be due to inherent defects in the sperm themselves, but more often is the result of chronic cervical infection or cervical stricture.

The rate of travel of spermatozoa is comparatively rapid, for within an hour or two after their deposition in the vagina they have been found at the ampullar portions of the fallopian tubes, and also may often be detected in the peritoneal fluid. Transport through the tube is incompletely understood. Despite the peristaltic activity and ciliary activity being directed toward the uterus, spermatozoa have little difficulty in their ascending migration. It is likely that the tubal secretions, enhanced during late follicular phase, aid in this migration since tubal fluid moves toward the peritoneal cavity. Moreover, ciliary activity and tubal

peristalsis have been shown to be efficacious primarily in the transport of larger objects such as the fertilized ovum with its corona. The spermatozoa are able to survive some 24 to 48 hours after their arrival, and should ovulation take place during this time, fertilization is likely.

FERTILIZATION

The process of fertilization is very complex indeed and not completely understood as yet. What is known comes from many different laboratories and is derived from many different species. Although the basic phenomena are similar, it is striking to see in how many details species of mammals differ in the underlying enzymatic and physical phenomena of this event. Although a few descriptions of early fertilized human ova exist and despite a few experiments of experimental in-vitro fertilization in man with subsequent culture to 16 cell stages, relatively little is known about the biochemical events that occur in human fertilization. It is from isolated findings and inference only that the process can be described in some detail.

As indicated previously, the spermatozoa in the seminiferous tubules are immotile and reach the epididymis passively, by fluid secretion, ciliary activity, and tubular contractions in the efferent system. At ejaculation, a complex spinal reflex, they are ejected by muscular contraction and acquire motility upon being mixed with the alkaline secretions of the seminal vesicles. In the vagina the local acid secretion tends to destroy the favorable environment the spermatozoa have enjoyed and thence various forces reduce the number and viability of sperm capable of fertilization. In their upward migration there is a drastic reduction in number and, presumably, a selection against defective elements. In most species the spermatozoa acquire the facility to penetrate the ovum only during this migration, when in contact with uterine and tubal secretion; they undergo a "capacitation" reaction which is thought to be an enzymatic destruction of decapacitating factors. In most mammals and probably in man fertilization occurs in the ampullary portions of the fallopian tube into which the ovulated ovum has been transported. Under normal circumstances, the gametic encounter is restricted to only a few hours, either the ovum or the spermatozoa being too aged for effective fertilization thereafter.

The ovum has commenced first meiosis before birth and exists as a tetraploid cell in the dictyotene stage for between 15 and 45 years. During this time some maturation occurs; in particular, the cytoplasm acquires numerous granules not present before birth. In the resting stage the ovum measures approximately 40 microns in diameter but at the time of ovulation it has grown to measure between 100 and 150 microns. The nature of cytoplasmic structures is exceedingly complex; most are aggregated around the nucleus and their function is poorly understood. It has been suggested that some are of nutritive value, that others contain enzymes needed in early developmental processes, and that mitochondria have specific shapes that allow their identification from mitochondria of spermatozoa. Stimulation of oocytes and their granulosa cells to become graafian follicles proceeds in an orderly fashion; those at the corticomedullary junction are the first to enter meiosis before birth and these are also the first to become follicles. Growth of the oocyte is particularly evident when FSH has initiated multiplication of granulosa cells and a cumulus oophorus has formed with the appearance of an antrum. Several follicles at nearly similar stages are often seen in sections of an ovary, and, since multiple ovulation is not common in man, it is thought that only one follicle proceeds to full maturation, the others undergoing a specific degenerative event, atresia, that leaves different scars than result from a corpus luteum.

During follicular development the oocyte acquires a thin glassy membrane, the zona pellucida, which is rich in glycoproteins. Some granulosa cells are closely applied to this membrane, the so-called corona radiata cells, and evidence exists that processes of these cells penetrate both the zona radiata and the oocyte membrane. Granules from the corona cells have been observed to be "pumped" into the oocyte cytoplasm and the perivitelline space that now develops between these two membranes. For this reason these cells have been referred to as nurse cells. Their cytoplasm is connected by bridges. The former notion that follicular enlargement and rupture occur

because of increasing pressures developing within the antrum is no longer held accurate. Indeed, direct pressure measurements have failed to substantiate this concept. Instead, it is envisaged that an enzymatic (? collagenase) local process leads to the dispersal of elements in the ovarian cortex, with ovulation ensuing. The ovum emerges with numerous cumulus oophorus (granulosa) cells attached to the surface and this irregular bolus is swept into the tube by the mucosal ciliary activity of the highly motile fimbriated end. A considerable amount of evidence exists that the 4000 to 5000 cumulus cells that envelop the ovum for some time are now dispersed by enzymatic dissociation, perhaps by hyaluronidase of the sperm fluid. With its thin layer of corona cells still attached, the ovum is now ready for fertilization.

The first meiotic division has been completed at approximately the time of ovulation. Diakinesis is thought to be stimulated by the LH surge at midcycle whence first meiosis completes with the first polar body being placed in the perivitelline space next to the ovum. When observations of in-vitro fertilization are made it is seen that spermatozoa encounter the ovum at random, there being no specific attraction. Once they have touched, the spermatozoa orient at right angles to the ovum surface, the tail effecting continuous movement of the object. Corona cells subsequently begin to be dispersed, presumably under the influence of bicarbonate ions, if analogies with rabbit ova hold. This process is under the influence of carbonic anhydrase mediation of the tubal secretions. Just how the sperm penetrates the 8- to 10-micron-thick zona pellucida in man is not clear. Most likely it is aided by the trypsin-like enzymatic content of the acrosomal portion of the sperm head found in many species, including man. Once the head is through the zona pellucida and in the perivitelline space, the microvilli of the ovum surface fuse with the spermatozoal membrane and the sperm is more or less phagocytized by the ovum. In man and many species the entire sperm, including tail, enters the ovum cytoplasm, the sperm cytoplasmic membrane having fused with that of the ovum. In many studies elements of sperm can be observed through several cleavage divisions; eventually they degenerate. Of particular interest in this respect are the mitochondria. In several species the mitochondria of ovum and spermatozoon have distinctively different features that allow their identification. It can readily be seen in these species, including man, that the few mitochondria contributed by the spermatozoon soon swell and disintegrate. This raises an important point: since mitochondria are not made de novo but arise by division, it appears that all zygotic mitochondria are of maternal origin. Whether the male mitochondrial DNA survives is so far unknown.

Immediately after sperm entry the male nucleus becomes rehydrated and swells to the size of the female pronucleus, in man both being of the same size (Fig. 4). The second meiotic division of the ovum having been initiated by the fertilization event, the two pronuclei are now of haploid (n=23) chromosome content and the zygote as portrayed in Figures 4 and 5 is of diploid content and ready to begin cleavage. In this unique fertilized ovum of about 25

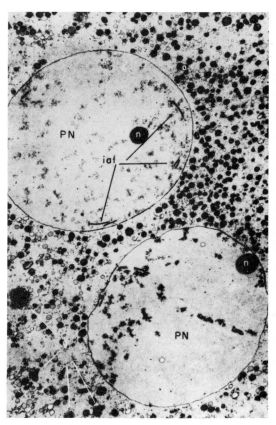

Figure 5. Electron micrograph of one of 300 serial sections of the penetrated human ovum shown in Figure 4. The two pronuclei (*PN*) contain one nucleolus (*n*) each. Note the extreme hydration of the pronuclei, their dispersed dark chromosomes, and the annulate lamellae (*ial*), whose function is unknown. The cytoplasm contains a very large number of granules of various kinds, particularly around the pronuclei. The Golgi complex is seen at *g*. Approx. × 2500. (From Zamboni, L., Mishell, D. R., Jr., Bell, J. H., and Baca, M.: J. Cell Biol., 30:579, 1966.)

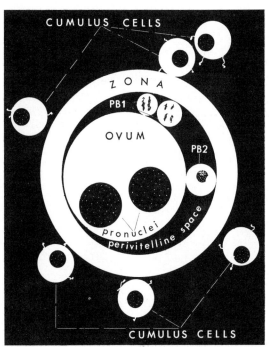

Figure 4. Diagram of penetrated human ovum shown in Figure 5. Few cumulus cells remain attached to the zona pellucida. The ovum contains two equal-sized pronuclei and remnants of sperm tail. No spermatozoa were seen in the perivitelline space, which contained three polar bodies: two were similar morphologically and were close together; the third (*PB2*) differed and was still attached to the ovum. Ovum aspirated from tube 26 hours post coitum. (From Zamboni, L., Mishell, D. R., Jr., Bell, J. H., and Baca, M.: J. Cell Biol., 30:579, 1966.)

hours age (or slightly less) the first polar body had undergone its second meiotic division, and the second polar body was just being discharged, as evidenced by still existing cytoplasmic bridges. Remains of sperm tail were found in serial sections within the ovum.

With fusion of the two pronuclei (synkaryon) fertilization is completed and marked changes occur in the organelles preparatory to the ensuing rapid cleavage divisions (mitotic divisions of the early zygote). In particular, DNA synthesis is rapidly resumed and clear evidence exists that this initiation is triggered by cytoplasmic factors and that the rehydration of chromosomes is an essential part. Similarly, ribosomal RNA synthesis commences almost immediately after fertilization and some evidence exists in mammals that it is in part directed by paternal genes. The origin of centrosomes of subsequent mitotic spindles is not clear as these have not been detected in the gametes or early zygote.

Just how long it takes before cleavage divisions commence in man is not certain. It has been suggested from in-vitro fertilization experiments that 30 hours elapse before this event. The penetrated ovum with two pronuclei shown in Figure 5 was found 26 hours after coitus and the two-cell cleavage ovum aspirated from the fallopian tube by Hertig (Figure 1 in Chapter 7) was estimated to be 36 hours old, coitus having occurred 60 hours before discovery. Thereafter cleavage proceeds rapidly, a 58-cell blastula being described at 96 hours. In this specimen with 5 embryonic cells and 53 trophoblastic, one polar body was still identified within the zona. This ovum was found at a time when the zona was presumably in the process of dissolution.

Timing of zona lysis is presumably important, lysis usually appears to occur only after cavitation of the developing ovum, i.e., after embryonic cells differentiate and trophoblast makes up the shell. The process is under delicate hormonal and enzymatic control and usually occurs in the uterus. Not only might late zona lysis prevent ectopic implantation but also it may well be instrumental in preventing fusion of zygotes and thus the formation of chimeras.

It is apparent, in summary, that gametogenesis and fertilization are highly complex processes. They involve numerous well regulated cellular and extracellular events that are efficiently safeguarded to insure effective selection and prevention of mishaps. Nevertheless, despite these mechanisms, abnormal fertilization, principally triploidy, is amazingly frequent. The possible events leading to this phenomenon have been summarized by Austin. Polyandry is spoken of when two male gametes participate, and polygyny when two female nuclear products (e.g., polar body suppression) partake. These appear to be the commoner events, the third possibility —aneugamy—being rarely incriminated. All of these events take place with much increased frequency in aging eggs and almost all subsequently end in abortion.

BIBLIOGRAPHY

Austin, C. R.: Anomalies of fertilization leading to triploidy. J. Cell. Comp. Physiol., 56:1, 1960.

Baker, T. G.: A quantitative and cytological study of germ cells in human ovaries. Proc. Roy. Soc. B., 158:417, 1963.

Blandau, R.: Anatomy of ovulation. Clin. Obstet. Gynec., 10:347, 1967.

Block, E.: Quantitative morphological investigations of the follicular system in women. Acta Anat., 14:108, 1952.

Brown, R. L.: Rate of transport of spermia in human uterus and tubes. Amer. J. Obstet. Gynec., 47:407, 1944.

Clermont, Y.: Renewal of spermatogonia in man. Amer. J. Anat., 118:509, 1966.

Edwards, R. G.: Are oocytes formed and used sequentially in the mammalian ovary? Phil. Trans. Roy. Soc. B., 259:103, 1970.

Edwards, R. G., Steptoe, P. C., and Purdy, J. M.: Fertilization and cleavage in vitro of preovulatory human oocytes. Nature, 227:1307, 1970.

Federman, D. D.: Abnormal Sexual Development. A Genetic and Endocrine Approach to Differential Diagnosis. W. B. Saunders Co., Philadelphia, 1967.

Gillman, J.: Development of gonads in man, with consideration of role of fetal endocrines and histogenesis of ovarian tumors. Contrib. Embryol., 32:83, 1948.

Greene, R. R., and Burrill, M. W.: Experimental intersexuality: effects of combined androgens and estrogens on prenatal sexual development of the rat. Amer. J. Physiol., 29:368, 1940.

Heller, C. G., and Clermont, Y.: Spermatogenesis in man: an estimate of its duration. Science, 140:184, 1963.

Hertig, A. T., and Adams, E. C.: Studies on the human oocyte and its follicle. I. Ultrastructural and histochemical observations on the primordial follicle stage. J. Cell Biol., 34:647, 1967.

Hertig, A. T., Rock, J., Adams, E. C., and Mulligan, W. J.: On the preimplantation stages of the human ovum: a description of four normal and four abnormal specimens ranging from the second to the fifth day of development. Contrib. Embryol., 35:199, 1954.

Jost, A.: Hormonal factors in development of fetus. Cold Spring Harbor Sympos. Quant. Biol., 19:167, 1954.

Lillie, F. R.: The freemartin; study of the action of sex hormones in the foetal life of cattle. J. Zool, 23:371, 1917.

MacLeod, J.: Metabolism of human spermatozoa. Amer. J. Physiol., 132:193, 1941.

Manotaya, T., and Potter, E. L.: Oocytes in prophase of meiosis from squash preparations of human fetal ovaries. Fertil. Steril., 14:378, 1963.

Mastroianni, L., and Noriega, C.: Observations on human ova and the fertilization process. Amer. J. Obstet. Gynec., 107:682, 1970.

McLaren, A.: The fate of the zona pellucida in mice. J. Embryol. Exp. Morph. 23:1, 1970.

Pinkerton, J. H. M., McKay, D. G., Adams, E. C., and Hertig, A. T.: Development of the human ovary. A study using histochemical technics. Obstet. Gynec., 18:152, 1961.

Richart, R. M., and Benirschke, K.: Diagnosis of gonadal dysgenesis in newborn infants. Obstet. Gynec., 15:621, 1960.

Roosen-Runge, E. C.: The process of spermatogenesis in mammals. Biol. Rev., 37:343, 1962.

Ruby, J. R., Dyer, R. F., Gasser, R. F., and Skalko, R. G.: Intercellular connections between germ cells in the developing human ovary. Z. Zellforsch., 105:252, 1970.

Shettles, L. B.: The living human ovum. Amer. J. Obstet. Gynec., 76:398, 1958.

Solari, A. J., and Tres, L. L.: The three-dimensional reconstruction of the XY chromosomal pair in human spermatocytes. J. Cell Biol. 45:43, 1970.

Szollosi, D.: The fate of sperm middle-piece mitochondria in the rat egg. J. Exp. Zool., 159:367, 1965.

Weisner, B. P.: Postnatal development of genital organs in albino rat with a discussion of new theory of sexual differentiation. J. Obstet. Gynaec. Brit. Emp., 41:867, 1934; 42:8, 1935.

Wells, L. J., and van Wagenen, G.: Androgen-induced female pseudohermaphroditism in the monkey (*Macaca mulatta*); anatomy of the reproductive organs. Contrib. Embryol., 35:93, 1954.

Williams, W. W., and Simmons, F. A.: Intracervical survival of spermatozoa. Amer. J. Obstet. Gynec., 43:652, 1942.

Zamboni, L., Mishell, D. R., Bell, J. H., and Baca, M.: Fine structure of the human ovum in the pronuclear stage. J. Cell. Biol., 30:579, 1966.

Chapter 7

Implantation. Placental Development. Uteroplacental Blood Flow

After fertilization in the distal portion of the fallopian tube, the ovum is propelled toward the uterine lumen, presumably by a combined effort of the tubal ciliary activity and rhythmic muscular contraction. It is thought that these forces act primarily upon the sparse fluid and that these activities are partially dependent upon steroid stimulation. During this progress mitotic activity commences in the large (100 to 150 μ) object, which is sustained mostly by the energy supplies contained within. A certain amount of evidence exists, however, that some nutrients and oxygen from tubal fluid are important during these early cleavage stages. From the original morula the blastocyst with its cavity is formed by the third day after fertilization, at about the time when it is expected to enter the uterine cavity. Here too, the glandular secretions, the "uterine milk" or "embryotroph," support the developing organism prior to the time of implantation, which is thought to occur six to seven days after fertilization, i.e., the 20th to 21st day of the normal menstrual cycle.

In most fundamental aspects early embryogenesis follows closely that of other placental mammals except for the timing of events and type of placentation. The fundamental studies by Hertig and Rock, however, brought closer insight into early human development. These investigators studied approximately 200 human uteri with knowledge of timing of intercourse and ovulation and were thus able to describe the developmental sequence in accurate detail, although such critical specimens as that of actual implantation are still missing.

PREIMPLANTATION STAGE

The initial morphologic features of a segmenting two-cell ovum have been studied in a specimen of perhaps 24 to 36 hours' fertilization age that was recovered from the fallopian tube 60 hours after coitus (Fig. 1). The two blastomeres are of equal size and presumably equipotential. They are contained within the zona pellucida and two diminutive polar bodies are also seen. The latter presumably degenerate, as they are no longer seen in older specimens. The zona pellucida is not quite intact in this specimen and at the next stage depicted here (Fig. 2) it has disappeared. This is achieved probably by enzymatic lysis immediately after the blastula stage is reached. The earliest blastula found, i.e., a mass of cells containing a cavity, is the 58-cell stage, estimated to be 96 hours old and recovered from the endometrial cavity. At this stage already an "inner cell mass" of five cells, clearly separated from the mantle of 53 cells, is set aside. The former cells are thought to represent the progenitor cells of the embryo, the latter the future trophoblastic cells. Thus, at this early age, differentiation, i.e., irrevocable directional change of the blastomeric elements, has taken place. Presumably the mantle of cells is capable of developing only into trophoblast and the inner cell mass only into embryonic tissue proper. At four days of age

179

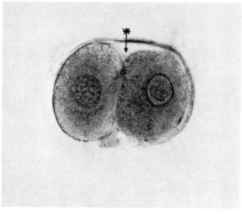

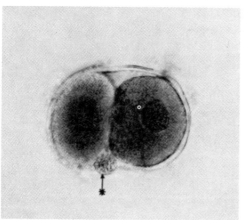

Figure 1. Two different serial sections from a two-cell human ovum recovered from fallopian tube, showing extrusion of two polar bodies. × 335. Polar bodies are indicated by stars. Coital date, 60 hours; probable fertilization age, 24 to 36 hours. (From Hertig, A. T., Rock, J., Adams, E. C., and Mulligan, W. J.: Contrib. Embryol., 35:199, 1954.)

(Fig. 2) the blastocyst cavity has greatly enlarged, and there are now 107 cells, eight of which are the larger embryonic cells at the top. With some imagination one may detect differences in the latter cells; perhaps the future germ cells are already set aside at this stage.

IMPLANTATION STAGES

Specimens are not available that depict the early stages of blastocyst attachment in man although the features in the rhesus monkey have been described and are thought to be essentially similar. Attachment may be envisaged as lying down of the blastocyst with inner cell mass toward the endometrial surface. It is likely that biochemical interaction occurs in these

initial stages of attachment between the endometrium and the embryonic trophoblast. Perhaps the latter differs in quality somewhat from that of the abembryonic pole. The regularity with which the process occurs in this manner and the regular differences among various species suggest complex biochemical interactions. In the human implantation occurs most often on the surface of the midportion of the posterior wall of the uterus.

Directional implantation as described has been suggested to be the reason for the eventually central position of the cord on the placenta, and "upside-down" implantation has been thought to be a possible reason for velamentous insertion. Other explanations are feasible and perhaps more attractive, as will be seen. After attachment there is rapid dissociation of endometrial surface cells, and trophoblastic cells can be shown to ingest some of these elements as the blastocyst invades the uterine lining. A recently implanted seven day ovum is seen in Figure 3, the blastocyst cavity presumably having collapsed artifactually. The vast difference in appearance of trophoblast is very apparent, that effecting the implantation (invasion) being very prominent and hyperplastic, and that covering the cavity toward the endometrial lumen having an

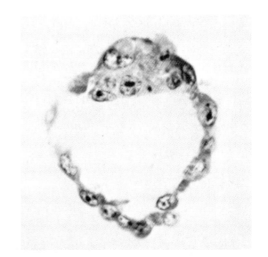

Figure 2. Cross-section of a normal human blastocyst approximately four days of age, recovered free in uterine cavity on 19th day of menstrual cycle. The smaller cells comprising the wall of the blastula are destined to become trophoblast and to form the chorion. The large cells in the upper portion constitute the inner cell mass. × 300. (From Hertig, A. T., Rock, J., Adams, E. C., and Mulligan, W. J.: Contrib. Embryol., 35:199, 1954.)

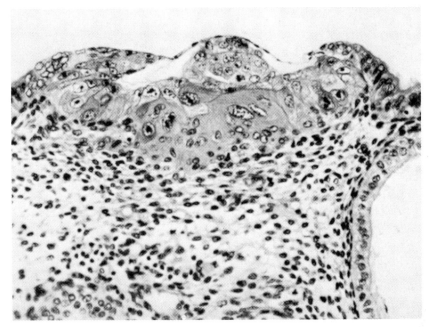

Figure 3. Seven day human ovum sectioned through its midplane and implantation site. The germ disc has a bilaminar appearance. The early amniotic cavity is seen between the maternal surface of the disc and the invasive trophoblast. The implantation endometrium on the 22nd day of the menstrual cycle reveals marked physiologic stromal edema adjacent to a secreting gland. Reepithelization of the endometrium is beginning over the implantation site. × 250. (From Hertig, A. T., and Rock, J.: Contrib. Embryol., 31:65, 1945.)

atrophic appearance. It is also seen that the lateral endometrial surface epithelium begins immediately to re-cover the defect caused by the invading blastocyst. Often a small coagulum is formed at this site and implantation bleeding may occur (Hartman's sign) but eventually the entire ovum becomes surrounded by endometrium.

By the 12th day (Fig. 4) important changes have occurred. The endometrial defect has been closed, the extracoelomic cavity is well delineated, and differentiation of embryonic structures has begun. The cells adjacent to the cavity represent the precursors to yolk sac and entoderm, and the larger cells of the disc are for the most part ectoderm beneath which begins to develop the amnionic space. On either side of the embryo mesodermal fibroblasts sprout to line the chorionic cavity and here may differentiate ultimately into the chorionic membrane. The trophoblast shell varies greatly in thickness, being the most hyperplastic below the embryo. Here an inner layer of cytotrophoblast (single nucleated cells) is surrounded by irregular columns and sprouts of syncytical cells. The interface between maternal and fetal organisms remains this layer of uninterrupted syncytium. In the latter some spaces or lacunae are now seen, the primitive intervillous space into which a few maternal cells have already gained entrance. At this stage one may consider that the rudiment of a placenta has been formed. It is assumed that chorionic gonadotropin is already secreted by trophoblast at this time, to reach the maternal blood in sufficient amounts to provide the message for the corpus luteum to continue and increase progesterone production.

In the succeeding days of development rapid changes occur. The trophoblast shell erodes maternal (decidual) blood vessels and in the lacunae the primitive circulation becomes established. Almost coincident with this development the invasive process stops, the reason for this limitation of expansion being unknown. Suffice it to say, normally there remains a layer of decidua between trophoblast and myometrium, but if the decidua is deficient or the erosive properties of the trophoblast are excessive a placenta accreta or increta may result. From the inside of the blastocyst cavity now fibrous tissue proliferates in finger-like projections into the trophoblast columns, thus providing the fibrous tissue core of the future villi (Figs. 5 and 6). Some consider

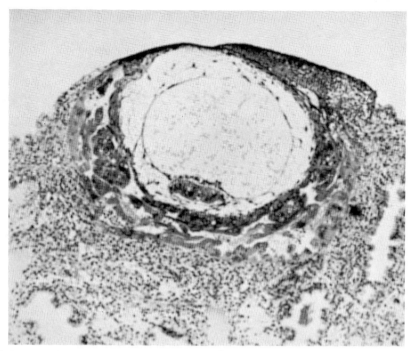

Figure 4. Midsagittal section of 12 day human ovum. The outer irregular syncytiotrophoblast forms the lacunar spaces containing maternal blood. The inner cytotrophoblast varies from a single differentiated epithelial layer to irregular masses of cells which project into syncytiotrophoblast and constitute the primordia of the chorionic villi. The exocoelomic cavity is lined by a membrane (Heuser's membrane), derived by delamination from the inner surface of the trophoblast and continuous with the edge of the embryonic disc. × 100. (From Hertig, A. T., and Rock, J.: Contrib. Embryol., 29:127, 1941.)

the villous fibrous tissue to delaminate from trophoblast but we do not consider the evidence for this concept convincing.

At approximately this time also the hematopoietic activity commences. Blood vessels and blood cells develop in the primitive yolk sac, which is undergoing rapid differentiation. Simultaneously, apparently, a vascular plexus develops within the chorionic membrane and the villi. The two vascular systems fuse to become the future villous circulation about the 24th day after fertilization when the embryonic axis measures no more than 4 mm. In these initial stages the entire chorionic membrane and the villi of the entire sphere possess a vascular system; however, as the placenta enlarges and begins to protrude from its interstitial implantation into the endometrial cavity, the abembryonic chorion and villi develop into the future "membranes," the villi and their vessels then undergoing atrophy.

The minute amnionic cavity seen between ectoderm and chorionic membrane in Figure 2 expands rapidly while the embryo enlarges, folds, and undergoes axia-

tion. Its epithelial lining, being contiguous with the ectoderm, if not derived from it, becomes cuboidal to cylindrical and fluid accumulates within the space. The origin of this fluid in these early stages is unknown; in later development much of it is derived from the fetal urinary tract. As the amnionic cavity enlarges and the embryo folds, the vascular stalk, the future umbilical cord, is formed, and it is perhaps easiest to understand the relationship if one envisages that the embryo herniates backward into the enlarging amnionic space. Thus amnion epithelium comes to cover the entire length of the umbilical cord and, when fully expanded, it lines the chorionic space, but this is not accomplished until the third month of pregnancy. Until then the chorionic cavity contains a gelatinous fluid in which amnion with embryo and yolk sac are suspended (Fig. 7). The amnion possesses no blood vessels and, although eventually it is firmly pressed onto the chorionic membrane, it never grows into intimate contact with the chorion, and therefore at delivery the amnion is often dislodged from the vascular chorion. Its

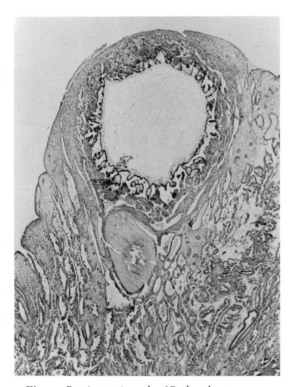

ectodermal derivation is betrayed by the frequent nodules of squamous metaplasia found, which are particularly common near the insertion of the cord onto the placenta. The yolk sac undergoes atrophy early, after having furnished the vascular system and primitive germ cells. Its remains can still be seen in Figure 7, lying between amnion and chorion. Subsequently it accumulates calcium salts and can often be identified as a 2 to 3 mm. yellow plaque in the term placenta. Rarely some of its structures remain, such as portions of the omphalomesenteric duct or vitelline vessels, and these may then be found in sections of the umbilical cord (Fig. 8).

The fetal circulatory system of the human placenta is known as the chorionic or allantoic vasculature. This term refers to the relationship of vessels to the allantois, a rudimentary structure in man but an important aspect of placentation in ruminants, such as cattle and other forms. The allantois makes its appearance as a diverticulum developing from the yolk sac into what will become the body stalk or umbilical cord. In subsequent development (Fig. 9) it may be considered an elongation of a hindgut structure and then becomes associated with the umbilical arteries of the fetus. It elongates sufficiently into the body stalk to meet the chorion, and the accompanying

Figure 5. Approximately 15 day human ovum, removed accidentally during hysterectomy for carcinoma in situ of the cervix. The endometrial defect (above) has been completely repaired by decidua. The embryonic mass is seen at 7 o'clock of the cavity. Into the dark masses of trophoblast finger-like projections of villous connective tissue extend from the chorionic membrane. Grossly this appeared as an endometrial polyp. H & E × 16. (Courtesy of Dr. R. J. Weaver, Athens, Georgia.)

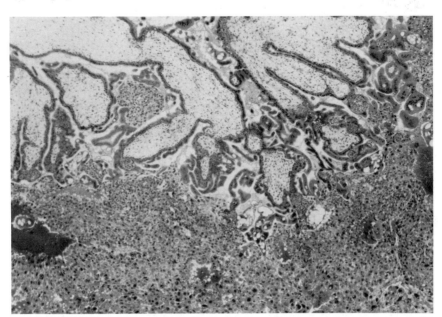

Figure 6. Site of attachment of immature placenta (30 days). Villous cores are edematous and light staining. Sheets of cytotrophoblast and vacuolated syncytium border the underlying decidua with its large number of pleomorphic placental site giant cells and few vessels. H & E × 40. (From Benirschke, K., and Driscoll, S. G.: The Pathology of the Human Placenta. Springer-Verlag, New York, 1967.)

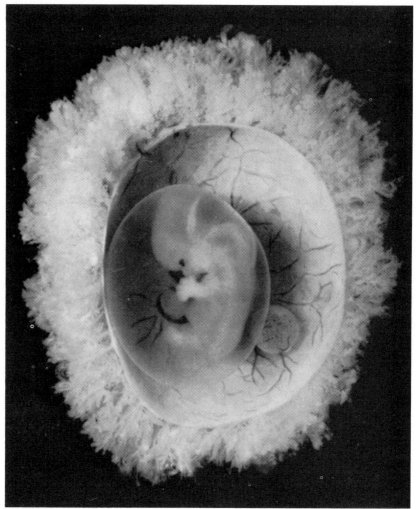

Figure 7.   Photographic reproduction of human pregnancy of approximately 10 weeks' gestational age. × 2. A portion of the chorion with its attached villi has been removed to expose the chorionic cavity, the yolk sac, and the amniotic sac with the fetus. (From McKay, D. G., Roby, C. C., Hertig, A. T., and Richardson, M. V.: Amer. J. Obstet. Gynec., 69:735, 1955.)

vessels then anastomose with the developing vasculature of the chorionic plate. In this sense the umbilical (allantoic) vessels represent the contribution of the embryo to its own placental circulation. At the end of the fourth week the primordial heart begins to beat and thence it furnishes the energy for the fetal placental circulation. Complete placentation may then be considered as established and only minor structural changes and general maturation processes shape the future development of the exchange organ of the fetus.

TROPHOBLAST

From the time of implantation to delivery it is possible to recognize the two principal types of chorionic epithelium. Toward the fetus develops the cytotrophoblast, the cellular trophoblast, or, as it is also known, the Langhans layer (Figs. 3 and 10). This cell is mitotically active until term but in the delivered placenta usually only few divisional figures are seen. The cells proliferate initially in broad columns that subsequently become invested by the ingrowth of fetal chorionic connective tissue and vessels. Thus the initial main stem villi are formed and their ramifications proceed subsequently in much the same fashion. These columns also "anchor" the placenta to the decidual floor and the respective villi are known as anchoring villi. Cytotrophoblastic cells have a single nucleus and well defined boundaries, their cytoplasm being relatively uncomplicated.

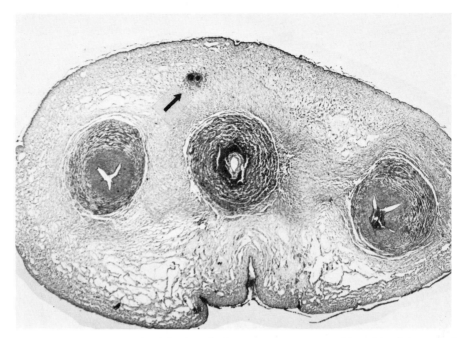

Figure 8. Cross-section of mature umbilical cord; the two arteries are on either side of the central vein. The edematous nature of Wharton's jelly is apparent from the spaces below. At the arrow are minute remains of vitelline (omphalomesenteric) vessels. H & E × 16. (From Benirschke, K., and Driscoll, S. G.: The Pathology of the Human Placenta. Springer-Verlag, New York, 1967.)

Figure 9. Diagrammatic representation indicating attachment of allantois to primitive hindgut. Segments of the umbilical vessels have coalesced with the vessels of the chorionic plate. Elongation of the body stalk will give rise to the definitive umbilical cord containing a single vein and two arteries. (From Cullen, T. S.: Embryology, Anatomy and Diseases of the Umbilicus, Together with Diseases of the Urachus. W. B. Saunders Co., Philadelphia, 1916.)

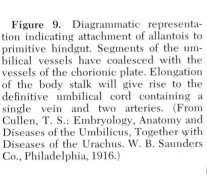

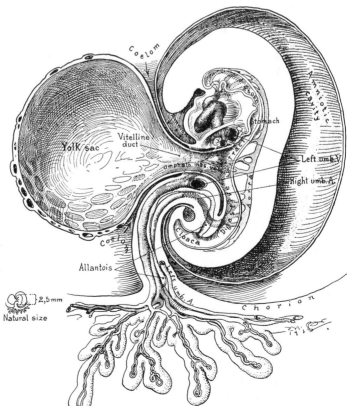

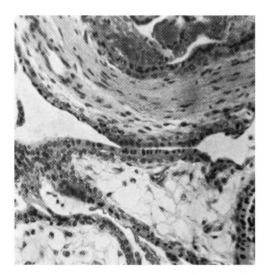

Figure 10. High-power photomicrograph of villus from 16 week placenta. The cells of the inner lining consist of well differentiated cytotrophoblast having delineated boundaries and vesicular nuclei. The outer syncytiotrophoblast has no limiting cell membranes and exhibits hyperchromatic nuclei. × 200.

They cover the limiting basement membrane of the villus, initially in a solid layer. As differentiation and growth proceed, however, they no longer form a continuous cover of the villi and the spaces between the Langhans cells are then occupied by syncytium.

The syncytiotrophoblast is multinucleate, there being no recognizable cell barriers between the nuclei. The cell never shows mitotic activity and various studies have shown clearly that nuclei and cytoplasm are derived from cytotrophoblastic precursors through an intermediary cell type. It is envisaged that daughter cells of dividing Langhans cells fuse to constitute the syncytium. This process of multiplication and fusion may be regarded as a regenerative process as it proceeds to term and adds constantly to the syncytial mass. The cytoplasm of the syncytiotrophoblast is highly complex (Fig. 13). In early stages of implantation it forms the vacuoles whence the labyrinth and, later, the intervillous space develop. Its maternal surface is endowed with an enormously complex microvillous structure (brush border) that enlarges the exchange surface manifold. The surface toward the fetus, that portion of syncytium which is exposed either to cytotrophoblast or to the villous basement membrane, has complex infoldings which presumably also enhance feto-maternal exchange. In con-

trast to the cytotrophoblast, the cytoplasm of the syncytium is very diversified. It contains an enormous number of vacuoles, lipid droplets, and ribosomes. By the fluorescent antibody technique of Coons it has been shown that this is the site of production of placental gonadotropin and lactogen (somato-mammotrophin). Indirectly it can be assumed also that it governs steroid metabolism and the various processes of active transport across this membrane. The syncytium then represents the fetal tissue that is directly exposed to the intervillous maternal blood and through which all feto-maternal exchange must take place (Fig. 14). At present it is not understood what regulatory forces control this tissue so as to allow different secretory phenomena at different times in gestation. Moreover, it is possible but not proved as yet that during the regular process of cell fusion in the histogenesis of the syncytium some alteration in its cell membrane occurs that renders it nonantigenic.

In the maturing placenta one regularly sees clumps of nuclei and cytoplasm budding off the villous surface. These "syncytial knots" or sprouts are known to break off frequently, to be swept away in the intervillous current, and sometimes to lodge in the maternal lung. Here they reside in the capillaries and, having no ability to replicate, they die. When defects are caused, by this means or otherwise, in the trophoblastic shell of villi a small fibrin coagulum seals the spot as in any defect. With increasing age, but principally after the first trimester, more and more fibrin thus accumulates throughout the placenta. The fibrin coagulum is often the site of dystrophic calcification in the last few weeks. There is no good evidence that these events have a deleterious effect on the efficacy of the placenta as an organ of transport.

Other syncytial cells migrate as so-called placental-site giant cells some distance into the decidua at the site of implantation. They furnish good evidence of uterine implantation in curettings absent of villi when the differential diagnosis of intrauterine abortion and ectopic pregnancy is considered. At this site also the layers of fibrin are found that are known as Rohr's and Nitabuch's layers. These discontinuous and irregular deposits of fibrin and debris have no known functional significance, and contrary to common belief, this is not the stratum at which

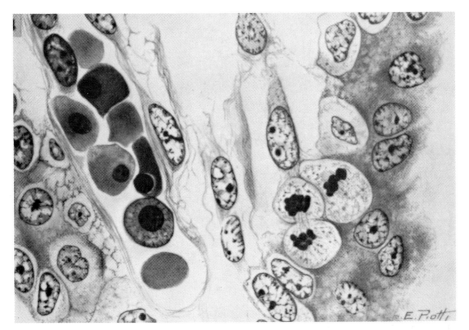

Fig. 11

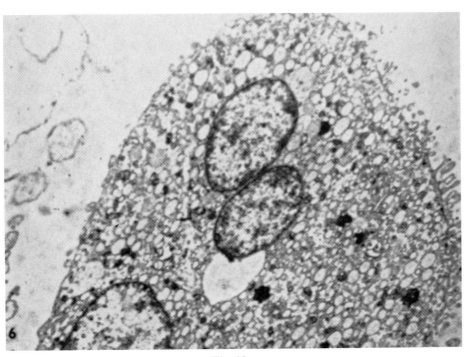

Fig. 12

Figure 11. Drawing of section of human chorionic villus of four weeks' gestational age. The inner Langhans layer, containing cells with distinct cell boundaries, is growing rapidly, and several mitotic figures are evident. The outer layer of syncytium contains thick, multi-nucleated cells without obvious cell boundaries. The villous core contains a thin-walled capillary with many nucleated erythroblasts. × 1600. (From Wislocki, G. B., and Bennett, H. S.: Amer. J. Anat., 73:335, 1943.)

Figure 12. Electron micrograph showing the character of the syncytial border. × 8000. Note protruding microvilli and ergastoplasmic sacs. Three nuclei are plainly visible.

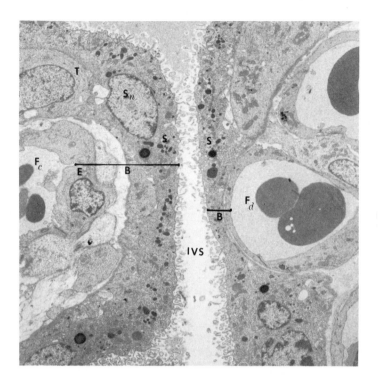

Figure 13. Electron micrograph of portions of two villi at 30 weeks' gestation. The intervillous space (*IVS*) in the center is bordered by the microvillous projections of syncytium (*S*). Transitional trophoblast (*T*) is considered an intermediary stage from Langhans cells to syncytium. F_c represents a contracted fetal capillary with endothelium (*E*); F_d is a dilated capillary of a villus with two red blood cells. S_n is the nucleus of a syncytial cell. Note the granularity and general complexity of the syncytial cytoplasm and the variable thickness of the "placental barrier" (*B*). × 3150. (From Wynn, R. M.: Morphology of the placenta. In Assali, N. S., ed.: Biology of Gestation. Academic Press, New York, 1968.)

the placenta detaches after delivery. The cleavage occurs deeper in the decidua basalis and Nitabuch's layer is shed with the placenta (Fig. 15). The endometrial stromal cells have changed during gestation to assume the plump shape of decidual cells,

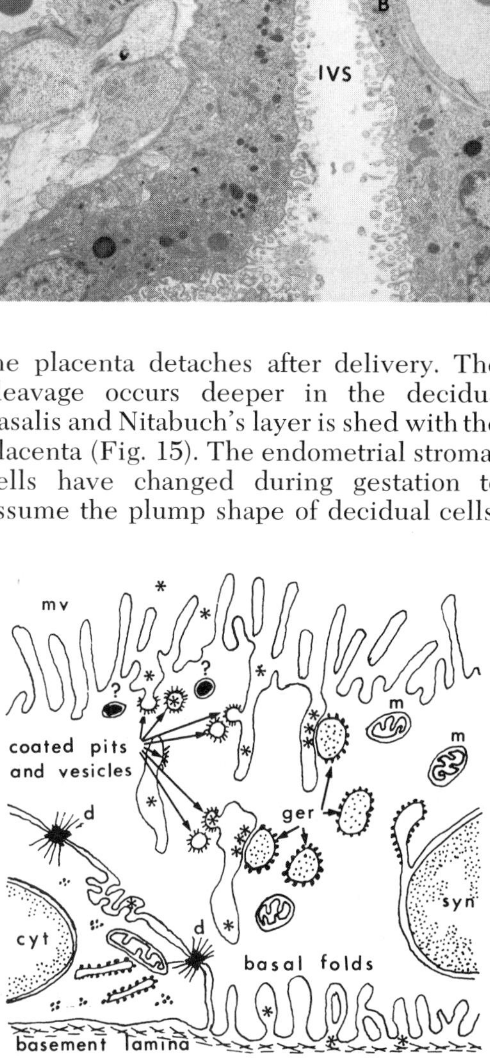

Figure 14. Diagram of trophoblastic membrane engaged in transport of ferritin (°). Absorptive pits form vesicles containing the transported substance which is discharged in the folds at the outer basement membrane of the villus. ger = granular endoplasmic reticulum; *m* = mitochondria; *mv* = microvilli; *d* = desmosomes connecting syncytium and cytotrophoblast (*cyt*). (From Ashley, C. A.: Study of the human placenta with the electron microscope. Arch. Path., 80:377, 1965.)

while the glandular epithelium has undergone atrophy.

When the columns of trophoblast proceed to invade the decidua there remain islands of endometrium between them. These subsequently form the placental septa and represent the boundary zones between the very irregular maternal cotyledons. The cells of these septa assume a peculiar basophilic appearance and, because of their unknown origin, they were termed the X-cells. Recent studies have shown that they have continued mitotic potential and that they are indistinguishable from similar decidual cells in the floor of the placenta. These septa partition the intervillous space irregularly and they may rarely span all the way to the chorionic plate, thus limiting intervillous blood exchange between cotyledons. Frequently, but particularly when much fibrin is deposited in a placenta, cysts form in the septa which contain a mucoid fluid and which often protrude on the chorionic surface.

VILLI

There is a pronounced difference in the histologic appearance of the chorionic villi from first-trimester placentas and those at term. These changes occur in an orderly

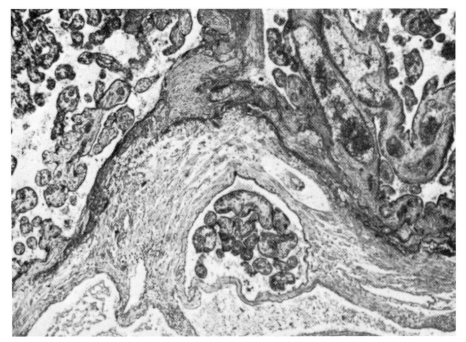

Figure 15. Photomicrograph of uteroplacental site near term. The presence of villi within a maternal sinusoid is a prominent feature. A dark-staining layer of fibrinoid material may be seen along the decidual margin of the placenta (Nitabuch's stria). Fibrinoid may also be seen in various contact areas of the fetal and maternal tissues within the intervillous space (Rohr's stria). × 100. (Courtesy of Dr. A. T. Hertig.)

progression, may be regarded as maturation processes, and most surely parallel changing parameters of placental exchange (Figs. 16 and 17). The most striking of these changes is the diminution in diameter of the terminal unit. In part this is accomplished by continued branching, and in part it is secondary to the loss of connective tissue fluid. Thus, in a mature placenta the villous core elements are more closely packed, and the fetal capillaries are relatively closer to the basement membrane surface and they are larger. Concomitantly the trophoblastic investment has thinned,

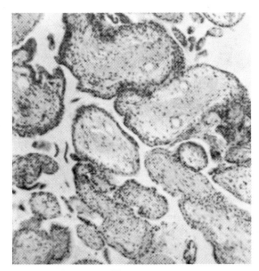

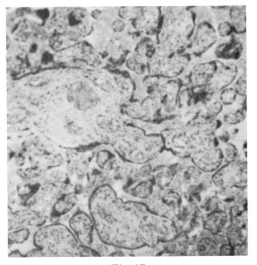

Fig. 16. Fig. 17.

Figure 16. Photomicrograph of placenta of approximately 16 weeks' gestational age. The villi are covered by both a layer of cytotrophoblast and syncytium. The stroma is cellular and contains few blood vessels. × 100.

Figure 17. Low-power photomicrograph of a term placenta. The stroma has been largely replaced by blood vessels. Secondary villi are markedly increased, while the overlying syncytial layer is thin. × 100.

more syncytial sprouts have developed, and within the connective tissue centers the unique Hofbauer cells have apparently decreased. Hofbauer cells are a prominent feature of immature placentas and hydatidiform moles. They have the general qualities of macrophages and phagocytic activity can be shown to have occurred in abnormal circumstances. What their function is in normal events, however, is not fully understood.

These maturational changes allow the experienced observer to estimate the approximate age of the organ. It must be noted, however, that these changes blur with pathologic changes and that they do not proceed uniformly throughout the organ. In any case, they are normal events and should not be equated with pathologic aging. Through their aegis the total area available for exchange increases continuously. The older notions that placental growth and maturation cease toward term are now considered incorrect.

INTERVILLOUS SPACE AND CIRCULATION

The initial intervillous circulation is established in the lacunae of the trophoblast shell at a time prior to the existence of actual villi. The process is accomplished by the erosion of myometrial veins, and it is not until the second month of pregnancy that the decidual spiral arterioles are tapped. The mechanics of placental circulation have been deduced from anatomic corrosion preparations and, more recently, from cineradiographic observations employing contrast dyes. They are clearly known only for the mature organ, in which between 20 and 30 spiral arterioles empty into the intervillous space. The force of this injected spurt drives the blood toward the chorionic plate, its energy gradually being dissipated. The current view of these relationships is represented in Figure 18. It will be seen that the blood gradually returns under this force to the decidual plate whence it is drained through endometrial veins. These veins are found throughout the floor of the placenta, and the older concept of principal drainage toward the margin is no longer acceptable. While there is a discontinuous "marginal sinus" present in the term placenta, it receives only a small proportion of the total intervillous blood flow (Figs.

19 and 20). Indeed, lateral dispersion of blood from one cotyledon to another is discouraged by the simultaneous (or nearly so) injection of blood in neighboring cotyledons and the presence of irregular baffles, the septa. It is thus also explicable how large infarcts may remain localized to one cotyledon when a spiral arteriole becomes occluded by pathologic processes, for the villous tissue depends for its integrity on the maternal circulation.

The usual histologic appearance of the intervillous space is misleading because of the fixation shrinkage of the villous tissue. When the fetal circulation is intact the villi are distended with blood and the intervillous space is reduced to slitlike sinusoidal spaces, as quick-frozen specimens have shown and as is also evident in electron microscopic preparations (Fig. 12).

FACTORS REGULATING MATERNAL UTEROPLACENTAL BLOOD FLOW

The anatomic organization of the intervillous space facilitates the ready passage of blood from the arterial to the venous system. Indeed, it has been proposed by Burwell that this uteroplacental blood channel is not unlike an arteriovenous fistula. Physiologic changes consistent with this theory are seen when there is an increase in cardiac output and blood volume and an elevation in femoral venous pressure in excess of any impediment to blood flow, due possibly to the weight of the pregnant uterus on the inferior vena cava.

Attempts have been made to measure directly and simultaneously the intervillous blood pressure and amniotic fluid pressure, with the reported values ranging between 8 and 20 mm. Hg and 5 and 33 mm. Hg, respectively. Studies on measurement of blood pressure in this vascular space are hampered by uncertainties regarding sampling sites and uterine tonus at the time the observation is recorded. Certainly the blood from the spiral arteries enters the intervillous space under substantial pressure, not appreciably reduced below the general systemic pressure. At cesarean section in the term patient, observations in this clinic indicate that the pressure in the uterine vein prior to delivery ranges from 20 to 30 mm. Hg. If blood is to leave the intervillous space, it must be at a pressure higher than that of the uterine vein.

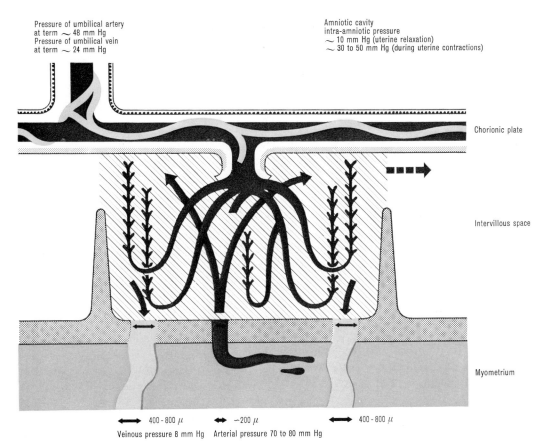

Pressure of umbilical artery
at term ∼ 48 mm Hg
Pressure of umbilical vein
at term ∼ 24 mm Hg

Amniotic cavity
intra-amniotic pressure
∼ 10 mm Hg (uterine relaxation)
∼ 30 to 50 mm Hg (during uterine contractions)

Chorionic plate

Intervillous space

Myometrium

←→ 400 - 800 μ   ←→ ∼200 μ   ←→ 400 - 800 μ
Veinous pressure 8 mm Hg   Arterial pressure 70 to 80 mm Hg

Figure 18.   Schematic presentation of maternal intervillous blood flow in one cotyledon, bordered by decidual septa, and various pressure relationships. *J.B.* refers to Borrel's jet, the spiral arteriolar spurt. (From Snoeck, J.: Physiological aspects of the human placenta. Triangle, 5:178, 1962.)

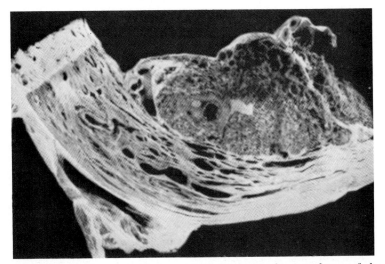

Figure 19.   Tangential section of intact uteroplacental site in region of marginal zone of placenta, showing the circular or marginal sinus and underlying dilated uterine sinusoidal blood spaces. There are porthole communications between the intervillous space and the marginal sinus. (From Spanner, R.: Z. Anat. Entwicklungsgesch., 105:163, 1935.)

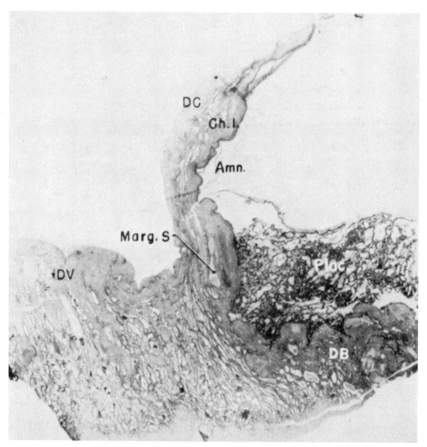

Figure 20. Low-power view of marginal zone of intact uteroplacental site (*Plac.*). Note the decidua vera (*DV*) on the left. The decidua capsularis (*DC*) overlies the regressing chorion laeve (*Ch.l.*), which is lined by the amnion (*Amn.*). The decidua basalis (*DB*), the decidua capsularis, and the decidua vera merge in the region of the marginal sinus (*Marg.S*).

Various factors have been assigned a role in promoting the flow of maternal blood through the intervillous space. These include increased uterine tonicity, villous movement, and the actual contractility of the placenta itself. Although the uterus exhibits a periodic contractility throughout pregnancy, the so-called Braxton Hicks contractions, it is doubtful whether these changes in uterine tonicity affect to any degree the rate of intervillous blood flow.

Disturbances of intervillous blood flow occur from a variety of causes, including excessive intrauterine pressure directed against the placenta. Chronic distention of the uterus, as in hydramnios, although rarely associated with an appreciable rise in intrauterine pressure, may, through distention and stretching of the myometrium, interfere with the normal patency of the arterial and venous blood vessels going to and from the intervillous space. A fall in systemic blood pressure, as in serious hemorrhage from placenta praevia or as a complication of conduction anesthesia, could result in a critical decrease in intervillous blood flow. It is conceivable that a similar result would accompany pregnancy toxemia, in which it is believed that there is constriction of the spiral arterioles. Violent uterine contractions may impede arterial and venous blood flow to and from the intervillous space. This effect is more likely due to constriction of the endomyometrial blood vessels than to an excessive increase in intrauterine pressure. The weight of the pregnant uterus on the inferior vena cava may possibly interfere with the normal venous drainage from the intervillous space. Pertinent to this discussion, however, it must be recalled that there are potential safeguards which serve to prevent excessive increases in intervillous pressure. These include the capacity of the uterine venous system to dilate and the ability of the marginal sinus to distend without necessarily rupturing.

In summary, the pressure and blood flow in the intervillous space are adversely influenced by the combined effect of the action of the myometrium on the blood vessels supplying and draining this space or by a decrease in systemic blood pressure. Abnormal uterine motility or myometrial distention may alter the arterial or venous channels so that the normal amount of blood fails either to enter or to leave the intervillous space. It is apparent that in any specific complication a variety or combination of factors may be operating to impede normal intervillous blood flow.

MACROSCOPIC APPEARANCE OF THE PLACENTA

The mature placenta is a discoid organ measuring 15 to 20 cm. in diameter and 2 to 3 cm. in thickness. It weighs between 500 and 600 grams and owes its dark color principally to fetal hemoglobin, most intervillous blood having drained before birth. Hence in fetal anemia (erythroblastosis) the color of the villous tissue is very light. In a majority of placentas the cord inserts near the center, and more rarely at the margin (Battledore type) (Fig. 21) or on the membranes (velamentous insertion), and measures about 50 cm. in length. Excessively long or short cords are uncommon and then often the cause of fetal complications (knots, thrombosis, disruption). The cord contains two arteries and one vein, and frequently insignificant remnants of transitory structures such as vitelline vessels and allantoic duct. The vessels are supported by Wharton's jelly, a gelatinous substance within fibrous stroma that also contains a large number of mast cells. The quantity of this ground substance varies remarkably and is particularly deficient in malnourished and postmature infants. The vessels often form redundant loops in the cord tissue, giving the appearance of false knots. Near the insertion of the cord the two arteries anastomose in 98 per cent of placentas and thence are distributed over the chorionic plate. Here they are supported in the chorionic membrane and lie uppermost, i.e., above the umbilical vein tributaries. In the fetal vascular districts usually a one-to-one relationship between artery and vein is found (Fig. 22). That is to say, a major district will receive one arterial input and be drained by a single vein. Occasionally so-called fetal cotyledons, i.e., vascular

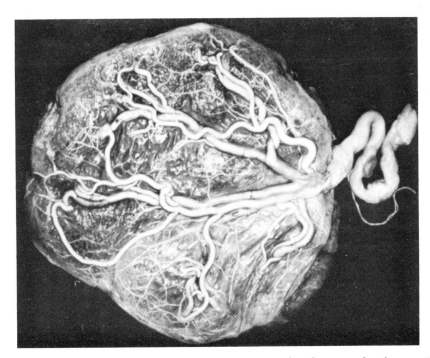

Figure 21. Chorionic surface of mature placenta, showing arterial and venous distribution. The umbilical artery and umbilical vein were injected simultaneously. The arteries are seen to course over the veins.

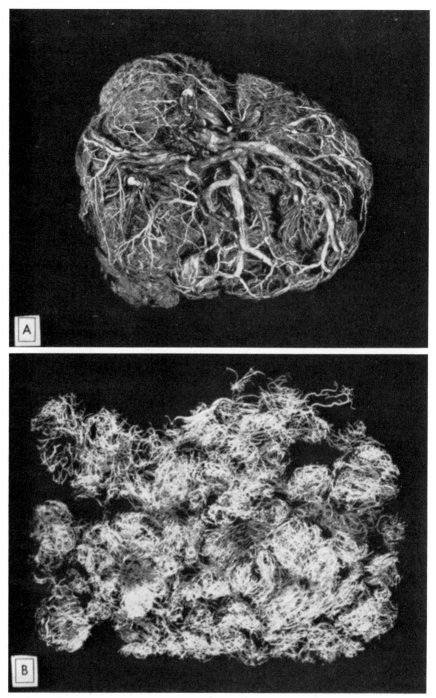

Figure 22. Corroded plastic preparations of the fetal placental vessels: A, chorionic, and B, decidual view. Note differences in caliber of arteries and veins. Smaller vessels are arteries. The decidual view reveals the extensive nature of the fetal vessels in this region. The cotyledonary distribution of the vessels is easily seen. (From Romney, S. L., and Reid, D. E.: Amer. J. Obstet. Gynec., 66:1104, 1953.)

districts, merge one with another. The vessels are covered by the translucent amnion which is readily peeled away from the chorion.

On the maternal surface an irregular number of cotyledons are separated by the persistence of decidual septa. When not disrupted by the manipulations at delivery, the maternal surface is covered by a grayish film, the small amount of decidua basalis that is shed with delivery, including Nitabuch's fibrin layer. This decidua is contiguous at the margin of the delivered organ with the decidua capsularis. The decidua capsularis derives from the "healing" regeneration of the endometrium after the initial interstitial implantation is accomplished (Fig. 5). Inasmuch as the progressive expansion of the chorionic cavity leads to an attenuation of this portion of the membrane, the decidua capsularis undergoes considerable regressive changes and is often necrotic (yellow). As the membranes become apposed to the decidua vera of the opposite side of the uterus in the second half of gestation, the two decidual leaves merge mechanically and the free space of the endometrial cavity is obliterated (Fig. 23).

PATHOLOGY OF THE PLACENTA

The placenta assumes many shapes and has many features, some of which may be dictated by hereditary phenomena, although the majority are doubtless reflections of happenstance of location and others are secondary to pathologic circumstances. Frequently an accurate analysis of these morphologic changes allows deductions of intrauterine life which are not possible once the organ has been discarded. For this reason a thorough inspection of this important organ should conclude every delivery and the findings should be charted. In case of prematurity, twins, or fetal death, the placenta should be sent to the pathologist.

Aside from the inspection of the maternal surface for completeness, various features should be looked for systematically. A cross-section of the umbilical cord should reveal the number of vessels. Absence of one artery, occurring in up to 1 per cent of consecutive newborns, correlates to a high degree (30 to 40 per cent) with fetal abnormalities of one kind or another. It represents a signal to the pediatrician to search for possible congenital anomalies. It is also more common with velamentous insertion of the cord, which has the same frequency. In this condition there is an increased chance of vascular thrombosis of the vessels that course in the membranes, and, of course, possibly disrupted vasa praevia with consequent fetal blood loss must be detected immediately to be of assistance to the newborn. Next most important is the detection of chorioamnionitis, which makes its macroscopic appearance by an opacification of the usually shiny, blue fetal surface. Other macroscopic features of importance to immediate neonatal care are the less common angiomatous tumors of the placenta and infarctive changes in the vil-

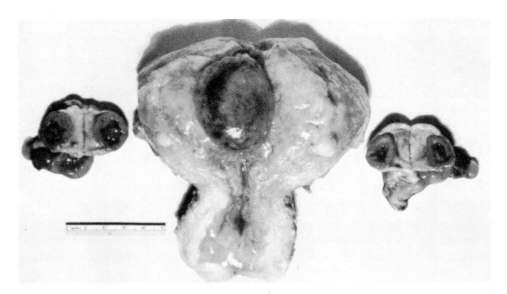

Figure 23. A five weeks pregnant uterus opened laterally and across the fundus to expose an intact chorionic vesicle covered by necrotic hemorrhagic decidua capsularis. Each ovary contained an active corpus luteum, although the uterus contained the ovisac of only a single pregnancy. (Courtesy of Dr. A. T. Hertig.)

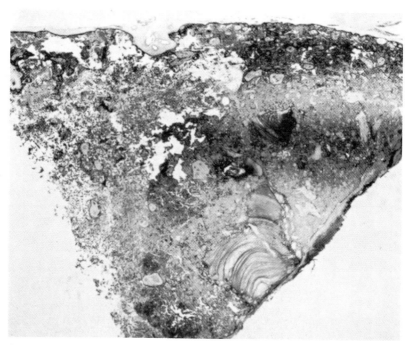

Figure 24. Photomicrograph of section of mature placenta containing a laminated fibrin thrombus. × 5. The thrombus appears to have deposited on the maternal surface of the placenta, with degeneration of villi and trophoblast. The thrombus in the intervillous space has deprived this area of the placenta of normal blood supply, producing a wedge-shaped infarct. (From Hertig, A. T., and Gore, H.: Diseases and anomalies of the ovum. In Davis-Carter Gynecology and Obstetrics, W. F. Prior Co., Hagerstown, 1959.)

lous tissue. Chorioangiomata are at times bulky, solid tumors in the placental villous tissue that have a tendency to infarction. They have been correlated with hydramnios, fetal heart failure, and angiomata in the newborn. They are benign and probably best regarded as hamartomas. Infarcts are firm, often yellow or red areas within the villous tissue and are commonly associated with toxemia of pregnancy. They result from occlusion of a maternal spiral arteriole and when excessive in size or number they may limit drastically the area of exchange. Fetal malnutrition in patients with pregnancy toxemia may be correlated with such vascular changes. Somewhat similar in appearance is the laminated intervillous thrombus (Fig. 24) whose pathogenesis is not fully understood. Other macroscopic changes are perhaps striking but not necessarily correlated with fetal pathologic conditions. Thus, a circumvallate placenta may present evidence of repeated prenatal hemorrhage or, at times, prolonged leakage of amniotic fluid, but fetal growth may proceed undisturbed. Similarly, the various form anomalies such as the bipartite placenta and the succenturiate lobe are merely evidence of some peculiarities of prenatal life and have no important implications for the management of the newborn.

BIBLIOGRAPHY

Benirschke, K., and Driscoll, S. G.: The Pathology of the Human Placenta. Springer-Verlag, New York, 1967.

Boving, B. G.: The biology of trophoblast. Ann. N.Y. Acad. Sci., 80:21, 1959.

Bourne, G. L.: The Human Amnion and Chorion. Lloyd-Luke, London, 1962.

Boyd, J. D., and Hamilton, W. J.: The Human Placenta. Heffer & Sons, Cambridge, 1970.

Hertig, A. T.: Human Trophoblast. Charles C Thomas, Springfield, Ill., 1968.

Ramsey, E., and Harris, J. W. S.: Comparison of uteroplacental vasculature and circulation in the rhesus monkey and man. Contrib. Embryol., 38:59, 1966.

Wilkin, P.: Pathologie du Placenta. Masson et Cie, Paris, 1965.

Chapter 8

Multiple Pregnancy

"Everyone is or should be interested in twins."
(H. H. Newman, The Biology of Twins, 1917)

Multiple pregnancies, with the birth of twins, occasionally of triplets, and more rarely of quadruplets, quintuplets, and so on, are of interest and importance not only because they have practical significance in terms of patient management (with an inherently greater fetal loss), but also because they have contributed to the understanding of fetal physiology and endocrinology. Further, twins have been used in many studies directed toward unraveling the question of whether certain diseases are of environmental or genetic origin. In addition to the immunologic phenomena exhibited by twins, the possibility of transplanting tissues and organs from one twin to the other has rekindled interest in the biology of twinning.

INCIDENCE

The exact incidence of multiple gestations is difficult to assess, and that recorded in birth statistics does not reflect accurately the distribution of multiple pregnancy. Numerous factors lead to an underestimation of the frequency of this interesting phenomenon. For example, twins are more frequently aborted than singletons, and one of a set of twins, triplets, or more is often delivered stillborn, as a malformed fetus or as compressed fetus papyraceus, incidents that never appear in the birth record.

Multiple pregnancies are principally of two types, "fraternal" and "identical." In triplets and higher orders of multiple births these two types may be admixed and, contrary to common belief, triplets and quintuplets may be of "identical" (monozygous) origin, the uneven number notwithstanding. The Dionne quintuplets are an example. There is good evidence that various factors control the frequency of "fraternal" (dizygous—DZ) twinning, whereas "identical" (monozygous—MZ) twins occur apparently at random, once in about 200 pregnancies. Dizygous twinning is the result of double ovulation (and fertilization), a form of littering. It is subject principally to pituitary FSH secretion and is influenced by many factors, especially ethnic. Thus, among African Negroes, fraternal twinning is infinitely more common than among whites, and the lowest frequency occurs in Orientals. In families with increased frequencies of multiple births it is this variety that is affected. Presumably such families, or races, have a somewhat higher FSH secretion rate that leads to polyovulation in the twin-bearing mother (although the trait may be inherited through her father), but accurate measurements to support this assumption have not been made. On the other hand, most of the multiple births, up to octuplets, recently reported from all parts of the world are the result of treatment with hormones. Human FSH treatment for infertility ranks first in this respect; treatment with clomiphene and withdrawal of the "pill," with consequent release of stored FSH, are other causes. One may conjecture that nutrition and sunlight are possible additional determinants since these are known to cause polyovulation in many mammals. Finally, dizygous twinning increases with increasing maternal age, up to age 39, and then its frequency falls.

No such predisposing factors are known to affect the frequency of monozygous twinning; its occurrence seems to be sporadic. With the exception of the quadrupling nine-banded armadillo, monozygous births are uncommon among other mammals.

It is thus important that, when citing twinning frequencies, the population sample be accurately defined. Over the past three decades there has been a gradual slight decline of the frequency of multiple births in the United States; this may reflect changes in racial composition or maternal age, but it has not been completely explained. National vital statistics are available up to 1958, when 10.8 twins were recorded for 1000 deliveries. The incidence in whites was 10 per 1000, and in Negroes, 13.8/1000, the difference being entirely due to fraternal twins (Fig. 1).

These statistics do not portray an accurate picture, however. The obstetrician deals with twins more often than in 1 per cent of his patients. Many multiple pregnancies end before the point of legal viability, and this underreporting leads to an underestimate of the magnitude of the problem. For practical purposes, the American obstetrician encounters twins once in 80 pregnancies; his Japanese counterpart, on the other hand, encounters them only once in about 150 pregnancies.

The incidence of multiple offspring can be approximated by Hellin's hypothesis, which states that if twinning occurs with a frequency of N, triplets occur in N^2, quadruplets in N^3, and quintuplets in N^4 pregnancies. Assuming that the termination of a viable twin pregnancy (after 20 weeks) occurs approximately once in 80 deliveries, the incidence of triplets is, therefore, 1 in 6400 pregnancies (80×80), the incidence of quadruplets is 1 in 512,000 pregnancies

($80 \times 80 \times 80$), and so on. Although this calculation has often been criticized, it allows for a practical estimation of the incidence of multiple births.

Weinberg is credited with drawing attention to the possibility of differentiating identical from fraternal twins on a statistical basis by employing the sex ratio. The "Weinberg differential method" is derived by the suggestion that if twins were all dizygotic, the distribution of sexes in these twins would, of necessity, follow a pattern similar to that in single pregnancies; that is, there should be approximately 51 males and 49 females among 100 twins (or whatever the sex ratio at birth happened to be in the population studied), the distribution of sexes among the pairs being governed by the same chance factors that affect fertilization of single ova. Thus, the expected sex distribution, if all human twins were dizygotic, would be approximately 25 FF, 50 MF, and 25 MM twins. There is, however, an excess of like-sexed pairs amounting to 20 to 30 per cent over the expected 50 per cent. This number is regarded as representing monozygous twins—a ratio of 1 in 3.

The problem has been admirably stated and discussed by Neel and Schull:

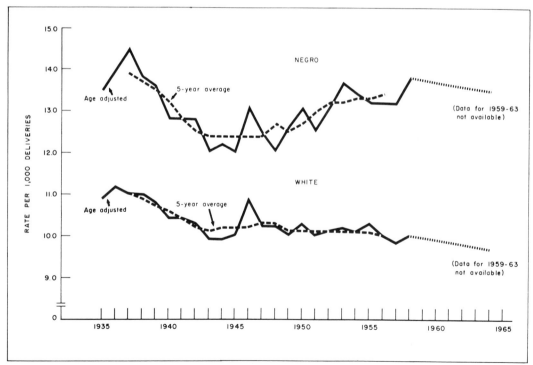

Figure 1. Twin rates, age-adjusted, per 1000 deliveries, by race for the United States. (From Multiple Births United States—1964, National Center for Health Statistics, Series 21, Number 14. Washington, D.C., 1967.)

If we assume that fertilization is a random process and that p and q are the frequencies of male and female births in the total population, respectively, then the frequencies of DZ twins with respect to sex are given by:

$$p^2(\male\ \male) + 2pq(\male\ \female) + q^2(\female\ \female) = 1.$$

Of these three groups of DZ twins, only those which are of unlike sex can be differentiated from MZ pairs. It may be noted, however, that

$$\frac{\text{Unlike-sexed DZ}}{\text{all DZ}} = \frac{2pq}{p^2 + 2pq + q^2} = \frac{2pq}{1};$$

whence

$$\text{All DZ} = \frac{\text{unlike-sexed DZ}}{2pq}$$

and

$$\text{All MZ} = (\text{total twins} - \text{all DZ}).$$

A similar approach and one which constitutes a satisfactory approximation to the proportion of MZ twins in most instances may be calculated by merely subtracting from the total number of like-sexed twins the observed number of unlike-sexed twins. The difference between these latter numbers is attributed to MZ twins. This procedure amounts to assuming that the sexes are equally frequent at birth, and, although this generally does not obtain, the departure from 1:1 is sufficiently small to justify this as an approximation procedure.

These calculations, however, have only statistical validity. In an individual set of twins they are of little help in establishing the diagnosis of zygosity, a quest rightly conferred upon the obstetrician, and it should be carefully noted that the only time when the diagnosis of monozygous twinning can be made with certainty is at birth, when the placenta is still available. After it is discarded, various so-called likeness studies can achieve very high probabilities that a given set of twins is monozygous, but it always remains merely a probability that is fraught with many problems. Also, the high mortality of at least one twin in the perinatal period, as well as many biologic problems to be discussed in the succeeding pages, makes it imperative that the fleeting opportunity to examine the placenta be fully exploited. The results of such study must be made an entry in the patient's chart. It is also desirable that the parents, and thus ultimately the twins, be informed of these findings, if only for the possible reason of ultimate organ transplants. Knowledge of placentation thus is critical and it is most easily comprehended after a brief review of the method of true twinning, i.e., MZ twinning.

THE TWINNING EVENT

Dizygotic ("fraternal") twinning represents simply the result of double ovulation and fertilization; the same applies to higher orders of dizygotic multiple births. The ova may be shed from one ovary or both, and the blastocysts may implant at any place. When they are near each other a certain amount of competition for endometrial space may ensue during the subsequent development of the placenta. This chance location, of course, ultimately determines the shape of the twin placenta in dizygous twins. Two entirely separate discs may be delivered or, when the blastocysts implant side by side, an intimately fused organ develops. In any event, the result is *always* a dichorionic structure in which the "dividing membranes" are made up of two amnions, two chorions, and, in between them, some atrophic villi. The structures are usually quite opaque. Villous or vascular connections are not established between the two organs. Parenthetically, it may be noted that of course one or both of these blastocysts may implant in an ectopic site, for instance the fallopian tube.

Monozygotic ("identical") twinning is an event that may take place at different times in embryonic development; presumably it occurs usually before the eighth day. In rare cases the division may proceed as late as the 14th day after fertilization. From the embryologic data collected by Hertig and Rock it is possible to construct an approximate timetable for early human development. Thus, it is known that an "inner cell mass," destined to become the embryo, is first visible on day 3. Presumably, then, at this time the blastocyst shell is programmed to become the chorion, and the inner cell mass will become the embryo. When a twinning impetus, as we may call it, occurs at this time, the cavity, that portion which becomes chorion, cannot be split any longer, and only the inner cell mass will divide. Similarly, after the amnion becomes established, about day 8, it will not be capable of being split, and once an embryonic axis appears after day 14, true twinning is presumably no longer possible at all or, at most, conjoined twins develop. These relationships are drawn in Figure 2 and the resulting type of placentation is indicated at the bottom of that schema. It will be seen that a majority (two thirds) of MZ twins

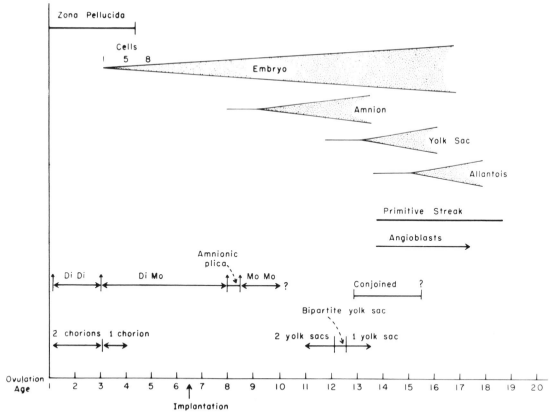

Figure 2. Embryonic and placental differentiation with fertilization age. At the bottom of the diagram are indicated the types of placentation that will result when monozygotic twinning occurs on specific days of development.

would be expected to have a diamnionic, monochorionic placenta, only one third, a diamnionic, dichorionic placenta; in fact, such is the distribution of monozygous twin placentas in consecutive series. It is apparent also that after day 8 few twins are formed, for monoamnionic twinning is not common and double monsters are very rare. Implicit in these deductions is the idea that, whatever the twinning impetus, it takes place at random in the early phases of development, quite unlike the event in the nine-banded armadillo where it follows implantation regularly.

The timing of the twinning event has a profound influence upon the subsequent development of the twins. As will be seen, the mutual exchange of blood in mono-chorionic twins often determines fetal growth, and the coexistence in a single cavity of monoamnionic twins leads to their very high mortality because of entangling of cords. These determinants are fairly well understood. From a theoretical

point of view, though, one must also consider the possibility that splitting of, say, two embryonic cells may yield more nearly equal fetuses than splitting of some 50 or 100 cells later in development. Although such assumptions have been verified in the often very disparate organ development of conjoined twins, no good observations have been made for completely separate twins. Investigations have been hampered by the lack of accurate recording of twin placentation, a prerequisite for such studies. This is but one reason why such documentation is a sine qua non of obstetrics without which many biologic and genetic studies are greatly hampered.

DETERMINATION OF ZYGOSITY

The establishment of zygosity has taken on even greater importance with the introduction of organ transplantation. Aside from this aspect, parents wish to know whether their twins are "identical" or not, and the obstetrician is the appropriate person to furnish this information. In fact, it cannot be emphasized sufficiently that, once the placenta has been discarded, all subsequent (and more cumbersome) studies furnish only probabilities about zygosity that are never completely decisive as far as the diagnosis of monozygosity is concerned. Not only should the findings be recorded, but also they should be explained in detail to the parents.

The practical aspects are simple. After the twin (or triplet, or whatever) placenta is delivered, the cords having been identified with a single clamp for infant 1, two clamps for infant 2, and so on, the original shape of the placenta and membranes is re-created. The important next step is the study of that portion of membranes that divides the two fetal cavities. It is completely irrelevant whether one or two discs are found; only the membranes matter. In the rare instances of monoamnionic twins with a single sac, all are monozygous. When two sacs exist, the "dividing membranes" are composed of either (1) two amnions or (2) two amnions and two chorions (Figs. 3 to 6). The former are all monozygous twins. The latter are mostly dizygous (fraternal) twins but a few are monozygous, a point often overlooked by obstetricians. In practice, of this latter group those twins with different sex can be excluded; they are dizygous. There remains a group of perhaps 45 per cent of like-sexed twins with a diamnionic, dichorionic placenta. Indeed, many of these placentas will be separate organs, and still the twins may be monozygotic. At the time of birth this group of twins can readily be studied further by blood-group determination of a

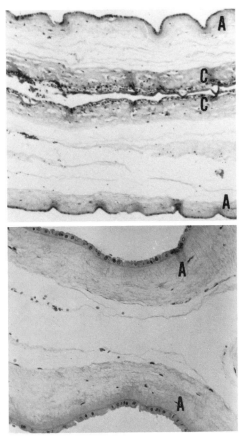

Figure 4. The histologic appearance of the "dividing membranes" of two main types of twin placentation. Above is the diamnionic, dichorionic type; below, the diamnionic, monochorionic type. A, amnion; C, chorion.

sample of cord blood. When different blood groups are found, the twins are dizygous. To assess the relationship of twins with similar blood groups and like sex, one must await differentiation of phenotypic characters (hair, eye color, finger prints, and so forth) that are useful for the so-called likeness methods. Moreover, extensive blood-group determination that includes parents and sibs may ultimately have to be undertaken by a pediatrician or geneticist. Observations on switch skin grafts have also been employed for this difficult diagnosis.

In a large series of twin births (668 pairs) conducted in Birmingham, England, this method yielded the following results:

20 per cent of twins had a monochorial placenta and were hence MZ

35 per cent of twins were of unlike sex (and had dichorial placenta) – DZ

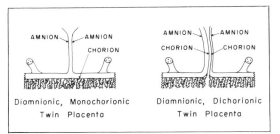

Figure 3. The two principal types of twin placentation, monochorionic and dichorionic. All twins with the type shown at left are single ovum-derived, monozygotic.

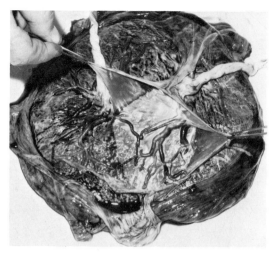

Figure 5. A diamnionic, monochorionic twin placenta (monozygotic twins). The dividing membranes are separated, being composed of two amnions only. The confluent chorionic plate with fetal vascular anastomoses is seen after the amnions are separated. (From Benirschke, K., and Driscoll, S. G.: The Pathology of the Human Placenta, Springer-Verlag, New York, 1967.)

45 per cent of twins were of like sex and had dichorial membranes; upon genotyping (blood groups, etc.) 37 per cent were found to be DZ, and 8 per cent MZ

In this connection it must be appreciated that the physical development of twins at birth is of no help at all in assigning zygosity. It is well known that serious malformations such as anencephaly and cleft palate may affect only one of "identical" twins and also, because of placental vascular connections, MZ twins as a group are more unlike in

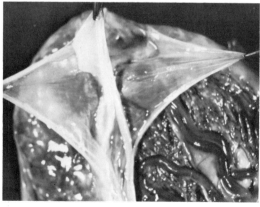

Figure 6. A diamnionic, dichorionic fused twin placenta is examined in the same way as the specimen in Figure 5. After the amnions are separated (left and right), there remains a membrane in the center that is composed of two chorions.

physical parameters at birth than are dizygous twins as a group. Finally, it should be possible, theoretically at least, to ascertain at times of cesarean section or at the occasional postpartum oophorectomy from the number of corpora lutea what type of twinning exists. This method has proved very unreliable and should not be considered unless one is willing to split the ovary and examine it histologically for the presence of corpora lutea. In a personal experience with a triplet pregnancy that required delivery by cesarean section, inspection of the one remaining ovary (one having been previously removed) revealed no gross corpora lutea although gross and microscopic study of the membranes indicated that the three newborns originated from three ova.

PERINATAL MORTALITY

Plural births have a much higher perinatal mortality than single births; this is most easily assessed in twins. When only pregnancies of more than 20 weeks' duration are considered, approximately 14 per cent of twins die in the perinatal period, as opposed to, at the most, 3 per cent of singletons. Many factors contribute to this excessive loss but all authors agree that the major reason is the much greater prematurity rate among multiple births. When twin mortality is compared with that of singletons of the same birth weight, however, twins fare, if anything, slightly better.

The most meaningful correlation exists when the mortality is related to the type of twin placentation. In a series of 250 consecutive twin sets from Boston Hospital for Women the following figures were obtained.

	Monochorionic Twin Placenta		Dichorionic Twin Placenta	
	Mono-amnionic	Di-amnionic	Fused Placenta	Separate Placenta
Total Twins	6	148	170	176
Dead	3 (50%)	37 (25%)	14 (8.2%)	17 (9.6%)
	40 of 154 = 25.9%		31 of 346 = 8.9%	
	250 twin pairs			
	71 dead of 500 = 14.2%			

It will be seen that monoamnionic twins have the highest mortality, and it is usually related to the entangling of their cords with interruption of the circulation (Fig. 7). The numerically largest contribution to the perinatal deaths is made by the MZ twins with a diamnionic, monochorionic placenta. As a group, these infants are born the most prematurely, often because of the development of hydramnios. The reason for their poor prognosis probably lies in the consequences of vascular communications between the two fetal placental vascular beds, of which the so-called transfusion syndrome is the most important.

The question is often debated whether the second-delivered twin has a poorer prognosis as a result of prolonged exposure to anesthesia, uterine contractions, or the frequency of breech extraction. Statistics for large numbers of births have shown that no significantly greater hazards exist for the second twin; however, in a numerical analysis of survival the second twin is more often found disadvantaged merely because a stillborn fetus, macerated or not, is almost always born last.

Aside from these considerations, the physician must be aware of the fact that velamentous insertion of the cord occurs more commonly in twins (7 per cent vs. 1 per cent in singletons). This anomaly of placental growth raises the possibility of vasa praevia with rapid fetal exsanguination during delivery. Blood loss must also be prevented by clamping the placental end of the cord of each delivered twin. Instances have been described of exsanguination of the second twin, because of large anastomoses, through the unclamped cord of the first twin. Furthermore, congenital anomalies are more common in twins and the severest anomaly that can be envisaged, the acardiac monster, occurs only as one of MZ twins. This twin, like the fetus papyraceus coexisting with a normal twin, probably is most often not even registered as a twin delivery. Cord prolapse and dystocia or interlocking are rare causes of perinatal death of twins in competent hands. Finally, maternal complications such as toxemia and hydramnios contribute to the excessive loss of plural births. To reduce this high figure is a difficult task as there are few ways by which the often significant hydramnios can be treated, let alone prevented. The goal is to bring the pregnancy beyond a point where each twin weighs 2000 grams by preventing toxemia and premature dilatation of the cervix, and by giving adequate rest, nutrition, and antenatal care. In the delivery room skilled pediatricians should be available to care for all multiple births.

Not only have multiple offspring a much

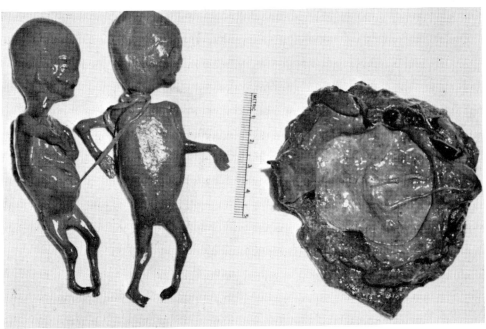

Figure 7. Frequent fate of monoamnionic twins; entanglement of cords with cessation of circulation. (From Benirschke, K.: New York J. Med., 61:1499, 1961.)

increased perinatal mortality, but also various studies indicate that the neonatal morbidity is greater (hyaline membrane disease, pneumonia) than that of singletons and that, as a group, their intellectual performance is less. Studies of verbal reading performance indicate that twins do less well than singletons, and triplets fare worse still. Whether this is due to their prematurity or because of special prenatal problems such as the transfusion syndrome is at present unknown. Similarly, one of twins is more likely to suffer from cerebral palsy than singletons, but it is again not known whether placentation or prematurity is the predisposing cause. It appears that like-sexed twins are more often affected, and hence the suspicion exists that MZ twins suffer greater handicaps. Such studies are greatly hampered in the absence of placental data, another reason for requiring entry of the findings of a placental study in the patient's chart.

In summary, there is increased mortality of MZ twins, and prenatal handicaps may be greater for surviving MZ twins. When twin studies are undertaken in later life in efforts to unscramble hereditary from environmental factors, these built-in biases of the twin population must be borne in mind.

SPECIAL FETAL COMPLICATIONS OF MULTIPLE PREGNANCY

Probably the most important and most interesting condition peculiar to multiple pregnancy is the *transfusion syndrome.* The German obstetrician Friedrich Schatz accurately described this consequence of special interfetal anastomotic vascular connections. It is limited to monochorial, and hence MZ twins. During the development of the single placenta, some blood vessels frequently, almost regularly, join. These anastomoses may be of the artery-to-artery, vein-to-vein, or arteriovenous type. The latter kind is diagrammatically shown in Figure 8 and is readily identified by injection study or merely by inspection. Arteries characteristically occupy a superior position on the fetal surface of the placenta and thus are easily distinguished from veins, and shared, common cotyledons such as shown become evident. The most significant degree of the transfusion syndrome ensues when a single arteriovenous communica-

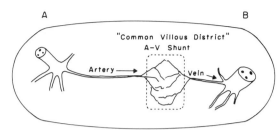

Figure 8. The interfetal anastomosis of monochorionic twins that forms the basis of the transfusion syndrome.

tions exists. Here one fetus (A, the donor) continuously loses blood to the other (B, the recipient). As a consequence, hypervolemia and presumably hypertension, cardiac hypertrophy, and occasionally edema develop in B and he grows generally larger. Presumably also this leads to excess urination by B and resultant hydramnios. In contrast, the donor shows runting, microcardia, anemia, dehydration, and perhaps oligohydramnios, and even amnion nodosum. Depending on the size of these communications, their number, and their directions, as well as other unknown factors, this very common syndrome is seen in a broad spectrum of dissimilar twins. Several such cases are shown in Figures 9 to 11. Good studies exist now to indicate that the sometimes remarkable differences in growth and development seen at birth persist for many years, and perhaps such "identical" twins always remain different because of this prenatal developmental disturbance. The syndrome has its onset in the first trimester when cardiac size may already be much different, and it often becomes symptomatic with hydramnios at around 20 weeks. The polycythemia, partly engendered by the transfusion, partly perhaps because of supply of erythropoietin from the donor, poses a threat postnatally. It may lead to severe jaundice with kernicterus and also to coagulative processes. Infarctive necrosis in limbs, as well as of internal organs, has been observed in the survivors, and intelligent pediatric care is essential in this syndrome.

At times, one of twins succumbs from this syndrome before birth. Gradually his fluid constituents are resorbed and, with the growth of his cotwin, the dead fetus becomes a shriveled, compressed appendage, the *fetus papyraceus* or *compressus* (Fig.

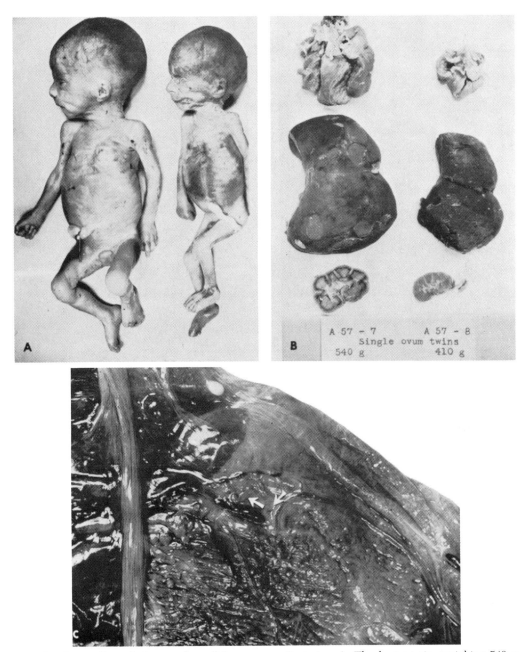

Figure 9. Severe "transfusion syndrome" in monozygotic twins. A, The larger twin, weighing 540 grams, is slightly edematous; the smaller, weighing 410 grams, is dehydrated. B, The viscera of the twins, showing marked hypertrophy of the heart of the larger twin, which weighed three times the expected amount. C, Close-up of portion of the placenta, showing an arteriovenous fistula from right to left at arrows. (From Gestation, Transactions of the Fifth Conference, sponsored by the Josiah Macy, Jr., Foundation, 1958.)

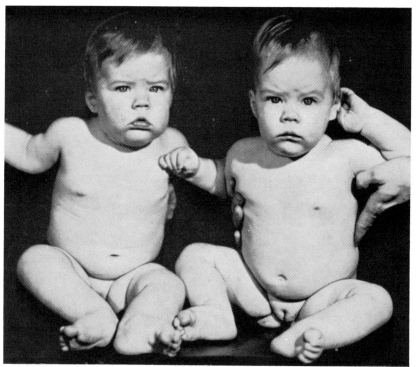

Figure 10. Monochorial twins with "transfusion syndrome" (birth weights 6 lb. 3 oz. and 3 lb. 13 oz.), shown here at age 6 months. Although monozygotic, they still show many phenotypic dissimilarities.

12). At times, fetal death occurs at such an early age that the very small mummified mass is overlooked in the membranes and is not registered as a twin pregnancy at all.

One of the most interesting conditions is the twin pregnancy with one fetus developing as an *acardiac* monster (Fig. 13). In man this occurs only in monochorial twins, and thus this most remarkable congenital anomaly, which occasionally simulates an inside-out teratoma, is one of "identical" twins. This should be reason enough to avoid the term "identical" twin whenever possible. Acardiacs result from the presence of an artery-to-artery plus a vein-to-vein anastomosis in twins. Early in development one twin has a circulatory advantage and reverses the blood flow in the other. The latter therefore fails to develop a heart and is nourished as an appendage to the donor, but with deoxygenated blood flowing in the reversed direction of normal. Hence a host of abnormalities can be found; usually the legs develop best because their blood supply is most adequate in this circulatory situation. Acardiacs may become quite large and represent obstacles to vaginal delivery. Chromosome studies have shown that they are not the result of gross genetic errors. Recently, their pathogenesis has been verified in cattle, where fraternal twins frequently have anastomotic connections; a female acardiac was found connected to the placenta of a normal male fetus.

A variety of other features are peculiar to twins. It has been mentioned that vela-

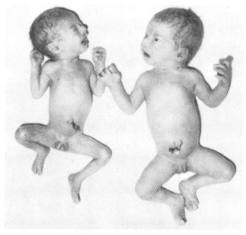

Figure 11. Moderate degree of "transfusion syndrome" in monozygotic twins.

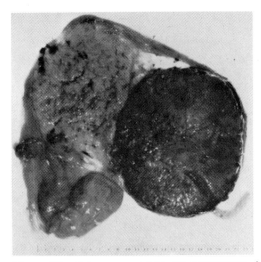

Figure 12. Fetus papyraceus or compressus in dichorial pregnancy at term. Note massive infarction of placenta.

mentous insertion of the cord occurs more often in one of twins, and in higher numbers of multiple births it is practically the rule. Similarly, one of twins more often lacks one umbilical artery in the cord, perhaps because of prenatal atrophy. This is a regular feature of acardiac twins and is explained by the competition for space during placental development. In a few cases of monochorial twins a peculiar generalized thrombotic event has been observed that is believed to result from prenatal infusion of thromboplastic material from a dead twin into the other through large anastomoses to elicit in the recipient a generalized coagulative process with dire consequences. Finally, there are peculiar immunologic consequences of twin gestation that warrant attention.

It has been found that many ruminants have dizygous twins whose placental blood vessels communicate freely. The phenomenon is best known from Lillie's work on freemartinism. In freemartinism, there are placental vascular anastomoses between a male and a female cattle twin and the female is sterilized prenatally by the male cotwin. She becomes a barren freemartin. After Owen's discovery of the permanent nature of the admixture of blood groups in such twins, the stage was set for the concept of acquired tolerance. It turns out that not only are primitive blood precursor cells transferred through these vessels to become permanent residents in the new host, but

also this early embryonic exposure to the twin's tissue antigens leads to his complete tolerance of all the cotwin's tissues. In the human placenta, anastomoses usually exist only in the monochorionic organs of MZ twins, who would be expected to be tolerant to one another on a genetic basis anyway. In only a very few sets of dizygous twins has such blood chimerism been detected and, although their placentas have not been studied, it must be inferred that on very rare occasion dichorial placentas may develop anastomoses in man as well. The reasons for this unusual behavior are completely unknown; surely they are not related to crowding since in intimately fused, crowded, quadruplet placentas no communications have been found. In any event, there are now on record at least 11 human twin blood *chimeras*, some of whom have also been tolerant of skin exchange. Generally, they are discovered by inexplicable blood grouping results. Their blood admixture varies greatly in extent and it has a tendency to change with age. What is the most interesting aspect of such unusual twins in man is the fact that in a heterosexual set of chimeras the female partner is not sterile or infertile, unlike the findings in ruminants. Indeed the twins are entirely normal.

Heterokaryotic monozygotic twins are another fascinating group of exceptional twins. It has been discovered that MZ twins may differ in chromosome number, at first sight a contradiction since "identical" twins should surely have the same genetic complement. The paradox becomes explicable when one remembers that the origin of chromosomal mosaicism, so often found now in karyotypic studies of individuals with sex chromosome errors, is the result of mitotic nondisjunction of chromosomes. In other words, during mitosis of cells in the developing embryo a chromosome may be lost or it may reach the wrong daughter cell. If the twinning event occurs at about the same time, one twin may be composed of, say, XO cells, and the other of XXX cells. Likewise, one may be XY and a boy, and the other XO and phenotypically a girl when a Y chromosome is lost on the spindle. Twelve such instances of heterokaryotic MZ twins have been described in the short span of time that cytogenetic study has been available and the frequency of this occurrence cannot at

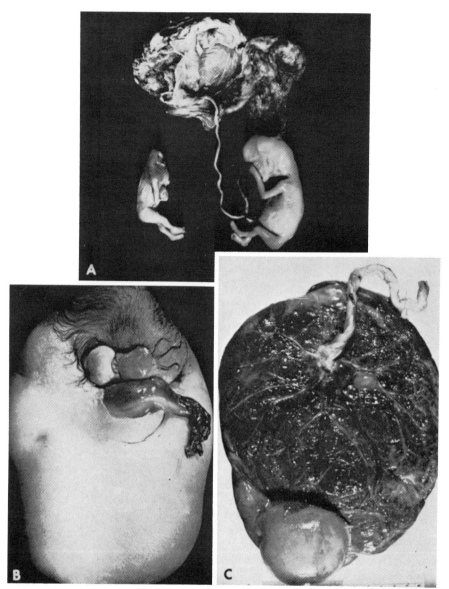

Figure 13. Forms of acardiac monsters. A, Twin abortus at 14 weeks: acephalic monster with prominent omphalocele at left; normal fetus at right, with placenta and umbilical cord of normal fetus above. B, Holoacardius amorphus from pregnancy at term. C, Monochorial twin placenta with holoacardius amorphus attached, showing also umbilical cord of normal fetus delivered at 39 weeks' gestation. (From Benirschke, K.: Obstet. and Gynec., 14:72, 1959.)

present be estimated. The evidence that such exceptional twins are in fact monozygotic comes from the study of their placenta, from blood-group analysis, and from successful exchange skin grafts. These surely are the most divergent MZ twins and they form a distinct category. The phenomenon of discordance for specific anomalies of MZ twins, other than chromosomal, is discussed in the section on teratology; the pathogenesis leading to that disturbance in embryonic growth pre-

sumably differs from the cytogenetic events just described.

MANAGEMENT OF MULTIPLE PREGNANCY

The patient with a multiple pregnancy deserves special consideration until she is safely delivered. Reference has been made to the increase in fetal wastage inherent in the twinning process itself. Pregnancy toxemia, desultory and unproductive labor, and postpartum hemorrhage are a few of the major complications characteristic of a multiple pregnancy. Triplets pose all of the problems and complications of twins, with more frequent recourse to cesarean section as a means of delivery.

A multiple pregnancy is suspected when there is a discrepancy between the size of the uterus and the duration of gestation, assuming that the menstrual history is accurate. Owing perhaps to the small size of the fetuses the heart tones are less likely to be audible at a time when the size of the uterus would indicate that they should be heard. The Doppler method is useful, as is ultrasound, in establishing the presence of twins. X-ray examination of the maternal abdomen may be unrevealing until the end of the fifth month of gestation. Prior to this period of pregnancy, if one fetus moves at the time of x-ray exposure, it may not be visualized and, hence, a singleton pregnancy may be erroneously diagnosed. By the sixth to seventh month of pregnancy, routine abdominal palpation should reveal the presence of multiple small parts and more than two fetal poles. X-ray examination at this time may be required if the diagnosis of multiple pregnancy is in doubt. Also, the relationship of the presenting parts to each other may be useful information in the conduct of labor and delivery.

The presence of twins is all too often not suspected or diagnosed until after birth of the first infant when the uterus is found to be nearly as large as before. Failure to palpate the uterus routinely immediately post delivery has led to administration of an oxytocic drug in an undiagnosed twin pregnancy, adding to both the fetal and the maternal hazard. Not only will the effect of the oxytocic drug invite fetal hypoxia and placental separation, but it will also interfere with the obstetrician's efforts to deliver the second fetus. When this accident occurs, if a breech or vertex is presenting the infant can be extracted promptly without harm, but if the second fetus is in a transverse position swift steps must be taken to relax the uterus by a properly selected and administered anesthetic to permit the fetus to be delivered promptly by internal podalic version.

Patients with a multiple pregnancy should be placed on a more rigid prenatal régime directed toward the prevention of the two major complications, pregnancy toxemia and premature labor. This means scrupulous weight control, including a careful review of the diet, and provision must be made for the mother to secure added periods of daily rest. Near-complete bed rest during the crucial period of 28 to 36 weeks has been advocated in an attempt to reduce the hazards of premature birth. The prenatal visits should be more frequent than in the average case, and the patient should be familiar with the cardinal signs and symptoms of pregnancy toxemia. In addition to the problem of its prevention, there is the question of how best to manage and deliver the patient should toxemia develop. At times one must await medical viability, if this is not at the expense of the mother's welfare. One is hesitant to attempt to induce labor, because desultory labor is known to occur more often in multiple pregnancy than in single pregnancy. Oxytocin stimulation, although not strictly contraindicated, must be used with great caution and is potentially more dangerous in the presence of more than one fetus. Thus, the obstetrician must be aware of the limitation of procedures to induce labor in the case of multiple pregnancy, and be prepared to do a cesarean section if induction fails or labor is unproductive.

The spontaneous onset of labor is awaited, and the first stage is conducted according to the usual routine. The type of anesthesia used must take into account the distinct possibility that the second twin may have to be delivered by internal podalic version. Pelvic delivery of the first infant differs little from that of a singleton pregnancy. Opinions differ regarding the time that should be permitted to elapse from the birth of the first infant to the birth of the next. Some favor allowing the patient to resume labor for at least an hour or more, hoping that a spontaneous delivery will occur. Many clinicians consider this more hazardous to the fetus than immediate delivery, for as the uterus contracts and reduces in size after the birth of the first baby, the placental site becomes constricted, and this favors placental separation. Also, the presenting part of the second twin is usually above the pelvic inlet or occasionally in a transverse position, and in either event prolapse of the cord and dystocia are more likely to occur. These constitute sufficient reasons to proceed with immediate delivery of the second twin rather than to wait. A vaginal examination is performed, and the position and presentation of the second twin are determined. The membranes are artifically ruptured, and the subsequent obstetric procedure will depend on the presentation. If the fetus is in a transverse position, an internal podalic version is performed. If the vertex presents, the presenting part may settle into the pelvis following rupture of the membranes to permit a comparatively easy forceps delivery; otherwise, an internal podalic version, which is not difficult to perform under these circumstances, may expedite the delivery.

Interlocking twins can occur in which the vertex of the first twin presenting by the breech interlocks with the second twin presenting by the vertex. If by chance the x-ray reveals that the lower limbs of the first twin and the vertex of the second twin are attempting to enter the pelvis simultaneously, then a cesarean section must be considered. Unfortunately, the complication is usually not recognized until the process of delivery has begun. With the breech delivered, traction is disastrous. If the interlocked vertices are above the inlet, an attempt is made, with the patient under deep inhalation anesthesia, to dislodge the first twin by displacing the vertex upward and rotating the chin by 90 to 180 degrees. If this fails and the fetus is obviously dead, the vertex is decompressed and delivery completed in the hope of salvaging the second twin.

If the vertex of the second twin has entered the pelvis together with the compressed body of the first twin, again under deep inhalation anesthesia the second twin must be dislodged if at all possible and the first twin delivered. Partial dislodgment with decompression of the vertex of the first twin may allow salvage of the second twin. Whatever else, the mother must not be subjected to possible trauma, i.e., uterine rupture, in a frantic attempt to accomplish delivery in this unusual but serious complication.

BIBLIOGRAPHY

Allen, G.: Twin research: problems and prospects. In Steinberg, A. G., and Bearn, A. G., eds.: Progress in Medical Genetics. Grune and Stratton, New York, 1965, p. 242.

Benirschke, K.: Spontaneous chimerism in mammals, a critical review. In Current Topics in Pathology, vol. 51. Springer-Verlag, Heidelberg, 1969, p. 1.

Benirschke, K., and Driscoll, S. G.: The Pathology of the Human Placenta. Springer-Verlag, New York, 1967.

Cameron, A. H.: The Birmingham twin survey. Proc. Roy, Soc. Med., 61:229, 1968.

Cohen, M., Kohl, S. G., and Rosenthal, A. H.: Fetal interlocking complicating twin gestation. Amer. J. Obstet. Gynec., 91:407, 1965.

Conjoined Twins. Birth Defects Original Article Series, Vol. 3. National Foundation, New York, 1967.

Edwards, J. H.: The value of twins in genetic studies. Proc. Roy. Soc. Med., 61:227, 1968.

Friedman, E. A., and Sachtleben, M. R.: The effect of uterine overdistension on labor. I. Multiple pregnancy. Obstet. Gynec., 23:164, 1964.

Guttmacher, A. F., and Kohl, S. G.: Cesarean section in twin pregnancy. Amer. J. Obstet. Gynec., 83:866, 1962.

Jonas, E. G.: The value of prenatal bed rest in multiple pregnancy. J. Obstet. Gynaec. Brit. Comm., 70:461, 1963.

Kaelber, C. T., and Pugh, T. F.: Influence of intrauterine relations on the intelligence of twins. New Eng. J. Med., 280:1030, 1969.

Lillie, F. R.: The free-martin; a study of the action of sex hormones in the fetal life of cattle. J. Exp. Zool., 23:371, 1917.

MacDonald, R. R.: Management of the second twin. Brit. Med. J., 1:518, 1962.

Moore, C. M., McAdams, A. J., and Sutherland, J.: Intrauterine disseminated intravascular coagulation: a syndrome of multiple pregnancy with a dead twin fetus. J. Pediat., 74:523, 1969.

Multiple Births United States — 1964. National Center for Health Statistics, Series 21, Number 14. Washington, D. C., 1967.

Naeye, R. L.: Human intrauterine parabiotic syndrome and its complications. New Eng. J. Med., 268:804, 1963.

Neel, J. V., and Schull, W. J.: Human Heredity. University of Chicago Press, Chicago, 1954.

Owen, R. D.: Immunogenetic consequences of vascular anastomoses in bovine twins. Science, 102:400, 1945.

Price, B.: Primary biases in twin studies. A review of prenatal and natal difference-producing factors in monozygotic pairs. Amer. J. Hum. Genet., 2:293, 1950.

Ross, G. T., Tjio, J. H., and Lipsett, M. B.: Cytogenetic studies of presumptively monozygotic twin girls discordant for gonadal dysgenesis. J. Clin. Endocr., 29:440, 1969.

Ryan, R. R., and Wislocki, G. V.: The birth of quadruplets, with an account of the placentas and fetal membranes. New Eng. J. Med., 250:755, 1954.

Schatz, F.: Die Gefässverbindungen der Placentakreisläufe eineiiger Zwillinge, ihre Entwicklung und ihre Folgen. Arch. Gynaek., 58:1, 1899.

Weinberg, W.: Beiträge zur Physiologie und Pathologie der Mehrlingsgeburten beim Menschen. Arch. Ges. Physiol., 88:346, 1901.

Wharton, B., Edwards, J. H., and Cameron, A. H.: Mono-amniotic twins. J. Obstet. Gynaec. Brit. Comm., 75:158, 1968.

Chapter 9

Immunologic Interactions in Pregnancy

The conceptus in all but inbred lines of mice must be considered genetically different from its host, the mother. Inasmuch as placentation affords intimate contact between these diverse organisms, one must expect that an immunologic reaction should be forthcoming of the kind that ensues when skin from a child is transplanted to its mother, i.e., an allograft rejection. No such event takes place at the site of placental attachment and the explanation of this apparent deficiency has been a baffling challenge ever since sophisticated transplantation experiments began around 1950.

The possible reasons for this unexplained phenomenon have been examined in innumerable experiments and reviewed by the most competent biologists. They still elude us to some extent despite the continuous creation of novel hypotheses. We have learned that the uterus does not represent a "privileged site" such as the cornea, and of course abdominal pregnancies could not be explained by such a hypothesis anyway. Immunization, as it were, of the mother during pregnancy (by injecting fetal parts, which are destroyed) or prior to pregnancy (by exposure to paternal antigens) does not alter placental survival. The fetus has been found to possess transplantation and other antigens in early life. Indeed red blood cells and presumably lymphocytes are often passed from fetus to mother; they should be recognized by her and presumably are, as the Rh-incompatibility events indicate, yet placental attachment remains unperturbed. Although the hormonal changes of pregnancy may be responsible for the slight prolongation of some experimental grafts, they are unable to support their survival for the duration of pregnancy in long-gestational species. Moreover, it must be borne in mind that among the animal species studied there exists a wide variety of hormonal patterns

in pregnancy, none completely specific or universal for pregnancy except progesterone. One of the earlier concepts held that the anatomic separation of mother and fetus is the basis for the apparent immunologic nonreactivity, a concept that has recently been modified to encompass fibrin as an important barrier between the two systems. It must be appreciated, however, that fibrin does not develop in the placenta until approximately the 10th week of gestation and that, cellularly speaking, no true barrier exists. Indeed, the histologic picture of the human placental site (and that of rodents, but by no means of all placental types) shows an extremely intimate admixture of fetal and maternal cells. The placental giant cells, usually considered to be of syncytial origin, intermingle with decidual cells, and some are regularly deported, but at their sites no equivalent of a rejection reaction is seen.

It is possible that several unique factors of placentation act in concert to provide the immunologically secure position of normal placentation. Thus, despite the intimate intermingling of trophoblast and decidua, no true vascularization of this placental site by either maternal or fetal vessels takes place. As Simmons has pointed out, such is the usual event in allograft rejection although it does not necessarily ensue in a second-set graft, of which many of course occur in placentation. It is indeed a peculiar finding of placental pathology that true granulation tissue, i.e., the ingrowth of fibrous tissue and capillaries as in the process of "organization" of thrombi, infarcts, and so forth anywhere else in the body, does not take place in any type of placental lesion, least of all in the placental site or the excessive fibrin deposits.

More recently investigators have become interested in the sialomucin coat of trophoblast, following a suggestion by Currie and

Bagshawe. It is now recognized that tropho-blastic cells are enveloped by a thin layer of this sulfated mucopolysaccharide, not unlike malignant cells. This secretory product of the syncytium is considered to increase the hydration of the trophoblast cell surface and thus obscure its transplantation antigens to recognition by maternal lymphocytes, the latter being common mediators of a transplant rejection. This coat, the glycocalyx, may be selectively destroyed by neuraminidase, in which case the cellular antigens are unmasked and subject to transplant rejection. These findings are disputed by others (Urbach) and it is necessary to indicate here that the last word has not been spoken in this extremely complex field. This is emphasized by a new hypothesis recently formulated by Swinburne, suggesting that antigenic stimulation proceeds normally throughout pregnancy by minute fetal-to-maternal transplacental blood leakage. The maternal response is thought to be "mopped up," as it were, by the placental "sponge," the ever increasing fibrin deposits testifying to this event.

Not only is the lack of allograft rejection of the placenta during normal pregnancy ill understood, but also obscure is the reason why in successive pregnancies even less reactivity occurs. Moreover, contradictory but interesting findings have been made in pregnancies of rodents, comparing inbred lines with outbred ones. In mice placental and fetal weights are smaller in the former, and the increased size of hybrid litters and their placentas is considered to be related to immunologic interaction of mother and hybrid placenta. This does not hold true of all such crosses and the complexity of the experiments is not yet understood. Suffice it to say that termination of pregnancy surely is not an immunologic event although such was once considered possible.

These studies all relate importantly, however, to the suggested etiology and treatment of choriocarcinoma. This tumor of trophoblast has been found spontaneously only in man and the rhesus monkey. The frequency of its occurrence varies geographically for unknown reasons, it being much more prevalent in the countries of the Far East (China, Philippines) but not the Asians of this country. Since the chemotherapy of choriocarcinoma is highly successful, and even spontaneous regressions are on record, and because such is not the

case with choriocarcinomas in males or ovaries deriving from germ cells, it has been assumed that gestational choriocarcinoma differs because of its genotype. Gestational choriocarcinoma is likened to an F_1 "hybrid," possessing paternal as well as maternal genes; hence if it were "recognized" by the mother as foreign, i.e., as an allograft, then it might be rejected more readily. Conversely, if it derived from closely related parents, greater similarity of antigens could be assumed and hence the tumor might be more aggressive or more common in such inbred populations.

Support for all these suggestions has been forthcoming. In inbred populations the tumor is thought to be more common (but it does not occur in inbred animals) and in a few instances immunotherapy, employing immunization of the afflicted woman with paternal antigens, is thought to have been successful. In such women paternal skin grafts have, at times, also enjoyed increased survival. These findings may relate to the observations mentioned in the discussion of choriocarcinoma in Chapter 14 that those tumors which are surrounded by plasma cells have a better prognosis than those which do not elicit the cellular response. Transplantation antigens are expressed by choriocarcinoma, but also the same sialomucins that coat normal trophoblast are present on malignant trophoblastic cells. Finally, Scott has furnished evidence that the tumor is more common in older women but disproportionally in first pregnancies or with fresh matings.

These observations have at present little practical relevance, as immunotherapy of gestational choriocarcinoma is difficult and can only be regarded as an experimental adjunct to the standard chemotherapeutic measures. Nevertheless, careful documentation is desirable to increase our understanding of the still mysterious placental allograft immunity.

Other aspects of immunologic interactions between mother and fetus are better understood, particularly the effects of rhesus-antigen immunization. It is clear now that maternal antibodies are transferred transplacentally to the fetus to initiate hemolytic anemia with the possible end-result of fetal heart failure and hydrops fetalis. Only secondarily does the placenta become involved in this edematous process, the primary immunologic target being the fetal red blood cells. In a similar vein it appears that the factors responsible for idiopathic thrombocytopenic purpura in the mother, presumably IgG globulins, are often transferred to the fetus in whom they may initiate hemorrhage attending traumatic delivery. Hence Scott makes the plea that women with this disease, at present or in the past, should be delivered most gently and that the possibility of transient thrombocytopenia in the newborn be borne in mind. Neonatal mortality in such circumstances is reported between 13 and 25 per cent. While leukoagglutinins also cross the placenta, no specific ill effect has been ascribed to their presence. Other maternal antibodies pass the placenta in effective amounts; best known perhaps are those to insulin in women with treated diabetes, which may inactivate fetal insulin to some extent until their disappearance after some days into neonatal life. And similar effects may be secondary to maternal isoimmune disorders such as thyroid disease and myasthenia and perhaps others. In general, the disturbance is transitory in neonatal life and must be understood by the neonatologist, because effective therapy may depend on the recognition of these rare disorders.

Little evidence exists that permanent "grafting" of maternal cells onto the fetus occurs regularly. To be sure, fetal and neonatal disseminated melanoma, originating in the mother and passed after placental metastasis, has been witnessed a few times, as has disseminated fetal and maternal choriocarcinoma. These are exceptional circumstances, however, and only these two tumors are implicated. The more common maternal leukemia and fetal malignant tumors (leukemia and neuroblastoma) are not known to produce such transplacental chimerism. If their cells are transferred, we assume they are rejected by immunologic means.

Finally, in recent years the suggestion has been made that normal maternal lymphocytes might enter the fetus via the placenta to colonize his hematopoietic system. The experimental evidence firmly rejects such a hypothesis now, and of course the anticipated XX/XY cell chimerism in the blood that would be expected in males is not detected in the vast number of chromosome studies now on record. Only once, when a fetus suffered an inborn immunologic deficiency, is such engrafting presumed to

have taken place. Usually, if such transfer does occur at all, the cells are rejected by the immunologically competent conceptus.

In the past it was believed that the fetus was incapable of immunologic response, primarily because this response was sluggish or absent until the second month of neonatal life. It is now recognized that this relative inertia is normally due to the fact that the fetus is nearly completely protected against the common antigens. If antigenic stimulation occurs, however, either experimentally or by infection, then a specific immunologic response may be mounted surprisingly early in fetal life. This was early recognized by the massive cellular response (mostly plasma cells) in congenital syphilis, e.g., the pneumonia alba, or in toxoplasmosis. Indeed, according to Silverstein, who initiated investigations in this field, it may be this very cellular response that causes the recognized disease states. In its absence and with large amounts of antigen present, relatively little pathogenicity may be recognized. In experimental animals, and presumably in man, a very orderly but unpredictable pattern of immunologic maturation (given an antigenic stimulus) occurs in fetal life. Suffice it to say that after midgestation the human fetus might be considered completely matured in this respect. He is capable of rejecting transplanted tissues and cells and of producing humoral antibodies of all types. Given some antigens, such as reproductive hematopoietic cells from a cotwin through placental anastomoses early in embryogenesis, a fetus may grow up to be tolerant of these foreign cells. He will develop permanent blood cell chimerism, as is the case in freemartinism in bovine twins and in the 10 or so pairs of human fraternal twins with blood chimerism. In adult life this tolerance then extends to other tissues from the same donor.

This recognition of the capacity of the fetus to respond to antigenic stimulation has considerable clinical importance (see Chapter 22, Prenatal Infections). Because of the usual freedom from antigenic stimulation the antibodies of the normal fetus are acquired in large measure by transplacental passage from the mother. Some antibodies, because of their structure, do not pass readily. However, if substantial levels of such IgM globulins are detected in neonatal blood it is permissible to infer that fetal infection has preceded. Such is the case in congenital rubella, cytomegalovirus infection, toxoplasmosis, syphilis, and so forth. Indeed, specific types of antibodies are thus detected whose existence allows the diagnosis of certain types of prenatal illness, even if the antigen cannot be recovered.

See Placental Transfer, in Chapter 3.

BIBLIOGRAPHY

Billingham, R. E.: Transplantation immunity and the maternal-fetal relation. New Eng. J. Med., 270:667, 720, 1964.

Bradbury, S., Billington, W. D., Kirby, D. R. S., and Williams, E. A.: Surface mucin of human trophoblast. Amer. J. Obstet. Gynec. 104:416, 1969.

Currie, G. A., and Bagshawe, K. D.: The masking of antigens on trophoblast and cancer cells. Lancet, 1:708, 1967.

Furth, R. van, Schuit, H. R. E., and Hijmans, W.: The immunological development of the human fetus. J. Exp. Med., 122:1173, 1965.

Galton, M.: Immunological interactions between mother and fetus. In Benirschke, K., ed.: Comparative Aspects of Reproductive Failure. Springer-Verlag, New York, 1967, pp. 413–416.

Gross, S. J.: The current dilemma of placental antigenicity. Obstet. Gynec. Survey, 25:105, 1970.

Mathé, G., Dausett, J., Hervet, E., Amiel, J. L., Colombani, J., and Brule, G.: Immunological studies in patients with placental choriocarcinoma. J. Nat. Cancer Inst., 33:193, 1964.

Mogensen, B., and Kissmeyer-Nielsen, F.: Histocompatibility antigens on the HL-A locus in generalised gestational choriocarcinoma: a family study. Lancet, 1:721, 1968.

Scott, J. S.: Choriocarcinoma. Amer. J. Obstet. Gynec. 83:185, 1962.

Scott, J. S.: Immunological diseases and pregnancy. Brit. Med. J., 1:1559, 1966.

Silverstein, A. M.: Ontogeny of the immune response. The development of immunologic responses by the fetus has interesting pathobiologic implications. Science, 144:1423, 1964.

Silverstein, A. M., and Lukes, R. J.: Fetal response to antigenic stimulus. I. Plasma cellular and lymphoid reactions in the human fetus to intrauterine infections. Lab. Invest., 11:918, 1962.

Simmons, R. L.: Histoincompatibility and the survival of the fetus: current controversies. Transpl. Proc., 1:47, 1969.

Swinburne, L. M.: Leucocyte antigens and placental sponge. Lancet, 2:592, 1970.

Urbach, G. I.: Fetal-maternal-placental immunologic relationship. Fertil. Steril., 21:356, 1970.

Chapter 10

Cytogenetics. Amniocentesis

The chromosome complement of man and many mammals is well understood as a result of large numbers of studies carried out in the last decade. Because of the frequency of numerical or structural alterations—1 in 200 newborns—and because these so often play an important part in the reproductive functions, it is necessary to review this subject in some detail.

From a technical point of view it is easiest to assess chromosome number and structure from short-term lymphocyte cultures. Lymphocytes are stimulated by the addition of the red bean extract phytohemagglutinin to tissue culture fluids and within three days of culture hundreds of mitoses may be observed, photographed, and karyotyped. The usual technique employs merely a few drops of blood and, through the commercial availability of "kits," the technique is accessible to anyone whose laboratory possesses but a minimal amount of equipment. Photography and interpretation of results, however, require greater facility and training. Nevertheless, slides may be sent and can be interpreted elsewhere so that a patient whose condition requires cytogenetic study can be evaluated without the necessity of travel to a genetic counseling center. Information is available from the National Foundation, 800 Second Avenue, New York, New York 10017. Another source of dividing cells, sterilely obtained fibrous tissue or skin biopsy, can be immersed in tissue culture fluid and shipped without great precautions to a laboratory equipped for the more tedious task of fibrous tissue culture. The same applies for amniotic fluid cells.

Through an international agreement (the Chicago Conference) the human karyotype is set out in a uniform manner (Fig. 1) which allows easy reference to pinpoint possible errors. Principally two types of chromosomes are distinguished, biarmed (so-called metacentrics and submetacentrics) and single-armed (so-called acrocentrics). Chromosomes are thus grouped according to their length and configuration. Pairs of chromosomes, one element derived from the paternal and one from the maternal gamete, are thus arranged in seven groups (A to G) plus the sex chromosomes, XY or XX. Within certain limits, and with special techniques, many chromosomes may be distinguished specifically. Those that present difficulties in identification because of similar-sized elements are grouped in Figure 1 and connected by lines. The reason that the elements of individual pairs in karyotypes such as shown have somewhat different shapes, i.e., are more curved, thicker, and so forth, relates to preparatory artifacts and not to actual differences in structure. Although these elements are made up of DNA, it is impossible to distinguish individual genes visually and, therefore, a chromosomal (i.e., macroscopic structural) analysis in individuals with specific gene defects, for instance phenylketonuria, yields normal results.

As can be seen, the total amount of chromosomal material of females is greater than that of males. That is to say, the XX pair is greater in DNA quantity than XY. Such imbalance does not seem feasible in mammalians and nature has evolved a mechanism by which the excessive amount of DNA contained in the second X of the female becomes inactivated in normal cellular events. It is rendered "heterochromatic"; i.e., it becomes darker-staining and its DNA is not employed for genetic transcription, in contrast to the "euchromatin" of the rest of the chromosomal set. The condensed X is visually identifiable as the "Barr body," the sex chromatin body seen at the nuclear membrane of women's cells. It is readily identified in smears from the buccal mucosa or in vaginal smears (Fig. 2), so long as the smear is fixed rapidly in a manner like that for Papanicolaou preparations. Any laboratory stain colors this sex chromatin, and in normal females, at least 20 per cent of well preserved cells should be "chromatin-positive," i.e., have one Barr body. When

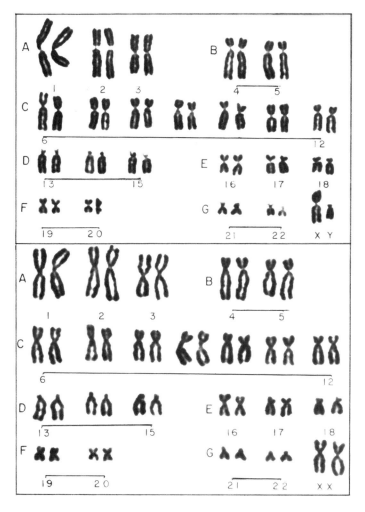

Figure 1. Karyotype of normal male (top) and female (below) lymphocytes arranged according to the Chicago Conference. Those chromosomes connected by lines (groups C, D, F, and G) cannot be critically differentiated one from another. (From Hsu, T. C., and Benirschke, K.: An Atlas of Mammalian Chromosomes, Vol. I. Springer-Verlag, New York, 1967.)

more than two X chromosomes are present, additional Barr bodies are found (XXX, two Barr bodies; XXXX, three Barr bodies, and so on). Normal males are chromatin-negative and persons with the typical Klinefelter's syndrome (XXY) have one Barr body. This condensation of the additional X is called "dosage compensation" and follows a rule that is commonly referred to as the Lyon hypothesis, after its inventor, Mary Lyon.

It is suggested by this hypothesis, and there is a good deal of confirmatory evidence, that the female embryo, endowed with one X from the father and one from the mother, starts out his cellular divisions with both sex chromosomes active. Soon the individual cells, at random, "decide" whether to inactivate father's (X^P) or mother's (X^M) X chromosome, and all their successors fall into this now fixed pattern (Fig. 3). Thus, a female's body is functionally a 50/50 mosaic. Half the cells express those gene codes (enzymes and so

forth) on the paternal X, and half express those on the maternal X.

Barr bodies, while easiest detected in buccal or vaginal smears, are found throughout all tissue cells, may be detected in sec-

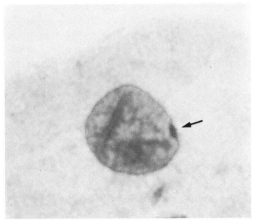

Figure 2. Vaginal epithelial cell from Papanicolaou smear. At arrow, the Barr body (sex chromatin) pressed against the nuclear membrane. × 3500.

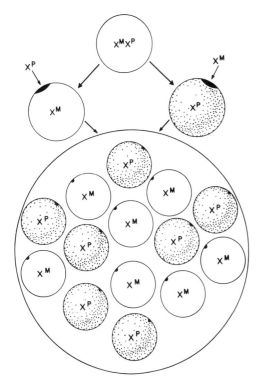

Figure 3. The Lyon hypothesis. An uncommitted embryonic cell at top divides and its decendants inactivate either paternal (X^P) or maternal (X^M) X chromosome. This becomes the Barr body and the pattern becomes fixed for the subsequent progeny of these cells. Thus, the female organism (bottom) is a mosaic composite of two functionally different cell types. (From Benirschke, K.: Mosaicism and chimerism. In Yearbook of Science and Technology. McGraw-Hill Book Co., New York, 1967, pp. 248–251.

tions of well fixed organs, and indeed were discovered in neuronal cells. In polymorphonuclear leukocytes they assume the shape of a "drumstick" (Fig. 4), but because of its low frequency (2 to 3 per cent) their analysis is not usually helpful.

Although males have no sex chromatin in their nuclei, a recently developed technique allows visualization of the Y chromosome. This is possible because the Y chromosome has only few functional genes, the major portion of its long arms being constructed of a special type of DNA. This "constitutive" heterochromatin (as opposed to the "facultative" heterochromatin of the second X making up the Barr body) has a particular affinity for the antimalarial Atabrine. The bound quinacridin can then be identified as a fluorescent spot in cells of normal males. Men with two Y chromosomes, 47,XYY as their official designation is, would have two such fluorescent spots but no Barr bodies.

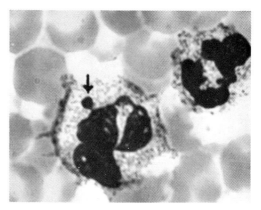

Figure 4. Peripheral leukocyte with "drumstrick" at arrow, indicating presence of two X chromosomes. Patient with Klinefelter's syndrome. Wright stain. × 3500.

These techniques have all been employed in the study of abnormal babies, infertile patients, and abortions, and also in surveys of consecutive newborns. A particularly large study by Lubs and Ruddle of 4500 consecutive newborns is presumably representative of the minimal expected frequency of numerical chromosomal errors. They detected 22 major errors plus some minor variations which will here be neglected (Table 1).

The first group in Table 1, the translocations, require comment. Best known among chromosomal errors are the trisomies, particularly trisomy G, (trisomy 21, mongolism,

TABLE 1. MINIMAL EXPECTED FREQUENCY OF NUMERICAL CHROMOSOMAL ERRORS IN NEWBORNS*

Types	Number in 4500 Consecutive Births	No./1000 Births
Translocations†	6	1.37
Trisomy D	1	0.23
Trisomy E	1	0.23
Trisomy G	3	0.69
XYY†	3	0.69
XXY	4	0.93
XXX†	3	0.69
XO	1	0.23

*Modified from Lubs, H. A., and Ruddle, F. H.: Science, 169:495, 1970.

†Conditions that are phenotypically not identifiable at birth, the infant appearing normal. In the remainder of the conditions the infant would have various and typical anomalies. Of parenthetic interest is the finding that several of the infants with the XYY and XXY anomaly were "small-for-dates" babies.

Down's syndrome). Various evidence exists that this error occurs at gametogenesis through nondisjunction of one element. In other words, one chromosome fails to reach the proper daughter cell at division and the resulting gamete receives 24 instead of the normal 23 elements. Because increased maternal age so often correlates with these errors, and because overripe ova in other species can be shown to suffer similar defects frequently, it is inferred that most often faulty maternal gametogenesis is the cause although direct evidence is difficult to obtain.

The situation is different with translocations. As is evident from Table 1, the event is frequent, and it is also one occurring perhaps at gametogenesis; at least evidence of it is present in the gametes. In this event two chromosomes bind together permanently after breaks have occurred and the chromosome number is reduced by one. Such individuals lose virtually no chromosomal material in the process and, although they possess only 45 elements, most commonly they are phenotypically normal. Translocations occur most often in the groups D and G chromosomes, the acrocentrics. They may be D/D, G/G, or D/G in type and karyotyping quickly identifies these abnormalities. From studies of affected families, particularly those in which children with mongolism have been born, it has been learned that (1) the translocation is heritable and (2) an increased frequency of trisomies occurs because of faulty gametogenesis in the phenotypically normal "translocation carriers." Moreover, at times such patients are found among those classified as habitual aborters. A review of a large number of individuals with Down's syndrome identifies the problem in Table 2.

It is seen that the frequency of the two types of translocation commonly leading to the trisomy 21 syndrome (D/G and G/G) is about the same, and that in both types, sporadic (i.e., de-novo) translocations exceed the number of inherited types. Also, mongolism of the translocation type is more often ascertained in younger mothers.

It is the latter patients — those with known translocation carrier state, whose risk of having a child with this disease is great — who might benefit the most from prenatal chromosome analysis. In other words, if the exact chromosome structure of her child could be learned prior to fetal viability then a decision could be reached on some rational basis as to whether or not to allow the pregnancy to continue, for such analysis might predict precisely whether the child would be afflicted by the disease, would be a phenotypically normal translocation carrier, or would have entirely normal chromosomes. Similarly, in such sex-linked disorders as hemophilia the fetal sex may be anticipated accurately, and more recently a variety of enzymatic studies have become available which aid immeasurably in what is now called prenatal counseling. Some have even suggested that pregnant women older than 35 years should have such studies routinely because of their much enhanced risk of carrying a trisomic fetus.

Amniocentesis for genetic counseling has gradually evolved from the experience gained in the management of Rh sensitization. It was anticipated by Fuchs and Riis who early demonstrated that the desquamated cells of the amniotic fluid could be used to establish the fetal sex by the Barr body method. Their transvaginal approach has been replaced by the much more pre-

TABLE 2. TRISOMY VS. TRANSLOCATION*

| Maternal Age | No. | "Regular" Trisomy 21 | Translocation Mongolism | | | | | | Trans-location |
| | | | D/G | | | G/G | | | |
			Sporadic	Inherited	?	Sporadic	Inherited	?	
Under 30 years	722	658	16	11	6	23	2	6	8.9%
Over 30 years	660	646	5	2	–	6	–	1	2.1%
Total	1,382	1,304	21	13	6	29	2	7	5.7%

*From Wright, S. W., Day, R. W., Muller, H., and Weinhouse, R.: The frequency of trisomy and translocation in Down's syndrome. J. Pediat., 70:420, 1967.

ferable transabdominal route, and the procedure is now best performed between the 14th and 16th weeks of pregnancy for the purposes of genetic advice. From the extensive experience of a few laboratories certain important observations have been made.

Needless to say, it is imperative that amniocentesis for counseling purposes be undertaken only if there exists a clear understanding that definite treatment can and will be undertaken, that is to say, that termination of pregnancy in the case of a positive finding is acceptable to all parties. This condition limits the procedure to a time prior to fetal viability and may necessitate the performance of repeat taps in case of failure. While failure to obtain liquid is rare, the failure rate of successful tissue culture varies, is at times 40 per cent, and has led to repeat taps in several cases. Ideally the placenta is localized by ultrasound, a feasible technique after 13 weeks of gestation, and the transplacental approach is then avoided by suitable direction of the needle. Puncture of fetal placental vessels could cause exsanguination; moreover, contamination of the fluid by blood may render the specimen useless for chemical or cytogenetic analysis. In all cases the possibility of a twin pregnancy must be borne in mind when the results are interpreted. Of course, in case of fraternal twins, study of the amniotic fluid of one fetus predicts nothing of the other's status.

The procedure is performed under sterile conditions, not unlike a spinal fluid puncture. The bladder is emptied immediately before the tap, the skin is cleansed and infiltrated with a local anesthetic. A 22-gauge spinal needle (5 inch length) is used with stylet in place. It is aimed directly into the center of the uterus, the stylet is removed, and between 2 and 10 ml. of fluid is withdrawn. While complications have been reported (fetal injury, placental injury, fetal-maternal bleeding with possible sensitization, abortion), their frequency is not great. Nevertheless, the risk must be clearly understood. The fluid obtained may be used for cellular, cytogenetic, and biochemical techniques, and shipment to one of the centers that is equipped for the analysis has proved feasible. After centrifugation the cellular sediment is suspended in culture medium and within two to four weeks, occasionally earlier, sufficient cellular growth has occurred to allow karyotypic analysis.

The origin of the cells grown in culture is still in doubt. Cytologic examination indicates that a mixture of cells is obtained. Some clearly derive from skin and amnion, others are macrophages, and others still are perhaps derived from the urogenital and respiratory tract. Suffice it to say, in a tap containing no blood, all may be considered of feto-placental origin and if adequate precautions are taken, contamination with decidua or intervillous (maternal) blood cells is avoidable. If twins are excluded and contamination is avoided, correct cytogenetic evaluation can be expected within four weeks, and often earlier. The Barr bodies may be evaluated immediately.

Cytogenetic evaluation serves two principal purposes, the detection of trisomy 21 (mongolism) in fetuses of mothers of advanced age, and the detection of trisomics or unbalanced translocation carriers in offspring of parents with known balanced translocations. It is now known that the risk of having an unbalanced, i.e., trisomic, infant when one parent possesses one of the common balanced translocations is much lower than expected from theoretical considerations. Hamerton finds the highest frequency for the commonest type (D/G) to be only 9 per cent and for other types even less. Prenatal karyotyping from cells obtained by amniocentesis then becomes a most important tool in managing such families.

Aside from cytogenetic studies, amniotic fluid is used for a variety of other studies. One may determine the ABO blood groups of the fetus, estimate the volume, assess fetal maturity in later pregnancy by means of chemical and cytologic studies, and seek to identify homozygous biochemical defects (inborn errors of metabolism) in fetuses of known heterozygous parents. It has thus been suggested that the adrenogenital syndrome may be detected from the steroid content, and that analysis for a variety of amino acids can be made. Biochemical analysis of cultured cells and, at times, of uncultured cells may provide diagnostic evidence of fatal fetal disorders. Thus, the diagnosis of Pompe's disease (glycogen storage disease, type II), Tay-Sachs disease, some mucopolysaccharidoses, metachromatic leukodystrophy, galactosemia, and other disorders has been made successfully, to be proved when therapeutic abortion was performed. There is intense research activity in this field and no doubt many other rare disorders will be found to be detectable by this means. The complexity of biochemical studies is great in some cases and it is apparent that only a few centers should be allowed to undertake the task. Efforts are being made to establish a central registry for prenatal genetic analysis.

BIBLIOGRAPHY

Creasman, W. T., Lawrence, R. A., and Thiede, H. A.: Fetal complications of amniocentesis. J.A.M.A., 204:91, 1968.

Chicago Conference: Standardization in human cytogenetics. In Birth Defects: Original Article Series *II*:2, The National Foundation, New York, 1966, pp. 1–21.

Fuchs, F., and Riis, P.: Antenatal sex determination. Nature, 177:330, 1956.

Hamerton, J. L.: Fetal sex. Lancet, 1:516, 1970.

Jacobson, C. B., and Barter, R. H.: Intrauterine diagnosis and management of genetic defects. Amer. J. Obstet. Gynec., 99:796, 1967.

Lubs, H. A., and Ruddle, F. H.: Chromosomal abnormalities in the human population: estimation of rates based on New Haven newborn study. Science, 169: 495, 1970.

Lyon, M. F.: Sex-chromatin and gene action in the mammalian X-chromosome. Amer. J. Hum. Genet., 14:135, 1962.

Nadler, H. L., and Gerbie, A. B.: Role of amniocentesis in the intrauterine detection of genetic disorders. New Eng. J. Med., 282:596, 1970.

Ostergard, D. R.: The physiology and clinical importance of amniotic fluid. A review. Obstet. Gynec. Survey, 25:297, 1970.

Wright, S. W., Day, R. W., Muller, H., and Weinhouse, R.: The frequency of trisomy and translocation in Down's syndrome. J. Pediat., 70:420, 1967.

Yunis, J. J.: Human Chromosome Methodology. Academic Press, New York, 1965.

Chapter 11

Anatomic and Physiologic Changes of Pregnancy

The bodily changes and alterations in function that result from pregnancy become recognizable shortly after the first missed period. It is generally regarded that pregnancy imposes a "load" on the maternal organism, particularly upon the circulation, and that many of the changes represent the response of the body to additional metabolic demands. The physical and functional alterations of pregnancy involve all the body systems, some to a greater extent than others.

ALTERATIONS IN VARIOUS SYSTEMS AND ORGANS

Reproductive Tract

UTERUS. Although increase in uterine size is in response to the growing conceptus, evaluation of uterine enlargement in the early weeks of pregnancy must be made with regard to the parity of the patient. The uterus that has undergone a previous pregnancy is slightly larger that that in the nulliparous patient. Therefore, a slight increase in size of the uterus soon after the first missed period may be of value in the primipara, but is of less significance in the multigravid patient.

By the end of the second month of pregnancy, the uterus triples in size and weight; this may cause the organ to shift its position so that exaggerated anteflexion or retrocession and retroversion are not uncommon. By the end of the third month, the uterus occupies most of the pelvic cavity and, when in the normal anterior position, can usually be palpated suprapubically. At the end of the fourth month the uterus has become an abdominal organ, and midway through pregnancy the upper uterine pole has reached the level of the umbilicus. With continuous growth, by the 36th to 38th week the fundal portion of the uterus reaches nearly to the ensiform process. During the last three or four weeks of gestation, the superior pole of the uterus may recede slightly, provided there is descent of the presenting part of the fetus into the pelvis, a phenomenon referred to as "lightening." In the majority of pregnancies the uterus tends to rotate from left to right and, in the event of extreme rotation, were the abdomen opened, the left round ligament would be found near the midline.

During the early weeks of pregnancy the contour of the uterus changes from its typical flat, pear shape of the nonpregnant state to a more rounded form, an outline that it retains until the sixth month. At the beginning of the last trimester, the uterus assumes an ovoid shape with its vertical axis lengthening more rapidly than either the transverse or anteroposterior diameter.

Mitotic activity is rarely noted in the myometrium, and the enlargement that occurs is most probably due to hypertrophy rather than to hyperplasia. Hypertrophy of the existing muscle cells begins in the early weeks, and during the course of pregnancy their size increases five- to ten-fold. With this hypertrophy, the uterine cavity enlarges at a rate that is at first in excess of the growth rate of the conceptus—a neat arrangement, for one might speculate that were it otherwise, degrees of placentation would occur through the endometrial surface and placenta membranacea of some form would be the rule rather than the extremely rare exception. In the early weeks of pregnancy the uterine cavity is filled mostly with a luxuriant growth of decidua (Fig. 1). Injection of the intact specimen with a latex mass makes it possible to visualize the spiral arterioles throughout the decidua vera (Fig. 2).

221

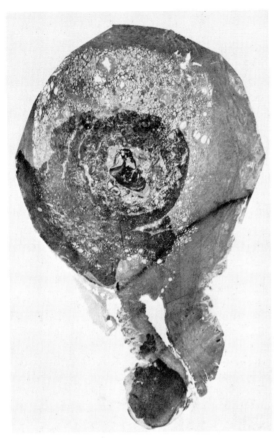

Figure 1. Section of a uterus at 10 weeks' gestation. At this stage much of the uterine cavity is occupied by decidua vera only. (Courtesy of Dr. S. L. Romney.)

A question that has long been considered but not conclusively answered is: What properties of the uterus permit it to expand and accommodate the growing conceptus? It has been suggested that this expansile behavior is due not to any rearrangement of the muscle bundles, but rather in part at least to the collagenous framework of the uterus. Undoubtedly the collagen content of the myometrium at different stages of pregnancy has clinical relevance as the uterus accommodates the growing conceptus, or at least until placentation is completed. Apparently the expansile property of the myometrium appears greatest in the first half of pregnancy and following delivery.

Although the myometrium is supposedly rich in mast cells compared to other tissues of the body, the prevalence of these cells is no greater in the uterus in pregnancy than in the nonpregnant uterus. This is mentioned as one seeks a reason why the myometrial blood vessels are conspicuously free of thromboses despite the fact that they are often subject to a degree of external trauma from uterine massage by physician or nurse for the purpose of promoting myometrial contractility and avoiding postpartum bleeding. It is equally remarkable that this never occurs in, or is a sequel to, cesarean section, when these vessels can be seen as gaping

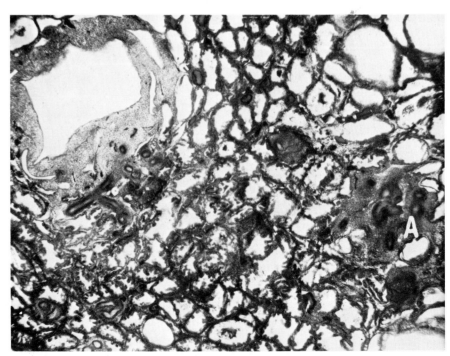

Figure 2. Photomicrograph of a section of intact uterus injected with a latex mass, showing the spiral arterioles (A) in the decidua vera. (From specimen shown in Figure 1; courtesy of Dr. S. L. Romney.)

sinusoids in the uterine wound. Thrombi in the postpartum patient originate from the pelvic or leg veins, not from the uterus. Also, the status of uterine mast cells may be raised in cases of obstetric hemorrhage associated with a clotting defect, where the question may arise as to the possibility of heparin-like action being present or desirable.

The myometrium of the corpus in early pregnancy measures 2 to 3 cm. in thickness, but in late pregnancy it is reduced to 1 to 2 cm. In multigravid women, or in the presence of hydramnios or multiple pregnancy, this thinning of the uterine wall may become exaggerated. The patient who has had many children may present such a readily palpable fetus that the examiner might wonder if he is dealing with an abdominal pregnancy. In case of serious question, recourse to soft tissue x-ray examination will outline the uterine wall and demonstrate the location of the fetus within the uterus. In one of the writer's patients, the pulsating umbilical cord within the uterus could be palpated through the abdominal wall. This startling experience was verified by a second observer, who detected with a fetoscope an abrupt fall in the rate of fetal heart tones simultaneous with the application of pressure to the abdomen over the cord. The patient subsequently had a normal pelvic delivery, and exploration of the uterine cavity at the time revealed no defect or diverticulum of the myometrium.

During the early weeks of pregnancy, the isthmic portion of the uterus undergoes hypertrophy similar to the process taking place in the corpus. The point of demarcation between the isthmus and corpus, known as the anatomic internal os, is represented by a thinning of the endometrium (Fig. 3). The lower boundary of the isthmus is known as the obstetric or histologic internal os, and at this point the endometrium and the endocervical mucosa meet. The hypertrophy of the isthmus during the first trimester triples the distance between these two anatomic landmarks, and the isthmic canal becomes approximately 3 cm. in length. In the early weeks of pregnancy this area feels softer than either the cervix or the corpus. This softness, referred to as Hegar's sign, can be detected readily at vaginal examination by bimanual compression and is a reliable diagnostic indication of pregnancy. Between the 12th and 16th weeks, the uterine cavity becomes totally occupied by the growing conceptus. The isthmus now becomes incorporated into the main body of the uterus and the isthmic canal becomes part of the uterine cavity (Fig. 3). For purposes of emphasis, it is again mentioned that the isthmus becomes a major portion of the lower uterine segment and that its inner surface is covered by less luxurious and much thinner endometrium. This favors the belief and finding that the trophoblast has a greater chance to become attached to the myometrium than elsewhere in the uterus, resulting in what is referred to as a placenta accreta—a complication that appears more common when implantation occurs in the lower uterine segment, i.e., placenta praevia. Until about the last trimester of pregnancy, the walls of the isthmus and the corpus are of approximately the same thickness, and direct inspection at laparotomy fails to reveal a conspicuous junction between these two portions of the uterus.

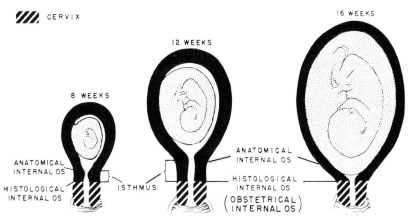

Figure 3. Schematic diagrams of the uterus at different stages of pregnancy, illustrating formation of the lower uterine segment.

However, near term a definite transverse linear depression develops on the surface of the uterus slightly below the vesico-uterine fold of peritoneum. This marks the union between the corpus and the former isthmus, or the upper and the lower uterine segment, respectively (Fig. 4). The level at which this line of demarcation appears, known as the "physiologic retraction ring," is believed to be identical to the anatomic internal os. The uterine musculature above this ring is decidedly thicker than the wall of the lower uterine segment. With labor, the latter widens and the physiologic retraction ring rises to a higher level. Following delivery, internal palpation of the well contracted uterus will reveal a ring as a marked constriction between the corpus and what is ostensibly the lower uterine segment or the isthmus.

In some cases of prolonged labor the physiologic retraction ring may be palpated as a ridgelike structure above the upper margin of the symphysis, and, in the extreme, it may rise midway to the level of the umbilicus. Especially in the presence of rupture of the fetal membranes with nearly a complete loss of amniotic fluid, the physiologic retraction ring may so constrict the fetus as to impede labor. In this circumstance the structure is referred to as a pathologic contraction ring (Bandl's ring).

The portion of the cervix lying above the fibromuscular junction is composed mostly of muscle, and this also becomes part of the lower uterine segment, but much later in pregnancy. This phenomenon may explain the effacement or "taking up" of the cervix, which is an important change during late pregnancy and the first stage of labor. The portio vaginalis of the cervix, being composed principally of fibrous tissue, dilates by stretching during labor in response to the forces imposed by advancement of the presenting fetal part or by the intact fetal membranes. Certainly the cervix has neither the morphologic characteristics nor the physiologic behavior of a sphincter, a fact to recall when considering those factors which may influence labor. Further evidence of this is the fact that immediately after delivery, and in the early puerperium, the cervix is found in redundant folds lying loosely in the upper vagina.

Any increase in size of the vaginal portion of the cervix is the result of increased vascularization and not of hypertrophy. With growth, the cervical glands tend to obliterate

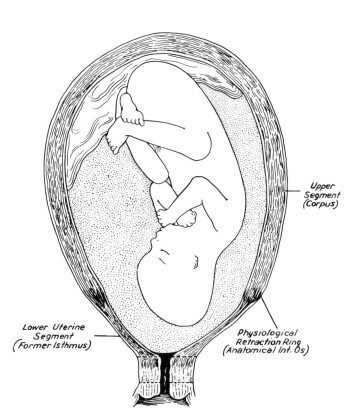

Upper
Segment
(Corpus)

Lower Uterine
Segment
(Former Isthmus)

Physiological
Retraction Ring
(Anatomical Int. Os)

Figure 4. Drawing of the pregnant uterus, showing demarcation of the upper and lower uterine segments.

the canal, and the excessive mucus from these glands gives to the endocervix a spongelike appearance. At the onset of labor, some, or at least the outer portion, of these glands and the mucus are extruded as a gelatin-like structure, the so-called "mucus plug."

Changes in both the columnar and the squamous cervical epithelium in pregnancy have more than descriptive interest because of the possibility that they may relate to cervical eversion and erosion and carcinoma in situ, or the genesis of cervical cancer. Before these lesions are considered more specifically, it might be well to reemphasize the embryonal origin of the types of epithelium covering the cervix and vagina. At about the 70 mm. stage of the embryo, the primitive epithelium lining the müllerian duct system, and resembling columnar epithelium, begins to differentiate in its more distal portion. Undergoing stratification, it fuses with the stratified epithelium of the urogenital sinus, a union that is apparently easily discernible microscopically. The stratification extends upward well into the cervical canal. During the latter half of intrauterine development, the columnar epithelium that lines the upper part of the cervical canal is said to proliferate and grow downward. Coincidentally, the surface squamous epithelium recedes, leaving a layer of basal cells which become covered by the advancing columnar epithelium. The squamous epithelium may recede to such an extent as to allow the columnar epithelium to grow downward and cover the portio vaginalis about the external os. In essence, this is what constitutes so-called congenital erosion, or, more accurately, congenital eversion of the cervix. In the region of the external os of the cervix, these two types of epithelium meet at the so-called squamocolumnar junction. This junction changes location during childbearing, as the endocervical or columnar epithelium undergoes growth and regression. But more important is the fact that it is in this vicinity that nearly all cancers of the cervix are found.

Until rather recently, it has been more or less accepted that the squamous epithelium, or that covering the infravaginal portion of the cervix, changes little during pregnancy. It may become slightly thickened as the basal cells may increase from the usual one cell to two to four cells. The cell nuclei maintain their normal polarity and the mitoses, which are infrequent, are restricted in the main to the cells in the basal layer. The extent of the so-called "basal cell" hyperactivity of the cervix in pregnancy has been the subject of some controversy. It is stated that one third to one half or more of the thickness of the squamous epithelium shows cellular activity with some degree of anaplasia and mitoses in cells a considerable distance away from the basal layer. In contrast to its low incidence in the nonpregnant state, basal cell hyperactivity has been reported to occur more frequently in pregnancy.

Attempt has been made to grade the degree of basal cell hyperactivity in accordance with the amount of squamous epithelium involved. The intention is to determine whether these changes regress following delivery, or persist to arouse suspicion of carcinoma in situ (stage O). Others have failed to find any higher incidence of these changes, and if they have found changes, question whether they regress. Hence, the basic issue would seem to be not whether basal cell hyperactivity occurs with greater frequency in pregnancy, but rather whether the lesion has the potential to reach a stage consistent with a diagnosis of carcinoma in situ. (See Disorders of the Reproductive Tract in Relation to Pregnancy, in Chapter 30.)

The endocervical epithelium shows marked growth and proliferation during pregnancy and, with deepening of the cervical glands and surface growth, the columnar epithelium is thrown into folds. The everted endocervical tissue, located at the external cervical os, may appear quite hyperemic to inspection, and the slightest trauma may occasionally cause surface bleeding. This effect about the external os is often erroneously referred to as an erosion, whereas in fact it is a cervical ectropion or eversion. Obviously, one will not routinely biopsy the cervix with these apparent normal changes, but lurking among all obstetrical patients will be those who have or who are destined to develop carcinoma in situ (8 per 1000). Hence, the value of cytologic examination as a routine in prenatal care is apparent.

Normally, in the course of the puerperium the endocervical epithelium tends to regress and the squamocolumnar junction recedes toward the cervical canal. Such regression may fail to occur, however, and the endocervix remains exposed to the vagina. Also, during the dilatation of normal labor, the vaginal portion of the cervix sustains unavoidable minute lacerations and the external os loses its nulliparous circular outline and presents as a transverse slit with a somewhat gaping appearance. With the resultant exposure of the distal portion of the endocervix to the vaginal environment, the endocervical columnar epithelium may become infected, a condition referred to as acute or chronic cervicitis. Ulceration may occur on the surface of the everted columnar epithelium, as well as on the squamous epithelium of the vaginal portio. These lesions can be correctly referred to as cervical erosions. On occasion, the opening of the cervical glands may become occluded; they are distended by their own secretion, and appear about the external os as raised cystic areas, known as nabothian cysts.

Atypical epithelium is frequently observed in the endocervix in pregnancy as a result of the process known as epidermidalization, or squamous metaplasia. Characteristically, the cylindrical or columnar epithelium becomes replaced by squamous-like epithelium. The degree of metaplasia may vary from isolated foci to instances in which the columnar epithelium is almost entirely replaced by pseudostratified squamous epithelium. In 40 to 80 per cent of surgically removed uteri, squamous metaplasia will be found somewhere in the cervical canal. It is found with even greater frequency in pregnancy.

The source of the cells that participate in the process of squamous metaplasia has been the subject of controversy and debate. The earliest view favored the belief that endocervical squamous metaplasia was due to a horizontal ingrowth of basal cells from the squamous epithelium of the ectocervix into the stroma beneath the endocervical glands. The fact that squamous metaplasia is found high in the endocervix in isolated areas and within cervical polyps speaks against this idea. Rather evidence has accumulated to favor the concept that squamous metaplasia is derived from the infraepithelial cells normally located beneath the basement membrane of the columnar epithelium.

A number of names have been applied to these infraepithelial cells, but they are now known appropriately as "reserve cells." Although they were at one time believed to be basal cells left behind during the recession of the squamous epithelium during intrauterine life, they are now believed to be an inherent constituent of the endocervical epithelium. These more or less cuboidal cells, with vesicular nuclei and scanty cytoplasm, appear in a continuous line above an indistinct basement membrane and below the columnar cells lining the endocervical glands (Fig. 5A). The "reserve cells" are evident in all ages: transiently in the newborn owing presumably to the effect of placental estrogens, during the reproductive period, especially in pregnancy, and even after the menopause, particularly in patients on estrogen therapy.

It is thought that as the basal or reserve cells proliferate, the overlying columnar epithelium is pushed upward and becomes detached from the basement membrane, and is shed (Fig. 5B). The growing reserve cells accumulate more cytoplasm, and those near the surface become squamous-like in appearance (Fig. 5C).

Although squamous metaplasia or epidermidalization occurs in many parts of the body, and is said to undergo malignant changes occasionally, most authorities have maintained that this does not apply to the cervix and that squamous metaplasia is not a precancerous lesion. Such a conclusion is supported by some experimental evidence. Although not necessarily comparable to similar changes in the epithelium of the human endocervix, squamous metaplasia has been observed in the endometrium of the mouse after administration of estrogen and chorionic gonadotropin, but the process never became malignant. More closely related perhaps has been the production of squamous metaplasia in the endocervix of the young and castrated female monkey following estrogen therapy. With cessation of the treatment, the lesions regressed; interestingly, the latter occurred when progesterone was administered together with estrogen. At no time did the lesions show any invasive properties, although treatment was prolonged.

VAGINA. Changes in the vagina are restricted to hyperemia and edema, for the tissues themselves undergo little or no morphologic transformation. The vaginal mucosa, through venous engorgement later in pregnancy, may become bluish in color (Chadwick's sign). The pressure of the presenting part of the fetus within the birth

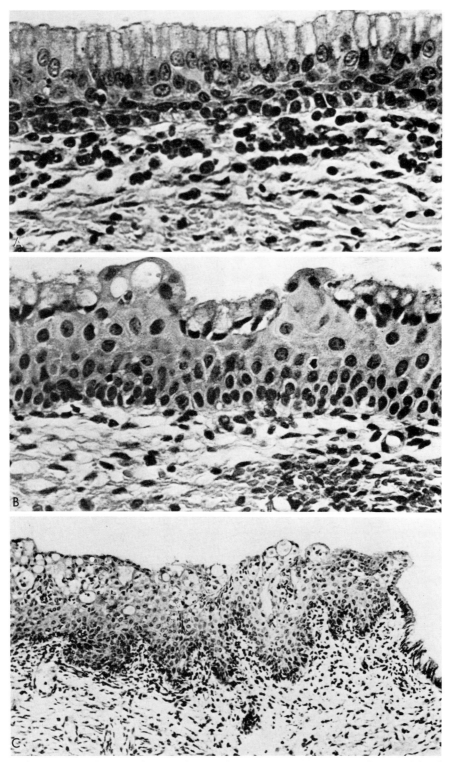

Figure 5. Photomicrographs of endocervical epithelia of nonpregnant cervix, showing (A) columnar cells beneath which are infraepithelial cells, now referred to as "reserve cells"; (B) proliferation of the infraepithelial, or "reserve," cells; and (C) squamous metaplasia, or so-called epidermidalization. A and B, × 275; C, × 80. (From Carmichael, R., and Jeaffreson, B. L., J. Path. Bact., 52:173, 1941.)

canal during the latter weeks of pregnancy often interferes with venous emptying, and thus accentuates this sign.

OVARIES. During the early weeks of pregnancy the ovaries become somewhat enlarged. In response to chorionic gonadotropin during this period, the corpus luteum flourishes and, rising well above the surface of the ovary, usually is easily recognized on inspection at laparotomy. Grossly, the corpus luteum measures about 2 to 2.5 cm. in diameter at the period of maximum growth, whereas the convoluted border is nearly 0.5 cm. thick. After the sixth to eighth week of gestation, the ovaries become smaller and even atrophic in appearance, and may resemble those seen after the menopause. The surface of the ovary is often covered by islets of reddish-appearing tissue that represents a decidual reaction of the underlying stroma. This finding can be important in establishing the diagnosis of pregnancy, should the question initially arise during the course of a laparotomy.

The corpus luteum, during the days of the free blastocyst, is grossly and histologically identical to the corpus luteum of the luteal phase of the menstrual cycle, but, beginning with the time of implantation, the wall of the structure becomes much thicker and the infolding of the granulosa layer is more marked. The criteria that are accepted as denoting functional activity of the corpus luteum of the menstrual cycle are applicable to the corpus luteum of pregnancy. These include dilated capillaries within the theca and granulosa layers, sudanophilic substance, and, as revealed by histochemical methods, ketonic lipid and alkaline phosphatase within the cytoplasm of the lutein cells.

In the early life of the corpus luteum of pregnancy, there is marked vacuolization of the theca and granulosa cells, and the boundaries of the latter cells become very indistinct. At six to seven weeks after the last menstrual period, or three to four weeks after implantation, the corpus luteum reaches its maximum stage of development. By this time the coarse lipid deposits seen in the theca lutein cells become finely granular. Although in the corpus luteum of the menstrual cycle these lipid deposits are mainly in the theca lutein cells, during pregnancy the lipid material has been noted in greater amounts in the granulosa cells. The alkaline phosphatase content is also increased in the granulosa cells. The presence of increased lipids and alkaline phosphatase in the granulosa cells of the corpus luteum of early pregnancy may mean that these cells have a much more active endocrine role than that which has been assigned to them during the menstrual cycle (see the section on endocrinology).

Ketonic lipid-containing cells have been described, to which is attributed a major role in the endocrine activity of the corpus luteum. These cells, having small, irregularly hyperchromatic nuclei and homogeneous eosinophilic cytoplasm, appear to originate in the theca interna and become distributed among the granulosa lutein cells. Whether these specialized cells, referred to as K cells, are responsible for the production of progesterone awaits further evidence. Until such evidence is presented, however, the granulosa cells must be considered a likely source of progesterone secretion during the life cycle of the corpus luteum of pregnancy.

Regressive changes are seen in the corpus luteum as early as the 35th to 40th day after the missed period, or within two to three weeks after implantation. From the morphologic appearance of the corpus luteum, the transfer of steroid function from the ovary to the placenta probably occurs at about the sixth or seventh week after the last menstrual period, which is somewhat earlier than had been generally thought. The pregnancy is known to continue when the corpus luteum is removed as early as the 41st day of gestation. However, it is best, when possible, to postpone ovarian surgery until after the 10th to 12th week of pregnancy. (See Disorders of the Reproductive Tract in Relation to Pregnancy, in Chapter 30.)

As the corpus luteum regresses, the theca interna soon disappears, but the granulosa lutein portion persists as a definite structure until the middle of pregnancy. The corpus luteum eventually becomes a connective tissue structure, i.e., a corpus albicans.

Maternal and Fetal Body Fluids

Before proceeding further it seems appropriate to consider the alterations in maternal body fluids. Although the vascular component of the extracellular fluid compartment, the plasma volume, appears to have the most clinical relevance, perhaps this is due to a greater certainty as to the extent of measurable change.

Human pregnancy is characterized by a

state of progressive hydration which may become excessive and lead to complications. This fact has stimulated numerous studies which have had as their purpose the delineation of the fluid increase in the various body compartments. The portion in the vascular compartment, the plasma volume, will be considered with the hematopoietic system. However, both interstitial and extracellular fluid must be dealt with in concert with total body water. These in turn cannot be divorced from the fetal fluids.

The introduction of deuterium oxide (D_2O) and the dilution technique, together with the antipyrine method, has made possible studies of the increase in total body water in pregnancy. The total body water in the normal nonpregnant person ranges in value from 53 to 72 per cent, and 52 to 55 per cent, of the total body weight as determined by the deuterium oxide and antipyrine methods, respectively. The deuterium space is of order of 50 to 55 per cent of body weight throughout pregnancy, remaining relatively constant for each patient.

The increase in total body water is paralleled by an almost equal increase in total body solids. A similar relationship between body water and body solids has been demonstrated by the antipyrine method. However, a study using the antipyrine method for measurement of total body water, and mannitol for measurement of extracellular fluid, revealed that the increase in total body water exceeded the gain in total body weight. Because total body water and lean body mass have a constant ratio, this means there was a loss of solids. In view of the positive nitrogen balance in pregnancy, which would exclude loss of protein as the source of weight loss, it has been suggested that the loss is most likely due to conversion of fat. Some recent metabolic studies on the sources of energy in pregnancy fail to support this contention. Except for a brief period of decreased water consumption during labor and the diuresis of the early puerperium, the water turnover rates in pregnancy are normal. Whatever increase occurs is restricted to the first week of the puerperium.

In attempting to assess the body water within the various compartments, the limitations of the methods must be considered, particularly as they pertain to the measurement of the volume of the extracellular fluid. These influencing factors include the possibility that test substances may enter the cell, or become involved in the general metabolism, or be excreted at a rate too rapid to permit valid determinations to be made. Sucrose and mannitol have been criticized on the grounds that they may not be completely recovered in the urine, owing to their possible degradation. Sodium, chloride, sulfate, and thiocyanate may enter some of the body cells to a variable degree. Because it is lipid-insoluble and has a relatively large molecular weight, inulin is presumed not to penetrate the cell membrane. Although it is rapidly excreted, the difficulty of maintaining a plasma level has been overcome by the administration of a constant infusion.

Account must be taken of the fact that during pregnancy there are additional subdivisions of the extracellular compartment, and these may not be readily permeated by the tracer. For instance, inulin does not enter the amniotic sac nor does it pass from the amniotic fluid to the maternal circulation. Hence, the fetal extracellular fluid and the amniotic fluid are excluded from measurement when inulin is used. Similarly, only a small amount of radiosodium reaches the amniotic sac in 30 minutes, and the degree to which sodium penetrates fetal tissues with respect to time is uncertain. Consequently, with the above methods the results will reveal relative rather than absolute changes in the extracellular space during pregnancy.

One of the first attempts to measure extracellular fluid changes in pregnancy was the determination of the volume of the thiocyanate space in a large number of patients picked at random. The mean increase in the volume of the extracellular space was 6.3 L., of which 1.5 to 2.0 L. was assigned to the fetus, placenta, and amniotic fluid. When mannitol was used to measure the extracellular fluid space in serial determinations from early pregnancy onward, this showed changes of the same order of magnitude—about 6 L. Single determinations in patients near term, by the inulin and radiosodium methods, revealed that the extracellular compartment accounted for 14 per cent and 29 per cent, respectively, of the body weight. These values are within the range considered normal for nonpregnant persons, as determined by these methods.

On the basis that the sodium space of the newborn constitutes 40 to 45 per cent of its body weight, the average-sized infant of

3200 grams would contain approximately 1200 ml. of extracellular fluid. With the amniotic fluid amounting to 800 ml. at term, and plasma volume increasing by 1500 ml., the remaining 2500 ml. represents the increase in maternal interstitial fluid. Thus, in pregnancy, as in normal healthy persons, the ratio of cell mass to extracellular fluid remains quite constant. This speaks for the belief that whatever water is retained in excess in pregnancy is extracellular and not intracellular in location.

When plasma volume and extracellular fluid space are measured simultaneously, it can be shown that the maternal vascular and interstitial spaces retain fluid at different rates and in varying amounts in each trimester. This relationship, illustrated in Figure 6B, is the ratio between the volumes of these two fluid spaces. Although the volume of each is increasing during early gestation, plasma volume is increasing at a greater rate than the extravascular or interstitial fluid volume. The difference in the

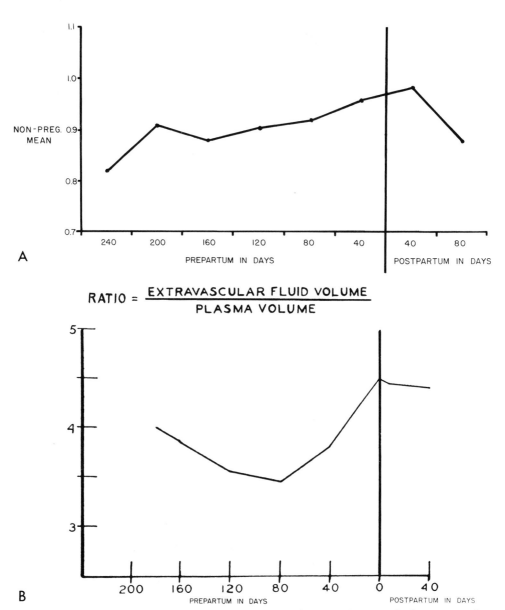

Figure 6. Physiologic changes in pregnancy. A, Changes in the ratio of average body to venous hematocrit during normal pregnancy and the puerperium. (From Caton, W. L., et al., Amer. J. Obstet. Gynec., 61:1207, 1951.) B, Changes in the ratio of extravascular fluid to plasma volume during pregnancy and the puerperium. (From Caton, W. L., et al., Amer. J. Obstet. Gynec., 57:471, 1949.)

rate of change is reflected by a decrease in the ratio between the volumes of the two compartments. Approximately 80 days prior to the onset of labor there is a definite reversal of this ratio, resulting from an accelerated increase in interstitial fluid volume and further augmented by the prelabor decrease in plasma volume. Could it be that the increase in interstitial fluid accounts for the prelabor decrease in plasma volume? It has been shown that interstitial fluid increases and the plasma volume falls in pregnancy toxemia, which may represent an exaggeration of the normal pregnancy changes in fluid volumes of these two compartments. Regardless of speculation, in the early puerperium a slow return of interstitial fluid volume to normal is in sharp contrast to the rapid decrease of plasma volume that follows delivery.

The factors that regulate the expansion of the extracellular fluid space must still be clarified. Although the plasma proteins are reduced to a degree in normal pregnancy, they rarely fall to levels where their oncotic pressure would permit edema formation. The capillary filtration rate is slightly increased in the latter weeks of pregnancy. Except in the femoral vessels, venous pressure is not elevated.

If indeed the intervillous space is an arteriovenous fistula, the blood volume changes might simply be the body's response to its presence. But as stated previously, the changes are those of total hydration with several body compartments involved; hence there must be a strong endocrine component and most likely a renal factor concerned (see the section on endocrinology).

In considering the fetal fluids, the chorionic fluid compartment, or the fluid contained within the extraembryonic coelom, is present for only a brief period, for by the ninth week it is completely obliterated and replaced by the expanding amniotic fluid compartment. Chorionic fluid, on analysis, appears to be similar in most respects to interstitial fluid, with its osmotic activity falling somewhere between that of maternal serum and that of amniotic fluid.

During the 16th to 20th week, the amount of amniotic fluid apparently varies between 150 and 400 ml. and increases steadily in amount, to reach a maximum volume of 1000 to 1500 ml. at the seventh month of pregnancy. After this there is a steady decline, and at term the uterus contains about 700 to 800 ml. of amniotic fluid. During this latter phase of gestation the fetal mass increases by some 1600 grams, which accounts for 600 to 700 ml. of extracellular fluid, with a total of some 1200 ml. in term fetus of average weight; consequently, the extracellular fluid space of the uterus and its contents change little in the last 8 to 10 weeks of pregnancy. Rather, in the mother, extravascular volume increases and plasma volume decreases. In the fetus the sodium space increases, and the amniotic fluid decreases. In the truly postmature state, i.e., 43 weeks, the fluid may decrease from 600 ml. to as low as 100 ml. In death in utero, the fluid may diminish to 200 ml. or less.

The source, the character, and the regulation of amniotic fluid in the various stages of pregnancy have long received attention. Investigations are being directed toward determining whether amniotic fluid is derived entirely or partially from active secretion by the amniotic epithelium, from passive transudation through the fetal membranes, or by way of the fetus and the placenta. Investigations at the beginning of the present century led to the conclusion that amniotic fluid originated from a dual source via the fetal membranes and fetal urine. It was found that the freezing point of amniotic fluid averaged $-0.482°$ C., while those of fetal and of maternal serum were identical, $-0.537°$ C. Translated into terms of osmolar concentrations on the basis that 1.86 osmols of solute depresses the freezing point $1°$ C., this means that the maternal serum contained 289 milliosmols per liter, and the amniotic fluid contained 259 milliosmols per liter. Further, it was observed that the bladder urine of the fetus at birth had a freezing point depression ranging from $0.148°$ to $0.340°$ C., with an average of $0.203°$ C., or 109 milliosmols per liter. A later study substantiated these findings in a large series of cases extending throughout pregnancy. Again, fetal urine had a lower osmolar concentration than maternal serum, of the order of 85 milliosmols per liter. It was concluded that in early pregnancy the amniotic fluid is almost a protein-free dialysate in near equilibrium with maternal serum but resembling interstitial fluid. In later pregnancy, the amniotic fluid was found to become hypotonic, presumably being diluted with significant amounts of fetal urine.

As indicated, the chemical constituents

of amniotic fluid differ somewhat at various periods of pregnancy. The protein content of amniotic fluid, similar to that of interstitial fluid, is low, ranging between 100 and 500 mg. per 100 ml. The nonprotein nitrogen of amniotic fluid is subject to rather wide fluctuations, but has an average value similar to that of the maternal serum. The glucose content is low, with an approximate value of 40 mg. per 100 ml., but will rise following intravenous administration of glucose to the mother or in uncontrolled diabetes, when the value may rise to 100 to 150 mg. The sodium content is somewhat lower than that of maternal serum but has a wide range, from 75 to 165 mEq. per liter. The potassium content fluctuates, with an average value of 4.2 mEq. per liter reported. The chloride is appreciably higher in amniotic fluid than in maternal serum. The inorganic phosphorus and alkaline and acid phosphatase are distinctly higher than in maternal serum, whereas the calcium values are nearly equal.

With the introduction of isotope techniques, current investigations have been directed toward determining more precisely the amount of fluid contributed or exchanged by the fetus and the fetal membranes. With a double tracer technique, wherein one tracer is injected into the maternal circulation and its rate of appearance in the amniotic fluid is measured, and the second is deposited into the amniotic fluid and its disappearance time is measured, the turnover rate of amniotic fluid has been calculated to be about 600 ml. per hour in the human. It was further calculated that the major portion (at least 75 per cent) of water exchange occurs through the fetus. Only a small amount of amniotic fluid was exchanged through the fetal membranes, the vast amount returning through the fetus and placenta. The electrolytes, sodium and potassium, exchange at their own rates, and several hours are required for the amniotic fluid sodium to be totally exchanged.

It is evident that the fetus swallows and absorbs amniotic fluid and excretes a urine with a lower osmolar concentration than the imbibed fluid. In considering the physiology of the fetus, the fetal kidney tubule responds little to the antidiuretic hormone and consequently fetal urine resembles a glomerular filtrate, with its low osmolar activity. It is apparent that the fetus plays a major role in the delicate steady state

necessary to maintain a normal amount of amniotic fluid in the latter half of pregnancy.

Hematopoietic System

The hematopoietic system in pregnancy has been the subject of rather extensive investigation. The observed changes apply to a variety of clinical states. The pattern and magnitude of blood volume change has been a subject of some controversy, undoubtedly owing in large measure to the fact that too few determinations were made on the same patient throughout pregnancy. It is apparent that the degree of blood volume change differs from patient to patient. The increase in plasma volume appears to relate to the eventual size of the fetus, with the largest increment in a twin pregnancy. There is some indication that the increase in red cell mass may be influenced by whether an anemia is present or in the offing or, more precisely, by the status of the patient's iron stores. Although some absolute values will be cited, it is recognized for the reasons just listed that these may vary quite widely.

The plasma volume enlarges throughout pregnancy by some 1200 to 1400 ml. (45 to 50 per cent), reaching its maximum two to six weeks prior to term (Fig. 7). There is a prelabor decrease in the late weeks of pregnancy of some 20 per cent of the maximum increase. With delivery there is a rapid return to normal so that at the end of the first postpartum week, the plasma volume is near nonpregnant values.

The red cell mass or volume was determined originally by indirect measurement and later by red cells tagged with radioactive iron (^{55}Fe), phosphorus (^{32}P), and chromium (^{57}Cr) (Fig. 7). The red cell volume increases from 300 to 500 ml. (20 to 40 per cent) (Fig. 7). The rate of red cell production is accelerated in pregnancy, but the cells' life span is not altered, for after taking into account blood loss with delivery, it is some months before the red cell mass reaches nonpregnant values. Considering the increase in plasma volume and red cell mass, the average increase in total or whole blood volume is 40 to 45 per cent. Together with the increase in cardiac output these changes represent a load on the circulation that may become crucial to patients with medical diseases, especially those with a damaged heart.

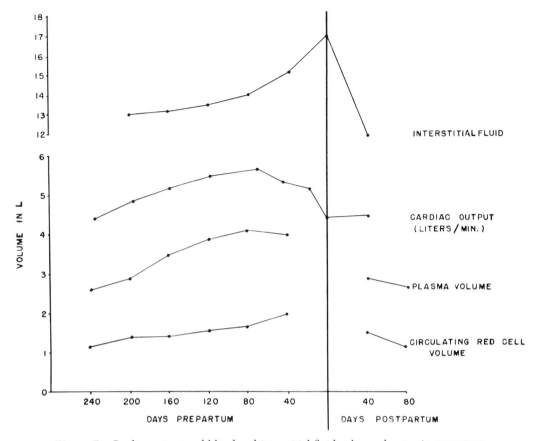

Figure 7. Cardiac output and blood and interstitial fluid volume changes in pregnancy.

With a proportionately greater increase in plasma volume over red cell mass, the venous hematocrit falls by some 15 per cent. The body hematocrit, which is the average cell-to-plasma ratio of the total circulating blood, decreases to about 8 per cent. The ratio of the body hematocrit to the large-vessel or venous hematocrit is dependent upon the distribution of whole blood between the large vessels and the capillaries. In the nonpregnant, about 20 per cent of the total blood volume circulates in the capillaries and 80 per cent in the large transport vessels. Because of the effect of vessel caliber, the hematocrit of capillary blood is lower, while the larger vessels have a higher cell-to-plasma ratio. If more than 20 per cent of the total blood volume is in the capillaries, therefore, the ratio of body to venous hematocrit will fall. Conversely, a redistribution of blood that results in the presence of more than 80 per cent of the volume in the larger vessels will be reflected in an increase in the ratio of body to venous hematocrit. It follows that the ratio between body and venous hematocrit is an index of the distribution of blood in the vascular bed.

As stated before, there is a decline in both body and venous hematocrit, but of different degrees, resulting in an increase in the ratio of body to venous hematocrit (see Fig. 6A). The progressive increase in the ratio as pregnancy advances indicates that the greater portion of the new blood volume is contained within the larger transport vessels including the intervillous space and less than the normal 20 per cent of the circulating blood is being accommodated in the capillary bed.

More recently it has been stated that the ratio of body to venous hematocrit does not differ from the values observed in the nonpregnant. Whether the results are comparable is open to question, for the approach was rather different. In the first instance the conclusion was based on serial determinations made throughout pregnancy and the puerperium on the same patients. In the more recent study, single determinations were made on patients at term and compared to an equal number of patients delivered some 48 hours prior to the determination.

With a greater increase in plasma volume

to red cell mass there is a relative fall in hematocrit and hemoglobin values. However, the mean corpuscular volume, the mean corpuscular hemoglobin, and the mean corpuscular hemoglobin concentration change insignificantly. There is a moderate increase in reticulocytes from the fourth to the sixth month.

The leukocyte count rises to a level of 9500 per cu. mm. at the second month and thereafter remains fairly constant at 10,500 per cu. mm. until delivery. During labor there is a further increase to 12,500 to 16,000 per cu. mm., values that persist through the first week of the puerperium. The increase occurs mainly in the polymorphonuclear leukocytes. This normal rise places limitations on the leukocyte count in the diagnosis of infectious conditions during pregnancy and the early puerperium. Myelocytes and metamyelocytes have been observed in the blood of normal pregnant women. It was concluded that these forms found in primary blood dyscrasias are simply the bone marrow response to normal pregnancy and have no pathologic significance.

The total eosinophil count varies between 130 and 150 during pregnancy, with a sharp decrease to between 25 and 40 in labor and the early puerperium. By comparison, therefore, with the normal nonpregnant woman whose total eosinophil count is approximately 200, the eosinophil count decreases by almost 20 per cent in early pregnancy, 30 to 40 per cent in late pregnancy, and 85 per cent in labor and parturition. In pregnancy the platelets are fewer in number, owing presumably to hemodilution, but in the puerperium values rise above the normal average.

The procoagulants, especially factor VIII, are increased in pregnancy, as is fibrinogen. The clotting time is speeded up as expressed in the ratio of glass-to-silicone clotting time. In the normal nonpregnant, the average ratio is 3.0, and in normal last trimester pregnancy it is 2.4. The prothrombin time as measured by the Quick method is likewise shortened, as is the partial thromboplastin time.

In the majority of studies of iron metabolism in pregnancy, serum iron is reported to decrease from an average value of 100 to 200 mcg. per 100 ml. to 80 to 60 mcg. per 100 ml. Coincident with this decrease is a rise in protoporphyrin from 40 to 90 mcg. per 100 ml. Although a serum iron below 80 mcg. per 100 ml. is generally regarded as being consistent with an iron-deficiency anemia, in pregnancy it is not until the concentration falls below 60 to 70 mcg. per 100 ml. that the values are pathognomonic. It has been found that when the hemoglobin values are below 10 grams the serum iron is also below 60 to 65 mcg. per 100 ml. Several reports have appeared that present evidence that it is possible to arrive at a fair approximation of the iron stores by determination of the hemosiderin content of aspirated bone marrow. Effort has been made to apply this method to the assessment of the iron stores in pregnancy. The response of serum iron concentration to a standard dose of an iron preparation might serve a useful purpose in such an assessment.

There is general agreement that iron-binding capacity is appreciably increased during pregnancy. In contrast to other states, in pregnancy the iron-binding capacity is not necessarily regulated by the serum iron level. Presumably, the elevation of iron-binding capacity is a response to an increased rate of iron absorption, mobilization, and possible placental transport, and to fetal iron needs.

During pregnancy the total iron requirements approximate 1 gram, of which 300 to 400 mg. is needed by the fetus, while the remainder is required for the increased circulating red cell mass. It has been established that the normal adult body is capable of storing 600 to 1000 mg. of iron. Consequently, it would appear that the normal woman should be able to mobilize sufficient iron to meet the demands of pregnancy. The iron requirements differ in the various trimesters of pregnancy, but reach their maximum in the third, when 10 to 12 mg. per day is needed, much of it for fetal requirements. It is during this period that the fetus fulfills its iron stores.

The hematologic response of the individual patient to pregnancy, however, is unpredictable, owing to the inability to quantitate accurately the iron stores. If perchance they are low, or if iron absorption is impaired, the red cell count, hemoglobin concentration, hematocrit, and serum iron will fall to levels that are compatible with the findings in iron-deficiency anemia. A hemoglobin of less than 11 grams and a hematocrit below 34 per cent have been arbitrarily taken to delineate between a "physiologic anemia," produced by the disproportionate increase in plasma volume to red cell mass, and a true anemia. Accordingly, if these are correct standards, iron-deficiency anemia will be found frequently in many patients and, in some clinics, in most.

Cardiovascular System

The cardiovascular system during pregnancy is subject to a variety of changes that in some instances are progressive. Any apparent increase in the transverse diameter of the normal heart in pregnancy must be attributed to changes in its position rather than to alterations in its size. Elevation of the diaphragm as the uterus enlarges causes a counterclockwise rotation and a lateral upward displacement of the heart. X-ray studies during normal pregnancy have revealed indentation of the esophagus and a straightening of the left border of the heart. This variation in contour represents a change in position of the left atrium rather than dilatation.

The electrocardiographic pattern is altered by the new position of the heart, with changes most notable in lead III in which the Q wave is prominent and often deep. The T wave is occasionally inverted, but the remaining components are normal. Left axis deviation accompanies the displacement of the heart, but these changes are variable and often can be detected only after careful axis plotting.

In the examination of the pregnant woman account must be taken of these changes. Palpation of the precordium may reveal an obscure or diffuse apical beat, and percussion of the heart size is less reliable. At auscultation, apical systolic murmurs are audible in 50 per cent of normal pregnant patients, whereas pulmonic systolic murmurs, often transmitted into the neck, are heard in nearly all patients. The presence of these murmurs is attributed to the displacement of the heart, slight torsion of the great vessels, and the blood dilution resulting from the increase in plasma volume. The most significant peripheral circulatory finding is a collapsing pulse and often a demonstrable capillary pulsation of the nail beds. The superficial veins of the body, particularly those of the breast, become prominent and serve to contain some of the increment in blood volume (Fig. 8).

Venous pressure in pregnancy is of more than casual interest for it may well influence directly or indirectly uterine and renal blood flow, diuresis and antidiuresis, and the overall regulation of extracellular fluid volume. Undoubtedly, bodily position plays a role in edema formation and other complications of pregnancy due in part to alterations in venous pressure. Certainly, it is more than a clinical impression that weight control as it pertains to extracellular fluid volume is more readily maintained in patients who avail themselves of periods of bed rest in the course of the day and are not unduly active, especially in the last few months or weeks of pregnancy.

The venous pressure in the upper portion of the body as measured in the antecubital

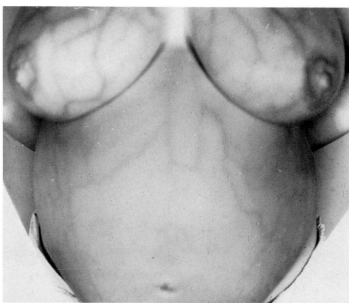

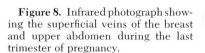

Figure 8. Infrared photograph showing the superficial veins of the breast and upper abdomen during the last trimester of pregnancy.

vein is not elevated and averages 7 to 8 cm. H₂O or less in the latter half of pregnancy, but the femoral venous pressure increases as pregnancy progresses from a normal of 8 cm. to 25 cm. H₂O. Consistent with the increase in venous pressure is a considerable retardation of rate of venous flow in the legs of women at term.

Initially the increase in femoral venous pressure was attributed mostly to the inflow of relatively large amounts of blood from the uterus into the iliac-femoral system. Subsequent observations indicate that the weight of the uterus on the inferior vena cava may account for some of the rise, at least in the last trimester. But to determine the relative contribution of each, more studies are needed of femoral venous pressure in the upright, supine, and lateral positions at various stages of pregnancy in the same patient.

It has been shown that prior to removal of the fetus at cesarean section, the venous pressure in the inferior vena cava was 20 to 25 cm. H₂O. By lifting the uterus forward prior to delivery or with removal of the fetus it falls to a normal of 4 to 8 cm. These changes have relevance to monitoring the central venous pressure in the undelivered patient. This obstruction to the inferior vena cava has been elegantly demonstrated by caval angiograms (Fig. 9). It is clearly evident that substantial quantities of blood from the lower portion of the body can be returned by the azygos and vertebral veins. This offers an explanation why patients who have had ligation of the inferior vena cava to combat pulmonary emboli arising from the veins of the pelvis and lower extremities are relatively free of vascular sequelae and are subsequently capable of successful childbearing. Also, this ready access of blood to the azygos and vertebral veins poses the question whether one can be certain of disrupting the journey of emboli from the pelvis and lower limbs in every instance by ligation of the inferior vena cava and left ovarian vein, at least in pregnancy.

Occasionally, near term, the patient may feel faint when in the supine position for any length of time. There is associated pallor, sweating, and tachycardia and the blood pressure may drop. Turning the patient on her side usually will relieve the symptoms immediately.

These hypotensive episodes in pregnancy

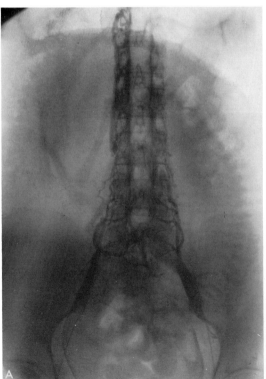 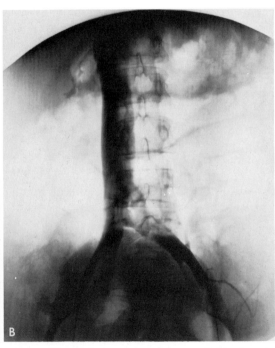

Figure 9. A, Caval angiogram at cesarean section. Supine position before opening abdomen. B, Caval angiogram at cesarean section. Supine position after delivery of fetus and placenta. (From Kerr, M. G., J. Obstet. Gynaec. Brit. Comm., 72:513, 1965.)

have been likened to those induced by spinal anesthesia with pooling of the blood in the lower extremities. Although lifting the undelivered uterus forward manually results in sharp fall in inferior cava venous pressure, caval occlusion apparently does not cause a fall in systemic blood pressure. As indicated, the collateral veins are capable of delivering substantial amounts of blood from the pelvis and lower extremities if the occasion demands.

An alternate explanation is the possibility that the syndrome is a reflex vagal affair caused by uterine pressure on the diaphragm. Certainly, syncope in pregnant patients in the supine position is more commonly seen when the uterus has attained unusual size, as in multiple pregnancy or polyhydramnios, but again there is probably a greater effect on the inferior vena cava pressure.

This impediment to caval venous return by the weight of the uterus has been applied to those clinical situations in which one might envision the effect of a decrease in venous drainage from the uterus. Experimental evidence has been offered in species other than the human that the back pressure created by the caval obstruction might be sufficient to detach the placenta by pressure transmitted to the uterine venous system. It may well be a factor, among others, in the causation of this complication. But there are compensatory mechanisms present to maintain the pressure relatively constant in the intervillous space, to wit, the ability of the broad ligament veins to dilate and the adequacy of the venous return through the azygos and vertebral veins.

There is a minimal increase in the filtration rate in the forearm of normal pregnant patients. The mean filtration rate is 0.160 ml. per minute per 100 cc. forearm in the pregnant woman, whereas it is 0.111 ml. in normal controls. A somewhat related subject is limb volume. The normal increase in leg volume on rising from the supine to the upright position occurs within 10 to 15 minutes. The change in leg volume from the supine to the upright position in normal pregnant women does not exceed the 3 to 5 per cent increase observed in the nonpregnant healthy female. Under some circumstances there may be a two- to three-fold increase. Many factors influence this increase in volume, ranging from venous pressure and environmental temperature to the general physical fitness of the subject.

The rate of blood flow is accelerated during pregnancy; although the circulation time is within the normal limits for nonpregnant women, when it is determined serially some decrease is shown between the 17th and 36th weeks of pregnancy. The average arm-to-carotid sinus circulation time in early pregnancy is 17 seconds, whereas at the 37th week it is 14 seconds. The increase in blood velocity is somewhat greater in the peripheral than in the pulmonary circulation, for there is a proportionately greater decrease in the arm-to-carotid sinus time than in the external jugular-to-carotid sinus time.

By contrast, the rate of peripheral blood flow through the upper extremities, particularly the hands, is increased in normal pregnancy (Fig. 10). These changes probably account for the erythema of the palms commonly seen in pregnancy and the increase of skin temperature of these areas.

The cardiac rate is increased ante partum by an average of 10 beats per minute in most patients, whereas bradycardia is occasionally observed in the puerperium. A decrease in blood pressure occurs during the fourth to ninth months, with the diastolic pressure declining to a slightly greater degree than the systolic pressure. The tendency to feel faint on standing for a period of time in pregnancy may be akin to postural hypotension. However, during labor the systolic blood pressure may rise to 140 to 150 mm. Hg with uterine contractions, being accentuated further by the bearing-down effort of the second stage of labor.

The cardiac output is significantly increased in pregnancy (see Fig. 7). The earliest attempts to measure the cardiac output utilized the nitrous oxide method of Krogh and the acetylene technique of Grollman. More recently the techniques used have included cardiac catheterization and the dye dilution and the pulse pressure methods. One of the earliest studies using the acetylene method was performed on six women throughout the course of pregnancy and the puerperium. In these serial observations, the peak increase in cardiac output was 50 per cent or more. With the introduction of the catheter technique, isolated observations were made on 68 normal pregnant women. A composite plotting of the results revealed a maximum output of 5.7 L. per minute in the period from the 26th to the 29th week, which was an increase of 27 per cent above the non-

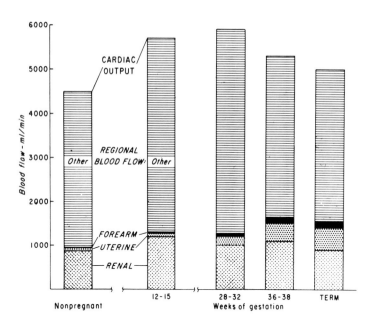

Figure 10. Comparison of cardiac output and regional blood flow during pregnancy with nonpregnant values. (From Metcalfe, J., Peterson, E. N., and Novy, M. J., in Conn, H. L., and Horwitz, O., eds.: Cardiac and Vascular Disease. Lea & Febiger, Philadelphia, 1971.)

pregnant level. A similar type of study revealed an increase from 4.6 L. in the nonpregnant to 5.8 L. in the pregnant. In this study it was shown that the cardiac output virtually returned to early pregnancy values by the 38th to the 40th week. These earlier catheter studies have been criticized on the grounds that the investigators had no fluoroscopic control over the placing of the tip of the catheter. Subsequent observations employing this refinement revealed the cardiac output in pregnancy to be 40 per cent in excess of normal nonpregnant values, substantiating the earliest measurements with the acetylene method. With the catheter in situ, the heart exhibited a normal myocardial response to exercise. The right atrial, ventricular, and pulmonary pressures were those of the normal nonpregnant person, and in nearly all cases remained within the normal range during exercise.

Attempt has been made to estimate the cardiac output in labor, using the so-called pulse pressure method. It was believed that the method would permit measurement of percentage change in output and provide an index of the workload on the heart during labor. Many variables that might influence cardiac output, such as pain, anxiety, and events connected with labor, including the bearing-down effort of the second stage, were appraised. Although all these caused some rise in cardiac output, the most significant factor was the strength of the myometrial contractions. During contractions of active labor, there was a 31 per cent increase in cardiac output as calculated by this method, with a 37 per cent rise in the first hour of the puerperium. The increase was thought to reflect the return of uterine blood to the systemic circulation with the uterus emptied and completely contracted. Similarly, the increase in cardiac output during labor was also believed to be the result of the blood being squeezed out of the uterus, thus increasing momentarily the effective blood volume. This idea is in keeping with the observations that the right atrial pressure rises slightly with a uterine contraction. Further, the amount of blood returning to the right heart during labor remains relatively constant, perhaps through the ability of the broad ligament veins to dilate and act as blood reservoirs. The bearing-down effort of the second stage of labor, comparable to the Valsalva test, did not diminish cardiac output.

If the cardiac output were increased significantly during labor, one could expect cardiac failure to develop with some frequency at this time in patients with damaged hearts. This is not, however, in accordance with clinical experience. The fact that the damaged heart rarely fails initially during labor perhaps reflects the finding that the cardiac output near term is receding to near-nonpregnant levels. But if the cardiac output is temporarily increased in labor, it seems prudent in dealing with a cardiac patient to avoid excessive hours of labor and eliminate as much of the second stage as is consistent with the overall safety of both mother and fetus. One is left with the problem of the validity of methods when concurrent or repeated measurements of cardiac output are desired. Undoubtedly only the accuracy of the cardiac catheter technique would be acceptable universally. Since it is not without dangers, good and substantial medical reasons should be at hand to warrant the procedure. These should include the firm belief that the correct management of the patient is dependent upon knowing the exact type of cardiac lesion, and that the diagnosis can be established only by cardiac catherization. At present no data on the cardiac output during labor are available by this method. Until a completely safe but equally accurate method is developed, the status of the cardiac output in labor perhaps should remain an open question.

No single factor seems to explain adequately why the cardiac output returns to normal prior to term. Neither the oxygen consumption nor the metabolic rate increases proportionately to the cardiac output, nor does either fall prior to labor—in fact, they increase. Further, the prelabor decrease in blood volume is only some 25 per cent of the maximum increase.

One possibility suggested to explain the prelabor decrease in cardiac output is that the intervillous space, which may act physiologically like an arteriovenous fistula, closes partially near term because of morphologic changes in the placenta. No definitive changes are demonstrable to support this idea. Moreover, in normal pregnancy the rate and amount of intervillous blood flow reach their maximum near term. It is also interesting that in a few studies utilizing an isotope technique it has been shown that, despite the diminished uterine blood flow in pregnancy toxemia, the cardiac output is greater in most patients with this syndrome than it is for comparable periods in normal pregnancy.

Whatever determines its distribution in the body, in pregnancy the blood is diverted to the uterus, apparently in increasing amounts up to term. In determining the rate and minute volume of uterine blood flow, three methods have been used: (1) the application of the Fick principle using nitrous oxide, (2) introduction of radiosodium into the intervillous space, and (3) introduction of radiosodium into the uterine wall, with measurement of the disappearing half-time of the isotope.

With a modification of the Kety method for measuring cerebral blood flow, the uterine blood flow at cesarean section has been measured in normal term pregnancies. Briefly, the technique consists of placing a small polyethylene catheter in the uterine vein at the time of operation. The mother, under spinal anesthesia, breathes a 17 per cent nitrous oxide mixture. After a short waiting period to allow for equilibration, blood samples are taken from the brachial artery and the uterine vein. The uterine blood flow is calculated from the difference in nitrous oxide content of the two samples. The average rate of uterine blood flow is 500 ml. per minute, and appears to be related to the weight of the newborn. This is supported by the finding in one study that in a twin pregnancy, with the infants having a combined birth weight of 7 kg., the uterine flow was 1150 ml. per minute.

The isotope method with the tracer introduced transabdominally into the choriodecidual area has yielded blood flow values for normal pregnant patients comparable to those found with the nitrous oxide method. This technique involves localization of the placenta by determining with a Geiger counter the area of greatest radioactivity over the uterus after injection into the antecubital vein of a small amount of radioactive sodium. When the placenta is found implanted on the anterior uterine wall, a known amount of radiosodium is deposited transabdominally into the choriodecidual or intervillous space. A Geiger counter is placed over the area of injection and, with continuous recording, the disappearance time of the isotope is determined. Rather than a determination of the rate of uterine blood flow, this may be regarded as a direct measurement of maternal-placental intervillous blood flow. By calculation, however, the values can be shown to be nearly identical. Although the observations were few in number, it is important to note that the rate of blood flow was significantly reduced in patients with various forms of hypertension encountered in pregnancy.

In summary, the distribution of the newly created blood volume and the cardiac output in pregnancy are depicted in Figure 10. Renal blood flow decreases somewhat, perhaps at the expense of the expected increase in uterine blood flow.

Respiratory System

Changes in the respiratory system begin early in pregnancy. The alteration in the dimensions of the chest is detectable in most patients even before there is any significant increase in the size of the uterus or elevation of the diaphragm. The circumference of the chest enlarges by 5 to 7 cm., and the transverse diameter increases by 2 cm., accompanied by a 35 degree, or 50 per cent, increase in the subcostal angle. The increase in size of the thoracic cage is brought about in part by relaxation of the ligamentous attachments of the ribs. Other joints show increased mobility, and this is particularly apparent at the junction between the sternum and manubrium. The pulmonary markings are accentuated, as observed on x-ray examination, possibly as

the result of an increase in blood volume within the pulmonary vessels. Comparison of roentgenograms in early and later pregnancy shows about a 4 cm. elevation of the diaphragm but, when observed under fluoroscopy, the excursion appears normal.

During pregnancy respiratory function is measurably altered. Figure 11 illustrates the values of the various components of total lung volume of nonpregnant and pregnant women. The point of demarcation between the two main phases of respiration, i.e., inspiratory capacity and functional residual capacity, is represented as the midposition. The inspiratory capacity is the volume of air that can be inspired forcibly at the end of a resting expiration, whereas the functional residual capacity is the volume of air that remains in the lungs after a normal resting expiration. The latter is equal to the sum of the expiratory reserve (volume of air that can be expired forcibly after a normal expiration) and the residual volume (volume

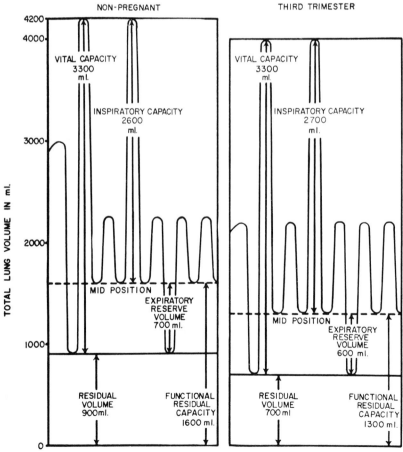

Figure 11. Changes in ventilatory pattern and lung volumes in normal pregnancy.

of air remaining in the lungs after maximum expiration). The vital capacity involves both the inspiratory and the functional residual capacity and is the volume of air that can be expired with maximum effort after a maximum inspiration. The tidal volume is the amount of air that is exchanged with each breath at any level of respiratory activity.

The definitive changes in the ventilatory pattern during pregnancy are an increase in inspiratory capacity (100 ml.) and a decrease in both the expiratory reserve (100 ml.) and the residual volume (200 ml.). The reduction in functional residual capacity is believed due to an elevated diaphragm. The decrease in the functional residual capacity is greater than the increase in the inspiratory capacity, so that the net result is a diminution in total lung volume by approximately 4.5 per cent (200 ml.). That the tidal volume is increased some 45 per cent supports the clinical observation that during pregnancy women breathe more deeply under basal conditions than they do in the nonpregnant state.

The vital capacity has been found to remain unchanged or to be increased (200 to 300 ml.). The upward displacement of the diaphragm might be expected to decrease vital capacity during pregnancy, but such an effect fails to occur because of the increased circumference of the chest. The vital capacity in the standing position during pregnancy is slightly more than in the sitting position. Even in marked hydramnios and multiple pregnancy, in which the enlarged uterus might restrict the excursion of the diaphragm, the vital capacity is not diminished. It is clinically important, therefore, to realize that, if a reduction in vital capacity is detected during pregnancy, it must be interpreted as pathologic.

Other tests have been recommended as an aid in the evaluation of respiratory activity. The most informative of these, and the one that furnishes an almost complete analysis of ventilatory function, is the determination of maximum breathing capacity. The value of this test lies in the fact that the success of its performance requires a normal vital capacity, the absence of bronchial obstruction, and integrity of the entire neuromuscular and skeletal respiratory apparatus. During normal pregnancy there is no significant variation in the ability of the patient to perform this test.

The rate of respiration in pregnancy is accelerated, and this, combined with the increase in tidal volume, results in a near 50 per cent increase in the minute ventilation (hyperventilation). Furthermore, even though oxygen consumption increases during pregnancy, ventilation is augmented even more, as evidenced by the change in the ventilatory equivalent. The latter is defined as the number of liters of air that must be breathed for the absorption of 100 ml. of oxygen. The increase in the ventilatory equivalent is offered as additional evidence that a state of hyperventilation exists during pregnancy (Table 1).

Although it has long been recognized that pregnant patients do hyperventilate, the reason for this remains obscure. Certainly the alveolar exchange of oxygen is not impaired during pregnancy, for oxygen saturation is normal. Therefore, one may conclude that an increase in ventilatory equivalent is an effect rather than a cause of hyperventilation. Further, the decrease in residual volume and the increase in tidal volume should improve the efficiency of the ventilatory system during pregnancy. Hence, there is no evidence that there is any anatomic reason for hyperventilation. The earlier explanation held that hyperventilation occurs to compensate for the reduction in the concentration of available base. The reduction in plasma bicarbonate, without a significant fall in plasma chloride, necessitates the lowering of the carbon dioxide tension to maintain normal blood pH. According to this concept, therefore, the hyperventilation of pregnancy is a manifestation of a compensated acidosis due to the

TABLE 1.   RESPIRATORY FUNCTION IN
PREGNANCY*

Value	Change	Percentage Change
Tidal Volume Increase	487 to 678 ml.	+39%
Respiratory Rate Increase	15 to 16	+10%
Minute Volume Increase	7.2 to 10.3 L.	+42%
Ventilatory Equivalent Increase	3.0 to 3.3 L./100 ml.	+10%
Breathing Reserve	92 to 89 per cent	−3%
Walking Ventilation	14.7 to 19.1 L./min.	+30%
Walking Dyspnea Index	15 to 21 per cent	+40%
Maximum Breathing Capacity	102 to 91 L./min.	−11%

*From Cugell, D. W., et al., Amer. Rev. Tuberc., 67:568, 1953.

slight alkali deficit, the cause to be established. The elevation of blood pH from 7.39 to 7.42 during pregnancy indicates that there is an adequate compensation, and, in reality, a state of mild respiratory alkalosis supervenes. It is now recognized and accepted that progesterone is responsible for the hyperventilation, through its influence on the respiratory center. Hence the above findings reflect the response of the body to the hyperventilation rather than a cause. This conclusion is supported by the demonstration that there is a lowering of the alveolar pCO_2 and a reduction in the concentration of serum sodium during the luteal or progestational phase of the menstrual cycle, which continues into pregnancy.

Hyperventilation must not be mistaken for dyspnea or difficult or conscious breathing. The common causes of dyspnea in pregnancy include severe anemia, pulmonary edema, severe acidosis, and those conditions which may markedly elevate the diaphragm.

Persons with low hemoglobin values on occasion can be surprisingly free of symptoms. One patient seen in the last trimester of pregnancy exhibited no dyspnea on ordinary activity, despite the fact that her hemoglobin was 2.5 grams. In general, however, when the hemoglobin falls below 5 grams the patient is dyspneic unless at complete rest. The dyspnea from pulmonary edema of cardiac origin or severe pregnancy toxemia varies in intensity but is usually severe.

Whether dyspnea appears without a detectable cause and can be a normal physiologic accompaniment of pregnancy is debated. Perhaps the threshold for effortless breathing of hyperventilation is exceeded in certain pregnant patients. The awareness of the effort to breathe would be surprising, however, in view of the small increase in ventilatory equivalent and the presence of a normal vital capacity. Further, the normal ratio of 2:5 between the functional residual capacity and the total lung volume is exceeded during pregnancy, and this should eliminate any tendency toward a sensation of respiratory distress or dyspnea. The increase in metabolic rate, or the reduction of available base in pregnancy, is so slight as to preclude these as causative factors of dyspnea. It is possible, perhaps, that an increase in pulmonary blood volume or some other factor might affect the compliance of the lungs and create a conscious effort to breathe. The walking dyspnea index, which is the percentage of maximum breathing capacity required for a standard exercise, showed that the values in pregnant patients remained well below 35 per cent, the level at which clinical dyspnea appears. Therefore, one must regard dyspnea in pregnancy as having an organic rather than a functional cause, and search as diligently for an explanation of this symptom in pregnant patients as in the nonpregnant.

Gastrointestinal Tract

A generalized softening of the gingiva, associated with bleeding on mild irritation, is observed in many pregnant patients. This hypertrophic change in the gums is referred to as gingivitis of pregnancy. On occasion this hypertrophy may reach proportions sufficient to produce tumor-like masses at the gum margins. Usually these lesions are the size of a pea, but they may become so large as to interfere with mastication and therefore require surgical removal. The tumors regress after parturition, and failure of them to do so warrants investigation.

The enlarging uterus causes the stomach to rotate to the right and become displaced upward to a more or less horizontal position. Concomitant upward displacement of the large bowel, the cecum, and the appendix also occurs. These changes in position of the viscera are significant when the physical signs of abdominal disease are being evaluated.

Gastric motility is reputed not to be altered in normal pregnancy. In one study made during pregnancy and uncomplicated labor, the emptying time of the stomach did not appear to be delayed. With respect to labor, this limited evidence is at variance with clinical experience. Vomiting in labor is frequent, especially in the second stage, and the vomitus often contains food eaten many hours before. The vomitus may contain duodenal contents, particularly in patients with prolonged labor. This would indicate decreased motility of the stomach and duodenum and relaxation of the pyloric sphincter.

Although constipation is a common symptom, there is no good evidence that the motility of the large bowel is diminished during pregnancy. Caution should be exercised in interpretation of diarrhea in pregnancy. It should never be considered functional. There is a reduction in biliary tract motility with a delay in the emptying time of the gallbladder. This biliary stasis is believed to be a factor in the production of cholelithiasis, and may account for the higher incidence of gallbladder disease in women who have borne children.

Although there is general agreement that in most patients a hypochlorhydria is present during normal pregnancy, opinions differ as to its etiology. Based on use of an alcohol test meal, serial determinations of the acidity of the gastric contents reveal an acid secretion below normal in 75 per cent of pregnant patients, with a rapid return to normal after delivery. The assumption is generally made that decreased hydrochloric acid production accounts for the hypochlorhydria. The normal chloride content of the gastric secretions during pregnancy, however, indicates that the condition may be due to neutralization by the duodenal contents rather than to an actual diminution in hydrochloric acid secretion. A rise in blood pepsin which supposedly parallels gastric pepsin levels has been noted in the last three months of pregnancy. This finding has been advanced to explain the frequent presence of heartburn in a situation where achlorhydria has been presumed to be present.

Despite the latter, iron absorption as measured by the radioactive isotope (^{59}Fe) reveals no impairment of uptake. By contrast, however, carbohydrate appears to be assimilated at a slower rate during pregnancy than in the nonpregnant state.

The liver during the late stages of pregnancy is displaced upward, backward, and to the right by the enlarging uterus. The pressure so exerted may account for the vague right upper abdominal discomfort of which patients commonly complain during the last trimester of pregnancy. Hepatic blood flow is unaltered, and the various liver function tests are within normal limits in nearly all pregnant women. Actually, in a few, thymol turbidity, cephalin flocculation, direct bilirubin, and urine bilirubin are elevated over the values accepted for normal nonpregnant persons.

Urinary System

Although there are anatomic changes in the urinary tract during pregnancy, the renal function is normal. The most striking change is the dilatation of the ureters, which may be readily demonstrated by pyelography (Fig. 12). This dilatation is often apparent before the uterus exerts any mechanical pressure, which suggests that an endocrine factor may be responsible for the effect. This theory is supported by observation in the monkey that pyelo-urethral dilatation persists after removal or death of the fetus, if the placenta remains in situ and continues to function. In addition, the sheath of Waldeyer, which encloses only the lower third of the ureter, hypertrophies during pregnancy, favoring urinary stasis and thereby increasing the dilatation of the upper portion of the ureter and the kidney pelvis. In conjunction with dilatation, the ureter becomes displaced lateralward (Fig. 12A). From a functional point of view, there is a marked decrease in ureteral motility, with the peristaltic waves being less frequent and intense. These anatomic alterations in the ureter and the kidney pelvis may persist for three or four months after parturition. To attain maximum information, it is wiser to postpone x-ray investigation of the urinary tract until after this interval. These anatomic and functional changes in the ureter and kidney pelvis, with the resultant urinary stasis, are sufficient reason for the increased frequency of urinary tract infection during pregnancy.

The clinical tests of kidney function, such as urea clearance, are normal, and the ability of the kidney to concentrate remains unchanged during pregnancy. Filtration rate, measured by phenol red, inulin, or creatinine clearance, is generally elevated over the value for the nonpregnant female. The effective renal blood flow is likewise increased, but in evaluating and comparing the values of the filtration rate and renal blood flow, consideration must be given to the time in pregnancy that the measurements are made. It has been shown that both renal blood flow and filtration rate reached their peak values at the 15th to 16th week, returning toward normal after the 32nd week (Table 2).

Apparently renal blood flow may decrease in the presence of large abdominal tumors or as the result of abdominal compression; the question has arisen whether this is relevant in pregnancy. It was reasoned that renal function might vary with the patient in the upright position, in contrast to the supine position in which the uterus might cause pressure on the structures and larger vessels lying over the pos-

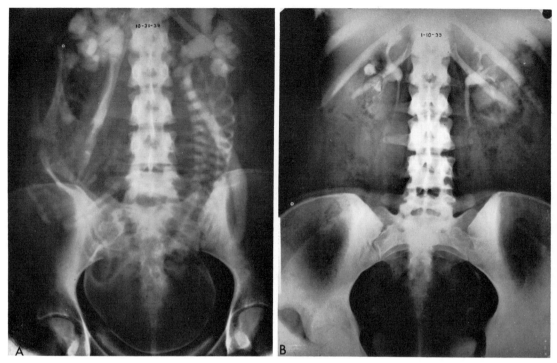

Figure 12. Pyelograms showing (A) normal changes in the urinary tract during normal pregnancy, and (B) urinary tract several weeks after delivery.

terior abdominal wall. Of the pregnant patients studied, lying supine for an hour, significant change in renal blood flow and glomerular filtration rate was noted in only two. It is interesting that in one of these, with a ureteral catheter inserted above the

TABLE 2.   RENAL BLOOD FLOW—
GLOMERULAR FILTRATION RATE IN
PREGNANCY AND THE PUERPERIUM[°]

Mean Time Weeks	Number of Patients	Clearance Inulin ml./min.	Clearance PAH ml./min.	F.F.[†] × 100
Ante Partum				
16.2	5	166	820	20.3
24.1	7	158	784	20.2
29.4	8	154	722	21.2
32.9	9	158	751	21.4
37.5	11	146	589	23.1
Post Partum				
6.7	8	97	448	21.2
13.0	6	96	525	18.7
25.0	6	103	430	24.1
Normal nonpregnant	9	108	623	17.3

[°]From Sims, E. A. H., and Krantz, K. E., Clin. Res. Proc., 4:142, 1956.

[†]F.F. = Filtration fraction (i.e., clearance of inulin/clearance of PAH).

pelvic brim to eliminate possible uterine compression, the renal blood flow and glomerular filtration rate were reduced by 24 and 18 per cent, respectively. In all of the patients sodium and water excretion fell 42 and 44 per cent, respectively.

In an attempt to assess further the possibility that vena cava congestion is a factor in reducing renal excretion, tourniquets placed high on each thigh with the patient on her side caused some temporary decrease in excretion of urine, which had a low sodium content. This decrease in renal excretion was not of the same magnitude as when the patient was in the supine position. The observations revealed that shifting the patient to her side from the supine position not only restored the urine output to normal but actually produced a rebound or excessive excretion for a time. It was concluded that the lag in urine output was due to compression of the ureters by the uterus rather than to a significant decrease in renal blood flow. Renograms confirm the marked ureteral stasis in pregnancy and that it can be relieved by postural changes.

It is a common clinical observation that the patient with excessive extracellular fluid will lose several pounds in weight within a few hours at bed rest. The influence of postural attitudes in human pregnancy directly on renal blood flow and indirectly on the size of the extracellular fluid space must not be minimized in patient management.

Endocrine System

See Adenohypophysis and Parathyroid in Chapter 3, and Endocrinology of Human Pregnancy, in Chapter 4.

Skin

Certain changes that are considered physiologic occur in the skin and the mucous membrane of the mouth and nasopharynx. The increased estrogen activity of pregnancy is believed to be the stimulus for many of these changes. Hyperemia of the mucous membrane of the nasopharynx is often present, sometimes to a degree that the patient may experience some difficulty in breathing. Nosebleeds are frequent and, in most instances, are not a symptom of underlying medical disease. Dermatographism is accentuated during pregnancy and is commonly seen at this time. Asymptomatic erythema of the palmar surfaces, particularly of the thenar and hypothenar eminences, is encountered. The absence of erythematous changes in the lower portion of the body indicates that the normal vasomotor gradient is essentially unaltered by pregnancy.

The phenomenon of hyperhidrosis of the surfaces of the feet, hands, folds of the skin, anus, vulva, and even the scalp may occur early and persist throughout pregnancy. Although not to be entirely disregarded as a symptom, night sweats in the early puerperium are a frequent complaint of the patient.

Hair growth may be stimulated or retarded, but for the most part usually remains unchanged during pregnancy. Excessive hair growth existing prior to pregnancy, however, is often accelerated. Varying degrees of hirsutism may arouse the suspicion that the patient is suffering from an endocrine disorder with an androgenic component. Patients will complain of loss of hair within weeks after delivery. There is no ready explanation why this occurs. The patient, however, may be reassured that the process will stop within a short time and will not reach serious proportions.

Telangiectasia associated with gestation is so common that careful examination will reveal these vascular manifestations in nearly all patients. They tend to appear suddenly and are usually distributed over the upper portion of the body and upper extremities. No relationship has been demonstrated between telangiectasia and hepatic disease, and its appearance in pregnancy is attributed to the high level of estrogen in the body fluids.

Striae of some degree occur in the skin on the buttocks, abdomen, thighs, and breasts, and once they appear they persist for life. These skin blemishes are several centimeters in length, curved, and somewhat irregular in outline; they are usually singular but may be confluent. Initially, they are pale pink in color and may give rise to some itching. Later, these striae tend to become white and scarlike, and are annoying for cosmetic reasons. New deposits of melanin tend to appear in those abdominal scars which already contain the pigment, whereas the scars of wounds created during pregnancy are apt to be more heavily pigmented. Freckles are intensified, and chloasma, the so-called "mask of pregnancy," which is characterized by a winglike pigmented area over the malar eminences and brownish discoloration over the forehead, may be prominent in some patients. This pigmentation fades and usually disappears after delivery.

Breast

See Mammary Gland and Lactation, in Chapter 4.

ALTERATIONS IN METABOLISM AND CHEMICAL CONSTITUENTS OF THE BODY

Although it has long been appreciated that the basal oxygen consumption (Fig. 13) is increased in pregnancy, as is also the basal metabolic rate, especially in the last trimester (plus 15 to 20 per cent), only recently has an attempt been made to establish the source of energy required for the development of the conceptus. Subject to some controversy and perhaps at variance with certain endocrine changes in pregnancy, it appears that carbohydrate is a major source of energy, particularly in the last half of pregnancy (Fig. 14), as meas-

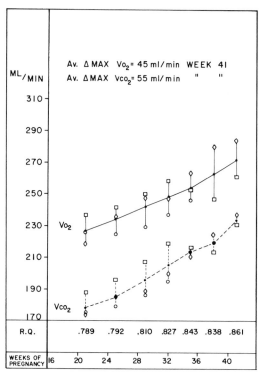

Figure 13. Average 24 hour oxygen consumption (V_{O_2}) and CO_2 production (V_{CO_2}) during pregnancy. (Courtesy of Dr. Kendall Emerson, Jr.)

ured by hourly determinations of oxygen consumed and carbon dioxide produced, and the resultant respiratory quotient (Fig. 15). Protein sparing is evident, consistent with favoring nitrogen retention. Both human growth hormone and human placental lactogen are generally postulated to suppress glucose oxidation by insulin and to mobilize maternal fat to provide the needed energy for the mother's daily metabolic requirements, thus conserving carbohydrate and protein for energy require-

ments and structural demands. This apparently is not entirely the case, although there is a rise in free fatty acids and increase in blood insulin levels. In certain clinical states, the oxygen consumption and respiratory quotient may start to fall some weeks before term, and this may be physiologic evidence that in terms of survival, the fetus is at risk (see Diabetes Mellitus, in the chapter, Medical and Surgical Diseases of Pregnancy).

When subjected to standardized tasks, pregnant women are as efficient as nonpregnant in terms of energy cost, certainly up to the 35th week. The amount of energy expended during labor is believed to be comparable to that of mild or moderate exercise.

Acid-Base Balance

The acid-base balance shifts to a new equilibrium during pregnancy. The most consistent change is seen in the decrease in the concentration of total base from the nonpregnant level of about 155 mEq. per liter to 145 to 147 mEq. per liter. This is reflected in the fall in serum sodium from 142 mEq. per liter to 135 to 137 mEq. per liter, and an accompanying drop in plasma bicarbonate from 25 to 22 mM. per liter. Blood chlorides or fixed bases are not elevated in normal pregnant patients. Reference has been made to the influence of progesterone on the respiratory center.

The maternal organism is in a moderate state of respiratory alkalosis and metabolic acidosis. The compensatory effect of the latter is apparently not influenced by metabolic products from the fetus for it remains rather stationary throughout pregnancy. The blood gas tension of the maternal blood

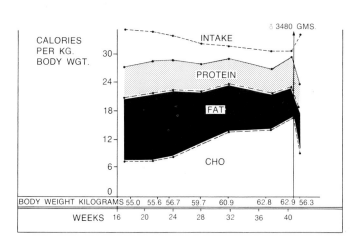

Figure 14. Caloric consumption in pregnancy per kilogram body weight: 3480 gram male infant. (Courtesy of Dr. Kendall Emerson, Jr.)

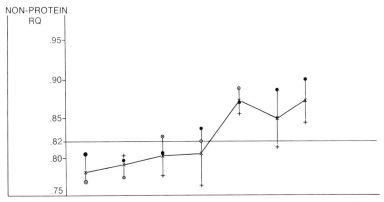

Figure 15.   Average 24 hour nonprotein respiratory quotient in pregnancy. (Courtesy of Dr. Kendall Emerson, Jr.)

in the intervillous space is favorable to fetal metabolism. However, induced hyperventilation as in labor can cause a lowering of maternal CO_2 (below 17 mm. Hg) and may cause delay of onset of respiration of the fetus at birth. Certainly CO_2 normally decreases during labor, reportedly from about 32 to 27 mm. Hg.

Protein

Characteristically, pregnancy creates a state of positive nitrogen balance. Not only does the maternal organism retain the nitrogen necessary for growth of the reproductive system and fetus, but nitrogen storage is so efficient during pregnancy that much of the needs of lactation are cared for as well. The most complete nitrogen balance study to date was one involving an individual patient throughout three pregnancies, which showed that on the average 446 grams of nitrogen was retained during the second half of pregnancy. Nitrogen loss associated with delivery was 114 grams, of which 58 grams was contained in the fetus, and the remainder was accounted for by the placenta and the blood loss in the third stage of labor. Fifty-three days after delivery, and while still lactating, the patient had a nitrogen credit of 250 grams.

Certainly nitrogen retention is in excess of 150 grams of calculated needs. Also, a daily intake of a gram of protein per kilogram of body weight, i.e., 60 to 75 grams daily, for most women would suffice to meet the metabolic needs. The pregnancy state of hyperinsulinism and increase in growth hormone together with placental lactogen affords protein sparing and promotes nitro-

gen retention, possibly to insure the most ideal milieu for the conceptus.

The value for plasma proteins ranges from an average of 7.0 grams per 100 ml. for the nonpregnant to approximately 6.6 grams per 100 ml. in the normal pregnant woman. The globulin fraction may be actually increased, whereas the albumin fraction is reduced, lowering the normal ratio between these two proteins from approximately 1.2 to 1.0. The fibrinogen levels increase from 250 mg. per 100 ml. in the nonpregnant state to 350 mg. per 100 ml. or higher in pregnancy. Irrespective of the percentile reduction in plasma proteins, the unit oncotic pressure remains well within normal limits. On the basis of the increase in plasma volume, there is an overall average increment of 80 grams of total circulating plasma proteins.

The electrophoretic pattern of the plasma protein fractions during pregnancy substantiates in more detail the well established values based on chemical analysis. Briefly, these more refined methods show that there is a mean decrease in total plasma proteins due mainly to a reduction in the albumin fraction and a slight fall in the gamma globulin. The α_1, α_2, and β globulins, as well as fibrinogen, are increased. The various plasma proteins return to nonpregnant values after the first week of the puerperium. Nonprotein nitrogen and urea values decrease, except prior to term, when a slight increase in these values is noted; perhaps the hydremia of pregnancy influences their concentration. Histidine has been found in the urine in normal pregnancy. Rather than an alteration in metabolism, it is thought that a lowering of the renal threshold is responsible for the histidinuria. This has been shown to be true for many of the amino acids.

Carbohydrate

Carbohydrate metabolism has received considerable attention, and the concept has been proposed that pregnancy imposes a diabetic effect on the maternal organism (see endocrinology section). Certainly excessive thirst, increased appetite, polyuria, and glycosuria are not uncommon in pregnancy. In this sense, pregnancy can simulate "chemical" diabetes. Many variables are involved in normal pregnancy, from elevated plasma insulin to increase in growth, thyroid, and adrenal hormones. Although its level is elevated, insulin, unlike the other hormones, also is degraded by the placenta. Further, it may be protein-bound and is not entirely in free form and metabolically active. The point is that attempts have failed to indicate that there is interference with peripheral utilization or storage of carbohydrate in pregnancy or that there is resistance to insulin or block in the glycolytic cycle.

The glucose tolerance test is modified, however, in pregnancy and is subject to interpretation. There is a delay in return of the blood glucose levels to normal when the glucose is given orally; instead of the conventional two hours for the level to return to normal in the nonpregnant, it takes three hours in the pregnant. This effect is not seen when glucose is administered intravenously. The delay seen in the oral glucose tolerance test is attributed to an alimentary hyperglycemia, for when the blood sugar was elevated glycosuria was common. Again, the latter was not commonly observed with the intravenous method, suggesting that the glycosuria of pregnancy said to occur in as many as 20 per cent of patients is due not to lowering of renal threshold for glucose, but rather to a decrease in the capacity for tubular reabsorption of glucose. The rapid return of the blood glucose levels to normal in the course of an intravenous glucose tolerance test supports the contention that carbohydrate metabolism is not altered appreciably. However, an abnormal oral glucose test demands a follow-up intravenous test, and if the latter is delayed beyond two hours, the patient indeed may have a deviation in carbohydrate metabolism.

Fats

Serum lipids apparently decrease slightly soon after the first missed period, but the free fatty acids rise progressively till delivery, and decline slowly during the puerperium. Total cholesterol may rise from 170 to 350 mg. or more per 100 ml., with a concomitant increase in the free cholesterol, so that a normal ratio between free and total serum cholesterol is maintained. Certainly blood cholesterol determination is less useful as an aid in the diagnosis of disorders of the thyroid in pregnancy. It has been stated that the increase in tissue mass about the trunk and upper thighs in the average woman up to the 30th week of pregnancy is due mainly to fat. Whatever enlargement occurs subsequently is due to extracellular fluid.

Sodium

Prior to application of isotope techniques to clinical problems, the sodium retention during pregnancy was variously reported to be between 70 and 385 mEq. per week. A retention of such magnitude would expand the extracellular fluid volume by 5 to 25 L., if sodium was stored in an osmotically active form. When measured with ^{24}Na, however, the increment in total exchangeable sodium is shown to amount to approximately 500 mEq. during the second and third trimesters, a value that is consistent with the increase in extracellular fluid volume. It has often been considered that in pregnancy sodium might be retained in relatively large amounts in bone as an osmotically inactive complex, as in the nonexchangeable form, but the bone sodium in pregnancy remains to be determined.

Calcium

The fetus at term requires 30 to 40 grams of calcium for the formation of its skeleton. (See Fig. 7 in Chapter 23.) This deposition occurs mainly during the last three months of pregnancy. The average present-day diet contains 1.5 to 2.5 grams of calcium per day, of which 400 mg. is supplied in a quart of milk. Of this amount, 0.2 to 0.7 gram of calcium per day is reportedly retained during pregnancy. This is obviously sufficient to supply the needs for fetal growth without drawing on the maternal stores. The serum calcium levels may decrease slightly, an effect that may be associated with the hydremia of pregnancy. Even under the most adverse nutritional circumstances, however, the concentration of serum calcium is maintained well above the levels associated with tetany.

Phosphorus, Magnesium, and Copper

Both phosphorus and magnesium have been found to be retained in excess of normal needs in the nonpregnant state. The serum inorganic phosphorus concentration decreases somewhat, while the peak of its positive balance is reached in the second trimester. Changes in the copper content are restricted to the plasma, 109 to 222 mcg. per 100 ml., there being no change in the copper content of the erythrocyte.

Enzymes

In view of the growth requirements imposed by pregnancy, it is reasonable to assume that enzyme activity is augmented during this period. The placenta contains oxidizing, reducing, and hydrolytic enzymes, and is especially rich in monamine oxidase and diamine oxidase, which inactivate tyramine and histamine, respectively.

The enzymes that have been most extensively studied in pregnancy include diamine oxidase (histaminase), pitocinase, glucuronidase, angiotonase, and alkaline phosphatase, and elevated levels of all of them are found in maternal serum.

Soon after the missed period there is a sharp rise in diamine oxidase from nonpregnant levels of 3 to 6 units to 200 units by six weeks of gestation. Peak levels, of 400 to 500 units, are reached by the 16th week and are maintained throughout pregnancy; they drop to 50 units by the second or third postpartum day and to nonpregnant levels after 10 to 14 days. It is important to note as an aid to diagnosis that diamine oxidase did not rise in a patient with choriocarcinoma in the presence of high levels of chorionic gonadotropin.

The serum alkaline phosphatase is increased by some four times (12 to 15 units) over nonpregnant values of 1.5 to 4.0 Bodansky units per 100 ml. of serum. There is a steady rise from the fourth or fifth month onward to term. The fetal level is approximately one half that of the mother but twice that of the nonpregnant. The maternal level may reflect the functional state of the placenta, being lower in pregnancy toxemia. The higher level in the maternal blood, at least, is accounted for by alkaline phosphatase of placental origin; this is proved by the fact that it is partially inactivated by an acute human placental alkaline phosphatase antibody. No such inactivation was observed in sera from nonpregnant subjects and, interestingly, not in the blood of newborn infants.

Pitocinase, an enzyme capable of inactivating oxytocin, appears in the blood early in pregnancy, and from the 14th to the 38th week of pregnancy a thousand-fold increase has been reported.

BIBLIOGRAPHY

Adams, J. Q.: Cardiovascular physiology in normal pregnancy; studies of dye dilution technique. Amer. J. Obstet. Gynec., 67:741, 1954.

Bader, R. A., Bader, M. E., Rose, D. J., and Braunwald, E.: Hemodynamics at rest and during exercise in normal pregnancy as studied by cardiac catheterization. J. Clin. Invest., 34:1524, 1955.

Baird, D. T., Gasson, P. W., and Doig, A.: The renogram in pregnancy. Amer. J. Obstet. Gynec., 95: 597, 1966.

Browne, J. C. M., and Veall, N.: Maternal placental blood flow in normotensive and hypertensive women. J. Obstet. Gynaec. Brit. Emp., 60:141, 1953.

Burwell, C. S.: Circulatory adjustments to pregnancy. Bull. Johns Hopkins Hosp., 95:115, 1954.

Carmichael, R., and Jeaffreson, B. L.: Squamous metaplasia of the columnar epithelium in the human cervix. J. Path. Bact., 52:173, 1941.

Carrow, L. A., and Greene, R. R.: Epithelia of the pregnant cervix. Amer. J. Obstet. Gynec., 61:237, 1951.

Caton, W. L., Roby, C. C., Reid, D. E., Caswell, R., Maletskos, C. J., Fluharty, R. G., and Gibson, J. G., II: Circulating red cell volume and body hematocrit in normal pregnancy and the puerperium—by direct measurement, using radioactive red cells. Amer. J. Obstet. Gynec., 61:1207, 1951.

Caton, W. L., Roby, C. C., Reid, D. E., and Gibson, J. G., II: Plasma volume and extravascular fluid volume during pregnancy and the puerperium. Amer. J. Obstet. Gynec., 57:471, 1949.

Charles, D., and Jacoby, H. E.: Preliminary data on the use of sodium aminohippurate to determine amniotic fluid volume. Amer. J. Obstet. Gynec., 95: 266, 1966.

Chesley, L. C., Kellerman, H., Lenobel, A., and Uichanco, L.: Placental permeability to sucrose: A source of error in measuring volumes of sucrose distribution in gravidas. Obstet. Gynec., 23:795, 1964.

Chesley, L. C., and Sloan, D. M.: The effect of posture on renal function in late pregnancy. Amer. J. Obstet. Gynec., 89:754, 1964.

Coryell, M. N., Beach, E. F., Robinson, A. R., Macy, I. G., and Mack, H. C.: Metabolism of women during the reproductive cycle; XVII. Changes in electrophoretic patterns of plasma proteins throughout the cycle and following delivery. J. Clin. Invest., 29: 1559, 1950.

Cox, L. W., and Chalmers, T. A.: Exchange of sodium between plasma extracellular compartments in pregnant women as determined by Na^{24} tracer methods. J. Obstet. Gynaec. Brit. Emp., 60:195, 1953.

Cugell, D. W., Frank, N. R., Gaensler, E. A., and Badger, T. L.: Pulmonary function in pregnancy; I. Serial observations in normal women. Amer. Rev. Tuberc., 67:568, 1953.

Danforth, D. N., and Chapman, J. C. F.: Incorporation of the isthmus uteri. Amer. J. Obstet. Gynec., 59: 979, 1950.

Fay, J., Cartwright, G. E., and Wintrobe, M. M.: Studies on free erythrocyte protoporphyrin, serum iron, serum iron binding capacity and plasma copper during normal pregnancy. J. Clin. Invest., 28:487, 1949.

Fox, J. E., and Abell, M. R.: Mast cells in uterine myometrium and leiomyomatous neoplasms. Amer. J. Obstet. Gynec., 91:413, 1965.

Gadd, R. L.: The volume of the liquor amnii in normal and abnormal pregnancies. J. Obstet. Gynaec. Brit. Comm., 73:11, 1966.

Goodland, R. L., Reynolds, J. G., McCoord, A. B., and Pommerenke, W. T.: Respiratory and electrolyte effects induced by estrogen and progesterone. Fertil. Steril., 4:300, 1953.

Gray, J. J., and Plentl, A. A.: Variations of sodium space and total exchangeable sodium during pregnancy. J. Clin. Invest., 33:347, 1954.

Gryboski, W. A., and Spiro, H. M.: Effect of pregnancy on gastric secretion. New Eng. J. Med., 255:1131, 1956.

Haley, H. B., and Woodbury, J. W.: Observations on body composition and body water metabolism in normal pregnancy. J. Clin. Invest., 31:635, 1952.

Hamilton, B. E., and Thomson, K. J.: The Heart in Pregnancy and the Childbearing Age. Little, Brown and Co., Boston, 1941.

Hamilton, H. F. H.: Symposium on haemodynamics in pregnancy; I. Cardiac output in pregnancy. Tr. Edinburgh Obstet. Soc., pp. 1–9, 1949–1950; Edinburgh Med. J., March, 1950.

Hendricks, C. H., and Barnes, A. C.: Effect of supine position on urinary output in pregnancy. Amer. J. Obstet. Gynec., 69:1225, 1955.

Hendricks, C. H., and Quilligan, E. J.: Cardiac output during labor. Amer. J. Obstet. Gynec., 71:953, 1956.

Howard, B. X., Goodson, J. H., and Mengert, W. F.: Supine hypotensive syndrome in late pregnancy. Obstet. Gynec., 1:371, 1953.

Howard, L., Jr., Erickson, C. C., and Stoddard, L. D.: Study of incidence and histogenesis of endocervical metaplasia and intraepithelial carcinoma. Cancer, 4:1210, 1951.

Hunscher, H. A., Hummel, F. C., Erickson, B. N., and Macy, I. G.: Metabolism of women during the reproductive cycle; VI. A case study of the continuous nitrogen utilization of a multipara during pregnancy, parturition, puerperium and lactation. J. Nutr., 10: 579, 1935.

Hurwitz, D., and Jensen, D.: Carbohydrate metabolism in normal pregnancy. New Eng. J. Med., 234:327, 1946.

Hutchinson, D. L., Plentl, A. A., and Taylor, H. C., Jr.: Total body water and water turnover in pregnancy studied with deuterium oxide as isotopic tracer. J. Clin. Invest., 33:235, 1954.

Hytten, F. E., and Paintin, D. B.: Increase in plasma volume during normal pregnancy. J. Obstet. Gynaec. Brit. Comm., 70:402, 1963.

Hytten, F. E., Paintin, D. B., Stewart, A. M., and Palmer, J. H.: The relation of maternal heart size, blood volume and stature to the birth weight of the baby. J. Obstet. Gynaec. Brit. Comm., 70:817, 1963.

Hytten, F. E., and Taggart, N.: Limb volumes in pregnancy. J. Obstet. Gynaec. Brit. Comm., 74:663, 1967.

Hytten, F. E., and Thomson, A. M.: Water and electrolytes in pregnancy. Brit. Med. Bull., 24:15, 1968.

Hytten, F. E., Thomson, A. M., and Taggart, N. R.: Total body water in normal pregnancy. J. Obstet. Gynaec. Brit. Comm., 73:553, 1966.

Israel, S. L., Rubenstone, A., and Meranze, D. R.: The ovary at term; I. Decidua-like reaction and surface cell proliferation. Obstet. Gynec., 3:399, 1954.

Jacobson, H. N., Burke, B. S., Smith, C. A., and Reid, D. E.: Effect of weight reduction in obese pregnant women on pregnancy, labor and delivery, and on the condition of the infant at birth. Amer. J. Obstet. Gynec., 83:1692, 1962.

Kerr, M. G.: The mechanical effects of the gravid uterus in late pregnancy. J. Obstet. Gynaec. Brit. Comm., 72:513, 1965.

Kuvin, S. F., and Brecher, G.: Differential neutrophil counts in pregnancy. New Eng. J. Med., 266:877, 1962.

Kydd, D. M.: Hydrogen-ion concentration and acid-base equilibrium in normal pregnancy. J. Biol. Chem., 91:63, 1931.

Lahey, M. E., Gubler, C. J., Cartwright, G. E., and Wintrobe, M. M.: Studies on copper metabolism; VII. Blood copper in pregnancy and various pathologic states. J. Clin. Invest., 32:329, 1953.

Lund, C. J.: Studies on iron deficiency anemia of pregnancy, including plasma volume, total hemoglobin, erythrocyte protoporphyrin in treated and untreated normal and anemic patients. Amer. J. Obstet. Gynec., 62:947, 1951.

MacRae, D. J., and Palavradji, D.: Maternal acid-base changes in pregnancy. J. Obstet. Gynaec. Brit. Comm., 74:11, 1967.

Makepeace, A. W., Fremont-Smith, F., Dailey, M. E., and Carroll, M. P.: The nature of the amniotic fluid; a comparative study of human amniotic fluid and maternal serum. Surg. Gynec. Obstet., 53:635, 1931.

McKay, D. G., Roby, C. C., Hertig, A. T., and Richardson, M. V.: Studies on the function of early human trophoblast; I. Observations on chemical composition of fluid of hydatidiform moles. Amer. J. Obstet. Gynec., 69:722, 1955.

McKay, D. G., Roby, C. C., Hertig, A. T., and Richardson, M. V.: Studies on the function of early human trophoblast; II. Preliminary observations on certain chemical constituents of chorionic and early amniotic fluid. Amer. J. Obstet. Gynec., 69:735, 1955.

McLennan, C. E.: Further observations on capillary filtration rates in pregnancy. Amer. J. Obstet. Gynec., 52:837, 1956.

Mendleson, C. L.: Disorders of the heartbeat during pregnancy. Amer. J. Obstet. Gynec., 72:1268, 1956.

Metcalfe, J., Romney, S. L., Ramsey, L. H., Reid, D. E., and Burwell, C. S.: Estimation of uterine blood flow in normal human pregnancy at term. J. Clin. Invest., 34:1632, 1955.

Morris, N., Osborn, S. B., and Wright, H. P.: Effective circulation of the uterine wall in late pregnancy measured with $^{24}NaCl$. Lancet, 1:323, 1955.

Nesbitt, R. E. L., Jr., and Hellman, L. M.: The histopathology and cytology of the cervix in pregnancy. Surg. Gynec. Obstet., 94:10, 1952.

Page, E. W.: The value of plasma pitocinase determinations in obstetrics. Amer. J. Obstet. Gynec., 52:1014, 1946.

Peters, J. P., Heinemann, M., and Man, E. B.: The lipids of serum in pregnancy. J. Clin. Invest., 30: 388, 1951.

Plentl, A. A., and Hutchinson, D. L.: Determination of deuterium exchange rates between maternal circulation and amniotic fluid. Proc. Soc. Exp. Biol. Med., 82:681, 1953.

Pritchard, J. A., and Adams, R. H.: Erythrocyte production and destruction during pregnancy. Amer. J. Obstet. Gynec., 79:750, 1960.

Pritchard, J. A., Barnes, A. C., and Bright, R. H.: Effect of the supine position on renal function in the near-term pregnant woman. J. Clin. Invest., 34:777, 1955.

Pritchard, J. A., and Rowland, R. C.: Blood volume changes in pregnancy and the puerperium. Amer. J. Obstet. Gynec., 88:391, 1964.

Pritchard, J. A., Wiggins, K. M., and Dickey, J. C.: Blood volume changes in pregnancy and the puerperium; I. Does sequestration of red blood cells accompany parturition? Amer. J. Obstet. Gynec., 80:956, 1960.

Rath, C. E., Caton, W. L., Reid, D. E., Finch, C. A., and Conroy, L.: Hematological changes and iron metabolism in normal pregnancy. Surg. Gynec. Obstet., 90:320, 1950.

Reid, D. E., Frigoletto, F. D., Tullis, J. L., and Hinman, J.: Hypercoagulable states in pregnancy. In press.

Rose, D. J., Bader, M. E., Bader, R. A., and Braumwald, E.: Catheterization studies of cardiac hemodynamics in normal pregnant women with reference to left ventricular work. Amer. J. Obstet. Gynec., 72:233, 1956.

Rovinsky, J. J., and Jaffin, H.: Cardiovascular hemodynamics in pregnancy. Amer. J. Obstet. Gynec., 93:1, 1965.

Seitchik, J.: Body composition and energy expenditure during rest and work in pregnancy. Amer. J. Obstet. Gynec., 97:701, 1967.

Seitchik, J.: Total body water and total body density of pregnant women. Obstet. Gynec., 29:155, 1967.

Seitchik, J., and Alper, C.: Estimation of changes in body composition in normal pregnancy by measurement of body water. Amer. J. Obstet. Gynec., 71:1165, 1956.

Serum alkaline phosphatase in pregnancy: An immunological study. Preliminary communications. Brit. Med. J., 1:1210, 1966.

Severinghaus, A. E.: The cytology of the pituitary gland. In The Pituitary Gland: An Investigation of the Most Recent Advances. Williams and Wilkins, Baltimore, 1938.

Sims, E. A., and Krantz, K. E.: Serial studies of renal function throughout pregnancy and the puerperium in the normal woman. Clin. Res. Proc., 4:142, 1956.

Singh, H., Ramakumar, L., and Singh, I. D.: Serum proteins in pregnancy at term. J. Obstet. Gynaec. Brit. Comm., 74:254, 1967.

Sjostedt, S.: Acid-base balance of arterial blood during pregnancy, at delivery, and in the puerperium. Amer. J. Obstet. Gynec., 84:775, 1962.

Southren, A. L., Kobayashi, Y., Sherman, D. H., Levine, L., Gordon, G., and Weingold, A. B.: Diamine oxidase in human pregnancy. Amer. J. Obstet. Gynec., 89:199, 1964.

Stevens, A. R., Jr., Coleman, D. H., and Finch, C. A.: Iron metabolism; clinical evaluation of iron stores. Ann. Intern. Med., 38:199, 1953.

Strauss, M. B., and Castle, W. B.: Studies of anemia in pregnancy; I. Gastric secretion in pregnancy and the puerperium. Amer. J. Med. Sci., 184:655, 1932.

Theobold, G. W., and Lundberg, R. A.: Changes in limb volume and in venous infusion pressures caused by pregnancy. J. Obstet. Gynaec. Brit. Comm., 70:408, 1963.

Thomson, K. J., and Cohen, M. E.: Studies on the circulation in pregnancy; II. Vital capacity observations in normal pregnant women. Surg. Gynec. Obstet., 66:591, 1938.

Thomson, K. J., Hirsheimer, A., Gibson, J. G., II, and Evans, W. A., Jr.: Studies on the circulation in pregnancy; III. Blood volume changes in normal pregnant women. Amer. J. Obstet. Gynec., 36:48, 1938.

Thomson, K. J., Reid, D. E., and Cohen, M. E.: Studies on circulation in pregnancy; IV. Venous pressure observations in normal pregnant women, in pregnant women with compensated and decompensated heart disease and in the pregnancy "toxemias." Amer. J. Med. Sci., 198:665, 1939.

Traut, H. F., and McLane, C. M.: Physiological changes in the ureter associated with pregnancy. Surg. Gynec. Obstet., 62:65, 1936.

van Wagenen, G., and Jenkins, R. H.: Pyeloureteral dilatation of pregnancy after death of the fetus; an experimental study. Amer. J. Obstet. Gynec., 56: 1146, 1948.

Vosburgh, G. J., Flexner, L. B., Cowie, D. B., Hellman, L. M., Proctor, N. K., and Wilde, W. S.: The rate of renewal in women of the water and sodium of the amniotic fluid as determined by tracer techniques. Amer. J. Obstet. Gynec., 56:1156, 1948.

Wallraff, E. B., Brodie, E. C., and Borden, A. L.: Urinary excretion of amino acids in pregnancy. J. Clin. Invest., 29:1542, 1950.

White, R. F., Hertig, A. T., Rock, J., and Adams, E.: Histological observations on the corpus luteum of human pregnancy with special reference to corpora lutea associated with early normal and abnormal ova. Contrib. Embryol., 34:55, 1951.

Willson, J. R., Carrington, E. R., Hadd, H. E., and Boutwell, J.: Pregnancy edema; chemical and hormonal constituents of blood, urine, and edema fluid in patients with fluid retention and pre-eclampsia. Obstet. Gynec., 3:651, 1954.

Wood, C.: The expansile behavior of the human uterus. J. Obstet. Gynaec. Brit. Emp., 71:615, 1964.

Zangemeister, W., and Meissl, T.: Vergleichende Untersuchungen uber mutterliches und kindliches Blut and Fruchtwasser nebst Bemerkungen uber die fotale Harnsekretion. Munchen. Med. Wschr., 1: 673, 1903.

Zuckerman, H., Sadovsky, E., and Kallner, B.: Serum alkaline phosphatase in pregnancy and puerperium. Obstet. Gynec., 25:819, 1965.

Zuspan, F. P., and Goodrich, S.: Metabolic studies in normal pregnancy. Amer. J. Obstet. Gynec., 100:7, 1968.

PART III

Pathology of Reproduction

Chapter 12

Abortion

Spontaneous abortion is a common event and constitutes a major segment of what has been called "pregnancy wastage." The term has been defined in many different ways but it must be stated that no universally satisfactory definition has been arrived at. All attempts at limiting "abortion" to a specific time period of pregnancy are fraught with many biologic, statistical, and medical, not to mention religious, problems that cannot always be satisfactorily resolved.

The Third World Health Assembly in 1950 recommended that fetal death be defined as "death prior to the complete expulsion or extraction from its mother of a product of conception, irrespective of the duration of pregnancy"; it did not arrive at a definition of abortion but recommended that fetal deaths be placed into three major categories: (1) early fetal deaths with less than 20 weeks of gestation; (2) intermediate fetal deaths, 20 to 28 weeks of gestation; and (3) late fetal deaths of 28 weeks or more, commonly considered stillbirths. Whatever definition one chooses, the choice has a pronounced influence upon the statistical assessment of perinatal mortality and also on the abortion rate. Hence, comparable reporting of these various events is mandatory when such figures form the basis for comparing national or geographic incidence figures. The legal determination of a "viable" pregnancy, and hence often abortion, is a rather arbitrary point in time of development. It is quite variable in different regions of the world, and even in different states of this country, and as its basis weeks in gestation after last menstrual period is often used, or in other contexts, size or weight of the fetus.

All these considerations that are so important from a statistical and public health point of view have relatively little biologic validity. This has become even more evident in recent years when more sophisticated methods were applied to the study of the abortion product, "the abortus."

From a biologic point of view there exist no sharp borders between these categories; they form a spectrum of diseases that blend imperceptibly at different times of development.

In monotocous species, such as man, spontaneous abortion constitutes a frequent, clinically obvious, and hence important event. This is not necessarily the case in other mammals. Although the percentage of pregnancy wastage is probably very similar in polytocous mammals, the death of one or more embryos usually goes unnoticed, the remainder of live embryos assuring the continuation of pregnancy. The study of such mammals, particularly the pig and rabbit, has aided materially in our understanding of many aspects of zygotic loss and from such comparisons has come the notion that spontaneous abortion may be an important selective mechanism that eliminates the "unfit" products of conception. That this view has much merit has become more acceptable with the recent discovery of numerous chromosomal errors in abortuses, both in man and in polytocous mammals. Therefore, an understanding of the difference in reproductive mechanisms of various species is necessary if one wishes to comprehend the nature of this event. On the other hand, to view spontaneous abortion in all its forms as a selective, and thus species-protective, mechanism is surely unwarranted since, as will be seen, the composition of abortuses is so heterogeneous.

TERMINOLOGY

For the purposes of this discussion an abortion is considered the termination of pregnancy before 20 weeks of gestation, counting from the first day of the last menstrual period. It may be spontaneous or induced, the latter category being composed of what might be considered legal, medical (therapeutic), and also criminal, or illegal. As has been indicated, this is arbitrary but it does coincide with the definitions of many legislatures and has the merit of at least some medical justification. At this age the normal fetus weighs approximately 500 grams, has a crown-to-rump (CR) length of 16.5 cm., and, at least occaionally, is capable of extrauterine survival – it is then said to be "viable." Viability, though, is a changing concept. Medical advances in the treatment of the premature make it possible to anticipate that even these very small abortuses of 20 weeks' gestation may soon have a greater chance of survival and one surely does not then wish to describe a surviving fetus as an abortus.

The term miscarriage is often used by the layman, and the physician may use it when discussing the process with his patients. From a medical standpoint, though, it is best avoided. Many other terms are in common usage for the process of abortion — habitual, threatened, inevitable, incomplete, missed, and so forth. These usually refer to the clinical aspects of the event and the terms will be discussed under that heading. It is also important, at least conceptually, to bear in mind that good evidence exists that "fetal wastage" includes a presumably large number of fertilized ova that may never implant or that are expelled at the time of the menstrual period following conception, which may then be somewhat excessive. Since these "pregnancies" have not been clinically appreciated as such, these conceptuses are usually not considered in this context and, of course, they cannot be enumerated. Nevertheless, it appears that this is an appreciable number of potential pregnancies and they should be included as conceptions when such parameters as the "sex ratio" are considered.

Finally, from a cursory overview of the total population of spontaneous abortuses it appears that it is made up of two major segments; they may be called the "early" abortions (before 12 weeks and comprising the majority) and the "late" abortions (from 12 to 20 weeks). This differentiation is only partially justified, but it would seem that the early abortuses are more commonly the chromosomally deranged conceptuses (the old term "germ plasm defect" describes this variety), whereas the late abortions overlap with the category of premature labor. From a clinical and therapeutic point of view the latter would seem to contain more often salvageable pregnancies and their maternal complications are often of greater magnitude.

INCIDENCE

It is estimated now that at least 15 per cent of known pregnancies terminate in spontaneous abortion, but the true incidence is unknown for various reasons. When defined populations are studied in detail, as was done recently in a Hawaiian island, estimates of the abortion ratio up to 25 per cent are valid; they may hold for the general population. A useful graphic representation of the distribution of fetal losses for the United States in 1964 has been presented by Stickle (Fig. 1). It is estimated from that compilation that in the United States 1,537,000 abortions occur in 5,712,000 annual conceptions, approximately 27 per cent, abortions occurring most often in the first three weeks, and the incidence of loss declining rapidly after the 15th week of gestation.

The evidence for abortion loss greater than the 10 per cent usually quoted comes from various observations other than the specific population surveys quoted. Thus, among elective hysterectomies studied by Hertig and Rock numerous clearly defective ova were observed, some so deranged that implantation could not be anticipated. Clinicians observe frequently patients who state that their last period was delayed by one or two weeks, and then the menstrual flow was unusually profuse. Occasionally at least, early implantations have been recovered in such circumstances. Moreover, cytogenetic considerations and a comparison of events in other mammals enhance the suspicion that spontaneous abortion is a more common event than heretofore believed.

ETIOLOGY

It is generally agreed that spontaneous abortion usually takes place many days after the embryo has died; perhaps most commonly this interval is two weeks, and it is much longer in the case of hydatidiform moles and "missed abortions." During these early stages of development the embryo is a very delicate structure that is very prone to disintegration. Hence, the pathologic

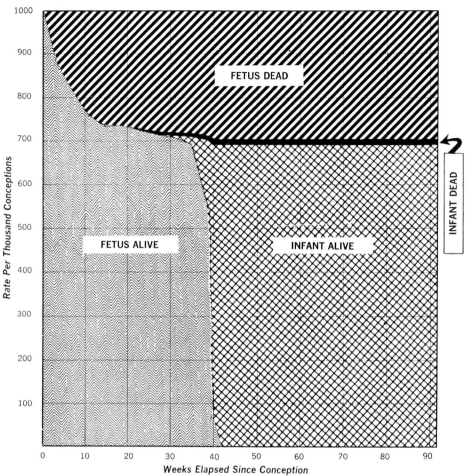

Figure 1. Cumulative outcome of pregnancy by numbers of weeks elapsed from conception. It is evident that the greatest "pregnancy wastage" occurs during the first 10 weeks of gestation, the total loss of zygotes amounting to approximately 30 per cent. (From Stickle, G., Amer. J. Obstet. Gynec., 100:442, 1968.)

study of the abortus, i.e., the embryo and placenta, may not reflect their morphologic status at the time of death. For instance, important autolytic changes take place that hamper the anatomic and genetic study of such conceptuses. Despite these restrictions, much has been learned from such pathologic investigations even though they do not always answer the questions of etiologic mechanism underlying the event.

The reasons for the lack of success of an implanted pregnancy can be placed in several broad categories, including genetic or structural deficiencies in embryo or uterus, infection, trauma, circulatory deficits, and others. To ascertain the specific causes for individual cases is the aim of pathogenetic studies, and doubtless the recent investigations concerning the chromosome complement of the abortus have

shed the most light on the disputed nature of the old concept of "germ plasm defect," a chapter of investigation that has not been closed. On the other hand, it is now evident that additional major causes must be identified before the largest proportion of spontaneous abortions may be explained satisfactorily.

The *pathologic findings* in abortuses are extremely varied and it is doubtful that the old classification of Mall and Meyer into their groups I to VI serves much purpose any longer. One reason of course is that many specimens are incomplete, either because portions have been expelled and lost, or because the specimen has been disrupted by curettage. Another reason is the frequent postmortem autolytic change that renders a critical study impossible, particularly of the embryo. Therefore, the group formulating the Geneva Report on Chromosome Studies of Abortuses adopted the simplified anatomic classification proposed by Fujikura, Froehlich, and Driscoll. It is descriptive and also practical since it may ultimately prove useful in an etiologic context. This study proposes the following subdivisions:

Group I: Incomplete specimens; villi, decidua and trophoblast, amnion, or chorion, but not a complete sac (22 per cent).

Group II: Ruptured empty sac; (a) with cord stump (4 per cent), (b) without cord stump (23.5 per cent).

Group III: Intact empty sac (5.5 per cent).

Group IV: Specimens containing an embryo: (a) normal embryo or fetus (35.8 per cent), (b) deformed embryo, e.g., stunted, amorphous (4 per cent), (c) embryo with specific localized anomalies (1.8 per cent), (d) embryo whose examination as to normality is impossible by virtue of fragmentation or autolysis (3.4 per cent).

The percentages are based on the authors' analysis of 327 abortuses and exclude moles and ectopic pregnancies. A study of the fetal size and gestational age of these specimens showed the abortuses to be smaller than those expected from Streeter's tables but technical differences may be the explanation. As might be expected from other studies, a majority of Group I to III abortions (the older group of "blighted ova") occurred in the first trimester, while relatively more Group IV specimens were observed later in pregnancy.

An obvious criticism of this classification might be that it is largely oblivious to possible placental anomalies. Many structural changes are observed in the placentas of spontaneous abortuses. Thus, aside from the fact that the cord may be absent or that it may lack an artery, the chorion and villi often lack fetal vessels. The villi are often swollen ("hydatid change"), their number is reduced ("hypoplasia"), and the trophoblast is atrophied (Fig. 2). Unfortunately, it is impossible at present to assign these pathologic changes any specific significance. It is well known that blood vessels of the placenta disintegrate rapidly after the embryo dies and they may disappear completely. Equally possible is that, for cytogenetic or other reasons, the trophoblast fails to grow or differentiate properly, with inevitable decidual necrosis and abortion ensuing. But why the decidua under-

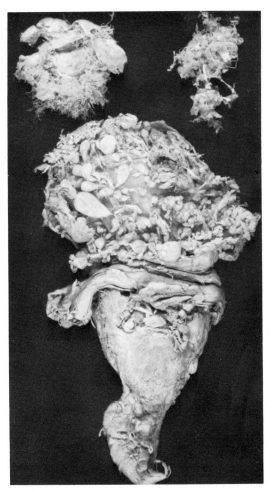

Figure 2. Progressively greater degree of hydatidiform change in a series of three abortuses. A degree of underdevelopment—sparse distribution of vesicular villi—may be seen in the complete uterine cast below. (From Benirschke, K., and Driscoll, S. G., The Pathology of the Human Placenta. Springer-Verlag, New York, 1967.)

goes these changes is unknown and one can only assume that local hormonal factors may be at fault.

Many authors assert that structural changes of the placenta are principal determinants of abortion and hold a defective implantation (too deep or too shallow) responsible. This is a fruitful area of future study as now some seemingly specific pathologic changes have been described in the placenta associated with specific chromosomal errors (Philippe and Boué). A relatively common form of placental pathologic change in abortions is the so-called Breus' mole (Fig. 3). Under the chorionic plate masses of intervillous hematomas accumulate that project into the chorionic space; hence its designation "subchorionic

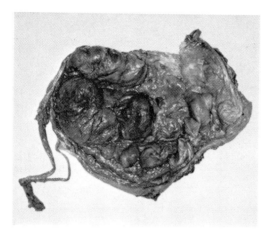

Figure 3. Subchorionic tuberous hematomas (Breus' mole) in missed abortion. The fetal surface of the placenta shows characteristic hemorrhagic protrusions. The anomaly is often associated with chromosomal errors.

tuberous hematoma." This condition is found most often in the so-called "missed abortions" and often it is apparently associated with chromosome errors.

On the basis that uterine rather than fetal conditions favor the development of placenta praevia, low implantation has arbitrarily been placed in the category of maternal pathogenesis of abortion. Were it not for the tendency of patients with low implantation to abort (Fig. 4), the incidence of placenta praevia, as encountered in the last trimester, would be significantly greater.

In recent years it has been learned that *chromosomal errors* are common among abortuses, and it can now be safely assumed that they are responsible for the spontaneous termination of the pregnancy. The justification for this assumption comes from the cytogenetic findings in abortuses on the one hand, and those in consecutive newborns and induced abortions on the other. Among 358 induced abortions studied in Japan by Makino et al. chromosomal errors were found in 1.7 per cent of the abortuses and of these errors many are considered to be compatible with normal survival. When consecutive newborns are studied the frequency of detectable chromosome errors is in the neighborhood of 0.5 per cent (Sergovich et al.) and many of these also are compatible with normal development, e.g., reciprocal translocations.

This contrasts sharply with the cytogenetic anomalies detected in spontaneous abortions. Approximately 1000 of these abortuses have now been analyzed in unselected series by tissue culture of embryonic fragments, amnion, or chorion, and approximately 25 per cent show chromosomal anomalies. The largest percentage (about half) are trisomic for a chromosome, a third monosomic X (45, XO), and a third are polyploid (usually triploid, but tetraploidy occurs also).

Among the trisomic specimens it is to be noted that (1) these abortions occurred earliest in gestation, and (2) many trisomies involved chromosomes whose trisomic state is not seen among live offspring, e.g., groups A, B, C and E. In particular, trisomy 16 is often encountered (Fig. 5). These findings suggest that such genetically deranged embryos cannot survive long. It is possible that placental development is faulty, particularly since occasionally structurally normal embryos are encountered. Of the XO embryos it is remarkable that the vast majority are aborted; few reach term and demonstrate Turner's syndrome. It is of further interest that detailed study of the XO fetuses shows their ovaries to possess a normally developed follicular complement. It is inferred that, if such embryos were to have survived to term, their germ cells would have degenerated so as to render the gonads the typical "streak" type. It is of course not certain whether XO abortuses would have become boys or girls; in any event, in surveys of sex chromatin they would have been counted as chromatin-negative and, hence, as boys. This type of abortion tends to occur later than those associated with trisomies. The polyploid conceptuses also tend to abort later in pregnancy than do those with trisomies,

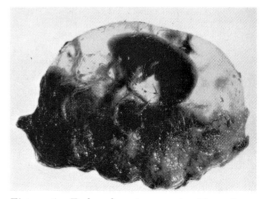

Figure 4. Early placenta praevia. Normal conceptus. A portion of the placenta on the left was contained within the upper cervix and lower uterine segment.

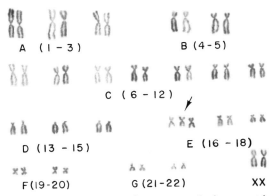

Figure 5. Karyotype of a seven week abortus with trisomy 16. Trisomies are the commonest anomalies in early abortuses; trisomy 16 is especially common and is apparently lethal to embryonic development.

A (1 – 3)   B (4 – 5)

C (6 – 12)

D (13 – 15)   E (16 – 18)

F (19 – 20)   G (21 – 22)   XX

and the most common sex chromosome distribution in this group is XXY, next most often, XXX, and least common, XYY. The frequent and striking hydatidiform degeneration of this group is to be noted, many specimens impressing as "transitional moles," i.e., with immature placentas whose villous tissue is in part as grapelike as that of true hydatidiform moles.

A very small number of abortuses is found to possess a mosaic chromosome constitution, autosomal monosomy, and even less commonly structural alterations of chromosomes have been found in abortions. At one time it was thought that the abortuses of patients with habitual abortion might show specific types of anomalies, but inquiry into such families has not been very rewarding. A few specific translocations have been identified when the abortus had an unbalanced genetic set, but by and large they are normal.

It must be cautioned that these investigations are all quite recent and larger series may well uncover new parameters. In order to standardize future studies the Geneva Conference of WHO reviews the published results and techniques and makes suggestions for future studies. How important such future prospective studies may be can be appreciated from the recent controversy over the suggested increased frequency of polyploid conceptuses occurring within six months after cessation of oral contraceptive therapy. Obviously, if confirmed, these studies may have important social implications, but since these anomalies all terminate in abortion and because no higher incidence of viable trisomies has

been noted, the danger seems limited.

From what has been said, it is apparent that spontaneous abortion may well represent a selective mechanism. Among the youngest abortions the highest rate (50 per cent) of chromosomal anomalies occurs; the longer the duration of pregnancy when it is aborted, the less significant is this cause.

Inasmuch as most abortuses are not mosaic, one must assume faulty gametogenesis to be responsible and, broadly speaking, parallels with trisomies discovered at birth can be found. Thus, trisomic abortuses are associated with higher maternal age than nontrisomic abortuses, as is the case for mongolism. This does not hold for trisomy 16 – a common finding among trisomic abortuses – for polyploidy, and for the XO anomaly. It is thus likely that other mechanisms are responsible for these aneuploidies than those leading to the most common trisomies seen in the newborn population. Delayed ovulation, aging of the ovum, and perhaps viral or physical alterations of the ovum are considered etiologic factors at present but there are no good clues for the ultimate etiologic determinants. It should also be mentioned that the cytogenetic techniques are successful in only perhaps 50 per cent of abortuses cultured, although Carr has brought forth cogent arguments that the chromosome constitutions of the unsuccessfully cultured specimens would be the same as those of successfully cultured ones.

Events of faulty gametogenesis and thence leading to aneuploid (trisomic) zygotes require the theoretical possibility that the other segregation product of meiosis should often also lead to autosomal monosomy. The fact that such abortuses have only rarely been observed, and also that not all chromosomes are found in trisomic states (notably group F), suggests that some zygotes fail to implant or are aborted so early as to be clinically inapparent as pregnancies. Implicit in this assumption is the notion that the total zygotic loss may much exceed the abortion ratio described, a suggestion that is enhanced when comparison with other mammals is made (Fig. 6). Some of the extremely abnormal implantations discovered by Hertig and Rock may belong in this category (Fig. 7).

These considerations are pertinent to the so-called primary *sex ratio*. It is well known

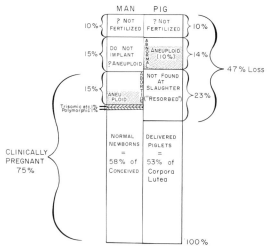

Figure 6. Graphic comparison of the timing and identified causes of spontaneous losses of 100 conceptuses in man and a polytocous species, the pig. (Data from Hertig, A. T., 1967, and Corner, G. W., 1923.)

that the sex ratio is not 1:1 at birth, there being an excess of males. Previous studies of aborted conceptuses has suggested that there were also more males in spontaneous abortions, findings largely derived from chromatin surveys of placental membranes. With more accurate sex determination by karyotyping it has become clear, however, that more XX than XY abortuses are found. Furthermore, when the XO abortuses, representing a large proportion as will be re-

membered, are arbitrarily assigned as males, a sex ratio of near unity is obtained. This again must be considered highly circumstantial, though, since the triploids cannot be placed properly and since nothing is yet known about the unimplanted but wasted conceptuses.

In some instances of spontaneous abortion distinct *maternal factors* may be held responsible. These include various uterine structural abnormalities, leiomyomata, and a plethora of other conditions. Numerically speaking, these factors account for only a small group of spontaneous abortions. Trauma, a commonly implicated cause, accounted for only one case of the 1000 specimens analyzed by Hertig and Sheldon, and specific uterine anomalies were detected in eight. Only 20 cases of febrile illnesses were thought to be responsible for abortions in their series. It must be said, however, that opinion is divided as to the importance of an infectious etiology of spontaneous abortions. There is little doubt that severe viral and bacterial infections may be responsible at times, rubella, smallpox, and listeriosis serving as good examples. The pathologist is rarely able, however, to verify such agents in the causation of abortion, at least in the first trimester of pregnancy. Similarly, toxoplasma organisms, while often incriminated, have rarely been directly identified in this mate-

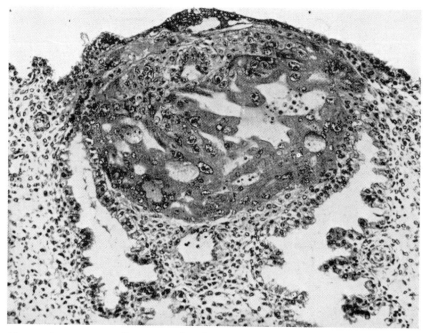

Figure 7. Abnormal ovum—germ disc present but chorionic cavity absent. × 200. (From Hertig, A. T., Rock, J., and Adams, E. C., Amer. J. Anat., 98:435, 1956.)

rial. The picture is somewhat different in the second trimester. Pathologic study of placenta and fetus near 20 weeks shows in a preponderance of abortuses significant chorioamnionitis, fetal vasculitis, and aspirated pus in lung and stomach of the fetus. The implication of these findings is that ascending placental membrane infection is common in this group, and that it leads to amniotic sac infection and to premature labor. Chromosomally and structurally these abortuses are otherwise normal and the process blends imperceptibly with, or can be regarded as, "premature labor." Repetitive abortion at this gestational age is not uncommon in such women, and it may occur for the same reason. Recently it has been found that Mycoplasma endocervicitis (and male urethritis) may be a cause of this wastage and prophylactic antibiotic treatment has been efficacious in some affected couples (Kundsin et al.). From a therapeutic point of view this is the most gratifying group of patients and this etiology should be carefully considered when the diagnosis "incompetent os" is entertained.

An abortion may occur as the result of a laceration of the cervix, but only when it is extensive to the point of producing cervical incompetence. These cases should be rare with the abolition of manual dilatation and operative delivery through the undilated cervix, and with routine inspection of the cervix after every difficult labor and delivery, with the immediate repair of any cervical laceration.

Surgical amputation of the cervix resulting in marked shortening of the canal may cause abortion or premature labor. Heretofore this was a method of treatment for the extensively lacerated or infected cervix, or as part of the technique of the Manchester-Fothergill operation for procidentia. Fortunately, surgical amputation of the cervix is rarely performed today, at least in women who hope to have more children. In the extreme, when the vaginal portion is removed completely, the fetal membranes may be seen rather early in pregnancy on speculum examination. This situation predisposes to spontaneous rupture of the membranes, invites infection, and results in fetal loss.

Abortion and premature labor occur with much greater frequency when the uterus is incompletely formed. Fetal wastage is the highest when there is either failure of fusion or extensive septate formation of the body of the uterus. In this instance, only half of the uterus may be available for the purpose of gestation, with the blood supply derived from a single uterine artery and a limited amount of myometrium to accommodate the growing conceptus. A fetal wastage rate of 40 per cent from abortion and premature labor has been reported when the uterus is double or bicornuate. When the cervix, of either the double or septate variety, presents the major anomaly, the abortion rate is no higher than normal, and any increase in fetal wastage that does occur revolves about labor and delivery.

More recently, considerable importance has been attributed to a possible defect in the cervix as a cause of habitual abortion and repetitive premature labor. This defect, now more generally referred to as an incompetent cervix and occurring in about 0.2 per cent of pregnancies beyond 20 weeks, is thought to be due primarily to the forces and trauma of labor or possibly forceful dilatation of the cervix attending curettage. In rare instances it may be congenital.

Other determinants of spontaneous abortion are most difficult to define. Clearly, it is likely that the male may contribute to this wastage of conceptuses. In the occasional habitual aborter this has been found to be the case when the male carried some specific chromosome translocation or a mosaic population of diploid/trisomic cells. Also, of course, he may be the source of infection but, by and large, no numerically important contribution can be assigned to male factors. Maternal nutritional, immunologic, toxic (drugs), and psychosomatic factors have all been incriminated but they too seem to play no numerically important role. Similarly, there is no convincing evidence that "endocrine imbalance" is an important etiologic factor and certainly the replacement therapy attempted in many threatened abortions can no longer be held to be efficacious in their salvage. Inasmuch as the so frequent chromosomal errors found represent de novo mutations, it has been suspected that specific genic (single lethal autosomal genes) mutations may make up a segment of this fetal wastage. Although this is an attractive concept, there has been no support for it from investigations. Indeed, among highly inbred populations where such genes might be accumulated, no higher abortion rate is found.

In summary, it may be said that perhaps 40 per cent of the early abortions and 30 per cent of all abortions can be explained satisfactorily. The remainder constitute a challenge to future investigators.

TYPES OF ABORTION

The clinician recognizes a variety of situations associated with abortion, and to define them has clinical usefulness. The classification of the various types of abortion follows:

1. A threatened abortion is here defined as an episode of painless uterine bleeding, usually brownish in color. When associated with spasmodic lower abdominal or suprapubic discomfort attributed to uterine contractions, and bright red bleeding occurs, the condition is approaching that of an inevitable abortion.

2. An inevitable abortion is the persistence of vaginal bleeding with uterine contractions of sufficient intensity to produce cervical dilatation. The products of conception may or may not present at the partially dilated cervical os.

3. An incomplete abortion is one in which the products of conception have not been expelled in their entirety.

4. A complete abortion occurs when the conceptus with its placental components has been expelled in toto.

5. A habitual abortion is a sequence of three or more abortions. It is sometimes referred to as "primary" when all previous pregnancies have resulted in abortion, and "secondary" when one or more earlier pregnancies have proceeded to a period of fetal viability.

6. A missed abortion exists when the conceptus has died in utero and is retained and not delivered for weeks or even months after its death.

7. A septic abortion is any abortion complicated by infection of the uterus and the products of conception; it may be either inevitable or incomplete, spontaneous or induced.

8. A criminal abortion is the unlawful and artificial premature termination of pregnancy.

9. A therapeutic or medical abortion is the deliberate and lawful termination of pregnancy prior to the period of viability for defined medical indications.

DIFFERENTIAL DIAGNOSIS

Differential diagnosis takes into account those conditions associated with uterine bleeding and lower abdominal discomfort, which means the exclusion of local vaginal and cervical lesions and extrauterine pelvic pathologic conditions. At times the diagnosis seems unnecessarily confusing, principally because the history is unreliable, as in cases of septic abortion. In general, a tubal pregnancy, and tubal infection, or coincidental ovarian disease gives the clinician the most concern. Implantation bleeding always raises the question of a threatened abortion. Frequent gentle pelvic examination will assure the clinician that the uterus is enlarging in size consistent with a normal pregnancy, the diagnosis being implantation bleeding. Such an approach will identify or exclude the possibility of a developing ectopic pregnancy.

MORBIDITY AND MORTALITY

Except for the occasional patient who may be weakened from excessive blood loss, the recovery from spontaneous abortion is rapid. Although many patients resume their normal activities within three or four days, a longer recuperative period is recommended. However, a septic abortion may result in a prolonged illness, and many months may elapse before the pelvic inflammatory exudate is completely absorbed, and the uterus and adnexa become freely movable and essentially normal at pelvic examination. Pelvic infection in association with a septic abortion may occasionally result in infertility, but this supposedly occurs less frequently than it does after a Neisseria infection. The infection may extend from the decidua through the lymphatics to cause parametritis, pelvic peritonitis, pelvic abscess, thrombophlebitis, and possible septicemia. Salpingitis may develop by direct extension.

Maternal death from abortion ranges between 0.25 and 2.0 per cent, the difference being largely accounted for by the number of criminal abortions in a given series. Death may follow directly as a consequence of septic shock, peritonitis, or acute renal failure from either bilateral cortical necrosis of the focal type or acute tubular necrosis.

MANAGEMENT OF THE VARIOUS TYPES OF ABORTION

The form and extent of the preventive and definitive treatment of an abortion will depend on its type and status when the patient is initially observed. Because of articles in medical and lay literature associating uterine bleeding in the early weeks of pregnancy with congenital malformation, some patients who bleed in early gestation are concerned about what this may mean to the fetus. These patients may be assured that the chance of the baby's being abnormal is not increased by the bleeding episode, and if the conceptus is abnormal, they will eventually abort regardless of the treatment used. If the patient is on sex steroids and other therapy, the question arises whether the treatment should be continued when there is uncertainty about the normalcy of the conceptus. Both the physician and the patient would unquestionably agree that it is undesirable to prolong a pregnancy if the conceptus is abnormal. If, for example, a hydatidiform mole is the ultimate stage of a blighted ovum, considerable harm might accrue from retaining an anomalous conceptus. The incidence of hydatidiform mole and malformation appears no higher since the introduction and extensive use of sex steroids and vitamins in the therapy of abortion and repetitive premature labor.

The various forms of treatment may, in general, be placed into one of three categories; all overlap to a degree, but all aim to treat the patient completely and with sympathetic understanding. The first incorporates only the use of sedatives and the limitation of activity. The second stresses the importance of nutrition and supplementary vitamins, alone or in combination with psychotherapy. The third therapeutic regimen places emphasis on those endocrine factors which control the reproductive cycle. The first form of treatment is concerned mainly with the management of a threatened or initial abortion, and, although the latter two regimens may

also be instituted in the course of a threatened abortion, they are more logically applicable to the prevention of a repeat or habitual abortion.

Threatened Abortion

Restriction of the patient's activities, plus mild sedation to allay her anxiety, is the treatment of the patient with a threatened abortion. With the full realization that there is evidence to indicate that the restriction of activity has no appreciable influence on the abortion rate, the patient is nevertheless placed on bed rest for a few days. The rationale of such treatment is to permit any shed blood within the uterus to become clotted and thus retard further bleeding about the implantation site. Although reportable, a small amount of painless bleeding does not always necessitate immediate hospitalization; when the bleeding persists, however, the patient is usually hospitalized even though additional therapy may not be contemplated.

Were it possible to establish definitely the condition of the conceptus, the management of threatened abortion could be more intelligently applied.

Of the various procedures proposed to determine the condition of the conceptus, all are directed toward evaluating the status of the syncytiotrophoblast and cytotrophoblast. Considerable reliance has been placed on the urinary values of pregnanediol and chorionic gonadotropin as an index of the viability of the conceptus, but this is more applicable to patients with repeat or habitual abortion.

A gentle vaginal examination under sterile precautions is the most useful procedure to determine whether the pregnancy is normal, but this, too, is not infallible. The failure of the products of conception to develop in the case of a blighted ovum means that the uterus rarely enlarges beyond the size of a six to seven weeks' pregnancy. The discrepancy between gestational age and uterine growth is discernible on vaginal examination, and discovery of a cervix beginning to dilate is consistent with an inevitable abortion. To the experienced examiner, the uterus of the patient destined to abort is, at times, firm rather than soft, the result of hyperirritability. Exceptions to these findings are seen on occasion. On vaginal or abdominal examination, the uterus may appear enlarged for the gestational period. Although there is a possibility that the patient has a hydatidiform mole, it is possible that the excessive enlargement is the result of concealed hemorrhage. In either case the patient will continue to bleed, and in amounts that demand that the pregnancy be terminated.

In résumé, the management of threatened abortion rests on the philosophy that, with a normal conceptus, symptoms are likely to subside and the pregnancy continue without supplementary therapy, and that, in the presence of an abnormal conceptus, abortion will eventually occur spontaneously. Before the patient is permitted to resume her normal activities, as the vaginal staining subsides and disappears a sterile vaginal examination is performed to exclude the possibility of a tubal pregnancy. A speculum examination is performed at this time to exclude local lesions that might account for the bleeding, such as polyps, cervical ectropion or erosion, and the rare possibility of carcinoma.

Although a brownish discharge may linger for several days, subsequent vaginal examination will demonstrate whether the uterus is growing and is consistent in size with the gestational age. If the uterus fails to enlarge, the amount of brownish discharge usually increases, low abdominal cramps and bleeding develop, the cervix dilates, and the abortion enters the inevitable stage. In a few instances, although the uterus recedes in size, the cervix remains closed and the bleeding is insignificant. In this event the provisional diagnosis is a blighted ovum, and, should the condition continue beyond a few weeks, it is regarded as a missed abortion.

Inevitable Abortion

The conceptus is usually expelled spontaneously in part or in whole within a few hours after the abortion reaches the inevitable stage, although at times it may be retained for several days. In the hope that the pregnancy will terminate spontaneously and completely, there are those who prefer that the treatment be one of watchful expectancy unless the vaginal bleeding becomes excessive, in which event the uterus is emptied immediately. This method of therapy is based on the belief that surgical interference might precipitate serious hemorrhage, and introduce infection. It is now appreciated that the presence of dead

and necrotic placental tissue invites infection which may result in septic shock, a most serious complication. In recent years, therefore, earlier operative evacuation of the uterus has been practiced, and accumulated experience has shown it to be safe; in addition, the period of convalescence is materially shortened.

This statement should not be construed to mean that the patient is curetted immediately after entrance to the hospital. In fact, if the bleeding is minimal and the abortion is adjudged inevitable by clinical signs and symptoms, an oxytocic may be administered. Pitocin, by the intravenous drip method, may cause complete expulsion of the usually blighted conceptus. If, after a few hours, this treatment fails or bleeding becomes excessive, curettage is performed. In the interim, the patient is given adequate amounts of sedation, the hematocrit value is determined, and the patient's blood is cross-matched. If there is evidence of infection the cervix is cultured and antibiotic therapy is initiated.

Because the pregnant uterus is perforated more easily than the nonpregnant, the products of conception are removed by sponge or ovum forceps, followed by a gentle exploration with a large, blunt curette. As the products of conception are removed and the uterus begins to regain its nonpregnant size, a more vigorous curettage may be attempted to insure that the uterus is empty of its contents. The aspiration curette has its enthusiasts. Hemorrhage from uterine atony is lessened by a constant Pitocin drip infusion. The abortion specimen should be carefully saved and referred to the laboratory for pathologic examination.

Even when the conceptus is expelled spontaneously in toto, many clinicians favor routine curettage to avoid subsequent postpartum bleeding. Although a rare patient may at some later date bleed and require readmission to the hospital and subsequent curettage, this hardly justifies submitting all patients who spontaneously abort to even the slight risk of an anesthetic, and the outside chance of uterine infection that has been known to follow a seemingly benign curettage. It is a personal view that when the specimen appears grossly complete and the bleeding is hardly more than with a period, curettage is unnecessary. Because fetal erythrocytes can be present in the maternal circulation from the second month of gestation, anti-Rh$_0$ immunoglobilin must be considered for the Rh-negative patient with an abortion. Transplacental hemorrhage increases in accordance with uterine manipulation, and certainly when artificial termination occurs the risk of Rh immunization is enhanced.

Septic Abortion

In most cases of septic abortion it may be taken for granted that there has likely been some interference with the pregnancy. Most cases occur not in the unmarried but rather in multigravid women. Vaginal bleeding, exquisite uterine and lower abdominal tenderness, chills, fever, and leukocytosis comprise the clinical signs and symptoms of a septic abortion.

Although septic abortion is a serious complication of pregnancy, a favorable prognosis can be offered provided the patient is managed correctly. Even those patients who develop septic shock should be salvageable if seen before they are in a terminal state. This is in contrast to the reported mortality of over 50 per cent for bacteremic shock associated with surgical and medical conditions. There are at least two reasons why survival favors the obstetric patient with septic shock. One is her relatively young age and the second is that the infection is more clearly defined, being largely restricted to the uterus and its immediate environs. Hence the infection can be brought under control by hysterectomy when medical measures appear to fail.

Over 90 per cent of patients with septic abortion will respond favorably to antibiotic therapy and evacuation of the products of conception, the major nidus of the infection. In those who fail to respond to this treatment, septic shock with all of its hazards may develop, and in a few, tubo-ovarian abscess(es) with possible septic shock in the event of rupture. It cannot be too strongly stated that in the case of the latter, immediate laparotomy and pelvic cleanout should be performed. It has been amply documented that the mortality is at least 60 per cent or greater if this approach is not pursued.

In the management of septic abortion, recognition must be given to etiologic factors other than infection, that is, chemical substances such as Lysol and soap. These agents can create great havoc when introduced into the uterus, causing myometrial necrosis; and should they gain entrance to the maternal circulation may cause hemolysis and a marked disturbance in the clotting mechanism with secondary effects on the kidney, lung, and other organs. Thus, in the initial assessment of the patient suffering from the aftermath of a nonmedical and possible septic abortion, the methods used to procure the abortion should be elucidated at the time of hospital admission. Because of the social onus of a nonmedical or criminal abortion, these patients seek help only when they become seriously ill, often several days or a week after the event. Hence, prompt diagnosis, evaluation, and early treatment are imperative.

Diagnostic and laboratory examinations should be performed in an orderly fashion. Blood should be drawn for hematocrit determination, leukocyte and platelet counts, and blood urea nitrogen and electrolyte determinations. Arterial blood lactic acid determination and repeated hematocrit readings may afford some index of the severity of the patient's condition, including evidence of hemolysis. Bacteriologic studies include repeated blood cultures and cultures of the cervix, the uterus, and its contents. Immediate Gram staining of the material will usually identify the offending organism, i.e., gram-negative bacilli, streptococci, and clostridia. The exotoxins of the latter may be associated with hemolysis and tissue necrosis, but otherwise, if septic shock occurs, it is similar to that encountered with the endotoxin of the gram-negative bacillus. Because clostridial organisms are found rather commonly about the cervix, it has been emphasized that to be etiologically meaningful, these organisms must be found within the uterus or its contents.

An upright x-ray examination of the abdomen should be performed to exclude free air and hence uterine perforation. Urine output is recorded hourly with an indwelling catheter. The significance of central venous pressure monitoring in these patients is subject to interpretation. Knowing the central venous pressure undoubtedly is helpful in the prevention of overloading the circulation in the presence of pulmonary hypertension and a low cardiac output. Actually, a fall in central venous pressure may herald recovery and permit the judicious use of blood replacement in restoring the effective circulating blood volume to normal.

Except perhaps for the early removal of

the source of infection, the treatment is similar to that of sepsis encountered in other conditions. Therapy begins with penicillin (10 million units), streptomycin (0.5 gram), or kanamycin (1 to 2 grams), depending on the urinary output. Subsequent sensitivity studies may demand a more specific approach to antibiotic therapy. Fluid therapy, with lactated Ringer's solution, must be maintained in balance. Should septic shock intervene, adrenal steroids in appropriate dosage are indicated. With a falling urine output and a rising hematocrit, indicating a hypovolemic state, mannitol (12.5 grams) may prove temporarily useful both therapeutically and prognostically. Lack of renal response may imply deterioration of the patient in the hours ahead. Isoproterenol may assist in improving cardiac output.

Within 6 to 12 hours after medical therapy is initiated, the infected products of conception should be removed from the uterus. Indeed, a Pitocin drip may be started soon after hospital admission in the hope that spontaneous uterine evacuation may occur or that at least the cervix will dilate sufficiently to permit ready removal of the infected uterine contents. A gentle finger exploration at the end of the procedure will assure the operator that the uterus is emptied of its contents and there is no evidence of previous trauma. A dramatic fall in blood pressure in the absence of blood loss is occasionally encountered during or immediately following the curettage. The writer has chosen to call this the "D & C" test for the presence of or impending septic shock. It is envisioned that the manipulation required in evacuating the infected products of conception causes a further release of endotoxin in the maternal circulation.

Failure of the blood pressure to return to near normal and, if suppressed, the urine excretion to increase following uterine evacuation suggests that the infection is not under control and that the remaining decidua is harboring the offending organism in lethal quantities. Indeed, it is the patients in whom the conventional measures just mentioned fail that the mortality resides. It is in these patients that hysterectomy can be lifesaving, albeit not a pleasant conclusion to contemplate in the nonparous patient. But to procrastinate may lead to further deterioration of the patient to the point that she reaches a state of irreversible shock. Additional candidates for a hysterectomy are those patients who have been aborted by chemical means and those in whom renal failure is a prominent feature. Also, there will be the rare patient in whom the uterus cannot be safely emptied vaginally and recourse to hysterectomy is necessary. Inferior vena cava and ovarian vein ligation should be considered at the time of hysterectomy for prevention of subsequent pulmonary embolism. Certainly at the time of hysterectomy, thrombosis of the neighboring veins is commonly seen.

As mentioned, a coagulopathy may be encountered, and hence the clotting mechanism should be checked periodically in the course of caring for the patient. Here, and in renal failure, the underlying pathophysiology can be based to a degree on a common denominator, i.e., the Shwartzman phenomenon that is characterized by a widespread deposition of fibrin. In both situations, heparin therapy should be considered. Heparin may protect against intravascular clotting. Fibrinogen may be required, however, to restore the clotting mechanism to normal. Exchange transfusion has been introduced to combat the effects of a continuing hemolysis.

In cases associated with anuria, a dramatic renal response has followed heparin therapy, resulting in a sharp fall in the elevated urea nitrogen level and a rise in previously depressed blood platelet values. However, the kidney is subject to a variety of lesions. Should the infection be due to *Clostridium welchii*, the resultant renal damage may be from a toxic effect, hemolysis, or both. Varying degrees of bilateral cortical necrosis have been encountered, and here the prognosis must be guarded. When the anuria is due to tubular necrosis, recovery is the rule with the assistance of hemodialysis.

In summary, the septic uterus is a life-threatening state that may be encountered in any period of pregnancy, but the majority of cases follow a nonmedical abortion. Those who show evidence of septic shock or chemical abortion deserve all that an intensive care unit can provide. These patients can present a wide spectrum of clinical symptoms and may require a variety of therapeutic aids from assisted respiration to hemodialysis. An aggressive policy of management is recommended, in the hope of preventing septic shock rather than having to treat it.

Evacuation of the uterus is recommended

within 6 to 12 hours after the onset of medical treatment. A favorable response and prompt recovery is anticipated. Should this fail, hysterectomy should be considered, especially if there is a strong renal component involved. Reference has been made to serious consequences of chemical abortion, which, together with tubo-ovarian abscess, is an indication for exploratory laparotomy with possible hysterectomy, preferably with conservation of at least one uninvolved ovary.

Missed Abortion

In cases of missed abortion, an ineffective attempt is made by the uterus to expel the products of conception as evidenced by episodes of cramps, usually without bleeding but sometimes with brownish discharge. Clinically, there is regression in the breast changes and in the symptoms and signs of pregnancy, as well as in the uterine size.

Clinicians of previous days have been heard to remark that patients with missed abortion had a tendency to bleed excessively at the time of delivery. Because of this they were loath to interfere. In retrospect, with the conceptus dead and retained in utero for a period of time, the possible appearance of a coagulation defect may have been a major factor when the degree of bleeding was life-threatening. Because of this possibility, the question has been raised regarding early interference in the treatment of missed abortion.

Actually this is rather theoretical, for several weeks may have elapsed before the condition is recognized or the physician is convinced the uterus is not enlarging at a rate consistent with normal pregnancy. However, once it is diagnosed, blood samples and the clotting mechanism should be checked at least weekly. In the interim of three to four weeks a spontaneous abortion may ensue. Moreover, should a bleeding defect develop it is manageable.

Once the patient is aware that she has a missed abortion, understandably she may be emotionally upset, and may request and indeed implore that the (defective) pregnancy be terminated. In fact, pregnancy has been known to continue in these patients beyond the calculated date of confinement—a rather difficult experience for the patient. Although the physician should not be influenced unduly, when the uterus has receded in size to that of an 8 to 10 week pregnancy, uterine evacuation is probably less hazardous than letting the pregnancy continue indefinitely. When the uterus is beyond 12 weeks' size and particularly when bony fetal elements are identifiable, despite the threat of a coagulation defect, unless one is prepared to perform a vaginal or abdominal hysterotomy one should await the spontaneous onset of labor and termination of the pregnancy. But again, the introduction of saline infusion and prostaglandin to initiate labor may permit artificial termination of pregnancy without undue risk. One should be aware of a coagulation defect that may not be clinically apparent, and hence the clotting mechanism should be carefully checked prior to any interference. Pitocin drip to precipitate or initiate labor is not without its complications, for the resultant uterine activity, possibly somewhat excessive, may contribute to the coagulation defect, as reflected in a lowering of the blood fibrinogen level. Careful administration of intra-amniotic saline is highly effective, labor ensuing within a few hours.

Habitual Abortion and Repetitive Premature Labor

The treatment of habitual abortion begins before conception has occurred, with a search for nutritional and metabolic disturbances and pelvic disease or defects in the reproductive tract that might contribute to the condition. Besides a careful nutritional history, determination of the basal metabolic rate, or of thyroxin levels, and of blood cholesterol, and routine blood examinations constitute the minimum of laboratory procedures. Despite the probability that the quality of the semen may relate only to infertility, examination of a postcoital specimen is commonly performed. Artificial insemination with a donor's sperm is sometimes considered when low counts and many immotile and abnormal forms of sperm persist despite treatment.

In the course of a vaginal examination, when the cervix is found to be extensively lacerated, surgical repair may be indicated. Perhaps intermittent antibiotic therapy throughout pregnancy, based on sensitivity studies of the organisms present, should be considered in some patients in whom difficulty is encountered in controlling the cervicitis by prepregnancy cauterization and other means.

If hysterography during the preconceptional investigation reveals the uterine cavity to be distorted by uterine fibroids, a myomectomy is considered justifiable. It is well to emphasize, however, that patients with extensive leiomyomata do remarkably well in the course of childbearing.

Although most anomalies of the reproductive tract are identifiable by pelvic examination, all too often they go unrecognized. It is apparent that nearly half of the cases of congenital anomalies of the female generative tract remain undiagnosed until pregnancy complications have already occurred. Further investigation, either by uterine exploration at the time of delivery or by hysterography three or six months later, will usually identify any abnormality of the uterus. In patients prone to late or repetitive premature labor, it is well to explore the uterus manually at delivery to determine whether there is any anatomic abnormality.

Digital exploration of the uterus at delivery may be enlightening. A ridge may be felt in the midline of the corpus, suggesting incomplete fusion, but equally impressive is the detection of a thinning of the anterior and the posterior wall at the midline, again suggesting incomplete müllerian duct fusion. What appears to be near-complete myometrial fusion need not necessarily mean normal vessel cross-anastomosis. Figure 8 shows a specimen in which myometrial fusion is not quite complete (arcuate uterus), and there is a failure of cross-anastomosis of the uterine vessels. Although it may not necessarily prevent a successful pregnancy, such a vessel arrangement offers the possibility that the blood supply is inadequate to maintain the pregnancy. This is particularly so if the supposedly relatively avascular anterior or posterior uterine wall is the site of implantation. Whether these patients, like those with double and bicornuate uteri, can benefit by surgery in accordance with the principles of the Strassmann procedure remains an unanswered question. Surgical resection of the ischemic area of the myometrium and coaptation of the divided uterus conceivably might establish a normal cross-anastomosis of the uterine vessels. Regardless of all else, in patients with late abortion or repetitive premature labor, the clinician must bear in mind that failure of therapy may result from an ana-

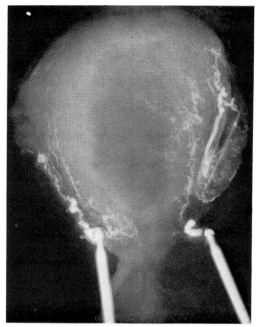

Figure 8. Arcuate uterus with absence of cross-uterine anastomosis. Injected specimen. (Courtesy of Dr. S. L. Romney.)

tomic rather than an endocrine or other deficiency.

A conclusion of some significance is that endocrine therapy has produced less favorable results in the treatment of repetitive premature labor than in habitual abortion, suggesting that in the former some other factor is at fault. In these patients, repeatedly in the middle trimester or early part of the last trimester, the cervix dilates without apparent cause and the conceptus is lost. On questioning, the patient may state that while the uterus was contracting she experienced little discomfort until delivery became imminent. She has afterward been told by her physician that the fetus was grossly normal. Endocrine therapy has not provided the complete therapeutic answer. Encouraging results are now being reported with a surgical procedure complementing sex steroid therapy. Although the procedure to be described is discussed in the etiology and management of repetitive premature labor, it is assigned here for it involves late abortion and is usually performed prior to the 20th week of pregnancy.

Reference has been made to the incompetent cervix (Fig. 9) as a possible cause of these pregnancy failures and this is now regarded as a clinical entity. Originally it was thought that the internal os only was incompetent. The lesion was defined as a

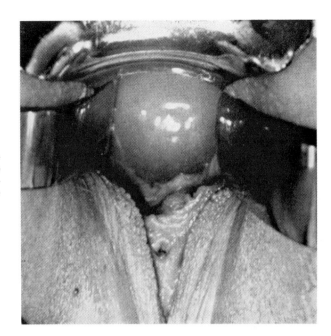

Figure 9. Incompetent cervix with membranes exposed at 26 weeks' gestation. The cervix was closed according to technique described (Fig. 10), and the pregnancy was salvaged.

thin scarlike defect situated in the anterior cervical wall in the region of the internal os.

It is believed by many that the history is sufficient to make a diagnosis. The history often reveals that the first and sometimes the second pregnancy proceeded to near term, and was followed by a series of nonviable pregnancies. This has been interpreted to mean that the cervical lesion is acquired by the impact of labor and is not congenital in origin. Such an inference is not necessarily correct, however. In an occasional case the condition appears to be primary, the patient never having experienced a viable pregnancy, albeit several pregnancy losses.

Several methods have been recommended to identify the possible defect, none of which up to the present have been entirely convincing. Recently, however, a more scientific approach to the diagnosis and treatment of patients with this syndrome when seen in pregnancy may be through ultrasound, which may make it possible to demonstrate the relationship of the growing conceptus to the internal os. Redundancy of this structure may indicate its incompetency and justify surgical management and correction.

It has been recommended that these cervical defects be repaired prior to pregnancy. In brief, the technique of Lash consists of a transverse anterior incision of the vaginal mucous membrane overlying the cervix with an upward displacement of the bladder. This is followed by wedge excision of the cervix. The cervix is closed and the vaginal mucous membrane is sutured in place. This may be the preferred method when the patient is not pregnant, but it does not meet the needs of the patient with this syndrome who is already pregnant.

Several methods of surgical closure of the incompetent cervix in pregnancy have been recommended, differing only in detail and mainly in the type of suture material used. When the pregnancy appears normal the procedure is carried out at about the 16th week, or later if at weekly speculum examination the cervix is observed to be dilating. The principle is to approximate and close the upper part of the cervical canal. The original technique employed fascia lata as the suture material (Shirodkar method). With the cervix exposed according to the method to be described, and by means of an aneurysm needle, the fascial strip is placed about the cervix, medial to the descending branches of the uterine arteries. A not difficult, relatively avascular procedure, which follows the basic principles advocated by others, is briefly described here (Fig. 10).

The anesthetized patient is placed in a moderate degree of Trendelenburg position to encourage the fetal membranes to recede into the uterus. The cervix is exposed and grasped carefully and gently by DeLee cervical forceps. After a solution

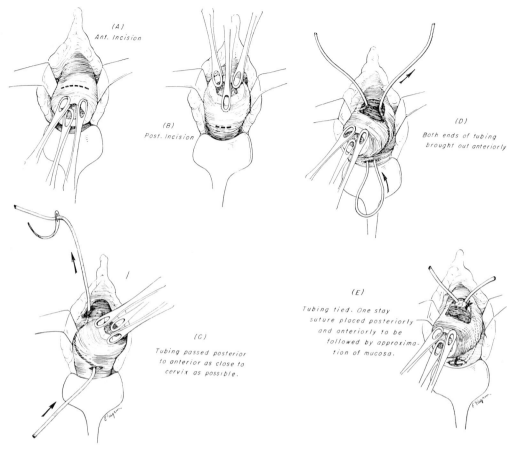

(A)
Ant. Incision

(B)
Post. Incision

(D)
Both ends of tubing
brought out anteriorly

(C)
Tubing passed posterior
to anterior as close to
cervix as possible.

(E)
Tubing tied. One stay
suture placed posteriorly
and anteriorly to be
followed by approxima-
tion of mucosa.

Figure 10.

containing epinephrine is injected locally about the cervix to reduce blood loss and facilitate dissection, an incision is made transversely on the anterior surface of the vaginal portion of the cervix, and the bladder is displaced upward, as in a vaginal hysterectomy. Next, a small transverse incision is made in the vaginal mucous membrane of the posterior fornix where the uterosacral ligaments join the cervix. Through the posterior incision the end of a small polyethylene tube containing a thin silver wire suture is passed forward close to the cervix to emerge anteriorly at the level of the upper end of the cervix. The other end of the suture is passed in similar manner around the opposite side of the cervix, thereby forming a sling or mattress suture about the cervix. One or two other sutures are simultaneously placed either distal to or above the first. The anterior and posterior incisions are closed, and the procedure is completed.

Near term, in most cases, the sutures are removed and the patient is allowed to deliver vaginally. The sutures can be satisfactorily replaced in a subsequent pregnancy. In some cases, however, circumstances will demand that the patient be delivered by cesarean section, in which event the sutures can be left in place. Other forms of suture are used, some permanent in nature, in which case delivery must be accomplished by abdominal hysterotomy.

Should the membranes rupture and labor ensue before the fetus reaches a state of medical viability, the sutures as here described can and should be removed promptly to obviate the hazard of infection or serious trauma to the cervix. The suture material used in the technique described can be readily removed. The incidence of success in pregnancies so managed has been approximately 85 to 90 per cent in patients with repeated pregnancy losses when the conceptus has been otherwise normal.

In an attempt to report on the results of

treatment of habitual abortion from a voluminous literature, criticism may be leveled at all forms of treatment, for rarely is attention given to providing proper controls. Moreover, when specific medication is administered the patient is usually receiving more personal obstetric supervision and care. Until the factors that control pregnancy are known, the treatment of habitual abortion will remain in the realm of empiricism.

In summary, the treatment of habitual abortion begins with a careful medical evaluation of the patient, with a search being made for local or systemic conditions that might contribute toward accidents of pregnancy (see Etiology). Personal problems should be recognized and discussed prior to pregnancy, and a regimen that gives careful attention to proper nutrition and weight control should be outlined for the patient. The recommendations should include daily periods of rest, and, in special cases, the restriction of activity to the point of a bed-and-chair existence.

In the evaluation of the status of the pregnancy in patients with recurrent and habitual abortion, study of urinary pregnanediol and the vaginal smear karyopyknotic index and the cervical mucus appear useful. Infection may distort the latter two examinations. This can be avoided in the case of the karyopyknotic index by preparing the smear from urine. Progesterone deficiency is indicated if the predominantly navicular cells observed in the vaginal smear in normal pregnancy disappear and if there is an increase in cornification from 10 to 15 per cent to 30 to 40 per cent. A progesterone lack and unopposed estrogenic effect is also denoted by the presence of ferning. Low cornification and absence of ferning indicate a normal progesterone secretion.

Normally, urinary excretion of pregnanediol at the onset of pregnancy is approximately 10 mg. per 24 hours, increasing by 10 mg. each month. This represents about 10 per cent of the daily progesterone secretion and affords an index of the amount of the hormone required when substitutional therapy is being considered. Hence, pregnanediol values below 10 or 20 or 30 mg. per 24 hours for the first three months of pregnancy may connote impending abortion. Thus, in the management of the patient with previous repetitive abortion, assuming previous cytogenetic studies were normal, replacement therapy of progesterone or progestational steroids, in physiologic amounts, should be considered.

The patient is seen frequently throughout pregnancy, to give her the benefit of the reassurance derived from the fact that the pregnancy is progressing normally. When the history suggests that the patient may have an incompetent cervix syndrome, speculum examination is performed at each visit and, if the cervix appears closed, a gentle vaginal examination is made to verify the fact that the cervix is not effaced or dilated. Should there be any question, the patient is hospitalized for observation to determine the status of uterine motility and the desirability of closing the cervix surgically. Granted that it is difficult to evaluate the patient's description of her symptoms, attention must be given to a history of uterine irritability, and sometimes hospitalization for a period of observation is advisable. Only in this way is it possible to appraise the patient's symptoms, and experience attests to the fact that the uterus seems to become quiescent under the apparent security of hospital environment without any specific treatment. This is cited to illustrate how individualized the treatment and the evaluation of results attributed to specific therapy must be.

Therapeutic or Artificial Abortion

Conventionally referred to as a therapeutic abortion when it was performed mainly to save the life and reason of the mother, the broadening of the indications for the procedure suggests that this is an outmoded term. Perhaps the terms artificial and medically induced abortion would be more appropriate. These terms would be used when the procedure is performed in accordance with established medical standards and policy, whereas criminal abortion would continue to be applied when the procedure is performed under conditions where these stipulations are not fulfilled.

There is perhaps no medical procedure that is receiving greater scrutiny by both the profession and society than that of artificial or medically induced abortion. Society is aware that the statutes governing medical abortion are in the process of revision or have been revised in many states. Society anticipates and indeed intends that medicine, like the law, will respond to social needs whether or not the profession is of like mind. This is certainly applicable here, where it is plainly evident that there is a rising tide of social and professional sentiment to have the indications for abortion extended to meet whatever is the social need. In fact, the opinion has been expressed both in and out of the profession that all statutes governing the procedure should be rescinded.

The major reason cited for liberalization of the statutes is to reduce criminal abortion with all its health hazards, certainly a laudable objective. The more extreme view is that abortion should be available to any woman who does not wish the pregnancy to continue. The latter is obviously more a social than a medical issue or indication.

Reliable information and facts on this controversial issue are difficult to obtain. For example, in any society or nation, the true incidence of criminal abortion is uncertain. The frequency may be crudely estimated from the assumption that perhaps 20 per cent of those undergoing criminal abortions are admitted to the hospital, that is, only those who develop complications. Also, the prevalence of artificial abortion compared with the number of live births is often difficult to determine from state to state and in many nations. When abortion is available to any woman the incidence to that of live births may range from 10 to more than 100 per cent. When the procedure is used as a method of population control, the incidence will vary depending on the birth and death rate and the availability and desire to use methods for conception control. At present in the United States if the annual birth rate (18 per 1000) were reduced to match the annual death rate (12 per 1000), despite conception control some one and a half million abortions would have to be performed in order to stabilize the population. This is mentioned for logistic purposes in the event this procedure is utilized as a method of population control, to show what is required to stabilize the population at its present level.

There is no uniform legal statute governing this procedure for the United States. Many states have highly restrictive laws; a few have no statute on therapeutic or artificial abortion, although they define criminal abortion. Regardless of the statutes it is how the courts interpret them that is basic, for that is indeed the law.

By contrast, many nations, if not most, have permitted abortion on medicosocial indications, beginning with Sweden in 1938. The Abortion Act of 1967 of the United Kingdom extended the indications, as did the American Law Institute in the United States. Their influence is recognized in the following statement by The American College of Obstetricians and Gynecologists:

Termination of pregnancy by therapeutic abortion is a medical procedure. It must be performed only in a hospital accredited by the Joint Commission on Accreditation of Hospitals and by a licensed physician qualified to perform such operation.

Therapeutic abortion is permitted only with the informed consent of the patient and her husband, or herself if unmarried, or of her nearest relative if she is under the age of consent. No patient should be compelled to undergo, or a physician to perform, a therapeutic abortion if either has ethical, religious or any other objections to it.

A consultative opinion must be obtained from at least two licensed physicians other than the one who is to perform the procedure. This opinion should state that the procedure is medically indicated. The consultants may act separately or as a special committee. One consultant should be a qualified obstetrician-gynecologist and one should have special competence in the medical area in which the medical indications for the procedure reside.

Therapeutic abortion may be performed for the following established medical indications:

1. When continuation of the pregnancy may threaten the life of the woman or seriously impair her health. In determining whether or not there is such risk to health, account may be taken of the patient's total environment, actual or reasonably foreseeable.

2. When pregnancy has resulted from rape or incest: in this case the same medical criteria should be employed in the evaluation of the patient.

3. When continuation of the pregnancy is likely to result in the birth of a child with grave physical deformities or mental retardation.

In the interpretation of this statement, the second sentence of the first indication is ostensibly from the recent British law and takes into account the medical status of the patient in terms of her socioeconomic environment. This is written into the second indication also. In addition, the writer suggests that the teenager be here included, on the assumption that the immature person may not have the capability to apply critical discrimination and judgment. The same reasoning might apply in making a determination and decision as to the advisability of an artificial abortion for psychiatric reasons.

The statutes in most states are being considered and revised and several states have removed or are now removing their statutes. It would be rather meaningless to list the statutes in the various states in this period of change. Indeed the issue may well be resolved at the federal level, the constitutionality being within the framework of the "general welfare." Thus, Congress and the Supreme Court might determine and decide whether or not there should be a statute for any state or a uniform statute for all states.

Irrespective of how and to what degree the statutes are changed, including elimination of all statutes governing artificial or medical abortion, the complications, be they medical or psychologic, and related issues must be carefully and periodically assessed. For example, although the incidence apparently declines, criminal abortion is not eliminated, however liberal may be the statutes governing medical or artificial abortion, and even where there are no statutes. There are apparently several reasons for this. Believing that an extensive social and medical investigation may be made—and in many countries with liberal laws this is so, to wit, Sweden—some women may be reluctant to apply for a legal abortion and hence will seek the criminal abortionist. In a married couple, the desire of the husband may differ from that of the wife. There is the possibility that the request may be declined. This raises the question of whether or not this may lead to suicide, especially when the patient threatens it. In the absence of psychiatric illness there is no good evidence the patient will destroy herself. Finally, patients who have had one or more artificial abortions in those nations where they are always available may be reluctant and embarrassed to return repeatedly to the clinic and will resort to other ways of terminating the pregnancy.

It is commonly held that artificial or medical abortion is without appreciable risk prior to the 10th to 12th weeks, if performed as a hospital or medically supervised procedure. Also, it is frequently stated that the death rate is less than the maternal mortality. However, the latter includes deaths from abortion, and these should be removed for purposes of valid comparison. In assessing risk it must be recognized that the criminal

abortionist tends to avoid the nulliparous patient, particularly if the pregnancy is beyond the 10th to 12th week.

Unfortunately many patients come under surveillance only after that period, and here a more formidable procedure than a cervical dilatation and curettage must be considered. The immediate risk and sequelae rise and the influence on future childbearing may be substantial. Intra-amniotic saline infusion is not without its dangers. Abdominal hysterotomy requires a recovery period and leaves the patient in a less favorable state for future childbearing. These patients acquire the risk of uterine rupture in a later pregnancy and the possible need for delivery by cesarean section. Forceful dilatation of the cervix, particularly if repeatedly performed, may cause a state of relative infertility through the syndrome of the incompetent cervix and less well understood factors such as tubal dysfunction. The vacuum method of abortion can cause myometrial disruption, and uterine perforation by the curette is always a hazard. If the Rh-negative patient is not protected by immunoglobulin, sensitization may follow. With the instrumentation and manipulation required, fetal red cells may gain entrance to the maternal circulation in artificial abortion more frequently and in greater quantity than in spontaneous abortion.

The psychology overlay and residual in patients who have had therapeutic or artificial abortion for indications beyond those of strict medical reasons has not yet been determined in sufficient numbers of such women to warrant convincing conclusions. It should follow that when the public is sufficiently informed and realizes that artificial abortion is subject to complications immediate and remote even when performed under proper supervision and surgical environment, there will be a greater incentive toward conception control. This is supported by the decrease in recent years of the number of abortions performed for population control in Japan.

The pregnancy is terminated by a variety of methods, depending on the gestational age and uterine size. Up to the 8th to 12th week, this is usually accomplished by dilatation of the cervix and curettage or vacuum aspiration. Later in pregnancy (13th to 20th week) recourse must be made to intra-amniotic hypertonic saline solution or abdominal or vaginal hysterotomy. The surgical methods may in the future give way to medical methods of terminating pregnancy, with the introduction of prostaglandin or agents that may interfere with the endocrine activity of the corpus luteum or placenta.

When patients are referred for therapeutic abortion, the physician who is to perform the operation is well advised not to be unduly influenced by the medical opinion of the referring physician. In other words, from his medical conscience, knowledge, and experience, he must be convinced that the procedure is warranted. Although the opinions are sought of consultants who are medical experts in the disease from which the patient suffers, and although the advice is in most instances followed, the final decision must rest with the physician who is to perform the procedure.

It might well be asked whether the physician is in neglect if he fails to perform a therapeutic abortion when accepted medical practice dictates such a course. It is presumed that if in the physician's opinion the patient's life is not in imminent danger, he cannot be held in neglect. Otherwise, he could be performing an abortion contrary to conscience and in some states this might be an illegal abortion.

In summary, therapeutic or artificial abortion for purely medical reasons, i.e., vascular, renal, or heart disease, and so forth, is rarely indicated in current medical practice. With liberalization of the statutes governing the procedure the indications are being extended in the socioeconomic sphere and in some countries for purposes of population control. Regardless of indications or the methods and procedures, the physical and psychologic risks are real, even under the most careful scrutiny and medical supervision, and the long-term effects are not entirely clear.

Criminal Abortion

Any person who advises or participates in a criminal abortion is criminally liable. It is mandatory in some states that the physician report to the proper authorities any case in which criminal interference is definitely established.

The majority of criminal abortions are said to be self-induced. Catheters, bougies, intrauterine pastes, Lysol, and soap are commonly introduced into the uterus. Intrauterine pastes and soap are particularly dangerous, for when injected into the uterus under pressure the substance may gain entrance into the maternal circulation by way of the endomyometrial veins, causing shock, anuria, and death, or the material may pass directly through the fallopian tubes into the abdominal cavity, producing a peritonitis. Douches, too, containing Lysol and potassium permanganate solution are commonly employed as abortifacients and may result in extensive local tissue damage. Potassium permanganate crystals deposited into the vagina can excoriate the vaginal mucous membrane to the point of causing serious bleeding from the areas so denuded.

The criminal abortionist terminates the pregnancy either by cervical dilatation and curettage or occasionally by uterine pack, wherein a small gauze pack is introduced into the uterus and removed some hours later with the hope that it will cause the patient to abort. The products of conception are often only partially removed, and the patient is frequently discharged, being told that the abortion has been completed. In these patients uterine cramps, lower abdominal pain, and vaginal bleeding will eventually occur, and when the patient seeks medical advice she will have the clinical signs and symptoms of an incomplete septic abortion and should be treated accordingly.

Perforation of the Uterus

The uterus may be accidentally perforated during the course of a curettage in a therapeutic abortion, in the completion of an inevitable abortion, or for purposes of diagnosis. The myometrial wall, being soft and having less substance in the presence of pregnancy, is easily perforated, especially when the uterus is retroverted or acutely anteflexed. The most serious perforation may be encountered in patients who have had an illegal abortion. Here infection is often present and the extent of the perforation is unknown.

In accidental perforation of the uterus incidental to a diagnostic or a therapeutic curettage in the nonpregnant, no treatment is necessary provided there is no further instrumentation at the time. If the operator believes that he has perforated the uterus in the pregnant patient a laparotomy is indicated and the uterus is emptied by hysterotomy. Further vaginal instrumentation would be extremely hazardous. The perforation is usually more extensive in the pregnant patient, with a greater danger of hemorrhage or subsequent peritonitis if the rent is not surgically closed. When there is accompanying infection, particularly in association with an illegal abortion, hysterectomy must be considered as the safest method of management to prevent death from peritonitis or septic shock.

Sexual Sterilization

Because the clinical problems surrounding its indications are so closely related to those of therapeutic or artificial abortion, sexual sterilization is discussed here. The majority of states have statutes pertaining to sexual sterilization, which may include eugenic and, in the case of criminals, punitive sterilization, or relate to voluntary therapeutic sexual sterilization. It appears that the operation, like therapeutic abortion, is permissible as a medical necessity, and the physician must defend his position on this basis. This could be subject to broad interpretation, for it could be argued that voluntary sexual sterilization in the female is prophylaxis against criminal abortion.

Most states have legislation providing for the sterilization of those regarded as morally and mentally inadequate, which includes the feeble-minded, insane, and epileptic. The permission to perform such an operation is derived through consent and due process of the law. History of the era of World War II testifies to the grim fact that the state should never delegate the authority to the physician to be the judge or force him to participate in what is defined as eugenic sterilization. The same applies to medical abortion and a democratic society should be wary of such terms as abortion on demand.

In general, the indications for therapeutic sexual sterilization follow those for therapeutic abortion, and several previous cesarean sections, recurrent toxemia, and cardiovascular renal disease are examples of the more frequent obstetric reasons. Recognition must be given to the possible effect of multiparity on maternal mortality, and this effect may be considered in women who have completed their childbearing. Thus, the procedure is permissible provided the patient and her husband have given their consent and are clearly aware of its meaning. The procedure is usually performed in conjunction with an abdominal hysterotomy or immediately post partum.

In the latter circumstance the delivery is performed in the operating room with provisions made for laparotomy, and the anesthesia is planned accordingly. If it is to be done during the postpartum period, it is best to perform the procedure immediately at the time of delivery for several reasons, the most important being that it eliminates the need for further anesthesia and removes the remote risk of infection. Following uncomplicated labor and delivery and with the uterus well contracted, the abdomen is prepared and draped. The abdomen is opened through a 5 cm. midline incision, beginning about 4 to 5 cm. below the umbilicus. The tubes are readily identified and treated according to the Pomeroy or Irving technique, and the abdomen is closed. The postoperative care is routine, and the patient is allowed to go home per schedule. (See Chapter 29, Operative Obstetrics.)

BIBLIOGRAPHY

Boronow, R. C., McElin, T. W., West, R. H., and Buckingham, J. C.: Ovarian pregnancy. Amer. J. Obstet. Gynec., 91:1095, 1965.

Carr, D. H.: Cytogenetics of abortions. In Benirschke, K., ed.: Comparative Aspects of Reproductive Failure. Springer-Verlag, New York, 1967, p. 96.

Carr, D. H.: Lethal chromosome errors. In Benirschke, K., ed.: Comparative Mammalian Cytogenetics. Springer-Verlag, New York, 1969, p. 68.

Clarkson, A. R., Sage, R. E., and Lawrence, J. R.: Consumption coagulopathy and acute renal failure due to gram-negative septicemia after abortion. Ann. Intern. Med., 70:1191, 1969.

Corner, G. W.: The problem of embryonic pathology in mammals, with observations upon intrauterine mortality in the pig. Amer. J. Anat., 31:523, 1923.

Diggory, P., Peel, J., and Potts, M.: Preliminary assessment of the 1967 Abortion Act in practice. Lancet, 1:287, 1970.

Easterday, C. L., and Reid, D. E.: The incompetent cervix in repetitive abortion and premature labor. New Eng. J. Med., 260:687, 1959.

Finn, W. F.: The outcome of pregnancy following vaginal operations. Amer. J. Obstet. Gynec., 56:291, 1948.

Fujikura, T., Froehlich, L. A., and Driscoll, S. G.: A simplified anatomic classification of abortions. Amer. J. Obstet. Gynec., 95:902, 1966.

Geneva Conference: Standardization of procedures for chromosome studies in abortion. Bull. WHO, 34:765, 1966.

Green-Armytage, V. B., and McClure Browne, J. C.: Habitual abortion due to insufficiency of internal cervical os. Brit. Med. J., 2:128, 1957.

Heer, D. M.: Abortion, contraception and population policy in the Soviet Union. Demography, 2:531, 1965.

Hertig, A. T.: The overall problem in man. In Benirschke, K., ed.: Comparative Aspects of Reproductive Failure. Springer-Verlag, New York, 1967, p. 11.

Hertig, A. T., and Sheldon, W. H.: Minimal criteria to prove prima facie case of traumatic abortion or miscarriage; analysis of 1000 spontaneous abortions. Ann. Surg., 117:596, 1943.

Huldt, L.: Outcome of pregnancy when legal abortion is readily available. Lancet, 1:467, 1968.

Indications for termination of pregnancy. Report by B.M.A. Committee on Therapeutic Abortion. Brit. Med. J., 1:171, 1968.

Jones, W. S., Delfs, E., and Jones, G. E. S.: Reproductive difficulties in double uterus; the place of plastic reconstruction. Amer. J. Obstet. Gynec., 72:865, 1956.

Kundsin, R. B., Driscoll, S. G., and Ming, P. M. L.: Strain of Mycoplasma associated with human reproductive failure. Science, 157:1573, 1967.

Litwak, O., Taswell, H. F., and Banner, E. A.: Transplacental fetal bleeding in spontaneous abortion. Lancet, 2:1161, 1969.

Makino, S., Awa, A. A., and Sasaki, M.: Chromosome studies in normal human subjects. Ann. N.Y. Acad. Sci., 155:679, 1968.

Mall, F. P., and Meyer, A. W.: Studies on abortions; survey of pathologic ova in Carnegie embryological collection. Contrib. Embryol., 12:1, 1921.

Matthews, C. D., and Matthews, A. E. B.: Transplacental haemorrhage in spontaneous and induced abortion. Lancet, 1:694, 1969.

McDonald, J. A.: Suture of the cervix for inevitable miscarriage. J. Obstet. Gynaec. Brit. Comm., 64: 346, 1957.

McKay, D. G., Jewett, J. F., and Reid, D. E.: Endotoxin shock and the generalized Shwartzman reaction in pregnancy. Amer. J. Obstet. Gynec., 78:546, 1959.

Philippe, E., and Boué, J. G.: Le placenta des aberrations chromosomiques létales. Ann. Anat. Path. (Paris), 14:249, 1969.

Prystowsky, H., and Eastman, N. J.: Puerperal tubal sterilization; report of 1,830 cases. J.A.M.A., 158: 463, 1955.

Reid, D. E.: Assessment and management of the seriously ill patient following abortion. J.A.M.A., 199: 805, 1967.

Reid, D. E.: Population Control—Medical and Public Policy. Harvard Med. Alumni Bull., 45:4, 1970.

Ricciardi, I., and Kupperman, H. S.: Management of threatened early abortion. In Reid, D. E., and Barton, T. C., eds.: Controversy in Obstetrics and Gynecology. W. B. Saunders Company, Philadelphia, 1969, p. 23.

Sergovich, F., Valentine, G. H., Chen, A. T. L., Kinch, R. A. H., and Smout, M. S.: Chromosome aberrations in 2159 consecutive newborn babies. New Eng. J. Med., 280:851, 1969.

Shirodkar, V. N.: New method of operative treatment for habitual abortions in second trimester of pregnancy. Antiseptic, 52:299, 1955.

Spangler, J. J.: Population problem: in search of a solution. Science, 166:1234, 1969.

Stickle, G.: Defective development and reproductive wastage in the United States. Amer. J. Obstet. Gynec., 100:442, 1968.

Strassmann, E. O.: Plastic unification of double uterus; a study of 123 collected and five personal cases. Amer. J. Obstet. Gynec., 64:25, 1952.

Studdiford, W. E., and Douglas, G. W.: Placental bacteremia; a significant finding in septic abortion accompanied by vascular collapse. Amer. J. Obstet. Gynec., 71:842, 1956.

Wilkens, L., Jones, H. W., Jr., Holman, G. H., and Stempfel, R. S., Jr.: Masculinization of female fetus associated with administration of oral and intramuscular progestins during gestation; nonadrenal female pseudohermaphrodism. J. Clin. Endocr., 18: 559, 1958.

Chapter 13

Ectopic Pregnancy

DEFINITION

Ectopic, extrauterine, and tubal pregnancy are terms to designate pregnancies occurring outside the uterine cavity. The former two terms include ovarian and abdominal pregnancies, as well as those implanting in the oviduct, which are commonly referred to as tubal pregnancies. Approximately 98 per cent of extrauterine pregnancies are tubal in type.

TUBAL PREGNANCY

The various conditions suggested for the causation of tubal pregnancy are the following:

1. Congenital anatomic variations in the oviduct, including diverticula, defective cilia formation of the tubal epithelium, and embryonal deposition of endometrial stroma with the potential to form decidua.

2. Anatomic alterations of the oviduct resulting from pelvic inflammatory disease, which may follow gonorrheal and, more rarely, postabortal infection and pelvic tuberculosis. The usual incidence of tubal pregnancy is listed from 0.25 to 1.0 per cent of all pregnancies, but where pelvic inflammatory disease is prevalent, tubal pregnancy has been reported to occur once in 30 pregnancies and hence can be the commonest surgical emergency.

3. Endometriosis of the oviduct, with the transplanted endometrium providing a possible site for nidation.

4. Plastic operation for restoration of tubal luminal patency. Whatever type of operation is performed, ectopic pregnancy occurs with disturbing frequency following these procedures.

The impression has been gained that the frequency of tubal pregnancies has increased since the advent of antibiotics and chemotherapeutic agents. It is proposed that the therapy prevents tubal occlusion, but the mucosa fails to escape injury; this causes a disturbance in normal migration of the ovum. Patients who have had one ectopic pregnancy appear to be more prone to have another in the remaining tube, as frequently as 10 per cent where the incidence of pelvic inflammation is high. It should also be noted that tubal pregnancy can occur in the presence of an intrauterine device (IUD).

The pathology of tubal pregnancy finds the ovum implanting in either the interstitial, the isthmic, or the ampullary portion of the oviduct with the trophoblast invading the mucosa and muscularis, eventually penetrating to the serosa. On histologic examination decidual cells are sometimes observed at the implantation site. Whether the penetration of the tube is facilitated by the lack or absence of decidua is speculative, for the decidua has been assigned the function of determining the extent of the effect of the proteolytic or invasive capacity of the trophoblast. However, many ectopic pregnancies have the histologic quality of a placenta accreta and a placenta percreta. The sudden onset of pain may be the result of intratubal abruptio.

The embryo is often absent and when present it may be stunted. The fact that the ovum is rarely normal and is frequently "blighted" in tubal pregnancy offers evidence that conditions associated with implantation or environmental factors may cause deviations in normal ovular development. The villi in the conceptus of a tubal pregnancy commonly show hydatid change. In fact, molar pregnancy may occur and choriocarcinoma may be the sequela of a tubal pregnancy.

It is well to consider separately the pathology of the various types of tubal pregnancy, for the signs, the symptoms, and the clinical course of extrauterine pregnancy depend in some measure on the portion of the tube where implantation occurs.

The *interstitial* or *cornual* type has features of both intrauterine and extrauterine pregnancy. Like other portions of the uterine corpus, the cornual area containing the tube hypertrophies, permitting the conceptus to reach sizable proportions before it penetrates the uterine and tubal wall and causes rupture. In the cornual form, therefore, the pregnancy may reach the beginning of the middle trimester before signs and symptoms appear. In fact, rupture may occur unheralded by uterine bleeding or any complaints except those of a normal pregnancy. As pregnancy advances, a portion of the conceptus expands and grows into the uterine cavity, and a considerable amount of the trophoblast becomes nourished by the uterine decidua. The sex steroid output may be comparable to the amount secreted in a normal intrauterine pregnancy. Consequently, in contrast to other forms of tubal pregnancy, the uterine decidua is not likely to regress in the cornual type, thereby accounting for the absence of vaginal bleeding. Accordingly, neither the patient nor the physician is forewarned of impending rupture. Cornual pregnancy, therefore, is the most dangerous type of tubal pregnancy, for the diagnosis is often not made prior to rupture, and the intra-abdominal hemorrhage is sudden, usually massive, and an immediate threat to life.

The *isthmic type* is more common, with the patients presenting the classic signs and symptoms attributed to this condition. Owing to the small caliber of the tube, the trophoblast may penetrate to the peritoneal surface within two or three weeks after the first missed period (Fig. 1). Rupture usually occurs on the abdominal surface, but occasionally the tube may rupture into the broad

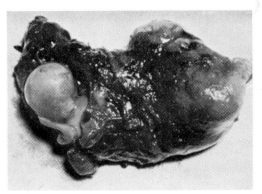

Figure 2. Tubal pregnancy with extrusion of the fetus through the ampullary portion of the tube.

ligament. In the latter case a hematoma may form, causing only mild abdominal or systemic complaints, and the patient may not consult a physician for some time. There may be no symptoms for several weeks, but with further growth of the pregnancy, together with enlargement of the hematoma, the broad ligament may finally rupture, its contents being extruded into the abdominal cavity. Again, the pregnancy may remain quiescent in the broad ligament and be regarded as a broad ligament mass other than an ectopic pregnancy. The latter situations may be referred to as a *chronic type* of ectopic pregnancy. Emphasized here is the fact that the physician should not discard ectopic pregnancy from the differential diagnosis of a pelvic mass simply because the patient's last normal period occurred many months rather than only a few weeks before.

The *ampullary type* possibly occurs more frequently than any of the other forms of tubal pregnancy. When implantation occurs near the fimbria, the ovum may be extruded into the peritoneal cavity without injury to the tube. The symptoms of so-called *tubal abortion* may be so mild that the patient may not consult a physician; hence, the incidence of ampullary implantation is not accurately known. Transient pelvic pain, lasting only a few hours, is often the only symptom. Following tubal abortion, however, bleeding from the implantation site may become accentuated, leading to the signs and symptoms of intra-abdominal hemorrhage. Further, when implantation occurs medial to the fimbria, the clinical course is comparable to that of the isthmic type, leading to eventual rupture (Fig. 2).

Ovarian pregnancy is mentioned here, for

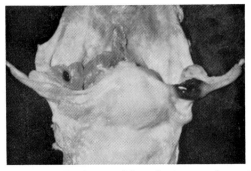

Figure 1. Fatal case of the isthmic type of ectopic pregnancy. Corpus luteum in the right ovary evidences transmigration of the egg with implantation in the left tube. (Courtesy of the Department of Legal Medicine, Harvard University Medical School.)

the preoperative diagnosis is usually between tubal pregnancy of the ampullary type and an ovarian tumor. To qualify for a diagnosis of ovarian pregnancy, the egg must be fertilized and implant within its follicle and not upon the surface of the ovary (Fig. 3). The latter would be an abdominal pregnancy. The majority of cases come to surgery by the end of the first trimester with the exact diagnosis usually being established at laparotomy.

Diagnosis of Tubal Pregnancy

Cases of ectopic pregnancy continue to appear in maternal mortality statistics with three to four deaths per 1000 cases. The deaths are in the women who fail to consult the physician on the question of pregnancy until after the second or third missed period. The history reveals that the patient has disregarded vaginal staining for several days or weeks, and is suddenly seized with abdominal pain, collapses, and dies before she can receive surgical attention. Fortunately, most patients who have reason to suspect that they are pregnant and who have vaginal bleeding are anxious to know if they are pregnant and whether the pregnancy is normal.

Because some degree of vaginal bleeding is common in early pregnancy, the diagnosis of ectopic pregnancy must be considered frequently. To establish the diagnosis of ectopic pregnancy before the event of rupture, it is imperative that certain of these patients with vaginal staining be examined at frequent intervals until the physician is satisfied that ectopic pregnancy can be excluded from the differential diagnosis.

The diagnosis of ectopic pregnancy prior to rupture is never certain short of an exploratory laparotomy or laparoscopy, and following rupture the diagnosis is usually obvious. Thus, the diagnosis should be considered under two categories—the suspected or unruptured and the ruptured state.

With regard to patient history, some consideration should be given to age, parity, and previous reproductive performance. Women with a history of longstanding sterility are more apt to initiate their reproductive careers with a tubal pregnancy. Although the characteristic history reveals one or more missed periods or a scanty menses, cases are encountered in which the *reliable* patient is unaware of any abnormality of the menstrual cycle. In retrospect, it may be said that the patient furnished an inaccurate story, but the practical fact remains that *a history of a normal menses does not exclude the possibility of ectopic pregnancy*, however the physician wishes to interpret the patient's story.

A history of amenorrhea or a disturbance in the normal menstrual cycle, vaginal staining beginning a few days or two to three weeks after the missed period, the sudden onset of abdominal pain, often while straining at stool, and syncope are the characteristic symptoms in nearly all cases. The latter two symptoms may indicate beginning or frank tubal rupture. Often the patient has an urge to urinate or defecate when blood is present in the pelvis.

Before rupture, the symptoms of lower abdominal and pelvic discomfort may be vague. Frequently in the earlier stage there are no abdominal findings, although some suprapubic tenderness and spasm should develop eventually. Vaginal examination reveals a uterus that is not appreciably enlarged over the nonpregnant state. Movement of the cervix commonly elicits sharp, rather localized, pelvic pain. This is regarded as a common but not necessarily a universal response in ectopic pregnancy. Early in the disease an adnexal mass may be described as cylindrical and finger-like in shape, but later it becomes more oval in outline and may increase in size to several centimeters in diameter.

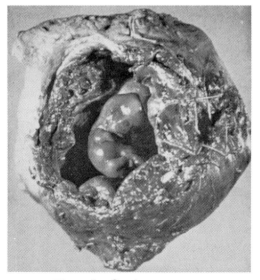

Figure 3. Ovarian pregnancy.

The diagnosis of *unruptured ectopic pregnancy* involves a series of diagnostic tests and procedures, including leukocyte count, which is commonly elevated (10,000 to 20,000), hemoglobin and hematocrit determinations, and routine urinalysis. The sedimentation rate is useful in differentiating between ectopic pregnancy and pelvic infection, showing only a modest increase in the presence of a pregnancy, and being considerably elevated in acute pelvic infection. Depending on the viability of the chorionic elements, the biologic test for pregnancy is positive in no more than half of the cases of ectopic pregnancy. In other words, a positive test is helpful, but a negative test does not exclude the diagnosis of ectopic pregnancy.

A generous amount of endometrium showing complete decidual change might be expected in ectopic pregnancy, but *this is rarely found* either by endometrial biopsy or at curettage. If the patient has bled for any appreciable time the endometrium will have been shed, and the amount of tissue obtained at curettage may be meager. Also, in only about 20 per cent of cases will there be typical decidua; of the remainder, about half will have proliferative endometrium, and in the rest the endometrium will be in various periods of the secretory phase (Fig.

4). Like the biologic test for pregnancy, the presence or absence of decidua will depend on the viability of the syncytium and its ability to secrete a normal amount of gonadotropins and sex steroids. *Thus, a scanty endometrium or its lack of decidual reaction does not exclude the diagnosis of ectopic pregnancy.* Endometrial atypia is sometimes associated with ectopic pregnancy, the so-called Arias-Stella reaction.

With a convincing history, a positive biologic test for pregnancy, the presence of an adnexal mass, a uterus that is only slightly enlarged over the nonpregnant state, and nonclotting blood on culdocentesis, the diagnosis of ectopic pregnancy is tenable. Before laparotomy is performed, however, the uterus should be curetted to exclude an incomplete abortion or a "blighted ovum," conditions that can on occasion closely simulate an ectopic pregnancy, with minimal bleeding and approximately normal size of the uterus.

When the diagnostic evidence is less definite, namely, when the biologic test is negative and the presence of an adnexal mass is questionable, rather than resorting immediately to exploratory laparotomy, it is recommended that the cul-de-sac be explored either by culdoscopy or by colpo-

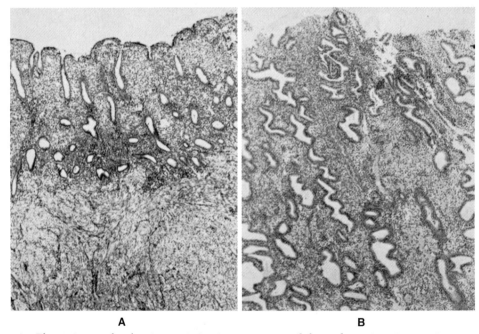

A   **B**

Figure 4. Photomicrographs showing variation in appearance of the endometrium in ectopic pregnancy. A, Proliferative endometrium. ×35. B, Secretory endometrium associated with tubal pregnancy. The glands are moderately tortuous with basal vacuolization and extensive stromal edema. ×50. (B from Romney, S. L., Hertig, A. T., and Reid, D. E.: Surg., Gynec. Obstet., 91:605, 1950.)

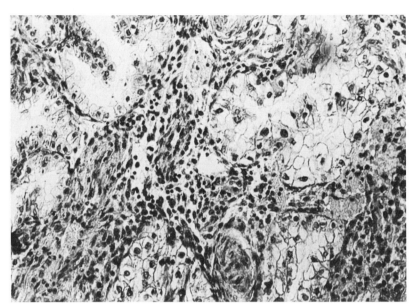

Figure 5. The Arias-Stella reaction of the endometrium observed in association with an ectopic pregnancy. Nuclear enlargement, pleomorphism, and hyperchromatism are characteristic and should not be mistaken for neoplasia.

tomy. In the hands of the experienced operator, the peritoneoscope or culdoscope will furnish valuable information about the type of pelvic pathologic change present.

Equally effective is a surgical colpotomy, that is, incision and opening of the posterior cul-de-sac. This relatively simple and safe procedure is carried out in the following manner. After the patient has been anesthetized, prepared, and draped, with traction the cervix is brought downward and forward, and the posterior fornix of the vagina is exposed. Posterior to the cervical insertion of the uterosacral ligaments a small transverse incision is made in the vaginal mucous membrane and the peritoneum is opened. If tubal rupture has occurred, free blood will be encountered, in which event the peritoneum can be quickly closed and laparotomy performed. If the cul-de-sac does not contain blood, the tubes and ovaries can be exposed and inspected to rule out adnexal disease or the possibility of an unruptured ectopic pregnancy. If no abnormality is found, a few stitches will close the peritoneum and vaginal mucous membrane. The patient can leave the hospital in a day or two without the risk and discomfort of an exploratory laparotomy. Furthermore, some prefer this procedure to needle aspiration of the cul-de-sac or culdocentesis, for the latter may fail to locate free blood in the peritoneal cavity.

In other words, a negative culdocentesis does not exclude the diagnosis; only when it is positive is the procedure of value.

In résumé, when the history reveals a disturbance in the menstrual cycle a suspected ectopic pregnancy must be considered if the diagnosis is to be made prior to frank rupture with its consequences. When the diagnosis of pregnancy or the normalcy of the pregnancy is being equated against the possibility of an ectopic pregnancy, repeated vaginal examination (at times biweekly) is indicated. If in the course of these examinations an ectopic pregnancy becomes more than a suspicion because of the development of a questionable or definite adnexal mass, and there is pelvic tenderness on movement of the cervix and the uterus is not appreciably enlarged, a culdocentesis as an office procedure, together with a biologic test for pregnancy, should be performed. If either is positive, hospitalization and further investigation are indicated. The diagnosis is not excluded if these procedures are negative, and the patient should be followed closely. If the uterus fails to enlarge to a size consistent with a normal pregnancy or an adnexal mass becomes definable, the patient should be hospitalized and examined under anesthesia with preparations made for laparotomy. Culdoscopy or culdotomy should be performed to confirm or exclude the diagnosis. The question arises whether a curettage should be performed prior to culdostomy, the fear being that the patient might be normally pregnant. If the uterus is only slightly enlarged and definitely smaller in size than for the gestational period, a curettage is indicated on the possibility that it may reveal a blighted ovum. If the latter is encountered, culdotomy may still be indicated if there is any question concerning the status of the adnexa, for simultaneous intrauterine and extrauterine pregnancy is a possibility, albeit rare.

Finally, in the case of a cornual or interstitial pregnancy, the pelvic examination reveals an asymmetric uterus. Also, in the early weeks of a normal pregnancy, the uterus may feel somewhat asymmetric, but by the 10th week the uterus becomes symmetric as elicited on repeated vaginal bimanual examination. A pregnancy in a bicornuate uterus will reveal asymmetry also. Because of the hazards of cornual pregnancy, an exploratory laparotomy or laparoscopy should be performed if there is any doubt regarding the diagnosis.

The diagnosis of a ruptured ectopic pregnancy is more obvious, with the extent of the signs and symptoms being governed largely by the amount of intraperitoneal hemorrhage. The pertinent physical findings are those of abdominal pain, tenderness, and rigidity with evidence of fluid in the abdomen. Bluing of the skin about the umbilicus is a late sign and is present only when the peritoneal hemorrhage is extensive. When the blood extends to the diaphragm, there may be shoulder pain. Varying degrees of shock are usually present, commensurate with the amount of blood shed.

Differential Diagnosis of Tubal Pregnancy

The differential diagnosis of tubal pregnancy includes the following conditions. (1) Corpus luteum cyst is by all odds the most frequent cause of transient amenorrhea in normal healthy women. Failure of the corpus luteum to undergo normal regression following ovulation may delay the menses indefinitely, usually for two to three weeks at least. The endometrium may show predecidual or decidual changes. The biologic test for pregnancy is negative, however, and the pelvic findings are consistent with a small ovarian cyst. Pelvic tenderness is not elicited on motion of the cervix, and there are no other signs to suggest ectopic pregnancy. These patients should be examined frequently until a normal period occurs or until the physician is convinced that the ovarian enlargement has disappeared. The cysts usually regress, rarely requiring definitive surgical therapy, and the menstrual periods return to normal. (2) Besides causing a mass, tubal infection may upset the menstrual flow, but this usually takes the form of hypermenorrhea. Several other pelvic conditions must also be considered in the differential diagnosis, the most important being (3) degeneration of a leiomyoma, particularly when it is located in the broad ligament; (4) an ovarian cyst, especially with pain due to torsion; and (5) appendicitis, especially when the appendix has a pelvic location. These various pelvic conditions may mask the presence of an extrauterine pregnancy, and here the biologic test for pregnancy has its greatest value.

Treatment of Tubal Pregnancy

The patient who enters the hospital with tubal rupture requires immediate surgery. Since shock is a constant threat, the anesthesia should be of the inhalation type. Rather than attempt to restore blood volume prior to surgery, it has been advocated, and wisely so, that transfusion be started simultaneously with the abdominal incision and, as soon as hemostasis is achieved, the blood should be administered rapidly in amounts to restore the volume to normal. Attempts to raise the blood pressure preoperatively can result in further abdominal hemorrhage. In patients who approach surgery in shock, venous cut-downs should be used to ensure an uninterrupted flow of blood during transfusion. As a gauge in restoring the blood volume to normal, central venous monitoring is essential.

The laparotomy should be performed with dispatch for the sole purpose of establishing hemostasis. Valuable time should not be lost in attempting to pack off the abdominal contents and to expose the uterus in the conventional manner. In the presence of any degree of hemoperitoneum this procedure will not give adequate exposure and will only disturb whatever clotting has occurred about the bleeding site. Rather, the operator should grasp the uterus and bring it into the wound and quickly identify the involved tube. When a hemostat is placed at the area of the utero-ovarian anastomosis and beneath and parallel to the involved tube, hemostasis is effected. Salpingectomy is performed, with preservation of the ovary whenever possible. When a hematoma has formed in the broad ligament it may be necessary to perform a salpingo-oophorectomy.

If one tube has previously been removed, an attempt to preserve the remaining tube by resection and reconstruction may be warranted. In cases of tubal abortion, when the implantation site is on the fimbria, the bleeding may be controlled by suture ligatures and the tube preserved. In interstitial pregnancy, the cornua may be resected and the uterus left intact. Such a procedure may weaken the myometrial wall, however, and cesarean section is undoubtedly the safer method of delivery for a subsequent pregnancy.

SIMULTANEOUS INTRAUTERINE AND EXTRAUTERINE PREGNANCY, OR COMBINED PREGNANCY

Simultaneous intrauterine and extrauterine pregnancy occurs once in the course of several thousand pregnancies. Extrauterine pregnancy is masked initially in the presence of a pregnant uterus consistent in size for the gestational date. Pelvic pain and tenderness in the presence of adnexal discomfort raise a question of an abnormality and the suspicion of so-called combined pregnancy. The appearance of the signs and symptoms of peritoneal irritation forces the issue, and the diagnosis is established by exploratory laparotomy. With removal of the involved tube, every precaution is taken to preserve the intrauterine pregnancy. Sedatives in generous amounts, in conjunction with intensive progesterone therapy, may prevent an abortion in the postoperative recovery period.

The simultaneous occurrence of an intra-

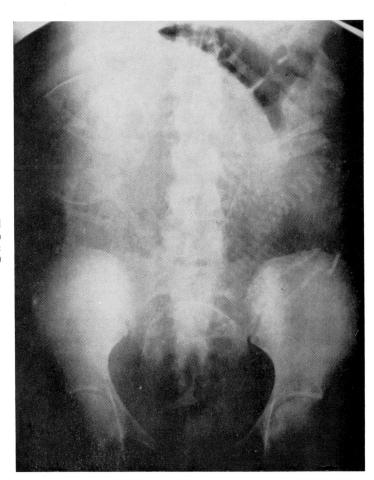

Figure 6. Simultaneous abdominal and uterine term pregnancies. (From Vasicka, A. I., and Grable, E. E.: Obstet. Gynec. Survey, 11:603, 1956.)

uterine and an abdominal pregnancy (Fig. 6) has been recorded, with both fetuses reaching the stage of medical viability. The problem is primarily that of the abdominal pregnancy and the patient is treated accordingly.

ABDOMINAL PREGNANCY

Abdominal pregnancy is extremely rare and, although it may occur as a primary implant, it may develop secondary to tubal abortion. The site of implantation may be anywhere within the abdominal cavity or on its contents, but more often implantation occurs on the surface of the pelvic peritoneum or the structures of the reproductive system. The condition may go undetected and the fetus succumb and become a lithopedion, being identified years later incidental to abdominal exploration or necropsy.

The history will sometimes include slight vaginal staining of a few days' duration, sometime after the missed period. The bleeding presumably coincides with the time of tubal abortion and secondary implantation, and is attributed to a transient decrease in sex steroid production resulting therefrom. However, many of the cases of early abdominal pregnancy are diagnosed at laparotomy, the preoperative diagnosis having been tubal pregnancy.

Pain is the universal symptom, its origin and the location of the associated tenderness being related to the area of implantation. A fluctuant mass may be outlined on either vaginal or abdominal palpation, and, should the fetus be sizable, it may be palpated with great ease, which, indeed, gives the examiner the impression that it lies beneath the skin of the abdomen. On bimanual examination, the uterus is not appreciably enlarged and is sometimes difficult to outline, being displaced by the abdominal conceptus. Examination under anesthesia may prove helpful, and, if the uterus is approximately normal in size, probing of the uterus and curettage will assure the clinician that the pregnancy is extrauterine. Finally, by the use of the soft tissue technique of x-ray examination, a procedure similar to placentography, it should be possible to demonstrate that the fetus is not contained within the uterus.

Once the diagnosis has been made, the wisdom of waiting until the fetus matures must be considered in planning the management of the case. Regardless of the type of management used, the fetal mortality is high. Further, the placenta may detach at any time, a serious complication even with the patient in the hospital under observation. Thus, many authorities feel that the condition should be dealt with surgically as soon as the diagnosis is made. However, if the diagnosis is made in the latter weeks of pregnancy and the patient is free of symptoms, the pregnancy may be allowed to continue until the viability of the fetus is assured. The patient is kept under constant hospital surveillance.

Adequate amounts of blood must be available, for the blood loss is unpredictable and is usually substantial. The surgeon should be prepared to resect vital structures if they are involved in the implantation site and become the source of uncontrolled bleeding. Further, secondary hemorrhage requiring reoperation is always a threat for the two weeks following delivery, for although the placenta is absorbed if left in situ, it may separate before the vessels of the placental site completely thrombose. Methotrexate in one half the doses given in the management of trophoblastic disease might encourage placental regression.

At laparotomy, the abdomen should be carefully inspected to determine the site of implantation before any attempt is made to remove the fetus. Should the placenta become inadvertently detached, serious hemorrhage may ensue. It follows that the fetus should be removed with great care so that the placenta is not disturbed. It has been recommended that the edges of the fetal membranes be carefully preserved by placing suitable clamps along their cut edges at amniotomy and subsequently suturing them to the peritoneal opening of the abdomen after the fetus is removed (marsupialization). The amniotic cavity may then be packed firmly with gauze so that pressure is applied to the placenta to prevent it from separating. The gauze pack can be removed gradually during the early postoperative period. Should the implantation be on the uterus or broad ligaments, salpingectomy together with hysterectomy may be the safer and preferable treatment.

BIBLIOGRAPHY

Baden, W. F., and Heins, O. H.: Ovarian pregnancy; case report with discussion of controversial issues in the literature. Amer. J. Obstet. Gynec., 64:353, 1952.

Beacham, W. D., and Beacham, D. W.: Culdocentesis. Clin. Obstet. Gynec., 1:607, 1958.

Beacham, W. D., Hernquist, W. C., Beacham, D. W., and Webster, H. D.: Abdominal pregnancy at Charity Hospital in New Orleans. Amer. J. Obstet. Gynec., 84:1257, 1962.

Boronow, R. C., McElin, T. W., West, R. H., and Buckingham, J. C.: Ovarian pregnancy. Amer. J. Obstet. Gynec., 91:1095, 1965.

Breen, J. L.: A 21-year survey of 654 ectopic pregnancies. Amer. J. Obstet. Gynec., 106:1004, 1970.

Cross, J. B., Lester, W. M., and McCain, J. R.: Diagnosis and management of abdominal pregnancy, with review of 19 cases. Amer. J. Obstet. Gynec., 62:303, 1951.

Decker, A.: Culdoscopy. Amer. J. Obstet. Gynec., 63:654, 1952; Culdoscopy; A New Technic in Gynecologic and Obstetric Diagnosis. W. B. Saunders Co., Philadelphia, 1952.

Douglas, C. P.: Tubal ectopic pregnancy. Brit. Med. J., 2:838, 1963.

Eberhardt, C. L., and Jacobziner, H.: Ectopic pregnancies and spontaneous abortions in New York City—Incidence and characteristics. Amer. J. Publ. Health, 46:828, 1956.

Evans, G. E., and Goyanes, E.: Bilateral ectopic gestation. Amer. J. Obstet. Gynec., 64:444, 1952.

Hyams, M. N.: Unruptured interstitial pregnancy. Amer. J. Obstet. Gynec., 65:697, 1953.

Lathrop, J. C., and Bowles, G. E.: Methotrexate in abdominal pregnancy. Obstet. Gynec., 32:81, 1968.

O'Leary, J. L., et al.: Rudimentary horn pregnancy. Obstet. Gynec., 22:371, 1963.

Stander, R. W.: Abdominal pregnancy. Clin. Obstet. Gynec., 5:1065, 1962.

Vasicka, A. I., and Grable, E. E.: Simultaneous extrauterine and intra-uterine pregnancies progressing to viability; review of literature and report of two cases. Obstet. Gynec. Survey, 11:603, 1956.

Webster, H. D., Jr., Barclay, D. L., and Fischer, C. K.: Ectopic pregnancy; a 17 year review. Amer. J. Obstet. Gynec., 92:23, 1965.

Chapter 14

Gestational Trophoblastic Disease

Gestational trophoblastic disease refers to the pathologic entities of hydatidiform mole, chorioadenoma destruens or invasive mole, and choriocarcinoma. Excluded by this terminology are the trophoblastic tumors arising from nongestational sources of the ovary, testes, and other structures.

A hydatidiform mole is a hydropic swelling or "degeneration" of the stroma of the immature chorionic villi, resulting in segmental, grapelike accumulations of fluid within the villous branches. Although these villous swellings may be seen microscopically in the chorion laeve and in some blighted ova, they are grossly visible in a hydatidiform mole, reaching a centimeter or more in diameter, and comprise all of the villous tissue.

The prodromal or formative stages of a hydatidiform mole are seen in two thirds of all blighted or pathologic ova. However, since most blighted ova abort by the 10th to the 12th week of pregnancy, nearly all potential hydatid moles are expelled before they have the chance to develop. In most clinics a fully developed hydatidiform mole occurs about once in 1500 pregnancies. For some unexplained reason the incidence of hydatidiform mole is much greater in the Orient, especially China, the Philippines, and Malaya, where its frequency is at least four times greater than in other areas of the world.

The earliest view of the pathogenesis of a hydatidiform mole favored the belief that the hydatid change was a degenerative process, resulting from an endometritis. Later, it was proposed that a hydatidiform mole originated through faulty villous development. It is now recognized that hydatid change occurs because the villous circulation fails to develop normally. Although blood vessels are present occasionally in the villous core, they tend to disappear, and only a few are encountered on microscopic examination of molar tissue. In the absence of a circulation, the villous stroma becomes edematous and eventually forms a cystic structure.

The hydatid process is occasionally visible under the dissecting microscope in normally developing chorions at the junction of the chorion frondosum and the chorion laeve, and, as stated previously, it is commonly seen in blighted ova in which the embryo is absent, nodular, or stunted. A further gradation of hydatid change is seen in the so-called *transitional hydatid mole* where only the essential form of the ovisac is preserved, and the remaining placental tissue consists of a mass of large, swollen, vesicular villi. A hydatidiform mole, therefore, might be considered the ultimate stage in the natural history of a blighted ovum that failed to abort at the usual time, but that continued to grow and undergo further hydatid change.

Histologically, most villous vesicles are covered by the normal double layer of epithelium, an outer syncytiotrophoblast, and an inner cytotrophoblast or Langhans' layer. The thickness of the covering syncytiotrophoblast and cytotrophoblast varies considerably, and, where the villi are markedly distended with fluid, these epithelial layers are noticeably attenuated. Proliferation of the syncytium and Langhans' layer is present in most moles, but the relative proportions of these epithelial elements are inconsistent. The microscopic appearance, therefore, differs from specimen to specimen and in different areas of the same specimen. The smaller vesicles are filled with mesenchyme containing mucoid material, whereas the larger vesicles have a central cystic cavity filled with a clear fluid.

On the theory that the condition begins to develop early and prior to a functioning fetal circulation, it may be assumed that the trophoblast of a hydatidiform mole retains some of the invasive qualities that characterize the trophoblast during the period of implantation. Indeed, a hydatidiform mole may on occasion realize its malignant potential. It may restrict its neoplastic behavior to local invasion of the myometrium, in which case it is referred to as chorioadenoma destruens or invasive mole. On occasion, an otherwise benign mole may reach sites outside the uterus. Finally, a hydatidiform mole may develop into a highly invasive tumor—a choriocarcinoma.

Chorioadenoma destruens (invasive mole) may be only microscopic, with villi found between myometrial bundles, or plainly visible as large hemorrhagic areas extending to the serosa. Actually, the condition can simulate a cornual pregnancy, its presence being heralded by sudden and severe intra-abdominal hemorrhage if the molar tissue perforates through the serosa.

Tissue consistent with a diagnosis of a mole rather than choriocarcinoma has been encountered in distant areas from the uterus, notably the vagina and lungs, and this has

led to the term *metastatic mole.* If it is undiagnosed or inadequately treated, death may follow because of interference with cardiopulmonary function, the ultimate result being a state of *cor pulmonale.* A similar consequence can occur in choriocarcinoma.

Choriocarcinoma, a rare, highly malignant tumor that until the introduction of chemotherapy in 1955 was associated with at least a 90 per cent mortality, is composed only of cytotrophoblast and syncytiotrophoblast. One third of the cases are derived from normal pregnancies of over 20 weeks, one third from pregnancies of less than 20 weeks, including ectopic gestations and abortions, and the remaining third from molar pregnancies (Fig. 1). Because of its tendency to metastasize, when sudden hemoptysis or evidence of spontaneous cerebral hemorrhage occurs in a woman having experienced a recent pregnancy, the diagnosis of unrecognized metastatic gestational trophoblastic disease should be considered.

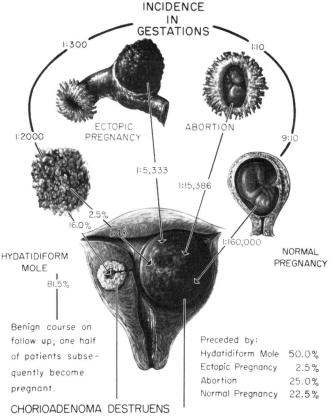

INCIDENCE
IN
GESTATIONS

1:300

1:10

ECTOPIC
PREGNANCY

ABORTION

1:2000

1:5,333

1:15,386

9:10

2.5%

16.0%

1:40

1:160,000

NORMAL
PREGNANCY

HYDATIDIFORM
MOLE

81.5%

Benign course on
follow up; one half
of patients subse-
quently become
pregnant.

Preceded by:
Hydatidiform Mole   50.0%
Ectopic Pregnancy   2.5%
Abortion   25.0%
Normal Pregnancy   22.5%

CHORIOADENOMA DESTRUENS

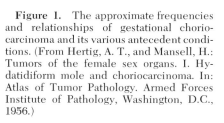

Figure 1. The approximate frequencies and relationships of gestational choriocarcinoma and its various antecedent conditions. (From Hertig, A. T., and Mansell, H.: Tumors of the female sex organs. I. Hydatidiform mole and choriocarcinoma. In: Atlas of Tumor Pathology. Armed Forces Institute of Pathology, Washington, D.C., 1956.)

For purposes of patient management, assessment of therapy, and follow-up, it has proved useful to classify the various forms of gestational trophoblastic disease as metastatic or nonmetastatic disease. Subject to differences of classification, as defined here, metastatic disease exists when the process extends beyond the uterine cavity. (See Pathology.)

Lutein Cysts

Hydatidiform mole is associated with ovarian enlargement due to lutein cyst formation. In some cases the ovary may reach grapefruit size or larger (Fig. 2), but, regardless of size, these cystic structures regress spontaneously after delivery and require no surgical treatment. Generally the ovary is normal in size within two or three weeks post delivery, but occasionally the larger cysts are palpable abdominally many weeks postpartum. The fluid in the lutein cysts is rich in chorionic gonadotropin, and contains estrogen and some progesterone as well. This disease is characterized by low estriol synthesis because of the absence of fetal adrenals.

Composition of Molar Fluid

The fluid within the hydatid vesicles is similar to ascitic and edema fluid, but with notable exceptions. Like edema fluid, mole fluid has a low sodium and protein content, these being approximately 123 mEq. per liter and 1.0 gram per 100 ml., respectively. Molar fluid has a higher concentration of potassium, inorganic phosphate, and alkaline and acid phosphatase than does maternal serum, a relationship similar to that of the fetal and the maternal serum of normal pregnancy. Molar trophoblast, like that of a normal placenta, appears to have specific transport function and is not simply a semipermeable membrane. This may be taken as evidence that transport across the trophoblast membrane is not regulated exclusively by fetal needs.

PATHOLOGY OF TROPHOBLASTIC DISEASE

Hydatidiform Mole

Macroscopically the appearance of a mass of translucent vesicles is characteristic and unmistakable (Fig. 3). The vast majority of placental villi have swollen to such an extent that they assume a grapelike appearance, the usual diameter of these vesicles measuring between 2 and 5 mm. They are attached by fibrous strands one to another and distend the entire uterine cavity. In between these grapelike vesicles clotted blood, masses of fibrin, and degen-

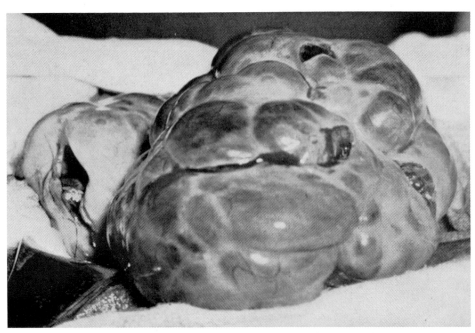

Figure 2.   Lutein cysts of ovary at laparotomy associated with a molar pregnancy.

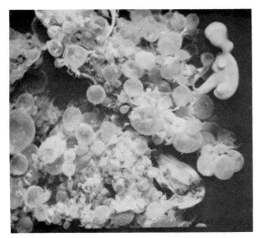

Figure 3. Hydatidiform mole with stunted embryo. ×2. (From Hertig, A. T., in Meigs, J. V., and Sturgis, S. H., eds.: Progress in Gynecology, vol. 2. Grune & Stratton, New York, 1950.)

erated material of various origin are frequently found. For a proper pathologic analysis and, more importantly, for attempts at prognostication, these masses of clot and debris must not be discarded but should be sampled for histologic interpretation. When the entire specimen is available and when very meticulous study is undertaken then one may find on occasion the remains of a degenerating fetus, as in Figure 3, and more rarely a chorionic cavity. This finding is important because it suggests that molar transformation of placental villous tissue is a secondary phenomenon and that embryo-

genesis may have proceeded normally at least for a while.

This macroscopic appearance of the fully developed mole, usually expelled after 12 weeks of gestation, is not suddenly developed. It is preceded by a gradual swelling of villi here and there in placental tissue. When such abortuses are expelled, and usually this occurs at earlier gestational ages, the picture of a "transitional hydatidiform mole" is found. In general, there is less obvious and less diffuse distension of villi with fluid, and more often a macerated embryo and chorionic cavity are found. Even earlier in this temporal sequence, in the abortus expelled spontaneously, "hydatid degeneration" of villi is found only on the microscopic investigation.

It is thus envisaged that perhaps initially normal placentas undergo this pathologic event of villous fluid imbibition when fetal death occurs (with consequent failure of fetal vascular development) and that it becomes most pronounced when prompt abortion does not take place (Fig. 4). Hence most moles are detected and delivered after 12 weeks of gestation.

The microscopic appearance betrays the gross findings. Villi are enormously distended, their fibrous tissue cores often showing empty spaces, formerly filled with fluid. The fibrocytes are dissociated, Hofbauer cells scattered, and fetal capillaries absent or degenerating (Fig. 5). At the same time, the villous surface remains covered

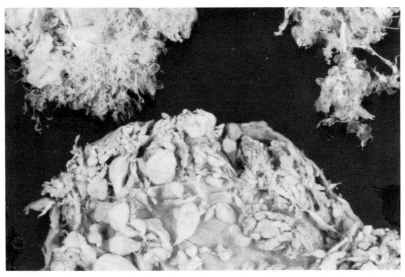

Figure 4. Three stages of progressive hydatidiform change in spontaneous abortion. Above left: the mildest degree, and visible only microscopically. Above right: transitional molar villous change. Below: the classic grape-like vesicles of a mole with their filamentous strands attached to each other.

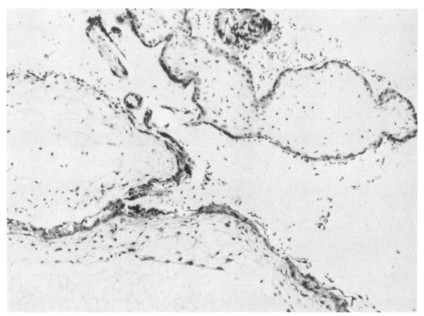

Figure 5.   Histologic picture of a benign mole with only minimal trophoblastic proliferation. H & E ×100.

with trophoblastic cells, or else it is covered with fibrin and maternal clot. Some of the latter deposits doubtless accumulate because of the markedly altered pattern or absence of intervillous circulation, and some of it may be due to the denudation of villous tissue after trophoblastic degeneration. The most variable feature is the extent of trophoblastic proliferation. In some moles a thin layer of cytotrophoblast and syncytium is found (Fig. 5), while in others the intervillous space contains islands of apparently proliferating trophoblast (Fig. 6), which may occasionally be seen connecting to villi. A wide spectrum between these two extremes is found and by no means is the appearance of one section from a mole similar to that of another. This variability has led authors,

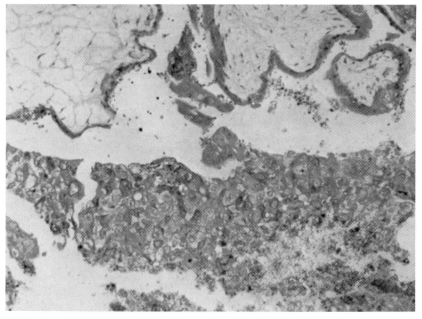

Figure 6.   Hydatidiform mole with vesicles above and central core of proliferating cytotrophoblast. Very little syncytium is present. Death from choriocarcinoma. H & E ×200.

in particular Hertig, to attempt assigning prognostic grades to individual specimens. Thus, a "benign mole" (Grade I), as seen in Figure 5, would not be expected to be followed by the development of a choriocarcinoma, whereas in a more "malignant" one (Fig. 6), perhaps Grade V to VI, there was a significant chance of its development. This controversial issue has not been resolved but seems to us an eminently practical approach. It must be stressed, however, that it rests upon thorough study with mul-

A

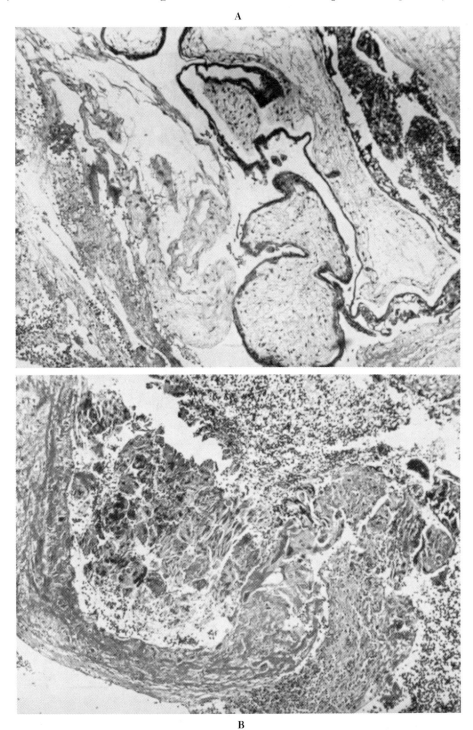

B

Figure 7. A, Benign mole (Grade II), showing degenerating villi and trophoblast. ×80. Normal pregnancy completed 16 months later. B, Molar tissue from a vigorous curettage immediately following vaginal delivery of the benign mole (Grade II). Sheets of trophoblast are seen surrounded by fibrin and strips of myometrium. ×200.

tiple sections. In this regard it is important to recognize that usually the most significant area studied is the curettings obtained after evacuation, i.e., the molar placental site in the decidua, which is often also the most malignant-appearing area (Fig. 7).

Unlike normal trophoblastic growth, malignant trophoblast has a tendency to be composed of more proliferating cytotrophoblast with only little syncytial maturation, well shown in Figure 6. Electron micrographic study has supported the similarities between trophoblast from moles and that of normal placentas. An abundance of cytotrophoblast with few cytoplasmic organelles, typical "intermediary cells" (transitional to syncytium), and syncytium with its highly complex structure are found. In the latter there is an abundance of pinocytotic vesicles and other organelles and the suggestion has been made that the prevalence of the latter cells only correlates with hormone production and degree of villous swelling.

Chorioadenoma Destruens

By definition, the invasive mole is a destructive (i.e., invasive) lesion composed of trophoblast *and* villous tissue. It is a lesion that can be diagnosed accurately only by microscopic examination. Irrespective of how plentiful and malignant-appearing the trophoblast may be, so long as villi are present the diagnosis is not choriocarcinoma. Macroscopically such lesions are usually composed of hemorrhagic nodules in the muscular substance of the uterus and, at times, they may only represent an exaggerated placental site of a mole. An analogy to the placenta increta might be drawn. Histologically, a much greater abundance of trophoblast is usually evident and multiple sections may be required before villous tissue is detected. The propensity of trophoblast to invade blood vessels and to proliferate in blood clot is well expressed in these lesions. Hence they are usually very hemorrhagic. By and large less "fibrinoid degeneration" is associated with the invasive trophoblast, which otherwise does not differ histologically or electron microscopically from that of moles.

Choriocarcinoma

Whether in the uterus or metastatic, whether gestational or derived from germ cells in males or nonpregnant women, choriocarcinoma has a singular appearance. Macroscopically it is a hemorrhagic, nodular lesion, frequently with much clot associated. The amount of blood and fibrin may so exceed the trophoblastic cause of the lesion that histologic sections may fail to encounter the malignant cells. There is an abundance of cytotrophoblast, often in large sheets and with numerous mitoses, and usually only a small component of differentiated multinucleated syncytial cells (Fig. 8). The latter is often extensively vacuolated. Growth occurs preferentially within vascular spaces but metastases may be found in any tissue (lung, brain, liver, nodes, gut, and so on). Electron microscopic studies of choriocarcinoma from patients and of that transplanted and carried in hamsters or in tissue culture shows that it differs from normal placental trophoblast in no important detail. As expected, more irregular anaplastic nuclei and larger vacuoles are seen in the syncytium. The intermediary type of cell was first described in this tumor, to be seen subsequently in other trophoblast. No virus

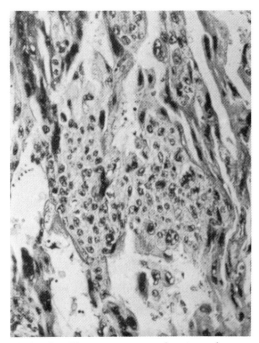

Figure 8. Choriocarcinoma showing the cytotrophoblast surrounded by syncytiotrophoblast. The latter in some places is vacuolated as seen in early implantation. ×200. (From Hertig, A. T., and Mansell, H.: Tumors of the female sex organs. I. Hydatidiform mole and choriocarcinoma. In: Atlas of Tumor Pathology. Armed Forces Institute of Pathology, Washington, D.C., 1956.)

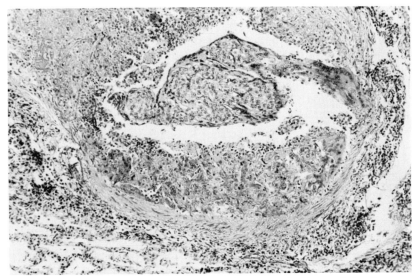

Figure 9. Pulmonary artery occluded by proliferating malignant trophoblast and clot, four years after delivery of mole. Death from cor pulmonale. In places where trophoblast penetrates into arterial wall an intense lymphocyte and plasma cell reaction has taken place. H & E ×160. (From Benirschke, K., and Driscoll, S. G.: The Pathology of the Human Placenta. Springer-Verlag, New York, 1967.)

particles have been identified despite extensive search. Villi are absent.

It is usually not safe to make the diagnosis of choriocarcinoma in the presence of molar tissue, and yet some moles obviously eventuate in this lesion. Are the anaplastic components of a highly malignant-appearing mole already choriocarcinoma or are they still to dedifferentiate into this lesion? These questions cannot be answered at present, but they are even more pertinent with respect to choriocarcinoma following — rarely — an apparently normal pregnancy. Numerous such cases are recorded, some in which the destructive metastatic disease became apparent simultaneously in mother and child. Did it arise from a dizygotic twin that, unnoticed, underwent degeneration? Probably not. Driscoll's important chance discovery of a histologically typical choriocarcinomatous island within a normal placenta (no sequelae in mother or baby) clearly indicates that indeed the disease may derive by mutational events from a normal trophoblastic precursor.

The different response of gestational choriocarcinoma upon treatment with cytostatic drugs when compared in particular to that of choriocarcinoma in males (developing from testis) has led to an inquiry of immunologic factors. Briefly, it can be argued that the genotype of a gestational choriocarcinoma, differing from that of the mother (approximating that of a fetus),

might lead to immunologic "recognition" of the tumor by the mother and hence more rapid destruction, i.e., rejection in immunologic terms (see Chapter 9, Immunologic Interactions in Pregnancy). Indeed, the occasionally verified spontaneous regression of metastatic lesions can best be so explained. Commensurate with this assumption, the systematic study by Elston showed that the survival was much greater in those patients whose choriocarcinoma had caused a plasma cellular reaction in the invaded tissues than when none was present. This phenomenon is shown in Figure 9 in a patient who died from cor pulmonale four years after removal of a hydatidiform mole. All pulmonary artery branches were occluded by trophoblast and clot and only at those sites where the vascular wall was invaded was there an active round-cell infiltration such as one might expect to find in the rejection phenomenon. That the tumor expresses some transplantation antigens is supported by the regular rejection when it is transplanted into the hamster cheek pouch or into monkeys.

CYTOLOGY AND CHROMOSOMES

The findings of cytogenetic studies of molar material and their pathologic relatives are still contradictory at the time of this writing. It is apparent that approximately 80 per cent of typical hydatidiform moles have a single Barr body and, so far as can be judged from microspectrophotometry, they are diploid. Although only a few specimens have been adequately karyotyped, most are 46,XX. Nevertheless, typical moles with a 46,XY genotype have been reported, an important observation relative to our understanding the pathogenesis. A few moles have been found to be aneuploid (e.g., 47,XXX), and the suggestion has been made by some that these may become the "malignant" ones. Thus, karyotyping may ultimately aid in assessment of the prognosis.

This is in striking contrast to what has been considered a precursor condition, hydatid degeneration in a spontaneous abortus. In particular when a fetus (often abnormal) is associated, such transitional moles or abortuses with significant hydatid degeneration of villi are commonly found to possess a polyploid complement. Triploidy (69,XXY and 69,XXX) is the more common genetic set but tetraploidy is also seen. This necessitates as a causal mechanism either double fertilization (two spermatozoa) or failure of the second polar body to be extruded, and it becomes thus doubtful that this condition is indeed a precursor to a true mole. A relationship to preceding hormonal therapy, that is, "the pill," is suspected but detailed confirmatory studies are still outstanding.

In all cases of chorioadenoma destruens and choriocarcinoma an aneuploid karyotype has been found. That is to say, the chromosome complement was irregular, often 50 to 80 in number and without any specific pattern. This is not dissimilar to other malignant tumors and supports the contention that karyotypic analysis of any of these lesions may provide valuable prognostic clues.

DIAGNOSIS OF TROPHOBLASTIC DISEASE

The diagnosis of hydatid mole is not always certain for there is always the possibility that one is dealing with a multiple pregnancy or a threatened abortion with concealed hemorrhage, causing the uterus to enlarge beyond the size expected for the gestational age. In a twin pregnancy the uterus is disproportionately large, and the fetuses, being smaller, may not be visualized as early on x-ray examination, while the chorionic gonadotropin titer is higher than in a single pregnancy. Finally, the uterus may recede in size over a period of some weeks, leading to the mistaken diagnosis of a blighted ovum or missed abortion when in fact the patient has a "missed" mole.

The following is a list of the established clinical symptoms and signs and the laboratory and radiographic methods employed in the diagnosis of gestational trophoblastic disease:

I. Nonmetastatic and Benign Disease
   A. Clinical symptoms and signs
      1. Vaginal bleeding of uterine origin
      2. Uterine size in excess of gestational data or the period of amenorrhea
      3. Early toxemia, possibly severe
      4. Passage of hydatid villi
   B. Specific diagnostic tests and procedures
      1. Markedly elevated chorionic gonadotropin titers
      2. Increase in protein-bound iodine (PBI) on occasion
      3. Absence of fetal heart tones by auscultation and fetal electrocardiography
      4. Ultrasound
      5. Radiographic studies
         a. Absence of fetal skeleton
         b. Characteristic x-ray findings by intrauterine dye injection

II. Metastatic or Persistent Trophoblastic Disease
   A. A spectrum of symptoms and signs
   B. Elevated gonadotropin titers
   C. Roentgenogram and arteriography
   D. Encephalogram and brain scan

Vaginal bleeding is usually the first symptom that directs the clinician's attention to the possibility of a molar pregnancy. Occasionally, however, the disproportionate size of the uterus based on the gestational age is the most striking finding, and the vaginal bleeding may not appear until later. The bleeding occurs because with placental disarray the intervillous space lacks functional structure. In the absence of chorionic plate and marginal sinus, the maternal blood in the intervillous space arriving from the spiral arterioles is not directed back into the veins of the placental site, but rather some is retained within the molar tissue, from which it eventually escapes into the vagina. The blood shed is variable in amount and in appearance. It can be brownish to bright red in character, and although it can be less than that of a normal menstrual period, the bleeding may also be profuse.

In the early stages of the disease there is usually a discrepancy between the expected and actual size of the uterus. The uterus is disproportionately large for the stage of pregnancy, although there is the occasional exception. In patients first seen after several missed periods, the molar process may have regressed and the uterus receded in size. The uterus may be that of an 8 to 10 week pregnancy and the mole mistaken for a blighted ovum or a missed abortion. Also, the uterus is reputed to have a characteristic soft, doughy consistency, but this finding is difficult to evaluate, for the same may be said of a normally pregnant uterus, particularly in a woman who has borne many children, or of the uterus with a multiple pregnancy.

Proteinuria and hypertension develop frequently, reportedly in more than half the cases. The degree of toxemia is variable, from mild to severe, and although extremely rare, eclampsia or convulsions have been reported. In fact, death from pregnancy toxemia has been known to occur in association with a hydatidiform mole. At this early stage of pregnancy, in the presence of hypertension, edema, and a urinary sediment showing red cells and casts, one might favor the diagnosis of acute glomerular nephritis. The latter occurs very infrequently in pregnancy, however, and these signs and symptoms appearing in the first half of pregnancy are more likely due to a hydatidiform mole.

An occasional patient with a molar pregnancy may show evidence of a temporary hyperthyroidism and a hypermetabolic state. There is tachycardia, the systolic blood pressure is elevated, and the patient may complain of weight loss. The protein-bound iodine has been observed to be elevated above that for normal pregnancy, ranging between 12 and 20 mcg. per 100 ml. These values return to normal, as will the vital signs listed, within 24 to 72 hours after the molar pregnancy is terminated.

Much is made of the possibility that the patient may expel from the vagina grapelike hydatid villi, which, of course, if recovered and identified are pathognomonic of the condition. Unless the patient is in labor, the appearance of the hydropic villi is so rare that it offers little assistance in the diagnosis of hydatidiform mole.

An elevated titer of chorionic gonadotropin, exceeding 50,000 international units (I.U.), in the early weeks of pregnancy, or values of 20,000 to 100,000 I.U. after the 90th day of pregnancy are highly suggestive of a hydatidiform mole (see Fig. 7 in Chapter 2). It will be recalled that in normal pregnancy the daily urinary values for chorionic gonadotropin reach their peak about the 12th week and range from 20,000 to 50,000 I.U. Thereafter, the value declines to 4000 to 12,000 I.U. daily.

It is evident that a quantitative test prior to the 80th to 90th day of pregnancy is of less diagnostic value and, indeed, may be misleading, particularly in a twin pregnancy. Further, when the molar degeneration is marked, the chorionic gonadotropin levels may be low from the onset and throughout the patient's clinical course.

Consistent with x-ray examination of the abdomen, auscultation and the Doppler technique reveal absence of fetal heart tones, and this finding is substantiated by lack of electrocardiographic activity. Ultrasound reveals a characteristic speckled appearance of the mole similar to the honeycomb pattern seen in intrauterine dye injection. Ultrasound unquestionably is equally specific diagnostically.

In normal pregnancy a roentgenogram of the abdomen should reveal a fetal skeleton with the uterus consistent in size with a four or five month gestation. With the exceptions to be noted, the fetus is absent on x-ray examination in a molar pregnancy. One may be deceived in the presence of a multiple pregnancy in which the fetuses may not be identified either because of movement during the exposure or because the gestation may actually be less than is indicated by uterine size. Also, there is the rare possibility that the fetus may coexist with a mole. The majority of these have been associated with a single placenta. However, somewhat more than a third have been cases of dizygotic twins, with a normal placenta and fetus and the molar tissue separate. Chromosomal abnormalities within the fetus and molar tissue have been reported, particularly triploid cell lines.

Cytologic study has shown a preponderance of sex chromatin–positive cells.

The most definitive diagnosis of an undelivered molar pregnancy prior to evacuation can be obtained radiographically with injection of radiopaque material into the uterine cavity. Having had a preliminary x-ray of the abdomen, the patient is catheterized and the lower abdomen is surgically prepared and draped. A No. 18 spinal needle is introduced transabdominally into the uterine cavity at a point in the midline 3 to 5 cm. below the umbilicus. After aspiration of fluid to verify intrauterine location of the needle, 20 to 30 ml. of radiopaque material is injected rapidly. The needle is then withdrawn and anteroposterior and lateral radiographs are taken within five minutes after the injection of the medium. A "moth-eaten" or "honeycomb" pattern is consistent with a diagnosis of a hydatidiform mole (Fig. 10).

Special diagnostic procedures for metastatic or apparent persistent disease that fails to respond to systemic chemotherapy include both radiographic and arteriographic examination for diagnosis and decisions as to therapy. Patient survival may depend on localization of the lesion(s) and a more direct chemotherapeutic attack. When the disease is identified in the myometrium, having gone unrecognized on previous curettage, or in the broad ligament areas, it may be possible to salvage the reproductive system for future childbearing by effective localized chemotherapy (Fig. 11). Thus, metastatic disease in the reproductive and cardiopulmonary systems and liver may be identified by arteriography and so treated. When brain involvement is suspected, encephalogram and brain scan may localize the lesion(s).

MANAGEMENT OF NONMETASTATIC AND METASTATIC DISEASE

Whenever the diagnosis of hydatidiform mole is established, rather than await the onset of labor definitive treatment is indicated because of the hazards of toxemia, recurrent and serious bleeding, local invasion with perforation of the uterus, and the more remote possibility of the development of choriocarcinoma.

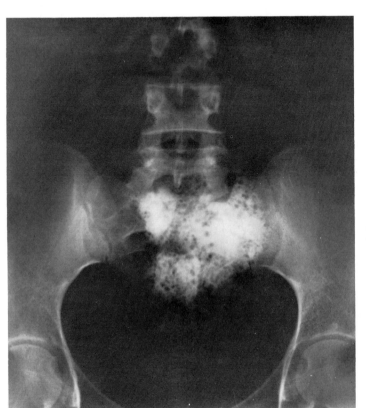

Figure 10. A suspected molar pregnancy (11 to 12 weeks gestational age, 20 weeks by size) confirmed by intrauterine radiopaque material. Note the excess size of the uterus, reaching to the umbilicus. Pregnancy successfully terminated by suction curette following prophylactic chemotherapy.

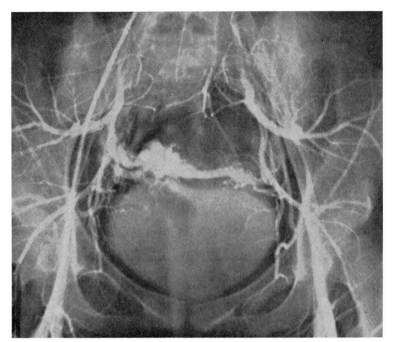

Figure 11. Pelvic arteriogram indicating persistent metastatic disease in uterine wall and right broad ligament, confirmed at laparotomy. (From Goldstein, D. P., Gore, H., and Reid, D. E.: GP, 35:124, 1967.)

The management of a patient with non-metastatic or molar pregnancy should begin with a roentgenogram of the chest and with routine blood studies; two units of compatible blood should be available for transfusion.

The methods of uterine evacuation include: dilatation and curettage, with the suction curette, with or without an initial period of oxytocin stimulation; and abdominal hysterotomy or hysterectomy. Hysterectomy has a definite place in the initial management of molar pregnancy in women who have completed their childbearing. Prior to the introduction of the suction curette abdominal hysterotomy was regarded by some as safer than dilatation and curettage because it avoided undue blood loss and sepsis and insured complete removal of the mole. This applied especially to patients with the larger moles with the uterus consistent in size with a four or five month pregnancy. Certainly the conventional method of cervical dilatation and curettage is not without its dangers from uterine perforation and excessive blood loss. Also, the cervix must be open sufficiently to allow rapid evacuation of the uterus, for serious hemorrhage can occur during the curettage that will not subside until the uterus is emptied of its contents. After careful dilatation of the cervix, the

mole is removed by placental forceps; one first extracts the central part or core without disturbing the more vascular portion in contact with the uterine wall. The myometrium may be especially friable, at least in some areas. In the efforts to avoid perforation, the necessity for a relatively gentle curettage incurs the risk that some molar tissue may remain. It has been advocated that a second curettage be performed four or five days later when the uterus has involuted and there is less risk of perforation. This is especially desirable in the parts of the world where patient follow-up is difficult or less likely. This approach may well serve as a prophylaxis against possible local invasion of residual molar tissue, a factor to keep in mind when assessing the value of chemotherapy administered prior to curettage in patients who have spontaneously delivered a mole a few days previously.

The suction curette has replaced other methods, particularly abdominal hysterotomy, and it permits even large moles to be removed with relative safety. After the mole has been evacuated by the suction curette, the uterus is gently curetted. Digital exploration of the uterus may also be included. The cure rate of molar pregnancy, once the mole is removed, is approximately 85 per cent. To reduce sequelae and improve the cure rate, prophylactic chemotherapy prior to the evacuation of the mole has been advocated. It is envisioned that with prophylaxis there is less likelihood of deportation and dissemination of tumor by manipulation at the time of curettage or subsequent local invasion of trophoblastic tissue. Methotrexate in doses of 15 to 20 mg. is administered intramuscularly for three to five days prior to removal of the mole.

The patient must be observed closely for at least a year, even though the findings of the initial follow-up examination are entirely normal and gonadotropin activity is no longer identifiable. The urinary gonadotropin titer or serum HCG by radioimmunoassay (which in the normal postpartum patient should be negative within a few days post delivery) in the patient recently delivered of a mole should be negative within six weeks after evacuation.

For patients with trophoblastic disease, a mouse uterine weight method of assaying the gonadotropin titer appears essential to avoid the false assumption that the patient is free of disease when the routine immunoassay for pregnancy becomes negative. The mouse uterine weight method measures total gonadotropins — that is, follicle-stimulating hormone (FSH), luteinizing hormone (LH), and human chorionic gonadotropin (HCG) — and although the test takes four days, it measures values as low as 0.5 I.U. or 5 M.U.U. per 24 hours. This level indicates the total absence of HCG, for whatever the gonadotropin activity present, it is pituitary in origin. In childbearing women, that is to say, those with functioning ovaries, the normal values for pituitary gonadotropins by this method are less than 200 M.U.U. or 20 I.U. The immunoassay utilized for the diagnosis of pregnancy is equivocal or negative at 20,000 M.U.U. and 2000 I.U., and at 5000 M.U.U. and 50 I.U. for urinary gonadotropin levels per 24 hours, respectively. Gonadotropin levels below these values as measured by the mouse uterine method have been detected in patients with residual trophoblastic tissue recovered at secondary curettage sometime (six to eight weeks) after evacuation of the mole.

In the immediate follow-up of patients treated for molar pregnancy, gonadotropin assay determinations should be performed weekly and a chest x-ray obtained every two weeks. After the bioassay becomes negative, the gonadotropin titer should be determined at monthly intervals for six months and every two months for the remainder of the year. X-ray examination of the chest and pelvic examination should be done periodically every two to four months during the year of follow-up. At the end of this time, with the tests negative and examinations normal, the patient if she desires may attempt a pregnancy with every hope of success. There is the rare patient who has had more than one molar pregnancy.

The chance of signs and symptoms of residual or metastatic disease developing after a molar pregnancy increases in relation to the duration of time that it takes the gonadotropin titer to become negative. What, then, about the patient who has subsequent vaginal bleeding other than menses or whose gonadotropin titer fails to recede to normal within six weeks after evacuation of a mole? These occurrences should be less frequent with prophylactic chemotherapy, and there is some indication that this is the case.

Before the patient is considered to have metastatic disease and treated, a second curettage with chemotherapy coverage should be performed to remove any benign trophoblastic tissue that had perchance been left behind at the time of evacuation. One must appreciate the possibility that little will be accomplished by curettage if the trophoblastic tissue resides in the myometrium. However, residual molar tissue may be obtained, and the procedure may be followed by cessation of bleeding and apparent cure as reflected by continuous and complete regression of the gonadotropin titer. In the event that the gonadotropin titer fails to regress — remains the same or increases — the patient must be regarded as having metastatic disease and so managed.

The initial treatment of metastatic disease, irrespective of its origin, is chemotherapy, and a remission and probably cure can be anticipated in over 90 per cent of patients. The failures are more likely to occur in patients with liver and brain metastases. Other factors that influence the prognosis unfavorably are (1) the height of the initial gonadotropin titer, (2) duration of the disease prior to treatment, (3) previous inadequate treatment, and (4) drug toxicity that precludes the usual therapeutic dosage. The outlook is less hopeful when the patient fails to receive treatment in the early stages, or before the third or fourth month from the apparent onset of the disease.

The chemotherapeutic treatment is based on the fundamental observations that uterine response (i.e., growth and weight increase) to administered estrogen fails to occur in the absence of folic acid, and that fetal tissues are apparently more sensitive than maternal tissues to folic acid antagonist. This led to the possibility that, being of fetal origin, trophoblast tissue, a rich source of estrogen, might show a regressive response to treatment by these compounds without harm to the host. Of biologic interest is the fact that the administration of anti-folic acid compounds will cause regression of choriocarcinoma in the female but apparently not in the male.

A careful medical work-up is essential prior to chemotherapy. Besides a roentgenogram of the chest and blood studies, liver and renal function should be assessed. Blood urea nitrogen and serum creatinine should be determined, and intravenous pyelogram should be performed, especially when there is pelvic extension of the disease. Serum glutamic, oxaloacetic, and pyruvic transaminase determinations should be done for evaluation of liver function.

Methotrexate is administered intravenously or intramuscularly in a dose of 0.4 mg. per kilogram daily for five days; the total for any one day should not exceed 25 mg. Actinomycin D may be used rather than methotrexate and is the preferred drug if there is any evidence of hepatic dysfunction. The dosage is 10 mcg. per kilogram daily for five days, administered intravenously.

During the period of therapy with either agent, clinical toxicity should be recognized, as evidenced by nausea, vomiting, stomatitis, conjunctivitis, skin rash, alopecia, and vulvitis. Bone marrow depression may occur and may reach dangerous proportions whenever the blood platelets are less than 100,000 and the leukocyte count is reduced to 3000 with the actual polymorphonuclear count less than 1500 per cu. mm. Serious thought must be given to discontinuing the chemotherapy when these symptoms occur, especially if there is evidence of abnormal liver function as indicated by a rise in transaminases. Thus, during the period of therapy the status of the liver, renal and hematopoietic systems is checked almost daily for evidence of drug toxicity.

A favorable response is indicated by a recession of the gonadotropin titer within a week after the onset of therapy, and in the case of metastatic disease of the lung, by regression of the lesion as determined by repeated roentgenograms. Each patient should receive at least two courses of methotrexate, the number influenced somewhat by the patient's tolerance to the therapy and the time it takes the signs and symptoms to regress. In the absence of toxicity, the course of therapy is repeated every 7 to 21 days until such time as the gonadotropin levels are below 50 to 200 M.U.U. or 5 to 20 I.U., i.e., pituitary levels (see Fig. 8 in Chapter 2). Failure to respond after two or three courses might call for a change from methotrexate to actinomycin D.

The patient is considered to be in remission when the gonadotropin titer does not exceed pituitary values as determined by the mouse uterine method for three consecutive weekly determinations, and in permanent remission if it remains within this range for a year. These patients should be followed indefinitely on a six-month basis. If there is to be a relapse, it will usually occur within the first three to six months after the initial treatment. In the event this occurs, chemotherapy is reinstituted.

Patients whose disease is resistant to the above régime may require specialized and adjunctive therapy, which includes: (1) triple therapy with methotrexate, actinomycin D, and Cytoxan, or possibly chlorambucil; (2) adjunctive x-ray therapy; (3) intra-arterial infusion therapy to bypass systemic toxicity; or (4) surgery.

Because of its toxicity, combined or triple therapy should be used only by the most experienced chemotherapist. Given simultaneously with actinomycin D, adjunctive x-ray therapy appears to have a place in the treatment of metastatic lesions to the brain and possibly liver, i.e., 1000 to 2000 rads spaced over several days.

Intra-arterial infusion finds its greatest usefulness when serious drug toxicity arises and when on arteriography the lesions are found in areas that can be approached by arterial catheterization—the liver and cardiopulmonary system and also the uterus and its environs in the case of persistent disease, especially in patients who are desirous of retaining their reproductive function (at some risk, it might be added).

Methotrexate or actinomycin D in roughly 25 per cent or less of the usual systemic dosage is administered daily through the intra-arterial catheter. In the case of the reproductive system, the catheter is placed preferably in the hypogastric artery and a high concentration of the chemotherapeutic agent is thus delivered to the area of persistent disease.

Since the advent of chemotherapy, the indications for adjunctive surgery have become markedly limited. However, when there is persistent pelvic disease following systemic chemotherapy, especially when future childbearing is not a consideration, or failure to respond to intra-arterial chemotherapy, hysterectomy has a distinct place in patient management. The uterus will often reveal intramural trophoblastic disease. Also, surgery may be required to control uterine bleeding and possibly sepsis. Preoperative chemotherapy coverage has been recommended. In the event the gonadotropin titer fails to fall to pituitary levels during the postoperative follow-up, a careful search must be made for metastatic disease elsewhere.

In summary, nonmetastatic molar pregnancy is free of sequelae in approximately 80 to 85 per cent of patients. Whether the rate can be further increased by chemotherapy coverage instituted prior to the evacuation of the mole remains a subject of some controversy. The suction curette finds its greatest usefulness here and has replaced the need for abdominal hysterotomy in the presence of a large mole. Hysterectomy and chemotherapy coverage have a place in the therapy of a molar pregnancy in those patients in whom further childbearing is not a consideration. The meticulous follow-up of patients with molar pregnancy is mandatory, with gonadotropin titers determined by a more sensitive assay than is conventionally used for the diagnosis of pregnancy.

Metastatic trophoblastic disease may occur rarely in association with a benign mole and somewhat more frequently with an invasive mole. While choriocarcinoma may arise from hydatidiform moles, normal pregnancy of both early and late gestation and pregnancy in ectopic sites account for two thirds of the cases. The clinical features of metastatic disease are variable and at times bizarre, contributing to delay in diagnosis that in turn affects adversely the cure rate. When metastases occur in vital structures, failure to cure is more likely, but even here brilliant therapeutic results have followed chemotherapy in otherwise hopeless cases.

With chemotherapy and adjunctive therapy, the overall cure rate of 90 per cent is reported, and cure may be anticipated in patients with metastatic trophoblastic disease. Systemic single-agent chemotherapy with methotrexate or actinomycin D is the primary therapy. The latter is the agent of choice if hepatic function is in question or if drug resistance or toxicity to methotrexate develops. Patients must be carefully monitored for evidence of toxicity by those experienced in the management of this disease.

To bring maximum effect to bear on localized lesions and to avoid toxicity, arterial infusion chemotherapy can be highly effective, but the complications of this approach must not be minimized. Adjunctive radiotherapy of 2000 rads to hepatic and cerebral lesions administered over a 5- to 10-day period and in the course of chemotherapy may add to the effectiveness of the latter. The place of adjunctive therapy is becoming more clearly defined in the hands of the experienced and patient salvage has improved.

Hysterectomy is now restricted to cases in which metastatic disease is suspected to reside in the myometrium (possibly identified by radiography) despite adequate chemotherapy or when uterine bleeding may become life-threatening. It is clearly evident that the treatment of these so-called high-risk patients must be highly individualized, and their interests are best served if they are treated in oncology centers especially prepared both by experience and facilities to care for these women.

BIBLIOGRAPHY

Baggish, M. S., Woodruff, J. D., Tow, S. H., and Jones H. W., Jr.: Sex chromatin pattern in hydatidiform mole. Amer. J. Obstet. Gynec., 102:362, 1968.

Barlow, J. J., Goldstein, D. P., and Reid, D. E.: A study of *in vivo* estrogen biosynthesis and production rates in normal pregnancy, hydatidiform mole and choriocarcinoma. J. Clin. Endocr., 27:1028, 1967.

Beischer, N. A., Fortune, D. W., and Fitzgerald, M. G.: Hydatidiform mole and coexistent foetus, both with triploid chromosome constitution. Brit. Med. J., 3:476, 1967.

Benirschke, K., and Driscoll, S. G.: The Pathology of the Human Placenta. Springer-Verlag, New York 1967.

Brewer, J. I., Gerbie, A. B., Dolkart, R. E., Skom, J. H.,

Nagle, R. G., and Torek, E. E.: Chemotherapy in trophoblastic diseases. Amer. J. Obstet. Gynec., 90:566, 1964.

Carr, D. H.: Cytogenetics and pathology of hydatidiform degeneration. Obstet. Gynec., 33:333, 1969.

Chesley, L. C., Cosgrove, S. A., and Preece, J.: Hydatidiform mole, with special reference to recurrence and associated eclampsia. Amer. J. Obstet. Gynec., 52:311, 1946.

Chun, C., Braga, D., Chow, C., and Lok, L.: Treatment of hydatidiform mole. J. Obstet. Gynaec. Brit. Comm., 71:185, 1964.

Cockshott, W. P., Evans, K. T., and Hendrickse, J. P. de V.: Arteriography of trophoblastic tumors. Clin. Radiol., 15:1, 1964.

Delfs, E.: Quantitative chorionic gonadotropin prognostic value in hydatidiform mole and chorionepithelioma. Obstet. Gynec., 9:1, 1957.

Douglas, G. W.: Diagnosis and management of hydatidiform mole. Surg. Clin. N. Amer., 37:379, 1957.

Driscoll, S. G.: Choriocarcinoma: An "incidental finding" within a term placenta. Obstet. Gynec., 21:96, 1963.

Elson, C. W.: Cellular reaction to choriocarcinoma. J. Path., 97:261, 1969.

Goldstein, D. P., Couch, N., and Hall, T. C.: Infusion therapy in the treatment of patients with choriocarcinoma and related trophoblastic tumors. Surg. Forum, 13:426, 1967.

Goldstein, D. P., Gore, H., and Reid, D. E.: Management of gestational trophoblastic disease. GP, 35:114, 1967.

Goldstein, D. P., and Reid, D. E.: Recent developments in the management of molar pregnancy. Clin. Obstet. Gynec., 10:313, 1967.

Hammond, C. B., and Parker, R. T.: Diagnosis and treatment of trophoblastic disease. Obstet. Gynec., 35:132, 1970.

Hendrickse, J. P. de V., Willis, A. J. P., and Evans, K. T.: Acute dyspnoea with trophoblastic tumours. J. Obstet. Gynaec. Brit. Comm., 72:376, 1965.

Hertig, A. T., and Sheldon, W. H.: Hydatidiform mole, pathologico-clinical correlation of 200 cases. Amer. J. Obstet. Gynec., 53:1, 1947.

Hertz, R., Bergenstal, D. M., Lipsett, M. B., Price, E. B., and Hilbish, T. F.: Chemotherapy of choriocarcinoma and related trophoblastic tumors in women. J.A.M.A., 168:845, 1958.

Hertz, R., Lewis, J., and Lipsett, M. B.: Five years experience with the chemotherapy of metastatic choriocarcinoma and related trophoblastic tumors in women. Amer. J. Obstet. Gynec., 82:631, 1961.

Hertz, R., Ross, G. T., and Lipsett, M. B.: Primary chemotherapy of nonmetastatic trophoblastic disease in women. Amer. J. Obstet. Gynec., 86:808, 1963.

Klinefelter, H. F., Jr., Albright, F., and Griswold, G. C.: Experience with a quantitative test for normal or decreased amounts of follicle-stimulating hormone in urine in endocrinological diagnoses. J. Clin. Endocr., 3:529, 1943.

Knoth, M., Hessedahl, H., and Falck Larsen, J.: Ultrastructure of human choriocarcinoma. Acta Obstet. Gynec. Scand., 48:100, 1969.

Lewis, J., Jr., Gore, H., Hertig, A. T., and Goss, D. A.: Treatment of trophoblastic disease, with rationale for the use of adjunctive chemotherapy at the time of indicated operation. Amer. J. Obstet. Gynec., 96:710, 1966.

Llewellyn-Jones, D.: Trophoblastic tumours. J. Obstet. Gynaec. Brit. Comm., 72:242, 1965.

McCorriston, C. C.: Racial incidence of hydatidiform mole. Amer. J. Obstet. Gynec., 101:377, 1968.

McKay, D. G., Roby, C. C., Hertig, A. T., and Richardson, M. V.: Studies of function of early human trophoblast; I. Observations on chemical composition of fluid of hydatidiform moles; II. Preliminary observations on certain chemical constituents of chorionic and early amniotic fluid. Amer. J. Obstet. Gynec., 69:722, 1955.

Odwell, W. D., Bates, R. W., Rivlin, R. A., Lipsett, M. B., and Hertz, R.: Increased thyroid function without clinical hyperthyroidism in patients with choriocarcinoma. J. Clin. Endocr., 73:658, 1963.

Park, W. W.: Occurrence of sex chromatin in chorionepitheliomas and hydatidiform moles. J. Path. Bact., 74:197, 1957.

Ross, G. T., Goldstein, D. P., Hertz, R., Lipsett, M. B., and Odell, W. D.: Sequential use of methotrexate and actinomycin D in the treatment of metastatic choriocarcinoma and related trophoblastic diseases in women. Amer. J. Obstet. Gynec., 93:223, 1965.

Ross, G. T., Hammond, C. B., and Odell, W. D.: Chemotherapy for nonmetastatic gestational trophoblastic neoplasms. Clin. Obstet. Gynec., 10:323, 1967.

Spellacy, W. N., Meeker, H. C., and McKelvey, J. L.: Three successful pregnancies in a patient treated for choriocarcinoma with methotrexate. Obstet. Gynec., 25:607, 1965.

Thiele, R. A., and de Alvarez, R. R.: Metastasizing benign trophoblastic tumors. Amer. J. Obstet. Gynec., 84:1395, 1962.

Tow, W. S. H., and Cheng, W. C.: Recent trends in treatment of choriocarcinoma. Brit. Med. J., 1:521, 1967.

Wynn, R. M., and Davies, J.: Ultrastructure of hydatidiform mole: correlative electron microscopic and functional aspects. Amer. J. Obstet. Gynec., 90:293, 1964.

Wynn, R. M., and Harris, J. A.: Ultrastructure of trophoblast and endometrium in invasive hydatidiform mole (chorioadenoma destruens). Amer. J. Obstet. Gynec., 99:1125, 1967.

Zondek, B.: Importance of increased production and excretion of gonadotropic hormone for diagnosis of hydatidiform mole. J. Obstet. Gynaec. Brit. Emp., 49:397, 1942.

Chapter 15

Hyperemesis Gravidarum

Some nausea and occasional vomiting occur in approximately half of all pregnancies. The duration of these annoying symptoms varies greatly, and patients may experience nausea with or without vomiting in one pregnancy and not in another. For the most part the symptoms are mild and transient, and tend to disappear by the end of the first trimester; but, if the vomiting persists and materially interferes with fluid balance and the other phases of nutrition, it is potentially dangerous and must be regarded as abnormal. When the disturbance is this severe, it is referred to as hyperemesis gravidarum, or pernicious vomiting of pregnancy.

Rarely does one see the severe form in current practice and one must turn to the older literature to appreciate the severe nutritional changes that have been encountered in this pregnancy complication. Although with current methods of treatment death from this disease is rarely if ever reported, it must be recognized that patients with hyperemesis gravidarum have a potentially serious condition.

The specific etiology of hyperemesis gravidarum is unknown, but several possibilities have been suggested, including endocrine and toxic factors and reflex and neurotic or psychosomatic causes.

In the consideration of endocrine factors attention has been called to the parallelism that exists between the chorionic gonadotropin values and the occurrence of vomiting. The titers of chorionic gonadotropin in the urine and serum have been reported significantly elevated in patients with nausea and vomiting of pregnancy. These values are regarded as an actual increase over the normally high values of the early weeks of pregnancy and are thought to denote an upset in hormone balance. However, the serum and urine titers of chorionic gonadotropin seem more in keeping with a state of dehydration than with any increase in secretion. It has been suggested that the condition is caused by a progesterone deficiency, but progesterone therapy has never relieved the vomiting with any greater consistency than other forms of therapy. Also, the urinary pregnanediol excretion has never been demonstrated to be diminished in this syndrome. If the corpus luteum or the developing syncytiotrophoblast failed to secrete adequate amounts of progesterone during the critical period of implantation and placentation, a greater incidence of abortion could be anticipated. The spontaneous abortion rate in hyperemesis gravidarum is not increased and may actually be lower than the usual incidence. Perhaps the maternal organism is experiencing difficulty in adjusting metabolically to the relatively large quantities of estrogen present in pregnancy. Certainly a symptom commonly associated with estrogen overdosage in the nonpregnant is that of nausea and vomiting.

Although no foreign or specific protein substance has been identified in the blood and urine of these patients, the idea has been expressed that the developing ovum may elaborate a substance that causes toxic manifestations in the mother, one of which is vomiting. Chorionic elements, to be sure, have been identified in the lungs of pregnant patients at autopsy, affording evidence that substances can escape from the uterus and enter the maternal circulation. Whether the deportation of chorionic tissue from the uterus may cause toxic symptoms in the mother is highly debatable.

The term *reflex* as it applies to the cause of hyperemesis gravidarum connotes that somewhere within the body, presumably the reproductive tract, a stimulus arises that will cause vomiting. Some believe that uterine displacement may furnish the stimulus, and that its correction will relieve the vomiting. However, no cause-and-effect relationship has ever been established between uterine retroversion and nausea and vomiting of pregnancy.

The commonly held explanation for the cause of nausea and vomiting of early pregnancy is that it is a psychosomatic condition, which earlier was termed neurotic vomiting. It must be granted that factors that create a sense of insecurity and anxiety may accentuate the patient's vomiting. The life situations that may secondarily contribute to the condition are multitidinous, from not wanting the pregnancy to the many social, economic, and family problems that are part of human existence. It is difficult to acquire data, except in narrative form, that could establish the probability that the condition is psychologic in origin. In ascribing the cause of the vomiting, repression of the feminine role, conscious or unconscious repudiation of the pregnancy, excessive mother attachment with repressed aggressive tendencies toward her, and immaturity are terms used by those who are psychiatrically inclined. Nevertheless, when the etiology is regarded as psychosomatic and the relief the patient receives is attributed to psychotherapy, data are lacking on the duration and severity of the vomiting, the physical status of the patient, the laboratory findings, and the supplementary therapy used.

Unquestionably a systematic study of the psychologic elements involved in the syndrome is warranted. Except for the condition of hysteria, there is no documentation to substantiate the belief that patients who develop nausea or vomiting have a greater incidence of psychiatric difficulties than other pregnant women. The impression has been gained, however, that patients with hysteria are more likely to vomit, and in these patients characteristically the vomiting is more or less sporadic throughout pregnancy. These patients are difficult to treat, requiring great patience and understanding by the physician, and they usually experience multiple hospital admissions in the course of pregnancy.

Regardless of the controversy relative to etiology, when symptoms persist one should be alert to the possibility that there may be physical causes for vomiting that are not necessarily related to pregnancy. Moreover, there are limitations to all forms of psychotherapy. In fact, the psychiatrist may have little success in "reaching" the patient who is seriously ill until sometime in the puerperium. It is possible, therefore, even under competent medical and psychiatric supervision, for the occasional patient to continue to vomit and reach a nutritional state bordering on irreversibility.

In conclusion, the specific etiology of hyperemesis gravidarum remains to be determined, despite the number of theories that are offered. Although environmental conditions may arouse emotional conflicts that may accentuate the vomiting, it may be hazardous to regard the condition primarily of psychogenic origin. The possible exception is the vomiting associated with hysteria, but here the history and symptoms that characterize hysteria readily establish the diagnosis. The fact remains that the vomiting of pregnancy may persist to a point where the patient succumbs from the effects of malnutrition and electrolyte loss.

PATHOLOGY

The pathologic changes are those produced by starvation. The liver may show many fat-laden cells, and on occasion there may be actual necrosis. Earlier descriptions of the liver included necrosis of the central area of the liver lobule, which was regarded as pathognomonic of the disease. Although the necrosis is usually midzonal in type, any portion of the liver may be involved.

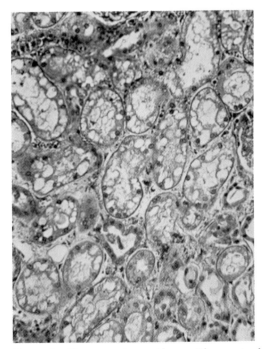

Figure 1. Hyperemesis gravidarum. The proximal convoluted tubules show cytoplasmic vacuolation, a lesion presumably reflecting potassium depletion, that is, "hypokalemic vacuolar nephropathy." ×225. (From Ober, W. B., Reid, D. E., Romney, S. L., and Merrill, J. P.: Amer. J. Med., 21:781, 1956.)

Other changes throughout the body are those which result from vitamin deficiency, particularly of vitamins B and C. There may be myelin degeneration of the peripheral nerves, and scurvy-like lesions may appear in various areas of the body. Renal lesions similar to those in potassium depletion, consisting of vacuole formation in the tubular epithelium (Fig. 1), are found. Petechial hemorrhages and degeneration in areas involved in Wernicke's encephalopathy and Korsakoff's syndrome have been observed in the brain.

SYMPTOMS

Symptoms vary greatly in their intensity. They are relatively mild in patients with the nonpathologic type of pregnancy vomiting. Often there may be only the sensation of nausea without vomiting; however, vomiting usually occurs sporadically at various times of the day, especially when the stomach is empty. Hence, the patient is aware of these symptoms on awakening in the morning, which accounts for the lay term for this condition, "morning sickness." Although the patient may lose some weight, it is only a few pounds, and is quickly regained with treatment. In the majority of instances the weight remains stationary, for the patient is able to retain food in adequate amounts at some period of the day. Lassitude is often an associated symptom, but this is almost pathognomonic of pregnancy, occurring in most patients within a few days after the first missed period and persisting until the end of the third month.

In hyperemesis gravidarum, or pathologic vomiting, the symptoms are markedly exaggerated. In discussing the treatment of this disease, it is helpful to divide the patients into two groups, with the severity and duration of the vomiting as a basis.

The *moderately* severe group includes patients who have had unrestrained vomiting for two to four weeks. The pulse is slightly elevated but below 100 beats per minute, and although there is often a weight loss of 10 or more pounds, there may be little evidence of serious nutritional change. There is moderate to severe dehydration, and the patient is generally miserable and anxious to have relief from her symptoms. The condition is entirely reversible, however, and, with rare exceptions, patients respond to corrective therapy and are free from symptoms within a few days.

The *severe* or neglected group, rarely if ever seen today in most countries and societies, includes patients who have been vomiting continuously for over four weeks. There is marked weight loss, even to the point of emaciation. The pulse is elevated to 110 or more beats per minute, and in the seriously ill patient jaundice may be present. The patient is severely dehydrated, and the effects of nutritional depletion are evident. Vitamin C lack is evident by scurvy-like lesions of the gingiva, which are soft and spongy and bleed easily; subperiosteal hemorrhages are suggested by pain over the anterior surface of the tibia. Folic acid depletion in longstanding vomiting is associated with a macrocytic nutritional anemia and characteristic oral and rectal lesions. In fact, a personal failure to appreciate the significance of the development of diarrhea in a patient with severe hyperemesis gravidarum in which constipation is a universal complaint, delayed the diagnosis of this nutritional deficiency until it was demonstrated by careful and complete hematologic examination. The lesions that were revealed by sigmoidoscopic examination disappeared rapidly with administration of folic acid. The ocular hemorrhages that have been reported in the severe form of this disease may be a manifestation of vitamin C deficiency. This rare finding consists of areas of retinal hemorrhage about an otherwise normal disc.

Vitamin B deficiency in hyperemesis gravidarum is usually seen in the form of a polyneuritis, with marked muscular weakness and wasting of the extremities. The neurologic findings are more frequently seen in the lower extremities and rarely in the upper extremities. The deep reflexes are absent, while some, but rarely all, of the abdominal reflexes are difficult to elicit. Symptoms of a psychosis may be present, with hallucinations and confabulation, as seen in Korsakoff's syndrome.

LABORATORY OBSERVATIONS

The laboratory observations frequently reflect the patient's state of dehydration and the findings must be so interpreted. The erythrocyte count and the hematocrit and hemoglobin values are often normal or abnormally high. With proper hydration these values decrease and it will be evident in many of these patients that a hypochromic anemia or a macrocytic nutritional anemia has been masked by the dehydration. Likewise, the blood urea nitrogen and uric acid values may be temporarily increased, but these usually return to normal following the restoration of body fluids. The appropriate function tests may denote parenchymal liver damage. In the beginning of vomiting there is a loss of chloride and an excess of available base. With protracted vomiting tissue catabolism is increased, and with glycogen depletion a metabolic acidosis develops. The urine consistently contains acetone bodies, and bilirubinuria reflects liver involvement. Proteinuria is usually present in the initial specimens, but generally disappears after the correction of dehydration.

TREATMENT

The treatment of nausea and vomiting of pregnancy has both a medical and an obstetric component, but is mostly medical. The physician should display a sympathetic and understanding attitude and exhibit a convincing desire to relieve the patient of her symptoms. Too often these patients are regarded as emotionally unstable, supersensitive individuals. If the physician holds such a view and bases his treatment accordingly, the patient may sense the fact and regard herself as queer or different and resent the implication. Information sometimes unfortunately gained from the physician or from casual remarks of the husband may connote to the patient that the condition is due to psychologic rather than pathophysiologic reasons. All of this contributes to a sense of insecurity and, in her attempt to carry on, the patient's symptoms become unnecessarily aggravated and more difficult for her to control.

The medical treatment of mild nausea and transient vomiting of early pregnancy is largely empiric and supportive. In fact, there is perhaps no condition in medicine in which so many pharmacologic, endocrine, and vitamin preparations have been offered as a specific remedy. These reports are usually without adequate controls, and subsequent experience has failed to substantiate the original therapeutic claims.

In effect, treatment must be considered a part of the routine of prenatal care. To avoid the consequences of an empty stomach, a time-honored regimen is to prescribe frequent small meals. Actually, the patient should be allowed to choose whatever foods may appeal to her, for it is reasonable to suppose that foods of her own choice may be more acceptable to her than those suggested by the physician. It is more likely that the patient will eliminate fats from her diet, and it is hoped that she will retain adequate amounts of carbohydrates and proteins. Constipation is the rule, requiring a mild cathartic or occasionally an enema for its correction.

The vomiting may be diminished by the use of various sedatives in small doses. Phenobarbital is a longstanding remedy, and is usually given in one half grain doses in midmorning, in midafternoon, and at bedtime. Dramamine and the various tranquilizer drugs also have their supporters. Because of the threat of liver damage, prolonged administration of certain of these medications should be avoided.

The usually energetic person is disturbed, however, by the lassitude, lack of energy, and the desire for additional sleep. To suggest sedatives to such a patient for the control of her nausea seems paradoxical, and indeed may be impractical by making her so drowsy that she will be unable to carry on a minimum of household duties. A compromise must be reached in such patients, and the unpleasantness of the symptoms must be weighed against the desire for relief. The patient must be made aware that the condition will usually disappear spontaneously sometime during the third month of pregnancy. In the interim she should be given a schedule which should include periods of rest. These simple remedies, plus the assurance that this condition is common to normal and otherwise stable women, usually suffice to control the symptoms of most patients.

The immediate problem in the management of patients with hyperemesis gravidarum is to combat dehydration and starvation with the treatment directed toward correcting the metabolic deficiencies. The treatment should always be conducted in the hospital, for these patients need expert nursing care and medical supervision. On admission, and as needed thereafter, an enema should be given to correct the ever present constipation. Liberal amounts of sedatives should be administered, rectally if necessary, to decrease the impulse to vomit and to ensure rest.

Following effective sedation a regimen should be initiated to correct the nutritional deficiencies, the most immediate being the dehydration. Two or three liters of potassium-containing solutions, alternating 5 per cent glucose in water and physiologic saline solution, should be administered parenterally daily until such time as the patient is retaining normal amounts of fluid and the urine is consistently free of acetone bodies. Hypokalemia may develop on occasion with severe hyperemesis, since potassium is lost in large amounts in gastric vomitus. In years past sudden death was observed in patients with severe hyperemesis gravidarum following apparently adequate hydration and some clinical improvement. It is conjectural, in retrospect, whether a hypokalemia with resultant respiratory failure may have been the basis for these deaths, since microscopic appearance of the kidney is consistent with a severe potassium deficiency in some of the fatal cases. Marked muscular weakness and the disappearance of the deep reflexes should arouse suspicion of a possible potassium depletion. Certainly in the seriously ill patient an electrocardiogram should be performed at intervals to detect, at the earliest moment, potassium deficiency should it develop. Parenteral potassium-free solutions of glucose and sodium can and will aggravate the effects of its depletion. If the electrocardiogram shows evidence of potassium depletion, potassium should be added to the intravenous fluid, in amounts of 20 to 40 mEq. per liter, until the patient is taking and retaining food and fluids.

If vomiting continues, the patient should be fed by gavage. A small tube is passed into the stomach 1 hour after the rectal administration of 3 to 6 grains of Sodium Amytal. The tube is connected to a side-arm flask through which the patient can be given, at hourly intervals, alternate feedings of 4 to 6 oz. each of milk, eggnog, and orange juice, containing supplementary vitamins. In addition, supplementary vitamins including folic acid are administered either parenterally or intramuscularly. This type of therapy is continued for an 8- to 12-hour period daily, until the patient ceases to vomit for at least 24 to 48 hours. Once this has occurred, the patient may be started on frequent small feedings by mouth, begin-

ning with a soft-solid diet; usually within two or three days the patient is retaining sufficient food to begin to replenish her depleted nutritional stores.

After one or two days of careful medical management, and at a time when the patient is feeling appreciably better, there should be several friendly personal interviews between the patient and her physician. The worries and troubles of these patients follow no special pattern. The social, economic, and personal problems may be complicated and relevant in some patients, and entirely absent or unimportant in others. Sympathetic guidance and understanding will contribute to the patient's ultimate recovery.

Therapeutic abortion has a place in the management of hyperemesis gravidarum, although with present-day treatment it is the rare patient who requires this procedure. In the moderately severe case therapeutic abortion must be considered should medical therapy fail, that is to say, in the event that vomiting persists despite careful medical treatment of some five to seven days' duration, or if bile appears in the urine, jaundice develops, or the pulse rate increases above 110 to 120 beats per minute. Continuation of the pregnancy may prove fatal in these situations.

Although therapeutic abortion soon after hospital entrance was regarded at one time as the only hope of recovery in the severe or neglected case, it is now realized that the procedure should be postponed at least for a time. The patient's condition may be so critical that any surgical procedure at this time would only decrease the chance of recovery. Hence, therapeutic abortion should be considered only after some progress has been made in combating the nutritional deficit, which may require one or two weeks of intensive medical treatment. The procedure can then be performed without undue risk. Personal experience supports the view that in the patient with the neglected or severe form of this disease recovery will be hastened by termination of the pregnancy. This is particularly true if there are neurologic changes, for these seem to improve more rapidly with termination than with continuation of the pregnancy.

In summary, with the supportive treatment as outlined, therapeutic abortion is infrequently needed and is restricted mainly to the rare patient with the moderate form of hyperemesis gravidarum who fails to respond to medical therapy. However, the patient's condition must be evaluated daily, and, if therapeutic abortion is to have a favorable effect, it should be performed before the situation becomes critical and the patient enters the severe or neglected stage.

BIBLIOGRAPHY

Adams, R. H., Gordon, J., and Combes, B.: Hyperemesis gravidarum; I. Evidence of hepatic dysfunction. Obstet. Gynec., 31:659, 1968.

Berkwitz, N. J., and Lufkin, N. H.: Toxic neuronitis of pregnancy; clinicopathological report. Surg. Gynec. Obstet., 54:743, 1932.

Combes, B., Adams, R. H., Gordon, J., Trammell, V., and Shibata, H.: Hyperemesis gravidarum; II. Alterations in sulfobromophthalein sodium-removal mechanisms from blood. Obstet. Gynec., 31:665, 1968.

Harvey, W. A.: Psychological findings in patients with vomiting during pregnancy. Arch. Neurol. Psychiat., 66:659, 1951.

Kroger, W. S., and DeLee, S. T.: Psychosomatic treatment of hyperemesis gravidarum by hypnosis. Amer. J. Obstet. Gynec., 51:544, 1946.

McGaugan, L. S.: Severe polyneuritis due to vitamin B deficiency in pregnancy. Amer. J. Obstet. Gynec., 43:752, 1942.

Ober, W. B., Reid, D. E., Romney, S. L., and Merrill, J. P.: Renal lesions and acute renal failure in pregnancy. Amer. J. Med., 21:781, 1956.

Purtell, J. J., Robins, E., and Cohen, M. E.: Observations on clinical aspects of hysteria; quantitative study of 50 hysteria patients and 156 control subjects. J.A.M.A., 146:902, 1951.

Reid, D. E., and Teel, H. M.: Treatment of vomiting of early pregnancy. New Eng. J. Med., 218:109, 1938.

Robertson, G. G.: Nausea and vomiting of pregnancy; study in psychosomatic and social medicine. Lancet, 2:336, 1946.

Romney, S. L., Merrill, J. P., and Reid, D. E.: Alterations of potassium metabolism in pregnancy. Amer. J. Obstet. Gynec., 68:119, 1954.

Schoeneck, F. J.: Gonadotropic hormone concentration in hyperemesis gravidarum. Amer. J. Obstet. Gynec., 43:308, 1942.

Sheehan, H. L.: Pathology of hyperemesis and vomiting of late pregnancy. J. Obstet. Gynaec. Brit. Emp., 46:685, 1939.

Strauss, M. D., and McDonald, W. J.: Polyneuritis of pregnancy; a dietary deficiency disorder. J.A.M.A., 100:1320, 1933.

Chapter 16

Obstetric Hemorrhage in Late Pregnancy and Post Partum

Some 5 to 6 per cent of patients experience vaginal bleeding or staining in the last half of pregnancy. Roughly one third will prove to have placenta praevia or will develop premature separation of the placenta of sufficient severity to require investigation and definitive treatment. In those patients in whom the diagnosis is not established, and in the absence of local lesions of the vagina and cervix, it is assumed by exclusion that the bleeding is due to slight placental separation or a small rupture of the marginal sinus of the placenta. Presumably the involved blood vessels thrombose and the bleeding ceases. The clinical problem is to identify and properly manage those patients with placenta praevia or a degree of placental separation that may threaten fetal existence and become hazardous to the mother.

Rigby, in 1776, was the first to distinguish between cases of placenta praevia and those of premature separation of the normally implanted placenta. In descriptive terms, he chose to call the latter "accidental hemorrhage," in contrast to the "unavoidable hemorrhage" associated with placenta praevia.

PLACENTA PRAEVIA

Definition

Placenta praevia develops when the ovum implants on or near the isthmic portion of the uterus, and the placenta, in its subsequent growth and development, covers a portion of the lower uterine segment (Fig. 1). Cases have been reported in which implantation occurred within the upper

cervix and were accordingly designated *cervical pregnancy.*

Incidence

Placenta praevia is encountered in approximately 1 per cent of patients who are beyond the 20th week of pregnancy, but the diagnosis must be considered more frequently for reasons stated. The incidence would be even greater were it not for the fact that a number of pregnancies in which placenta praevia is destined to develop abort in the early weeks of gestation. Indeed, some 5 per cent of spontaneous abortions show gross evidence of low implantation of the placenta. (See Abortion.) The incidence of the condition is higher in multiparous than in primiparous patients,

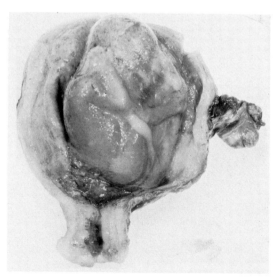

Figure 1. Uterus with central placenta praevia and fetus in situ.

and the greater the parity the more frequently is placenta praevia found.

Pathogenesis

The etiology of placenta praevia is still a subject of speculation, but a number of explanations have been offered for its genesis. The morphologic material on which these concepts are based is meager, and in some instances different interpretations have been placed on the gross specimens.

The original concept, dating back to the time of Soranus, but popularized near the turn of this century by German obstetricians, asserted that on occasion the decidua was unsuited for placental development, but the ovum during its descent through the uterine cavity might by chance encounter an area of healthy endometrium in the lower portion of the uterus and implant there (Fig. 2). Exhaustion of the endometrium with its failure to regenerate fully was believed to follow a rapid succession of pregnancies, trauma, and what was termed chronic endometritis.

Later, it was proposed that a placenta praevia could develop after implantation in the upper segment owing to a faulty and poorly vascularized endometrium. In the presence of relative ischemia, the placenta, in order to be an effective organ of transport, must possess a greater decidual surface than normal. Accordingly, during its growth and development, the placenta spreads over a large area and presumably extends on occasion into the lower uterine segment. Certainly in some cases of placenta praevia the placenta is thin with a large surface area, and additional cotyledons in the form of succenturiate lobe formation are not uncommon, lending support to this hypothesis (Fig. 3).

In one well preserved in-situ specimen of a placenta praevia the decidua basalis in the upper segment was found to be scanty compared with the other areas of the uterine lining. If this concept is valid, that the condition develops because of the need, through lack of normal decidual blood supply, for an excessively large surface area for effective fetomaternal exchange, the placenta would tend to develop eccentrically to the site of implantation, and, therefore, the marginal insertion of the umbilical cord should be a common finding in placenta praevia. Actually, marginal insertion of the cord is not uncommon in placenta praevia.

The term "chemotropism" was introduced to indicate that, if the endometrium of the upper segment is inadequate, by preference the ovum will implant somewhere in the lower uterine segment, that is to say, on the most suitable endometrium available. However, characteristically the uterine isthmus is covered with significantly less endometrium than is the uterine corpus. Indeed, the scantiness of the endometrium over the isthmus favors the development of placenta accreta, a complication that occurs with some frequency in placenta praevia.

A third concept proposed that a placenta praevia may develop from the portion of the decidua reflexa or capsularis located near or

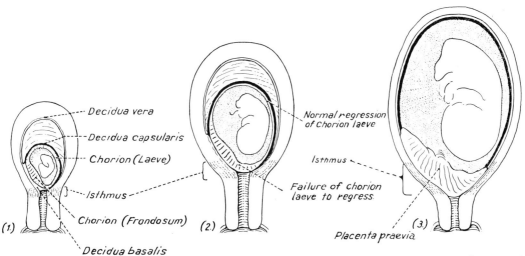

Figure 2. Implantation on the uterine isthmus or future lower uterine segment, with schematic demonstration of the development of a placenta praevia.

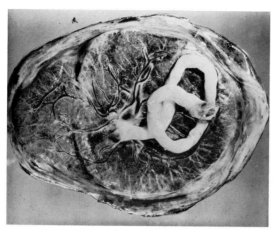

Figure 3. Placenta in a case of placenta praevia, due to succenturiate lobe. Note the chorionic vessels to the extrachorionic portion. If such vessels are found ruptured at routine inspection of the placenta after delivery, the uterus should be explored promptly and the succenturiate lobe recovered.

in contact with the lower uterine segment. Were a placenta praevia to form, the villi of the chorion laeve beneath this particular area of the decidua capsularis would have to persist. In accordance with this concept of the pathogenesis, the chorion laeve adjacent to the lower segment presumably fails to outgrow its blood supply as in normal placentation and the villi continue to flourish to form a placenta praevia. In fact, the belief was expressed that the decidua capsularis and decidua vera not only come in contact with each other but actually form an attachment, but the fusion is delayed until the fourth or fifth month of pregnancy. There is no evidence to show that the vessels of the decidua capsularis anastomose with those of the decidua vera. Certainly if the decidua capsularis becomes involved in placental formation, this must occur in the early weeks of placentation, and cannot be delayed beyond the 10th or 12th week. Further, one would expect the portion of the placenta comprising the praevia to develop beyond the chorionic plate and be devoid of a marginal sinus. Circumvallate placenta, however, occurs with no greater frequency in placenta praevia than in normal implantation.

According to this hypothesis a placenta praevia would in fact be a variant of placenta membranacea. The latter, an extremely rare condition of unknown etiology, develops from the failure of the chorion laeve to regress completely. Consequently the placenta fails to become the usual discoid organ limited to the chorion frondosum and decidua basalis. Rather, areas throughout the chorion, and involving the decidua capsularis, basalis, and vera, participate in the formation of the placenta, causing the amniotic sac to be covered with large islands of placental tissue.

Whatever it may mean in terms of etiology, the incidence of placenta praevia is related to high parity. Rather than any deficiency of the reproductive process, a high fertility index appears to be a factor in the development of placenta praevia. Perhaps highly fertile patients retain the ovum when it implants low within the uterus, whereas under similar circumstances less fertile women abort.

Classification of Types of Placenta Praevia

The clinical course of patients with placenta praevia is governed largely by the extent and location of the placenta within the lower uterine segment. The amount of the placenta involved in the praevia becomes an important factor in decisions of management, methods of delivery, and the evaluation of the results of therapy. It is clinically helpful, therefore, to classify cases of placenta praevia into several groups on the basis of the relationship of the placenta to the internal os of the cervix as determined at vaginal examination or at the time of cesarean section.

Over the years several classifications have been presented of the various types of placenta praevia, and attempts have been made to develop one that would be acceptable to all. The most commonly used classification is as follows: (1) total placenta praevia—the internal os is covered by placenta; (2) partial placenta praevia—the internal os is partially covered by placenta; (3) low implantation of placenta—the margin of the internal os is encroached upon by the placenta so that the placenta does not extend beyond the margin of the internal os.

Although this classification describes the position of the placenta, it fails to provide the criteria necessary to establish in every instance the amount of placenta involved in the praevia. In other words, the type of placenta praevia diagnosed is determined to a degree by the extent of cervical dilatation at the time of examination and not necessarily by the extent of the praevia. For example, when the placenta abuts on the edge of the cervix at the time it is 2 cm. dilated, as determined by vaginal examination, the amount of placenta included in the praevia is considerable. On the other hand, if the placenta is at the edge of the internal os when the cervix is 8 cm. or more dilated, the extent of the praevia is obviously much less. According to the classification, in both instances the findings fulfill the definition of a marginal or a low implantation type of placenta praevia, but the clinical course and management in the two instances are quite different.

In order to establish in each case the extent of the placenta praevia, it seems basic to compare the pelvic findings under standard conditions. Certainly the treatment and the anticipated clinical course of the patient depend on a precise description of the amount of placenta involved, as well as its location.

The following classification, based on the pelvic findings *when the cervix is approximately 2 cm. dilated,* is proposed (Fig. 4). This standard for cervical dilatation is selected because it represents the clinical situation that exists in the majority of patients with placenta praevia when they are examined in the latter weeks of pregnancy and before the onset of labor. Four types are distinguished: (1) complete, or central, type —the placenta covers the opening of the internal os; (2) partial type—the placenta covers the lower uterine segment beyond 8 cm. dilatation and sometimes a portion of the internal os; (3) marginal type—the placenta is at or within 3 cm. of the circumference of the 2 cm.-dilated internal os, a circumstance in which the placenta would abut on the internal os were the cervix about 8 cm. dilated; (4) low attached type— the placenta is within 4 to 5 cm. of the circumference of the internal os. In other words, the examining finger, when introduced through an internal os dilated 2 cm., can barely palpate the placenta. This is commonly referred to as a low implantation of the placenta.

Although it does not take into account the pelvic findings under standardized conditions, a classification has been introduced

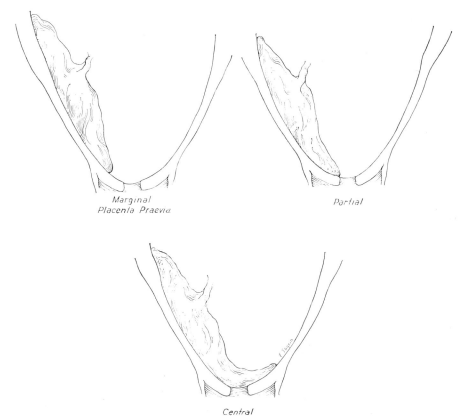

Marginal
Placenta Praevia

Partial

Central

Figure 4. Schematic demonstration of the three more extensive types of placenta praevia as identified with the cervix 2 cm. dilated.

into British obstetrics that also recognizes four degrees or types of placenta praevia (Fig. 5).

Diagnosis

The diagnosis of placenta praevia is based on a reliable history and observation of painless uterine bleeding appearing in the latter half of pregnancy. Characteristically the bleeding occurs without warning and in the absence of trauma, and unless the patient is experiencing labor the bleeding is not accompanied by pain. Owing to the presence of the placenta in the lower uterine segment, abnormal presentations are rather common. For example, should a transverse fetal position be recognized in the course of a routine prenatal examination in the latter weeks of pregnancy, the possibility of a placenta praevia should be realized and the diagnostic procedure is placental local-

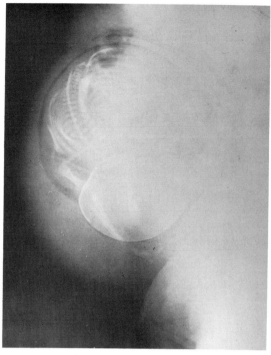

Figure 6. Placentography revealing central placenta praevia with an associated transverse presentation.

ization before the patient has experienced her initial bleeding (Fig. 6).

Placentography or localization of the placenta in situ is especially useful in the period prior to the 35th to 36th week of pregnancy. After that period, vaginal examination under "double set-up" precautions will definitively establish the diagnosis. Vaginal examination is contraindicated before this time, for it may precipitate serious bleeding and demand immediate termination of the pregnancy.

The critical period is up through the 34th to 35th week. If the diagnosis can be excluded by placental localization and bleeding has ceased and the fetal condition is apparently normal, the patient can be discharged from the hospital, after a short period of observation, to await the ultimate onset of labor. Presumably the bleeding was due to a mild placental separation or a small rupture of the marginal sinus. In either case the mother is without risk, as compared to the situation in placenta praevia. If placental localization indicates a placenta praevia, this would justify and indeed demand that the patient be hospitalized until delivery and expectant treatment instituted.

The methods of placental localization include:

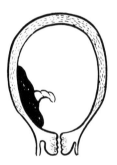

First Degree

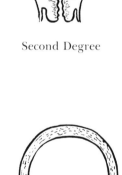

Second Degree

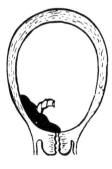

Third Degree   Fourth Degree

Figure 5. Various degrees of placenta praevia. (From Browne, F. J.: Antenatal and Postnatal Care. J. & A. Churchill, Ltd., London, 1947.)

1. Cystography, with the use of contrast medium of sodium iodide or air in the bladder. A demonstrating upward displacement of the fetal vertex from the bladder can be seen if the placenta is present in the lower segment. This method has been largely discarded.

2. Retrograde femoral angiography. This technique involves passing a small catheter through an 18 gauge needle previously introduced under local anesthesia, into the femoral artery about 10 inches distal to the aortic bifurcation. A contrast medium—25 ml.—is injected and a film taken within two or three seconds. The placenta is localized through the outline of the intervillous space.

3. Isotope localization. Radioactive iodinated (^{131}I) human serum albumin is the medium commonly used. A scintillation detector connected to a count rate meter is placed over the uterus, and the counts are recorded on a schematic diagram representing the uterus. To minimize or prevent thyroid uptake of the ^{131}I, especially by the fetus, Lugol's solution is prescribed for two weeks following the test and, if possible, a few days prior to the test. In any case, the total maternal irradiation with this method is stated to be less than 10 millirads.

4. Ultrasonic technique. This method is said to outline the precise boundaries of the placenta. It has the advantage that radiation hazard is not a consideration. In the hands of the experienced this is proving to be a highly accurate and useful method.

5. Soft tissue technique. Placental localization utilizing the soft tissue technique has been widely used. When performed during the last six to eight weeks of pregnancy by a skilled technician, this technique can locate the placenta in 95 per cent of the cases of suspected placenta praevia. With the patient lying on her side on the x-ray table, a lateral view is taken with a Potter-Bucky diaphragm and conventional 14 by 17 inch film. Also, a standing lateral film of the abdomen aids in establishing the relationship of the fetal head to the pelvis.

In reading the film, a gooseneck lamp is found useful to demonstrate the contrast between the uterine wall and the placenta. In a satisfactory film, the wall of the uterus stands out in sharp relief to the abdominal and amniotic sac contents, and it becomes significantly thicker in the area where the placenta is implanted. In addition, when the placenta is located on the posterior wall, the presenting part will lie several centimeters away from the sacral promontory.

When the film is being interpreted it should be realized that the anterior uterine wall is several centimeters longer than the posterior (Fig. 7). In a posterior implant a tentative diagnosis of placenta praevia can be made whenever the upper margin of the placenta is below the fundal portion of the uterus (Fig. 8). To warrant a diagnosis of probable placenta praevia in an anterior implant, however, the upper margin of the placenta should be below the junction of the upper and middle thirds of the uterine wall. In other words, in an anterior wall implant the diagnosis of placenta praevia is excluded if any portion of the placenta is implanted in the upper third of the fundal portion of the uterus. Although the uterine wall is well outlined, the placenta occasionally will not be seen. These findings are consistent with the diagnosis of a complete placenta praevia, for it is assumed that the placenta is totally contained within the lower uterine segment and cannot be visualized.

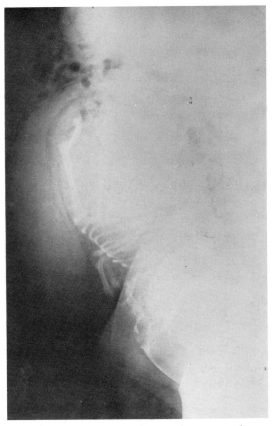

Figure 7. Placentography revealing a normal anterior wall implant. No placenta praevia.

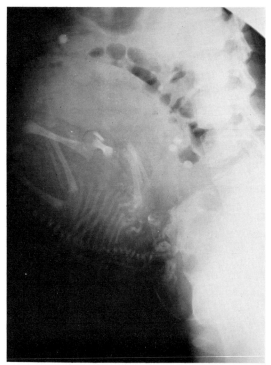

Figure 8. Placentography showing low-attached or first-degree placenta praevia, despite high posterior implant.

In résumé, all the methods have a 95 to 98 per cent accuracy, within certain limits. Presumably the angiographic and ultrasonic techniques are accurate by the early and middle portion of the third trimester. The soft tissue technique is less accurate before the 34th week of pregnancy, as is the isotope technique. With the latter there may be difficulty in recognizing a posterior implant. It may be that the ultrasound technique can permit identification of the placenta in the last 10 weeks of pregnancy, or even earlier, and with total accuracy.

As to abdominal findings, in the patient suspected of placenta praevia, on palpation the presenting part is usually found above the pelvic inlet, and, except in the milder forms, the presenting part does not enter the pelvis when pressure is applied by the examining hand over the fundal area of the uterus. When the placenta praevia is located on the posterior uterine wall, the presenting part is displaced forward and overrides or protrudes above the superior or upper margin of the mother's symphysis pubis. Conversely, the fact that on abdominal palpation the presenting part appears to be engaged does not exclude the possibility of a placenta praevia. The placenta may be thin and occupy little space, allowing the presenting part to enter the pelvis.

Although placentography is helpful, *the definitive diagnosis of placenta praevia is made by vaginal examination performed according to a definite technique. Rectal examinations must never be performed on patients who bleed in the last trimester of pregnancy if placenta praevia is a possible diagnosis.* The examination will furnish little information and may dislodge the placenta sufficiently to produce a dangerous hemorrhage when the examiner is not prepared to arrest it.

If a patient in whom a placenta praevia is suspected is to be examined vaginally, it should always be in the operating room, which is previously made ready for whatever obstetric procedure may be indicated. To avoid any delay in institution of the appriate treatment should bleeding recur at the time of the vaginal examination, both pelvic and abdominal kits should be available for immediate use. The examination requires an obstetric team composed of a suture nurse and operating assistants properly scrubbed and gowned in the event that abdominal hysterotomy becomes necessary. This arrangement of the operating room has become known as the *double set-up* preparation for the diagnosis and management of patients suspected of having placenta praevia.

The patient is anesthetized in the operating room by a highly skilled, experienced anesthesiologist. The type of anesthesia should be individualized, with the facts kept in mind that blood loss is unpredictable and that fetal distress is common. After preparation of the vulva and adjacent areas, the patient is draped and the cervix is inspected for any local lesion that might account for the bleeding. Next, a bimanual vaginal examination is performed. Initially, the vaginal fornices are carefully palpated, and with the abdominal hand the examiner attempts to impress the presenting part into the pelvis. If it can be brought into close apposition to the lower uterine segment, this is suggestive evidence that the patient does not have a placenta praevia, at least of the complete type. Also, this maneuver indicates the possible location and extent of the placenta praevia when the presenting part is easily palpable in one of the fornices and not in another. Some clinicians believe that palpating the vaginal fornices and estimating the thickness of the tissue between the examining fingers and the presenting part is sufficient to either exclude or establish the diagnosis of placenta praevia. Although the difference in the thickness of the lower uterine segment is helpful information and may be useful as a guide, the unequivocal diagnosis depends on locating the placenta within the lower uterine segment (Fig. 9).

The final step in the examination, therefore, is to insert the examining finger gently through the cervical canal and beyond the internal os to verify the presence or absence of the placenta within the lower uterine segment. To avoid recurrent bleeding, the examiner should be cautious and gentle and attempt to locate the placenta without dislodging it. If initially the placenta is not encountered, the diagnosis of placenta praevia cannot be excluded until the examining finger has been swept around the inner surface of the lower uterine segment, to cover an area comparable to the internal os when the cervix is completely dilated (10 to 12 cm.).

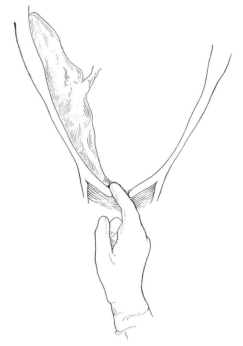

Figure 9. The ultimate in diagnosis of placenta praevia, in this instance the partial type.

Differential Diagnosis

After local lesions of the cervix, premature separation of the normally implanted placenta and rupture of the marginal sinus are the other causes of late obstetric hemorrhage. The differences in signs and symptoms between premature separation of the more severe type and placenta praevia are listed in Table 1.

In marginal sinus rupture the diagnosis is one of exclusion and can be confirmed only at delivery. The blood clot that can be observed at the placental margin often extends onto the fetal membranes. The bleeding is painless and simulates that in placenta praevia. When first seen, the patient often

TABLE 1.   FEATURES DISTINGUISHING PLACENTA PRAEVIA AND PREMATURE SEPARATION OF THE PLACENTA

Placenta Praevia	Premature Separation of the Placenta
1. Bleeding is mostly external	1. Bleeding is external, but much of it is often concealed within the uterus
2. Pain and tenderness are absent unless the patient is in labor	2. Uterine pain is usually present; areas of uterine tenderness can be elicited
3. Uterus is soft and relaxed	3. Uterus is firm in consistency in certain areas and occasionally throughout
4. The uterus has a normal contour	4. The uterus may enlarge and change in contour depending on the amount of concealed hemorrhage
5. The presenting part is usually not engaged	5. The presenting part may or may not be engaged
6. The bleeding is often bright red in color	6. The bleeding is usually venous in appearance
7. The fetal heart tones are usually normal	7. The fetal heart tones may be irregular or absent
8. Shock is not present unless the amount of external bleeding is excessive	8. Shock is moderate to severe, depending on the extent of concealed as well as external hemorrhage
9. Urine examination is negative	9. Urine may contain a significant amount of albumin, and the sediment may contain casts
10. Vaginal examination reveals a placenta in the lower uterine segment	10. Vaginal examination reveals no palpable placenta—blood clots may be mistaken for the placenta

shows signs of impending labor; at least the uterus is irritable and contractions are evident on palpation. Artificial rupture of the membranes will usually suffice to control bleeding from this source. Amniotomy should be conducted in the operating room with the double set-up preparation.

Fate of the Placenta during Labor

Obviously in the complete form of placenta praevia extensive placental detachment occurs with cervical dilation. Although in the lesser forms the placenta may become detached (Fig. 10), in some instances it apparently can retract upward and remain attached. This phenomenon has been reported only in isolated observations; its incidence has never been determined in any series of cases. Certainly this is not a universal effect, for according to the British fetal distress and recurrent bleeding develop in at least 50 per cent of the partial and marginal types of placenta praevia treated by artificial rupture of the membranes, necessitating cesarean section in some cases. This fact alone places limitations on use of amniotomy and pelvic delivery in the conservative management of placenta praevia when the fetus is medically viable.

Perinatal Mortality

In recent years the fetal and neonatal mortality rate in cases of placenta praevia has been reduced to approximately 15 per cent, and in patients beyond the 35th week of pregnancy the perinatal mortality should not exceed 5 per cent. This improved perinatal mortality has been credited largely to the policy of expectant treatment. Undoubtedly some babies have been salvaged when delivery has been delayed until the fetus has reached a more mature state. Other factors deserving recognition include an overall improvement in anesthesia, adequate blood replacement prior to termination of the pregnancy, and expert care of the premature infant.

Fetal and neonatal deaths are due largely to the effects of intrauterine asphyxia and so-called hyaline membrane disease, especially in the premature group. Monstrosities are said to be relatively more common in cases of placenta praevia, providing an added indication for an x-ray film of the abdomen to ascertain the appearance of the fetus.

Owing to the position of the placenta, interference with the fetal circulation is an increased hazard, while the low-lying cord can more easily prolapse or become compressed by the presenting part. Like other organs of the body, the placenta has considerable functional reserve. Clinical experience gained at the time of cesarean section in cases of premature separation of the placenta supports the belief that approximately one half of the organ may become detached and the infant be liveborn. This may apply to placenta praevia although it is not entirely possible to relate the degree of praevia and perinatal mortality.

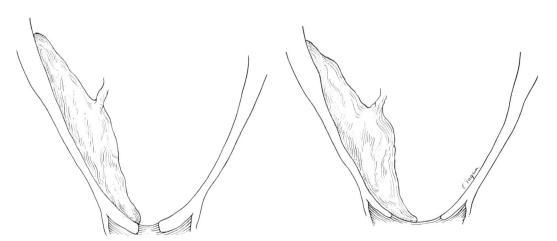

Figure 10. Partial placenta praevia. The placenta may become detached in the course of labor, and cause serious bleeding if untreated.

Treatment

The obstetric treatment of placenta praevia is either *expectant* or *immediate*. The course to be followed will depend on the *extent of the bleeding, whether it is continuing*, and the *maturity and condition of the fetus*.

Immediate treatment is indicated whenever the bleeding threatens the mother's welfare, *regardless of the stage of pregnancy or the maturity of the fetus*. If the patient is within four to five weeks of term, obstetric treatment should not be postponed, even though the bleeding may be slight or has ceased altogether. At this stage of pregnancy recurrent bleeding is more hazardous to both mother and fetus.

At least half of the patients with placenta praevia are within four to six weeks of term so that immediate treatment is warranted and usually mandatory when the patient is first seen. Some 20 per cent of patients seen prior to this period demand the same treatment because the magnitude of the bleeding is a serious threat to the mother.

This leaves about a third of the patients, in whom the fetus is still immature (i.e., prior to the 35th week) and the bleeding has subsided or ceased; here expectant treatment is preferable.

For the patient who enters the hospital within five to six weeks of term, bleeding actively and with the fetal heart tones normal, discovery of the cause of the bleeding becomes secondary to prompt definitive obstetric treatment. Valuable time must not be lost on placental localization. The diagnosis can be made on vaginal examination at this stage of pregnancy.

Although an acquired defect in the clotting mechanism is not expected in cases of placenta praevia, a clot observation test may be made on blood drawn for cross-match. Although the obstetric team should not sacrifice safety for speed, in a well conducted obstetric service, patients with serious degrees of bleeding should receive the benefit of definitive treatment within 30 minutes after hospital entrance. Otherwise, shock may supervene from needless blood loss, and any delay may result in the loss of the fetus or in birth of a severely hypoxic infant.

Although it is doubtful whether artificial rupture of the membranes will control bleeding of any magnitude when it originates from placenta praevia, the procedure will usually check hemorrhage from marginal sinus rupture and often from abruptio placentae, at the same time initiating productive labor and avoiding the necessity of cesarean section. The efficacy of the procedure will become obvious within a short time after the membranes have been ruptured. During the interim the patient should be kept in the operating room for any eventuality, and an immediate abdominal hysterotomy should be performed in the event of fetal distress or recurrence of bleeding.

On occasion the patient enters the hospital near exsanguination from late pregnancy hemorrhage. The immediate problem is to treat the shock and restore the blood volume by several rapidly administered blood transfusions. There should be one or more venous cut-downs to ensure a free flow of blood at transfusion, for in cases of this type complete vascular collapse is a constant threat. Central venous pressure should be monitored. Here, the preferential treatment is abdominal hysterotomy, regardless of the condition of the fetus or the amount of placenta involved, and vaginal examination is better deferred. In this precarious circumstance, if amniotomy failed to arrest the hemorrhage, irreversible shock could well supervene. In all likelihood bleeding of this severity is indicative of placenta praevia of the complete type.

In most patients with placenta praevia, however, the initial bleeding is not so alarming, often being described by the patient as a cupful or less. Frequently bleeding has ceased by the time of admission to the hospital, or there is only a trickle of blood exuding from the vagina. As indicated above, under these circumstances, preparations may be made for immediate obstetric treatment if the patient is within five weeks of term; otherwise expectant treatment is indicated.

The *expectant treatment* of placenta praevia is to delay delivery whenever possible in order to enhance fetal maturity and improve the fetal prognosis. This may mean a prolonged period of hospitalization for some patients. In the interim both the mother and fetus are at risk. The fetus may die in utero and the mother is subject to recurrent bleeding requiring supportive transfusion. At what point is the maternal risk unacceptable? Episodes of bleeding in which the blood loss reaches or exceeds 500 ml. would preclude the further pursuance of expectant treatment.

Another disturbing feature of expectant treatment is the possible effect of recurrent bleeding on the fetus if it survives. Evidence can be mustered to indicate that central nervous system damage, presumably from hypoxia, in these smaller infants is significantly increased, perhaps by some three times over the normal incidence (1.5 to 5 or 6 per cent). Although expectant treatment has permitted the salvage of some of these infants, it requires careful hospital observation and management and fortuitous timing of delivery.

Although conservative or expectant treatment should be employed through the eighth month of pregnancy, the mother's welfare must never be jeopardized in a desperate, and sometimes futile, effort to salvage the immature infant. Even those who advocate expectant treatment believe that definitive treatment should be instituted once the 36th to 37th week of pregnancy has been reached, and further delay is unwarranted.

The *definitive obstetric treatment* of placenta praevia is influenced by the following considerations: the extent of the bleeding, the degree of placenta praevia encountered, and the maturity and condition of the fetus. Ample amounts of compatible blood must be available for patients suspected of having placenta praevia, and no patient should be examined for placenta praevia except with *double set-up* precautions under which prompt treatment can be instituted.

The obstetric treatment is either cesarean section or artificial rupture of the membranes with vaginal delivery. No longer are methods of tamponade of the placenta used.

Patients with complete and partial placenta praevia are delivered by cesarean section. Most patients with marginal placenta praevia, and those with low-attached placenta praevia as defined can be treated by amniotomy unless there is a history of longstanding infertility or some other obstetric or medical indication for delivery by cesarean section. This form of treatment presupposes that the release of amniotic fluid will allow the presenting part to enter the pelvis, tamponade the portion of the placenta comprising the praevia and thus produce effective hemostasis. Slight traction on the fetal scalp by a special instrument, the Willett forceps, will ensure a more uniform pressure on the area of the placenta involved in the praevia. Oxytocin to stimulate labor must be given

with great care if at all, for the lower uterine segment is especially vascular and friable and subject to easier rupture.

It has been shown that when the placenta is implanted on the posterior uterine wall the presenting part is less likely to enter the pelvis after artificial rupture of the membranes. Engagement is presumably prevented by the interposition of the placenta between the presenting part and the sacral promontory. Here amniotomy in marginal or low-attached types of placenta praevia is more apt to fail as a therapeutic measure. Thus, cesarean section is the preferred treatment when the placenta is implanted posteriorly, regardless of the extent of the praevia.

When vaginal delivery is elected, interference with fetal circulation by pressure of the presenting part against the placenta or impingement of the cord is a distinct hazard. The patient therefore must be under constant surveillance by the physician throughout labor, and the fetal heart tones must be constantly monitored. The operating room must be kept in readiness for immediate cesarean section, in case fetal distress develops or bleeding of an alarming character recurs. A summation of reported clinical experience would indicate that in approximately one half of the patients with marginal or low-attached placenta praevia treated by amniotomy, fetal distress or recurrent bleeding may develop during the course of labor and necessitate abdominal delivery. Moreover, infection is a distinct hazard when the fetal membranes have been ruptured for several hours. Consequently, when amniotomy fails to produce effective labor in these cases, it may be unwise to postpone cesarean section indefinitely.

Some controversy exists concerning the type of cesarean section employed in the treatment of placenta praevia. The lower segment operation seems to be favored in most clinics. Besides the advantage of restricting the incision to the lower segment, it is proposed that it offers an opportunity to locate the source of bleeding should it occur in threatening amounts from the placental site once the placenta is delivered. Owing to the friability of the tissues involved, the placing of mattress sutures in and about the vessels of the placental site may fail, and the time so spent markedly augments the blood loss. The lower uterine segment contracts less well than the upper segment, a factor to be considered in the control of bleeding from the large uterine sinusoids beneath the portion of the placenta comprising the praevia.

In the belief that to avoid incising the placental site will minimize blood loss, the classic type of cesarean section is advocated. If the bleeding continues from the placental site despite the use of oxytocin, uterine packing should be considered, although this procedure is controversial. Failure to use a uterine pack on occasion is to disregard the principles involved in placental site hemostasis (see Postpartum Hemorrhage). One end of a gauze strip, 3 yards long and 1½ inches wide, is passed through the cervix, and the uterus is packed and closed. Placing one end of the gauze through the cervix first aids in identifying the pack and removing it some 24 hours after operation. In the patient with several children, when the uterus fails to contract and uterine atony is a threat, supracervical hysterectomy is performed immediately. See below.

Complications

PLACENTA ACCRETA. Probably because the uterine isthmus has less decidua, placenta accreta, usually of the focal type, occurs with greater frequency in placenta praevia than in upper segment implantations (Fig. 11). This is a formidable complication requiring prompt and energetic treatment. Valuable time should not be spent in attempting to remove the placenta piecemeal, for the blood loss can mount quickly. A rapid supracervical hysterectomy should be performed, with the cervix amputated as low as possible. Complete hysterectomy requires additional time and frequently leads to annoying ooze about the vaginal cuff, which, in a patient who has usually already experienced considerable blood loss, may be enough to initiate serious shock. Rather, with low cervical amputation bleeding can be brought under control by a series of overlapping mattress sutures through the remaining cervix. The area is then peritonealized in the conventional manner. A vaginal cervicectomy a few months later is a simple procedure.

ANTEPARTUM UTERINE INFECTION. Antepartum uterine infection is a threat in patients with placenta praevia, enhanced by the close approximation of the placenta to the cervix. Uterine infection poses a formidable clinical problem in the undelivered patient, regardless of the avail-

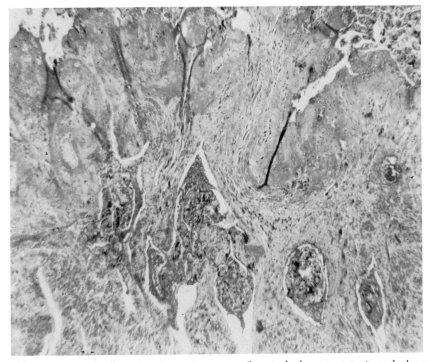

Figure 11. Photomicrograph of uterine tissue in a case of central placenta praevia and placenta accreta or increta. Note placental tissue adherent to the myometrium and penetrating into the substance of the myometrium. Failure to remove uterus at cesarean section resulted in a fatal hemorrhage.

ability of antibiotic and chemotherapeutic agents. In the extreme, abscesses may be encountered between the lower portion of the placenta and the myometrium.

The anterior location of the placenta praevia precludes use of the extraperitoneal type of cesarean section. The least hazardous procedure in this circumstance would be cesarean section followed by hysterectomy.

CERVICAL PREGNANCY. Cervical pregnancy is an extremely dangerous and serious complication, for it carries the risk of complete placenta praevia together with placenta increta. The initial diagnosis is more likely to be a complete placenta praevia, but further exploration at the time of cesarean section will reveal that implantation is deep in the lower uterine segment and on the inner surface of the cervix (Fig. 12). In the absence of decidua, the placenta becomes firmly attached to the fibrous and muscular elements of the cervix, causing the formation of a placenta accreta. The activity of the trophoblast may be such that it invades and eventually penetrates the cervix, producing a so-called *placenta increta*, or even a *placenta percreta*, with involvement of the vagina immediately adjacent to the cervix.

The cardinal symptom of bleeding appears early in the course of pregnancy, and in nearly every instance, by the middle of pregnancy, recurrent bleeding is of such magnitude that therapeutic intervention is required.

The management follows that for placenta praevia. After a period of observation, during which the patient usually requires and receives several transfusions, the bleeding becomes so alarming that the pregnancy must be terminated. Vaginal examination under a *double set-up* preparation reveals a cervix considerably dilated and what feels like a complete placenta praevia. A suprapubic mass consistent in size with a pregnancy dating from the time of the last normal menstrual period is outlined. Somewhere on its surface should be a small, nonpregnant corpus which can be mistaken for a fibroid. In other words, the body of the uterus is not involved in the pregnancy, and the cervix and lower segment become markedly attenuated.

Although cases have been reported in which the conceptus was removed vaginally and packing controlled the bleeding, pelvic delivery, which may be considered preferable because of the nonviable state of the fetus, is contraindicated because of the likelihood of the presence of a placenta accreta. Any manipulation is likely to precipitate

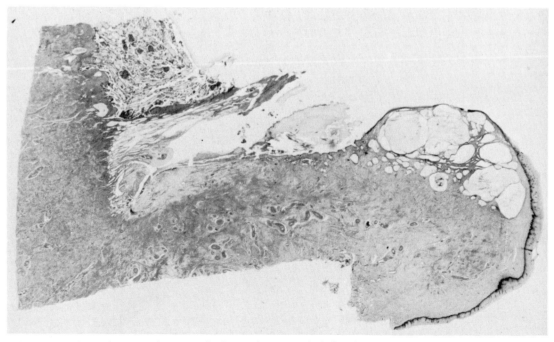

Figure 12. Sagittal section of cervix with placental tissue included in the upper cervix. Note the large nabothian cysts.

furious and uncontrolled hemorrhage. Rather, the vagina should receive additional surgical preparation and an immediate abdominal hysterotomy should be performed. After the fetus is removed, failure to recognize the condition may lead to serious error. Piecemeal attempt to remove the placenta will precipitate uncontrolled bleeding. Instead, a complete abdominal hysterectomy should be performed without delay. Some difficulty may be encountered in establishing the cleavage planes between the bladder, cervix, and vagina if there is a percreta, making effective hemostasis the subject of some concern. The effort to compromise with a supracervical type of hysterectomy may end in failure, however, for vaginal hemorrhage will continue from the placental site within the cervix. Proper preoperative preparation of the patient and maintenance of blood volume by multiple transfusion are paramount in the successful treatment of this extremely rare but serious condition.

PREMATURE SEPARATION OF THE NORMALLY IMPLANTED PLACENTA

Definition

Premature separation of the normally implanted placenta is the detachment of the placenta during the interval from the time the fetus reaches legal viability (the 20th week) until term. Abruptio or ablatio placentae and accidental hemorrhage, the latter term being that commonly used in British medicine, are used synonymously to describe this complication. When the placenta delivered prior to the 20th week shows premature detachment, the condition is regarded as incidental to an abortion and not as a separate clinical entity.

Premature separation of the placenta can be considered the most serious complication of pregnancy. Recorded experiences from several sources document the fact that in the more severe form of premature separation, which comprises 10 per cent of the cases, the maternal mortality may approximate 10 per cent. Fortunately, in 85 to 90 per cent of the cases only a relatively small area of the placenta is detached and the clinical course is comparatively benign. One must not fail to appreciate, however, the comparative risks in the severe versus the mild form of premature separation of the placenta.

In most patients who succumb from premature separation of the placenta, death is due to hemorrhagic shock. Renal and pituitary changes may occur which are themselves the result of hemorrhagic shock.

Incidence

Premature separation of the placenta of clinical significance occurs in approximately 1 per cent of all viable pregnancies. The general incidence, however, differs in the various series reported, with several factors accounting for this discrepancy. The frequency of the condition in any one clinic population will be influenced to a degree by the numbers of patients with pregnancy toxemia or vascular and renal disease, for there is a greater tendency for the placenta to separate in patients with these conditions. When the placenta is subjected to routine pathologic examination, the overall incidence of placental detachment is somewhat higher. This means that pathologic evidence of placental separation, either gross or microscopic, is present in some cases in which the condition had not been clinically diagnosed.

Etiology

Interference with the afferent flow of blood to the intervillous space has been the most popular premise for explaining the pathogenesis of premature separation of the placenta. By analogy, the decidual cells are the building blocks that support the structures of the placenta, specifically the villi and the maternal vascular channels of the placenta and placental site. These include the intervillous space and the vessels that enter and leave it, that is, the spiral arterioles with their accompanying veins and the marginal sinus. During the course of normal pregnancy, particularly in the last trimester, degeneration and necrosis of the decidua near its junction with the trophoblast are readily demonstrable. Should this process become pronounced, these vascular channels lose their support and collapse, causing bleeding from the placental site. The sequence of events might be compared to the morphologic alteration of the endometrium and its spiral arterioles that precedes and accompanies the menstrual bleeding. Whether the integrity of the spiral arterioles of the placental site is compromised by a critical fall in sex steroids must be regarded as speculative. Along the same vein, nutritional factors have been involved, more specifically, a folic acid deficiency. The latter remains in the realm of controversy with respect to etiology. Suffice to say patients with a megaloblastic anemia are seemingly no more prone to abruptio placentae or accidental hemorrhage than other patients.

It has been postulated that interference with the venous return of maternal blood from the uterus may cause placental separation. The weight of the term uterus on the inferior vena cava when the patient is in the supine position is thought to raise venous pressure in the uterine veins and intervillous space sufficiently to detach the placenta through the mechanism of a retroplacental hematoma formation.

However, one must recall that adaptive mechanisms exist to safeguard the stability of the uterine circulation, more precisely that within the intervillous space. The large medusae of veins in the broad ligaments have been commonly referred to as reservoirs for excess blood. Undoubtedly the venous pressure within the uterus and about the placental site is kept fairly constant through the dilation and contraction of these veins. At cesarean section these veins appear quite transparent, and by direct observation it is seen that the blood within them is in a state of turbulent flow. This would indicate that these vessels are capable of great accommodation, dilating and contracting at will. Under circumstances of acute vena cava stasis, therefore, any increase in venous pressure may become dissipated in the veins of the lower extremities and those contained within the broad ligaments.

Perhaps the most common type of abnormal placental development associated with premature separation is circumvallate placenta. A number of spontaneous abortions (5 per cent) show evidence of a developing circumvallate placenta, indicating that this is a frequent deviation in placentation. Moreover, besides playing a significant role in the etiology of late pregnancy bleeding, circumvallate placenta is the most common cause of uterine bleeding in the mid trimester. The chance of placental detachment in this type of anomaly is increased by the fact that the decidual necrosis in the extrachorionic area is more extensive, which favors placental separation in and about the periphery (Fig. 13).

Tension on a short umbilical cord during labor, or, for example, at the time of external version, by the mechanics involved may produce premature separation of the placenta. Such accidents are rare indeed, and the possibility need not contraindicate external version as an obstetric maneuver. Excessive intrauterine pressure from marked polyhydramnios or multiple pregnancy may lead to premature separation in one of two ways. Increased hydrostatic pressure presumably can produce pressure necrosis of the decidua and precipitate placental detachment. A sudden and marked decrease in intrauterine pressure may also cause the placenta to detach, as in the case of spontaneous rupture of the fetal membranes in the presence of polyhydramnios.

At no time in pregnancy will mild trauma cause premature separation of the placenta or other pregnancy accidents, and only rarely will a violent blow delivered over the abdomen cause the placenta to separate. Whenever physical violence occurs in any form, patients become fearful of their pregnancy and should be given a physical and obstetric examination, including auscultation of the fetal heart tones, to reassure them.

According to the literature, in 33 to more than 50 per cent of the cases of the more extensive type of premature separation there is some degree of proteinuria and hypertension. In view of the fact that only 5 to 10 per cent of all pregnancies are complicated by proteinuria and hypertension it is obvious that premature separation of the placenta occurs with much greater frequency in toxemic than in normal patients. It is postulated that the toxemic process, through constriction of the spiral arterioles of the placental site, causes more extensive decidual degeneration. The local vessel changes are considered part of the generalized arteriolar spasm that characterizes pregnancy toxemia. But the cause-and-effect relationship must still be established.

As previously stated, the diagnosis of premature separation in some cases has been made on pathologic findings rather than on clinical signs and symptoms. The histologic findings seem to indicate that the frequency of placental detachment increases with the severity of the toxemia. On the basis of available data, however, there appears to be no close relationship between the frequency of clinically manifested premature separation and the severity of the toxemia. In

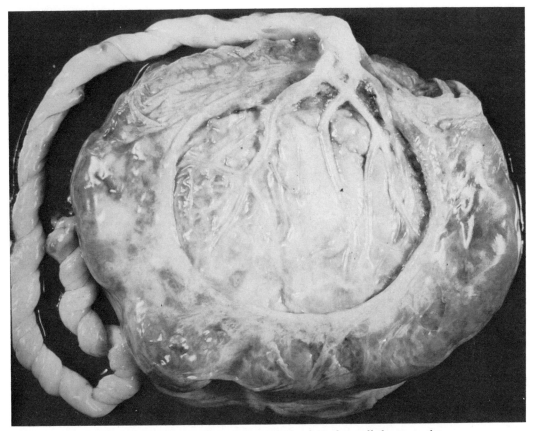

Figure 13.   A circumvallate placenta, with relatively small chorionic plate.

order to accumulate such data and to determine the influence that hypertension and albuminuria have on the production of placental separation, each case must be carefully diagnosed and categorized according to the classification of patients with pregnancy toxemia or vascular and renal disease.

Pathology

Degeneration and necrosis of the decidua basalis are considered to produce the earliest uterine lesion. Whether this is a mechanical effect produced by pressure of the growing conceptus or a functional disturbance of the blood vessels supplying the placental site remains obscure. Rare chance observation has revealed thromboses of the spiral vessels with degeneration and necrosis of the surrounding decidua. Also, degenerative changes in the placental site arterioles have been identified. In a few cases fat-laden phagocytes have been demonstrated beneath the tunica intima of the decidual arterioles (Fig. 14A). Fibrinoid deposition within the tunica media

of the vessel, followed by fibroblastic proliferation, has been observed. These changes may lead to obliteration of the vessel lumen with subsequent necrosis of the surrounding decidua (Fig. 14B). The various blood vessel changes thought at one time to be pathognomonic of the placental separation complicating pregnancy toxemia have been noted to occur predominantly in patients with antecedent vascular or renal disease.

Although in the circumvallate placenta the separation is limited to the periphery, in many instances separation is initiated by the formation of a retroplacental clot which mechanically detaches the placenta from the spongiosa layer of the decidua (Fig. 15). The process usually involves several, but sometimes only one or two, cotyledons. In the severe cases of partial to complete placental detachment, the measured clot volume at the time of delivery may be as much as 1000 ml. The retroplacental hematoma, together with the increased intrauterine pressure, may cause compression of the placenta, and removal of the hema-

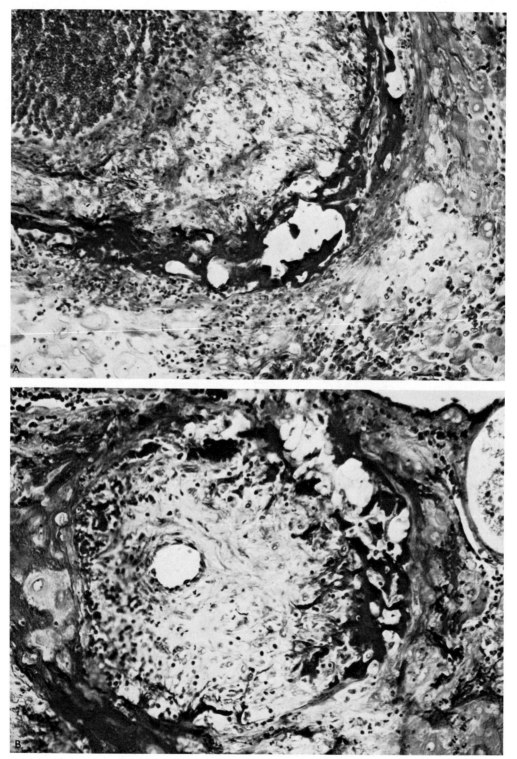

Figure 14.   Photomicrographs of tissue from placental site. A, Degenerative changes in an arteriole. Possibly seen only in patients with antecedent renal or vascular disease. B, End-result of arteriolar change with obliteration of the vessel by fibroblastic proliferation. (From Hertig, A. T., Clinics, 4:585, 1945.)

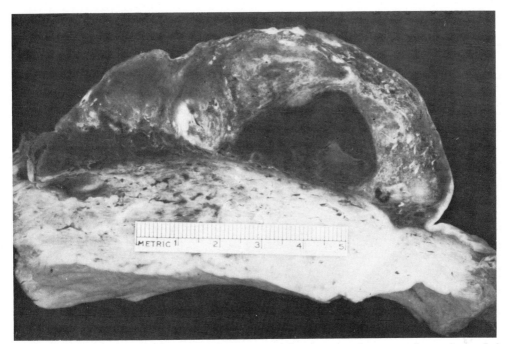

Figure 15. Sagittal section of uterus with placenta in situ, demonstrating formation of retroplacental clot and placental separation.

toma from the decidual surface of the placenta after delivery often reveals a characteristic saucer-like depression. Blood will dissect downward between the myometrium and the membranes, eventually escaping through the cervix. Seldom is the bleeding entirely concealed, and it is the rare patient who does not exhibit some external bleeding.

In the severe form of the disease the myometrium becomes infiltrated with blood that may involve the entire uterine wall. The serosa overlying the uterus assumes a mottled purplish appearance which tends to occur initially about the cornua and spread to other areas (Fig. 16). A uterus with this characteristic appearance is commonly referred to as a Couvelaire uterus. In addition, hematomas may form beneath the uterine serosa and within the broad ligaments, adding to the total amount of blood shed. In fact, considerable blood may be extravasated into the broad ligaments and retroperitoneal spaces of the lower abdomen. Cases are known in which hematoma formation was so extensive in the broad ligament as to cause ureteral obstruction and temporary mechanical anuria. The amniotic fluid is often seen to have a burgundy red color at the time of artificial rupture of the membranes or at cesarean section.

In fatal cases, pathologic changes may be evident elsewhere in the body but are restricted mainly to the liver and the kidney. Vascular lesions in the form of thrombosis and fibrin deposition have been reported throughout the body, and those occurring in the pituitary are particularly significant. Necrosis of the anterior pituitary and hypothalamic region has been observed. When liver lesions are present, there is usually an associated pregnancy toxemia. The liver may show small areas of peripheral necrosis consistent with those seen in convulsive toxemia.

When acute renal failure develops the kidney may show two types of lesions, bilateral cortical necrosis or acute tubular necrosis, the latter occurring when severe and prolonged shock has been a feature of the case. The renal lesions of bilateral cortical necrosis presumably are related to causes other than shock and renal ischemia, for the condition may develop in the patient when shock has at most been transient. A nephrotoxin has been evoked comparable to that associated with the crush syndrome. Whatever the exact etiology of the renal lesion, severe premature separation of the placenta accounts for the majority of cases of bilateral cortical necrosis encountered in medicine. However, this form of renal lesion is infrequent when considered in

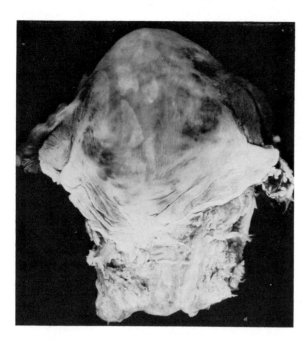

Figure 16. Uterus removed from a patient with the severe form of placental separation, showing the characteristic gross changes resulting from infiltration of the myometrium with blood (Couvelaire uterus).

relation to the total number of patients in whom severe premature separation of the placenta develops. Can there be any reason why this serious complication should occur in the rare patient and not in others? One study of a limited number of autopsies revealed that without exception nephrosclerotic changes were seen in the kidney. This is in accord with clinical experience that most cases of bilateral cortical necrosis in pregnancy occur in the older patients, in whom antecedent vascular and renal disease is more likely to be present.

There is another feature of the renal pathology that has clinical implications. The characteristic vascular lesion that accounts for the more extensive type of cortical necrosis is thrombosis of the intralobular artery, although thrombosis of the afferent glomerular arterioles is sometimes seen. There has been some debate as to whether the intralobular artery thrombosis is produced by propagation of the afferent glomerular arteriole thrombosis or originates as a separate lesion. In any event, intralobular artery thrombosis is rarely seen before 36 hours after the onset of severe premature separation. To the clinician, this should mean that indefinite delay in delivery enhances the chance that a patient with severe premature separation will develop this rare but possibly fatal renal complication, a fact that implies an element

of preventability in terms of patient management.

Diagnosis

The diagnosis of premature separation of the placenta presents no special difficulties, but evaluation of the extent of the disease poses an element of clinical uncertainty. Since the management and definitive treatment are governed largely by the amount of placental separation, the diagnosis should include some appraisal of the severity of the disease.

One of the earliest signs of premature separation of the placenta is vaginal bleeding, for, as stated, only rarely is the hemorrhage entirely concealed. Although abdominal pain and uterine tenderness may precede overt bleeding, they usually appear at its onset. In the severe form the uterus may increase in size, as determined by repeated measurement of the distance from the top of the fundus to the xiphoid process; it becomes exquisitely tender to palpation, and boardlike in consistency. When placental separation reaches this severe stage, the patient begins to reveal some degree of shock, and the fetal heart tones often disappear or are absent.

Proteinuria is present in some cases, but whether it is a precursor or an effect of the premature separation is debatable. Hence, it has been customary in these patients to make a diagnosis of toxic or nontoxic premature separation, depending on the presence or absence of proteinuria and hypertension. Thus, clinicians often view the patients with these findings as having the more severe form of premature separation. The severity of the disease, however, depends not so much on the presence or absence of toxemia per se, as *on the extent of the separation and the amount of concealed hemorrhage. It is unwise to assume that in the absence of demonstrable toxemia the patient's disease is necessarily mild, an important consideration with respect to treatment.*

The signs, symptoms, and laboratory findings enable one, with fair accuracy, to place patients into one of two groups, namely, the mild to moderately severe and the severe. In the former group, placental separation is generally not accompanied by shock, and, when present, shock is transient in character. The uterus is soft and relaxed, consistent in size with the length of gestation, and the fetal heart tones are usually of good quality. Uterine tenderness is restricted to a comparatively small area. If by chance cesarean section is performed, the serosal covering of the uterus may show slight localized discoloration, but otherwise the organ has a normal appearance.

By contrast, and stated previously, patients with severe premature separation reveal some, and at times an extreme, degree of shock. The uterus is tender to palpation. The fetal heart tones, although sometimes normal, may be absent or grossly slow and irregular in rate. When seen at cesarean section, the uterus has the characteristic bluish-purplish mottled appearance. Disturbances in blood clotting have been observed in patients with the severe form of premature separation of the placenta. Placentography may reveal moth-eaten appearing areas beneath the detached placenta, interpreted as large retroplacental hematomas. This is not a consistent finding, however, and hardly warrants placentography as an aid in diagnosis. However, ultrasound technique has described the same finding, and may aid in the diagnosis. The differentiation of this condition from the other major cause of late pregnancy bleeding will depend on vaginal examination performed with the proper precautions.

Table 2 lists the various features by which the severity and the amount of placental detachment can be estimated, and is proposed as a guide to clinical management.

Treatment

The obstetric treatment of premature separation of the placenta takes one of two forms. One is directed toward ultimate vaginal delivery; the other, abdominal hysterotomy. Regardless of which method is used, the seriousness of the complication necessitates close medical and constant nursing supervision of the patient until she has been safely delivered. Adequate amounts of blood for transfusion and other appropriate measures must be available to prevent or combat shock. The clotting mechanism is always evaluated.

TABLE 2.   FEATURES DISTINGUISHING MILD OR MODERATE AND SEVERE PREMATURE
SEPARATION OF THE PLACENTA

Mild or Moderate Type *(90 Per Cent of Cases)*	*Severe Type* *(10 Per Cent of Cases)*
1. Concealed hemorrhage, minimal; on abdominal palpation the uterus is relaxed, and existing tenderness is restricted to a small area	1. Concealed hemorrhage, extensive; on abdominal palpation the uterus is rigid, distended, and tender
2. Shock—absent or transient only	2. Shock of variable degree
3. Fetal heart tones usually within normal limits	3. Fetal heart tones often absent or irregular
4. Uterus may show localized areas of peritoneal discoloration at cesarean section, but myometrium is largely devoid of change	4. Uterine surface mottled and discolored; myometrium infiltrated with blood (Couvelaire uterus)
5. Proteinuria rare	5. Proteinuria frequent
6. Clotting mechanism always normal	6. Possible defect in the coagulation mechanism
7. On postdelivery examination of the placenta, 30 per cent or less of the maternal surface is found to be involved in the separation, with or without a small retroplacental hematoma	7. On postdelivery examination of the placenta, 50 to 100 per cent of the maternal surface is found to be involved in the separation; retroplacental hematoma is often of considerable size

With due regard for the individualization of patients, a general policy of management may be formulated on the basis of the estimated degree of placental separation. Like other organs, the placenta has a functional reserve. Clinical experience indicates that one third to one half of the placenta can be detached and the fetus survive. For the milder cases of premature separation induction of labor and pelvic delivery is the preferred method of treatment. The patient should be examined in the operating room with preparations for laparotomy should a placenta praevia be encountered or amniotomy or artificial rupture of the membranes fail to check the bleeding.

In addition to initiating labor, amniotomy is thought to immobilize the detached portion of the placenta. With judicious oxytocin stimulation in most instances labor will ensue and pelvic delivery may be anticipated. Careful observation must be continued during labor to detect any evidence of further placental separation or of fetal distress. Forceps delivery is performed soon after the first stage of labor is completed to avoid the risk of fetal hypoxia from further placental separation during the second stage of labor.

Cesarean section is performed in patients with the milder form of separation when effective labor fails to develop after artificial rupture of the membranes, if bleeding continues after amniotomy, or when clinical judgment indicates that further placental separation may be occurring and the fetus is in jeopardy. Rarely is it required for the treatment of continued bleeding after amniotomy. Accordingly, in this group cesarean section is performed primarily to salvage the fetus. Even so, prematurity, hyaline membrane disease, and the effect of hypoxia precipitated by the initial separation take their toll.

By contrast, the treatment of patients with the severe form of premature separation is directed primarily toward the interests of the mother. The summation in this group of the stillbirth rate and the neonatal morbidity and mortality from the extreme intrauterine asphyxia attests to the futility of designing treatment specifically to salvage the baby. Although one may be inclined to perform an immediate cesarean section if the fetal heart tone is perceptible at the time the diagnosis of severe premature separation is made, the relative maternal risk involved hardly justifies operation, at least as an immediate

procedure on hospital admission. However, it is recognized that cesarean section soon after the diagnosis is established continues to remain the method of choice in the treatment of severe premature separation of the placenta in many clinics. Recommendation of early surgical intervention is based on the belief that the so-called Couvelaire uterus is incapable of sufficient labor to accomplish pelvic delivery. According to this concept, cesarean section will provide prompt evacuation of the uterus and enable it to contract and thus control the bleeding. At the same time the procedure will allow the operator to perform a hysterectomy immediately, should uncontrolled postpartum hemorrhage ensue, presumably from atony.

Clinical experience attests to the fact that the quality of the uterine contraction is sufficient to effect pelvic delivery, although the myometrium may be markedly infiltrated with blood. Further, atony is not a special feature in patients so delivered. More significant is the possibility that the clotting mechanism may be insufficient for effective hemostasis. Cesarean section or, indeed, pelvic delivery under this circumstance may end in disaster from uncontrolled bleeding. As stated, however, postpartum hemorrhage rarely supervenes following pelvic delivery, and this suggests that a defect in blood clotting rather than uterine atony is responsible for such hemorrhage. Accordingly, hysterectomy will rarely be required in the treatment of postpartum hemorrhage associated with severe premature separation of the placenta, provided the deficiency in the coagulation mechanism has been corrected. Furthermore, the procedure could prove hazardous, indeed disastrous, should the clotting mechanism be abnormal at the time of surgery.

The treatment in severe premature separation, therefore, must take into account the possibility that the patient's blood is or is about to become incoagulable. The idea has been put forth that the clotting mechanism will deteriorate if the patient remains undelivered, and any delay in delivery is to be avoided. This reasoning must not disregard the possibility that the clotting mechanism may already be deficient when the patient is first observed, a not unusual clinical experience.

Instead of early delivery at the moment the diagnosis of severe premature separation is established, which would mean cesarean section except for the occasional patient who enters the hospital late in the first stage of labor, a more deliberate plan of treatment and study is recommended. The first step in the management of these patients is to determine whether a clotting defect exists, by performing a "clot observation test" and other determinations (see Coagulation Defects in Chapter 19). Immediately after the patient is admitted multiple transfusions are begun to combat shock and restore the blood volume to normal. With shock and circulatory collapse a constant threat, venous cut-downs are routine to ensure uninterrupted parenteral therapy. On the average, two to four transfusions are given during the first two hours. The clotting defect if present is treated. Morphine and atropine are given to quiet the patient and prepare her for an anesthetic if needed. The operating room is prepared for any eventuality.

One may gain the impression that the depth of the shock is out of proportion to the amount of blood shed. Consequently it has been proposed that some unknown factor, perhaps a toxic substance derived from traumatized tissue, is somehow responsible for the shock. It would seem unnecessary, however, to evoke reasons other than a decrease in effective blood volume to explain the shock, for the magnitude of the initial blood loss is often not fully appreciated. Reference has been made to hidden blood loss throughout the pelvis and uterus.

Early in the second hour after hospital admission a vaginal examination is performed in the operating room to verify the diagnosis and to determine the condition of the cervix. An amniotomy is performed, regardless of the degree of effacement and dilatation of the cervix. The fact that productive labor may ensue even when the cervix is regarded as unfavorable for induction justifies the routine rupture of the membranes before cesarean section. Moreover, there is the clinical impression that the process of defibrination seems to decrease and fibrinolytic activity diminishes following artificial rupture of the membranes.

During the third and fourth hours, additional blood and fibrinogen and possibly heparin are administered if indicated. It is anticipated that by this time the patient has recovered from her initial shock and her vital signs are normal. With the clotting mechanism known to be normal and the shock effectively treated, the patient may now face cesarean section without undue risk. Indeed, in the absence of effective labor some four to eight hours after artificial rupture of the membranes, cesarean section should be performed. A prolonged labor would seem unwise in a patient who has already experienced an episode of shock.

Experienced clinicians are aware that there is an occasional patient in whom separation of the placenta will occur in subsequent pregnancies. Also, too often this complication develops prior to the 35th to 36th week of gestation. These are trying cases, requiring the utmost in patient care. Restricted activity throughout pregnancy is mandatory for all these patients and for some, hospitalization by the 30th week. Repeated pregnancy failure justifies the delivery by cesarean section of these patients once the fetus has reached maturity, i.e., 35 weeks.

POSTPARTUM HEMORRHAGE

Definition

Postpartum hemorrhage denotes an abnormal amount of vaginal bleeding associated with delivery or the puerperium; a loss of more than 500 ml. of blood, either measured or estimated, is considered excessive.

Etiology

In considering the etiology of the condition, postpartum hemorrhage may be classified as immediate or late.

IMMEDIATE POSTPARTUM HEMORRHAGE. Immediate postpartum hemorrhage is associated with delivery and the early hours of the puerperium. The conditions causing such hemorrhage, in the order of their relative frequency, are discussed in the following paragraphs.

Lacerations of the birth canal, should they occur, usually follow operative vaginal delivery, but may on occasion be encountered in the absence of operative intervention. Bleeding caused by such lacerations may originate in the perineum, the vagina, the cervix, and, rarely, the lower uterine segment. More frequently involved are the vaults or lateral fornices of the vagina and the vaginal wall behind the pubic arch and lateral to the urethra.

Extension of the vaginal portion of the

episiotomy incision can result in considerable blood loss. Although it occurs only rarely after a median type of episiotomy, extension of the incision in the vaginal mucous membrane may be lateralward into the vaginal sulci but is more likely to be upward toward the vaginal-cervical junction posteriorly. In the latter event disruption of the branch of the vaginal artery located in this area may cause brisk bleeding. In a mediolateral episiotomy, the laceration will course upward into the lateral wall of the vagina.

Inept application of the forceps blades and poorly performed forceps procedures, particularly those involving rotation of the fetal vertex, may result in tissue trauma, especially of the vaginal fornices. The forceps extraction of the fetus when mid-pelvic or outlet contraction contraindicates pelvic delivery can severely damage the vaginal tissues anywhere.

Excessive pressure of the fetal occiput as it passes beneath the symphysis may injure the anterior wall of the vagina. Thus, during a forceps operation, extension of the vertex before the occiput has passed the symphysis may cause lacerations about the clitoris and anterior portions of the labia minora. A similar effect may follow when attempt is made to deliver the head by Ritgen's maneuver without first performing an episiotomy. Under these circumstances, as the operator attempts to deliver the vertex over the perineum without causing perineal lacerations, the anterior vaginal wall is subjected to undue pressure by the fetal occiput. Lacerations in this area can bleed copiously.

The cervix may lacerate during normal labor, but lacerations are more likely to follow operative delivery or tumultuous labor, which is a special hazard when labor is stimulated by oxytocic drugs. Disruption of cervical scar tissue from previous deliveries can be caused by the forces of labor and may extend upward, resulting in rupture of the lower uterine segment. In addition, tumultuous labor may produce multiple lacerations of the vagina from the rapid descent of the presenting part.

Atony of the uterus causes postpartum hemorrhage because the myometrium fails to constrict completely the endomyometrial vessels. Uterine atony is often precipitated by failure of the placenta to separate normally and to be extruded completely from the uterus. In some instances, either before or after delivery of the placenta, the uterus may fail to contract without obvious cause. Certain factors may adversely influence uterine contractility. Deep inhalation anesthesia for complicated operative deliveries, prolonged labor due to inertia, marked distention of the uterus by multiple pregnancy or polyhydramnios, and the presence of fibromyomata may interfere with the normal contractility of the uterus and contribute to the development of uterine atony.

The uterus tends to become atonic in the presence of hypotension. Thus, in a case of postpartum hemorrhage from sources other than the uterus, as in cervical and vaginal lacerations, and with the appearance of hemorrhagic shock, the uterus commonly becomes atonic. At this point there is a dual source of bleeding.

Retention of the placenta, sometimes the result of improper conduct of the third stage of labor, may lead to postpartum hemorrhage. The placenta may partially separate concurrent with delivery, but more frequently such partial separation follows attempts to hasten the completion of the third stage of labor by massage or compression of the uterus. In nearly all cases, within a period of 3 to 5 minutes after administration of a suitable oxytocic drug, the intact placenta will be expelled spontaneously with a blood loss of usually less than 100 ml. and rarely more than 200 ml. That is not to say that steps should not be taken to deliver the placenta if bleeding ensues.

Inversion of the uterus, although a rare cause of postpartum bleeding, is dramatic and serious, with shock out of proportion to the amount of blood lost. The method of treatment is dependent on the time at which the inversion is recognized.

Rupture of the uterus may occur from a variety of causes, but in nearly every instance one of the following circumstances is found: dehiscence of a previous cesarean section incision, prolonged and obstructive labor, ill advised or improperly performed operative pelvic delivery, or tumultuous labor, on occasion precipitated by oxytocic medication.

LATE POSTPARTUM HEMORRHAGE. Late postpartum hemorrhage is that occurring at any time during the puerperium after the first few hours, and it may be due to a variety of causes. There may be secondary bleeding from lacerations of the birth canal, usually on or about the 10th postpartum

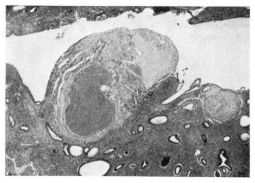

Figure 17. Photomicrograph showing subinvolution of the placental site, with partially thrombosed spiral arteriole in a remnant of decidua. Because of severe bleeding, hysterectomy was performed 10 weeks post partum, probably unnecessarily, for preliminary curettage, usually a curative procedure, was not performed. (Courtesy of Dr. William Ober and Dr. Hugh Grady.)

day. This coincides with the time of absorption of the sutures placed to control the primary hemorrhage. Retained placental tissue may cause delayed postpartum hemorrhage about 10 days after parturition, at a time when the decidua of the placental site undergoes maximal slough, or weeks and even months later. In the latter instance the retained placental tissue is commonly referred to as a placental polyp. In some of these cases a focal accreta formation may be the reason for the initial failure of the placental tissue to separate.

The placental site may be the source of abnormal uterine bleeding during the process of its repair. This is referred to as *postpartum hemorrhage from subinvolution of the placental site* (Fig. 17). The bleeding usually occurs between the 6th and the 10th week of the puerperium, the healing process being delayed perhaps because of low-grade endometritis. In accordance with normal repair of the placental site, the spongiosa layer of the decidua is lifted away from the implantation site by the regenerating endometrium. Occasionally, in this process, the thrombosed portions of the decidual blood vessels are sloughed away, leaving the proximal ends of the spiral vessels patent. The bleeding from these vessels may occur suddenly and can be rather profuse.

Diagnosis

The presence of brisk vaginal bleeding after delivery makes the diagnosis of post-partum hemorrhage obvious. Other symptoms of postpartum hemorrhage are those of impending or established shock. The most important aspect of diagnosis is determination of the source of the bleeding preliminary to definitive treatment.

Treatment

The successful management of postpartum hemorrhage involves early recognition of the cause and the ability to anticipate the need for and to institute promptly those procedures that are necessary to preserve and restore the circulating blood volume to normal. A preconceived plan should include supracervical hysterectomy performed before the patient enters a state of irreversible shock.

Inspection of the cervix and vagina, and palpation of the lower uterine segment should be performed routinely after every operative delivery. Even after a normal delivery when the bleeding is not alarming but continues as a small trickle, *the patient should never be removed from the delivery table until a careful search has been made and the cause of the bleeding explained.* Sometimes no reason will be found, and one must conclude that the bleeding is from the placental site. In this case the bleeding usually ceases within a few minutes after administration of additional oxytocic drugs. Occasionally, however, inspection may disclose an unsuspected cervical or vaginal laceration, with the bleeding readily controlled by surgical closure. Immediate attention to bleeding of any extent at the time of delivery, therefore, will eliminate the need for subsequent exploration of the reproductive tract an hour or two post partum with the requirement of additional anesthesia and transfusions to replace unnecessary blood loss.

In the initial search for the specific cause of postpartum hemorrhage, the placenta should be rapidly inspected for completeness. If a portion is missing, the uterus should be explored promptly and the retained tissue removed. In the event that the placenta is only partially separated and there is undue bleeding, it should be manually removed immediately to allow the uterus to contract. Forceful separation of the placenta should never be necessary; whenever the placenta appears adherent, placenta accreta should be strongly suspected and the patient treated accordingly.

Proper instruments should be available to provide adequate exposure of the reproductive tract. In most instances, when the assistant's hand abdominally compresses the uterus downward into the pelvis, the cervix will descend to the vaginal introitus and be easily visualized. With retractors placed in the lateral and posterior fornices of the vagina, the cervix is brought into view and in a clockwise fashion is inspected throughout its entire circumference. Lacerations are more frequently found laterally on the cervix where the descending branches of the uterine arteries are located. If the cervical laceration extends to the vault of the vagina, it may be difficult to visualize its apex, and exposure may be facilitated by a traction suture placed as near to the apex as possible. In lacerations of this type there is the danger that extensions into the lower uterine segment may go undetected. Hence, the uterine corpus and lower segment should be palpated at the time the cervix is repaired. If a uterine rupture is encountered, a small pack should be placed gently against the rent and an abdominal hysterectomy performed immediately.

Lacerations of the vaginal fornices are repaired under direct vision, but those that occur behind the pubic arch are extremely difficult to expose, even with the patient in a Trendelenburg position, and one may be forced to place the sutures by touch. The vagina is often extremely edematous and friable and venous ooze may continue along the suture line. At times a gauze pack placed in this area may prove more effective than further suturing.

Atony of the uterus should be anticipated when factors contributing to this condition are present. Thus, treatment of hemorrhage due to uterine atony begins with prevention of atony through the proper conduct of the third stage of labor. If atony is developing, additional oxytocic drugs should be administered by intravenous drip; this usually causes the uterus to regain its tone.

In the event that the uterus still fails to contract, and remains soft and flaccid, uterine packing or bimanual compression should next be considered. Controversy exists regarding the relative value of these procedures. Some, perhaps most, clinicians oppose packing of the uterus, believing that a uterine pack prevents the organ from contracting to a normal postpartum size. Accordingly, it is envisioned that the endomyometrial blood vessels remain patent and uterine bleeding continues. Therefore, bimanual compression of the uterus is recommended in preference to uterine packing.

The technique is to place one hand in the vagina and, making a fist, exert pressure against the anterior vaginal wall and uterus. With counter pressure being applied by the abdominal hand, the body of the uterus is thus firmly compressed between the two hands. The uterus is held until it begins to contract and regain its tone, and there are signs that the bleeding is controlled. This may take minutes or the better part of an hour.

Whether this method is more, or less, effective than uterine packing in the control of atony is judged on the basis of individual experience rather than on a series of cases treated alternately by the two methods. Reference has been made to the fact that postpartum hemostasis is not attained entirely as a result of constriction of the myometrial blood vessels by the myometrium. Clotting of the blood and thrombosis of the decidual vessels are necessary to complete uterine hemostasis. Similar to the effect of a pressure pack to control oozing from a body surface elsewhere, the irritation of the gauze is thought to promote thrombosis of the vessels of the uteroplacental site.

Further, uterine compression as a method of treatment of uterine atony is predicated on the concept of a single source for the bleeding. It is common clinical experience that prolonged labor and difficult forceps delivery are often associated; consequently, uterine atony and lacerations of the birth canal may occur together. Both need immediate attention, but simultaneous repair of lacerations and uterine compression are impossible. With a dual origin for the bleeding, it is recommended that the uterus be packed forthwith and the lacerations quickly closed with appropriate sutures. Finally, to ignore the value of a uterine pack means that, if the atony cannot be controlled by oxytocic therapy and a limited trial of uterine compression, the patient must be subjected to immediate supracervical hysterectomy. Furthermore the operation must be performed on patients who have experienced considerable loss of blood without ample time for replacement. This procedure is totally acceptable in patients with several children. But what about the patient of less parity desirous of further childbearing? If uterine packing will control the bleeding, and it will with rare exception, it would appear to be a more reasonable approach than to proceed to hysterectomy immediately. In the case of the exception, a rapid assessment of the clotting mechanism is in order. A deficiency in clotting may account for the bleeding rather than atony, in which case packing also will not help. However, ligation of the hypogastric arteries should be considered.

Since the ability of the uterus to contract is diminished with the onset of shock, an axiom that is believed wise is *"when in doubt, pack, pack early, and pack correctly."* To avoid defeating the therapeutic value of uterine tamponade, however, the operator should not use excessive amounts of gauze. It can be stated that the space occupied by one or possibly two gauze strips measuring 1½ inches wide and 3 yards in length will not exceed the immediate postdelivery capacity of the well contracted uterus. Even those who advocate uterine tamponade—and presumably they are in the minority—readily agree that the therapeutic value of the procedure is lost if the uterus is not packed correctly. The following technique is recommended.

The uterus is firmly compressed into the pelvis by pressure exerted by the operator's hand on the abdomen. The gauze strip is introduced from a sterile container held by the assistant, and the uterus is carefully packed from the top of the fundus downward (Fig. 18).

The pack remains in the uterus for 24 to 36 hours, and is always removed in the operating room under so-called "double set-up" precautions. Preparations are made to combat recurrent hemorrhage, an event that is extremely rare. The pack can be removed without appreciable discomfort to the patient. An anesthetic is rarely needed unless bleeding recurs and further treatment is required. Oxytocic drugs are administered in appropriate amounts during the period the pack remains in the uterus. Starting an oxytocin infusion some 30 minutes before the pack is removed is advised. Repacking is not desirable should bleeding continue or recur after removal of the pack. If the procedure has been correctly performed initially, there is no reason to expect that repacking will be more effective. Should bleeding recur, supracervical hysterectomy must be considered, and if

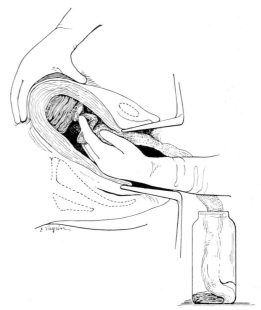

Figure 18. Packing of the uterus and vagina.

there is any doubt, the operation should not be postponed.

LATE AND RECURRENT POSTPARTUM HEMORRHAGE

Patients with subinvolution of the placental site require vaginal exploration and usually curettage. Sometimes a previous laceration may require resuturing. If retained placental cotyledons are present, they can usually be removed either by placental forceps or by a large dull curette, but a focal placenta accreta may necessitate supracervical hysterectomy. In patients with subinvolution of the placental site, curettage will traumatize the decidual arterioles, causing them to become thrombosed with a cessation of the bleeding. Characteristically, the amount of tissue obtained may often be meager.

Finally, there is the occasional patient in whom postpartum hemorrhage will develop in succeeding pregnancies. These patients obviously need special consideration, including limitation of family size.

BIBLIOGRAPHY

Baptisti, A., Jr.: Cervical pregnancy. Obstet. Gynec., 1:353, 1953.

Bonnar, J., McNicol, G. P., and Douglas, A. S.: The behaviour of the coagulation and fibrinolytic mechanisms in abruptio placentae. J. Obstet. Gynaec. Brit. Comm., 76:799, 1969.

Bysshe, S. M.: Premature separation of the normally implanted placenta. Amer. J. Obstet. Gynec., 62:38, 1951.

Cavanagh, D., Powe, C. E., and Gilson, A. J.: Placenta previa: Modern methods of diagnosis with special reference to isotopic placentography. Obstet. Gynec., 18:403, 1961.

Discussion of new ideas about the diagnosis and treatment of placenta praevia. Proc. Roy. Soc. Med., 44:121, 1951.

Doran, J. R., O'Brien, S. A., Jr., and Randall, J. H.: Repeated postpartum hemorrhage. Obstet. Gynec., 5:126, 1955.

Ferguson, J. H.: Rupture of marginal sinus of placenta. Amer. J. Obstet. Gynec., 69:995, 1955.

Gottesfeld, K. R., Thompson, H. E., Holmes, J. H., and Taylor, E. S.: Ultrasonic placentography—a new method for placental localization. Amer. J. Obstet. Gynec., 96:538, 1966.

Hibbard, B. M.: The role of folic acid in pregnancy with particular reference to anemia, abruption and abortion. J. Obstet. Gynaec. Brit. Comm., 71:529, 1964.

Hibbard, B. M., and Hibbard, E. D.: Aetiological factors in abruptio placentae. Brit. Med. J., 2:1430, 1963.

Irving, F. C.: Conservative treatment of premature separation of the normally implanted placenta. Amer. J. Obstet. Gynec., 34:881, 1937.

Johnson, H. W.: Conservative management of some varieties of placenta praevia. Amer. J. Obstet. Gynec., 50:248, 1945.

Kistner, R. W., Hertig, A. T., and Reid, D. E.: Simultaneously occurring placenta previa and placenta accreta. Surg. Gynec. Obstet., 94:141, 1952.

Laros, R. K., Jr., Thaidigsman, J. H., and Schulman, H.: Clinical application of placental scanning using RISA. Obstet. Gynec., 26:388, 1965.

Macafee, C. H. G.: Placenta praevia; study of 174 cases. J. Obstet. Gynaec. Brit. Emp., 52:4, 1945.

Macafee, C. H. G.: Modern views on management of placenta praevia. Postgrad. Med. J., 25:197, 1949.

Macafee, C. H. G., Millar, W. G., and Harley, G.: Maternal and foetal mortality in placenta previa. J. Obstet. Gynaec. Brit. Comm., 69:203, 1962.

McKelvey, J. L.: Vascular lesions in the decidua basalis. Amer. J. Obstet. Gynec., 38:815, 1939.

Mengert, W. F., Goodson, J. H., Campbell, R. G., and Haynes, D. M.: Observations on pathogenesis of premature separation of normally implanted placenta. Amer. J. Obstet. Gynec., 66:1104, 1953.

Menon, M. K. K., Sengupta, M., and Ramaswamy, N.: Accidental haemorrhage and folic acid deficiency. J. Obstet. Gynaec. Brit. Comm., 73:49, 1966.

Morton, D. G.: Anatomic description of case of marginal placenta previa, with discussion of etiologic implications. Amer. J. Obstet. Gynec., 33:547, 1937.

Ober, W. B., Reid, D. E., Romney, S. L., and Merrill, J. P.: Renal lesions and acute renal failure in pregnancy. Amer. J. Med., 21:781, 1956.

Page, E. W., King, E. B., and Merrill, J. A.: Abruptio placentae; dangers of delay in delivery. Obstet. Gynec., 3:385, 1954.

Pedowitz, P.: Placenta previa: an evaluation of expectant management and the factors responsible for fetal wastage. Amer. J. Obstet. Gynec., 93:16, 1965.

Reid, D. E.: Discussion on observations on pathogenesis of premature separation of normally implanted placenta (W. F. Mengert et al.). Amer. J. Obstet. Gynec., 66:1110, 1953.

Reid, D. E.: The acquired clotting defect (hypofibrinogenemia) in pregnancy. Amer. J. Obstet. Gynec., 87:344, 1963.

Reid, D. E.: Acquired coagulation defects in pregnancy. Obstet. Gynec. Survey, 20:431, 1965.

Sexton, L. I., Hertig, A. T., Reid, D. E., Kellogg, F. S., and Patterson, W. S.: Premature separation of normally implanted placenta. Amer. J. Obstet. Gynec., 59:13, 1950.

Sheehan, H. L., and Moore, H. C.: Renal Cortical Necrosis of the Kidney and Concealed Accidental Hemorrhage. Charles C Thomas, Springfield, Ill., 1953.

Stallworthy, J.: The dangerous placenta. Amer. J. Obstet. Gynec., 61:720, 1951.

Stevenson, C. S.: X-ray visualization of placenta; experiences with soft tissue and cystographic techniques in diagnosis of placenta previa. Amer. J. Obstet. Gynec., 58:15, 1949.

Tatum, H. J., and Mule, J. G.: Placenta previa. Amer. J. Obstet. Gynec., 93:676, 1965.

Visscher, R. D., and Baker, W. S.: Isotopic localization of the placenta in suspected cases of placenta previa. Amer. J. Obstet. Gynec., 80:1150, 1960.

Weinberg, A., Shapiro, G., and Bruen, D. F.: Isotope placentography. An evaluation of its accuracy and safety. Amer. J. Obstet. Gynec., 87:203, 1963.

Weiner, A. E., Reid, D. E., and Roby, C. C.: Coagulation defects associated with premature separation of normally implanted placenta. Amer. J. Obstet. Gynec., 60:379, 1950.

Weiner, A. E., Reid, D. E., and Roby, C. C.: Incoagulable blood in severe premature separation of the placenta; method of management. Amer. J. Obstet. Gynec., 66:475, 1953.

Chapter 17

Hypertensive (Toxemic) Pregnancy

DEFINITION

Pregnancy toxemia is a term applied to a syndrome characterized by excessive retention of extracellular fluid (edema) followed by the development of hypertension, proteinuria, and a complex of symptoms which, in the severe form of the condition, may culminate in convulsions, or eclampsia. Excluded by this definition are those women encountered in pregnancy who have underlying vascular or renal disease. Admittedly, these patients are difficult to distinguish from those with pregnancy toxemia, particularly in the last trimester. In fact, the correct diagnosis depends on observation of the patient before or in the early months of pregnancy.

Despite the possible inadequacies of descriptive terminology, a classification of the various types of hypertension and proteinuria in pregnancy is desirable. In addition to providing the indices for diagnosis, a suitable classification is essential if the answers to certain clinical questions relating to patient management are to be obtained.

Among other questions, those most commonly posed are: (1) What patients with vascular or renal disease can undertake pregnancy without undue risk and with a reasonable chance of delivering an infant of sufficient maturity to survive? (2) Conversely, because of the fetal and maternal risks involved, which women in this group should not attempt a pregnancy? (3) What are the clinical and laboratory criteria on which the physician will base his decision as to the advisability of pregnancy in patients with vascular and renal disease? (4) Will pregnancy accelerate the course of cardiovascular and renal disease in these patients? (5) Can pregnancy toxemia, either mild or severe, cause permanent damage to a previously normal vascular and renal system? (6) If so, what are the frequency and the severity of such sequelae? (7) What is the rate of recurrence of toxemia in subsequent pregnancies? (8) What is the incidence of the related medical and obstetrical complications in the different forms of hypertension and proteinuria in pregnancy? (9) Finally, what are the fetal hazards and survival rates in the various groups? Answers to these questions are necessary for any physician advising on the care of pregnant patients or those patients who desire to become pregnant.

CLASSIFICATIONS

In order to achieve uniformity of nomenclature, the American Committee on Maternal Welfare in 1940 proposed the following classification:

Group A. Disease not peculiar to pregnancy
    I. Hypertensive disease (hypertensive cardiovascular disease)
        a. Benign (essential hypertension)
           1. Mild
           2. Severe
        b. Malignant
    II. Renal disease
        a. Nephrosclerosis or chronic vascular nephritis
        b. Glomerulonephritis
           1. Acute
           2. Chronic
        c. Nephrosis
           1. Acute
           2. Chronic
        d. Other forms of severe renal disease (chronic pyelonephritis, etc.)

Group B. Disease dependent on or peculiar to pregnancy
 I. Pre-eclampsia
     a. Mild
     b. Severe (preconvulsive)
 II. Eclampsia
     a. Convulsive
     b. Nonconvulsive (i.e., coma, with autopsy findings typical of eclampsia)
Group C. Vomiting of pregnancy
Group D. Unclassified toxemia

Under this classification Group A includes patients whose vascular or renal disease is diagnosed prior to pregnancy, or before the 24th week of pregnancy. The latter time was arbitrarily selected as the period in pregnancy when toxemia may begin to develop, the only exception in the early weeks being a pregnancy toxemia in association with a hydatidiform mole.

Group B includes patients without apparent pre-existing vascular or renal disease in whom a specific disorder, designated "pregnancy toxemia," develops. Group B is further divided into mild or severe pre-eclampsia and eclampsia, depending on the degree to which the associated signs and symptoms are manifest. In addition to edema, albuminuria, and hypertension, the common symptoms include nausea, vomiting, and headaches. When the condition remains untreated, convulsions and coma may be added to the clinical picture, in which event the syndrome is referred to as eclampsia. Disregarding the classification for the moment, severe pre-eclampsia and eclampsia are often referred to as the "eclamptogenic syndrome," suggesting that the two conditions are the same disease, with concomitant morphologic changes.

Group C includes patients seen initially in the last trimester of pregnancy whose history, physical examination, and laboratory findings raise the suspicion that they may have cardiovascular or renal disease. This is impossible to prove if they have not sought care previously, and there are no observations on the status of their blood pressure and urine prior to or in the early months of pregnancy. If hypertension, proteinuria, or both persist post partum, the patient can ultimately be classified into one of the subgroups of Group A. It is emphasized, however, that these patients must be *excluded* from any study directed toward investigation of the question whether pregnancy toxemia will cause permanent damage to a previously normal cardiovascular or renal system. In other words, such a study should include only those patients whose cardiovascular and renal systems were known to be normal prior to the development of pregnancy toxemia. There are few studies in which this stipulation has been met, however, which accounts for the wide disparity in the reported incidence of residual hypertension and renal disease in patients in whom the diagnosis of pregnancy toxemia was made. (See discussion of sequelae, later in this chapter.)

This classification marked a milestone in the diagnosis and management of hypertension in pregnancy. It removed many terms that were unacceptable to medical nomenclature and permitted a greater understanding and a more accurate description of the patient's disease by both obstetrician and internist. There are several terms and entities that require further elucidation.

"Malignant" hypertension is a debated entity even in the nonpregnant, and the term is not entirely acceptable as a diagnosis in pregnancy. Because of its connotation with respect to ultimate prognosis, such a diagnosis in pregnancy may in fact prove to be erroneous. At first glance, the diagnosis of malignant hypertension may appear correct in the pregnant patient with hypertensive disease in whom cerebral, cardiac, or renal complications and a marked accentuation of the hypertension develop. The clinical situation is more accurately appraised, however, if the patient is regarded as a person with severe essential hypertension that is temporarily aggravated by pregnancy or perhaps with a superimposed pregnancy toxemia, for after delivery marked symptomatic improvement is the rule. The patient's blood pressure usually returns to its prepregnancy level, and the proteinuria may disappear. At this point, it is perhaps well to emphasize that, in terms of patient management, the physician should assume that the patient has a superimposed toxemia. Thus, the term "malignant hypertension," as it applies to pregnancy, serves no useful purpose. In fact, such a diagnosis may imply to some, and particularly to the internist, that the patient's condition is not likely to improve with termination of the pregnancy, although the opposite is usually true.

Regarding those conditions listed under renal disease, the terms nephrosclerosis and chronic vascular nephritis are not synonymous. In fact, the term chronic vascular nephritis is redundant and, therefore, need not be included.

Nephrosis is a purely descriptive term, rather devoid of specific etiologic connotations. As it might apply to pregnancy, it has definite limitations. As in the nonpregnant, the diagnosis may appear tenable in pregnant patients who present massive proteinuria, severe hypoproteinemia, refractory edema, and little or no hypertension. Experience reveals, however, that the patient has either an atypical pregnancy toxemia or a chronic glomerulonephritis in exacerbation or temporarily aggravated by pregnancy. In atypical pregnancy toxemia, the signs and symptoms will clear within a few days after delivery; in exacerbated chronic glomerulonephritis, the edema usually subsides, the proteinuria decreases, and the nephrotic-like syndrome becomes a less prominent feature of the disease. Further, as a "degenerative" condition of the kidney, as in amyloidosis, nephrosis is rarely encountered in pregnancy and is of secondary concern to the overall problems of the primary disease.

With regard to Group B, disease dependent on or peculiar to pregnancy, the division of the toxemia syndrome into mild and severe forms is clinically necessary and desirable. It may be questioned, however, whether a separate category should be made for patients in whom convulsions (that is, eclampsia) develop. Although it has come to represent a syndrome, eclampsia means nothing more and nothing less than *convulsion and coma*. Because of the necessity of categorizing patients who do not have convulsions but who die from pregnancy toxemia, the use of the term eclampsia has led to further semantic difficulties. For these cases the category "eclampsia," with a subheading, "(*b*) nonconvulsive," has been created. On examining this concept, the paradox of a nonconvulsive convulsion is obvious. Rather, pre-eclampsia–eclampsia might be classified in accordance with the definition of diabetes mellitus, for example, (*a*) diabetes, and (*b*) diabetes with coma. Viewed in this light, convulsions and coma

can be seen to represent an analogous situation in severe pregnancy toxemia and may be viewed as incidents in the course of a disease peculiar to pregnancy.

Hyperemesis gravidarum, or vomiting of pregnancy, is unrelated to toxemia; it need not be included in any classification concerned with albuminuria and hypertension in pregnancy.

Sufficient reasons have been offered to justify the following modification of the classification:

Group A. Disease not peculiar to pregnancy
    I. Essential hypertension
        a. Mild
        b. Severe — with or without cerebral, cardiac, or renal complications
    II. Renal disease
        a. Glomerulonephritis
          1. Acute
          2. Chronic
            i. Mild
            ii. Severe — with or without nephrosis
        b. Pyelonephritis
          1. Acute
          2. Chronic
            i. Mild
            ii. Severe
        c. Renal abnormalities — polycystic kidney, horseshoe kidney, unilateral renal agenesis, etc.

Group B. Diseases dependent on or peculiar to pregnancy
    I. Toxemia
        a. Mild
        b. Severe, with or without convulsions and/or coma

Group C. Unclassified, that is, Group A suspects. This group includes those patients in whom a definite diagnosis is not possible during pregnancy, for example, one in whom glomerulonephritis or essential hypertension is suspected. Because of insufficient data before or in the early months of pregnancy, it is imperative to exclude the patients in this group from the statistics, except when necropsy findings allow them to be placed into either Group A or Group B.

Through the recorded experience of patient performance in pregnancy it has been found clinically desirable to subdivide essential hypertension and the nephritides into mild and severe forms. This has proved invaluable in the assessment of whether or not the patient should attempt or continue a pregnancy. Admittedly, each patient must be individualized with respect to age, parity, and environment, but the physician's final decision and advice will be based primarily on the severity of her disease. As an example, even with the best of prenatal management and the newer hypotensive drugs, the fetal mortality rate in the severe form of essential hypertension is high—nearly 50 per cent— in contrast to the 5 to 10 per cent experienced in the mild form of the disease. Also, in the severe form the maternal risk is materially greater. In more recent years accumulated experience indicates that patients with the mild form of chronic glomerulonephritis under careful management will negotiate a pregnancy successfully and with a fetal mortality comparable to that experienced in cases of mild essential hypertension. By contrast, the fetal salvage rate is low in patients with the severe form of chronic glomerulonephritis.

Admittedly the definition of mild and severe essential hypertension must be rather arbitrary. The mild form of essential hypertension covers those patients whose initial blood pressure before or in the early weeks of pregnancy is less than 180 mm. Hg systolic and 100 mm. Hg diastolic, whose ocular fundi are essentially negative, and in whom there is no evidence of cardiac enlargement or impairment of renal function. In the severe form the blood pressure is increased over the above values, definite changes may be noted in the retinal vessels, and cardiac enlargement and renal damage may be evident.

As in essential hypertension, the diagnostic criteria of what constitutes the mild and the severe forms of chronic glomerulonephritis must of necessity be somewhat arbitrary, because one is unable to determine with consistent accuracy, by whatever means is used, the exact amount of renal damage. Patients who concentrate their urine to a specific gravity of at least 1.016, and have a maximal urea clearance of 70 ml. per minute or more, a blood urea nitrogen below 20 mg. per 100 ml. at the onset of pregnancy, and a blood pressure not exceeding 150 mm. Hg systolic and 100 mm. Hg diastolic are regarded as having the mild form of chronic glomerulonephritis. By contrast, those patients who have a greater impairment of renal function and possibly demonstrable vascular changes are classified as having the severe form.

The relationship of chronic pyelonephritis in the etiology of vascular disease is well established. Further, it is appreciated that in many cases of chronic pyelonephritis the initial acute episode has occurred in pregnancy. What is not so well known is whether patients with chronic pyelonephritis of whatever degree should be permitted to attempt a pregnancy, for there is a greater threat of an exacerbation of their disease at this time. Under careful urologic and obstetric management pregnancy is perhaps permissible in selected cases, but the risk involved must not be minimized. In general, the condition might be considered mild if renal damage is minimal, vascular disease is absent, and the infection is controllable. (See Medical and Surgical Diseases of Pregnancy.)

Again it is desirable to have subdivisions in Group B from the standpoint both of treatment and of the assessment or possible effect of the disease on the cardiovascular and renal systems. In brief, the mild form of toxemia is characterized by little or no visible peripheral edema, the blood pressure remains near or below 160 mm. Hg systolic, and the 24-hour urine contains less than 1 gram of albumin. The patient is comparatively free of symptoms.

Severe toxemia is characterized by generalized edema, reflected in a sudden and marked weight gain within a period of a few days or one to two weeks. The blood pressure is above 160 mm. Hg systolic, commonly 180 to 210 mm. Hg, or higher, and above 100 mm. Hg diastolic. The total daily urinary albumin is at least 1 gram, and, in the extreme, up to 10 to 30 grams. The urinary sediment has many hyaline and granular casts, and red cells are often present. The symptoms are variable. They include headache, usually frontal in location, nausea, vomiting, and epigastric pain. When the disease reaches this stage, convulsions or coma or both (eclampsia) may supervene. Exceptionally, convulsions may supervene when there is little or no edema and the degree of proteinuria and the blood pressure are within the range described for the mild form of toxemia.

INCIDENCE AND DIFFERENTIAL DIAGNOSIS OF HYPERTENSION AND PROTEINURIA IN PREGNANCY

The reported incidence of various forms of hypertension and proteinuria in pregnancy differs from clinic to clinic, but in general it is between 5 and 10 per cent. About 30 per cent of the total are patients with essential hypertension, chronic glomerulonephritis, and chronic pyelonephritis — Group A. Of these 30 per cent, about three fourths of the patients have essential hypertension; the remainder have renal disease. Thus, in the overall incidence of hypertension and proteinuria of pregnancy, about 5 per cent have chronic renal disease. Among the 70 per cent of hypertensive patients in Group B, the majority have mild toxemia. The incidence of the severe form of toxemia is influenced by many factors, including the pregnant patient's appreciation of the value of seeking early prenatal care and receiving it.

Attempts have been made to anticipate pregnancy toxemia by observing the blood pressure response of normotensive patients early in pregnancy to certain tests such as the "cold test." The test is of little practical value; and flicker photometry has also failed in forecasting toxemia.

To determine whether a patient with hypertension or proteinuria or both seen initially in the last trimester and prior to the 34th to 35th week has vascular or renal disease would be helpful in overall patient management and in postpartum follow up. One might feel more constrained to permit the pregnancy to continue to a stage of fetal maturity, recognizing that the chance of obtaining an infant that will survive will be no greater in a future pregnancy. At the same time, the degree of proteinuria and hypertension may demand termination of the pregnancy to avoid all the risks that a superimposed severe toxemia could incur.

Many tests have been applied to differentiate pregnancy toxemia from vascular and renal disease in pregnancy, but none have proved to be of special value clinically. Patients with pregnancy toxemia overreact to administration of minute amounts of Pituitrin as judged by an increase in blood pressure and a decrease in urine output. Patients with pregnancy toxemia appear to have a greater blood pressure response to administered angiotensin II than pregnant patients with essential hypertension. By contrast, in well controlled study, the peak urinary sodium excretion to salt loading in patients with essential hypertension was found to be three to five times greater than patients with pregnancy toxemia. This is somewhat at variance with previous observations.

The retina, its vessels, and the vessels of the bulbar conjunctiva have been extensively examined to ascertain whether such examination would permit a differentiation between pregnancy toxemia and hypertensive vascular and renal disease in pregnancy and whether the changes and their extent could aid in decisions of immediate patient management.

There is no question that narrowing and localized spasm of the retinal arterioles occur in pregnancy toxemia; in the severe form of the disease there may be some retinal edema, hemorrhages, exudate, and, rarely, detachment. These angiospastic changes vary in degree from hour to hour in the course of the toxemia, and the arterioles may regain their normal caliber if the blood pressure falls to near-normal levels. Vasospasm of the bulbar conjunctival vessels is seen in the severe form of pregnancy toxemia, but presumably because of their location these vessels are more subject to local stimuli, so that normal patients also reveal these changes. Considerable emphasis has also been placed on what is referred to as a "retinal sheen," which is described as a wet, glistening appearance of the retina. Although not necessarily regarded as a specific finding of pregnancy toxemia, it has not been seen in hypertensive vascular disease. Apparently these changes are commonly seen in young, healthy persons and are not necessarily related to pregnancy toxemia. Further, caution must be exercised in offering an opinion, based on retinal findings, as to the background of the hypertension and proteinuria, the fetal outcome, and the possibility of residual vascular or renal disease.

Certainly the retinal changes in severe pregnancy toxemia can mimic, albeit temporarily, those found in chronic vascular and renal disease. Further, it is difficult, if not impossible, to differentiate between the vessel changes in cases of mild hypertension and the vessel spasm of pregnancy toxemia. When there is definite arterio-venous compression and increased light reflex, however, the diagnosis of essential hypertension in pregnancy is tenable, although it should await confirmation by postpartum observations.

Like the degree of hypertension and proteinuria, the retinal findings would appear to reflect the severity of the toxemia, and could be helpful as a guide to patient management. The fetal mortality has been recorded as high when exudate and hemorrhages are present, but this is understandable, for these retinal changes are associated mainly with the severe form of the disease. Whether to terminate the pregnancy or permit it to continue will not be decided on the retinal findings alone. Rather, the degree of hypertension and proteinuria, the patient's response to therapy, and the stage of pregnancy will be the determining factors. Equally important, one cannot be completely certain whether observed changes are due to pregnancy toxemia or to vascular or renal disease until several weeks post partum.

In summary, many tests have been applied and by and large have been found wanting in the differentiation of the various forms of hypertension and proteinuria encountered in pregnancy. Actually, whether the patient has a pregnancy toxemia per se or underlying cardiovascular disease with or without superimposed pre-eclampsia may not be crucial in immediate management when the patient's signs and symptoms are of a magnitude that termination of the pregnancy is mandatory. Many diseases, not the least being lupus erythematosus and other renal and hypertensive states, must be considered in the differential diagnosis. (See Medical and Surgical Diseases of Pregnancy.)

NATURAL HISTORY OF PREGNANCY TOXEMIA

Pregnancy toxemia might be approached as a disease comprised of two phases. *Phase one* is regarded as preventable and reversible. *Phase two* constitutes a state wherein the disease is established clinically, and, although the condition may respond to therapy, recovery is dependent on the eventual termination of pregnancy. Thus, phase two may be considered irreversible, except with delivery, after which prompt recovery is the rule.

Although clinicians may speak of "fulminating" toxemia in the patient who is be-

lieved to have developed her disease over a brief period, perhaps a matter of days, this is undoubtedly rare and is difficult to prove unless the patient is seen at weekly or biweekly intervals.

The earliest sign of the *initial phase,* or, stated another way, the earliest indication that a patient may develop pregnancy toxemia, is a sudden weight gain beginning as early as the middle trimester, but usually after the 28th week, which is unexplainable on the basis of caloric intake alone. It must be assumed that the rapid weight gain is due to the accumulation of extracellular fluid in excess of that of normal pregnancy. *Generalized edema* becomes detectable clinically when the interstitial fluid has doubled in amount. In the woman weighing more than 60 kg. this would be approximately 5 to 8 L., or some 10 to 16 additional pounds of weight. It is recognized that generalized edema must be distinguished from postural edema. In pregnancy, edema localized to the lower extremities may have no pathologic connotations, and it generally responds to rest.

In the absence of postural edema, a weight gain of a few pounds must mean a comparable amount of edema, albeit occult. A useful clinical sign is the patient's inability to remove her rings from her fingers because of the presence of edema. The patient may volunteer the information that she fatigues easily and feels listless. Often she admits that she has an excessive thirst and drinks large quantities of fluid daily. One may surmise that she feels not unlike a person with beginning *water intoxication.* Up to this point, all of the symptoms and signs are usually reversible with bed rest, strict curtailment of daily activity, and careful nutritional control, including the avoidance of salt, with mild sedation to enforce the activity restrictions.

If the disease remains unchecked, the patient will soon enter the *second phase.* The blood pressure will become elevated; the urine is likely to contain significant amounts of protein; and the sediment may include various types of casts. The patient's disease will be regarded as mild or severe, depending on the degree of proteinuria and hypertension, and the presence or absence of further symptoms.

More commonly the disease will be the mild form as defined. However, despite treatment, the disease may suddenly accelerate, and the patient may develop the severe form with its additional symptoms and serious hazards. Also, and the more likely in those with the severe form, the disease may pass directly from the initial phase within hours or days. Irritability, insomnia, severe headache, scintillating scotomata, and anorexia are the classic symptoms. Epigastric pain is midline, and severe in character. The source of the pain is unknown. Negative electrocardiograms indicate that it is not associated with myocardial ischemia, and presumably it is not of coronary origin.

If the disease in its severe form is not quickly brought under therapeutic control, convulsions or coma, or both, will supervene, sometimes within a matter of hours. The blood pressure, unless reduced by hypotensive drugs, will rise rapidly (180 to 250 mm. Hg systolic, and 90 to 160 mm. Hg diastolic). The blood pressure is quite labile and, in fact, will vary considerably, with values differing as much as 30 to 50 mm. Hg in the systolic pressures recorded simultaneously in the two arms. The proteinuria may vary tremendously from hour to hour, usually ranging between 2 and 5 grams for 24 hours, but 30 grams has been measured. Besides many casts, red cells are commonly seen in the urinary sediment. The urine output may diminish to oliguric levels. The highly concentrated urine often becomes mahogany colored (see Fig. 7). At this stage, convulsions can be expected if they have not already occurred.

The convulsions are generalized and clonic in type, usually heralded by twitching of the face or mouth, sometimes of the arm, but eventually involving the entire body. There is frothing at the mouth, and the patient will bite her tongue if it is not protected. The convulsions last 30 to 60 seconds, often reappearing within a matter of minutes if steps are not taken to bring them under control. The patient either remains in a coma or appears stuporous for several minutes, and when she regains consciousness she is amnesic to the event. Actually, she may have been amnesic for a substantial period, sometimes days, before the onset of the convulsions.

If treatment fails, the agonal period before death usually lasts some 12 to 24 hours. The patient is oliguric and often anuric. The face and eyelids become markedly edematous. The skin of the face is rather florid, but at the same time the nail beds are often dusky and cyanotic. Fine to coarse rales may be elicited throughout the chest. The respiratory rate is elevated, and the pulse rate is commonly 120 or more per minute. The patient frequently at this stage has some fever (101 to 102° F.). The entire body becomes increasingly cyanotic, and, with gasping respiration, a rising pulse rate, and falling blood pressure, the patient succumbs.

The patient who recovers from severe toxemia after delivery usually does so rapidly and dramatically, barring complications. Within 24 to 48 hours it may be difficult to believe that the patient was so extremely ill. Her mental status improves, and the irritability or the stupor soon disappears. The blood pressure tends to recede to normal levels, although some hypertension may persist for several days to weeks. In fact, the blood pressure may remain somewhat elevated for several weeks or months, and finally return to normal, which is an important consideration in the assessment of residual hypertension. Proteinuria rapidly disappears, urine output increases, and a marked postpartum diuresis usually follows.

ETIOLOGY

The etiology of pregnancy toxemia remains unknown, and this may account for the many factors considered to be contributory to, if not causes of, the disease.

Environmental factors such as culture and climate, which in turn influence diet, activity, and health habits, appear to influence the incidence of the disease, though often appear contradictory. As an example, at one time it was believed that pregnancy toxemia occurred more frequently in the winter than in the warmer months. Many clinics, however, report the highest incidence in the summer.

The value of good nutrition in the prevention of toxemia has been stressed, but the exact relationship of poor nutrition to the development of pregnancy toxemia remains obscure. Although its frequency is reputedly low in many of the nonwhite populations of Africa and comparatively high in a similar ethnic group living in the United States, this may be partially explained by the fact that the diets of the two groups differ appreciably in both the basic composition and the total salt content.

The incidence of the disease was low in parts of Europe during both World Wars, at a time when it might be expected that acceptable standards of prenatal care would be difficult to maintain. War could be expected to impose unusual burdens on the pregnant woman through disruption of medical services, inadequate nutrition to the point of famine, and the necessity for the parturient to perform heavy manual labor to aid the war effort. However, society during wartime tends to guard its future generations by making special provisions for the pregnant woman by affording her additional foods in a time of general food shortage.

Toxemia of pregnancy has been considered to be possibly an autoimmune disease. This implies that the placenta is antigenic and may react immunologically to the maternal organism. (See Immunology of Pregnancy.) Also, for several decades it has been propounded that toxins from the placenta or decidua might be the cause of this disease. This concept is based on the production of toxemic-like lesions in the experimental animal by injection of various placental extracts. These substances are thought to arise from degradation of tissues resulting from either placental infarction or regression of the syncytium or the decidua. However, infarction of the placenta may well be an effect rather than a cause of severe pregnancy toxemia, and certainly placental infarct is present when the patient reveals no evidence of toxemia.

Uterine ischemia remains a popular theory of the etiology of pregnancy toxemia, but is based mainly on indirect evidence. In pregnancy toxemia the mean half-time clearance of isotonic radioactive sodium injected into either the intervillous space or the myometrium, regarded as an index of uterine blood flow, is prolonged over that in normal pregnancy. In pregnant patients with essential hypertension, the decrease in clearance was similar to the values obtained in pregnancy toxemia. This was interpreted to mean that uterine or placental ischemia was the result of rather than the cause of the hypertension of pregnancy toxemia.

More recently, experimental evidence has been introduced to support the uterine ischemia concept. It has been demonstrated in dogs that when the uterus is made chronically ischemic, the blood pressure will rise in the event of pregnancy. These experiments have been extended to reveal that the renin content of fetuses of hypertensive mothers is markedly higher than the fetuses of the normotensive pregnant dog. Interestingly, a renin-like enzyme has been found in substantial amounts in the amniotic fluid of human pregnancy. The major source of the amniotic fluid, certainly in the last trimester, is fetal urine.

These observations add relevance to the renin-angiotensin II-aldosterone system in the etiology of this disease. (See endocrinology section.) It is well established that angiotensinase activity is markedly elevated in normal pregnancy. Both angiotensin and renin levels are stated to be elevated in normal pregnancy but not in pregnancy toxemia. At the same time the juxtaglomerular cells are reported to be enlarged and increased in numbers in pregnancy toxemia. Aldosterone levels in pregnancy toxemia are not increased over the rise in normal pregnancy and indeed may be lower. If renin is a factor in the etiology of the disease, how should the failure of renin levels to rise in pregnancy toxemia be interpreted? This seems especially pertinent in the presence of a hypovolemic state observed in pregnancy toxemia that should stimulate renin output.

In the nonpregnant it has been postulated that angiotensinemia and secondary hyperaldosteronism, and certainly the latter applies to pregnancy, can develop only when angiotensin output exceeds its destruction. Thus, the suggestion has been made that the rise in renin and angiotensin levels in normal pregnancy may not always be held in abeyance despite the marked increase in angiotensinase activity. In other words, the source—the placenta or the erythrocyte or both—fails to maintain the plasma angiotensinase at a level necessary to keep in balance angiotensin production and destruction, with a resultant pressor effect. Of special relevance has been the observation that the blood of toxemic patients is unable to inactivate administered angiotensin to the same degree as the blood of normal pregnant women.

Also, the question is posed whether in human pregnancy the renin-angiotensin-aldosterone system of the kidney can be transferred or applied to the uteroplacental-fetal system. It is reported that the decidua contains a pressor substance designated hysterotonin. Whether this is renin or a renin-like substance must still be defined. The practical question in terms of patient management, however, is the observation that the blood pressure returned to normal more quickly post partum when the uterus was curetted at the time of delivery.

Attractive as this renin-angiotensin-aldosterone complex may be in the etiology of pregnancy toxemia, one is left inquiring, what is the mechanism that causes a normal pregnancy to embark on a pathologic career?

In consideration of the placenta and its possible etiologic role, an eminent physiologist has demonstrated antidiuretic activity without chloruresis in saline extracts from the placenta. With the isolation of additional protein hormones from the placenta, it may be unwise to exclude an antidiuretic hormone activity from that source in pregnancy toxemia. The diuresis immediately after delivery in the normal patient is impressive, and even more so within a few hours post partum in the toxemic patient.

Finally, in a recent experimental model in rats it has been possible by diet manipulation to produce a generalized Shwartzman reaction. Increased amounts of cryofibrinogen have been reported to occur in toxemic patients and this is cited as evidence of fibrin deposition. It is postulated that in the course of this disease fibrin deposition occurs slowly at first and, if unchecked, may lead to convulsions, coma, and death. Certainly Shwartzman-like lesions are observed at autopsy.

The early phase of pregnancy toxemia may be simply an accentuation of normal physiologic changes of pregnancy. The second phase is related to the severe form of the disease, which may progress if unchecked and may end in convulsions, coma, and possibly death. Such a division seems justifiable for the pathologic changes are restricted to the severe form, and are most marked when convulsions and coma occur.

To place certain of these normal changes of pregnancy, some of which are physiologically unique, into a schema that fulfills the pathophysiology of pregnancy toxemia, requires speculation that may extend beyond credibility. But, to begin at the beginning, progesterone secretion rises abruptly with the missed period and, with the resultant hyperventilation, serum sodium falls. The latter could lead to a modest increase in angiotensin and an aldosterone response accounting for the necessary enlargement in the extracellular fluid compartment. If such an endocrine symphony has validity or exists, it must be a carefully and delicately balanced phenomenon, the more so because of the ability of progesterone to promote sodium excretion and the antidiuretic hormone to participate in the overall economy of extracellular fluid. Although the stimulus might arise in the uterus, possibly by alterations of the trophoblast, local edema, nutrition, or other factors, should something occur in the kidney (i.e., a mild Shwartzman or an autoimmune reaction), with even a minor reduction in renal blood flow from minute amounts of fibrin deposition, renin might be released and ultimately angiotensin beyond the ability of a compromised placenta to inhibit these substances through failure to provide adequate amounts of angiotensinase. As outlined in summary form in Table 1 this would set in motion a hypertensive episode with all of its consequences.

PATHOPHYSIOLOGY

The pathophysiology of pregnancy toxemia is concerned mainly with those bodily functions that result in or are affected by edema and hypertension.

1. Progesterone — Hyperventilation — Serum Sodium 135 mEq.

2. Angiotensin — Aldosterone — Extracellular Fluid

3. Angiotensinase +   Renin ++   J.G. Cells +
   RBC   Kidney
   Placenta   ? Uterus
                             Amniotic Fluid
                             Fetus

4. Cryofibrinogen — Fibrin — Decrease R.B.F.
   Renin+++

Figure 1. An etiologic schema of pregnancy toxemia.

Although there may be agreement that edema must be generalized to be pathologic in pregnancy, it need not be visible to be present. Indeed, some 5 to 8 L. of extracellular fluid is said to be required before edema is visible. Hence, the edema may be occult; for example, edema of the brain is present in all patients who die with convulsive toxemia. Thus, it would appear unwise to regard edema as normal, although if truly restricted to the lower extremities it might not be harmful.

Since Lever in 1843 first observed that the urine from toxemic patients with convulsion contained albumin, the kidney has been implicated in the pathophysiology of this disease. Renal hemodynamics and filtration and tubular function have been extensively studied in hypertensive pregnancy. Although reduced from the increase of normal pregnancy, the glomerular filtration rate (170 ml. per minute) and renal plasma flow reported from several sources are within the range of normal for the nonpregnant female (Tables 1 and 2).

On the assumption that tubular reabsorption varies inversely with the glomerular filtration rate, it has been proposed that obligatory reabsorption might be increased in pregnancy toxemia, thus accounting for the edema formation. One is confronted with the possibility, however, that any reduction in glomerular filtration rate may be the result or the aftermath of the edema

TABLE 1. GLOMERULAR FILTRATION RATES OBSERVED BEFORE AND AFTER DELIVERY IN NONCONVULSIVE TOXEMIA AND HYPERTENSIVE PREGNANCY

	Nonconvulsive Toxemia		Hypertensive Pregnancy	
	Ante-partum ml./min./1.73m.²	Post-partum ml./min./1.73m.²	Ante-partum ml./min./1.73m.²	Post-partum ml./min./1.73m.²
Kariher and George, 1943	112	129.5	145	118
Dill et al., 1942	84	105	87	95
Corcoran and Page, 1941	90	102	106	104
Taylor et al., 1942	114	132	97	109
Odell, 1947	84	161	120	153
deAlvarez, 1950	103	99.5	100	—
Kenney et al., 1950	90	96	—	—
Sarles et al., 1968	120	—	110	—
Smith, 1951	Range in normal nonpregnant females 102–132 ml./min./1.73 m.²			

TABLE 2. RENAL PLASMA FLOW OBSERVED BEFORE AND AFTER DELIVERY IN NONCONVULSIVE TOXEMIA AND HYPERTENSIVE PREGNANCY

	Nonconvulsive Toxemia		Hypertensive Pregnancy	
	Ante-partum ml./min./1.73m.²	Post-partum ml./min./1.73m.²	Ante-partum ml./min./1.73m.²	Post-partum ml./min./1.73m.²
Kariher and George, 1943	555	582.5	613	521
Dill et al., 1942	680	482	515	465
Taylor et al., 1942	683	603	571	421
Corcoran and Page, 1941	464	417	—	—
deAlvarez, 1950	564.5	523	446	—
Sarles et al., 1968	550	—	625	—
Smith, 1951	Range in normal nonpregnant females 492–696 ml./min./1.73 m.²			

(such as thickening of the basement membrane of the glomerular tufts), rather than a cause of the edema formation. In fact, the modest decrease in glomerular filtration rate is consistent with the histologic changes observed in the glomerular unit.

If edema of pregnancy toxemia is of renal origin, it is due to endocrine influences and not directly to alterations in renal blood flow and glomerular function. That is not to exclude these in the causation of the disease. (See Etiology.)

Prerenal factors concerned with edema formation are not appreciably changed over normal pregnancy. The oncotic pressure of the plasma proteins is at times reduced but not to a crucial level, capillary filtration rate is not changed appreciably from normal pregnancy, and the protein content of edema fluid is not remarkable. Despite these findings, in the most severe form of the disease, especially with convulsions and coma, capillary physiology becomes severely compromised and transudation occurs, as reflected in hemoconcentration and a hypovolemic state (Fig. 2).

The hypertension is attributed to humoral or pressor substances. This is supported by the measured response of normal pregnant women and of those patients with pregnancy toxemia to high selective spinal anesthesia and ganglionic blocking agents, more particularly tetraethylammonium chloride (TEAC) testing. An exaggerated hypotensive response was observed in the normal pregnant patient when compared

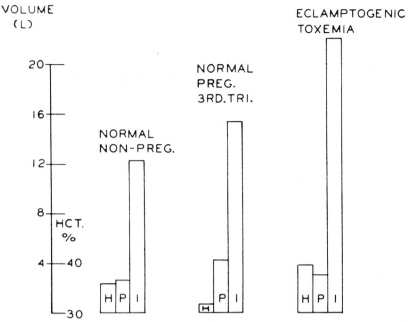

Figure 2. A comparison of hematocrit, plasma volume, and interstitial fluid volume in normal nonpregnant women, in the third trimester of normal pregnancy, and in eclamptogenic toxemia. *H*, hematocrit; *P*, plasma volume; and *I*, interstitial fluid volume. (From Freis, E. D., and Kenny, J. F., J. Clin. Invest., 27:283, 1948.)

with the nonpregnant, but there was a lesser response in patients with pregnancy toxemia. Marked drops in blood pressure were observed in a number of patients with pregnancy toxemia, however, making it difficult to accept without reservation the humoral concept of the etiology of the hypertension.

The cardiac output in severe toxemia is within the range of normal. Cerebral oxygen consumption is reduced in patients with convulsions, possibly accounting for the aberrations observed in electroencephalograms. With recovery, the slow high-voltage activity is replaced by a low voltage of the normal cerebral activity.

PATHOLOGY

The pathologic lesions described for pregnancy toxemia are those which are found in the most severe form of the disease, more particularly when convulsions or coma occurs. Although morphologic changes are found in severe toxemia without convulsions, they are less striking, and, in the event that a patient with the mild form succumbs for reasons other than toxemia, lesions associated with severe toxemia are not found.

In general, the lesions of severe pregnancy toxemia consist of hemorrhage and tissue necrosis, presumably the result of arteriolar and precapillary spasm and damage. The morphologic changes more often involve the liver, kidney, and brain, although they may be seen, but to a lesser extent, throughout the body. Fibrin deposition is seen resembling that encountered in the Shwartzman reaction.

Kidney

At necropsy the kidneys may be somewhat enlarged from the associated edema. The cortex on the cut surface may be moderately pale and interspersed occasionally with small areas of hemorrhage, or it may be dark red with the corticomedullary margins indistinct.

The most consistent lesions of this disease are found in the kidney. They are described as thickening, reticulation, and sometimes splitting of the basement membrane of the glomerular tuft, together with avascularity. Hyaline or fibrin thrombi are occasionally seen deposited within capillaries of the glomerulus (Fig. 3). If any lesion is pathognomonic of severe toxemia, it is generally agreed that it is thickening of the basement membrane of the glomerular

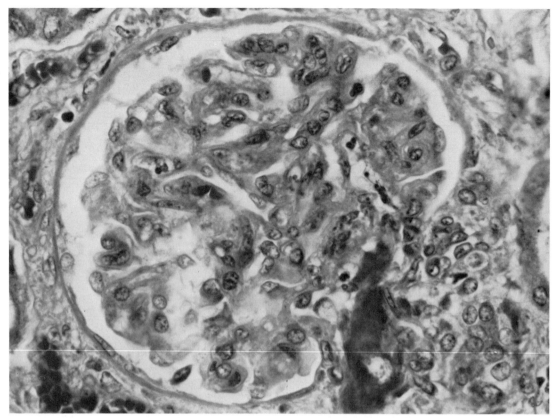

Figure 3. Glomerulus with thrombosis of afferent arteriole. × 450.

tuft, a reversible lesion. By use of the electron microscope, these findings have been verified in serial biopsies in severe toxemia, and it has been shown that these reversible changes in the glomerulus (Fig. 4) in no way resemble those observed in acute glomerular nephritis.

Renal lesions commonly associated with hypertension, such as hyalinization of afferent arterioles or muscular hypertrophy of interlobular arteries, have been noted in patients with toxemia who had a history of antecedent hypertension. In an occasional patient having severe toxemia with convulsions, whose urine and blood pressure were known to be normal prior to pregnancy, focal necrotizing arteriolitis, usually in the afferent glomerular arteriole, has been seen. The necrotizing arteriolitis is perhaps best interpreted as an effect of a sudden elevation of blood pressure, for similar lesions can be produced regularly in animals by abruptly raising the blood pressure.

Tubular lesions are not a conspicuous feature of this disease. "Hyaline droplet degeneration" is described in tubular epithelial cells, but this may merely represent the reabsorption of protein which is filtered in excessive amounts through slightly damaged glomeruli. Certainly there is no characteristic tubular lesion in pregnancy toxemia.

Liver

The liver is normal in size, and somewhat pale, with reddened areas of subcapsular hemorrhage often observed over the surface (Fig. 5A). On the cut surface (Fig. 5B) the hemorrhagic areas, although they may be widespread and distributed throughout the liver substance, are sometimes restricted to the right lobe. Microscopically these hemorrhagic areas are located more frequently in the periphery or periportal region of the liver lobule. The lesions extend toward the center of the lobule so that the mid and central zones may be involved, either together or separately. The degree of tissue damage varies, ranging from hemorrhage and deposition of fibrin in the sinusoids to necrosis of the surrounding paren-

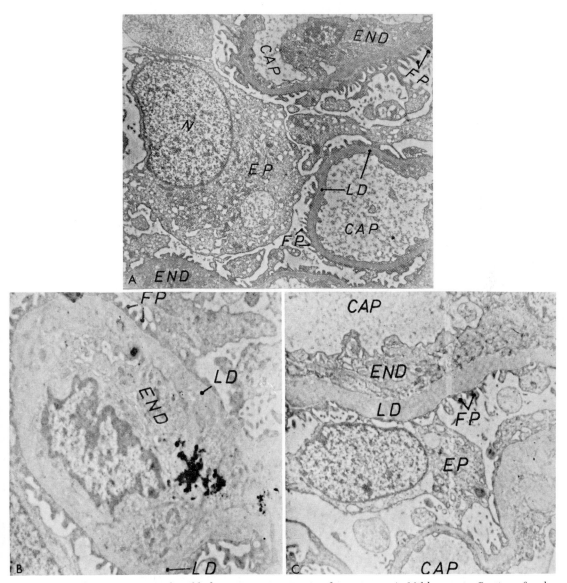

Figure 4. Electron micrographs of kidney tissue in toxemia of pregnancy. A, *Mild toxemia: Portion of a glomerulus*. Segments of three capillary loops (*CAP*) can be seen. The lamina densa (*LD*), or basement membrane, is normal. The endothelial cytoplasm is a thin, attenuated layer, as in the normal, except in two areas where there is an increase of endothelial cytoplasm (*END*), which is vacuolated. The epithelial cytoplasm (*EP*) is greatly swollen, with numerous vacuoles. The trabeculae appear to be distended. The foot processes (*FP*) are normal and discrete in most areas. The nucleus (*N*) of the epithelial cell is swollen. Reduced from × 10,000. B, *Severe toxemia: A single capillary loop*. The lamina densa (*LD*), or basement membrane, is normal. The foot processes (*FP*) are distinct and separated one from another. Note the very considerable increase of the endothelial cytoplasm (*END*), resulting in virtually complete occlusion of the capillary lumen. (The black smudges are artifacts.) Reduced from × 10,200. C, *Severe toxemia*. Note the vacuolation of the epithelial cytoplasm (*EP*). The foot processes (*FP*) are discrete in some areas but are fused in others. Note the increased deposition of basement membrane-like material in the endothelial cytoplasm (*END*) and the slight but definite thickening of the lamina densa (*LD*), or basement membrane. Reduced from × 6800. (From Pollack, V. E., and Nettles, J. B., Medicine, 39:469, 1960.)

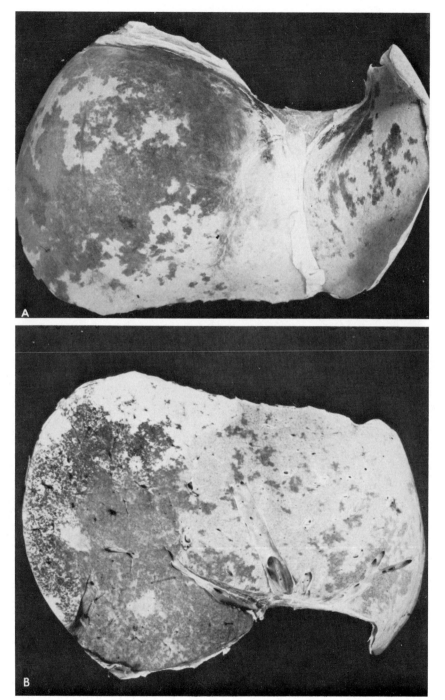

Figure 5.   The liver in toxemia associated with convulsions. A, Intact specimen. B, Cut surface.

chymal liver cells (Fig. 6A). In certain instances there may be complete fragmentation of the liver cords without actual necrosis (Fig. 6B). In liver biopsies obtained from patients with severe toxemia, in only two out of five cases was there evidence of necrosis and in the non-necrotic areas the glycogen content was normal.

Brain

The brain will show microscopic evidence of edema in nearly all cases of severe toxemia, and gross edema in about one half of the cases with convulsions. Hemorrhage may occur throughout the brain substance, varying widely in location and

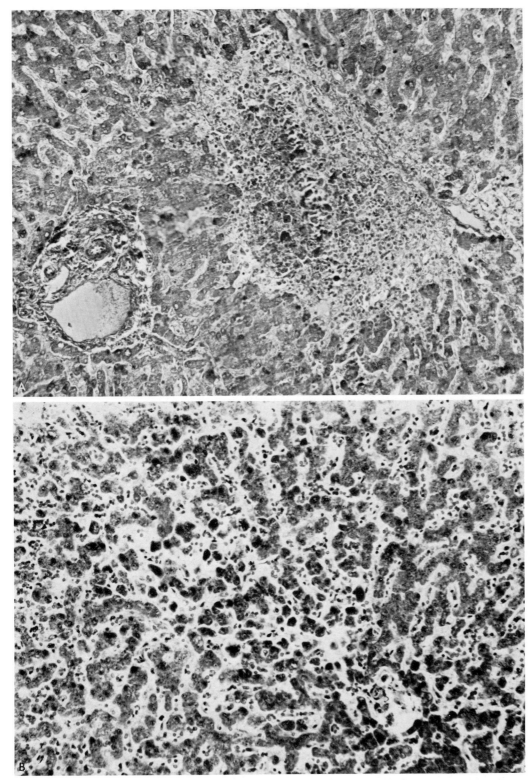

Figure 6. Micrographs of liver tissue in toxemia of pregnancy. A, Liver with focal necrosis. × 125. B, Fragmentation of liver cords in severe toxemia. × 125.

extent, from extensive subarachnoid hemorrhage to hemorrhage into the ventricles or basal ganglia. Of the deaths in pregnancy toxemia, 15 to 20 per cent are due to cerebral hemorrhage. There need be no antecedent vascular disease, as evidenced either symptomatically or at autopsy, and, in fact, in the majority of cases there is none.

Other Organs

Other organs, including the heart and lungs, may show small petechial hemorrhages, the evidence of generalized arteriolar involvement. Because some patients with severe toxemia develop acute pulmonary edema, a search has been made for evidence of myocarditis, both clinically and pathologically. Inflammatory lesions of the myocardium, however, have never been demonstrated in severe toxemia with convulsions. The lungs commonly show pulmonary congestion or edema, and there is usually some terminal bronchial pneumonia. The adrenals often reveal extensive petechial hemorrhages, thrombi, and subsequent necrosis in areas of the cortex.

Grossly, the reproductive organs usually reveal remarkably little change. Atheromatous changes have been seen occasionally in the decidual arterioles of the placental site. The question has arisen whether these findings are due to the toxemic process or if perchance they are the blood vessel changes that might be expected to occur in a patient who has vascular or renal disease — and the latter is probable.

Placenta

The placenta may reveal gross and microscopic changes, but these are by no means consistent. It is said that typically the syncytium shows regression and varying degrees of degeneration. There is autolysis and clumping together of the nuclei of the syncytial cells, which appear as dark-staining masses, leaving large areas of cytoplasm devoid of nuclei. Eventually the nuclei may disappear altogether. The older syncytium appears to be involved primarily, for the younger syncytial buds often fail to show these degenerative changes.

Histochemical techniques have demonstrated certain changes in the toxemic placenta many weeks prior to term that characteristically appear only at term in the normal placenta. It will be recalled that alkaline phosphatase and glycogen increase steadily in the syncytium throughout pregnancy, whereas acid phosphatase does not appear until late in pregnancy. In the premature toxemic placenta these substances are present in proportions similar to those observed in the normal term placenta.

Summary

In summary, the important pathologic features are those of generalized vascular changes and, sometimes, capillary fibrin deposition. Restricted to the severe form of the disease, the lesions that are seen are found most frequently in the kidney, the liver, the adrenal, and the brain, including the hypophysis. The most consistent findings are hemorrhages in the liver, usually periportal in location, and thickening of the tissue comprising the loops of the glomerular tufts of the kidney. Evidence favors the view that, in nearly all patients who survive pregnancy toxemia, tissue repair is complete and there is little or no residual morphologic damage. There is, however, the possibility that fibrin deposition about the hypophysis might cause necrosis and lead to panhypopituitarism, and certainly there are a few previously normotensive patients who reveal residual hypertension post partum. (See discussion of cardiovascular and renal sequelae, later in this chapter.)

LABORATORY EXAMINATIONS AND INTERPRETATION

In patients with the milder form of the disease, frequent clean-voided urine analysis is indicated and in the severe form this should be performed daily. The urinary sediment in the severe form may mimic the findings in renal conditions in the nonpregnant, with casts and red blood cells, and hence is not an aid in the differential diagnosis of the basis for hypertension and proteinuria.

The blood urea nitrogen may be moderately elevated during the severe form of the disease, reaching levels of 15 to 30 mg. per 100 ml. Often the highest levels are observed in the early phase of a postpartum diuresis. Uric acid values are commonly elevated, with levels above 10.0 mg. per 100 ml. Originally believed to reflect liver damage, the elevation in blood uric acid has since been attributed to increased renal tubular reabsorption.

The plasma carbon dioxide content in the convulsive form is often low (plus or minus 12 volumes per cent). The lacticemia associated with convulsions, together with diminishing urinary output, accounts for the metabolic acidosis.

Serum proteins with a reverse in albumin-globulin ratio are observed and although low albumin values are encountered, this is far from a consistent finding. Considerable credence has been given in the past to the hypoproteinemia. When serum albumin levels were low, salt-free albumin has been administered, but the therapeutic response has not been impressive.

Hyponatremia is commonly found, with serum sodium values ranging 120 to 130 mEq. or even lower in the severe form of the disease. Subject to interpretation, this does not reflect a low-salt syndrome—quite the reverse. In fact, the amount of sodium reputedly retained in pregnancy is far in excess of that required for the abnormal increases in the extracellular fluid. The question has been raised whether sodium is stored in an inactive form, as in bone, or intracellularly. There is no convincing evidence for either. Whatever the explanation for the hyponatremia, it is futile to try to correct the low sodium levels and indeed may be harmful and fraught with danger.

Other blood studies of special importance in the severe form of the disease are the hematocrit, blood platelets, and possible fibrinogen levels. In convulsive toxemia, the writer has observed the hematocrit to increase from 35 to 45 and in fatal cases up to 50 and 60 some hours prior to demise. Thus hematocrit may afford an index of the severity of the disease and the degree of hypovolemia. Moreover, following recovery, it is not unusual to find abnormally low hematocrits in patients with the convulsive form of the disease even when blood loss at delivery has been minimal. A decrease in blood platelets has been observed that is consistent with values found in a Shwartzman type of reaction. Indeed, in the preconvulsive period the clotting factor may be accelerated consistent with a hypercoagulable state. (See Chapter 11, Anatomic and Physiologic Changes of Pregnancy.) This may have practical implications for therapy and in the assessment of the disease. The disease at this stage might be reversible through heparin, sporadically advocated in the past in the treatment of pregnancy toxemia.

After the baseline studies as listed above have been secured, patients with the severe disease and certainly those with convulsion require daily blood urea nitrogen, uric acid, and plasma carbon dioxide content determinations. Hematocrit, blood platelet determinations and other clotting factors may be useful in assessing the course of the patient's disease, and several determinations may be indicated in the course of each 24 hours until such time as the patient is safely delivered and is recovering satisfactorily.

Generally serum glutamic oxalacetic transaminase (SGOT) and lactic dehydrogenase are not elevated appreciably over the slight rise of normal pregnancy and should be useful diagnostically in determining liver damage in pregnancy toxemia.

MATERNAL AND FETAL MORTALITY

In current practice, death is unexpected in the severe nonconvulsive form of the disease, although blood loss at delivery, shock, and renal failure are constant threats. (See Complications.) The maternal prognosis in severe toxemia with convulsions is influenced more by the elapsed time from the onset of convulsions to the beginning of treatment than by any special form of therapy. When medical treatment is not immediately available or the patient must be transported a long distance and arrives in the hospital some 24 to 48 hours after the convulsions began, the death rate is correspondingly high (5 to 10 per cent). When medical treatment has preceded or is instituted soon after the onset of convulsions, the mortality is comparatively low (0 to 2 per cent).

Reference has been made to the perinatal mortality in the various hypertensive groups. Suffice to say, the neonatal loss in toxemic patients is two to three times that encountered in normal patients, with prematurity accounting for much of the difference. Death in utero is equally high, so that the perinatal mortality is substantially increased.

COURSE IN PREGNANCY OF PATIENTS IN GROUP A

In general, patients with mild essential hypertension react favorably to pregnancy. In the severe form, however, not only is the risk of maternal complications substantially increased, but fetal death and the death rate from prematurity are high, the latter necessitated by early delivery in order not to subject the mother to undue hazards. Not only are these patients prone to develop "superimposed toxemia" with the threat of convulsions, but also cardiac and renal insufficiency and cerebral hemorrhage are increased hazards.

In both the mild and the severe form, during the course of pregnancy the blood pressure tends to fall during the middle trimester and to rise again in the last trimester, usually above the prepregnancy or first trimester level. Proteinuria commonly develops, and the hypertensive state may then be regarded as being aggravated by the presence of pregnancy or the additional rise in the blood pressure may represent a superimposed toxemia. Regardless of the point of view, all of the signs and symptoms of the toxemic state may develop, including convulsions, and the patient must be managed accordingly.

The treatment of patients with essential hypertension in pregnancy is no different from that for a nonpregnant patient with the disease. Therapy consists of the judicious use of a suitable antihypertensive agent alone or in combination with a thiazide diuretic. The possible ill effect of the latter on the fetus must be kept in mind.

It must be emphasized that, *even when the blood pressure is adequately controlled, the hazard to the fetus is not reduced, especially if there is renal involvement.* That is to say, the fetal risk is not favorably influenced simply by blood pressure control, and attention must be given to early delivery (i.e., from the 34th week onward) if the perinatal mortality is to remain low. There is no conclusive evidence that the course of the hypertensive disease is accelerated by pregnancy, but increasing age and parity may contraindicate further pregnancies.

Acute glomerulonephritis, like acute rheumatic fever, is rarely seen in pregnancy. Well documented cases in which the disease was known to begin during the course of pregnancy are few indeed. Unless the patient is seen in the early weeks of pregnancy, it is doubtful whether therapeutic abortion would aid in recovery. Certainly during the acute phase any abdominal procedure might well reduce the chance of recovery. The medical management of the pregnant patient is no different from that of the nonpregnant.

In patients with chronic glomerulonephritis, the advisability of continuation of pregnancy is a pertinent question. One has the impression that many authorities are inclined to advise against pregnancy. However, favorable results have been reported in sizable groups of patients with the milder form as defined in the classification, with a 90 per cent fetal salvage rate. On the other hand, in the more severe form, in at least half of the cases the fetus dies in utero or the pregnancy terminates spontaneously before the fetus is medically viable. Renal biopsy may be helpful in decision-making by determining the exact lesion and the degree of glomerular involvement. However, renal biopsy is said to carry a higher morbidity rate in pregnancy, and the conventional renal function tests and clinical status of the patient will usually suffice in determining whether pregnancy is permissible or should continue.

Like essential hypertension in pregnancy, the disease becomes temporarily aggravated. There is an increase in the daily amounts of protein in the urine, with a 24-hour loss of 5 grams or more of albumin in some cases. In the group with the milder form of the disease, careful prenatal management, together with hospitalization by the 32nd to the 34th week and delivery a week or two later, should result in fetal salvage. Whether pregnancy decreases the life expectancy of the patient with chronic glomerulonephritis is difficult to prove.

The question of therapeutic abortion arises in patients who have an exacerbation of their disease during pregnancy, or who have the severe form of the disease from the onset of pregnancy. Each patient must be individualized and carefully studied. These patients tend to react adversely to abdominal hysterotomy. Further, the patient is entirely likely to solve her own problem by spontaneous abortion as the urea nitrogen mounts.

With the constant threat of an exacerbation or a new urinary tract infection, the course of pregnancy in patients with chronic pyelonephritis is less predictable than in patients with chronic glomerulonephritis. Moreover, chronic pyelonephritis without evidence of bacterial infection adds another variable in establishing with certainty the diagnosis in pregnancy. In retrospect, this observation accounts for those patients dying of renal failure in pregnancy in whom the diagnosis of chronic glomerulonephritis was entertained but chronic pyelonephritis was found at necropsy. However, in the mild form, pregnancy is manageable as outlined for a patient with mild chronic glomerulonephritis, plus the necessary antibiotics to control the infection.

TREATMENT

Pregnancy toxemia can be curtailed or prevented to a degree by measures mentioned in the chapter on Conduct of Pregnancy. The highlights of these are weight control as it relates to extracellular fluid and generalized edema formation. In recalcitrant cases in which excessive weight gain continues despite a dietary régime and restriction of activity, diuretics might be added for a brief period. It is somewhat difficult to assess the value of diuretics in pregnancy, for bed rest alone commonly results in weight loss of 4 lb. or more in a 24-hour period.

Failure of the patient to respond to the above management should alert the physician to the strong possibility that she is destined to develop some form of pregnancy toxemia. The patient should be seen weekly or biweekly for recording of weight and blood pressure and urine examination, and on occasion hospitalized for a period of observation.

The definitive treatment of pregnancy toxemia is dictated by (1) the severity of the disease and (2) the gestational age of the pregnancy when the process develops. Obviously the clinical situation may demand a different approach to treatment if the patient is 30 weeks or 37 weeks pregnant or if she has mild rather than severe toxemia.

The management of mild toxemia is mainly in the interest of the fetus, on the assumption that the condition can be maintained in an arrested state and without jeopardy to the mother. In the mild form as defined, the pregnancy may be permitted to continue until the fetus is medically viable. Preferably the patient should be hospitalized or kept at near-complete bed rest. The blood pressure is maintained at near-normotensive levels often only by sedatives, and at other times by hypotensive agents. Clean-voided urine specimens should be examined frequently for the appearance or presence of albumin and casts. If the condition remains stationary, as described in the natural course of the disease, and the patient is relatively free of signs and symptoms, the pregnancy may be permitted to continue to the 35th to 36th week of gestation. In the interim, the status of the fetal condition may be followed by estriol determinations; should these fall to critical levels at the 32nd to 34th weeks, delivery may be advisable to avoid fetal demise. Ultrasound measurement of the biparietal diameter is especially useful here in assessing the rate of fetal growth.

Treatment of the patient with the severe form of pregnancy toxemia is primarily concerned with the mother, namely, to prevent convulsions or other serious complications that can arise in the course of this disease. Whether the pregnancy is permitted to continue to the stage of fetal maturity is dependent largely on the patient's response to treatment. Although on occasion the patient appears to improve markedly, this improvement often is only temporary. Whatever else, these patients should be under constant hospital surveillance until delivered, for the disease may suddenly worsen.

Should the disease develop early in the third trimester, and assuming that the disease can be medically controlled, the question arises whether allowing the pregnancy to continue for a matter of some weeks to permit the fetus to reach maturity may not increase the hazard of permanent vascular or renal damage. There is no convincing evidence in answer to this question, albeit the incidence of residual hypertension is low for patients in this group (see Sequelae, later in this chapter).

The aim in the treatment of the severe form is to control irritability, reduce the blood pressure by the appropriate agent, and promote renal excretion. As noted below, the selection of the hypotensive agent will depend on whether the patient is in or on the verge of a hypertensive crisis. The conventional diuretics, including mercurials, may be effective in the early stage of the disease. Mannitol may be used, but cautiously, with the threat of pulmonary edema borne in mind. Diuretics are of little avail when renal excretion drops to oliguric levels. Indeed, it is this fall in urine output plus the gross appearance of the urine that demands immediate termination of pregnancy lest the disease escape control and convulsions supervene (Fig. 7). Thus, in practice, continuation of the pregnancy is determined by the immediate response to medical measures and whether these are capable of holding the disease in abeyance. More commonly, termination of pregnancy is required to avoid progression of the disease, usually within days from the onset of treatment.

In the severe form of disease with convulsions (eclampsia), it is generally agreed that the patient should be delivered as soon as the disease is brought under medical control. But exactly what is meant by "medical control" in overall patient management and how much time should elapse from the onset of the convulsions until one

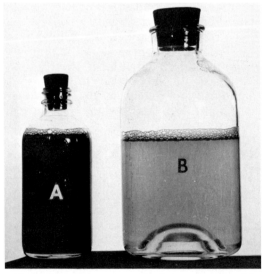

Figure 7. Appearance and relative amounts of the urine in a patient with severe pregnancy toxemia. *A*, Urine excreted in the 12-hour period preceding delivery, dark and scanty. *B*, Urine excreted in the 12-hour period immediately following delivery, light and plentiful.

takes steps to initiate labor are not easy questions to answer, for clinical experience teaches that the patient's condition can change hourly with this extremely labile disease. When seemingly under control, the patient may suddenly become irritable and unmanageable. The urine output may abruptly fall or convulsions recur. Moreover, there will be the exceptional patient in whom, despite hypotensive and anticonvulsive drugs, the blood pressure will fail to respond or the convulsions will continue. Thus, to state that termination of pregnancy by this means or that or at a designated time after the convulsions have apparently been brought under control is impossible except in general terms, for each patient must be therapeutically individualized. Rather, pregnancy should be terminated when one is convinced the patient has responded maximally to medical treatment or will fail to do so, and this is usually a matter of hours rather than days.

Supportive treatment includes placing the patient in a quiet room with a nurse in constant attendance. The patient should not be disturbed except when absolutely necessary, and such items as blood pressure observations should be made by the physician in charge. Commonly, the irritable patient may become less so following reduction of the blood pressure. In order to differentiate stupor caused by the disease from drug effects, these patients should receive the minimum of sedation. Also, in the selection of the drug to be used, and in determination of the dose, account must be taken of the fact that renal function is temporarily impaired and some degree of liver damage may be present. Some of the newer anticonvulsive drugs such as diazepam (Valium) have a place in therapy when other measures fail.

Oxygen is routinely administered with attention given to maintaining a clear airway. In the unconscious patient, this may be a problem and tracheostomy may be indicated. The amount of fluid administered must be balanced with urinary output. Some 1000 to 2000 ml. of 5 per cent dextrose in water is appropriate. Sodium lactate has been recommended in the correction of the acidosis.

Heparin therapy is mentioned, for it may influence renal function and the general course of the disease in accordance with its possible etiology. Actually, heparin has been considered periodically in the treatment of pregnancy toxemia. Recently some impressive responses have been encountered immediately following heparin administration, notably in patients with a markedly elevated blood urea nitrogen and thrombocytopenia. These findings suggest that renal fibrin deposition akin to the Shwartzman reaction might be present. Blood urea nitrogen was noted to fall and platelets to increase following heparin therapy, and this trend was enhanced by subsequent termination of the pregnancy. (See Etiology.) Hence, there well may be a place for heparin therapy in this disease, more particularly when renal output is seriously impaired prior to delivery, or when the kidney fails to recover functionally within a few hours after delivery.

In attempting to cover all conceivable contingencies, exchange transfusion might save the rare patient in whom liver involvement is the clinical feature. Certainly one can recall the eclamptic patient with rapidly mounting jaundice who at necropsy had extensive liver damage. Would exchange transfusion have salvaged such a patient?

Many drugs have been and may be used to control the hypertension and the list will grow. The time-honored drug has been magnesium sulfate, perhaps because of its rather wide margin of safety. The drug apparently has a dual action, with a depressant effect on the central nervous system, thus controlling irritability, and peripherally on neuromuscular transmission, with resultant vasodilatation.

Magnesium sulfate (U.S.P.), 4 grams in 20 per cent solution, is given intravenously over a period of five minutes. Simultaneously, 10 grams of the drug in 50 per cent solution is administered intramuscularly every four hours thereafter, unless the patellar reflexes become sluggish or the urine output falls below 25 ml. per hour. The magnesium plasma concentration is said to remain between 3.5 and 7.0 mEq. with this dosage, and no effect on labor is noted even at higher levels. Toxicity is revealed by the disappearance of patellar reflexes and this occurs before the blood magnesium concentration reaches 10 mEq. Respiratory failure can occur when the plasma concentration rises to 15 mEq. In the event that the blood pressure drops to alarming levels, the deep reflexes disappear, or signs of respiratory paralysis appear, 2 to 3 ml. of 25 per cent calcium chloride, a specific counteractant, should be given slowly intravenously. Although magnesium gains entry to the fetal blood, there is no apparent depression of the infant at birth.

The alkaloids of *Veratrum viride* or *V. alba* are the only known drugs that stimulate the afferent side of the reflex pathway responsible for the control of blood pressure. Nerve endings located in the left ventricle and carotid sinus, and about the aortic arch and pulmonary arteries, stimulated by these drugs, provide afferent impulses to the vasomotor center and cause a reduction in blood pressure and a slowing of the heart rate. It is accepted that the bradycardia is vagal in origin, but the efferent pathway of the stimuli that cause dilatation of the arterioles remains obscure. In addition to the peripheral vasodilatation, there is a decrease in cerebral and renal vascular resistance, apparently without a rise in cardiac output. Although toxic effects are comparatively rare, nausea, vomiting, and unacceptable degree of hypotension can develop. In contrast to many of the other hypotensive agents, protoveratrine has a time-limited effect so that the blood pressure tends to return to the initial levels within one or two hours after it is given.

Protoveratrine may be given orally, intramuscularly, or intravenously. For a sustained effect the drug is best administered by intravenous drip; 0.5 mg. of protoveratrine is added to a liter of 5 per cent glucose in buffered water, and the dosage is titrated from 10 to 40 drops per minute, depending on the blood pressure and pulse rate response. Any adverse effect such as marked bradycardia and a reduction of the blood pressure to shock levels may be rapidly corrected by the administration of atropine sulfate, 0.5 to 1.0 mg., either intravenously or intramuscularly.

Hydralazine (Apresoline) on theoretical grounds would appear to be the most useful drug for the control of hypertension in pregnancy when administered parenterally in 20 mg. amounts. It increases renal blood flow, which places it apart from all of the other ganglionic blocking agents, but this is done at the expense of an increase in cardiac output. Although the drug will reduce the blood pressure effectively, there is no evidence that it will increase urinary excretion in acute severe pregnancy toxemia, i.e., increase glomerular filtration. It would appear that some caution should be exercised in the use of this agent in the markedly edematous patient whose heart is laboring and in whom pulmonary edema is a threat.

Reserpine, an alkaloid from *Rauwolfia serpentina* with a sedative and a hypotensive effect, is used in the management of the patient with essential hypertension complicating pregnancy, as well as in pregnancy toxemia. Reserpine, 10 mg., may be given alone, or with hydralazine, 10 to 20 mg., the latter being used to produce a rapid initial response. In the mild form of toxemia, reserpine is administered parenterally, 5 mg. every one to two hours until the blood pressure is reduced to 140 mm. Hg systolic and 90 mm. Hg diastolic, and it is maintained at that level with a dose of 5 mg. each four to six hours. The side effects of drowsiness, weakness, and nasal congestion may apparently be prevented by decreasing the dosage of reserpine and using it in combination with other drugs. The drug causes nasal congestion in the newborn.

Methyldopate hydrochloride (Aldomet) causes a decline in blood pressure four to six hours after 250 to 500 mg. is given intravenously. Like reserpine, the drug may be administered orally for sustained therapy. It must be recognized that the drug is largely excreted by the kidney.

In summary, there are now available a number of hypotensive drugs that will reduce blood pressure rather effectively in the different hypertensive states of pregnancy. These agents may be used separately or in combination; the purpose of combining drugs is to eliminate undesirable side effects by using smaller doses of each drug and still to obtain a favorable hypotensive response.

A popular method is to start with magnesium sulfate and implement this drug with one or more specific hypotensive agents such as hydralazine should the blood pressure fail to come under control. Actually, one might consider these patients as being in a hypertensive crisis as observed in the nonpregnant patient with essential hypertension and treat her accordingly with the hypotensive agent most familiar to the physician. However, he should be cognizant of the transient nature of the condition being treated and of the fact that it is curable by termination of the pregnancy. This general principle applies to all drug therapy in this disease and suggests that only agents whose specific action and side effects are clearly known should be used.

When the patient shows improvement by cessation of convulsions, less irritability reduction of the blood pressure, preferably to a level of 140 to 150 mm. Hg systolic and 100 mm. Hg diastolic, and slowing of the pulse rate to less than 100 beats per minute, thought must be given to termination of pregnancy.

In the past, the view was commonly held that these patients were too ill to withstand whatever procedure was required to terminate pregnancy until such time as they respond fully to medical treatment. In the interim, the disease worsened and the patient reached a point of no return. Thus, in recent times there has been a tendency to deliver these patients as soon as they begin to respond to medical treatment, and this may be 6 to 18 hours after admission. This also suggests that there is some urgency in terminating the pregnancy, and labors extending beyond 12 hours in length are to be avoided lest the patient's condition become critical.

Labor frequently occurs spontaneously in these patients—in 25 to 30 per cent in some series. One may recall that certain of the factors considered in the etiology of the disease, not the least being renin, may promote myometrial activity. When required, induction of labor is carried out in the conventional way, and it may be stimulated by oxytocin infusion as in the nontoxemic patient. Undoubtedly some caution should be exercised in prolonging oxytocin administration in the edematous patient in whom water intoxication can be more easily provoked.

Lumbar epidural anesthesia is ideal for pain relief and may be used for both vaginal and abdominal delivery. This form of conduction anesthesia avoids the hazard of a hypotensive episode that is a possibility with spinal anesthesia. For labor, it affords total pain relief, a highly important consideration in these irritable patients subject to recurrent convulsions, and at the same time avoids the use of analgesic drugs whose action may make it more difficult to assess the patient's mental status, i.e., whether the somnolence or semi-comatose state is the result of the disease or is due to the effect of these agents.

Cesarean section is employed when immediate delivery is believed advisable. Also, abdominal delivery is required when effective labor, either spontaneous or induced, fails to ensue, and for other obstetric reasons such as cephalopelvic disproportion and breech presentation. As suggested, the method of anesthesia should be carefully chosen and the anesthetic carefully administered.

The postdelivery care of the eclamptic patient should continue to involve control of the blood pressure and irritability and attention to renal excretion. Rapid and spontaneous improvement can be anticipated in most cases, and the patient will require less of all medications. The blood pressure may return to near-normal levels within 24 to 48 hours. Diuresis may be impressive, although this may not occur for 24 hours post partum. The response to mannitol may be gratifying during this period.

However, the disease may show evidence of transient exacerbation, usually about the third postpartum day. The blood pressure may again rise, irritability may return, and convulsions have been observed. Hence these patients require careful medical supervision, especially during the first week or 10 days after delivery. When the blood pressure begins to recede the second time, it almost invariably returns to normotensive levels and the patient rapidly returns to a state of well-being.

COMPLICATIONS OF PREGNANCY TOXEMIA

In the severe form of the disease loss of vision, cerebral hemorrhage and thrombosis, acute pulmonary edema, and a hemolytic episode are the most disturbing complications encountered. Extremely rare, but recorded in the literature, are rupture of the liver and vertebral fracture, the latter in association with convulsions.

Disturbances of vision may vary from the loss of visual acuity to complete blindness. The blindness may be transient, with vision differing in degree from hour to hour, or it may last for several days. Transient blindness presumably is central in origin, depending perhaps on the degree of brain edema. Detachment of the retina is a common cause for continuing loss of vision, but, in contradistinction to the ominous significance of retinal detachment in nonpregnant patients with vascular or renal disease, complete spontaneous recovery within two weeks of delivery is the rule. This means also that retinal detachment, when it occurs in pregnancy, is due in most

instances to pregnancy toxemia, and not to vascular or renal disease.

In addition to cerebral hemorrhage, in which the presenting signs and symptoms are the same as when it occurs in the nonpregnant, cerebral thrombosis may be diagnosed in the rare patient who develops an aphasia or other localizing signs. Although in cerebral thrombosis the recovery may be delayed, a favorable prognosis may be given. Moreover, further pregnancies can be advised, depending on the patient's desires.

Acute pulmonary edema occurs in some 30 per cent of the patients who have convulsions, and its incidence is considerably higher in the fatal cases. This complication develops in severe nonconvulsive toxemia also. In these unusual cases (in which edema is marked), the toxemic patient while at bedrest, often without previous dyspnea or signs of embarrassment of the pulmonary circulation, is seized with a severe paroxysm of dyspnea associated with extreme orthopnea, cyanosis, and pulmonary edema. The suspicion might arise that hypertensive disease was present before the onset of pregnancy, and such may be the case, but after delivery the blood pressure and urine are normal in most of the patients who survive. Clinically, this syndrome is consistent with left ventricular failure.

A very important point to remember and differentiate in patient management is that recurrent attacks of paroxysmal dyspnea are the rule, and the prognosis must be guarded until the patient has been safely delivered, following which improvement is usually rapid and dramatic. This pattern of repetitive attacks is in contrast to the course of patients who have valvular heart disease with pulmonary edema in whom the pulmonary edema tends to disappear under proper medical management and usually not to recur. Thus, with rare exception, termination of pregnancy is avoided in the cardiac patient, at least during an episode of failure. In toxemia the pulmonary edema will persist to a degree until the patient is delivered (Fig. 8). Further, some consideration must be given to the danger of therapy which might mobilize the edema rapidly and thus precipitate an attack. The immediate treatment consists of morphine, venesection or peripheral cuff venostasis, oxygen therapy, and perhaps digitalis.

Improvement of pulmonary edema, at best, is only temporary; in fact, some fine rales can at all times be detected on ausculta-

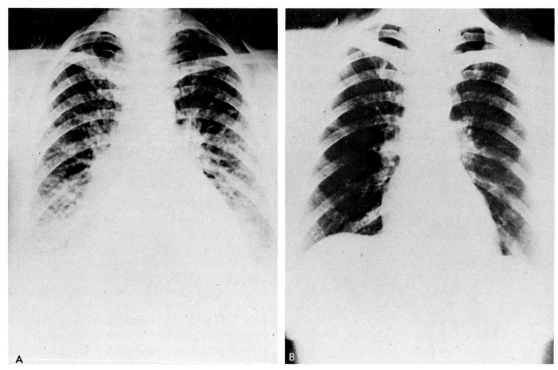

Figure 8.   Acute pulmonary edema, associated with severe nonconvulsive toxemia. A, Undelivered. B, A few days post partum.

tion. For this reason, unless the patient enters into labor spontaneously, pregnancy is terminated after a few hours of medical treatment, preferably by cesarean section. Again, it must be emphasized that the immediate prognosis must be guarded in the undelivered patient in whom pulmonary edema develops. Death may occur during an attack. However, it is equally important to realize that in the presence of pregnancy such attacks do not denote underlying vascular disease, but rather a burden imposed on the vascular system by the toxemia. In fact, nearly all of the cases studied had no vascular or renal disease, but marked generalized edema was a prominent sign. There is no reason to believe that this complication will arise in subsequent pregnancies, assuming that the patient is free of hypertensive disease.

A hemolytic episode has been encountered in pregnancy toxemia which could not be ascribed to other causes. The symptoms and findings include hemoglobinemia, hemoglobinuria, and thrombocytopenia, and the clotting time is prolonged. A positive tourniquet test may be elicited. Uterine hemostasis is not impaired and recovery is usual, although death has followed this

complication of toxemia, from cerebral hemorrhage or anuria resulting from the hemolytic crisis. This again may be a variant of the Shwartzman-like phenomenon.

RECURRENT INCIDENCE OF TOXEMIA AND CARDIOVASCULAR AND RENAL SEQUELAE

The recurrence rate of severe pregnancy toxemia can be low, owing to the probability that the patient with previous toxemia will seek early prenatal care. Also, her medical attendants will insist on a more rigid program to prevent the first phase of the disease from developing.

In the attempt to answer the question whether pregnancy toxemia initiates or causes cardiovascular or renal disease, in the earliest studies on the postpartum follow-up of patients diagnosed as having severe toxemia including eclampsia, hypertension persisted in nearly half of the patients. There was little evidence of residual renal involvement.

However, no distinction was made between patients in whom the urine and blood pressure were known to be normal prior to or in the early weeks of pregnancy and those in whom this could not be definitely established. In studies in which this distinction was made, it was found that in patients whose blood pressure and urine were normal prior to severe toxemia, including convulsions, the incidence of postpartum hypertension was low (2 to 10 per cent), and proteinuria was rare indeed. Also, it was concluded that no post-toxemic patient should be designated as having residual hypertension unless it is observed for 6 to 12 months after delivery. The blood pressure may remain elevated for many weeks or months, eventually to return to normal.

Approaching the question somewhat differently, the cause of death was studied in patients who died several years after convulsive toxemia. In a comparatively large group of such patients the death rate over a 1- to 20-year follow-up was 2.8 per cent in the primiparous and 13.6 per cent in the multiparous patients. In the latter, the majority of deaths were due to cardiovascular disease, which was not the case in the primiparous or younger patients. It was concluded that the increased mortality in the multiparous women could be attributed to a higher incidence of hypertensive disease antedating the pregnancy.

By contrast, it has been the writer's experience and that of others that in patients with mild toxemia, postpartum hypertension is more frequent and there is a greater tendency for the toxemia to recur. It is suggested that the milder form of toxemia reflects a tendency on the part of the patient to develop hypertension later in life. Further, in many patients the hypertension tends to develop earlier in each succeeding pregnancy, and by the age of 30 to 40 years the hypertension is likely to persist following delivery. This poses the practical question of how many children patients who react to pregnancy in this manner should be permitted to bear and how late in life. It is difficult to discard the possibility that repeated pregnancies, particularly after the age of 30 to 35, may hasten the development of hypertensive disease.

In summation, despite some differences of opinion in the literature on this subject, if cases are carefully documented with respect to the status of the cardiovascular and renal systems prior to pregnancy, there is evidence to support the belief that severe nonconvulsive and convulsive pregnancy toxemia, unless perhaps prolonged, rarely cause permanent damage to the vascular and renal systems. In contradistinction, patients with the mild form of pregnancy toxemia not only are more apt to have a recurrent mild toxemia in subsequent pregnancies, but they show a higher incidence of postpartum hypertension. By interpretation, this may mean that in a group of patients with mild toxemia there are many who are predestined to have hypertensive disease; hence the higher incidence of postpartum hypertension.

Finally, unilateral renal hypertension must always be considered in parturients with residual postpartum hypertension. This form of hypertension may well be reversible by appropriate treatment, especially in these relatively young women who are less likely to be afflicted with atherosclerotic changes. If searched for, the incidence of this form of residual postpartum hypertension could range as high as from 3 to 5 per cent. It is the responsibility of the obstetrician to make certain that the patient with persistent postpartum hypertension is studied and should the diagnosis prove to be renal hypertension, treatment may be instituted before the disease reaches an irreversible stage.

BIBLIOGRAPHY

Altchek, A., Albright, N. L., and Sommers, S. C.: The renal pathology of toxemia of pregnancy. Obstet. Gynec., 31:595, 1968.

Angell, M. E., Relman, A. S., and Robbins, S. L.: "Active" chronic pyelonephritis without evidence of bacterial infection. New Eng. J. Med., 278:1303, 1968.

Assali, N. S., Kaplan, S. A., Fomon, S. J., and Douglass, R. A., Jr.: Renal function studies in toxemia of pregnancy. J. Clin. Invest., 32:44, 1953.

Assali, N. S., Kaplan, S. A., Fomon, S. J., Douglass, R. A., and Tada, Y.: Effect of high spinal anesthesia on renal hemodynamics and excretion of electrolytes during osmotic diuresis in hydropenic normal pregnant women. J. Clin. Invest., 30:916, 1951.

Assali, N. S., and Prystowsky, H.: Studies on autonomic blockade; comparison between effects of tetraethylammonium chloride (TEAC) and high selective spinal anesthesia on blood pressure of normal and toxemic pregnancy. J. Clin. Invest., 29:1354, 1950.

Berger, M., and Langhans, J.: Angiotensinase activity in pregnant and nonpregnant women. Amer. J. Obstet Gynec., 98:215, 1967.

Berger, R. L., Liversage, R. M., Jr., Chalmers, T. C., Graham, J. H., McGoldrick, D. M., and Stohlman, F., Jr.: Exchange transfusion in the treatment of fulminating hepatitis. New Eng. J. Med., 274:497, 1966.

Borglin, N. E.: Serum transaminases in toxemia of pregnancy. J. Clin. Endocr., 19:425, 1959.

Bower, D.: The influence of dietary salt intake on pre-eclampsia. J. Obstet. Gynaec. Brit. Comm., 71:123, 1964.

Brain, M. C., Kuah, K. B., and Dixon, H. G.: Heparin treatment of haemolysis and thrombocytopenia in pre-eclampsia. J. Obstet. Gynaec. Brit. Comm., 74:702, 1967.

Brown, J. J., Davies, D. L., Doak, P. B., Lever, A. F., Robertson, J. I. S., and Tree, M.: The presence of renin in human amniotic fluid. Lancet, 2:64, 1964.

Brown, J. J., Davies, D. L., Doak, P. B., Lever, A. F., Robertson, J. I. S., and Trust, P.: Plasma renin concentration in the hypertensive diseases of pregnancy. J. Obstet. Gynaec. Brit. Comm., 73:410, 1966.

Browne, J. M. C., and Veall, N.: Maternal placental blood flow in normotensive and hypertensive women. J. Obstet. Gynaec. Brit. Emp., 60:141, 1953.

Bucht, H., and Werko, L.: Glomerular filtration rate in renal blood flow in hypertensive toxemia of pregnancy. J. Obstet. Gynaec. Brit. Emp., 60:157, 1953.

Chesley, L. C., and Cosgrove, R. A.: Remote deaths following eclampsia. Obstet. Gynec., 4:165, 1954.

Corcoran, A. C., and Page, I. H.: Renal function in late toxemia of pregnancy. Amer. J. Med. Sci., 201:385, 1941.

Crisp, W. E., Miesfeld, R. L., and Frajola, W. J.: Serum glutamic oxalacetic transaminase levels in the toxemias of pregnancy. Obstet. Gynec., 13:487, 1959.

de Alvarez, R. R.: Glomerular filtration rates, renal plasma flow, and sodium and water excretion in pregnancy toxemia. Amer. J. Obstet. Gynec., 60:1051, 1950.

de Bacalao, E. B., Kaunitz, H., Joseph, J., and McKay, D. G.: Lipid metabolism in toxemia and normal pregnancy. Obstet. Gynec., 24:909, 1964.

Dill, L. V., Isenhour, C. E., Cadden, J. F., and Robinson, C. E.: Glomerular filtration and renal blood flow in "normal" patients following toxemias of pregnancy. Amer. J. Obstet. Gynec., 44:66, 1942.

Freis, E. D., and Kenny, J. F.: Plasma volume, total circulating proteins and "available fluid" abnormalities in pre-eclampsia. J. Clin. Invest., 27:283, 1948.

Greiss, F. C., Jr., and van Wilkes, V.: Effects of sympathomimetic drugs and angiotensin on uterine vascular bed. J. Obstet. Gynec., 23:925, 1964.

Gibbs, F. A., and Reid, D. E.: The electroencephalogram in pregnancy. Amer. J. Obstet. Gynec., 44:672, 1942.

Ham, G. C., and Landis, E. M.: Comparison of pituitrin with antidiuretic substance found in human urine and placenta. J. Clin. Invest., 21:455, 1952.

Hamilton, H. F. H.: Cardiac output in hypertensive toxaemias of pregnancy. J. Obstet. Gynaec. Brit. Emp., 58:977, 1951.

Hayashi, T.: Uric acid and endogenous creatinine clearance studies in normal pregnancy and toxemias of pregnancy. Amer. J. Obstet. Gynec., 71:859, 1956.

Hayashi, T. T., Phitaksphraiwan, P., and Willson, J. W.: Effects of diet and diuretic agents in pregnancy toxemias. Obstet. Gynec., 22:237, 1963.

Hickler, R. B., Lauler, D. P., and Thorn, G. W.: Plasma angiotensinase activity in patients with hypertension and edema. J. Clin. Invest., 42:635, 1963.

Hodari, A. A.: The contribution of the fetal kidney to experimental hypertensive disease of pregnancy. Amer. J. Obstet. Gynec., 101:17, 1968.

Hodari, A. A., and Hodgkinson, C. P.: Fetal kidney as a source of renin in the pregnant dog. Amer. J. Obstet. Gynec., 102:691, 1968.

Hopper, J., Jr., Farquhar, M. G., Yamauchi, H., Moon, H. D., and Page, E. W.: Renal lesions in pregnancy. Clinical observations and light and electron microscopic findings. Obstet. Gynec., 17:271, 1961.

Hunter, C. H., and Howard, W. F.: Etiology of hypertension in toxemia of pregnancy. Amer. J. Obstet. Gynec., 81:441, 1961.

Imgerslev, M., and Teilum, G.: Biopsy studies on liver in pregnancy. Acta Obstet. Gynec. Scand., 25:339, 1945.

Jordan, W. K.: Apresoline (hydralazine hydrochloride) and its use in cases of hypertensive pregnancy. Amer. J. Obstet. Gynec., 68:618, 1954.

Kariher, D. H., and George, R. H.: Toxemias of pregnancy and inulin-Diodrast clearance tests. Proc. Soc. Exp. Biol. Med., 52:245, 1943.

Kellar, R. J.: Treatment of imminent eclampsia. J. Obstet. Gynaec. Brit. Comm., 62:683, 1966.

Kenney, R. A., Lawrence, R. F., and Miller, D. H.: Haemodynamic changes in kidney in "toxaemia of late pregnancy." J. Obstet. Gynaec. Brit. Emp., 57:17, 960, 1950.

Kirkendall, W. M., Fritz, A. E., and Lawrence, M. S.: Renal hypertension. New Eng. J. Med., 276:479, 1967.

Landesman, R., Biron, P., Castellanos, R., La Russa, R., and Wilson, K. H.: Plasma angiotensinase activity in normal and toxemic pregnancy. Obstet. Gynec., 22:316, 1963.

Llera, M. L.: Eclampsia, 1963–1966. J. Obstet. Gynaec. Brit. Comm., 74:379, 1967.

Luke, R. G., Linton, A. L., Briggs, J. D., and Kennedy, A. C.: Mannitol therapy in acute renal failure. Lancet, 1:980, 1965.

Mahran, M. M.: Water metabolism in pre-eclampsia and essential hypertension. J. Obstet. Gynaec. Brit. Comm., 71:218, 1964.

Massani, Z. M., Sanguinetti, R., Gallegos, R., and Raimondi, D.: Angiotensin blood levels in normal and toxemic pregnancies. Amer. J. Obstet. Gynec., 99:313, 1967.

McCall, M. L.: Cerebral circulation and metabolism in toxemia of pregnancy; observations on effect of Veratrum viride and Apresoline (1-hydrazinophthalazine). Amer. J. Obstet. Gynec., 66:1015, 1953.

McKay, D. G.: The placenta in experimental toxemia of pregnancy. Obstet. Gynec., 20:1, 1962.

McKay, D. G.: Clinical significance of the pathology of toxemia of pregnancy. Circulation 30(Suppl.2):66, 1964.

McKay, D. G., and Corey, A. E.: Cryofibrinogenemia in toxemia of pregnancy. Obstet. Gynec., 23:508, 1964.

McKay, D. G., and Goldenberg, V. E.: Pathogenesis of anatomic changes in experimental toxemia of pregnancy. Obstet. Gynec., 21:651, 1963.

McKay, D. G., Merrill, S. J., Weiner, A. E., Hertig, A. T., and Reid, D. E.: Pathologic anatomy of eclampsia, bilateral renal cortical necrosis, pituitary necrosis, and other acute fatal complications of pregnancy, and its possible relationship to the generalized Shwartzman phenomenon. Amer. J. Obstet. Gynec., 66:507, 1953.

Moore, J. G., Singh, B. P., Herzig, D., and Assali, N. S.: Hemodynamic effects of rauwolfia alkaloid (reserpine) in human pregnancy; results of intravenous administration. Amer. J. Obstet. Gynec., 71:237, 1956.

Moses, A. M., Lobotsky, J., and Lloyd, C. W.: Occurrence of preeclampsia in a bilaterally adrenalectomized woman. J. Clin. Endocr., 19:987, 1959.

Nash, H. A., and Brooker, R. M.: Hypotensive alkaloids from Veratrum album, protoveratrine A, protoveratrine B, and germitetrine B. J. Amer. Chem. Soc., 75:1942, 1953.

Ober, W. B., Reid, D. E., Romney, S. L., and Merrill, J. P.: Renal lesions and acute renal failure in pregnancy. Amer. J. Med., 21:781, 1956.

Odell, L. D.: Renal filtration rates in pregnancy toxemia; inulin and exogenous creatinine. Amer. J. Med. Sci., 213:709, 1947.

Pollak, V. E., and Nettles, J. B.: Kidney in toxemia of pregnancy; clinical and pathologic study based on renal biopsies. Medicine, 39:469, 1960.

Pollak, V. E., Pirani, C. L., Kark, R. M., Muehrcke, R. C., Freka, V. C., and Nettles, J. B.: Reversible glomerular lesions in toxaemia of pregnancy. Lancet, 2:59, 1956.

Pritchard, J. A., and Stone, S. R.: Clinical and laboratory observations on eclampsia. Amer. J. Obstet. Gynec., 99:754, 1967.

Pritchard, J. A., Weisman, R., Jr., Ratnoff, O. D., and Vosburgh, G. J.: Intravascular hemolysis, thrombocytopenia and other hematologic abnormalities associated with severe toxemia of pregnancy. New Eng. J. Med., 250:89, 1954.

Reid, D. E., and Teel, H. M.: Cardiac asthma and acute pulmonary edema complicating toxemias of pregnancy. J.A.M.A., 113:1628, 1939.

Reid, D. E., and Teel, H. M.: Nonconvulsive pregnancy toxemias. Amer. J. Obstet. Gynec., 37:886, 1939.

Reid, D. E., Frigoletto, F. D., Tullis, J. L., and Hinman, J.: Hypercoagulable states in pregnancy. In press.

Robinson, H. A., Schelin, E. C., and Davis Fort, W.: Postpartum curettement for hypertension. Amer. J. Obstet. Gynec., 88:788, 1964.

Sarles, H. E., Hill, S. S., LeBlanc, A. L., Smith, G. H., Canales, C. O., and Remmers, A. R.: Sodium excretion patterns during and following intravenous sodium chloride loads in normal and hypertensive pregnancies. Amer. J. Obstet. Gynec., 102:1, 1968.

Schewitz, L. J., Friedman, I. A., and Pollak, V. E.: Bleeding after renal biopsy in pregnancy. Obstet. Gynec., 26:295, 1965.

Seitchik, J.: Metabolism of urate in pre-eclampsia. Amer. J. Obstet. Gynec., 72:40, 1956.

Seitchik, J., and Alper, C.: Body compartments of normal pregnant edematous pregnant and preeclamptic women. Amer. J. Obstet. Gynec., 68:1540, 1954.

Smith, H. W.: The Kidney; Structure and Function in Health and Disease. Oxford University Press, New York, 1951.

Switzer, P. K., Union, S. C., Hester, L. L., Milam, J. W., and Ownby, F. D.: Edema fluid protein in patients with toxemia of pregnancy. Amer. J. Obstet. Gynec., 60:427, 1950.

Talledo, O. E.: Renin-angiotensin system in normal and toxemic pregnancies. Amer. J. Obstet. Gynec., 101:254, 1968.

Talledo, O. E., Chesley, L. C., and Zuspan, F. P.: Renin-angiotensin system in normal and toxemic pregnancies. Amer. J. Obstet. Gynec., 100:218, 1968.

Taylor, H. C., Jr., Wellen, I., and Welsh, C. A.: Renal function studies in normal pregnancy and in toxemia based on clearances of inulin, phenol red, and Diodrast. Amer. J. Obstet. Gynec., 43:567, 1942.

Teel, H. H., and Reid, D. E.: Eclampsia and its sequelae; clinical and follow-up study of all cases at Boston Lying-in Hospital over a 20-year period. Amer. J. Obstet. Gynec., 34:12, 1937.

Tenney, B., Jr., and Parker, F., Jr.: The placenta in toxemia of pregnancy. Amer. J. Obstet. Gynec., 39:1000, 1940.

Thomson, A. M., Hytten, F. E., and Billewicz, W. J.: The epidemiology of oedema during pregnancy. J. Obstet. Gynaec. Brit. Comm., 74:1, 1967.

Vassalli, P., Morris, R. H., and McCluskey, R. T.: The pathogenic role of fibrin deposition in the glomerular lesions of toxemia of pregnancy. J. Exp. Med., 118:467, 1963.

Venning, E. H., Dyrenfurth, I., Lowenstein, L., and Beck, J.: Metabolic studies in pregnancy and the puerperium. J. Clin. Endocr., 19:403, 1959.

Watanabe, M., Meeker, C. I., Gray, M. J., Sims, E. A. H., and Solomon, S.: Aldosterone secretion rates in abnormal pregnancy. J. Clin. Endocr., 25:1665, 1965.

Wellen, I.: Infant mortality in specific hypertensive disease of pregnancy and in essential hypertension. Amer. J. Obstet. Gynec., 66:36, 1953.

Wilner, G., Phillips, L. L., and McKay, D. G.: Platelet damage in experimental toxemia of pregnancy. Obstet. Gynec., 23:182, 1964.

Zuspan, F. P., and Bell, J. D.: Variable salt-loading during pregnancy with pre-eclampsia, Obstet. Gynec., 18:530, 1961.

Zuspan, F. P., Talledo, E., and Rhodes, K.: Factors affecting delivery in eclampsia. Amer. J. Obstet. Gynec., 100:672, 1968.

Chapter 18

Shock, Coagulation Defects, and Acute Renal Failure

Because they often interrelate through either cause or effect, or both, shock, coagulation defects, and acute renal failure are considered together in this chapter.

SHOCK

Shock in all its ramifications deserves to be considered the greatest risk of pregnancy. Not only is shock the leading cause of death in many maternal mortality reports, but hemorrhagic shock particularly is often a major factor, if not the actual cause, of obstetric deaths assigned to other conditions. For example, in pregnancy toxemia complicated by a severe form of premature separation of the placenta, it is not uncommon for profound hemorrhagic shock to develop, frequently as the result of a coagulation defect. Should death occur, it is usually reported as due to the toxemia, which is considered nonpreventable more often than is death due to shock. Furthermore, the most serious sequelae of pregnancy, namely, damage to the adenohypophysis and to the kidney, are related consequences of shock. In addition to foresight, judgment, and technical competence to prevent shock, the physician requires adequate assistance and facilities for treating a patient in shock. These are truly preventable deaths, and the responsibility for obstetric deaths from shock or its serious sequelae may rest with the hospital as well as the physician. This means that any hospital that accepts the care of the parturient must have certain basic facilities; for example, sufficient amounts of blood for transfusion must be close at hand *at all times.*

DEFINITION

Shock is here defined as a syndrome characterized by a decrease in effective blood volume associated with an insuffi-cient cardiac output leading to peripheral circulatory failure which, if uncorrected, will result in eventual progressive circulatory deterioration. Consequently, shock may be produced by reduction of the circulating blood volume, interference with normal cardiac action, or impairment of the function of the peripheral vessels themselves.

ETIOLOGY

Shock is attributed to either (1) hemorrhage, with or without trauma, (2) sepsis, or endotoxin shock or (3) myocardial infarction; and in some patients the causes are multiple. An example of an accumulation of causes is sepsis due to *Clostridium welchii*, in which, in addition to the toxic effect on the peripheral circulation or myocardium, there is often a significant reduction in effective blood volume through hemolysis.

It has been suggested that the hypotensive episode seen occasionally in the pregnant patient near term while in the supine position is a form of shock. It is envisioned that the pressure of the uterus interferes with the return of the blood to the right heart. This state has been considered to be similar to the hypotension induced by spinal anesthesia, and has been regarded as a form of syncope. This phenomenon has been commented on, with the observation that the symptoms are readily relieved by placing the pregnant patient on her side, as indeed they are. In contrast to shock, such prompt recovery indicates that the homeostatic mechanisms that regulate circulatory changes have not been compromised. It would appear then that this form of hypotensive episode seen in pregnancy is not comparable to the physiologic vascular deterioration associated with shock. It is conceivable, however, that shock in the undelivered patient could be aggravated by the supine position. Thus, the supine hypotensive syndrome of pregnancy is regarded as a form of syncope or loss of consciousness from an acute decrease in cerebral blood flow and not as a form of shock. In other words, a hypotensive state is not synonymous with shock, for shock denotes a physiologic state in which the body, unaided, cannot compensate sufficiently to restore the blood pressure to normal.

The term "obstetric shock" has been introduced to designate the circulatory change that may result from occlusion of the pulmonary arterial system by amniotic fluid and its constituents, or from fibrin deposition in abruptio placentae, supposedly from massive intravascular coagulation.

The idea that there is a separate entity that should be designated "obstetric shock" is further augmented by statements that connote the belief that in abruptio placentae the degree of shock is out of proportion to the visible blood loss. Actually, when shock develops in cases of abruptio placentae, the degree of blood loss is extensive and often is not fully appreciated. This is supported at autopsy, when marked extravasation of blood is usually found throughout the retroperitoneal spaces of the pelvis and abdomen. Further, in estimating blood loss it is well to recall that the observed grossly clotted blood represents no more than 40 per cent of the blood shed. It appears, therefore, that shock in abruptio placentae is the result of a significant decrease in effective circulating blood volume. According to the definition used here, therefore, shock in obstetrics is similar to that seen in medical or surgical conditions, and the patient is treated accordingly.

In summary, amniotic fluid embolism is a variant of pulmonary embolism and is not here considered in the etiology of shock except in the rare instance when a clotting defect develops secondarily, in which event it may be considered in the category of shock due to blood loss. Similarly, shock in abruptio placentae is not the result of pulmonary arteriole occlusion, but is nothing more or less than hemorrhagic shock and must be so treated.

CLINICAL FEATURES OF SHOCK

Since they are young and for the most part in a state of good health, obstetric patients can lose greater amounts of blood without exhibiting evidence of shock, in contrast to older patients in whom degenerative changes limit the capacity of the body to compensate. Consequently, when overt shock develops in the pregnant patient, she may be approaching a state of exsanguination.

In hemorrhagic shock, its severity is related to the degree of reduction in effective blood volume. In general, when the arterial pressure falls below 100 mm. Hg and the pulse rate is increased, indicating impending shock, the blood volume has already been reduced by some 30 to 35 per cent, or the equivalent of 1.5 to 2 L. of blood. The signs of a failing peripheral circulation soon appear, and the extremities become cold and moist. Should shock be extreme, the skin may become mottled; the blood pressure is usually unobtainable, and the radial pulse is barely perceptible. Because of cerebral tissue hypoxia, restlessness and mental confusion are prominent symptoms.

In an effort to maintain sufficient blood flow to the brain and myocardium in the presence of shock, vasoconstriction occurs, especially in the skin and kidney. Thus, renal blood flow is markedly reduced, actually out of proportion to the decrease in cardiac output. Experimentally, renal blood flow may nearly cease when the blood volume is decreased by 40 per cent, and at the same time the systolic blood pressure values may remain between 80 and 100 mm. Hg. Oliguria and anuria often follow and persist until the arterial pressure is restored and maintained at a normal level for several hours.

The term "irreversible" is used to describe the stage of shock in which the patient fails to respond to the known methods of treatment. Experimentally, when the blood volume remains below 50 per cent of normal for a period longer than four hours, the response to therapy diminishes appreciably, despite adequacy of the treatment. Although it has been the subject of much study and speculation, the body's loss of ability to respond to therapy in "irreversible" shock has never been entirely explained, and this clinical state has defied precise definition.

In animals in advanced hemorrhagic

shock, a circulating toxin has been demonstrated. Further, there is evidence to support the idea that the tolerance to hemorrhagic shock bears a relationship to the endotoxin-neutralizing potential of the reticuloendothelial system. That is to say, if injury to the reticuloendothelial system is previously induced, the endotoxin is free to paralyze the peripheral circulation, with the resultant systemic lesions resembling those of the generalized Shwartzman reaction. All of these experimentally produced changes appear related to the intensity and duration of the shock and possibly to the etiology of its irreversibility.

In septic shock, much of the pathophysiology remains to be elucidated. The total blood volume is not appreciably reduced except in cases of peritonitis with possible transudation of plasma, or in *Clostridium welchii* infection with destruction of red cells. The cardiac output falls, but vascular resistance fails to rise, presumably because of the effect of bacterial toxin on the peripheral blood vessels.

In patients who die from septic shock, thrombi may be found in many organs: lungs, adrenals (Fig. 1A), spleen, bowel, liver, kidney (Fig. 1B), and the hypophysis and its stalk. It would appear that these changes simulate those seen in the Shwartzman reaction where the disseminated thrombi consist of deposition of fibrin which is experimentally produced by the injection of an endotoxin. If death from septic shock is related to the Shwartzman reaction, it is proper that a more detailed description be given of this phenomenon to see if there are any features of this reaction which have pertinence to patient management.

The Shwartzman reaction is experimentally produced in the animal by the serial administration of two small doses of endotoxin given 24 hours apart. The first injection is referred to as the sensitizing dose; the second injection is presumably responsible for the disseminated fibrin deposition seen at autopsy. The pregnant animal apparently is more sensitive than the nonpregnant to endotoxin, for only one injection is necessary to produce a lethal outcome in the former. Of equal interest and perhaps of clinical significance is the fact that these lesions take several hours to develop following the second injection. When the animal is sacrificed within 8 to 12 hours after the second injection the pathologic changes are minimal. If it is permissible to transfer this observation to the management of the patient suffering from septic shock due to an infected uterus or its contents, it would seem proper to inquire whether, when the patient fails to respond to the usual conservative forms of therapy within a period of 6 to 8 hours from the onset of the hypotension, more radical treatment, that is, hysterectomy, may be indicated before the Shwartzman reaction is fully established.

Following endotoxin administration for the production of the Shwartzman reaction, there is an initial rise in the circulating fibrinogen, with a subsequent fall, as is also true of the platelets, which undoubtedly reflects disseminated fibrin thrombi formation. Fibrinolytic activity may develop in response to the latter and altogether a consumption coagulopathy may appear. The blood leukocyte levels fluctuate with first a leukopenia followed by a leukocytosis. Thus, the clinical laboratory data in septic shock must be interpreted in the light of the fact that values may differ depending upon the stage of the disease at which the observations were made.

Clinically, the patient with septic shock has fever, tachycardia, and hypotension, with the systolic blood pressure ranging from 60 to 80 mm. Hg. Hypothermia is sometimes observed, and also leukopenia, but usually there is a substantial leukocytosis. Failing to respond to treatment, the patient may die rather promptly as a consequence of an overwhelming "endotoxin injection" from the infected conceptus or decidua, or some days later from the effects of acute renal failure resulting from focal bilateral cortical necrosis, or, less frequently, acute tubular necrosis. Death may also occur from adrenal failure if fibrin deposition in the adrenal is profound, panhypopituitarism, or hemorrhage from a coagulation defect.

OBSTETRIC ENTITIES CONDUCIVE TO HEMORRHAGIC SHOCK

The obstetric entities that constitute the major causes of shock have been dealt with in appropriate chapters. In their listing here restatements are made for the purpose of emphasis. The more dangerous etiologic factors include ectopic pregnancy, late pregnancy bleeding, trauma of delivery, uterine atony, and inversion of the uterus.

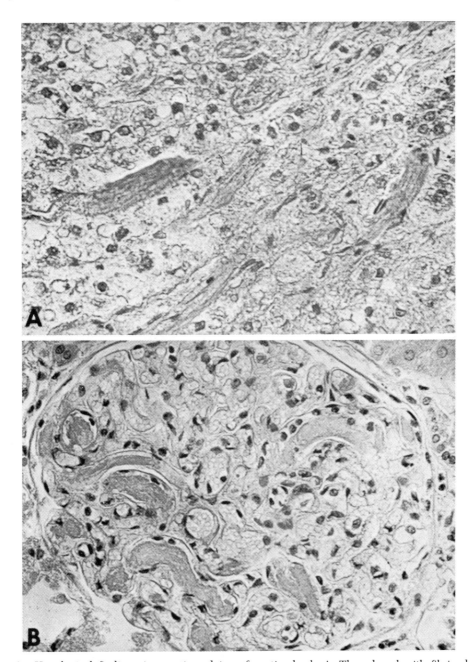

Figure 1. Histological findings in a patient dying of septic shock. A, The adrenal with fibrin deposition. ×200. B, Kidney glomerulus revealing extensive fibrin thrombi. ×200. Spontaneous premature rupture of the membranes 12 hours prior to a normal labor and delivery. Immediate postpartum septic shock—*Escherichia coli*. Patient not responsive to conventional medical therapy. Death followed 12 hours after delivery (?Shwartzman reaction). (Courtesy of Dr. Keith Russell.)

Ectopic Pregnancy

The prevention of shock from extrauterine pregnancy depends primarily on early diagnosis and treatment. Patients still succumb to ectopic pregnancy, dying at home or entering the hospital moribund. These catastrophes will continue until women realize the importance of early prenatal care, which, as the medical profession well knows, should begin within two or three weeks after the missed period.

Late Pregnancy Bleeding

In some respects, the management of patients who bleed in the last trimester of pregnancy is more difficult today. The patient is anxious to avoid prolonged costly hospitalization if possible, whereas the physician must be mindful of what is best for the patient. Actually, many patients who experience an episode of bleeding in late pregnancy will fail to demonstrate any cause for the bleeding. The problem, therefore, is to screen and carefully treat the patients who will prove to have placenta praevia.

Trauma of Delivery

Skill, experience, and judgment at delivery are factors that influence immeasurably the frequency and extent of trauma to the birth canal. Adherence to proper techniques of normal as well as forceps delivery may obviate soft tissue damage with its possible blood loss and gynecologic sequelae. Trauma at delivery has no place in modern obstetrics, and should it occur must be an admission of faulty judgment.

Uterine Atony

Most physicians are aware that atony is more likely to develop in conditions that interfere with normal uterine contractility. Whatever controversy there is concerns the definitive rather than the preventive treatment of uterine atony.

Retained Placenta

The problem of retained placenta affords a situation that serves to illustrate what is meant by providing maximal safeguards for the patient. As an example, because of the possibility of a placenta accreta the operating room should be prepared for performing an immediate hysterectomy. Some clinicians apparently regard manual removal of the placenta as a harmless procedure, but retention of the placenta is a major complication of delivery, the risk of which has been but partially eliminated through the chemotherapeutic control of infection.

Inversion of the Uterus

Although inversion of the uterus is commonly attributed to improper conduct of the third stage of labor, frequently there is no apparent cause. Failure to appreciate this fact may lead to a delay in diagnosis, particularly when the placental stage has been normal.

TREATMENT OF SHOCK

The preventive treatment of shock begins with the recognition and correction of iron deficiency and other forms of anemia in the pregnant patient, for certainly patients who enter labor with less than 10 grams of hemoglobin per 100 ml. are not suitably prepared for an anesthetic, are less resistant to infection, and are extremely vulnerable to the ravages of hemorrhage and shock.

The definitive treatment of hemorrhagic shock is to find the cause and control the bleeding, and to begin simultaneously to restore the blood volume to normal. Central venous pressure monitoring is essential and ideally repeated blood volume determinations unquestionably are useful in some cases.

The arterial pressure can be raised by pressor drugs, but their use is not without danger. In fact, the action of these drugs in hemorrhagic shock may mask blood volume deficiency. More significant, perhaps, is the fact that their therapeutic effect is at the expense of an increase in renal vasoconstriction. It is generally accepted that plasma and plasma expanders are not substitutes for whole blood. Furthermore, expander substances have no therapeutic advantage over plasma, and complications affecting the clotting mechanism have been reported following their use. When the blood loss is severe and the shock prolonged, one must suspect damage to the anterior lobe of the hypophysis (Sheehan's disease).

The dangers of prolonged restriction of sodium and use of diuretics must be recognized. Clinical experience attests to the fact that it is difficult to maintain the blood pressure in a patient with a salt-depletion syndrome. Electrolyte depletion in the pregnant woman, however, is extremely rare, and the administration of additional sodium, particularly to the patient with toxemia, must be viewed with caution. Furthermore, in the toxemic patient with low serum sodium, personal experience indicates that the depressed serum sodium level fails to rise following sodium chloride therapy.

Although the majority of obstetric patients with septic shock will recover, in a few the condition may very well become irreversible and lead to death unless the infectious process is quickly brought under control.

Thus, the active treatment of a patient with septic shock begins with an attempt to identify the offending organism. Before institution of antibiotic therapy, blood and uterine cultures are taken, and from a smear a search is made for *Clostridium welchii*. Antibiotic therapy is instituted. Blood loss should be replaced by transfusion, but in some cases the hematocrit will be normal. To combat the hypotension initially, the patient is placed on continuous intravenous infusion of a vasopressor drug, the amount used and the duration of administration being weighed against the possible harm that may accrue from prolonged administration. Although it is doubtful that the patients with this condition die primarily from adrenal failure, cortisone may be given as part of the therapeutic régime. If the patient responds to medical treatment, as determined by the vital signs and the restoration of the blood pressure to normal levels, evacuation of the uterus and further observation may be all that is indicated. If, on the other hand, the patient fails to react favorably to the above régime and remains in shock, consideration should be given to hysterectomy (see Septic Abortion). In patients with a viable pregnancy, the same hazards may arise in the presence of intrauterine infection. Prompt recovery is the rule once delivery occurs. Cesarean hysterectomy may be required if productive labor fails to ensue by the usual therapeutic means in order to accomplish delivery and bring the infection under control.

COAGULATION DEFECTS

From early in the present century discerning clinicians have been aware that shed blood appears not to clot in the occasional case of intrapartum and postpartum bleeding. In recent years it has become possible to relate an upset in the blood-clotting mechanism in cases of longstanding fetal death in utero, in the severe form of abruptio placentae, as a secondary effect of amniotic fluid embolism, and in association with some cases of sepsis or endotoxin shock.

The clotting defect is associated with a reduction in the plasma fibrinogen concentration and other clotting factors with a sharp fall in platelets. In rare cases no fibrinogen may be detected in the maternal blood, but usually the value is somewhere around 100 mg. per 100 ml. A fibrinogen concentration below 200 mg. per 100 ml. in the pregnant patient is now regarded as abnormal.

Referred to initially as an afibrinogenemia or hypofibrinogenemic state, these acquired clotting defects are now assigned other terms, reflecting the advances made in the understanding of the clotting mechanism. These include "the defibrination syndrome," "consumption coagulopathy," and "disseminated intravascular coagulation." The last term is perhaps the most commonly used to denote a generalized or systemic activation of the clotting mechanism beyond that of local clotting per se. The mere presence of local fibrin deposition need not connote a consumption coagulopathy, as in the case of pregnancy toxemia where the fibrinogen levels may exceed even the increase of normal pregnancy. Hence, a single term may be an oversimplification for a broad spectrum of clinical states. Moreover, the renewed interest in these states suggests that newer and ever changing approaches to the etiology and treatment may emerge.

INCIDENCE

The number of cases of coagulation defect seen will depend to a degree on the number of patients with Rh-negative sensitization, hypertension, and toxemia who are being cared for. These are the patients in whom fetal death in utero and abruptio placentae are more commonly encountered. A disturbance in clotting of some degree is estimated to occur in three to five instances in 1000 pregnancies.

DIAGNOSIS OF A COAGULATION DEFECT

The diagnosis of a clotting defect begins with an appreciation of those clinical conditions in which it may develop. As previously stated, a coagulation defect is hardly ever seen in the milder forms of premature separation of the placenta, and then it is restricted to patients who present a rather characteristic picture. This is illustrated by a patient in the latter weeks of pregnancy who, seized with moderate to severe abdominal pain, usually accompanied by vaginal bleeding, enters the hospital in some degree of shock. Physical examination reveals a spastic, tender uterus, indicative of extensive concealed hemorrhage. Fetal heart sounds are frequently absent or weak and irregular. If the uterus could be observed, it would present a mottled appearance owing to formation of hematomas beneath the serosa (Couvelaire uterus). There is often little or no urine in the bladder, and that which is present may contain protein and formed elements. The degree of shock seems out of proportion to the estimated amount of external bleeding. A clotting defect may be detected in these patients; but it must be remembered that some 90 per cent of the patients with abruptio placentae have the mild form and their blood clots normally.

A coagulation defect associated with fetal death in utero is often heralded by the appearance of ecchymoses and bleeding from the mucous membranes. For some unexplained reason the condition is rarely encountered before the 20th week of pregnancy. Also, it more often appears when the dead fetus has been retained for five or more weeks. Most patients with a dead fetus will deliver in this interim; but of those who retain the fetus beyond six weeks, 40 per cent have been known to develop a coagulation defect. Most cases of "dead-baby syndrome" are associated with Rh incompatibility, primarily because this is a common cause of fetal death in utero in the interval between the fifth and eighth month, when the spontaneous onset of labor is least likely. The clotting defect may develop before the onset of labor, or its appearance may be delayed until the intrapartum period.

Amniotic fluid embolism or amniotic fluid infusion, although a rare complication, is being reported with somewhat greater frequency. It can now be accepted that the sudden appearance of shock and severe respiratory distress during an otherwise normal labor is pathognomonic of amniotic fluid embolization. The factor that seems to be of etiologic importance is a rapid and tumultuous labor, which may be precipitated by the injudicious use of oxytoxic preparations to initiate or stimulate labor. If the patient survives the initial embolic insult, hemor-

rhagic manifestations may develop. It has been demonstrated that amniotic fluid contains a coagulant that behaves like a thromboplastin and will reduce the clotting time of hemophilic blood. In addition to uterine hemorrhage, which erroneously may be attributed to atony, there may be bleeding from mucous membranes, calling attention to the possibility that the patient may have a coagulation defect.

The clot observation test has proved to be a rapid and practical means of identifying the clotting defect. This simple test involves withdrawing 5 ml. of the patient's blood and placing it in a test tube, with frequent observation for clot formation and stability of clot. Normal blood will clot in 8 to 12 minutes, and the clot will remain intact for at least 24 hours. If a coagulation defect is present the blood may not clot, or, if it does so, the clot may undergo partial or complete dissolution within 30 to 60 minutes. Such clot fragmentation means a low fibrinogen level or fibrinolytic activity, or both. This has therapeutic implications, because what is desired in patient management is effective hemostasis, which, in the final analysis, requires a stable clot (Fig. 2). The fibrinogen may be reduced to hemorrhagic levels (less than 100 mg. per 100 ml.) and show a stable clot, or in the presence of lytic activity the clot may be unstable with a much higher and ordinarily nonhemorrhagic level of fibrinogen (Fig. 3). This test may be conducted entirely at the bedside; the blood taken for cross-matching may serve for the test. A more detailed laboratory analysis of the fibrinogen concentration of the patient's plasma, utilizing the estimation of tyrosine activity, is then instituted to confirm the diagnosis.

The differential diagnosis would include thrombotic thrombocytopenic purpura (Moschcowitz syndrome) and von Willebrand's disease.

ETIOLOGY

The etiology of acquired coagulation defects observed in pregnancy complications has been a subject of much controversy, centering around whether the reduction in the circulating fibrinogen is due to (1) direct effect of a primary fibrinolysis or (2) intravascular clotting with resultant activation of the fibrinolytic system.

Certainly the most consistent hematologic finding in acquired clotting defects

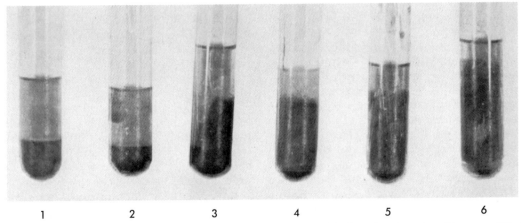

Figure 2. Clot observation test. (1) Soon after hospital admission; (2) after administration of 2 grams of fibrinogen and 500 ml. of blood, 2 hours after admission; (3) after administration of 8 grams of fibrinogen and 1000 ml. of blood, 3½ hours after admission; (4) second hour and (5) third hour after artificial rupture of membranes; (6) after administration of 10 grams of fibrinogen and 3500 ml. of blood, 1 hour after cesarean section. (From Reid, D. E., and Roby, C. C.: Clin. Obstet. & Gynec., 1:715, 1958.)

in pregnancy is a decrease in fibrinogen (hypofibrinogenemia) and plasminogen levels and varying degrees of thrombocytopenia.

Advances in hematology in recent years indicate that the condition, in some if not most cases at least, is one of disseminated intravascular coagulation or consumption coagulopathy with fibrinolytic activity appearing in response to fibrin deposition. Whether the event is triggered through the intrinsic pathway of coagulation by activation of factor XII (Hageman factor) or the extrinsic pathway by thromboplastin is not entirely certain and indeed it may be necessary to invoke both pathways to cover the various types of cases in which a clotting defect is encountered. For example, the development of the coagulation defect in

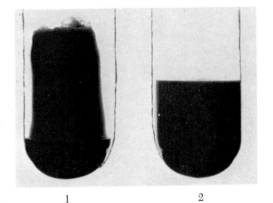

Figure 3. Clot observation test in a patient with "dead-baby syndrome." Blood samples taken several hours apart, and the fibrinogen levels revealed: (1) clot with 95 mg. per 100 ml., and (2) absence of clot with 180 mg. per 100 ml. (fibrinolytic effect?).

the case of amniotic fluid embolism or infusion presumably would involve the extrinsic mechanism, for amniotic fluid is known to contain a thromboplastin-like substance. The intrinsic mechanism might be involved in the dead-baby syndrome, where the coagulation defect develops slowly (and in this sense is chronic). In either case, the end result is the same, namely, a state of disseminated intravascular clotting with activation of the fibrinolytic system reflecting a decrease in plasminogen and the appearance of fibrin degradation or split products. In fact, one might inquire whether in normal pregnancy intravascular clotting is occurring, albeit not in detectable amounts, in the presence of a hypercoagulable state as indicated by a rise in factors VII, VIII, and X and fibrinogen. It has been suggested that this is a fortuitous arrangement in order to provide additional reserve in the coagulation system for the purpose of effective hemostasis at the time of delivery. Moreover the process of fibrin deposition may normally be required in order to maintain the integrity of the intervillous space, which is being constantly challenged by myometrial contractility and the pressure changes with the upright position and other postural changes, including vena cava compression, as well as to keep intact the placental surface wherein fibrin is found in varying degrees. Conceivably in the occasional instance fibrin deposition on the placental surface might reach pathologic proportions sufficient to interfere with placental transport. If indeed the intervillous space is a blood lake, some fibrin deposition might be anticipated in the event of episodes of stagnation.

A recent study of the coagulation system during labor and in the early puerperium of normal childbirth has relevance and should be recognized, as depicted in Figure 4. It was emphasized that the apparent rebound or secondary increase in levels of fibrinogen and factor VIII (antihemophilia factor, AHG) by the middle of the first week after delivery may also play a role in the thromboembolic states that are accepted as being increased in the puerperium. These observations represent local clotting in and about the placental site and within the spiral vessels in contradistinction to disseminated intravascular clotting.

As indicated above, whether the fibrinolytic system can be initiated without intravascular clotting and thus account for the destruction and reduction in the circulating fibrinogen must still be answered fully, as for example in the "dead-baby syndrome." Conceivably a proteolytic fibrinolysin might be liberated from the decomposed uterine contents and indeed so could thromboplastin. At any rate, it has been shown that fibrinolysin (streptokinase) will depress fibrinogen concentration in vivo. Moreover, an unstable clot (? lytic activity) has been observed preceding any decrease in fibrinogen levels in the case of a "dead-baby syndrome."

Finally, a clotting defect may appear in uterine sepsis caused by *Escherichia coli*, and it is postulated that plasma fibrinogen is reduced to a hemorrhagic level through widespread fibrin deposition that characterizes the Shwartzman reaction. Here fibrin split products fail to be cleared by the compromised reticuloendothelial system.

Regardless of contention, what is perhaps more important to patient management is the possible interplay between fibrinogen levels and fibrinolytic activity with respect to the production of unstable or stable clot (see Fig. 3). Certainly clot production is not dependent on fibrinogen levels alone. Moreover, besides lytic activity, fibrin degradation products may also contribute to the production of an unstable clot by acting as a powerful anticoagulant. Several hours must elapse before these products are cleared from the circulation after the shock has been corrected and the reticuloendothelial system and liver are functioning normally.

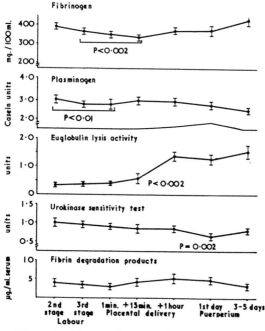

Figure 4. Plasma fibrinogen levels and the components of the fibrinolytic enzyme system during and after normal childbirth. (From Bonnar, J., McNicol, G. P., and Douglas, A. S.: Brit. Med. J., 2:200–203, 1970.)

TREATMENT

To correct the coagulation defect, it was initially recommended that fibrinogen (factor I) be administered together with whole fresh blood transfusion. In the acutely severe case, i.e., total abruptio placentae and amniotic fluid embolism, the minimal requirement to acquire a stable clot was 2 to 4 units of fresh blood together with 4 to 8 grams of fibrinogen. Under this régime, deaths from acquired hemorrhagic diathesis in these cases have become a rarity. In this earlier period, it was suggested by the writer that heparin might prove effective in amniotic fluid infusion to offset the lethal effect of thromboplastin-like substance present in the amniotic fluid. More recently, heparin therapy has been advised for all of the various forms of acquired clotting defect in pregnancy. Also, the administration of fibrinogen has been challenged, in the belief that the addition of this plasma protein will enhance the consumption coagulopathy and hence could be detrimental. Hepatitis following fibrinogen administration is listed as a contraindication to its use.

The source of the virus is open to question, for these patients receive several transfusions of fresh blood, ofttimes from donors perhaps not adequately screened.

But whether heparin with or without blood replacement can counteract or block intravascular coagulation and permit spontaneous restoration of the clotting mechanism in the patient previously described with the Couvelaire uterus must be demonstrated in a suitable number of patients. For in these acute states of an acquired coagulation defect there is a note of urgency regarding definitive obstetric treatment. Undue delay in delivering the patient may lead to further deterioration of the clotting mechanism. At the same time, one must take cognizance of the possibility that on hospital admission the patient's blood is incoagulable or on the verge of becoming incoagulable. Certainly operative intervention should not be instituted if there is a disturbance in the coagulation mechanism to this degree, else uncontrolled hemorrhage will ensue. Moreover, the bleeding in these severe cases that in past years has been attributed to atony in all probability is the result of a defect in the clotting mechanism. Whatever else, a stable clot is a requirement for any operative procedure, especially when an abdominal hysterotomy is deemed necessary to accomplish delivery. In order of sequence, fresh blood plus heparin may be instituted. If after an hour the clot remains unstable, fibrinogen should be considered.

In the case of amniotic fluid embolism the initial treatment is concerned with combating respiratory distress and shock. If the patient survives the initial insult, a delayed complication in the form of uncontrolled postpartum hemorrhage should be anticipated. If bleeding does ensue and an acquired coagulation defect is demonstrated, the patient with amniotic fluid embolism may survive if treated energetically.

How best to restore the clotting mechanism to normal promptly within two to three hours from the onset of treatment in the acute case in which prompt obstetric management is imperative remains to be clearly established in all cases. Fresh whole blood and fibrinogen has a record of being effective, despite the extremely rare adverse reaction attributed to fibrinogen administration. It may be that transfusion plus fibrinogen with coverage with heparin will prove to be the most appropriate treatment in the acute cases as in abruptio placentae and amniotic fluid embolism or infusion. The possible adverse effects of overheparinization in the presence of a clotting defect must be appreciated but this is readily controlled by protamine.

For the chronic state, i.e., a dead-baby syndrome, heparin alone may well restore the clotting mechanism to effectiveness. Indeed it has been so demonstrated even when epsilon-aminocaproic acid (EACA) had failed previously to combat the fibrinolytic activity and influence fibrinogen levels. This is evidence that the fibrinolysin is secondary rather than primary, for only in the latter should EACA be considered.

Fortunately the majority of patients with intrauterine fetal death will enter spontaneous labor and deliver within a few days or two to three weeks after disappearance of fetal activity or fetal heart tones by auscultation. As stated, the clotting defect develops usually one or two weeks later, or four or five weeks after fetal demise.

Hence, in the interim within two weeks after fetal demise labor should be initiated before a hemorrhagic diathesis develops. This is now readily done with intra-amniotic saline infusion. This method is especially effective in these cases with labor ensuing and delivery accomplished within a few hours or certainly within a day after the introduction of the saline. Thus, the necessity of hysterotomy some two to three weeks after fetal death to prevent the development of a coagulation defect in the "dead-baby syndrome" is no longer required unless there are pure obstetric indications, i.e., previous hysterotomy.

In summary, the acquired clotting defect encountered in pregnancy is accompanied by disseminated intravascular coagulation or a consumption coagulopathy. The clotting mechanism may be initiated by both the intrinsic and extrinsic pathways. The activation of plasminogen to plasmin is in response to fibrin deposition, and the resultant secondary fibrinolysin liberates fibrin split products and degrades fibrinogen, both of which are powerful anticoagulants. Heparin will inhibit the consumption coagulopathy, but whether together with fresh blood it can restore the clotting mechanism in a patient depleted or nearly so of fibrinogen and bleeding actively is open to question. This is the patient in whom it makes a difference where the clotting mechanism is in total collapse. The uterus must be evacuated of its contents to control the shedding of blood and presumably to remove the stimulus to clotting. Whatever else, this requires a stable clot for effective hemostasis at the time of delivery whether it be by the pelvic or abdominal route, else uncontrolled hemorrhage will ensue. Fibrinogen, 4 to 8 grams, administered simultaneously with fresh blood and heparin may be required in order to obtain a stable clot prior to surgery.

An equally uncertain situation is that of a patient in endotoxin shock from a septic uterus or its contents and with an evident consumption coagulopathy. Here again the patient's survival may depend either on evacuation of the uterus or its removal for control of the infection. The clotting defect must be restored preoperatively and promptly. The same sequence of therapy may be required before the effective hemostasis is restored to permit any operative procedure.

These therapeutic advances require careful scrutiny. Moreover, when assessing the changes in the clotting factors, a clear distinction must be made between systemic and local clotting.

ACUTE RENAL FAILURE

Oliguria and anuria are observed in pregnancy under a variety of circumstances. Some 20 to 40 per cent of cases of acute renal failure are associated with pregnancy complications. Stating it another way, of female patients with acute renal failure, about 50 per cent are, or have recently been, pregnant. However, these patients are seen with less frequency as traumatic pelvic delivery is eliminated, coagulation defects are energetically treated, and the incidence of toxemia is reduced.

Oliguria is here defined as a urinary output of 100 to 400 ml.; anuria as a urinary output of less than 100 ml. per 24 hours.

The depression of renal excretion to these pathologic levels may be transient in nature, lasting only a few hours or, at most, one or two days. Such temporary reduction of urine output may characterize the reaction of the kidneys to a brief hypotensive episode or to a severe pregnancy toxemia. When decreased urinary output persists beyond these limits, the condition must be regarded as acute renal failure, and the patient will pursue a protracted clinical course resulting either in recovery, with or without permanent renal damage, or, now rarely, in death.

Consideration must be given to those aspects which make acute renal failure preventable or, if not preventable, manageable. The clinician would like to know if it is possible, by a review of the patient's obstetric history, to interpret the nature of the renal lesion. As a practical corollary to this, is it possible to assess accurately the chance of total recovery or the likelihood of permanent renal damage, and are future pregnancies advisable?

An anatomic classification of the pathologic changes, and the more frequently encountered conditions that cause oliguria and anuria in pregnancy and that may result in acute renal failure, are presented in the following paragraphs.

SEVERE CONVULSIVE AND NONCONVULSIVE TOXEMIA

A state of oliguria often develops at some period in the course of the disease in the more severe forms of pregnancy toxemia. The most characteristic histologic renal change is thickening of the basement membrane of the glomerular capillary tuft. Tubular changes are minimal except when shock sufficient to produce acute tubular necrosis is superimposed. Although there is some decrease in glomerular filtration rate, a logical sequence to glomerular membrane change, could the suppression of renal function be due to generalized edema formation, the cause to be determined? Another characteristic of pregnancy toxemia is a redistribution of the extracellular fluid, which is decreased in the intravascular compartment (hemoconcentration) and increased in the interstitial compartment. Perhaps the kidney tissue, sharing in this increment in interstitial fluid, temporarily loses its function. Evidence that edema of renal tissue may influence the urinary output is gathered from experience in caring for patients with acute renal failure. Occasionally after marked oliguria the urine volume will increase suddenly to a daily output of 2 to 3 L. It is envisioned that this is due to the reabsorption of interstitial fluid of the renal parenchyma, resulting in decompression of the nephron and restitution of function, rather than to repair of damaged nephron tissue. Even if this were the mechanism for producing the oliguria in pregnancy toxemia, the factor responsible for edema formation must still be delineated. Whether the depression in renal function is extrarenal or intrarenal, the oliguria and anuria of pregnancy toxemia should not be expected to persist after delivery to the extent of acute renal failure unless there is an episode of prolonged shock or hemolysis resulting in acute tubular necrosis or an associated severe placental separation causing bilateral cortical necrosis. In other words, the histologic changes in the kidney attributed to pregnancy toxemia are, with rare exception, temporary and reversible.

SYMMETRIC BILATERAL CORTICAL NECROSIS OF THE KIDNEYS

Bilateral cortical necrosis of the kidneys is not entirely restricted to pregnant women, although about 80 per cent of the reported cases occur in association with severe premature separation of the placenta. The other cases, with a variety of etiologic backgrounds, are seen at random in adult males, nonpregnant women, infants, and children. It is now appreciated that in the obstetric patient bilateral cortical necrosis may develop in the course of septic shock, and the lesions are usually of the focal type comparable to those experimentally produced in the Shwartzman reaction. When associated with premature separation of the placenta, the lesions may be focal, patchy, confluent, microscopic, or gross (Fig. 5A). When the process is extensive and confluent, there is infarctive coagulation necrosis of the cortex in zones supplied by the thrombosed interlobar and intralobular arteries (Fig. 5B). Presumably the thrombosis is the result of the combined effect of prolonged intense arteriolar spasm and a nephrotoxin. Attention has been called to the possibility that antecedent nephrosclerosis may make the kidney more vulnerable to this complication (Fig. 6).

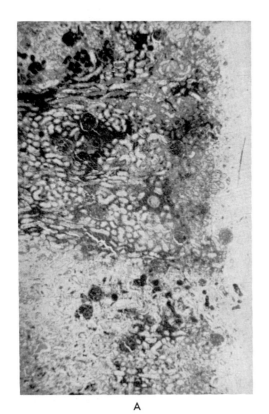
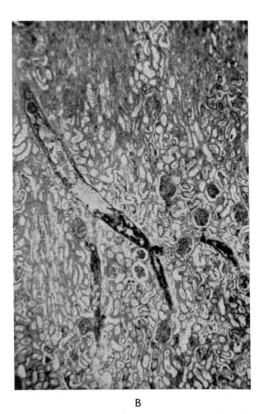

A   B

Figure 5. Bilateral renal cortical necrosis. A, Infarctive necrosis of the renal cortex. ×25. B, A branching thrombus in an intralobular artery and its subdivisions; the surrounding cortex shows coagulation necrosis. ×30. (From Ober, W. B., Reid, D. E., Romney, S. L., and Merrill, J. P.: Amer. J. Med., 21:781, 1956.)

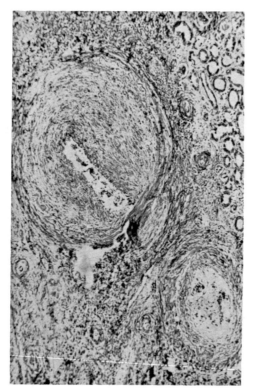

Figure 6. Extensive fibrous intimal proliferation of arcuate arteries, associated with bilateral renal cortical necrosis. ×70. (From Ober, W. B., Reid, D. E., Romney, S. L., and Merrill, J. P.: Amer. J. Med., 21:781, 1956.)

ACUTE TUBULAR NECROSIS

This type of renal lesion is the basis for the majority of cases of acute renal failure seen in pregnancy. Tubular damage with inability of the tubular cells to concentrate the glomerular filtrate with back-diffusion effect presupposes shock, prolonged ischemia with hypoxia, cast formation or red cell agglutination, or a direct toxic effect on tubular epithelium. Through meticulous microdissection of entire nephrons it has been demonstrated that the damage is not restricted to any one area of the unit. When toxins are involved, the tubular epithelium is impaired, but in renal ischemia both the epithelium and the basement membrane are damaged. In the first instance the affected tissues may be expected to regenerate earlier and more completely with less chance of residual renal dysfunction.

Acute tubular necrosis may be due to a hemolytic episode, as in *Clostridium welchii* infection (Fig. 7A), or shock, either hemorrhagic or septic; in some instances there is an element of both. The injection

of various sorts of pastes, Lysol, soap, and other such agents into the uterine cavity, with their chance entrance into the maternal circulation may cause hemolysis and tubular damage.

Acute tubular damage in pregnancy is more frequently caused by hemorrhagic shock, more especially from late pregnancy bleeding (Fig. 7B), and severe postpartum hemorrhage. A hemolytic reaction has been reported in the severe forms of pregnancy toxemia, resulting in acute tubular necrosis. Unfortunately, acute tubular necrosis is too often caused by the transfusion of incompatible blood.

URETERAL OBSTRUCTION

Ureteral obstruction complicating sulfonamide therapy or extensive retroperitoneal hemorrhage, usually from severe premature placental separation, is a possible cause of acute renal failure. If obstruction from retroperitoneal hemorrhage is suspected, retrograde cystoscopy will either exclude or substantiate the diagnosis.

MISCELLANEOUS CAUSES

Other causes of acute renal failure include allergic necrotizing arteriolitis with renal involvement, as may result from drug hypersensitivity, and recrudescence of chronic glomerulonephritis or pyelonephritis. Chronic pyelonephritis particularly may exacerbate in pregnancy with progression to death from renal failure before, at, or shortly after delivery.

MANAGEMENT OF ACUTE RENAL FAILURE

The prevention of acute renal failure is preferable to its treatment. An example is cited of the increased tendency of pregnant women with antecedent hypertension to develop placental separation, necessitating careful medical supervision of their vascular disease and a consideration of obstetric intervention for early delivery compatible with fetal viability. Such a program not only decreases intrauterine fetal loss but minimizes the risk of abruptio placentae and possible renal cortical necrosis.

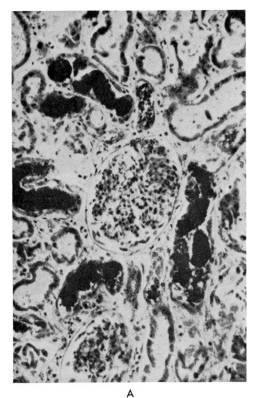
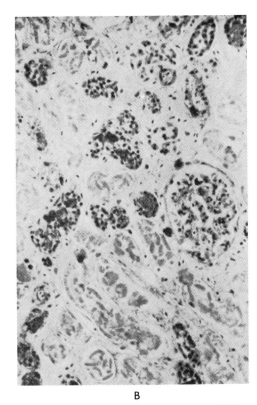

A   B

Figure 7. Acute tubular necrosis. ×125. A, Hemoglobinuric type. *Clostridium welchii* infection following spontaneous septic abortion. Severe hemolysis and uremia; death on 14th day, despite dialysis. B, Ischemic type, showing necrosis and desquamation of the tubular epithelium. This patient died 42 hours after massive hemorrhage from placenta praevia. (From Ober, W. B., Reid, D. E., Romney, S. L., and Merrill, J. P.: Amer. J. Med., 21:781, 1956.)

When the obstetrician is confronted with a patient with urinary suppression, the differentiation of acute tubular necrosis and renal cortical necrosis is important, not so much with regard to the immediate treatment but rather as it concerns the prognosis, the outlook being grave in cortical necrosis and encouraging in acute tubular necrosis.

Important in the history is the clinical background and sequence of events leading up to the oliguria and anuria. If the anuria is present before shock appears or if it develops coincidentally with the early stage of vascular collapse, the diagnosis of renal cortical necrosis is more probable. Conversely, if shock exists over a period of time prior to a reduction in the urine output, acute tubular necrosis is the more likely diagnosis. If, besides shock, there is an element of hemolysis, the kidney lesion is that of acute tubular necrosis, whereas premature separation of the placenta and sepsis are more likely to be associated with bilateral cortical necrosis. The two types of lesion can be definitely distinguished by

needle biopsy of the kidney, but this procedure is not without risk.

The general principles of the treatment of acute renal failure are now established. Such treatment consists of management of the oliguric and the diuretic phases. The oliguric phase covers a period of approximately 7 to 14 days, during which time tubular repair has begun (Fig. 8). During this period treatment is directed toward combating potassium intoxication and uremia. The diuretic phase (i.e., when the volume of urine excreted daily exceeds 1000 ml., and until the renal tubule is able to concentrate) covers the next several weeks. In the interim, water and electrolyte losses can be excessive. The parturient, with increased amounts of extracellular fluid and electrolytes, can better tolerate these losses, at least at the beginning of diuresis. It must be cautioned that the patient's life may still be at stake during the diuretic phase, and thus careful attention must be given to correcting any metabolic deficiencies.

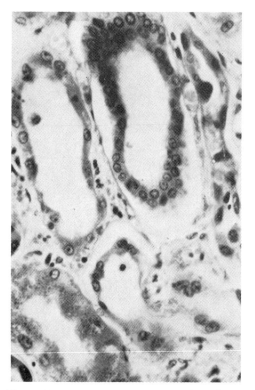

Figure 8. Acute tubular necrosis with evidence of beginning tubular repair. ×300. A mitotic figure is seen in regenerating tubular epithelium. (From Ober, W. B., Reid, D. E., Romney, S. L., and Merrill, J. P.: Amer. J. Med., 21:781, 1956.)

Besides general treatment, specific therapy is indicated in some cases in which acute renal failure is feared. An alkaline urine, achieved by administration of a few grams of sodium lactate intravenously, may give the kidney some protection. Mannitol, if given early, may reduce the hazard of tubular damage. The adverse effects of sulfonamides call for a counteraction of the sensitivity reaction or of obstruction to the kidney by the precipitation of sulfonamide crystals. Reference has been made to obstructive uropathy from retroperitoneal hemorrhage and the occasional need for ureteral catheterization to promote renal drainage.

In the general treatment of acute renal failure, overhydration should be avoided in the oliguric or anuric phase. The intake should never exceed the insensible water loss plus the urine output, which in the anuric patient means an intake of no more than 400 to 500 ml. daily. In the pregnant or, more appropriately, the recently delivered patient, in whom the extracellular fluid is in excess by at least 3 to 5 L., the intake should be even less. In fact, pulmo-

nary edema is a threat in the toxemic patient even when she is excreting a moderate amount of urine daily.

To maintain nutrition, 1000 calories should be provided daily in the form of protein-sparing substances. Whenever possible, this should include the oral administration of hard candy, Karo syrup, and ginger ale; if oral feeding is not possible, emulsified fat or glucose may be given intravenously, but for several reasons glucose is more suitable. Through a polyvinyl catheter, best tolerated and more likely to remain sterile in an arm vein, 50 per cent glucose solution in 400 to 500 ml. of fluid can be given continuously over a 24-hour period, thrombosis within the vein being minimized by the addition of a small amount of heparin to the parenteral fluid.

What constitutes electrolyte balance in the patient with acute renal failure is at times uncertain, and in the pregnant patient it is even more difficult to evaluate. In the anuric phase, the electrolyte requirement may be nil unless vomiting or sweating is a prominent feature. Low serum sodium values may be observed occasionally in the normal and more often in the toxemic patient (125 to 130 mEq.); despite this, however, sodium may be stored in excess. Regardless of pregnancy, low values of serum sodium and chloride are characteristic of the anuric phase. Potassium is elevated, owing to a shift from the intracellular to the extracellular compartment, glycogen depletion, and red cell destruction. The presence of a metabolic acidosis will accelerate the shift of potassium from the intracellular to the extracellular phase.

Thus, in the anuric phase the possibility of potassium intoxication is a particular hazard in the postpartum patient with acute renal failure. One must realize that such intoxication may develop earlier in the clinical course of the obstetric patient. For example, in abruptio placentae with concealed hemorrhage, large amounts of potassium are liberated because of the breakdown of red cells. Electrocardiograms should be taken at frequent intervals, beginning on the fourth day from the onset of acute renal failure rather than on the seventh or eighth day, as in the conventional management of the nonpregnant patient. It is conceded that serial electrocardiograms are more reliable as an index of developing potassium intoxication than are serum potassium determinations. With evidence of potassium intoxication, immediate steps should be taken to correct the hyperkalemia. The use of any of the cation-exchange resins in the sodium cycle has proved effective in removing potassium, but many of these are unpalatable and tend to cause fecal impaction. A new powdered exchange resin has been introduced, however, which the patients find more acceptable. The serum sodium has been observed to rise during resin therapy, although a possible danger of the sodium cycle resin is that it has been known to cause overhydration and pulmonary edema. Recently, sorbitol, which also removes potassium, has been combined with a sodium-exchange resin. Sorbitol aids the passage of exchange resin through the gastrointestinal tract and causes an osmotic diarrhea, with loss of body water, which presumably counteracts the threat of overhydration.

Most cases of acute renal failure, certainly those seen in association with pregnancy, can be successfully managed by cautious and careful medical treatment. If this fails, hemodialysis with the artificial kidney is lifesaving.

One must keep in mind the possibility that in the patient with anuria from tubular necrosis Sheehan's syndrome may develop as an aftermath of severe blood loss and shock. Recognition of this syndrome and institution of replacement therapy may mean the difference between recovery and death, especially in the diuretic phase. An associated diabetes insipidus may be encountered when pituitary destruction is extensive and there is hypothalamic involvement.

PROGNOSIS AND SEQUELAE OF ACUTE RENAL FAILURE

Recovery is the rule unless the anuria persists beyond three weeks. In patients who recover, kidney function may return to normal, although it may not become stabilized for several months. The majority show some 30 per cent persistent reduction in inulin and para-aminohippuric acid clearances. Residual damage is apparently not progressive and, if by 6 to 12 months after the acute failure renal function is reasonable, a future pregnancy may be contemplated. Under careful management such patients will successfully negotiate a future pregnancy.

BIBLIOGRAPHY

Beischer, N. A.: Intravascular defibrination in pregnancy with associated pituitary and kidney damage. Amer. J. Obstet. Gynec., 82:625, 1961.

Bernstock, L., and Hirson, C.: Thrombotic thrombocytopenic purpura, remission on treatment with heparin. Lancet, 1:28, 1960.

Bonnar, J., McNicol, G. P., and Douglas, A. S.: Coagulation and fibrinolytic mechanisms during and after normal childbirth. Brit. Med. J., 2:200, 1970.

Bonnar, J., McNicol, G. P., and Douglas, A. S.: The behavior of the coagulation and fibrinolytic mechanisms in abruptio placentae. J. Obstet. Gynec. Brit. Comm., 6:799, 1969.

Cavanagh, D., Rao, P. S., Sutton, D. M., Bhagat, B. D., and Bachmann, F.: Pathophysiology of endotoxin shock in the primate. Amer. J. Obstet. Gynec., 108:705, 1970.

Clarkson, A. R., Sage, R. E., and Lawrence, J. R.: Consumption coagulopathy and acute renal failure due to gram-negative septicemia after abortion. Ann. Intern. Med., 70:1191, 1969.

Deane, R. M., and Russell, K. P.: Enterobacillary septicemia and bacterial shock in septic abortion. Amer. J. Obstet. Gynec., 79:528, 1960.

Douglas, G. W.: Septic shock and acute renal failure. In Reid, D. E., and Barton, T. C., eds.: Controversy in Obstetrics and Gynecology. W. B. Saunders Co., Philadelphia, 1969, p. 271.

Fletcher, A. P., Alkjaersig, N., and Sherry, S.: Pathogenesis of the coagulation defect developing during pathologic plasma proteolytic ("fibrinolytic") states; I. The significance of fibrinogen proteolysis and circulating fibrinogen breakdown products. J. Clin. Invest., 41:896, 1962.

Fletcher, A. P., Alkjaersig, N., Sherry, S., Genton, E., Hirsh, J., and Bachmann, F.: The development of urokinase as a thrombolytic agent. Maintenance of a sustained thrombolytic state in man by its intravenous infusion. J. Lab. Clin. Med., 65:713, 1965.

Franklin, S. S., and Merrill, J. P.: Acute renal failure. New Eng. J. Med., 262:711, 1960.

Goldstein, D. P., and Reid, D. E.: Circulating fibrinolytic activity—a precursor of hypofibrinogenemia following fetal death in utero. Obstet. Gynec., 22:174, 1963.

Jimenez, J. M., and Pritchard, J. A.: Pathogenesis and treatment of coagulation defects resulting from fetal death. Obstet. Gynec., 32:449, 1968.

MacFarlane, R. G.: The development of ideas on fibrinolysis. Brit. Med. Bull., 20:173, 1964.

McKay, D. G.: Disseminated Intravascular Coagulation—An Intermediary Mechanism of Disease. Hoeber Medical Division, Harper and Row, New York, 1965.

McKay, D. G., Jewett, J. F., and Reid, D. E.: Endotoxin shock and the generalized Shwartzman reaction in pregnancy. Amer. J. Obstet. Gynec., 78:546, 1959.

McKay, D. G., and Muller-Berghaus, G.: Therapeutic implications of disseminated intravascular coagulation. Amer. J. Cardiol., 20:392, 1967.

McKay, D. G., and Shapiro, S. S.: Alterations in blood coagulation system induced by bacterial endotoxin. J. Exp. Med., 107:353, 1958.

Merskey, C., Johnson, A. J., Kleiner, G. J., and Wohl, H.: The defibrination syndrome: Clinical features and laboratory diagnosis. Brit. J. Haemat., 13:528, 1967.

Moloney, W. C., Egan, W. J., and Gorman, A. J.: Acquired afibrinogenemia in pregnancy. New Eng. J. Med., 240:596, 1949.

Ober, W. B., Reid, D. E., Romney, S. L., and Merrill, J. P.: Renal lesions and acute renal failure in pregnancy. Amer. J. Med., 21:781, 1956.

Oliver, J., MacDowell, M., and Tracy, A.: Pathogenesis of acute renal failure associated with traumatic and toxic injury; renal ischemia, nephrotoxic damage and the ischemuric episode. J. Clin. Invest., 30:1307, 1951.

Phillips, L. L.: Etiology of afibrinogenemia; fibrinogenolytic and fibrinolytic phenomena. Ann. N.Y. Acad. Sci., 75:676, 1959.

Phillips, L. L., Skrodelis, V., and Taylor, H. C., Jr.: Hemorrhage due to fibrinolysis in abruptio placentae. Amer. J. Obstet. Gynec., 84:1447, 1962.

Pritchard, J. A., and Brekken, A. L.: Clinical and laboratory studies on severe abruptio placentae. Amer. J. Obstet. Gynec., 97:681, 1963.

Pritchard, J. A., and Ratnoff, O. D.: Studies of fibrinogen and other hemostatic factors in women with intrauterine death and delayed delivery. Surg. Gynec. Obstet., 101:467, 1955.

Pritchard, J. A., Weisman, R., Jr., Ratnoff, O. D., and Vosburgh, G. J.: Intravascular hemolysis thrombocytopenia and other hematologic abnormalities associated with severe toxemia of pregnancy. New Eng. J. Med., 250:89, 1954.

Reid, D. E.: Acquired coagulation defects in pregnancy. Obstet. Gynec. Survey, 20:431, 1965.

Reid, D. E., Frigoletto, F. D., Tullis, J. L., and Hinman, J.: Hypercoagulable states in pregnancy. In press.

Reid, D. E., Weiner, A. E., and Roby, C. C.: Presumptive amniotic fluid infusion with resultant postpartum hemorrhage due to afibrinogenemia. J.A.M.A., 152:227, 1953.

Reid, D. E., Weiner, A. E., and Roby, C. C.: Incoagulable blood in severe premature separation of the placenta; a method of management. Amer. J. Obstet. Gynec., 66:475, 1953.

Reid, D. E., Weiner, A. E., Roby, C. C., and Diamond, L. K.: Maternal afibrinogenemia associated with longstanding intrauterine fetal death. Amer. J. Obstet. Gynec., 66:500, 1953.

Romney, S. L., Merrill, J. P., and Reid, D. E.: Alterations of potassium metabolism in pregnancy. Amer. J. Obstet. Gynec., 68:119, 1954.

Sheehan, H. L., and Moore, H. C.: Renal Cortical Necrosis and the Kidney of Concealed Accidental Haemorrhage. Charles C Thomas, Springfield, Ill., 1953.

Sherry, S.: Fibrinolysis. Ann. Rev. Med., 19:247, 1968.

Steiner, P. E., and Lushbaugh, C. C.: Maternal pulmonary embolism by amniotic fluid. J.A.M.A., 117:1245, 1941.

Studdiford, W. E., and Douglas, G. W.: Placental bacteremia; significant finding in septic abortion accompanied by vascular collapse. Amer. J. Obstet. Gynec., 71:842, 1956.

Tillett, W. S., Johnson, A. J., and McCarty, R. W.: Intravenous infusion of streptococcal fibrinolytic principle (streptokinase) into patients. J. Clin. Invest., 34:169, 1955.

Weiner, A. E., Reid, D. E., and Roby, C. C.: Hemostatic activity of amniotic fluid. Science, 110:190, 1949.

Chapter 19

Polyhydramnios and Oligohydramnios. Fetal Death

The amount of amniotic fluid may be abnormal in the presence of diabetes mellitus and other metabolic states and fetal malformation, but in at least half of the cases there is no discernible cause for such deviations from the normal amount. In both the experimental animal and the human female, it has been clearly demonstrated that the amniotic fluid is constantly changing, and that it is replaced completely every two or three hours. So rapid is the turnover of the fluid entering and leaving the amniotic cavity that a differential of a few milliliters in the to-and-fro rate of exchange would soon lead to a state of oligohydramnios or polyhydramnios. In oligohydramnios, rather than the normal 1000 to 1200 ml., only 100 to 200 ml. may be present. In polyhydramnios the amount of fluid may reach 4 to 6 L., or more.

Besides studies in which tagged materials were administered to the mother, some of nature's developmental mistakes have furnished supportive evidence on the question of regulation of amniotic fluid exchange. It is apparent that an upset in the normal equilibrium of amniotic fluid exchange may occur in one of several ways. The cells of the amnion appear to be secretory, and undoubtedly there is some exchange of fluid across this comparatively large area. Exactly how this membrane might be altered to upset the normal content of amniotic fluid is unknown. However, compared with normal pregnancy, in polyhydramnios more fluid is apparently exchanged over the fetal membranes than by way of the fetus and placenta, as measured by the isotope technique.

To maintain the amniotic fluid in a steady state, it is apparently necessary for the fetus to remove amniotic fluid by deglutition and to contribute to its formation through urination. This is supported by the finding that polyhydramnios develops in conjunction with esophageal and duodenal atresia, and oligohydramnios occurs with renal agenesis. It is possible that in anencephaly or, indeed, in hydrocephaly, there is a disturbance in the swallowing reflex through alterations in brain structure, accounting for the polyhydramnios commonly seen in these conditions.

Besides occurring in renal agenesis, oligohydramnios is observed in what are undoubtedly true cases of postmaturity, in which, characteristically, a very small amount of deeply meconium-stained amniotic fluid is found. Here, perhaps, the fetus is changing its physiologic behavior. For example, it is known that the renal tubule at birth is rather refractory to antidiuretic hormone (ADH); thus, the postmature fetus might be compared to the two or three week old newborn in some of its physiologic patterns, including response to ADH. Hence it may be that the postmature fetus fails to contribute the normal complement of urine to the amniotic fluid. Also, these infants may not have the normal amount of extracellular fluid, being in a comparative state of dehydration. The same may be encountered in the fetus with dysmature syndrome.

There is reason also to give some consideration to the possible alterations in the physiologic mechanisms of the trophoblast membrane in the etiology of these conditions. The edematous villi seen in erythroblastosis fetalis might interfere with exchange across the trophoblast membrane either directly by affecting water transport, or indirectly by interfering with osmolarity of the fetal blood.

Occasionally the excessive fluid recedes

spontaneously, and this perhaps can be taken as a sign that the fetus is normal. However, the accumulation of fluid may reach a state in which some form of treatment is required. Some physicians place considerable confidence in diuretics, but, given over a long period of time, these can cause serious electrolyte depletion without affecting the extent of the polyhydramnios. Transabdominal tapping of the uterus and the slow removal of 2 or 3 L. of amniotic fluid is of distinct value in selected cases. Rarely it is necessary to terminate the pregnancy to relieve the patient of her discomfort or any cardiovascular and respiratory embarrassment. Owing presumably to the marked uterine distention, the cervix is often found to be effaced and considerably dilated. If the membranes are artificially ruptured, the hand should be kept in the vagina for a short period to control the rate of escape of the fluid, and thus prevent possible placental separation or prolapse of the cord. As the presenting part settles against the cervix, the hand is withdrawn.

FETAL DEATH

The major causes of fetal death are erythroblastosis fetalis, hypertensive pregnancy, metabolic disorders, notably diabetes mellitus, congenital abnormalities, cord complications, and late pregnancy bleeding. It must not be forgotten that syphilis and malaria can be all too often associated with death in utero.

The incidence of death in utero will vary somewhat with the frequency of the complications listed above. However, in most series there is no apparent cause for the demise in about half the cases. Patients accept this misfortune if there is a cause or if the fetus dies before it is medically viable. It is difficult for the patient to be reconciled to this accident, however, when there is no reason for it, or when the fetus might have been saved by properly timed obstetric intervention. Further, when the fetus dies in utero the patient and her family may wonder about the wisdom of permitting the pregnancy to continue, and often go to some lengths to persuade the physician to do something about terminating the pregnancy.

Initially the diagnosis of fetal death is not always certain. The physician's attention is often first called to the possibility of fetal death by the patient's relating her failure to experience fetal motion. Absence of the fetal heart tones is strong evidence that the fetus is dead, corroborated by a fetal electrocardiogram. Overlapping of the skull bones of the fetus by x-ray examination is usually cited as a nearly infallible sign, but

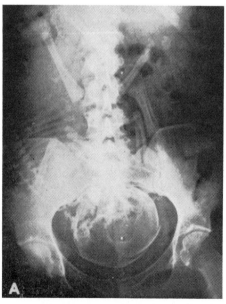 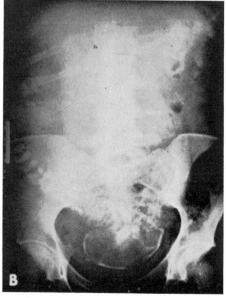

Figure 1. Overlapping of skull bones, apparent on roentgenography. A, A living fetus. B, A microcephalic fetus, subsequently delivered alive.

this phenomenon has also been seen in a living infant (Fig. 1A); conversely, when the fetus is dead overlapping may be absent.

Despite his suspicions that fetal death has occurred in utero, the physician must be certain of his position and be cautious in his remarks to the patient until there is overwhelming evidence that the fetus is dead. As time passes, however, the uterus will begin to decrease in size, and it becomes obvious to both the patient and the physician that the fetus is no longer alive.

Experience in general indicates that 75 to 90 per cent of patients will enter spontaneous labor after fetal demise. Introduction of hypertonic saline solution into the amniotic cavity is highly effective in initiating labor in these cases. Labor usually begins rather promptly, in a matter of hours, perhaps because the factors that maintain the pregnancy, presumably endocrine, are receding. It must be appreciated that ofttimes there is only a small amount of amniotic fluid present. Hence, certain safeguards should be considered to insure that the transabdominal needle or preferably the catheter has entered the amniotic sac. Normal saline can be first injected to demonstrate a free to-and-fro flow. In addition, a radiopaque material may be added to the normal saline solution and an x-ray taken to demonstrate that the needle is properly placed. It would seem reasonable that this procedure should be instituted and the pregnancy completed if by chance labor has not ensued two to three weeks after it has been determined the fetus has died. Development of a clotting deficiency rarely occurs before that period, but it may. (See Coagulation Defects in Chapter 18.)

A few exceptions can be listed in which pregnancy should be terminated when it is initially certain that the fetus has succumbed. A patient who has had several cesarean sections is undoubtedly safer delivered again by abdominal hysterotomy. Although pregnancy toxemia is reported to improve after the fetus dies, in an occasional patient the disease continues or even becomes worse.

BIBLIOGRAPHY

Goldstein, D. P., Johnson, J. P., and Reid, D. E.: Management of intrauterine fetal death. Obstet. Gynec., 21:523, 1963.

Hutchinson, D. L., Gray, M. J., Plentl, A. A., Alvarez, H., Caldeyro-Barcia, R., Kaplan, B., and Lind, J.: The role of the fetus in water exchange of the amniotic fluid of normal and hydramniotic patients. J. Clin. Invest., 38:971, 1959.

Lloyd, J. R., and Clatworthy, H. W., Jr.: Hydramnios as aid to early diagnosis of congenital obstruction of alimentary tract; study of maternal and fetal factors. Pediatrics, 21:903, 1958.

Yordan, E., and D'Esopo, D. A.: Hydramnios; a review of 203 cases at the Sloane Hospital for Women. Amer. J. Obstet. Gynec., 70:266, 1955.

Chapter 20

Dysmaturity-Postmaturity (Placental Dysfunction)

A pregnancy that extends beyond the calculated date of confinement has been the subject of controversy and debate, at least since the turn of the century. The questions asked have been (1) whether there is a clinical entity known as prolonged pregnancy and, if so, (2) whether a fetus can be adversely affected in this circumstance.

Prolonged pregnancy, although not uniformly defined, is one that extends to 290 to 300 days, or some four weeks beyond the period accepted for a term pregnancy. The postmature infant from such a pregnancy reveals several characteristic findings. Unlike the normal newborn, which has an abundance of vernix caseosa to protect its skin, these infants are nearly devoid of this substance, and that which is present is stained yellow or, in the extreme, dark green. The skin and the fingernails, the umbilical cord, and the fetal membranes take on a similar hue. The infants appear thin and malnourished with the skin ofttimes hanging in folds. As the infant's skin begins to dry following birth, it will show some degree of maceration. Various terms such as "parchment-like" and "collodion skin" are used to describe the appearance of the skin (Fig. 1).

The clinical features seen in the postmature infant have also been seen in infants born before term. A discrepancy appears to exist between gestational age and weight, the latter being less than established standards for the particular period of pregnancy. It is envisioned that there is a partial failure in the placental transport mechanism, leading to a state of fetal malnutrition. This is said in the face of the fact that no gross placental lesions are demonstrable in the majority of cases. From this background has emerged the term dysmature-postmature syndrome to apply to the state of the fetus and the newborn who appear to have suffered from the effects of placental dysfunction.

382

Evidence can be marshaled to indicate that the perinatal loss is higher (perhaps by four or five times) in infants weighing 1500 to 2000 grams whose stated gestational age is 37th week or beyond, i.e., those of the dysmature group, as compared to a group with a predicted weight of 2500 to 3000 grams or more for the identical stage of a normal pregnancy. Also, these dysmature infants emphasize the fact that prematurity must not be gauged by birth weight alone. In postmaturity, the perinatal mortality increases by two to three times that observed at the low figure at term, i.e., pregnancy of 38 to 41 weeks. To place the relative fetal risk in proper perspective, the perinatal mortality of normal pregnancy at term should be no more than 1 per cent or indeed less. The necropsy

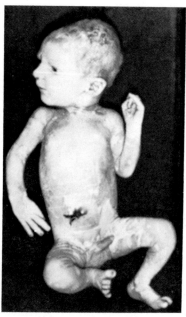

Figure 1. Baby born at 44 weeks gestational age, showing obvious skin changes. The facial expression is that of an older rather than a newborn child.

findings in the dysmature-postmature still-births reveal findings consistent with intra-uterine asphyxia.

Equally if not more disturbing is the possibility that the morbidity rate, or, more precisely stated, the incidence of neurologic deficits may likewise be higher in the post-mature-dysmature group, especially in the dysmature. Extremely low blood sugar or the hypoglycemic syndrome is encountered in some dysmature infants at birth and in the early days of life. One may inquire whether this is representative of a state of malnutrition that may interfere with the development of or cause damage to the central nervous system of the fetus. Once the diagnosis of the dysmature syndrome is considered, the clinical question is posed whether the possible ill effects from growth retardation are increased through the continuance of the fetus to exist in a presumably unfavorable nutritional milieu, or whether the infant should be delivered to face the known hazards of prematurity. The problem appears to be more than mere survival in utero. Hence, in determining the most favorable time to deliver the patient, the relative risks of dysmaturity, prematurity, and possible death in utero must be weighed and repeatedly evaluated.

As in the etiology of fetal death in utero, some 50 per cent of cases of dysmaturity must at the moment be considered idiopathic. Retarded fetal growth is associated with hypertensive pregnancy, chronic renal disease, recurrent late pregnancy bleeding, anomalies of the uterine corpus, and so forth; but in many cases there is no obvious cause. Also, in the idiopathic group the condition can recur, as well as in those with an apparent cause.

The diagnosis of fetal growth retardation begins with the clinical impression that the uterus is smaller than it should be for the gestational date. The maternal weight often remains stationary or decreases and the uterus on occasion appears to recede in size. The ultimate diagnosis of the dysmature-postmature-placental dysfunction syndrome employs all of the items listed in the assessment of the fetus in utero. One must assume that the fetus is in serious jeopardy if amniocentesis reveals meconium-stained amniotic fluid. If it could be measured accurately and with consistency, the volume of amniotic fluid would be found reduced in this syndrome. Measurement of the biparietal diameter of the fetal head by ultrasound may determine whether the fetus is growing at a normal rate. Urinary estriol and placental lactogen determinations may well reflect the condition of the fetus and its intrauterine environment and thus assist in the diagnosis. Values of 4 to 8 mg. per 24 hours for urinary estriol on repeated determinations in the critical period of the 32nd, 34th, and 36th week are indicative of placental dysfunction and a state of dysmaturity. In prolonged pregnancy estriol levels of 7.0 mg. or less have been used as the basis for artificial termination of pregnancy, usually by induction of labor. Placental lactogen may also provide an index of the status of placental function, particularly in the dysmature syndrome or altered fetal intrauterine growth rate. Certainly reduced values have been observed when there has been a discrepancy between birth weight and gestational age. As the amniotic fluid is studied in greater detail, it may be possible to determine that the fetus is reacting to stress and to anticipate fetal distress and growth retardation before these occur.

As previously stated, the management of patients suspected of having placental dysfunction is indeed difficult and each patient must be considered individually. The hazards of prematurity and the threat of death in utero make timing and method of delivery highly important in patient management. Associated conditions will dictate definitive obstetric treatment, e.g., recurrent bleeding from placenta praevia. When the etiology is obscure the method of management is the more uncertain and generalizations are hazardous. Only a few principles can be considered to serve as possible guidelines.

When dysmaturity is feared, delivery by the 32nd to 34th week must be considered, with estriol, placental lactogen, and ultrasonic determinations assisting in the ultimate decision. The method of delivery again is determined by obstetric circumstances.

Patients who are thought to be definitely two or more weeks overdue face the hazards of postmaturity and should be so managed. Special attention must be given to the "elderly" patient, 30 years or older, in her first pregnancy; in such a patient the dysmature-postmature syndrome appears to be more hazardous for the fetus. If the pregnancy continues 10 to 14 days beyond term the primiparous patient should be carefully evaluated and delivered if feasible by induction of labor. However, cesarean section must be considered, especially if the cervix is uneffaced and there is any doubt as to pelvic adequacy. If one decides to do a cesarean section, and the patient has truly a placental dysfunction syndrome, the amniotic fluid characteristically will be scanty in amount with a thick consistency and a pea-green color. It is difficult to believe the fetus would long survive in such an environment. When the gestational dates are believed accurate as determined by both history and early and repeated examination, induction of labor should at least be given consideration in the multiparous patient as well, once the pregnancy has exceeded 42 weeks.

Labor itself is an added hazard to a fetus whose mother's pregnancy is believed prolonged or who has the dysmature syndrome. Hence, the labor that might be in excess of normal both in time and quality is especially hazardous to these fetuses. This statement is cited not to exaggerate the risk of induction of labor, but rather to censure subjecting the mother with the placental dysfunction syndrome to excessive labor. Thus, if one decides to induce labor for dysmaturity and postmaturity, the obstetrician should be prepared to deliver the patient by cesarean section within 8 to 12 hours after amniotomy if productive labor fails to develop.

Some clinicians continue to disbelieve the possibility of the postmature syndrome, whereas others, while agreeing that it exists, justifiably question whether more harm may come to the fetus by the procedures necessary to terminate pregnancy than by allowing the pregnancy to continue and awaiting the spontaneous onset of labor. Whatever else, one must take a position, and to deny the existence of placental dysfunction and the associated dysmature-postmature syndrome is at variance with clinical observation and experience. It is hoped that in the future it will be possible to diagnose these conditions with total certainty, that the etiology of the dysmature syndrome will be uncovered, and that a method will be found to support the fetus nutritionally and avoid the possible hazards of intrauterine malnutrition. Moreover, in these victims of intrauterine stunting the possibility of central nervous system damage and other growth deficiencies must be kept in mind. It seems clear that postmaturity in mothers in the older age group, especially in the primiparous patient, warrants timely termination of the pregnancy, when the risks are balanced against the increase in the perinatal mortality and morbidity rate over that at term.

BIBLIOGRAPHY

Anderson, J. M., Milner, R. D. G., and Strich, S. J.: Pathological changes in the nervous system in severe neonatal hypoglycemia. Lancet, 2:372, 1966.

Ballantyne, J. W.: Problem of the postmature infant. J. Obstet. Gynaec. Brit. Emp., 2:521, 1902.

Brown, J. C. McC.: Postmaturity. Amer. J. Obstet. Gynec., 85:573, 1963.

Clifford, S. H.: Pediatric aspects of placenta dysfunction syndrome in postmaturity. J.A.M.A., 165:1663, 1957.

Elliott, P.: Relationship of liquor volume and placental insufficiency. Aust. New Zeal. Obstet. Gynaec., 4:113, 1965.

Elliott, P.: Foetal salvage in retarded intrauterine growth of the foetus. Aust. New Zeal. J. Obstet. Gynec., 7:13, 1967.

Gruenwald, P.: The fetus in prolonged pregnancy. Amer. J. Obstet. Gynec., 89:503, 1964.

Haworth, J. C., Dilling, L., and Younoszai, M. K.: Relation of blood-glucose to haematocrit, birthweight, and other body measurements in normal and growth-retarded newborn infants. Lancet, 2:901, 1967.

Lubchenco, L. O., Hansman, C., Dressler, M., and Boyd, E.: Intrauterine growth as estimated from liveborn birth-weight data at 24 to 42 weeks of gestation. Pediatrics, 32:793, 1963.

Macafee, C. H. G., and Bancroft-Livingston, G.: Studies in prolonged pregnancy; clinical assessment. J. Obstet. Gynaec. Brit. Emp., 65:7, 1958.

Nesbitt, R. E. L., Jr.: Postmature pregnancy; clinical and pathologic appraisal. Obstet. Gynec., 8:157, 1956.

Smith, K., Greene, J. W., Jr., and Touchstone, J. C.: The management of prolonged pregnancy through the use of urinary estriol. Amer. J. Obstet Gynec., 96:901, 1966.

Zuckerman, J. E., Fallon, V., Tashjian, A. H., Jr., Levine, L., and Friesen, H. G.: Rapid, quantitative estimation of human placental lactogen in maternal serum by complement fixation. J. Clin. Endocr., 30:769, 1970.

Chapter 21

Infections of Childbirth

PUERPERAL INFECTION

Puerperal infection is an infection incurred by way of the reproductive tract during the process of childbirth and the puerperium. The infection usually remains localized to the uterus but may extend to the parametrial and adnexal tissues, and on occasion may be manifest by a bacteremia.

As will be noted, there are two forms of puerperal infection: (1) the individual and (2) the epidemic type. The possibility of occurrence of the latter is influenced by the presence of Group A beta hemolytic streptococcal infection in the community. Fortunately the epidemic form is encountered rarely; sporadic outbreaks do occur but apparently fail to find their way into the scientific literature. A recent epidemic was observed and reported by the writer. In contrast to previous outbreaks, this epidemic was marked by at least two features: (1) for the first time the primary focus or source of the infection was identified, and (2) the hazard of death was avoided by prompt and massive administration of antimicrobial agents.

Actually, the diagnosis and control of the epidemic form of puerperal sepsis, or childbed fever, marks a milestone in the evolution of medicine. Not only did it reduce immeasurably the maternal mortality from this dread disease, but it also contributed to an understanding of the origin, the dissemination, and the contagion of infectious disease generally. Among others, Charles White, Oliver Wendell Holmes, and Ignaz Philipp Semmelweis deserve special recognition for identifying the factors that influenced the spread of this scourge which took the lives of countless women in their prime and left many children motherless. White, in 1773, demanded cleanliness in the care of the parturient. Holmes, in 1843, and Semmelweis, in 1861, contended that puerperal fever was carried from patient to patient by the physician or others in attendance at delivery or during the puerperium.

Certain complications of puerperal sepsis have already been considered in the discussion of abortion, septic shock, anuria, and coagulation defects. This discussion will be restricted principally to the identification of the causative organism or organisms, the mode and extent of infection, the diagnosis and clinical course of the disease, previously unmentioned complications, and treatment.

Etiology and Pathogenesis

The organisms causing puerperal infection are those associated with infections generally. In a consideration of these organisms, it is useful to divide them into two groups—those responsible for individual infection and the organism responsible for the epidemic form. The first group comprise the organisms normally present in the vagina and about the perineum, including the inhabitants of the lower bowel, such as *Clostridium welchii* and the coliform or enterobacterial group, that is, *Escherichia coli*, Proteus, *Aerobacter aerogenes*, *Pseudomonas aeruginosa*, and enterococcus. In addition, *Streptococcus viridans* is a rather frequent inhabitant of the vagina.

Staphylococcus pyogenes is more likely to be implicated in infections of the breast, of surgical and episiotomy wounds, and of the newborn. Of the many types of pathogenic staphylococci, type 80/81 is of the greatest concern because of its resistance to antibiotic therapy.

The second type is attributed to beta hemolytic streptococcus Group A, the organism responsible for the epidemic form of puerperal infection brought about by transmission from patient to patient, for whenever epidemics have been studied, the disease has been found to spread by contact and not from the general hospital environment. Thus, those in attendance should be suspected as being the source of infection and the nursing and medical techniques should receive critical review.

The portal of entry of all forms of puerperal sepsis is likely to be the placental site, which is in effect an open wound. As an endometritis, the infection spreads by way of the lymphatics to the parametrial tissues. An exudative process may form within the broad ligaments that may eventually resolve completely or produce a pelvic abscess, or, by continuity, cause a thrombophlebitis of the neighboring pelvic veins. In some instances the infection may extend through the myometrium or the fallopian tubes to cause a peritonitis, or gain entrance to the blood stream, resulting in a bacteremia.

The organism may have been introduced into the genital tract during a vaginal examination, sexual intercourse just prior to the onset of labor, operative delivery, or exploration of the uterus following delivery, or through faulty postpartum care. Occasionally, however, puerperal infection will develop when the labor and delivery have been entirely normal, and there is no reason to suspect a breach in the technique of postpartum care.

The cardinal signs and symptoms of uterine sepsis include fever, sometimes preceded by a chill, a rise in pulse rate, leukocytosis, tenderness of the uterus extending laterally over the broad ligament areas, and, depending on the organisms, a foul to nonodorous serosanguineous lochia.

In the diagnosis, fever developing in the puerperium must be regarded as due to uterine infection until proved otherwise. There are four common causes of fever in the puerperium other than that due to puerperal sepsis. Firstly, a low-grade fever on the second or third postpartum day is commonly due to retention of the lochia. Secondly, during the same period of the puerperium a temperature rise may result from saprophytic infection of the fetal membranes, if by chance they were not completely expelled at the time of delivery. Again, the pulse rate remains near normal, there is a minimal rise in temperature, and the patient does not appear ill. Characteristically the lochia has a foul odor, which persists for several days. The uterus fails to involute at the normal rate and appears larger than normal on palpation. In both of these circumstances the temperature quickly returns to normal following im-

provement of uterine drainage by the administration of additional oxytocic drugs. Thirdly, on the second to the fourth day of the puerperium there may be a slight rise in temperature, without an increase in pulse rate, due to breast engorgement. Fourthly, another likely cause of the pyrexia is a urinary tract infection.

In uterine sepsis the temperature usually rises to 102 to 103° F. or more, although this is not a universal finding. In fact, a discrepancy between pulse rate and temperature is an ominous sign. Certainly the pulse rate is the better index of the degree of toxicity, and 120 beats or more per minute is in keeping with a seriously ill patient.

Once the infection has extended beyond the uterus, thus giving rise to a parametritis, a rectal or sterile vaginal examination from the third or fourth day of the puerperium onward will reveal exquisite tenderness in the lateral vaginal fornices and a sensation of induration in the region of the broad ligaments with spasm and guarding by the patient.

In the epidemic form, characteristically the patient develops signs and symptoms within 24 to 72 hours after known exposure to the organism. Chills, fever, flushed cheekbones, glassy eyes, abdominal distention, absence of bowel sounds, and exquisite tenderness of the subinvoluted uterus and the adnexa are the classic signs of patients with epidemic puerperal sepsis from beta hemolytic streptococcus Group A. The scanty lochia is serosanguineous and free of odor. The infection spreads rapidly through the lymphatics and unless antibiotic therapy is initiated early, a bacteremia is common, as verified by blood culture. As the patient responds to therapy, the temperature falls, usually more rapidly than the pulse rate, but within a week or 10 days these have usually returned to normal, and the uterine and lower abdominal tenderness has subsided. Prior to the antibiotic era, the maternal mortality was at least 30 per cent in the epidemics reported.

Clostridium welchii and gonococcal infections at the time of childbirth have certain features which deserve special comment. *Cl. welchii* infection has been considered in the discussion of abortion, but, for purposes of emphasis, some of its features are again mentioned. When it occurs in association with labor and delivery, with rare exception it is the consequence of a poorly performed or ill advised obstetric procedure, with pelvic lacerations and resultant devitalized tissue.

This type of infection is evident soon after delivery—in fact, within a few hours. Characteristically, the patient reveals evidence of toxic shock. The signs and symptoms include a rapid pulse, falling blood pressure, rising temperature, possible hemolysis, and anuria. Evidence of gas formation as indicated by crepitation of the tissues appears later or not at all. An immediate attempt should be made to identify the organism with culture and smears of material taken from the cervix and uterus.

Gonococcal infection as a complication of the lying-in period should be suspected when mild fever and pelvic tenderness develop later, near the end of the first postpartum week. Although a bacteremia can occur, this is rare indeed in the obstetric patient. Unless one can identify the organism from Skene's ducts and by cervical culture, the diagnosis can only be suspected. In most instances the patient is not particularly ill and, after a few days of penicillin therapy, appears to have recovered.

Treatment

The most effective treatment of puerperal infection is prevention by the avoidance of traumatic delivery and by careful aseptic technique in patient management during labor, delivery, and the puerperium. Also, prevention begins by cautioning the patient of the dangers of self-infection by indulging in intercourse during the last six to eight weeks of pregnancy. A vaginal examination, when indicated during this period, should be done only under sterile precautions.

With the diagnosis of puerperal infection suspected in a patient, isolation precautions are in order. Patient management begins with the identification of the responsible organism. Besides a blood culture, material is taken from the uterus for bacteriologic studies. After proper preparation of the patient, a small sterile glass tube some 8 to 10 inches long is passed, with the aid of a bivalve speculum, through the cervix into the lower uterine segment; with a small syringe attached to the distal end of the tube, lochia is drawn into the tube. This material is planted on the various media; culturing for anaerobic organisms is included. As previously stated, direct smears may be helpful, as in the case of *Clostridium welchii*. In the case of staphylococcal infection, the coagulase test and phage typing may be required.

Before the causative organism is known and its antibiotic sensitivities are determined, it would seem prudent to give the patient broad-spectrum antibiotic coverage. Once the organism or organisms are identified, the current specific antimicrobial therapy may then be started. Supportive or general therapy should include the forcing of fluids, with parenteral administration when necessary, transfusions as indicated, and treatment of any complications which may appear. In cases of clostridium infection that fail to respond to antimicrobial therapy, serum, and open drainage, or when hemolysis and liver involvement are extreme, hyperbaric oxygen therapy and exchange transfusions must be considered.

Of the complications, the most common is a parametritis. At times it may be possible to identify the upper margin of the broad ligament as a shelflike structure extending from a somewhat enlarged tender uterus to the side walls of the pelvis. The process need not be bilateral; in fact it is frequently unilateral.

The natural history of a parametritis is for the exudate to undergo absorption, which may take several months, or for the process to go on to abscess formation. The latter may be in the form of multiple small (millimeter-sized) abscesses, which obviously are not amenable to drainage. They can be recognized only by needling the lateral vaginal fornices, a procedure that may prove helpful if for no other reason than to obtain material for further bacteriologic study, to permit reappraisal of the organism(s) involved and dictate the appropriate antibiotic to be used. A single abscess is more likely to form and, being retroperitoneal, it may spread in several directions, into the flank or over Poupart's ligament, or it may dissect posteriorly into the cul-de-sac of Douglas. The latter development is by far the most common.

Usually not until the second week of the patient's illness is the abscess likely to declare itself. Performed always under sterile precautions, a *gentle* pelvic examination will reveal a space-occupying mass in the posterior cul-de-sac. The cervix and the uterus are displaced upward. The process may at first be firm, indicating that it obviously has not reached the stage of suppuration. In the interim, the patient may reveal wide swings of temperature. By repeated vaginal examination performed two or three days apart and by the same examiner, it may be detected that an abscess is forming. A rectovaginal examination is helpful in estimating the size and the extent of the mass. When the clinician is convinced that the abscess is "ripe," as indicated by a soft mass bulging from the posterior vaginal fornix, it should be drained. With the patient anesthetized and prepared, the posterior fornix is exposed. A needle may be passed into the abscess to substantiate the diagnosis and obtain material for bacteriologic examination. Held by two Allis hemostats, the vaginal mucous membrane is incised transversely within 1 or 2 cm. of the cervix and a curved 8-inch hemostat is introduced directly into the abscess. Finger exploration will identify any pocketing of pus and break any barrier without damage to the surrounding vital structures such as the bowel. A Penrose drain is sutured in place, to be removed in two or three days. It is, of course, possible for the abscess to drain spontaneously into the rectum. Should the abscess rupture abdominally, the outlook is serious and the prognosis must be guarded. Immediate laparotomy and pelvic clean-out is mandatory to include total hysterectomy and unilateral or bilateral salpingo-oophorectomy depending on the extent of ovarian involvement.

Bacteremia in association with a puerperal infection presents all of the problems and hazards of a bacteremia originating from other sources and in other medical or surgical conditions. Bacterial endocarditis, embolic phenomena, empyema, and formation of abscesses in remote areas of the body are the complications to be anticipated.

The appearance of septic emboli may be the initial evidence that pelvic thrombophlebitis is present. Important in patient management is the fact that septic embolization may be controlled only by ligation of the inferior vena cava and ovarian veins.

Infection of the Episiotomy Wound

Infection of the episiotomy wound should occur most infrequently; this is remarkable when one considers the area of the body involved, which not only lends itself to easy contamination but is difficult to maintain completely sterile. Whether the episiotomy wound becomes infected depends to a degree on the circumstances of the case — whether the patient had fever and, presumably, intrauterine infection at the time of delivery, and whether the delivery was difficult, with possible trauma to the surrounding tissues and a lowering of the resistance of the tissues to local infection.

Routine inspection of the perineum on the third or fourth day after delivery commonly reveals a tissue reaction about the perineal incision and sutures. Careful perineal care is all that is required. What is a matter of more concern is infection of the deeper tissues involved in the episiotomy, that is, the pubococcygeus muscle and the fascia. The fever is usually low-grade, and although the patient is disturbed by the local discomfort, she is not seriously ill. Initially sinus tracts may be seen penetrating into the depth of the wound, occasionally leading to areas of suppuration. At the onset the treatment is heat to the area, and possibly antibiotics after material has been taken for cultures. In a few instances the question will arise whether the wound should be opened wide and permitted to drain adequately, with the realization that a secondary closure will be required. In most instances, with local heat and antibiotic therapy, the infection will subside. If it is not a gaping wound, sufficient granulation tissue will form to afford the perineum good support. Necessity of a secondary closure will be less likely in the median than in the mediolateral type of episiotomy.

If it is decided to remove the deep sutures, the wound should be cleansed and material for culture taken from the area every two or three days; when the cultures reveal little or no growth of a pathogenic organism the wound may be closed secondarily. This treatment is preferred, rather than requiring the patient to return several weeks later for such a procedure, for there is likely to be less distortion of the normal tissue relationship. In the closure, catgut sutures are permitted in the vaginal mucosa, but through-and-through, nonabsorbable sutures are used for the main body of the tissues involved in the episiotomy. These are removed 7 to 10 days later.

Puerperal Breast Infections

Acute infections of the breast, seen infrequently now in the obstetric patient, usually occur in the earlier weeks of the puerperium, soon after the onset of lactation, or at the time of weaning when the flow of milk has been disrupted. The organism most frequently responsible is the staphylococcus; streptococcus and coliform infections are rare. Several studies point to the fact that most of the staphylococci cultured are coagulase-positive.

The predisposing factors in the development of a lymphangitis of the breast, which, if it fails to respond to therapy, will eventuate in a breast abscess, include the establishment of portals of entry, such as fissure of the nipples, and stagnation of the flow of milk with entrance of the organism through the nipple.

It must be recognized that the milk of many nursing mothers contains *Staphylococcus aureus*. Further, although they are asymptomatic, most infants harbor the same organism in the nasopharynx within a week after birth. In routine cultures of the nasopharynx of mothers, babies, and hospital personnel, 40 per cent have been positive for *Staphylococcus pyogenes*, but rarely are types 42B/52/80/81 found.

The endemic form of staphylococcal breast abscess may be derived from either the hospital or the home environment. The epidemic form, however, is regarded as originating from nursery contamination. The literature is replete with reports of hospital outbreaks in which a number of mothers developed breast abscesses and infant deaths occurred, with the staphylococci cultured in any given epidemic belonging to the same strain.

The sources of contamination within the hospital environment are many, and thus determination of the origin of the infection is a baffling task. There seems little doubt that nursery contamination is more often by a carrier among the hospital personnel, and rarely by a baby whose mother is a carrier. Once the infection is introduced into the nursery, breast infection may follow in a substantial number of nursing mothers whose infants become infected. Moreover, in an epidemic, cases of breast abscess may be seen in patients who do not breast-feed their infants.

An outbreak of staphylococcal infection in a nursery calls for drastic measures. Because all infants in the nursery are suspect, breast feeding must be discontinued and no new babies should be admitted until the nursery has been meticulously cleaned

following discharge of the existing population. The nursery techniques employed should be generally reviewed, and a scrupulous search must be made for carriers. This includes culturing of the nose and throat of the nursing and medical personnel, as well as of the patients. The most important principle in the control of staphylococcal infections in hospitals is general cleanliness.

Ideally, each nursery should have its own nursing personnel and should house no more than eight newborns. Rooming-in is a further safeguard. It is assumed that those handling the infants in the nursery wash their hands with a solution containing hexachlorophene after caring for or examining each baby. Before each nursing the mother's breasts should be washed in toto and the area about the nipple cleansed with sterile water before the infant is placed to breast. All hospital personnel coming in contact with the mother or her infant should be carefully screened daily, and removed from duty if there is any evidence of body surface or respiratory infection. If these procedures are followed, the incidence of any infection of the infant in the first six to eight weeks of life should be nil. Infections occurring after that period can be assumed to be derived from the home surroundings rather than the hospital.

The symptoms of a breast infection are usually sudden in onset, with an elevation of temperature to 101 to 103° F. and diffuse tenderness of the breast which becomes localized within a few hours, accompanied by redness of the skin and followed by painful induration of the breast tissue. The symptoms may vary somewhat, depending on whether the infection is in the subareolar tissue or deep in the breast itself.

As noted, prevention of breast infection requires careful breast hygiene, and the appropriate treatment should be instituted if a fissure of the nipple develops in the course of nursing. A nipple shield may allow nursing to continue on the affected breast.

The specific therapy depends somewhat on the duration of symptoms and the amount of localization present. Early acute cases with minimal involvement of either the breast parenchyma or the subareolar tissue (lymphangitis) may be aborted by the application of ice, suppression of lactation, and the use of breast binders and antibiotic therapy. One does not wait for fluctuation to occur before incising the breast; otherwise much of the breast tissue may be destroyed. Pitting edema over the involved area is a relatively early and more useful sign that pus is present. Once an abscess has formed, surgical therapy with adequate drainage is the only treatment.

Infections of the subareolar tissue around the nipple may be opened with a small circumareolar incision, the pocket drained, and a small rubber wick or iodoform gauze pack left in place. Infections involving as much as one fourth of the breast require more extensive surgical drainage. Abscesses occurring in the upper half of the breast may be drained by radial incision, with an extra incision made in the dependent portion of the breast and through-and-through drains left in place. Abscesses located in the lower half of the breast are usually drained adequately through a radial incision over the abscess. Once an incision is made, it is necessary to break up the various loculi and pockets by blunt finger dissection. Antibiotics are administered according to sensitivity reports on cultures of material that is obtained at the time of drainage. Because many infections are caused by virulent organisms, cephalosporins and semisynthetic penicillins are often chosen. Methicillin and oxacillin are effective for penicillinase-producing bacteria.

Postoperative care requires careful cleansing of the surrounding skin to prevent additional infection, and the application of binders for suppression of lactation. At this time the use of various endocrine preparations for the suppression of lactation has little value. Recurrence or extension of the infection may necessitate secondary drainage. Recovery is often delayed, and several weeks may elapse before the patient has regained her usual strength and energy.

INDICATIONS FOR, AND GENERAL PRINCIPLES OF, ISOLATION TECHNIQUE

Isolation of the infected or the potentially infected obstetric patient has two purposes: (1) to provide her with the extra needed care, and (2) to protect the uninfected patient from cross-infection. It is preferable that isolation policies be developed by a committee composed of members representing both the obstetric and the nursing staff, and consultants who are familiar with all aspects of infectious disease; that all cases of infection be reviewed by the committee at stated intervals to make certain that the policies are being respected by all personnel; and that the committee be constantly alert to development of improved techniques that will afford maximal safety to the mother and her infant.

Patients may be isolated on individual precautions in single rooms, or transferred to an isolation unit for infectious cases in which they are individually isolated. In the interest of keeping the hospital free of infection, certain types of cases are best transferred to an area designated the isolation unit. This may be done on the basis of the clinical type of infection or the organism responsible for the infection, or both. The patient may be placed on individual precaution and not moved to the isolation unit in the case of a common cold, bronchitis, pyelonephritis, or idiopathic diarrhea of no longer than 24 hours' duration. Patients with a specific communicable bacterial or viral disease, and those with draining wounds, whether an abdominal or an infected episiotomy incision, or a breast abscess, must always be cared for in the isolation unit.

Under no circumstance is the baby permitted contact with the mother when she has any infection or harbors any organism that causes her to be placed in the isolation unit. To place further safeguards on the baby it, too, is transferred to the isolation unit and should be placed in an Isolette as additive insurance against cross-infection. The ideal isolation unit should provide an individual nursery, that is, a rooming-in arrangement, where the mother can take over the care of the infant when she is sufficiently recovered and is no longer considered capable of transmitting infection.

Certain minimal techniques must be followed by physicians and all those caring for the patient in isolation. Wrist watches and rings are removed before gown, mask, and shoe coverings are put on. The physician should wash his hands with a detergent containing hexachlorophene for one or two minutes before and after examining the patient. The stethoscope and other pieces of equipment should not be taken from one patient to another. Patients in the isolation unit must be delivered in a special delivery room outside the obstetric delivery suite. The physician must never leave the isolation delivery area without thoroughly scrubbing his hands and changing his scrub suit. It must be stressed that the physician must set the standards and tone in the isolation techniques of the infected patient. He must never be the one who offends by violating them.

In summary, safety in childbirth gained a new horizon with the introduction of antimicrobial drugs. At the same time there is the blithe belief that if infection occurs it can be readily controlled by appropriate antibiotics. Such a position tends to blunt the surgical conscience of all who come in contact with a patient in childbirth. The fear of infecting the parturient by cross-contamination tends to be forgotten as limited numbers of ancillary personnel must be shared by other hospital services and so-called "clean gynecologic" patients are housed on the floor with obstetric patients. The same casual approach is observed when the vaginal examination is performed in late pregnancy and labor without acceptable sterile precautions. Rather, the "clean-glove" technique is believed to be adequate but this slovenly approach is hardly consistent with the highest standards of patient care.

Indeed, ideal obstetric care must be practiced in surroundings that will not expose the parturient to traffic areas shared by other types of patients and in fact she should not be housed on a floor other than one reserved for obstetric patients. Facilities for ready isolation of infected or potentially infected patients and careful scrutiny of possible carriers of infection continue to be basic considerations. Standards of excellence must not be relaxed in favor of unlimited visiting hours and permitting the presence of nonprofessional personnel in the delivery room areas.

BIBLIOGRAPHY

Caswell, H. T., Schreck, K. M., Burnett, W. E., Carrington, E. R., Learner, N., Steel, H. H., Tyson, R. R., and Wright, W. C.: Bacteriologic and clinical experiences and methods of control of hospital infections due to antibiotic resistant staphylococci. Surg. Gynec. Obstet., 106:1, 1958.

Deane, R. M., and Russell, K. P.: Enterobacillary septicemia and bacterial shock in septic abortion. Amer. J. Obstet. Gynec., 79:528, 1960.

Gibberd, G. F.: Puerperal sepsis, 1930–1965. J. Obstet. Gynaec. Brit. Comm., 73:1, 1966.

Gillespie, W. A., Simpson, K., and Tozer, R. C.: Staphylococcal infection in a maternity hospital; epidemiology and control. Lancet, 2:1075, 1958.

Holmes, O. W.: The contagiousness of puerperal fever. New Eng. Quart. J. Med. Surg., 1:503, 1843.

Jewett, J. F., Reid, D. E., Safon, L. E., and Easterday, C. L.: Childbed fever – a continuing entity. J.A.M.A., 206:344, 1968.

Meleny, F. L., et al.: Epidemiologic and bacteriologic investigations of the Sloane Hospital epidemic of hemolytic streptococcus puerperal fever in 1927. Amer. J. Obstet. Gynec., 16:180, 1928.

Montgomery, T. L., Wise, R. I., Lang, W. R., Mandle, R. J., and Fritz, M. A.: A study of staphylococcic colonization of postpartum mothers and newborn infants. Amer. J. Obstet. Gynec., 78:1227, 1959.

Pedowitz, P., and Bloomfield, R. D.: Ruptured adnexal abscess (tuboovarian) with generalized peritonitis. Amer. J. Obstet. Gynec., 88:721, 1964.

Studdiford, W. E., and Douglas, G. W.: Placental bacteremia; significant finding in septic abortion accompanied by vascular collapse. Amer. J. Obstet. Gynec. 71:842, 1956.

Watson, B. P.: An outbreak of puerperal sepsis in New York City. Amer. J. Obstet. Gynec., 16:157, 1928.

Watson, B. P.: Practical measures in the prevention and treatment of puerperal sepsis. J.A.M.A., 103:1745, 1934.

Wysham, D. N., Mulhern, M. E., Navarre, G. C., La Veck, G. D., Kennan, A. L., and Giedt, W. R.: Staphylococcal infections in an obstetric unit; epidemiologic studies of pyoderma neonatorum. New Eng. J. Med., 257:295, 1957.

Chapter 22

Teratology

An insight into the causation and nature of congenital anomalies is important for the obstetrician for, frequently, the first question a mother will ask after the birth of her infant is whether it is normal or, if by chance it is abnormal, what is the cause. The second question often directed to the physician is whether the condition might recur in a subsequent pregnancy. Hence, obstetric management and neonatal care are significantly influenced by a competent understanding of the character and prognosis of malformations.

INCIDENCE

Estimates of the incidence of congenital anomalies vary widely, from 0.7 per cent to 4 per cent of newborns. It must be realized, however, that such estimates provide but the roughest approximation of the actual incidence. They are significantly influenced by a variety of factors: For example, epidemics of rubella will increase the incidence periodically; there is no general agreement as to what exactly is to be called congenital anomaly, and consequently statistics vary; specific studies to identify certain anomalies (e.g., chromosomal) will lead to increased incidence figures in a given population; and there exist significant racial and geographic differences in the incidence of certain anomalies.

While grossly recognized congenital anomalies are seen in approximately 2 per cent of newborns, many others go undetected and are discovered only in later life. Indeed, it has been found that in 10 per cent of adults some type of congenital anomaly is detected at autopsy. Malformations are the cause of approximately 13 per cent of the deaths in children under the age of 15, and 72 per cent of them are lethal within the first year of life, according to national statistics collected in 1961.

ETIOLOGY

Until recently the cause of most congenital anomalies was obscure. The recognition by the Australian ophthalmologist Gregg of a relationship between infantile cataract and deafness and maternal rubella infection marked the beginning of an era of intensive search into the etiology of congenital anomalies. The known factors may now be grouped under the following headings: (1) infections; (2) teratogens; (3) mutations; (4) hereditary basis; (5) multifactorial basis; and (6) radiation.

Infections

In the usual connotation of "malformation," only the rubella virus is implicated as a causative agent. When the virus is transmitted to the fetus within the first trimester, and if abortion does not occur, at least 25 per cent of the infected infants will have a multiplicity of congenital anomalies. Among these cataract, deafness, and congenital heart disease are the most prominent, but many other organs may be affected to a lesser extent.

On the basis of direct isolation of the rubella virus from affected organs (e.g., the lens) of the fetus two weeks after maternal infection, and even from infants who died in the neonatal period after prenatal infection, it is now accepted that the virus passes through the placenta. Töndury has traced the infection successively in abortions after verified maternal infection. He described inclusion bodies in fetal villous endothelium as the first event; subsequently, fetal viremia and often embolism of the necrotic material from the villous vasculature are thought to cause the inflammatory and degenerative events in the embryonic organs, there being no specific tropism for any one tissue. Myocardial necrosis is seen particularly frequently. In general, cellular necrosis is the most important event when viruses cause damage in early embryonic life; only later an inflammatory component participates and complicates interpretation of the pathogenetic mechanism. It is envisaged that the viral infection of rapidly dividing embryonic cells causes cell death not unlike that seen as cytopathogenicity in tissue cultures. Thus, when forming organs are involved during the process of organogenesis, defects may occur that represent true anomalies (e.g., interventricular septal defect). As the fetus matures and this so-called critical, organogenetic period of the first three months has passed, virus infections take a more conventional course, with cell necrosis, inflammation, and scarring. It is apparent, though, that a fluid transition between these events exists, and this is one reason for speaking of virus "embryopathy."

To differentiate clearly between the effects of infection, with respect to their production of typical anomalies, and fetal disease is even more difficult in other diseases. Thus, cytomegalovirus infection causes significant destructive events, particularly in the fetal brain, with calcification and microcephaly resulting, among its many other manifestations; yet it is not usually regarded as a virus causing congenital anomalies. The same may be said of the effects of the protozoon *Toxoplasma gondii*.

Among infectious diseases unequivocal anomalies are caused only by the rubella virus. In addition, significant destructive lesions simulating some type of malformation (e.g., hydrocephaly, microcephaly) are caused by cytomegalovirus and Toxoplasma. It is possible but not proved beyond doubt that infection with Coxsackie B virus and mumps bear a causal relationship to some types of congenital heart disease. Hepatitis virus, influenza A virus, and perhaps a few others have similarly been incriminated, and destructive lesions in embryos from such pregnancies have been recorded. Nevertheless, in infants with anomalies no such fetal infection has been demonstrated unequivocally. A variety of other infections (vaccinia, poliomyelitis, variola, herpes) have fetal manifestations without being the cause of anomalies (see Infectious Diseases in Chapter 30).

Teratogens

Thalidomide (Contergan and a variety of other names) is a mild sedative that has been clearly implicated as the cause of anomalies in a large number of infants. Classically, it is responsible for phocomelia (defective or rudimentary development of limbs) but closer scrutiny has revealed abnormalities in many organ systems as well. The most remarkable feature about this drug is that a single tablet, if taken during the critical period, has this destructive effect, and the effect can be precisely reproduced in rhesus monkeys. This critical period extends from approximately 34 to 50 days after the last menstrual period and about 100 per cent of embryos are deleteriously affected. In older teratologic terminology the time would be referred to as the "teratogenetic determination period," a period differing for each organ system and essentially delineating its most active time of differentiation. One would think that the extensive investigations initiated after the European thalidomide tragedy of the early 1960s might have resolved the question of the pathogenesis in molecular terms of this drug effect. This is not the case. Several hypotheses (riboflavin antagonism, glutamine antagonism, nucleotide simulation) are being considered, and the similarities to the rubella-caused cell damage have been pondered. At present the answer is unknown; perhaps most remarkable is the fact that the drug is virtually insoluble.

Other drugs have teratogenic effect in man but few are as specific and deleterious as thalidomide, which is no longer marketed. Best substantiated is the destructive potential of antimetabolites, which occasionally are ingested to induce abortion. Some of these agents are therapeutic instruments in the treatment of choriocarcinoma and may be embryotoxic only through their destruction of trophoblast. Most, however, generally interfere with cell division and probably exert their effect simultaneously on embryo and trophoblast. Another known teratogen in man is iodine deficiency or its excess; both effectively interfere with fetal thyroid development and function. Likewise, propylthiouracil affects fetal growth by initiating cretinism. Vitamin D and perhaps vitamin A in excessive amounts interfere with normal embryonic growth. The latter is a favorite tool of experimental teratologists, particularly in causing neural tube defects, with anencephaly and similar anomalies resulting. Whether human malformations are so produced is still open to question. Vitamin D in excess has been held responsible for characteristic skeletal and aortic anomalies but is uncommonly recognized as being their cause.

Isolated case reports have incriminated a variety of other chemicals as teratogenic; however, since they are taken by many pregnant patients, the association may be fortuitous. Of historic interest only perhaps is the testosterone analogue 19-nortestosterone (and perhaps a few relatives), formerly used for their progestational effects in threatened abortions. In female infants they have produced moderate but self-limited clitoral hyperplasia not unlike that seen in some infants with familial adrenal hyperplasia ("adrenogenital syndrome") or in mothers with virilizing adrenal tumors. Although useful in experimental studies, neither cortisone nor insulin has a proved teratogenic effect in man.

It is remarkable that in experimental studies in animals a very large variety of chemicals are capable of inducing at times rather specific fetal anomalies and that no such effect has been observed in man. To be sure, mode of administration and, particularly, quantitative differences are great; nevertheless, this observed discrepancy has been a great handicap for those endeavoring to screen new drugs in animals prior to their use in pregnant women. The predictive value, especially from the commonly used rodent model, has not been great, and agents such as thalidomide would have passed screening procedures, while others, e.g., aspirin or insulin, might well have been withdrawn on grounds of animal teratogenicity. Good clinical judgment is necessary when making the decision to prescribe any drug therapy. By and large, only truly indicated medication should be administered during pregnancy, especially in the first months.

Mutations

Genetic errors play a very important role in defective development. Some of these are due to inherited gene defects with known or unknown hereditary (mendelizing) character; others arise de novo and may be considered as mutations. Mutations with significant developmental effect most commonly, if not always, take place in the parental germinal cells and express their effect after the zygote has formed. While of course a significant number of individual gene mutations occur, they are likely to be heterozygous in a zygote or else cannot

readily be distinguished in man from heritable gene defects. However, chromosomal abnormalities must be grouped with mutations and their effect on embryogenesis has recently been amply documented.

From study of abortion material it has been learned that 25 per cent of spontaneous abortions are associated with, if not due to, numerical chromosomal errors, trisomy, X monosomy, and triploidy being the most common (see Chapter 12). In newborns chromosomal errors are found in 0.5 per cent, and if the phenotypically normal translocation carriers are excluded (about 1 in 4), these errors have significant effect upon fetal development (see Chapter 10). The trisomies of larger chromosomes and of Nos. 13–15 and 17–18 are lethal in neonatal life because they cause a variety of fetal malformations (cardiac, cerebral, and so forth). Other chromosome anomalies have specific effects that can be recognized at birth (trisomy 21 — mongolism; XO — Turner's syndrome; deletion of short arm of No. 5 — cri du chat syndrome), and some (XXX, XXY, XYY) express their harmful effect only in later life. On the whole, however, the contribution of chromosomal numerical errors to the overall problem of congenital anomalies of newborns is a relatively minor one, accounting perhaps for 10 per cent of congenital malformations at birth. Prenatal selection by spontaneous abortion appears to be relatively efficient in this case.

In most instances the cause of the mutation is unknown, and rarely can radiation of germ cells be held responsible for the event even though it is the best known experimental tool in their production. In recent years it has become clearer that increased maternal age is strongly correlated with several chromosomal errors, notably trisomies. The exact pathogenesis is not clear. Experimentally it has been shown that postovulatory aging of the ovum, i.e., delayed fertilization, leads frequently to polyploidy and thus abortion (see Chapter 6). Whether the same mechanism is applicable to trisomies that are the result of chromosomal nondisjunction during meiosis is not certain. Equally tenable is the suggestion that preovulatory aging, with resultant exposure of the egg in meiosis to many viral and other teratogens, may be the deciding event. Conflicting results have been obtained in studies that were undertaken to implicate the role of maternal hepatitis in this respect. Finally, a correlation exists between the occurrence of fetal trisomies and maternal thyroid antibody levels.

Hereditary Basis

A vast number of congenital malformations have a hereditary basis. When the genetic mechanism is well understood, such anomalies can be traced to dominant or recessive genes in the families and genetic counseling becomes of great importance in the management of future pregnancies. Examples for dominant inheritance are achondroplasia, osteogenesis imperfecta (see Fig. 2), Marfan's syndrome, multiple polyposis, and many more. Recessive genes are held responsible for such anomalies as the Laurence-Moon-Biedl syndrome, some types of polycystic kidneys, and Morquio's disease. Moreover, diseases such as cystic fibrosis, Hurler's syndrome, and phenylketonuria follow a pattern of recessive inheritance and it is difficult to make a clear-cut distinction between congenital "abnormality" and "disease." It is important to realize also that although many anomalies or diseases follow some type of hereditary pattern, environmental circumstances interact prominently in their expression (see next heading) and thus pose difficulties for genetic counseling. The frequent anomaly cleft palate, for instance, belongs in this category and the same applies for an ever increasing number of syndromes as more knowledge is gained. Finally, some hereditary disorders are mimicked by environmentally caused diseases. A good example of such a "phenocopy" would be hydrocephaly (see Fig. 4), an anomaly occurring about once in 500 births. Forms exist with a fairly clear-cut mendelian basis, while others are due to fetal toxoplasmosis; the problem then lies with diagnosis.

Hereditary diseases thus account for a large number of the congenital anomalies. Because many are the result of specific gene errors leading to the formation of defective enzymes (e.g., the adrenogenital syndrome) these are more readily diagnosed biochemically. Our knowledge has increased remarkably concerning these defects and it is now possible to anticipate many defects from a detailed study of amniotic fluid (see Chapter 10). By this means chromosomal errors, the sex of the infant (important for sex-linked disorders, that is, those carried on the X chromosome), and many enzyme deficiencies can be ascertained. A recent survey by Milunsky et al. lists some 40 specific diseases in which diagnosis from amniotic fluid is now possible or soon will be. No doubt many more will be added to the list. Genetic counseling is currently performed in several university centers, and the National Foundation (800 Second Avenue, New York, New York 10017) plays a leading role in rendering assistance and giving information to physicians and families presented with these problems. The value of counseling is especially apparent when one looks at the frequency of mental retardation. Significant retardation (i.e., an I.Q. of less than 70) occurs in about 3 or 4 per cent of births. Of these children 25 per cent suffer this deficiency because of genetic errors. To be sure, in the majority (80 per cent) of the latter the retardation is caused by chromosomal anomalies; nevertheless, in a vast number of retarded children the cause is a specific hereditary gene defect. Some of these cases will be detectable by prenatal diagnosis and the affected families would clearly benefit from genetic counseling.

The frequency and approximate recurrence risks for some of the major anomalies are summarized in Table 1. It must be appreciated, though, that these figures help little in advising individual families, for, as has been said, many factors contribute in the overall picture—parental age, infections, race, locality, and others. A careful genetic history (pedigree), thorough diagnosis of the anomaly, and detailed knowledge of the type of malformation and its genetic basis are crucial requirements before any prognostication becomes meaningful. Counseling should be undertaken by specially trained personnel.

Multifactorial Basis

In the last few years it has become increasingly evident that a variety of congenital malformations are due to a combination of environmental and genetic factors whose individual contribution varies; indeed, it is currently held that most of the important anomalies have such a multifactorial basis. The evidence for this has been furnished principally by experimental teratologic studies but comes also from epidemiologic studies in man. An understanding of what genetic and what environ-

TABLE 1. RISK FIGURES FOR LATER SIBLINGS AFTER BIRTH OF A CONGENITALLY
MALFORMED INFANT*

	Incidence in Population	Risk Figure in Later Siblings
All malformations	1 in 65	1 in 20
Central nervous system malformations (35%)		
Anencephaly	1 in 450 ⎫	1 in 50 ⎫
Spina bifida	1 in 375 ⎬ 1 in 200	1 in 25 ⎬ 1 in 22
Hydrocephalus	1 in 550 ⎭	1 in 60 ⎭
Mongolism	1 in 600	1 in 20
Muscular-skeletal malformations (25%)		
Harelip with or without cleft palate	1 in 1,000	1 in 7
Cleft palate alone	1 in 2,500	1 in 7
Polydactylia	1 in 1,200	1 in 2
Syndactylia	1 in 2,000	1 in 2
Clubfoot	1 in 1,000	1 in 30
Malformed arms, hands	1 in 5,000	
Achondroplasia	1 in 7,000	
Congenital hip dislocation	1 in 1,500	1 in 20
Cardiovascular malformations (20%)		
All congenital hearts	1 in 200	1 in 50
Patent ductus	1 in 2,500	1 in 50
Genitourinary malformations (6%)		
Hypospadias	1 in 1,000	1 in 50 (?)
Polycystic kidney (infant)	1 in 15,000	1 in 4
Gastrointestinal malformations (3%)		
Exomphalos	1 in 4,000	less than 1 in 100
Diaphragmatic hernia	1 in 10,000	
Tracheoesophageal fistula	1 in 6,000	less than 1 in 100
Atresia ani	1 in 5,000	less than 1 in 100
Multiple malformations (11%)		
Miscellaneous		
Pyloric stenosis	1 in 350	1 in 17

*From Anderson, R. C., and Reed, S. C.: J. Lancet, 74:175, 1954.

mental factors interact in individual cases of human malformations is just beginning, and documentation by the obstetrician of various factors will be of importance in the future.

The mechanism of this important category can best be explained by the intensively explored model of cleft palate in mice (Fraser; Trasler). It has been learned that certain strains of mice respond to teratogens (principally cortisone, but many others as well) administered to the mother by expression of a high frequency of cleft palate in the offspring. Other strains are not susceptible at all or are affected only when very much higher dose levels are employed. Detailed embryologic studies showed that closure of the palate requires complex interactions between the medial movements of palatine shelves and the develop-

ment of the tongue, among other factors. Different strains of mice proceed in these crucially timed events at different rates, and significant interference with shelf movement may lead to failure of palatine closure and thus cleft palate development. Differences exist not only among strains but also among their hybrids, sexes, individuals, and of course species. For explanatory purposes it is easiest to envisage the so-called "quasi-continuous" or "threshold" nature of this process by using a diagram like that in Figure 1. Individuals of a strain with little genetic predisposition to cleft palate would be distributed along the solid line, while those in which cleft palate occurs spontaneously are represented on the dotted curve. Beyond a certain "threshold" (vertical line) a certain number of embryos of the susceptible group will develop the defect.

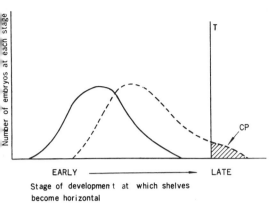

Figure 1. Model to explain the concept of multifactorial determination of congenital anomalies employing cleft palate in mice. The solid line represents population of relatively unsusceptible strain; interrupted line is composed of individuals of susceptible strain. T is threshold beyond which the defect is expressed and which may move with environmental circumstances; see text. (From Fraser, F. C.: in Nishimura, H., and Miller, J. R., eds.: Methods for Teratological Studies in Experimental Animals and Man. Igaku Shoin, Tokyo, 1969.)

When the threshold is moved by specific environmental interactions, either more or fewer embryos will be deleteriously affected. Thus, if shelf movement is retarded (the line may be moved toward the left) a larger percentage of susceptible embryos will manifest the disease, and few or none of the strain represented by the solid line will exhibit the cleft palate.

Such threshold characters presumably determine most human congenital malformations, and they have been explored notably for cleft lip (harelip). It emerges that parental facial shape significantly correlates with the probability of embryos to develop cleft lip. Thus, for example, a tendency for the anterior maxillary surface to be flatter and the mean dizygomatic and intraocular chin distances to be greater was found in the affected families. These findings make more explicable the knowledge that specific defects occur with greater frequency in certain families without having a clearly defined, mendelian background. The environmental factors that interact in such a fashion as to "push the embryo beyond that threshold" where an anomaly will be expressed, remain to be identified.

As in the case with experimental studies, it is possible that minor factors, not readily detected and of great diversity, will be implicated. For instance, it is possible that the great variation in the frequency of anencephaly (6 per 1000 in Dublin, Ireland; 0.5 per 1000 in the United States) relates to subtle local phenomena and that the preponderance in females (4:1) finds its reason in genetically controlled embryonal growth processes. In rare instances mothers who previously bore anencephalic infants repeatedly have had normal offspring after their own congenital heart disease was corrected. Thus, improvement of fetal oxygen supply may have moved the threshold in a more favorable direction for a genotypically susceptible embryo. Similarly position in the uterus may have a profound effect upon these relationships; this is well defined for the mouse model where the frequency of anomalies also increases with increased litter size. In man it is known that a velamentous insertion of the umbilical cord is much more frequently found with babies having a variety of congenital errors than with normal controls. This placental anomaly reflects, we believe, abnormal placental implantation and subsequent growth, factors perhaps sufficient to move the threshold beyond the critical level for susceptible individuals. It is perhaps convenient to study twins in this manner. An abundant literature shows that congenital anomalies occur approximately twice as often in twins as in singletons. Moreover, so-called identical (monozygous, MZ) twins often do not share the anomaly; they are discordant for it. For instance, only about 50 per cent of MZ twins are concordant for cleft palate (5 per cent of dizygous, or fraternal, twins are) even though the defect has a familial (hereditary) basis in some instances. It may be that the reason for the discordant expression of this genetic predisposition among MZ twins is a difference in the unequally shared uterine environment. One twin may have a placenta with velamentous cord, or he may lack one umbilical artery, and such factors possibly then serve as the deleterious environmental agents, not unlike cortisone in the mouse model. At present these multiple possible factors are poorly understood but detailed documentation of such circumstances will enable us in the future to have a more precise insight. Perhaps the reason for the doubled malformation rate among diabetic mothers' offspring relates to this multifactorial model as well.

Radiation

Radiation affects germ cells in several ways. In excessive doses it will cause lethal chromosomal errors which lead to death of germ cells and infertility. In lesser amounts it may cause mutations whose effects may be congenital anomalies in the embryos. The contribution of gonadal radiation to human malformations is difficult to assess but because of its mutagenic effect, so well known from animal studies, protection of gonads during diagnostic x-ray studies is widely practiced and should be encouraged even though little direct evidence exists in man that "routine" x-ray studies have specific mutagenic significance.

Irradiation of the developing embryo has various teratogenic effects and has been extensively studied in experimental animals. Accidental irradiation of human embryos has caused microcephaly, skull defects, blindness, and many other anomalies, and it is of course dose- and time-dependent. For these reasons, therapeutic irradiation is no longer practiced during pregnancy. Moreover, because of the uncertainties of the effect of ionizing radiation upon fetal development, it is good practice to abstain from pelvic and abdominal roentgenography during pregnancy as much as possible. Moreover, the effect upon the fetal gonads must be borne in mind, there being no doubt that the mutation rate is increased by the cumulative effect of radiation.

It is also possible that natural background irradiation and notably that caused by atomic reactions has a deleterious effect upon embryonic development. A large epidemiologic study in New York of the occurrence of significant malformations correlates these specifically with geologic strata. Thus, consistently higher rates of anomalies were found in regions where the geologic background leads to increased levels of local radiation acquired perhaps via the ingestion of drinking water.

THE OBSTETRIC MANAGEMENT

Considerable dimension has been added to the management of teratogenic diseases through the advances in intrauterine diagnosis (see Chapter 10). Many conditions may require decisions as to advisability of the continuation of pregnancy.

When any malformation or genetic condition is suspected and identified, preparation of the parents prior to delivery leads to a more ready acceptance of the situation at the time of birth. It is usually best to give the husband a detailed explanation, and

the mother should understand at least some of the facts as they are.

The more common gross fetal deformities encountered prenatally are hydrocephalus and anencephaly, and both may be suspected on the physical findings and verified by x-ray examination of the abdomen. The latter examination will also identify conjoined twins and abnormalities of the skeleton, including deformities of the spine, achondroplasia, and osteogenesis imperfecta (fragilitas ossium) (Fig. 2). Microcephaly is occasionally suspected from x-ray evidence but even at birth when the head size is borderline, caution must be exercised in drawing any conclusions concerning the possible diagnosis of this condition (Fig. 3).

Owing to the enormous size of the fetal head, hydrocephalus is generally detected by palpation prior to labor and readily demonstrated by x-ray examination (Fig. 4). When the cervix is 3 cm. or more dilated, the fontanelles will be found abnormally large on vaginal examination and the suture

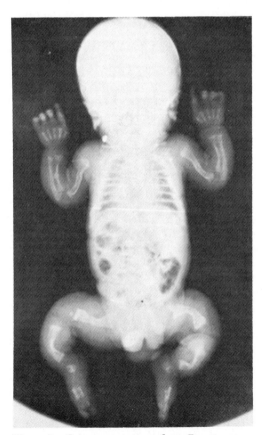

Figure 2. Osteogenesis imperfecta. Roentgenogram at birth shows presence of both old and new fractures. Note healing of spontaneous intrauterine fracture of left radius.

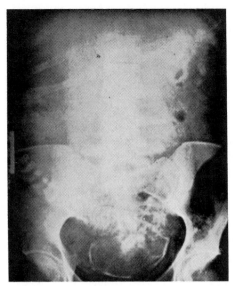

Figure 3. A microcephalic fetus, subsequently delivered alive.

lines widely separated, presumably from the pressure on the brain tissue exerted by the large amounts of intraventricular fluid. Characteristically, the bones of the calvarium are parchment-like in consistency, although they may vary markedly in this respect. Frequently spina bifida, with or without a meningocele or meningomyelocele, is an associated anomaly.

Anencephaly is one of the more common gross malformations and is characterized

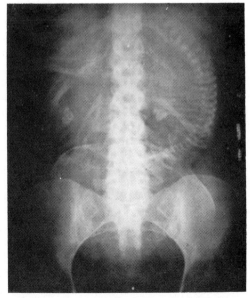

Figure 4. Roentgenogram showing hydrocephalic fetus.

by failure of skeletal enclosure of the brain. It is often associated by vertebral disturbances and may present as craniorachischisis, an open state of skull and spinal canal. Although central nervous system tissue was once normally present, it has degenerated because of the lack of osseous protection. The principal basic defect thus lies in the bony development, and not that of the brain. As a consequence the pituitary and adrenal glands are hypoplastic, and when polyhydramnios does not eventuate in premature labor, the pregnancy often terminates past term. The anomaly is often suspected in midpregnancy because of the frequency of marked hydramnios. One is unable to locate a cephalic pole. Compression by the examining hand of one of the fetal poles may produce a marked fetal bradycardia, apparently from pressure on the exposed medullary center of the anencephalic vertex. This is a useful diagnostic sign. X-ray examination is definitive in identifying the anomaly (Fig. 5). Hydramnios is also a frequent warning sign in cases of tracheoesophageal fistula and duodenal atresia.

Certain radiographic criteria have been suggested to establish whether twins may be conjoined. These include: (1) the heads are at the same level and plane; (2) in case of ventral fusion, the spines are usually in backward flexion; (3) in dorsal fusion, the spines are in close proximity; and (4) there is no change in the positions of the fetuses with movement, manipulation, or time.

In cases of hydrocephalic and anencephalic fetuses, the question arises whether the patient should be permitted to await the onset of labor, or whether intervention is warranted and preferable. In either type of malformation, complications of labor and delivery are frequent. When polyhydramnios coexists, if the membranes rupture prior to or early after the onset of labor, the sudden release of amniotic fluid may result in some placental detachment. Also, with rupture of the fetal membranes and the loss of their hydrostatic effect, the cervix may not dilate to permit pelvic delivery. In the anencephalic fetus, because of its contour, the head fails to fit snugly against the cervix, while in the hydrocephalic fetus, the large head is often unable to enter the pelvis and contact the cervix; in both instances the result is unproductive labor. In anencephaly, the pregnancy often continues for several weeks

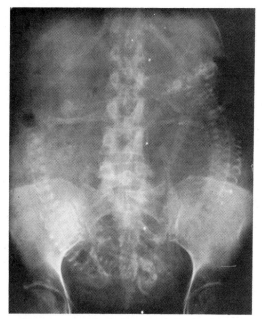

Figure 5. Anencephaly revealed by roentgenography. Twin pregnancy. Normal twin on patient's left side; anencephalic twin presenting.

beyond term, adding to the patient's emotional discomfort. It also raises the interesting speculation as to what the fetus may or may not contribute to the etiology of labor.

In the hydrocephalic fetus, the vertex may be decompressed by removing the excess cerebrospinal fluid. This requires that the cervix be at least 2 to 3 cm. dilated so that the appropriate needle can be introduced through the calvarium into the ventricles. After this procedure pelvic delivery is anticipated. When decompression has been accomplished, and with the cervix completely dilated, the vertex may be delivered spontaneously, by forceps, or by cranioclast, depending on circumstances (i.e., whether the fetus is alive or dead) and preference. With the cervix 2 or 3 cm. dilated and the membranes intact, an alternate procedure is to perform a Braxton Hicks version *after* the vertex has been decompressed, and allow breech delivery.

With conjoined twins, unless the infants are small enough to permit pelvic delivery, cesarean section is justified. The obstetric dangers in the delivery of such monsters must not be minimized, for, once the patient is committed to pelvic delivery, the procedure may lead from one difficulty to another unless the fetuses are dead, in which event embryotomy may avoid maternal trauma, including uterine rupture.

Other anomalous conditions that may give rise to obstetric difficulties are polycystic kidneys, various tumors of the abdomen, atresia of the urethra with markedly distended bladder, and sacrococcygeal teratoma. These latter malformations usually are not recognized before labor, but rather when the second stage is reached and delivery is attempted.

Besides the malformations that may cause dystocia, others that are recognizable or suspected at birth demand the obstetrician's immediate concern. These are the congenital defects that should receive early surgical attention, including cases of atresia of the esophagus, nearly all of which are in effect a tracheoesophageal fistula, imperforate anus, omphalocele, and extensive hernia of the diaphragm with displacement of the viscera into the thorax.

Certainly cyanosis and respiratory distress, together with the physical signs elicited on examination of the infant's chest, should arouse the suspicion of the presence of a large diaphragmatic hernia, with the diagnosis being established by an immediate x-ray. The thoracic cavity will be seen to contain some of the abdominal viscera, the amount depending on the size of the diaphragmatic defect. An imperforate anus may be recognized on the initial physical examination at the time of delivery, or the diagnosis may await the failure of the infant to pass meconium, or the obstruction may be found when an attempt is made to take the newborn's temperature. Omphalocele, a large umbilical herniation, is obvious at birth. A tracheoesophageal fistula is likely if there appears to be excessive salivation. In fact, when the newborn infant is first suspended at delivery for the purpose of clearing the nasopharynx, an excessive amount of fluid should arouse suspicion of the presence of this lesion. Should copious amounts of fluid exude from the nose and mouth when the infant is suspended a second time, further diagnostic procedures are mandatory, for early recognition of the anomaly is requisite to successful surgical correction. A small catheter passed into the esophagus will be met with obstruction, for in nearly all of these cases the upper esophagus ends in a blind pouch; the diagnosis can be confirmed by x-ray.

More common malformations that are identifiable, but in which surgical therapy is not urgent but may be indicated at some later date, include meningocele, meningomyelocele, harelip and cleft palate, clubbing of the feet, malformation of the appendages, congenital hydrocele, undescended testicles, and varying degrees of hypospadias or epispadias. A variety of skin lesions may be seen, many of which are referred to as birthmarks. It should be realized that some of these lesions are not evident at birth, but appear after the baby has left the hospital. Hence, if such is not recorded in the infant's hospital physical examination, it does not necessarily mean that the physician failed to recognize the lesion.

The question of whether the newborn's feet may be clubbed is occasionally raised, for the normal position of the feet in utero is that of a varus attitude with the plantar surfaces approximating each other. The two more common forms encountered are talipes equinovarus, with a downward and inward rotation of the foot due to shortening of the Achilles tendon, and talipes calcaneovalgus, with an upward and outward rotation as the result of gastrocnemius muscle paralysis.

Meningocele and meningomyelocele may be difficult to differentiate. In the former, the outlook is favorable; but in a meningomyelocele, the decision to attempt surgical correction will depend on the extent of the neurologic deficit, which in turn will be influenced in no small measure by the level or location of the defect. Thus, the obstetrician must give a guarded prognosis until the situation has been carefully evaluated by a neurosurgeon.

Other congenital anomalies may be suspected at birth. Failure to establish respirations in an otherwise normal infant, particularly when labor and delivery were normal, together with finding that the breath sounds are inaudible, should raise the question of pulmonary hypoplasia. In infants who prove to have cyanotic heart disease the question of the diagnosis may be raised soon after birth. It is a startling experience to witness a recently delivered infant who, having been well oxygenated at birth via the placenta, becomes cyanotic within one or two minutes after birth, even though he is respiring normally. Such an infant is likely to have a tetralogy of Fallot or some other form of congenital cyanotic heart disease.

The diagnosis of renal agenesis begins with the finding of oligohydramnios or almost total lack of amniotic fluid, which may be accurately ascertained provided the fetal membranes remain intact until after the patient enters the hospital; otherwise it must rest on the patient's history. The infant at birth has a peculiar appearance, with a flattened nose and a receding chin, and the ears, which are incompletely developed, are located somewhat lower than normally. In classic cases the amnion has a granular surface owing to the presence of numerous foci of debris; this is called amnion nodosum.

The cause of enlargement of the abdomen may run the gamut from a variety of tumors, including polycystic kidneys, to a distended bladder from urethral stricture. Further diagnostic procedures are needed after the infant has left the delivery room before the exact condition can be established. As with the congenital anomalies that may become evident later, the responsibility for the diagnosis and treatment of these conditions should be shared with the pediatrician and the pediatric surgical consultant.

An important clue to the early detection of anomalies is also provided by careful inspection of the cut surface of the umbilical cord. Normally two arteries and one vein are present; in 1 per cent of newborns, however, only one artery is found. This vascular anomaly is often associated with other visceral defects which have to be carefully searched for. Approximately 30 per cent of such babies will have one anomaly or another, some of which may require surgical correction at once.

Ambiguous development of external genitalia requires immediate and complete investigation. The condition most feared is familial adrenal hyperplasia, the "adrenogenital syndrome." Because of the hereditary (recessive inheritance) absence of an enzyme in the adrenocortical pathway leading to cortisol, infants with this condition lack a cortisol-pituitary feedback mechanism. Consequently, from perhaps as early as the 10th week of development an excessive amount of fetal ACTH drives his adrenal, which produces steroids, some of which are androgenic. In female fetuses this leads to clitoral hypertrophy and occasionally to fusion of labia (labioscrotal fusion). The small scrotum does not contain testes, and indeed the internal female genital organs are normal. Diagnosis begins with the identification of ambiguous external genitalia and proceeds promptly to an assessment of chromosomal sex by the search for Barr bodies in mucosal scrapings and lymphocyte culture. The elevated amounts of ketosteroids in the urine confirm the diagnosis and lead to institution of cortisone replacement therapy to prevent the neonatal crisis of adrenal insufficiency which otherwise occurs by the second or third week of life. In male infants the diagnosis is more difficult, there being only slight macrosomia of external genitalia.

Numerous sex chromosomal errors have minor or major developmental errors as one expression and an attempt should be made to make the diagnosis as soon as possible even though little therapeutic help can be rendered at this time. Of parenthetic interest in this respect may be the condition known as testicular feminization, or male pseudo-hermaphroditism. The external genitalia are female but slight clitoral hyperplasia may be present and bilateral inguinal hernias exist. In the hernia canals are situated the inguinal testes. This hereditary disease is manifest only in males, the karyotype being a normal 46,XY. Because of the inability of pubic areas to respond normally to fetal testicular androgens, the external genitalia remain female, the müllerian ducts undergoing atrophy. Individuals with this condition fail to develop sexual hair and remain amenorrheic and sterile. Nevertheless they often marry and lead otherwise normal female lives.

When the infant with an anomalous condition survives, the parents will expect an explanation regarding the immediate prognosis, the ultimate mental and physical status of the child, and what should be planned for its future medical care and management. Thus, the obstetrician should have some familiarity with the surgical procedures and the pediatric care of children with these various deformities. Patients tend to incriminate themselves and often attempt to relate the development of the malformation to something they may or may not have done. These ideas should be dispelled by the physician.

The question of the desirability of further pregnancies will eventually arise. After a careful review of the family history, in an effort to uncover genetic factors, and after eliminating any possible event in the pregnancy that might have contributed to the malformation, the discussion will turn to the general health of the parents. In recent years genetic counseling has become more than establishing a family tree, and is acquiring scientific exactitude. Repeated amniocentesis in the course of pregnancy has added substantially to diagnosis, and

indirectly to what may be the proper method of management of the pregnancy.

BIBLIOGRAPHY

Benirschke, K., and Hoefnagel, D.: Structural development of the placenta in relation to fetal growth. In Waisman, H. A., and Kerr, G. R., eds.: Fetal Growth and Development. McGraw-Hill Book Co., New York, 1970.

Carpenter, P. J., and Potter, E. L.: Nuclear sex and genital malformation in 48 cases of renal agenesis, with especial reference to nonspecific female pseudohermaphroditism. Amer. J. Obstet. Gynec., 78:235, 1959.

Carr, D. H.: Chromosomal errors and development. Amer. J. Obstet. Gynec., 104:327, 1969.

Carter, C. O.: Polygenic inheritance and common disease. Lancet, 1:1252, 1969.

Carter, T. C., Lyon, M. F., and Phillips, R. J. S.: Genetic hazard of ionizing radiations. Nature, 182:409, 1958.

Dwyer, P. J., and Ripman, H. A.: Delivery of thoracopagus twins after intra-uterine separation with some anatomical details of the monster, by P. L. Williams. J. Obstet. Gynaec. Brit. Emp., 66:437, 1959.

Fraser, F. C.: The genetics of cleft lip and cleft palate. Amer. J. Hum. Genet., 22:336, 1970.

Fraser, F. C., and Pashayan, H.: Relation of face shape to susceptibility to congenital cleft lip. A preliminary report. J. Med. Genet., 7:112, 1970.

Gentry, J. T., Parkhurst, E., and Bulin, G. V.: Epidemiological study of congenital malformations in New York State. Amer. J. Public Health, 49:497, 1959.

Gray, C. M., Nix, H. G., and Wallace, A. J.: Thoracopagus twins; prenatal diagnosis. Radiology, 54:398, 1950.

Kennedy, W. P.: Epidemiologic aspects of the problem of congenital malformations. In Birth Defects Original Article Series, Vol. 3. National Foundation, New York, 1967.

Lanman, J. T.: Delays during reproduction and their effect on the embryo and fetus. 2. Aging of eggs. New Eng. J. Med., 278:1047, 1968.

Lenz, W.: Thalidomide and congenital abnormalities. Lancet, 1:45, 1962.

Lock, F. R.: Human congenital anomalies—some current concepts. Obstet. Gynec., 20:867, 1962.

Marin-Padilla, M.: Morphogenesis of anencephaly and related malformations. Curr. Top. Path., 51:145, 1970.

Milunsky, A., Littlefield, J. W., Kanfer, J. N., Kolodny, E. H., Smith, V. E., and Atkins, L.: Prenatal genetic diagnosis. New Eng. J. Med., 283:1370, 1441, 1498, 1970.

Töndury, G.: Embryopathien. Über die Wirkungsweise (Infektionsweg und Pathogenese) von Viren auf den menschlichen Keimling. Springer-Verlag, Berlin, 1962.

Trasler, D. G.: Pathogenesis of cleft lip and its relation to embryonic face shape in A/J and C57BL mice. Teratology, 1:33, 1968.

Warkany, J., and Kalter, H.: Congenital malformations. New Eng. J. Med., 265:993, 1046, 1961.

Worcester, J., Stevenson, S. S., and Rice, R. G.: 677 congenitally malformed infants and associated gestational characteristics; parental factors. Pediatrics, 6:208, 1950.

PART IV

Clinical Obstetrics

Chapter 23

Diagnosis and Conduct of Pregnancy

DIAGNOSIS OF PREGNANCY

The possibility of pregnancy must always be considered when one is evaluating symptoms in the female during the childbearing age. At the same time, when pregnancy seems likely, one should not quickly assign to this cause the commonly accompanying symptoms of lassitude, malaise, nausea, vomiting, and sometimes lower abdominal and pelvic discomfort.

Amenorrhea, the absence or disappearance of the menstrual period, in patients whose menstrual cycles are regular is evidence of pregnancy until it is proved otherwise. Thus, in clinical situations in which pregnancy is suspected, one is concerned initially with differentiating this condition from other causes of amenorrhea. Amenorrhea could be the first symptom of a major medical illness.

Nonpregnant amenorrhea is of two types, primary and secondary. The former is the failure of the menses to occur prior to the 18th year of life, and secondary amenorrhea is the disappearance or cessation of the menses once they have occurred. The term secondary amenorrhea is often loosely used clinically, for it is commonly applied to patients who menstruate infrequently. Although infertility is more likely in such patients, they are not truly amenorrheic.

When not caused by pregnancy, amenorrhea is due to a disturbance in the pituitary-ovarian relationship and rarely to anatomic causes. The former cause is considered in the section on endocrinology.

Anatomically caused amenorrhea can appear as hematometra — accumulation of blood in the uterus — or as hematocolpos — accumulation of blood in the vagina. The former is due to a cervical stricture, either congenital or acquired as a sequela to trauma, infection, extensive cauterization, or some operative procedure on the cervix.

Hematocolpos results from the lack of an aperture in the hymen, with retention of the menstrual discharge at puberty. Besides absence of the menses, the presence of lower abdominal discomfort and a fluctuant suprapubic mass is characteristic of both conditions.

Another anatomic cause of amenorrhea is the absence of the endometrium. Here, one must visualize complete destruction of the endometrium by local disease or trauma. Irradiation might be included as a cause, but in this case the amenorrhea is due primarily to destruction of ovarian function and subsequent atrophy of the endometrium. Certainly in the presence of normal ovarian function only the smallest amount of endometrium is necessary to produce periodic vaginal bleeding.

Now referred to as Asherman's syndrome,* intrauterine adhesions, although infrequent, are the commonest anatomic cause for secondary amenorrhea. Following vigorous curettage, usually some weeks after abortion or term delivery, for excessive bleeding, intrauterine adhesions form that can lead to amenorrhea and sterility. Chronic endometritis and removal of the basal layer of the endometrium, in some areas at least, are factors in the etiology of the syndrome. The adhesions may be seen in the hysterogram (Fig. 1).

POSITIVE AND PRESUMPTIVE SIGNS IN THE DIAGNOSIS OF PREGNANCY

Of the physical signs in the diagnosis of pregnancy, the most useful is a softening of the uterus at the junction of the corpus and

---

*Jones, W. E., Amer. J. Obstet. Gynec., 89:304, 1964.

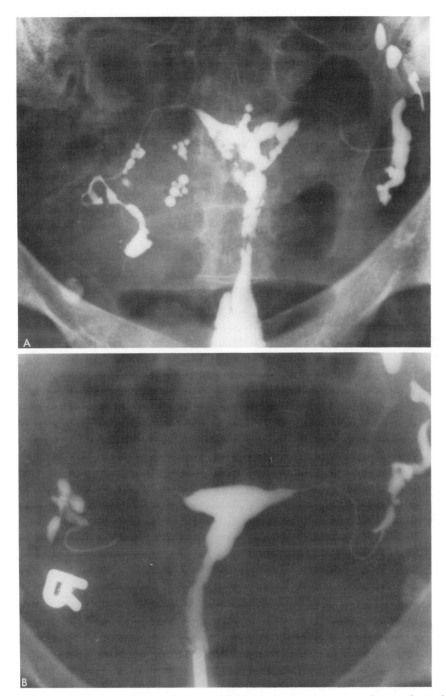

Figure 1. Asherman's syndrome. A, Intrauterine adhesions. B, Uterine cavity after mechanical rupture of adhesions. (Courtesy of Dr. Warren E. Jones.)

the cervix in the region of the uterine isthmus (Hegar's sign). This sign can be elicited usually within a week or two after the missed period (Fig. 2). Softening of the anterior portion of the corpus can also be detected early in pregnancy, and becomes more evident as pregnancy advances. Bluish discoloration of the vaginal epithelium (Chadwick's sign) is also a presumptive sign of pregnancy, but this may be observed in any condition causing pelvic congestion. At the onset, the breasts commonly are engorged

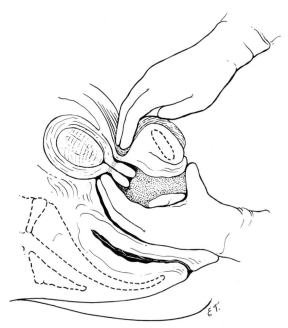

Figure 2. Hegar's sign; shaded area of the cervix is the isthmus.

and a clear liquid may be expressed from the nipples.

The fetal heart tones can often be detected as early as the 16th week by the head stethoscope and should be consistently heard by the 18th to 20th week of pregnancy. With the beginning of the last trimester, the fetus may be outlined and ballottement demonstrated. The latter is elicited when on vaginal examination the examiner's fingers experience the sensation of the return of the presenting part against the lower segment after it has been displaced by an upward thrust.

X-ray evidence of pregnancy can be obtained as early as the 14th to 16th week. An oblique view of the pelvis with the x-ray beam directed through the greater sacrosciatic notch (Fig. 3) will often reveal the fetus at an earlier age than will the routine anteroposterior view, in which the sacrum may obscure its shadow. Because of the undesirability of exposing the fetus to irradiation, x-ray diagnosis of pregnancy is used only when absolutely necessary. Indeed, this method undoubtedly will be replaced by the ultrasound method in diagnosis.

The biologic test for pregnancy may become positive within a week or two after the missed period (see endocrinology section). Basal body temperature, which

normally rises at the time of ovulation, remains slightly elevated for a time in early pregnancy and then falls, coinciding with the waxing and waning of the corpus luteum.

In summary, the positive findings in the diagnosis of pregnancy are the biologic test for pregnancy, the presence of the fetal heart tones, and x-ray visualization of the fetus. The presumptive signs include amenorrhea, Hegar's sign, and ballottement and palpation of the fetus.

The diagnosis of pregnancy in the earlier weeks may on occasion be uncertain for a variety of reasons. The most common of these is uterine retrodisplacement, which may not permit the examiner to outline the exact size and consistency of the uterus unless the corpus is replaced anteriorly. It is suggested that a pessary of the proper size and type be inserted and the patient asked to return for reexamination in one or two days, when the uterus is often found to be in an anterior position, which will favor a more accurate diagnosis.

Also, the conceptus may not be developing and growing normally, and consequently the uterine changes are so minimal that the diagnosis may be questionable. In addition, obesity of the patient, or her inability to relax her abdominal muscles and cooperate in the examination, will prevent the examiner from determining accurately the size, contour, and consistency of the uterus. Finally, other pelvic conditions may mask the presence of pregnancy. It is under these circumstances that the biologic test for pregnancy is more useful. Also, on occasion, a vaginal examination, with the patient anesthetized, may prove informative and, in fact, be required.

In the differential diagnosis of pregnancy, the clinician is concerned not only with determining whether the patient's symptoms are due to pregnancy, but also, if she is pregnant, with determining whether the pregnancy is normal. Thus, the differential diagnosis must include (1) deviations of the pregnancy from normal, and (2) diseases of the uterus, adnexa, and other pelvic organs. Included in the first category are normal intrauterine pregnancy with "implantation" bleeding; abortion, particularly associated with a blighted ovum; extrauterine pregnancy; pregnancy occurring in a congenitally anomalous uterus; and hydatidiform mole.

The primary concern in diagnosis is to assess the condition of a female patient of

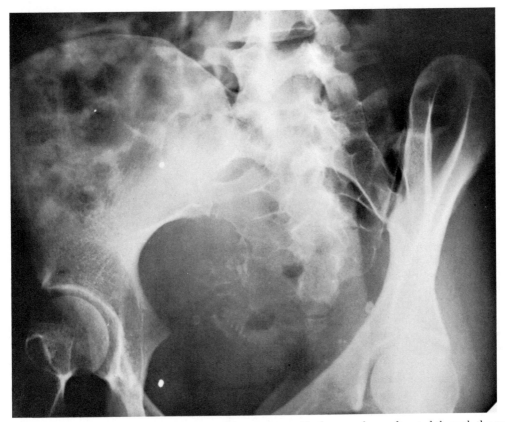

Figure 3. X-ray diagnosis of early pregnancy; oblique view, with the x-ray beam directed through the greater sacrosciatic notch.

childbearing age with amenorrhea when she is observed initially in the early weeks following a missed period. It is recognized that the ultimate diagnosis of the cause of the amenorrhea may depend on further observation and study.

If a generalization is permitted, it is essential that those patients with small amounts of vaginal bleeding or staining in the early weeks of pregnancy, who comprise 20 to 25 per cent of the total, should be followed carefully and deserve to be gently examined frequently to determine whether the pregnancy is normal. Subsequent examination should verify the fact that in over half of these patients, the uterus is enlarging at a rate compatible with a normal pregnancy. The remainder may eventually abort, or reveal the signs and symptoms of an ectopic pregnancy or, more rarely, a hydatidiform mole.

Further, the biologic test for pregnancy has diagnostic limitations and pitfalls. The test can be both falsely negative and falsely positive and altogether too much reliance

is placed on it in the diagnosis of pregnancy. Rather than rely on a laboratory test to exclude or diagnose pregnancy, as already suggested the physician should examine the patient at frequent intervals until he is convinced the patient is pregnant and that the pregnancy is normal, or that the situation demands further investigation.

When the uterus appears to be smaller than the gestational dates suggest, and even though the patient has not bled, a blighted ovum must be considered. In patients destined to abort, the conceptus usually fails to grow and the uterus to enlarge much beyond that of a six weeks' pregnancy. This is valuable information in a negative way, for should the patient develop the signs and symptoms of a threatened abortion, it is fair to assume the conceptus is abnormal and the patient should be treated accordingly (see Abortion).

Also, when the uterus appears smaller than gestational dates indicate, particularly in the presence of slight vaginal bleeding, one should consider the possibility of an ectopic pregnancy. Discomfort when the cervix is moved is regarded as an important finding. Tenderness in the adnexal region adds to the suspicion. Such a patient deserves careful attention, and if the signs and symptoms persist or progress, hospitalization is indicated (see Ectopic Pregnancy). To emphasize, the physician is truly guilty of neglect if he examines such a patient and fails to take every precaution to prevent the later occurrence of rupture in a tubal pregnancy. Culdocentesis as an office procedure to demonstrate free blood in the cul-de-sac is a useful procedure when positive, but the presence of a developing ectopic pregnancy is not excluded by a negative tap.

Pregnancy in an anomalous uterus may simulate a tubal pregnancy. Although the position of the round ligament is said to be a distinctive finding—medial to the mass in an ectopic pregnancy and lateral in the case of an anomalous uterus—this may be apparent only at laparotomy. Perhaps of more importance, it is conventionally thought that when the uterus is asymmetrically enlarged a pregnancy in an anomalous uterus or an intramural fibroid should be suspected. Not infrequently, in the early weeks of a normal pregnancy, the enlarging uterus feels asymmetrical at vaginal examination, presumably because implantation occurs somewhere away from the midline of the anterior or posterior uterine wall, the usual sites of implantation. The uterus will assume a symmetric shape by the end of the third month.

If the uterus appears larger than is normal for the gestational age and continues to enlarge at a rate that exceeds that of normal pregnancy, particularly if there is some bleeding, a hydatidiform mole is a strong possibility. The diagnosis is highly suggestive if fetal heart tones are not obtainable by any method in a uterus of the size seen after 16 to 20 weeks' gestation when the menstrual history is consistent with a pregnancy of three months. Absence of a fetal skeleton on x-ray is further strong evidence that the patient has a molar pregnancy and that hospitalization for further study is indicated (see Gestational Trophoblastic Disease). However, multiple pregnancy must be considered in such cases, the fetuses being too small to visualize by x-ray. It is in these situations that the ultrasonic Doppler cardioscope has practical useful-

ness by determining the presence or absence of fetal life, or again the ultrasound can assist in diagnosis.

Unquestionably the most common condition of the reproductive tract that causes a disturbance in the menses and raises the question of pregnancy is the steroid effect from a persistent corpus luteum and its failure to regress. Characteristically the menses is delayed for three or more weeks. On pelvic examination the uterus reveals no evidence of pregnancy and the involved ovary may actually be of normal size or slightly enlarged or cystic. Besides trying to decide whether the patient is pregnant, one must consider the silently developing ectopic pregnancy.

Other conditions involving the reproductive system which may lead to uncertainty in the diagnosis of pregnancy are uterine myomata and ovarian tumors. If the myoma is intramural or submucous in location, it may on vaginal examination simulate a pregnancy, or, in the early weeks, the tumor may mask the presence of pregnancy. In fact, a myoma in the early weeks may enlarge at a more rapid pace than the pregnant uterus and, at the same time, become exceedingly soft in consistency. When there is question as to whether a patient with uterine fibroid is pregnant, here is the one condition in which a biologic test for pregnancy is helpful, as is the Doppler technique and, on occasion, when in doubt ultrasound or x-ray examination to identify the fetus.

An ovarian tumor may disguise uterine enlargement in the early weeks of pregnancy and it might be difficult to differentiate it from a myoma softened by the increased vascularity of pregnancy. At the same time, ovarian tumors tend to become very mobile during pregnancy, and after the third month may often be displaced and found anywhere within the abdomen. The examiner may wonder whether he is dealing with a mesenteric cyst or some discrete abdominal tumor, and although further studies are indicated, in this age group the odds favor the diagnosis of an ovarian neoplasm. It is because of this increased mobility that an ovarian cyst is more prone to twist on its pedicle during pregnancy and create a surgical emergency.

In conclusion, the diagnosis of pregnancy on vaginal examination should be consistently and accurately made by the sixth week, or approximately three to four weeks after the missed period. The diagnosis may remain uncertain, at least by physical examination, for several weeks if the pregnancy is abnormal or if there is an associated pathologic condition of the uterus and adnexa; in the interim some patients should be followed closely and examined weekly until the physician is convinced that the pregnancy is normal or that the patient should be hospitalized for further study.

CONDUCT OF PREGNANCY

The medical supervision of pregnancy ideally should begin prior to conception, for, were it possible to take a complete history and perform a physical examination on the prospective mother before the onset of pregnancy, one could make a more intelligent appraisal of her medical status. A vaginal examination is also much more informative when performed on the patient prior to pregnancy, for the gravid uterus may conceal the nature and extent of any pathologic condition of the pelvis. Moreover, should such a condition be encountered, it might well demand surgical correction, and even the simplest abdominal operation performed after conception has occurred adds some degree of risk to the continuation of pregnancy. Thus, the worth of a so-called preconceptional examination must be emphasized, in the realization that most women who are contemplating a pregnancy have never been advised regarding its value.

Further, a well conducted obstetric program affords an unusual opportunity for the practice of preventive medicine, for disease may be recognized and either eradicated or controlled, so that complications that ordinarily might be expected to arise in later life can be avoided. From information derived during her prenatal supervision, the mother should become more aware of the value of preventive medical measures in maintaining the health of the family unit.

Ideally, patients should begin their prenatal care within two or three weeks after the missed period. Many patients, however, postpone seeking medical care until the third or fourth month of pregnancy, and, although in most instances little harm accrues, early prenatal medical supervision is desirable if certain of the complications of pregnancy are to be avoided or correctly treated.

Since the first prenatal visit is often the initial medical experience for many primiparous patients, it is natural for some to exhibit a degree of apprehension which a sympathetic attitude and gentleness in approach will usually dispel. Moreover, pregnant women are, in general, the most cooperative of all patients, principally because of the almost universal desire to do all they can for the unborn child. Even in the patient with an unwanted pregnancy, this attitude often comes to the fore as the pregnancy advances.

Understandably, a good deal of the patient's attention and thoughts will be focused on her pregnancy. Foremost in the minds of most pregnant women are questions that can usually be placed in one of four categories. Of primary interest are those factors which may affect the fetus. The list is long and ranges from the influence of vaginal bleeding to the effect of travel and household activities. Secondly, some patients are interested in the actual birth process. This may be explained to them without undue emphasis or dramatic detail. In addition, admission to a hospital may be a new experience for some pregnant patients, and they wish to know about the nursing procedures necessary to prepare them for labor. Finally, the majority of patients are interested in how the physician proposes to give them relief from the discomfort of labor.

Pregnancy offers an opportunity for attaining emotional maturity, and it becomes a period for recognizing and discarding some of the less desirable attitudes the patient may have had toward her social environment. Under medical guidance, it is possible for the patient to gain greater insight and emotional stability through the experience of pregnancy. It is within the ability of any sympathetic and understanding physician to identify and, through discussion, resolve most of the patient's personal problems. It is emphasized, however, that most women are calm and more emotionally stable in pregnancy, and, for some, life appears purposeful for the first time.

Patients exhibit greater degrees of uneasiness at certain times of pregnancy than at others. It is an impression that patients complain more of insomnia and, in general, are more irritable at or about the end of the seventh month, and, although not necessarily related, this is the time when physiologic changes appear to reach their maximum. It is a further impression that patients become more complacent as term approaches. Proper obstetric management must, therefore, consist of the regulation of the life and activities of the pregnant patient to conform with the changing tempo of both her metabolic and her emotional needs.

MEDICAL AND OBSTETRIC HISTORY

The history-taking follows the conventional pattern and should include a complete past and family history, an inventory by systems, and a detailed obstetric résumé. The latter should place emphasis on the menstrual history, evidence of infertility, and a careful inquiry into previous pregnancies. The menstrual history is principally concerned with determining the probable time of the onset of pregnancy by ascertaining the last normal menstrual period. Sometimes the last period is difficult to establish with certainty, particularly in patients whose periods vary in interval, duration, and quantity of flow. Not infrequently a patient may date the beginning of her pregnancy from a period that on careful questioning may have amounted to only slight vaginal staining. Justifiably, it may be concluded that the last normal period was undoubtedly some weeks prior to this particular episode. In such instances, the validity of the menstrual history will rest on the findings at vaginal examination. Under these circumstances, the gestational size of the uterus must take precedence over the menstrual history in the dating of the pregnancy.

The past obstetric history must be detailed to the point where the patient can be considered completely normal, or to the other extreme where her case must be set apart as a special obstetric problem or a pregnancy at high risk. Problems of infertility must be correlated with many variables, including the age and the parity of the patient and the history of previous obstetric disasters. A previous stillbirth is obviously important as it has relevance to pregnancy toxemia, Rh incompatibility, difficult labor, or any of the other complications that may have been responsible for the fetal death. The history of previous hypertension and proteinuria, premature labor, and uterine bleeding must be related to the period in pregnancy when these signs and symptoms were recognized. The time in gestation when labor occurred, its duration, the type of delivery, any complications, and the weight and the sex of the baby should be recorded routinely for all previous pregnancies. The indications and conditions surrounding operative deliveries, particularly with respect to forceps rotation, midforceps, breech extraction, and cesarean section, must be carefully reviewed and evaluated. An inquiry should be made regarding the postpartum course of both the mother and the infant, and the latter's subsequent well-being.

In eliciting the symptoms of the present pregnancy, inquiry must specifically be made as to the presence or absence of vaginal staining and whether the patient has experienced any pelvic discomfort. Although German measles (rubella) is the only infectious disease definitely known to produce disastrous effects on the fetus, one should inquire if the patient has been exposed to or has had any other viral or bacterial infection. In retrospect, this may be valuable information should the infant reveal evidence of malformation. Only by this means will it be possible to know the role that infection may play in the causation of malformations.

By tactful interrogation, the history-taking may prove to have therapeutic benefits as well. A previous illegitimate pregnancy or illegal abortion may have created many fears and phobias or a state of self-incrimination and guilt in the mind of the patient. The present pregnancy, if unwanted, may have led to the taking of abortifacients, causing the patient great anxiety and an unwarranted fear that the fetus may have been damaged by the drugs ingested.

PHYSICAL EXAMINATION

The physical examination is general and is not complete without the examination of the ocular fundi, the elicitation of the more important neurologic reflexes, and a rectal examination. The examination of the chest and heart deserves special consideration in pregnancy. Rather loud functional murmurs are frequent, whereas pathologic murmurs are softened and less easily detected.

The breasts should be very carefully palpated and a record made of the location and extent of any mass. A clear, watery secretion may be expressed from the nipples, but, except in primiparous patients, is not necessarily a sign of pregnancy, for this fluid may remain in the breasts for months following a delivery. At the time of examination of the breasts, the value of breast feeding may be suggested to the patient. Certainly if the patient's breasts and nipples are normal, it is an opportune time to impress upon her that she is probably capable of carrying out this function.

In the examination of the lower extremities, the venous pattern should be carefully recorded at the initial visit, since varicosities tend to appear or extend during pregnancy.

Vaginal Examination

In the early months, the purpose of the vaginal examination is to establish the diagnosis of pregnancy and to determine the presence or absence of pelvic or adnexal abnormality or disease. At a later time, preferably between the sixth and eighth months of pregnancy, one can measure and evaluate the obstetric pelvis. By then, the pelvic tissues have become more relaxed, the uterus is mainly an abdominal organ, and the presenting part of the fetus has not yet entered the pelvis. The pelvic cavity is thus comparatively empty, making it possible to palpate more easily the sacral promontory and the other pelvic landmarks without discomfort to the patient. Also, the patient is more accustomed to being examined and is less likely to be apprehensive.

The vaginal examination should always be performed with the patient on an examining table and in accordance with accepted techniques. The information gained by the examiner will be in direct proportion to the degree of gentleness of the examination.

Before proceeding, the physician must be certain that the patient is aware that a vaginal examination is to be performed, and for what purpose. For some women this means that the physician must explain the general information he seeks.

The vaginal examination should be performed systematically: inspection (Fig. 4) followed by palpation. Bluish discoloration of the vaginal epithelium from venous engorgement (Chadwick's sign), although commonly observed in pregnancy, is not regarded as pathognomonic and has little diagnostic value. After inspecting the vulva and describing any local lesions, the physician asks the patient to hold her breath, strain, and bear down for the purpose of demonstrating loss of urine from stress incontinence and the presence or absence of procidentia, and of urethrocele, cystocele, rectocele, and possibly enterocele formation. In addition to noting the presence or absence of such lesions, the examiner should observe whether the perineum is anatomically intact or lacerated.

Cytologic studies or screening for cervical cancer is now a routine in prenatal care. The speculum is inserted free of a lubricant that might contaminate the squamocolumnar junction and interfere with obtaining a meaningful cervical scrape. Next the cervix is inspected for local lesions in the form of occlusion cysts (nabothian cysts) of the endocervical glands, cervical ectropion or erosion, and endocervical or decidual polyps. By direct inspection, any cervical or vaginal lacerations are verified and their extent is more accurately assessed. If the cervix shows a suspicious lesion, besides the cytologic examination, Schiller's test and, if need be, a cervical biopsy are in order. Decidual and endocervical polyps are frequently seen, but their extremely low incidence of malignancy contraindicates their routine removal during pregnancy unless they bleed excessively, which rarely occurs. Rather, they tend to regress during the course of pregnancy and are seldom present after delivery.

Skene's ducts are next palpated by sweeping the index finger of the examining hand from right to left beneath the distal portion of the urethra; when infected, the ducts and the surrounding tissues become thickened and indurated, and an outward stripping

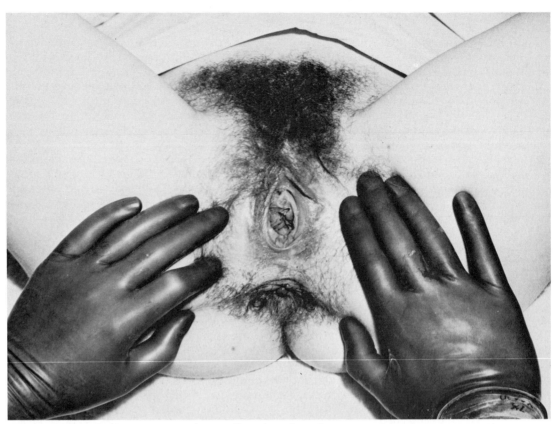

Figure 4. A multiparous patient with a small urethrocele and some scarring and relaxation of the perineum. A small hemorrhoid is visible.

motion along the duct may cause pus to exude from the gland orifice. Located off the midline near the posterior fourchette and deep within the perineum, Bartholin's glands normally are not palpable but become readily so when infected. The record should contain a reference to the fact that Skene's ducts and Bartholin's glands are negative to examination when this is so.

In performing the bimanual portion of the vaginal examination, the examiner should remember that the posterior portion of the vagina is less sensitive than the anterior. To avoid discomfort to the patient, the examining fingers should enter the vagina in sequence and not together. The second finger is first introduced through the introitus in the region of the posterior fourchette and the perineum depressed sufficiently to allow the ready insertion of the index finger (Fig. 5). In so doing, pressure on the sensitive areas, the anterior vagina, the clitoris, and the urethra, will be minimized. When dyspareunia or painful sexual intercourse is a symptom, the anatomic status of the hymen, scar tissue

formation about the introitus from previous lacerations, and the rigidity of the perineum should be noted.

The examiner now locates the position of the cervix, most commonly found in the area of the posterior fornix. When the cervix is located anteriorly, beneath the bladder and behind the symphysis, the cause is usually retroversion of the uterus. Otherwise, it is the result of a pathologic condition in the posterior cul-de-sac, displacing the cervix forward; but here the corpus is in an anterior position in contradistinction to its posterior position in retroversion. The consistency of the cervix should be elicited and pregnancy changes in the form of softening should be evident, including Hegar's sign. If present, the location and extent of cervical lacerations and vaginal scarrings, particularly of the lateral fornices, should be carefully described. It should be determined whether the lacerations involve the lower cervix only or extend upward to the vaginal fornix or the lower uterine segment. The amount of scarring or the extent of the lacerations in the cervix and vaginal vaults

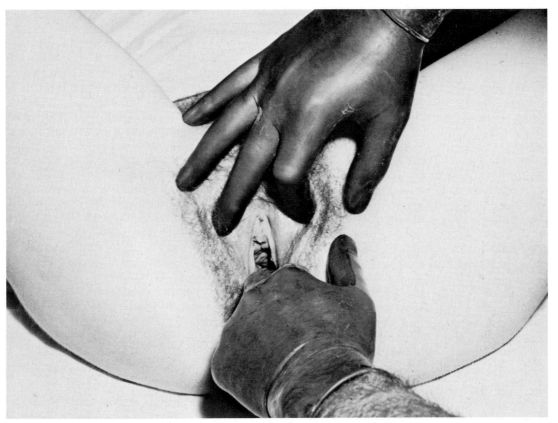

Figure 5. Middle finger has been introduced into the vagina and the perineum depressed. Index finger can now enter the vagina without causing pressure against the anterior portion of the vagina.

may dictate the type of delivery and furnish corroborative evidence of a history of previous difficult deliveries.

The next step is to outline the body of the uterus through bimanual examination and to describe its position, size, shape, consistency, and mobility. On palpation, the uterus often gives the impression of being softer and more prominent in one area, presumably where implantation has occurred. At this time the organ may have an asymmetric contour, but by the 8th to 10th week of pregnancy, with continued growth of the conceptus, the uterus regains its symmetry. In the interim, the possibility of a bicornuate uterus, cornual pregnancy, or uterine fibroid must be kept in mind. It should also be noted whether the uterus is consistent in size with the stage of pregnancy, a most helpful observation in the patient's management should she subsequently bleed and threaten to abort.

The clinical diagnosis of pregnancy in the early weeks is less accurate when the uterus is in a position of retroversion.

Under these circumstances the insertion of a Smith-Hodge type of pessary of the correct size will aid both diagnostically and therapeutically. Directing the cervix backward into the posterior fornix with a pessary is mechanically sufficient in most instances to cause the corpus to move forward. Reexamination even within one or two days after the insertion of the pessary will often disclose the corpus of the uterus in an anterior position, allowing for a more accurate diagnosis. This is by all odds the most comfortable method for the patient in correcting this common condition and is less traumatic and probably safer than bimanual replacement of the uterus into an anterior position.

Examination of the adnexa will normally reveal the ovaries near the lateral walls of the pelvis, freely movable, and somewhat tender to examination. Extending lateralward from the uterus and along the upper margin of the broad ligament, the normal oviducts are barely palpable. The parametrium, an area between the anterior and the posterior sheath of the broad ligament, is normally soft and pliable.

Rectal and Rectovaginal Examination

The physical and obstetric examination should include a rectal examination to evaluate the integrity of the perineum and the competence of the rectal sphincter, to detect the possible presence and extent of a rectocele, and to rule out any pathologic condition of the rectum. A rectovaginal examination may occasionally be indicated, consisting of the simultaneous introduction of the middle finger into the rectum and the index finger into the vagina. This examination allows ready palpation of the cul-de-sac and the lateral fornices, and is especially helpful in outlining and assessing the extent of any pathologic condition in the region of the rectovaginal septum, as in the case of endometriosis or the identification of an enterocele and its differentiation from a rectocele.

LABORATORY EXAMINATION

The laboratory examination at the initial prenatal visit includes hemoglobin and hematocrit determinations and, when indicated, a blood smear and red blood cell count. Blood should be drawn for typing, Rh determination, and serology. In some areas where syphilis is prevalent, repeat serology testing at the seventh month is recommended. Hemoglobin or hematocrit determination should be performed routinely at the 32nd week of pregnancy since in some patients an anemia may develop that was not evident before that time. In the case of an anemia, sufficient time remains before term to treat the patient adequately without recourse to transfusion.

The urine is examined for albumin and sugar, and a microscopic study is made of the urinary sediment from a so-called "clean-voided" urine specimen. Pyelonephritis is a constant threat to the pregnant patient, but this may be minimized by avoiding catheterization whenever possible. Despite meticulous technique, urinary tract infection may follow catheterization and, although in most instances the infection is readily controlled, it can be the beginning of a chronic pyelonephritis. In pregnancy, erroneous conclusions may be made regarding the source of erythrocytes

in catheterized specimens, particularly near term. When the presenting part of the fetus impinges against the urethra and bladder, the forceful introduction of a catheter into the bladder may produce microscopic or macroscopic hematuria through local trauma.

The following technique is used in obtaining the specimen for culture as well as for microscopic examination. Patients are instructed to wash the labia and urethral orifice with Zephiran sponges. Following this, the patient is moved to a commode or stool chair and instructed to hold the labia apart and void a small amount, which is discarded. The remaining portion of the voided specimen is collected in a sterile basin and is used for the examinations. A colony count of 100,000 ml. is indicative of a urinary tract infection and the question arises whether the patient should be treated prophylactically.

CHEST X-RAY EXAMINATION

The evidence is clear that whenever chest x-ray examination has been routinely performed in pregnancy, a significant number of patients have been found to have previously unrecognized pulmonary and cardiac disease. In cases of pulmonary disease, an x-ray examination provides a record for comparative purposes should there be an exacerbation of the condition, either during pregnancy or in the postpartum period. Although the roentgenogram examination of the chest is acceptable, as a routine measure it is expensive and less practicable. These objections are removed by restricting the x-ray examination to those who exhibit a positive tuberculin test (tine test).

PRENATAL INSTRUCTION

Prenatal instruction should enumerate those items needed to maintain a state of physical well-being throughout pregnancy. Environmental conditions will determine in some measure the ability of the patient to adhere to the instructions. Inquiry must, therefore, be made into the extent of her household duties and family responsibilities, and how these could be lessened should it be deemed advisable.

Nutrition and Weight Control

Of the various items in prenatal care, the most important are proper nutrition and weight control. Although the obstetric literature may contain statements to the contrary, most clinicians believe that complications of pregnancy are enhanced by obesity and excessive weight gain.

In normal pregnancy the weight loss during parturition and the first week of the puerperium is approximately 15 to 17 lb. Consequently, for patients whose weight is ideal this is a permissible amount of weight to gain during pregnancy. During the first and second trimesters, the patient should not gain more than 8 lb., for she tends to gain more weight in the seventh and eighth months, despite the fact that the caloric intake is not changed appreciably. Presumably this is due to a normal acceleration in the retention of extracellular fluid. Normally patients can be expected to lose 2 lb. or more in the two or three weeks before the onset of labor. This loss in body water is referred to as a prelabor diuresis.

In the event that the patient begins to gain weight in excess of the norm, the physician must decide whether this is due to protoplasmic growth or abnormal fluid retention. The patient's daily fluid intake and the extent of her physical activity should be reviewed, and the presence or absence of edema ascertained. To encourage the patient to participate fully in the program of weight control, it is helpful to obtain a commitment from her as to what she desires to weigh following completion of the pregnancy. This places a demand on the patient to play a more definitive role in maintaining ideal body weight, and will also make her conscious of the value of weight control later in life. Table 1 lists the ideal weight according to height and body build for women.

Although the diet of the average pregnant patient is not critically deficient, studies have shown that many fail to meet the necessary dietary recommendations. Socioeconomic factors, as they may reflect nutrition, have been carefully and intensively studied. Considerable importance must be attached to poor nutrition, not only in pregnancy but more particularly during childhood and the growing years, and its resultant effect in causing obstetric complications.

TABLE 1. DESIRABLE WEIGHTS FOR WOMEN OF AGES 25 AND OVER[*]

Height (with Shoes on) 2-inch Heels		Weight in Pounds According to Frame (in Indoor Clothing)		
Feet	Inches	Small Frame	Medium Frame	Large Frame
4	10	92– 98	96–107	104–119
4	11	94–101	98–110	106–122
5	0	96–104	101–113	109–125
5	1	99–107	104–116	112–128
5	2	102–110	107–119	115–131
5	3	105–113	110–122	118–134
5	4	108–116	113–126	121–138
5	5	111–119	116–130	125–142
5	6	114–123	120–135	129–146
5	7	118–127	124–139	133–150
5	8	122–131	128–143	137–154
5	9	126–135	132–147	141–158
5	10	130–140	136–151	145–163
5	11	134–144	140–155	149–168
6	0	138–148	144–159	153–173

[*]Metropolitan Life Insurance Company, 1960.

It is reasonable to suppose that malnutrition of the mother may have an adverse effect on the growth and development of the embryo and fetus. In the experimental animal, marked fetal abnormalities have resulted when the maternal stores were depleted of essential nutrients such as riboflavin. Also, teratogenic effects have been produced by a lack of vitamins A and E, and of pantothenic and pteroylglutamic acids. The fetal tissues are apparently more sensitive to the omission of these factors than are the maternal tissues, for in certain of the above deficiencies the maternal organism appeared outwardly normal although the fetus died in utero. Yet there is no real proof that malnutrition causes abnormalities in the human fetus. Actually, should malnutrition exist in the human comparable to that which was sufficient to cause fetal abnormalities in the experimental animal, conception would probably not occur owing to the resultant upset in the pituitary-ovarian function. It has been repeatedly observed in times of famine that amenorrhea is frequent and a state of relative infertility exists among the female populace.

When certain generally accepted nutritional standards for the mother are not fulfilled, however, there are measurable differences in the weight, the length, and the condition of the osseous system in the infant at birth. These studies are based on a careful record of the mother's food habits prior to and during pregnancy. According to their protein content, the diets were graded *good, fair, poor,* or *very poor*. The correlation between the caliber of the diet and the infant's weight, length, and general condition is shown in Figure 6. Besides these physical differences in the newborn, it was also believed that the incidence of toxemia and other obstetric complications was less in patients who had the benefit of a good diet, as defined.

An analysis of tissues of stillborn fetuses and infants dying soon after birth has furnished further evidence that an interrelationship exists between maternal diet and fetal nutrition. A correlation has been found between the vitamin A, riboflavin, and ascorbic acid content of the fetal liver and the maternal intake of these vitamins.

The question of limiting weight gain during pregnancy has recently been challenged by the reporting that the prematurity rate is lower in patients who gain in excess. The differences were more impressive when these patients were compared with underweight patients. Before conclusions are drawn, food intake data must be assessed and other variables considered such as prepregnancy weight in relation to body height and build. Actually, it has been

appreciated from carefully performed dietary intake studies already referred to (Fig. 6) that in underweight patients and those who failed to gain in pregnancy, the weight of the newborn is below the norm. It is evident that metabolic balanced studies are needed in many situations in pregnancy— for example, in the dysmature syndrome, repetitive premature labor, and the underweight patient.

Certainly it is unwise for the underweight patient to restrict her weight gain to the conventional 15 or 18 lb., assuming also that the daily food intake contains 90 grams of protein or more. But to accept weight gain when it might be in the form of increased extracellular fluid would be equally unwise and will result in increased incidence of pregnancy toxemia and other pregnancy complications.

Clinical evaluation of the patient's nutritional state is derived from the dietary history, the physical examination, and laboratory studies. In addition to listing the patient's food pattern, the dietary history should contain an appraisal of how her socioeconomic status may influence her nutrition. Certainly the diet may be poor because of faulty food habits and not necessarily as the result of a limited food

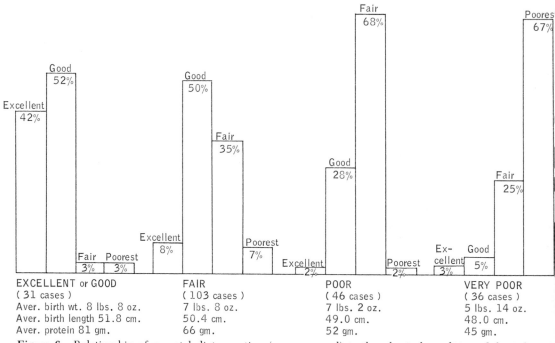

Figure 6. Relationship of prenatal dietary rating (mean general) to the physical condition of the infant at birth (four maternal dietary groups, 216 cases, first series). (From Burke, B. S., Stevenson, S. S., Worcester, J., and Stuart, H. C., J. Nutr., 38:453, 1949.)

budget. When there is flagrant nutritional deficiency, the findings at physical examination usually parallel the dietary history. The value of laboratory data in demonstrating a nutritional deficiency has limitations, and, for general clinical purposes, the hemoglobin content and total protein concentration of the blood are the most useful gauges in confirming the patient's nutritional status.

The nonpregnant adult is reputed to use 30 to 80 per cent of her total caloric intake for muscular and bodily activity. If the pregnant patient rests periodically and is less active in the last trimester, one would assume that her caloric requirements would be less. The caloric requirements will vary, therefore, with individual patients, depending on their particular life situations.

The prenatal patient whose weight is not ideal at the onset of pregnancy deserves special consideration. The underweight patient may be encouraged to gain up to 25 lb. or more. One must be certain, however, that the additional weight gain is not the result of an abnormal extracellular fluid retention. Patients who are overweight at the onset of pregnancy and in whom the dietary history indicates ample nutritional stores can afford to gain little or no weight during pregnancy. This aim can be accomplished by meeting the recommended requirements of essential nutritional substances and restricting the total caloric intake. Certain doubts may arise in the minds of these overweight patients as to the propriety of such a dietary régime, and they may question the effect of such extreme weight control on the development and eventual birth weight of the baby. It has been demonstrated that obese patients could lose 20 lb. or more during pregnancy without adverse effect to the pregnancy, while the weight and physical status of the newborn were well within the normal range. Moreover, if birth weight is influenced by maternal weight gain, it is related more to the last trimester of pregnancy, which coincides with the period of greatest fetal growth. Evidence for this belief is gained from a study conducted on the European continent near the end of World War II under conditions of near famine. It was shown that mothers who were in the last trimester of their pregnancy at the time when food became available in adequate amounts delivered infants whose birth weights were within the normal range. Some caution, however, must be exercised in the nutritional management of the overweight woman whose dietary history indicates a prolonged subminimal intake of essential food elements. Under such circumstances the correction of nutritional deficiency is of prime importance, while restriction of caloric intake must receive secondary consideration. Before a dietary prescription is formulated, therefore, the patient must be evaluated on the basis of her body weight and stature, individual energy requirements, the condition of her nutritional stores, the possible presence of underlying vascular, renal, or metabolic disorders, and the course of previous pregnancies.

On the basis of the above information, the physician may prescribe a diet containing 1700 to 3000 calories, depending upon the requirements of the individual patient. A basic 2000–calorie diet containing the essential food elements may be supplied in the amounts of 90 grams of protein, 90 grams of fat, and 200 grams of carbohydrate. The high protein intake is deemed necessary for fetal growth and the excess for maternal nitrogen storage for successful lactation. Meats, milk, and eggs provide not only protein but also inorganic constituents and vitamins or accessory food substances. For example, one slice of beef liver will supply 6 mg. of iron and 10,000 international units of vitamin A. Although there are no standards available for the fat intake requirements during pregnancy, nutritional principles require that at least 25 per cent of the total caloric intake be in the form of fats. Fats do serve as vehicles for the transport and absorption of fat-soluble vitamins (A, D, E, and K).

In the obese patients with adequate nutritional stores, it is unwise, particularly in pregnancy, to prescribe a diet of less than 1500 calories. The reduction in calories under that recommended for normal pregnancy would be at the expense of carbohydrate and fat intake. Before deciding the amount of carbohydrate in the diet prescription, some consideration must be given to the part it plays in the nutritional economy. The prevention of acidosis and ketosis requires the oxidation of at least 100 grams of glucose, and, in view of the pregnant patient's tendency to develop renal glycosuria and metabolic acidosis, the daily carbohydrate intake probably should never be curtailed below 150 grams. Recent studies yet to be reported indicate that carbohydrate is a major source of energy. (See Chapter 11, Anatomic and Physiologic Changes of Pregnancy.) The protein-sparing action of carbohydrate may also aid in increasing the maternal nitrogen stores during pregnancy. A diet containing 90 grams of protein, 150 grams of carbohydrate, and 60 grams of fat will allow the obese patient to lose weight and at the same time will meet her nutritional requirements.

FLUID AND ELECTROLYTE REQUIREMENTS. Pregnant patients often complain of thirst, particularly those who subsequently develop toxemia. Some attention, therefore, must be given to the patient's water and electrolyte intake. The daily water requirement of a normal nonpregnant adult subsisting on a diet of 2000 calories is approximately 3000 ml. The solid portion of the diet contributes 800 to 1000 ml. of water to the daily intake, when the ideal diet for pregnancy contains a high percentage of fruits and vegetables. The fluid intake in pregnancy, in the absence of sweat-

ing, need not exceed 2000 ml. daily. However, loss of up to 3000 ml., or some three times that lost normally through the skin and lungs, can occur in excessive sweating. The fluid and salt intake must be regulated accordingly.

To maintain the isotonicity of the approximate 6-L. increment in the volume of the extracellular fluid compartment in pregnancy, the body must retain 20 grams of sodium. In order to fulfill this requirement, the pregnant patient need accumulate only 0.1 gram of sodium per day. The average adult daily diet contains 3 to 8 grams of salt. It seems permissible, therefore, to adjust the diet in pregnancy so that it contains 2 to 4 grams of salt or 0.8 to 1.5 grams of sodium. A sudden gain in body weight or the appearance of gross edema calls for immediate review and, if necessary, drastic restriction in the sodium intake. The patient should be aware of foods with a high salt content and be cautioned to avoid adding salt to her food.

Supplementary iodine may be indicated in areas where goiter is endemic. This requirement is normally fulfilled, even when salt containing iodine is markedly reduced. The dietary standard for calcium

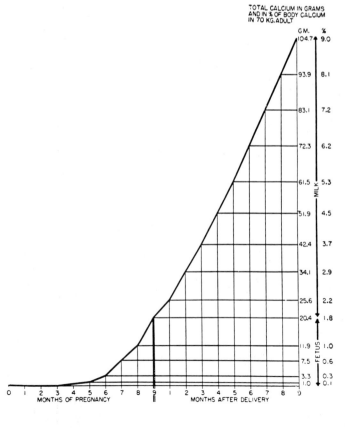

TOTAL CALCIUM IN GRAMS
AND IN % OF BODY CALCIUM
IN 70 KG. ADULT

Figure 7. Maternal loss of calcium during pregnancy and lactation. Note that calcium loss does not become appreciable until the seventh month of pregnancy; note also that the amount of calcium lost during nine months of lactation is more than four times that lost during pregnancy. (Data from Best and Taylor, 1940; Shohl, 1939; and Holt and Howland, 1922. *In* Albright, F., and Reifenstein, E. C., Jr.: The Parathyroid Glands and Metabolic Bone Diseases Williams & Wilkins, Baltimore, 1948.)

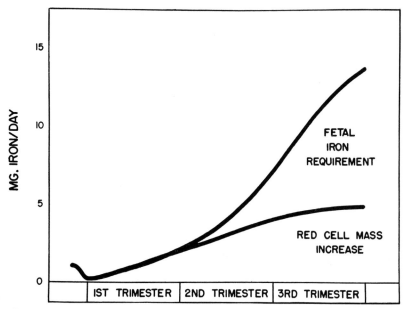

Figure 8. Daily maternal iron requirements during the various trimesters of pregnancy. (From Rath, C. E., Caton, W., Reid, D. E., Finch, C. A., and Conroy, L., Surg., Gynec. Obstet., 90:320, 1950.)

requirements during pregnancy is increased to 1.5 grams daily, with a further increase to 2 grams in lactation. A quart of milk will furnish 1.2 grams, so that, together with other protein in the diet, there is no need for supplementary calcium. To equal the amount of calcium in a quart of milk, however, some 4 to 6 grams of calcium lactate is required. As can be seen in Figure 7, the comparative amount of calcium deposited in the fetus is small, so that the additional calcium intake is directed toward meeting the subsequent demands of lactation. Besides, calcium in considerable amounts can be lost in the urine during prolonged periods of lactation.

The recommended increase in the daily iron intake is from 12 mg. in the nonpregnant to 15 mg. in the pregnant patient. As stated earlier, the bulk of the iron, in common with other minerals, is deposited in the fetus during the last three months of pregnancy, causing the iron requirements to rise (Fig. 8). Because iron deficiency is frequent, supplementary iron seems indicated for most patients during pregnancy. Folic acid supplement (5 mg.) should be considered routine in areas where macrocythemia is frequent.

VITAMINS. The water-soluble vitamin requirements for pregnant patients have been established at approximately 20 per cent above those for nonpregnant persons. Although often destroyed in the prepara-

tion of foods, vitamin C is supplied in sufficient quantities when there is a reasonable intake of raw fruits and vegetables. Vitamin B complex deficiency in pregnancy has been observed in this country only in prolonged hyperemesis gravidarum. However, in world areas where endemic beriberi exists, pregnancy may precipitate an exacerbation. In mothers with beriberi, apparently the newborn may also be afflicted.

The recommended requirements for the fat-soluble vitamins, A, D, E, and K, during pregnancy are likewise increased. When butter is being withdrawn from the diet for purposes of weight control, the intake of fruits and vegetables as sources of provitamin A or carotene should be high. Vitamin D or calciferol, essential to calcium-phosphorus absorption and metabolism, is seldom lacking in physiologic amounts for, although the diet may contain little vitamin D, ergosterol, a major source of the vitamin, is present in the skin and is activated by the ultraviolet light of sunshine. To ensure an adequate intake in the diet, most of the milk marketed is fortified with at least 400 I.U. of vitamin D to the quart, the estimated daily need. Raw, unfortified milk is still consumed in some localities, however, and under these circumstances it is conceivable that the vitamin D intake might be critically reduced if the patient were confined indoors.

In the experimental animal, fetal death and irreversible sterility have been produced by vitamin E deprivation, but no such effect has been known to occur in the human. Since the average diet contains large amounts of vitamin E, it is difficult to accept the belief that pregnancy accidents may be the result of a deficiency of this vitamin. Except when there is failure of absorption, there is no need for supplementary administration of vitamin K in pregnancy. Although vitamin K crosses the placenta readily, the fetus may not store the vitamin. It seems fair to conclude that when diets meet only subminimal standards or there is malabsorption syndrome, supplementary vitamins should be administered, but certainly there is no clear indication that they need be given routinely during the prenatal period.

In the prenatal patient who is thought to be storing excess extracellular fluid, as evidenced by abnormal weight gain or visible edema, recourse should first be taken to the palliative effect of bed rest and restriction of dietary salt. As is commonly observed in patients in this category, diuresis will frequently occur with loss of several pounds in 24 hours through the therapeutic effect of these simple measures alone.

Diuretic drugs have long been used as an adjunct to this therapy. Because of the availability of diuretics that can be prescribed with reasonable safety for ambulatory patients, these agents are being used as weight-control measures and sometimes for long periods of time. In the normal pregnant patient, as in the nonpregnant, diuretic drugs have the same value and limitations. These limitations include the development of a refractory state, metabolic acidosis, and electrolyte depletion. If diuretic drugs are to be utilized, they probably should be given for brief periods only, not to exceed three or four days.

Whenever control studies have been done, the thiazides when used prophylactically have not reduced the incidence of pregnancy toxemia. The more disturbing fact is that reliance is placed on these drugs for the purpose of weight control, rather than requiring the patient to restrict her activity and salt intake. The patient who gains in excess should have her weight and blood pressure checked weekly or biweekly and her dietary habits carefully reviewed. All too often the patient is given a diuretic rather than prenatal care and asked to return in a few weeks. By the time she returns or before, the patient may have an irreversible toxemia demanding immediate hospitalization.

By contrast, the patient who is carefully followed and gains excessive weight despite regular biweekly prenatal visits and instruction is either not following the régime as outlined or is developing a toxemic state despite it. The two situations may be readily differentiated by three or four days of bed rest and observation, preferably in the hospital. It is suggested that this approach, combined with a diet high in protein, is responsible wherever there has been a decrease in the incidence of pregnancy toxemia.

Drugs, Smoking, and Activity

The tragedy of thalidomide has reinforced the belief that extreme caution must be exercised in the administration of pharmacologic agents to a pregnant patient. Actually, in evaluating drug safety in pregnancy, the question is posed whether animal testing is sufficient to permit the use of drugs so studied to be used in human pregnancy. In fairness to the controversy, at the experimental level, in most instances comparatively large dosages are required to produce measurable effects on the fetus. However, iron, folic acid and vitamin supplements, and phenobarbital are the only agents required for most patients, and even these can be postponed until after the period of organogenesis.

The list of drugs that potentially might harm the fetus is endless. Anomalies and retarded development have been attributed to certain of the tranquilizers, cortisone acetate, sodium aminopterin, methotrexate, and chlorambucil. Tetracyclines administered to the mother are known to inhibit bone growth and cause discoloration of the teeth in the fetus. Chloramphenicol given to the mother may result in accumulation of the drug in the fetus and cause death shortly after birth, the result of bone marrow depression.

The long-acting sulfonamides may compete with bilirubin for albumin-binding, with serious consequence to the central nervous system from the free bilirubin. Neonatal bleeding from salicylates in large amounts has been reported from bishydroxycoumarin (Dicumarol). Thiazide diretics may result in thrombocytopenia in the newborn. Recently aspirin has been added to the list of causes of platelet adhesiveness in the mother and a bleeding tendency in the newborn.

Hence, in the administration of any drug or agent to a pregnant patient, it is well to ask the question whether the medication is truly necessary. No better example is found than the case of fluoridation; prenatal exposure to fluoride apparently does not reduce the incidence of dental caries in the deciduous teeth and permanent molars. The caries-inhibiting effects of this medication may be administered postnatally.

Vaccinia has been encountered in newborns, and fetal death is reported in patients initially vaccinated during pregnancy. Revaccination is probably without harm, but vaccination during pregnancy is best delayed. Certainly when live viruses are involved the immunization should be postponed in the first half of pregnancy. This would apply to poliomyelitis vaccination, in which a transient viremia is common. (See Chapter 30, Medical and Surgical Diseases in Pregnancy.)

Smoking has also been indicted as a health hazard in pregnancy, and all of the pharmacologic effects of nicotine must be considered. With the greater affinity of hemoglobin for carbon monoxide than for oxygen, theoretically extensive smoking would reduce the amount of oxygen available to the conceptus. Directly proportionate to the number of daily cigarettes, a doubling of the prematurity rate has been recorded in smokers when compared to nonsmokers. If there is controversy about the prematurity rate, there appears to be agreement that the infants of mothers who smoke weigh less than the infants of nonsmoking mothers. It obviously follows that patients with high-risk pregnancies should not smoke, and pregnancy is a particularly suitable time to discard the habit. One cannot help being impressed by the numbers of relatively young women who smoke excessively and have evident respiratory discomfort. These patients should be identified and if they continue to smoke should be subject to periodic x-ray examination of the chest. Also, they are at risk with respect to inhalation anesthesia. Briefly stated, prenatal care provides an excellent opportunity to emphasize the laws that govern health and a state of well-being.

It may appear paradoxical to the pregnant patient that she will tend to gain unduly if she is physically overactive. Excessive activity can lead to fluid retention, a common clinical observation. At the beginning this additional extracellular fluid may be restricted to the lower extremities and is not necessarily pathologic but eventually it may well become generalized. This is not to say that patients should not indulge in some exercise, but they should avoid long shopping tours and exhausting physical activity. One or two hours of rest is advisable during the day, particularly in the last trimester. Patients will frequently inquire as to the advisability of participating in sports. Although tennis, bicycling, and horseback riding should not disturb the pregnancy, it is perhaps best to avoid these because of the dangers of tripping or falling and the resultant possibility of severe lumbosacral and sacroiliac disability, to which the patient is more susceptible during this period when the ligaments supporting these joints are relaxed.

Until the last two months of pregnancy, the normal patient may travel at will, and the mode of transportation can be of her choosing. In patients with a history of previous abortions and premature labor, common sense dictates that they restrict their activity as part of preventive therapy but, at the same time, there is no convincing evidence to indicate that travel increases the incidence of spontaneous abortion.

General Instructions

The skin requires no special attention during pregnancy. Showers or sponge baths are preferable to tub baths in the later weeks of gestation to prevent the remote possibility of intrauterine infection. It is conceivable that water might enter the vagina, and, were the membranes to rupture or the patient to enter labor a few hours later, the chance of uterine infection might be increased.

It is a commonly held view that the teeth are more vulnerable to dental caries during pregnancy. There is evidence to refute this contention, however; the teeth are not demineralized during this or any other period of life. At the same time, the gingiva becomes soft and hypertrophic and may bleed easily from the slightest trauma. It is essential that dental caries and apical abscesses be recognized during pregnancy and treated promptly. The presence of pregnancy is no contraindication to the performance of dental procedures, and ideally the teeth should be checked and scaled at least twice during the course of pregnancy.

Although the breasts increase in size and weight and may require additional support, they demand no special care otherwise. Patients frequently inquire whether massage of the nipples and application of ointments will better prepare the breasts for nursing. Such therapy will not prevent fissures of the nipples, an occasional complication of breast feeding. Prepartal patients who are curious about such matters may inquire about the appearance of colostrum in the breasts which at times may be so copious that it stains the patient's clothing. No treatment is required, nor does its presence denote that the patient will necessarily lactate satisfactorily.

Sexual intercourse is permitted through the seventh month of pregnancy, but should be curtailed at this time because of the possibility of intrauterine infection should the membranes rupture or the patient enter labor soon after the act. Although some patients have the impression that intercourse at the time of the expected period is likely to cause an abortion, there is no evidence to support this view. The sexual desire during pregnancy may increase, diminish, or remain unchanged. In patients with high-risk pregnancy, condoms probably should be used to avoid the possible effect of seminal prostaglandin initiating premature labor.

The clothing during pregnancy need not be unusual. More important, in order not to impede venous return from the lower extremities, the stockings should be held in place by a garter belt and not by round garters. Except for the occasional patient, maternity corsets are not useful—why immobilize the muscles of the back and abdomen? Further, corsets detract from the patient's general appearance and they rarely relieve her discomfort. Hyperextending the back sometimes gives relief to patients who complain of backache in the lower region of the scapulae, and in such a case the maternity corset finds its greatest usefulness. Attention must be given to the feet in the causation of postural discomfort, and flat-heeled shoes are recommended to avoid tripping, a marked tendency during pregnancy.

PRENATAL VISITS

Prenatal visits are scheduled every three to four weeks during the first and second trimesters, at one to two weeks during the seventh and eighth months, and preferably weekly in the last month of pregnancy. At each prenatal visit the patient should be weighed, her blood pressure taken, and the urine examined for albumin and sugar. Periodically a hemoglobin or hematocrit determination should be done, and reference has been made to the desirability of repeating all of these tests at or about the 32nd week.

The patient should be questioned at each visit regarding vaginal bleeding, bowel habits, headaches, visual disturbance, edema of the face and hands, abdominal distress, discomfort on walking, bleeding gums, the degree of fetal activity, uterine irritability, respiratory infection, and the amount of rest and sleep that she is obtaining. An explanation should be sought for a weight gain in excess of ½ lb. per week. Specifically, this requires a review of the patient's diet, salt intake, and physical activity. In the patient who fails to follow prenatal instructions, a sobering effect is usually produced by insisting on weekly or biweekly visits for a time. If excessive weight gain is the problem, she can be reminded that should this continue there is a greater chance that toxemia will develop, requiring hospitalization. A systolic blood pressure of 140 or a diastolic blood pressure of 90 mm. Hg or a combination of the two in pregnancy is regarded as abnormal. With the tendency toward hypotension in normal pregnancy, an increase in the blood pressure of 10 mm. Hg, even if it falls within the range of normal, has significance. For these patients, and certainly for those with edema, the blood pressure and weight should be checked at frequent intervals. The patient should understand the importance of the vital signs and symptoms of toxemia and the hazards of bleeding in the last trimester.

At each visit the abdomen is palpated to ascertain that the uterus is consistent in size with the gestational age, that the fetal heart tones are present with a normal rate, and in the last trimester to establish the presentation. The fetal heart tones should be consistently heard by the 18th to 20th week. The uterine souffle, the rate of which is synchronous with the maternal pulse, may be so loud as to interfere with auscultation of the fetal heart. Detection of the fetal heart in the early months is facilitated by exerting a slight downward pressure with the examining hand over the fundus of the uterus, thereby displacing the small fetus upward toward the stethoscope. As the pregnancy progresses and the fetus attains polarity, the fetal heart is best heard in the area where the infant's chest or shoulder approximates the anterior uterine wall. Confirming the presence of the fetal heart tones is reassuring to the patient as well as to the physician.

The rather recent introduction of the ultrasonic Doppler cardioscope to clinical obstetrics has proved useful. The Doppler effect is produced by the change in frequency of sound waves, and the recorded frequency change will indicate the source of the movement producing the change. Alterations in the ultrasound are received by transducer and monitored through a suitable amplifier. By this method one can detect fetal life by the 12th to 14th week of pregnancy. It is equally definite in excluding fetal life, as in missed abortion, hydatidiform mole, and fetal death in utero.

The fetal heart rate is approximately 140 beats per minute, with 120 to 160 beats per minute regarded as the normal range. During an otherwise normal pregnancy, however, fetal heart rates of 200 beats or more per minute have been heard on routine abdominal examination, with the infant being quite normal at birth. Fetal heart rates as low as 60 to 70 beats per minute have also been detected in the course of a prenatal examination, but here the prognosis must be guarded, for congenital heart disease with heart block is a more likely possibility. Fetal systolic murmurs are audible at times, but, unless they are extremely harsh and loud, are generally unimportant.

The uterus is consistently palpable as an abdominal organ by the fourth month. For the purpose of establishing normal and abnormal rates of growth, the size of the uterus is recorded at each clinic visit. The age of pregnancy is expressed in terms of the assigned normal size of the uterus for the various weeks or months of gestation. Many clinicians prefer to record uterine growth by caliper measurement of the distance from the upper margin of the symphysis to the top of the uterine fundus, using the large Williams pelvimeter for this purpose. The size is expressed in centimeters. By palpating the fetus and the consistency of the uterus, a crude estimate is also made of the amount of amniotic fluid present.

In the last few weeks of pregnancy, particularly in a vertex presentation, the presenting part is likely to descend into the pelvis. This phenomenon, referred to as "lightening," occurs much more frequently in the primipara than in the multipara, for in the latter the abdominal muscles are often relaxed and only with labor does the presenting part enter into the pelvis. Having heard about this phenomenon, some patients hold the erroneous notion that labor will begin soon after the baby "drops," but not before.

External version should be considered if a breech presentation persists through the 35th week, and placental localization if the fetus is lying transversely at this period to identify or exclude a placenta praevia. Except in the latter instance, a rectal examination may be performed to verify the presentation and the status of the cervix.

The subject of vaginal examination is given considerable attention here, for the idea has been expressed that patients near term, or even in labor, may be examined vaginally with impunity and without exactitude of technique. Further, in recent years, elective induction of labor is being practiced with greater frequency. Besides depending on the expected date of confinement and the estimated size of the fetus, the day selected for elective induction of labor will be contingent on the status of the cervix. Regardless of the method used to initiate labor, its effectiveness will depend largely upon the degree of cervical effacement and dilatation, which can be determined more precisely perhaps by vaginal than by rectal examination. As an office or clinic procedure, however, the value and potential dangers of vaginal examination must be recognized. Under these semi-sterile conditions, invasion of the cervix by the examining finger to determine effacement and dilatation causes unavoidable contamination of this area of the birth canal, which is ordinarily relatively sterile. Although the mother may not reveal evidence of infection following the procedure, the question is asked whether the fetus may not become infected from fetal membrane contamination or amnionitis. It has been proposed that amnionitis may be the cause rather than the result of rupture of the fetal membranes prior to labor. Thus, in some patients this would invite premature delivery with its fetal hazards. It is concluded that vaginal examination in the latter weeks of pregnancy should be performed under sterile precautions. The same must apply in the conduct of labor.

Assessment of the Fetus in Utero

Assessing the status of the fetus in utero is an ever recurring problem in clinical obstetrics. In a variety of pregnancy complications where the fetus is at high risk, the advantages gained by premature delivery must be weighed against the risks of prematurity. Despite the relationship that exists between fetal age and fetal size, disparities occur and the practical question arises whether the fetus is growing at a normal rate. The problem is compounded when the validity of the last menstrual period is questioned. It is accepted that the ability of the fetus to survive in an extrauterine environment is determined more by gestational age than by weight. Once the 36th week of pregnancy has been attained, provided it is truly four weeks before term, extrauterine survival is comparable to that of the newborn delivered at the 40th week.

In addition to assessment of fetal maturity by roentgenographic evaluation of fetal bone age, examinations and tests of amniotic fluid and other means to determine fetal age are several, and the list is growing rapidly:

A. Amniotic fluid obtained by amniocentesis.

    1. Spectroscopic determination of bilirubin level: the test is based on the observation that the pigment disappears from the amniotic fluid rather abruptly around the 36th week. However, meconium and the presence of blood can influence the results.

    2. Creatinine levels: the creatinine content of amniotic fluid increases with fetal age; and maturity is regarded as assured when it reaches 2 mg. per 100 ml. However, exceptions to these levels limit the usefulness of this determination in decision-making, especially in patients with alterations in renal function, either temporary or permanent.

    3. Cytologic examination of the amniotic fluid: in the latter part of pregnancy measurable numbers of fat-staining cells appear in the amniotic fluid that differ morphologically from squamous epithelium. Thought to originate from sebaceous glands, these fat-laden cells are readily identified by a 0.1 per cent Nile blue sulfate solution. A fat cell count of less than 2 per cent of the total cells present is encountered prior to the 36th week or when the fetus weighs less than 2500 grams. After this period the numbers of fat cells increase and when they comprise 20 per cent or more of total cells examined, the fear of prematurity is reputedly no longer a consideration.

B. The recently introduced ultrasonic technique to determine the biparietal diameter of the fetal vertex shows great promise in determining both fetal age and rate of fetal growth. The measurements and their interpretation must be made by those familiar and working continuously with the method.

Although extrauterine survival is dependent on fetal maturity, this is only one side of the clinical coin; the other is the threat of death in utero and how to anticipate and avoid it. This is dependent on evaluation of the intrauterine milieu as it influences fetal growth and survival. In a sense the fetal environment is established indirectly by estriol assay, which measures the status of the fetoplacental axis, and human placental lactogen, which presumably reflects overall placental performance. Metabolic products of progesterone (urinary pregnanediol) could also be added to the list (see endocrinology section).

It is concluded that the current methods of determining fetal maturity become totally reliable about the 35th to 36th week of gestation, at least in the normal condition. The exception could be the measurement of the biparietal diameter of the fetal skull in the determination of fetal growth prior to this period, i.e., from the 28th week onward.

COMMON COMPLAINTS AND MINOR COMPLICATIONS OF PREGNANCY

During the first trimester of pregnancy, nausea and a sense of lassitude are the most frequent complaints of patients. The latter symptom is almost universally present, and nausea, with or without vomiting, occurs in over half of all pregnancies. The nausea of early pregnancy is often described as wave-like in character and is more apt to occur when the stomach is empty, as when arising in the morning, hence the term "morning sickness." If the nausea, with or without vomiting, continues after the ingestion of food, or is persistent after the first trimester, the possibility of hiatus hernia or some organic abnormality should be considered.

Although the cause of nausea and lack of energy of early pregnancy is unknown, there is a frequent tendency to interpret this condition as a neurotic manifestation. The idea that the patient should ignore her symptoms and become more active adds little to amelioration of the condition. Perhaps a more effective approach is to assure the patient that her discomfort is shared by the majority of pregnant women, and the symptoms represent a poorly understood physiologic adjustment to pregnancy, and these will disappear by the 10th or 12th week of pregnancy.

Many forms of treatment, including vitamins and various hormones, have been prescribed for the relief of the nausea of early pregnancy. There is no reason to believe that these substances have any specific influence in alleviating the symptoms. In the absence of definitive therapy, reliance must be placed on symptomatic treatment. Despite the newer drugs with tranquilizing and antispasmodic action, the most consistently effective and reliable drug seems to be phenobarbital, which can be given in doses of ½ grain in the mid-morning, the midafternoon, and usually an hour or two before bedtime. Unless given in excessive doses, this drug will not harm the fetus. Frequent feedings are helpful in decreasing nausea, and the patient should be encouraged to eat a small amount every two hours. These simple measures, combined with reassurance that the nausea will soon cease, will usually be sufficient to bring this symptom under control. The lassitude will end simultaneously, and the patient may feel more energetic than before she became pregnant.

Salivation is often increased during pregnancy and on occasion may become so excessive that it is decidedly uncomfortable. This abnormal state is often referred to as ptyalism. Although fortunately infrequent, when it does occur the patient is miserable. The patient will expectorate continuously and copiously, and the skin about the mouth may become excoriated. Atropine or similar drugs may be tried, but their results are far from satisfactory. The symptom dramatically disappears immediately with delivery.

Constipation is a frequent complication of both early and late pregnancy. Only the milder types of cathartics should be prescribed and an occasional enema resorted to when the constipation is severe. Because constipation is the rule in pregnancy, whenever diarrhea develops a diligent search should be made for its cause.

Owing to pressure on the bladder by the enlarging anteflexed uterus, frequency of micturition is a common complaint in the early weeks. This symptom tends to subside as the uterus becomes an abdominal organ, but may recur in the latter weeks of pregnancy, when the presenting part of the fetus begins to exert pressure against the bladder. Pressure about the internal sphincter of the bladder may cause urinary incontinence, which usually disappears with delivery. Because this may be confused with escape of the amniotic fluid after rupture of the fetal membranes, the patient requires careful observation to determine the source of the fluid.

During the third trimester, discomfort on locomotion is frequently experienced. This is more commonly about the symphysis, the sacroiliac joints, and the general area of the spine of the superior pubic ramus, and is usually precipitated by an attempt to rise quickly or to turn over when in a recumbent position. In addition, pregnant patients may develop backache and pain which is often referred to the region of the buttocks and down the thighs. Pain associated with muscle spasm is frequently present in the lower extremities, and patients will state that this cramplike sensation radiates even into their toes.

In these patients, one can often elicit considerable pelvic mobility and demonstrate by x-ray examination varying degrees of separation of the symphysis pubis and the sacroiliac joints. Although it is not always possible to relate the amount of discomfort to the demonstrable symphyseal separation, for occasionally there may be marked separation of the symphysis with very few associated symptoms, there is generally some correlation between the pain on locomotion and the degree of pelvic mobility.

Usually the symphysis pubis separates about 1 cm., but occasionally the separation is extreme.

Treatment in symphyseal separation is sometimes needed to relieve the local pelvic discomfort by immobilizing the pelvic joints and allowing the edema about the joints to subside. Personal experience has indicated that maternity corsets fail to prevent the development of discomfort from this source and give little aid in its relief. Rather, an easily made, inexpensive belt of heavy canvas, measuring some 8 inches in breadth posteriorly and 4 inches anteriorly, equipped with buckles, is helpful. When applying the belt, the upper margin should be placed at the lumbosacral junction posteriorly, allowing the belt to pass over the trochanters laterally and meet anteriorly over the symphysis (Fig. 9). When the belt is tightly drawn about the pelvis, the sacroiliac and symphyseal joints are brought back into normal alignment. After a few days of immobilization, combined with limited activity, the edema about the joints subsides, the patient is usually much more comfortable, and the belt may no longer be needed. Besides using the belt, the patient should sleep on a firm mattress reinforced by a bed board.

Noted more particularly on the right side, presumably because of the space-occupying effect of the liver, discomfort along the costal margins and the upper abdomen is common. This soreness and tenderness, due to pressure of the enlarging uterus, is probably aggravated by increased mobility of the ribs at their costochondral attachments. An unpleasant sensation in the upper abdomen seems to be more common in patients with breech presentation, probably because the presenting part is less likely to enter the pelvis until after the onset of labor.

Pregnant patients frequently complain of hemorrhoids, which are caused to a degree by the pressure exerted by the enlarging uterus and the resultant congestion of the pelvic veins. The treatment may include the application of cold compresses and various analgesic ointments; if constipation is present, measures should be taken to correct it. The pain may be so acute at times that opiates in some form may be required. In the extreme, it may be necessary for the patient to assume almost complete bed rest in order for the hemorrhoids to subside. The danger of pelvic infection contraindicates surgical removal during pregnancy; in fact, hemorrhoidectomy is best postponed until after the childbearing period, for a subsequent pregnancy may produce further hemorrhoids.

A vaginitis is often a minor complication of pregnancy and, although there are other causes, it is commonly due to either *Trichomonas vaginalis* or *Candida* (*Monilia*) *albicans*. The latter infections, commonly found together, are harbored by women

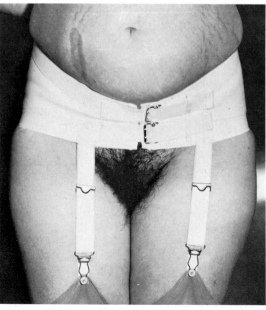 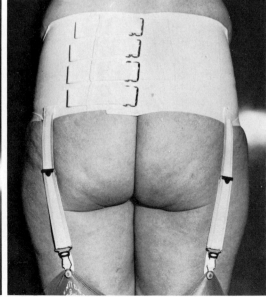

Figure 9.   Symphyseal belt in place.

who are often symptom-free except during pregnancy. Further, some patients during pregnancy may have a copious vaginal discharge from these infections and yet be relatively free from symptoms, whereas others complain bitterly of burning and a severe itching. With either type of infection, the discharge may occasionally cause the skin of the vulva and perineum to become excoriated.

In Monilia infection, the discharge has a characteristic white cheeselike appearance, and tends to adhere to the vaginal membrane; so distinctive is the vaginal secretion that it is generally unnecessary to resort to bacteriologic identification. In a Trichomonas infection, the discharge is typically foamy, and the vaginal epithelium contains small punctate, reddened areas. The ameboid organism may be readily identified by a fresh hanging drop preparation of the vaginal secretion.

Of the many types of treatment advocated for these forms of vaginitis, all are moderately successful in keeping the symptoms in abeyance, but it is doubtful that any are capable of cure. Topical application to the vaginal epithelium of gentian violet in 1 per cent aqueous solution will promptly bring a monilial infection under control. It has the advantage of avoiding the administration of pharmacologic agents in pregnancy. An antibiotic preparation derived from cultures of Streptomyces (Mycostatin) has also proved effective. Metronidazole (Flagyl) is apparently an effective method of treatment for a Trichomonas infection.

A mixed infection is not always evident clinically until after treatment has been instituted, for the discharge caused by the Monilia, which usually predominates, may conceal the presence of Trichomonas infection. With treatment for the Monilia, the vaginal discharge may assume the appearance consistent with Trichomonas infection. For some patients the form of treatment and the course of management must be changed to coincide with the prevailing type of infection.

The infant comes to no harm from either of these infections, except that it may develop thrush consequent to its exposure to Monilia during its passage through the birth canal. Also, the symptoms and the discharge, particularly in Monilia infection, frequently subside or disappear dramatically following delivery, suggesting a cause-and-effect relationship with the vaginal environment, possibly an alteration in the pH.

Incarceration of the Pregnant Uterus

On rare occasion (1:5000 pregnancies) a patient will develop symptoms of incarceration of the retroverted uterus in the earlier months of pregnancy. This is usually observed near the end of the fourth month, at a time when the uterus normally becomes an abdominal organ. The patient will be most uncomfortable, not from the incarceration, but rather as the result of her inability to void and the presence of a markedly distended bladder, which must not be mistaken for the uterus. Her history will reveal increasing difficulty in voiding, and even with straining she can release only a dribble of urine. The urinary retention is produced by pressure of the cervix against the bladder neck in the presence of an enlarged retroverted uterus.

The treatment obviously begins with catheterization of the patient with a small flexible catheter to avoid traumatizing the urethra. If vaginal or rectovaginal manipulation fails to dislodge the uterus, the patient should be hospitalized. With the patient anesthetized, manual replacement is usually successful. The literature reveals cases in which laparotomy was performed in order to bring the uterus out of the pelvis.

OBSTETRIC EXAMINATION AND MENSURATION OF THE PELVIS

From the time of Baudelocque in the 18th century until more recent times, it was believed that the size of the superior strait of the pelvis could be determined by means of certain external measurements. With the introduction of reliable methods of radiographic examination, it has been demonstrated that these bear no constant relationship to the size and shape of the pelvic inlet. Hence, external measurement of the inlet is no longer performed. Some patients continue to consider the taking of these measurements a necessary part of prenatal care. To avoid any misunderstanding on the patient's part, should she inquire, she is told why these measurements are not taken and is assured that, if there is any question about the adequacy of the pelvis, x-ray pelvimetry can be performed prior to or at the onset of labor.

After the physician performs a vaginal examination to determine the status of the patient's pregnancy, the obstetrically important anatomic landmarks of the pelvis are evaluated. It is preferable that the examiner train and use his less dominant hand to perform the examination, freeing the more adept hand for other manipulations if needed. Assuming that the examiner is right-handed, he would use the left hand to perform the vaginal examination.

In determining the pelvic architecture, the two fingers of the examining hand should first circle backward toward the sacrum. Palpating its anterior surface, reference is made to the contour of the pelvic curve

and the position and height within the pelvis where the sacrum terminates (Fig. 10A). Normally the sacrum may be described as having a normal curve to its anterior surface. It is positioned posteriorly, forming an angle of 90 degrees or more with the superior strait, and terminates at or below the level of the ischial tuberosities. (See Chapter 24, The Normal and Abnormal Obstetric Pelvis.) Together, these normal findings mean that the posterior segment of the pelvis has a normal capacity, and the pelvic bore is divergent from inlet to outlet. By contrast, the sacrum may incline forward, forming an angle of less than 90 degrees with the superior strait. Its anterior

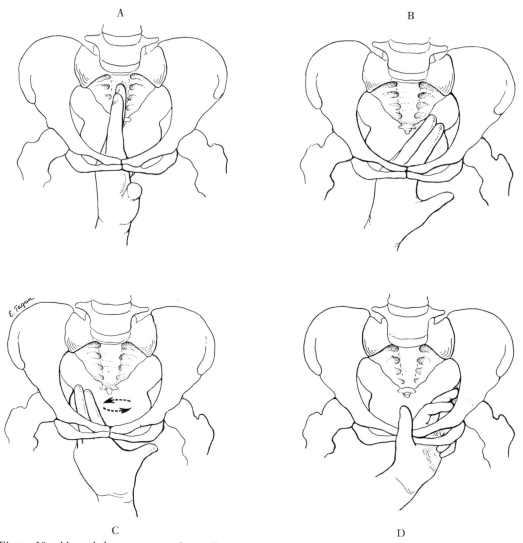

Figure 10. Manual determination of overall pelvic architecture. A, Determining the contour of the sacrum. B, Estimating the size of the sacrosciatic notch and the prominence of the ischial spines. C, Assessing the length of the bispinous diameter. D, Assessing the splay of the pelvic side walls.

surface may have little or no curve, and various areas may be extremely rough and irregular. The upper part only may be straight and the lower portion curved, or the reverse may be true. Further, the sacrum may end relatively high in the pelvis, not too distant below the level of the ischial spines. The above findings are consistent with a decrease in the normal capacity of the posterior segment of the pelvis with a pelvic bore that is convergent from inlet to outlet. The record, therefore, should contain a description of the length, the contour, and the position of the sacrum.

The examiner now locates the sacrospinous ligament by identifying its medial attachment to the sacrum above and adjacent to the sacrococcygeal joint. The examining fingers pass laterally along the inferior margin of the ligament until they come to rest on the ischial spine. The distance from the sacrum to the ischial spine affords an estimation of the size of the sacrosciatic notch, which is recorded in terms of 1, 2, or 3 fingerbreadths and is an index of the capacity of the posterior segment of the midpelvic plane (Fig. 10B). A distance of only 1 or 2 fingerbreadths between the sacrum and ischial spines denotes a forward-placed sacrum, whereas a distance of 2 fingerbreadths or greater is regarded as indicative of a normally placed sacrum.

The ischial spines are palpated to ascertain whether they are normal or unduly prominent. In some pelves the spines may have a broad base and are barely raised above the surface of the ischium, resembling the situation found in the subhuman primate. In the android pelvis particularly, the ischial spines may protrude one or more centimeters above their base and encroach upon the midpelvic plane. Although this is only an estimation, the experienced examiner can gain an impression of the length of the bispinous diameter by carrying the examining fingers across the midpelvis from spine to spine (Fig. 10C). X-ray pelvimetry has shown that should this diameter be less than 9.0 to 9.5 cm. (caused either by narrowing of the side walls, as in the occasional anthropoid pelvis, or by unusual prominence of the ischial spines, more commonly found in the android type) midpelvic contracture may exist. More specifically, if the sacrosciatic notch is less than 2 fingerbreadths and the bispinous diameter is decreased below 9.0 cm., a diagnosis of midpelvic contracture is warranted.

Before proceeding to measure the diagonal conjugate, some impression should be gained of the splay of the pelvis, a term used to denote the slope of the side walls of the pelvis as they extend from the iliopectineal line to the ischial tuberosities. Sweeping the examining finger over the lateral side of the vagina from the pelvic inlet downward, it may become apparent whether the bony side walls are normally straight or divergent or abnormally convergent (Fig. 10D). The latter, a so-called funneling effect, is consistent with possible midpelvic or outlet contracture.

The diagonal conjugate is now measured by bringing the examining fingers upward into contact with the sacral promontory. The patient should be told that, although this part of the examination may be uncomfortable, it lasts only a few seconds. During the examination it is important that the wrist, forearm, and index and middle fingers of the examining hand be kept in a straight line. This is more easily maintained if the examiner places his left foot on a low stool and rests the elbow of the examining hand on the inner aspect of his left knee, thereby providing a source of steady pressure necessary for his fingers to palpate the sacral promontory and anterior surface of the sacrum (Fig. 11). Further, a steady pressure offers less discomfort to the patient than intermittent pressure. When the second finger of the examining hand is felt to be touching the sacral promontory, the index finger of the right hand is used to mark the position on the left hand where it

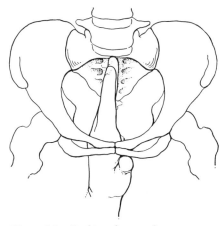

Figure 11. Seeking the sacral promontory.

touches the inferior margin of the symphysis. After the hand is removed from the vagina, the distance from the tip of the middle finger to the point where the hand contacted the symphysis is measured, and the value obtained represents the length of the diagonal conjugate (Fig. 12). The difference between the diagonal conjugate and the conjugata vera has been shown to vary from 1 to 3 cm. As will be noted, these differences are related to the width of the symphysis, and this must be taken into consideration when estimating the length of the conjugata vera. When the symphysis is unusually broad and inclined posteriorly, despite the fact that the diagonal conjugate may measure 11 to 12 cm. or more, the conjugata vera may be only 8.5 to 9.0 cm.

An estimation of the inferior plane or pelvic outlet begins by determining the width and the inclination of the symphysis (Fig. 13). Normally the width of the symphysis is 2.5 to 3.0 cm., but in heavily boned persons it is often wider. As previously stated, when the symphysis is unusually broad (more often a finding in the android type of pelvis), a normal diagonal conjugate of 12.5 cm. need not exclude the possibility of inlet contracture. Under these circumstances, the difference in length between the diagonal and true conjugates may be 3 to 4 cm. rather than the usual 1 to 2 cm. The inclination of the symphysis may likewise influence the size of the anteroposterior diameter of the superior strait. With the patient in the lithotomy position, the symphysis is normally tilted slightly posterior. On occasion the symphysis may be inclined more posteriorly so that its upper border encroaches into the superior strait and hence decreases the anteroposterior diameter sufficiently to produce inlet contracture (Fig. 14). The obstetric record should, therefore, contain some notation of the width and inclination of the symphysis.

In the remainder of the examination of the outlet, the patient should be placed in an exaggerated lithotomy position, for this allows the pubic arch to be more easily palpated. The pubic arch is outlined by touching the thumbs against the inferior margin of the symphysis with the palms of the hands flat against the patient's perineum and inner buttocks and thighs (Fig. 15A). The heels of the examiner's hands are now separated until the extended thumbs press firmly against the inner aspect of the pubic rami (Fig. 15B). The outline formed by the

two thumbs gives a visual impression of the shape of the arch, which is described as Roman or Gothic. More important for clinical purposes is whether the shape of the arch is such that it can be completely utilized by the fetal vertex. Consequently, the size of the subpubic angle and the flare of the pubic rami are the significant clinical features of the inferior plane, or the outlet.

The bi-ischial diameter affords some indication of the relative contour of the arch. It must be recalled that the lower portion of the pubic arch courses backward as well as laterally. If the examiner fails to appreciate this fact, he will make the mistake of measuring the bi-ischial diameter at some point along the arch (Fig. 16A), rather than from the ischial tuberosities. Such a measurement will obviously not represent the maximum width of the inferior plane. Tilting the pelvis forward by the extreme lithotomy position tends to avoid such a mistake by allowing the examiner to palpate more readily the ischial tuberosities. It will be found that the imaginary line connecting the ischial tuberosities, that is, the bi-ischial diameter of the outlet, will be situated approximately 1 to 2 cm. posterior to the anus. In the normal pelvis this diameter measures 9 to 11 cm.

This measurement is obtained by a specialized instrument, the Williams or the Thoms outlet pelvimeter. The former is a caliper, calibrated in centimeters, with rings attached at the ends. With the examiner's thumbs placed in the rings, the ends of the caliper are brought into contact with the inner surface of the ischial tuberosities, measuring the intervening distance, that is, the bi-ischial diameter (Fig. 16B). The Thoms pelvimeter permits simultaneous measurements of the bi-ischial diameter and the posterior sagittal diameter of the outlet (Fig. 17). The instrument has a sliding bar within a rod, both of which are calibrated in centimeters. An arm similarly calibrated is connected medially to the rod. The bi-ischial diameter is obtained when the outer ends of the bar and the rod are placed against the inner surfaces of the ischial tuberosities. At the same time, the posterior sagittal diameter can be measured by bringing the medial arm into contact with the sacrococcygeal joint. This diameter averages 7.5 to 8.0 cm.

The posterior sagittal diameter is measured equally well with a Williams pelvimeter by using some object to represent the

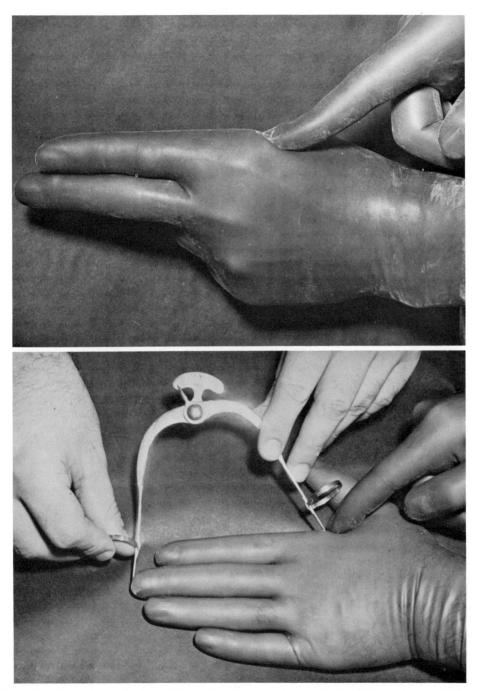

Figure 12.   Measuring the estimated diagonal conjugate with the aid of the Williams outlet pelvimeter.

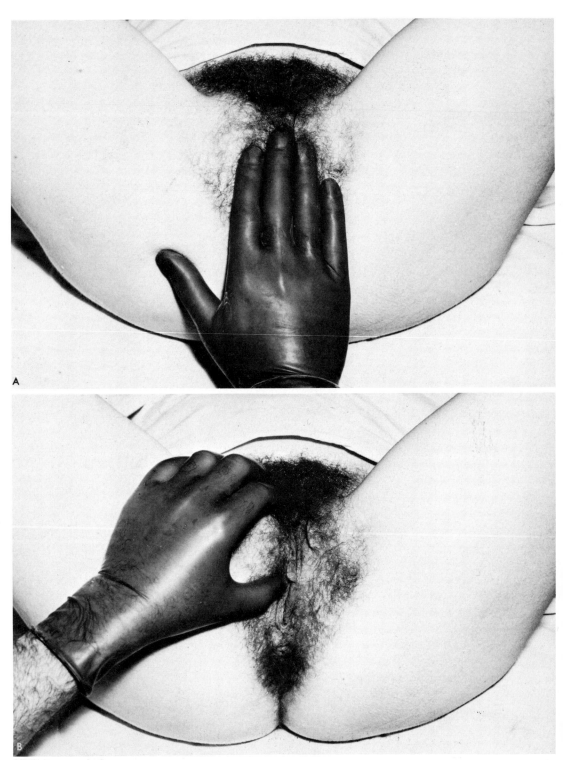

Figure 13. Estimating the inclination and width of the symphysis pubis. A, Assessing the inclination of the symphysis. B, Determining the width of the symphysis.

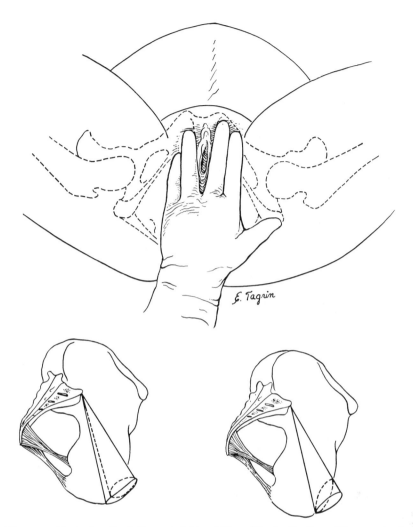

Figure 14. Diagrams illustrating the influence of the width and the inclination of the symphysis on the diagonal conjugate and the superior strait or inlet.

bi-ischial diameter. A tongue depressor serves the purpose and is held in place over the perineum by a nurse assistant in such a manner that it rests against the ischial tuberosities. The examiner places one arm of the Williams pelvimeter on the lower border of the tongue depressor at a point midway between the tuberosities, the second arm being placed at a spot overlying the sacrococcygeal joint. The posterior sagittal diameter of the outlet is thus obtained.

In résumé, the following information regarding the pelvic architecture should be obtained on vaginal examinations:

1. The contour, the position, and the length of the sacrum.

2. The width of the sacrosciatic notch.

3. The prominence of the ischial spines.

An estimation of the length of the bispinous diameter.

4. The slope or splay of the side walls of the pelvis.

5. The length of the diagonal conjugate and, indirectly, the true conjugate.

6. The width and the inclination of the symphysis.

7. The shape and the size of the pubic arch.

8. The bi-ischial diameter and the posterior sagittal diameter of the outlet.

9. The mobility of the coccyx.

It must be reemphasized that the vaginal examination, properly and systematically performed, can permit the clinician to establish that the pelvis is obstetrically normal in all respects, or, if it is abnormal, where the deviations exist.

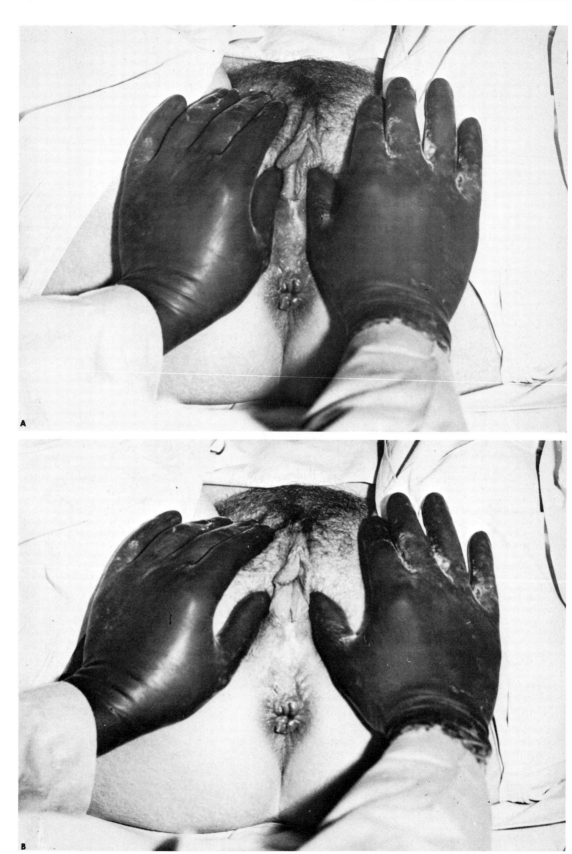

Figure 15.   Outlining the pubic arch. See text.

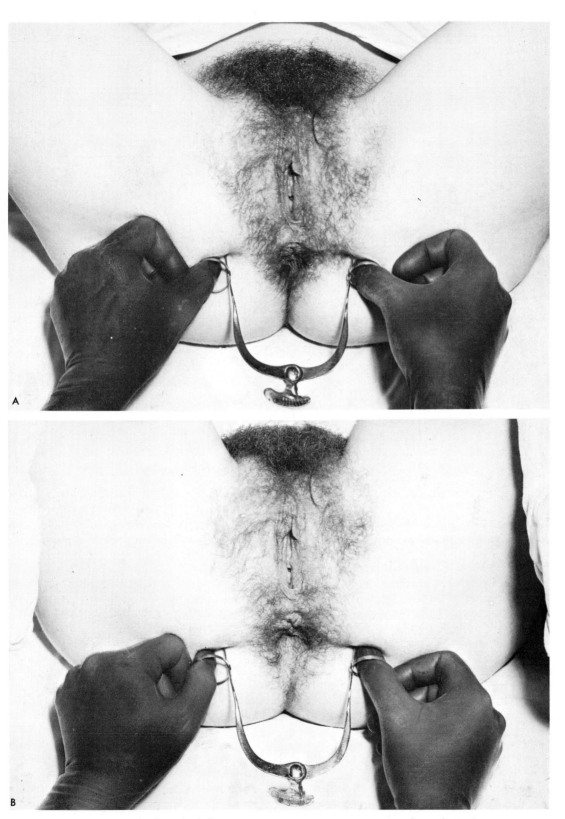

Figure 16. Measuring the bi-ischial diameter. A, Incorrect measurement on the arch. B, Correct measurement on the tuberosities.

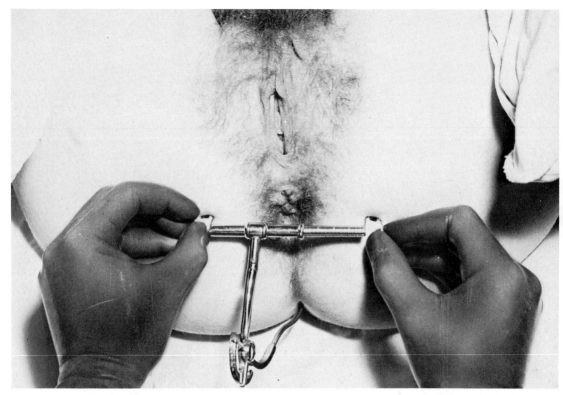

Figure 17. Simultaneous measurement of the bi-ischial and the posterior sagittal diameters of the outlet, using the Thoms instrument.

PRESENTATION

From the fourth or fifth month onward the patient is aware of fetal motions. In the last few weeks of pregnancy intrauterine activity diminishes to such an extent that the patient may show concern for the well-being of the fetus. This decrease in activity near term coincides with the attainment of a resting position within the uterus which the fetus usually maintains throughout the remainder of pregnancy and during labor. Prior to this time, the fetus has assumed many positions in utero, often being in breech presentation. In nearly all instances the final location finds the body of the fetus accommodating itself to the longest or vertical diameter of the uterus. This places the long axes of the fetal and maternal bodies parallel to each other, and the location of the fetus in utero is known as a longitudinal presentation. Deviations from this location are infrequent; but when the long axis of the fetus is found to lie at right angles to the axis of the pelvic inlet, it is designated a transverse presentation.

Etiology of Presentation

Since antiquity, it has been recognized that labor results in delivery of the infant head first in the great majority of cases, and there has been much speculation concerning why this is so. The student is referred to the numerous articles bearing on the etiology of breech presentation, for many of these enumerate the various theories and etiologic factors which have been proposed. It is apparent that the old concept based on the theory of accommodation offers the most logical explanation of why the fetus normally presents by the vertex. Accordingly, fetal presentation *at any time during pregnancy* is dependent upon a process of the mechanical adaptation of the fetus to the space available within the uterine cavity. This process is by no means static, but varies with progressive changes in size and contour of the enlarging uterus in relation to progressive quantitative changes in the several components that contribute to the aggregate bulk or mass of the products of conception.

In the second trimester of pregnancy the

uterine cavity as a whole is spherical in contour, its outline distorted to a mild degree by the flattened discoid mass of the placenta. At this stage the comparatively large amount of amniotic fluid to fetal mass allows the fetus a wide degree of motility within the membranes. During this period of pregnancy, therefore, the alleged theory of accommodation is not applicable, for the fetus may at any time assume a cephalic, breech, oblique, or transverse habitus.

During the third trimester the contour of the uterine cavity changes progressively from spherical to ovoid, demonstrated by abdominal palpation and readily verified by the outline of the uterus on lateral x-ray examination or ultrasound. The circumference of the corpus enlarges more rapidly than that of the lower uterine segment, producing a uterine cavity more spacious in its upper than in its lower portion. Simultaneously during the last weeks of pregnancy, the fetus grows rapidly, and the amniotic fluid decreases in amount. Consequently, the effect of the fluid as a buffer between fetus and uterine wall becomes diminished. Movements of the fetus exert an increased pressure on the uterine wall, which by now tends to contract with greater frequency. The combined effect is to align the longitudinal axis of the fetus with that of the uterus.

Little experience in abdominal palpation is necessary to ascertain that early in the last trimester, when the fetal parts can first be outlined consistently, the fetus is presenting by the breech or even transversely more frequently than it does at term. This observation is borne out by the fact that breech birth occurs more often when labor is premature in contrast to term.

Since space in the fundus normally exceeds that available in the lower uterine segment, the final presentation of the fetus is determined by the relative dimensions of its cephalic and caudal poles. Normally the caudal pole, comprising the breech augmented by the bulk of the attached lower extremities, exceeds the circumference of the fetal head. Consequently, if the fetal legs remain flexed, that is, the thighs flexed on the abdomen and the legs on the thighs, which they generally do, the effect of uterine contractions is to guide the head into the lower uterine segment and the podalic pole into the more spacious fundus, thus producing a cephalic presentation.

Types of Presentation

The part of the fetus that first enters the superior strait or pelvic inlet is known as the presentation. Cephalic presentation may be either vertex, brow, or face, depending upon the part presenting, and breech presentations are subdivided into frank breech, full breech, and footling. In a vertex presentation the fetal head is well flexed and near the junction of the lambdoidal and sagittal sutures the occiput becomes the leading point of the presenting part. Partial deflection of the fetal head will result in a brow or frontal presentation, while extreme deflection causes a face or mentum presentation. The subdivision of breech presentation into three types is on the basis of the position of the legs of the fetus in relation to its body. A frank breech presentation exists when the buttocks are presenting and the thighs are flexed upon the abdomen with the lower extremities extended, thereby lying parallel to the long axis of the body of the fetus. In the second type, or full breech presentation, the thighs are flexed upon the abdomen, with the lower extremities further flexed upon the thighs. When one is confronted with this type of presentation, it is found that both buttocks and feet constitute the presenting part. A variation of this type is seen in the footling, in which case one or both feet of the fetus have dropped into the pelvic cavity to produce a single or double footling presentation, respectively.

The physician must be able to describe the position of the presenting part as it relates to the areas within the pelvis at any given time. The superior plane of the maternal pelvis is, therefore, divided into four imaginary quadrants by the intersection of the anteroposterior and transverse diameters of the pelvis. The position of the quadrants in relation to the anteroposterior and transverse diameters determines their designation. Thus, the right posterior quadrant of the pelvic inlet occupies the region overlying the right sacroiliac joint (to the right of the anteroposterior diameter and posterior to the transverse); the left posterior occupies that overlying the left sacroiliac joint. The right anterior quadrant is located in an area beneath the right superior ramus of the pubis (to the right of the anteroposterior diameter and anterior to the transverse); the left anterior quadrant lies on the opposite side. To orient accur-

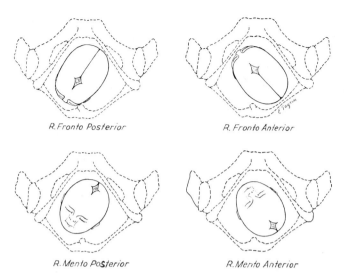

Figure 18. Various positions of brow and face presentation.

ately the presentation within the pelvis, it is necessary to designate some landmark on the presenting part that can be used for descriptive purposes. When the vertex is presenting, the occiput is designated as this point of reference, whereas in a brow or face, the sinciput or mentum, respectively, is used (Fig. 18). The location of the point of reference within a particular quadrant, therefore, defines the position of the presenting part. As an example, we may consider a vertex presentation in its various possible positions. Right occiput anterior (ROA) signifies that the occiput lies in the right anterior quadrant, and the fetal back

lies on the right side of the uterus. This would be reversed in left occiput anterior (LOA) (Fig. 19A). The posterior positions are designated right occiput posterior (ROP) and left occiput posterior (LOP) (Fig. 19B). Should the occiput coincide with the imaginary transverse diameter, its position would be either right occiput transverse (ROT) or left occiput transverse (LOT) (Fig. 19C), the right or left designation depending on the position of the occiput with respect to the anteroposterior diameter. Similarly, an occiput directed anteriorly or posteriorly along the anterposterior diameter is known as occiput anterior (OA) or occiput poste-

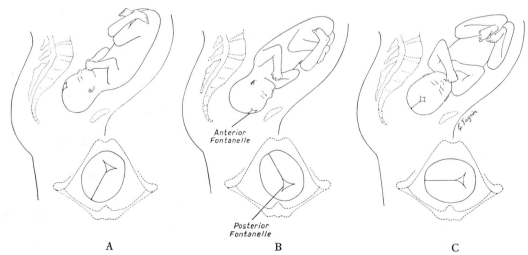

Figure 19. Three possible positions in vertex presentation. The findings on abdominal palpation and rectal or vaginal examination should be related to these diagrams. A, Primary position LOA. B, Primary position LOP. C, Primary position LOT.

rior (OP), respectively. These latter positions are not frequently observed when the vertex enters the superior strait but are seen in the terminal stage of labor as the fetal head accommodates itself to the pelvic outlet.

The various positions of breech presentation are described in a similar manner, the sacrum being used as the reference point. Likewise, in transverse presentations, the position is designated by the quadrant occupied by the presenting scapula or shoulder. The incidence of these various positions is shown in Table 2.

Prelabor abdominal palpation takes on special significance and is performed to determine (1) the presentation and position of the fetus; (2) whether, in the case of vertex presentation, engagement has occurred; and (3) if the vertex is in a normal state of flexion or at least is not deflexed, indicating a brow or face presentation. It is appreciated that complete flexion occurs with descent of the vertex into the pelvis. In addition, abdominal examination is con-

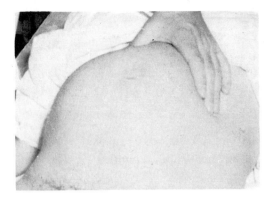

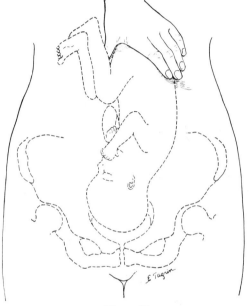

Figure 20.

TABLE 2. INCIDENCE OF FETAL POSITIONS COMMONLY FOUND IN VARIOUS TYPES OF PRESENTATION

Presentation	Per-centage
I. *Longitudinal Presentations*	99
A. Cephalic presentation	96
1. Vertex or occiput	95
Left occiput anterior (LOA)	
" " transverse (LOT)	
" " posterior (LOP)	
Right " anterior (ROA)	
" " transverse (ROT)	
" " posterior (ROP)	
2. Brow or frontal	0.5
Left fronto-anterior (LSinA)	
" " posterior (LSinP)	
Right " anterior (RSinA)	
" " posterior (RSinP)	
3. Face or mentum	0.5
Left mento-anterior (LMA)	
" " posterior (LMP)	
Right " anterior (RMA)	
" " posterior (RMP)	
B. Breech or pelvic presentation	<3
Left sacrum anterior (LSA)	
" " posterior (LSP)	
Right " anterior (RSA)	
" " posterior (RSP)	
II. *Transverse Presentation*	1
A. Scapula or shoulder	
Left scapula anterior (LScA)	
" " posterior (LScP)	
Right " anterior (RScA)	
" " posterior (RScP)	

cerned with the possibility of multiple pregnancy, polyhydramnios, hydrocephalus, and anencephaly, or previously unrecognized abdominal tumors.

Four maneuvers are ordinarily advocated to outline the habitus of the fetus. The first maneuver is designed to demonstrate which fetal pole is in the uterine fundus. The physician, by gently grasping the upper portion of the uterus, identifies the fetal pole (Fig. 20). A breech is likely if the fetal part is soft, rounded, and seems more continuous with the small parts. In general, it is not as freely movable as a vertex, which is readily ballottable, besides feeling spherical. The second maneuver is to ascertain the position of the small parts or fetal extremities and the fetal back and anterior shoulder which, together, confirm the position of the presenting part. One hand seeks the small parts, as the other supports the opposite side of the uterus. The back is located as a firm, smooth object opposite the side occupied by the extremities, and the shoulder is rather prominent to palpation (Fig. 21). In an anterior occiput position the fetal back approaches the mother's midline, and the fetal small parts are less obvious. In a posterior occiput position the small parts are readily felt anteriorly over most of the abdomen, and the fetal back is barely palpable at the side of the uterus.

The purpose of the third maneuver is to determine the portion of the fetus that is presenting at the inlet. This consists of placing the examining hand over the pelvic brim and gently grasping the presenting

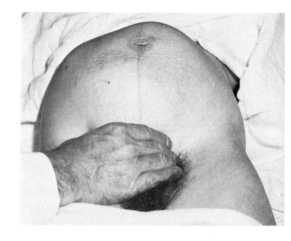

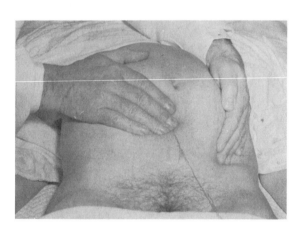

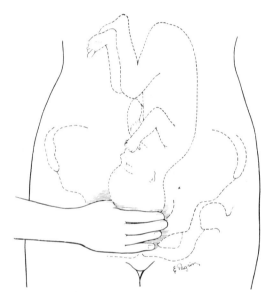

Figure 22.

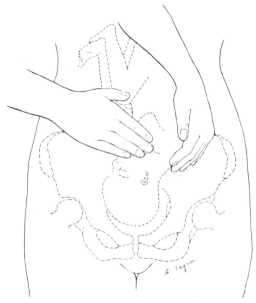

Figure 21.

part (Pawlik's grip) (Fig. 22). It is commonly taught that, when the vertex presents and is immobile, the head is engaged. This is not necessarily true, for in cases of prolonged labor or tests of labor when the cephalopelvic relationship is in doubt, it is erroneous to assume that the head is engaged because it is immovable. In the latter instance the vertex may be wedged in the inlet but not engaged, and as the result of prolonged labor the lower uterine segment may become so taut that the vertex becomes fixed but is not necessarily engaged. It is emphasized that fixation of a presenting part in the inlet is not synonymous with, nor does it qualify as a definition of, engagement.

The fourth maneuver confirms the findings of the third and, in addition, determines whether in a vertex presentation the vertex is flexed. The examiner reverses his position and faces the patient's feet. The tips of the extended hands are placed over the vertex and directed downward toward the symphysis (Fig. 23). It will be noted that one portion of the vertex is more easily felt than the other; when the vertex is flexed, it is the sinciput or brow. For example, if the position is left and the vertex is flexed, the head will be more prominent on the right of the midline of the mother's abdomen, and the examiner will observe that as his hands come to rest on the sinciput and occiput, respectively, the hand on the sinciput will be farther from the midline than the one on the occiput. The head is deflexed when the reverse is true, namely, when the most prominent part of the fetal vertex is opposite the small parts. This description of deflection is preferred, for

the usual definition, that is, when the most prominent portion of the vertex is encountered on the same side as the fetal back, is capable of creating a serious clinical error. As will be seen, one of the characteristics of a brow or face presentation is the extension of the infant's chest against the anterior uterine wall, in which event the chest may be mistaken for the fetal back. This will be discussed further in consideration of the management of a face or brow presentation. Finally, the fourth maneuver will exclude or raise the suspicion of possible cephalopelvic disproportion. If the anterior parietal bone of the vertex rises well above the level of the anterior margin of the mother's symphysis (the so-called overriding of the presenting part), the possibility of cephalopelvic disproportion must be considered in planning the patient's future management.

PRELABOR INSTRUCTIONS TO PATIENTS

The patient should be made familiar with the signs and symptoms of labor and the nursing procedures necessary for her management during labor. First, she should be advised to go to the hospital immediately at the onset of labor, and not wait until it is well established. This applies particularly to the multiparous patient, in whom the labor may be of short duration. The physician should describe the difference between the contractions which characterize the last weeks of pregnancy (Braxton Hicks contractions) and those associated with true labor. In the first instance they occur irregularly and without periodicity. Several contractions may occur in a matter of a few moments, with passage of an hour or more before their reappearance. Although these are generally not painful, the patient is aware of the contractions and volunteers the information that her abdomen becomes tense and firm. She is more conscious of these contractions when in a recumbent position, and in the latter weeks of pregnancy they may be so annoying that sedation is required for sleep.

True labor, by contrast, begins as a low, dull backache associated with uterine contractions usually occurring every 10 to 20 minutes at the onset. These contractions are regular and increase in frequency and intensity. Characteristically the discomfort will

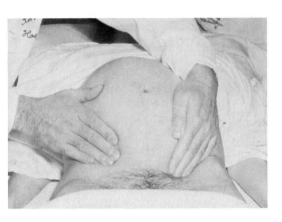

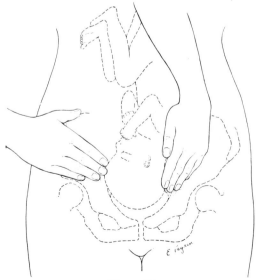

Figure 23.

shift anteriorly over the lower abdomen and become cramplike, often resembling that experienced with the menses. Once the contractions are occurring at intervals of 10 to 12 minutes, which in the average primiparous labor is one or two hours after the onset, the patient should proceed to the hospital. She should be forewarned, however, that labor may begin with contractions every two or three minutes. Early entrance to the hospital may occasionally avoid a disaster from a complication of labor, such as a prolapse of the umbilical cord, and will facilitate the program for pain relief in labor.

Second, the patient should be aware that labor is often heralded by the appearance of a slight bloody discharge ("show"). In patients near term, labor usually ensues within a few hours, and the patient should govern herself accordingly.

Third, spontaneous rupture of the fetal membranes may precede the onset of labor, in which event the patient should enter the hospital promptly. This applies particularly to the patient in whom cesarean section is being contemplated. The hazards of prolonged rupture of the membranes, with its potential danger of intrauterine infection, must never be minimized.

Fourth, if labor is impending or any of these signs or symptoms appear, the patient should restrict her diet to liquids. This will better prepare her for anesthesia should it be required. The patient should be impressed with the fact that a recent meal is a distinct hazard and limits the choice of the anesthesia to the conduction type.

Fifth, the patient should be told how she will be prepared for labor, how it will be conducted, and about the events surrounding delivery. The discussion should include the methods available for pain relief. This is as much a part of maternal preparation for parturition as the other aspects of the patient's psychologic and physical support.

Ideas have been expressed questioning the need for pain-relieving drugs during labor. Some have gone so far as to suggest that the pain of labor is psychologically necessary for the mother. Although these claims may differ in detail, their advocates conceive that perhaps more "natural" ways of childbirth might be desirable. They contend that antepartum exercises, concerned with breathing and relaxation techniques, and special class instruction regarding parturition will prevent much of the pain that is usually experienced, and that

a conscious delivery can be the source of a great sense of accomplishment, at least for the emotionally mature woman. Conduct of labor in accordance with these beliefs is referred to as "natural childbirth" or the "psychoprophylaxis" technique. However, the term natural childbirth has acquired several connotations, ranging from labor and delivery with no analgesia or anesthesia, to labor and delivery accompanied by some analgesia or anesthesia or both.

The success of psychoprophylaxis in preparation for labor is difficult to assess when either analgesia or anesthesia has been generally employed. Further, it is difficult to obtain the proper controls unless neither analgesia nor anesthesia is used. A study of 800 women undergoing labor without analgesia or anesthesia, 368 of whom served as controls, was conducted in a country comprised mainly of a single ethnic group of high socioeconomic standards (the Netherlands). Very satisfactory results in the first stage of labor were recorded in 80 per cent of the prepared patients, in contrast to 60 per cent of the controls, with a slightly greater difference in the response of the two groups in the second stage. The duration of the stages of labor was not significantly dissimilar in the prepared and the unprepared groups, averaging 17 hours and 12 hours for the first stage in primiparas and multiparas, respectively. The duration of the second stage was likewise the same in the two groups, averaging about 70 minutes in the primiparas and 20 to 25 minutes in the multiparas. The period of labor described as the "worst" was the end of the first stage (71 per cent), the incidence of the greatest discomfort being approximately the same in the second stage (14 per cent) and at the time of birth (15 per cent). Further, the average blood loss was slightly more than 300 ml., and either rupture of the perineum or episiotomy was recorded in approximately half of the primiparous patients and in 25 per cent of the multiparous patients. In an objective study it was concluded that antenatal exercises in a substantial series of patients (2675) had no influence on the length and character of the labor. Some 60 per cent received lacerations or episiotomy of the perineum which required repair, and the author cited other series in which prophylaxis methods were practiced and the incidence was 48 per cent and 87 per cent, respectively. It would appear that the length of normal labor is not reduced when patients are managed according to the psychoprophylaxis method.

Because the psychoprophylaxis method has been presented by its advocates in the popular press, however, and because it appears so transparently reasonable, it has become a subject of frequent discussion among the laity. Converts to this method have been led by their reading and discussions to believe that childbearing is essentially painless in the healthy female, and that the use of medication during labor compromises the welfare of the baby and may lead to mental retardation and perhaps cerebral palsy. This places the patient who accepts the implied tenets of psychoprophylaxis in the position that if she requests medication and anesthesia she at once demonstrates her inadequacy as a woman and may bring harm to her child, both of which are obviously repugnant to her. The issue is not necessarily whether a patient can deliver a baby by the precepts of psychoprophylaxis, but whether anesthesia of a high quality is constantly at hand.

Certainly sound obstetric care has always recognized the psychologic aspects of pregnancy, and offers emotional as well as physical support to the patient in labor. Patience, understanding, and personal interest, with an insight into the motivations, the psychologic behavior, and the personal problems of the obstetric patient, are essential qualities of any discerning and well trained obstetrician. Scientific psychology and scientific obstetrics are not incompatible, but it is hazardous to permit pure psychologic speculation to determine obstetric or medical decisions.

Currently there are a number of sensitive and inquiring patients who are confused by what they hear and read about the desirability of having the baby by the psychoprophylaxis method, which, to many, means without pain-relieving medication. The anxieties and unnecessary fears of these patients are greatly allayed when they learn that pain relief in labor contributes to achieving the best obstetric results. It is only fair, therefore, that the patient be told at an early prenatal visit how she is to be managed in the course of labor and delivery. The knowledge that the hospital has every facility to care for her and her infant, and that her obstetrician will do whatever is necessary during labor and delivery at the proper time and in the proper manner, will resolve any uncertainties the patient may have concerning pregnancy, labor, and delivery.

A plan for pain relief should be outlined and the forms to be used described — subject to change when indicated. The patient may be told that delivery will often include the use of episiotomy performed at the time, and that outlet forceps operation may be used to guide the vertex over the perineum and shorten the second stage of labor. Together, these result in the conservation of the pelvic tissues and the avoidance of fetal distress, which occurs most frequently in association with a prolonged second stage labor. She may be informed that when labor and delivery are conducted according to this method, and the episiotomy is properly repaired, the need for later gynecologic surgery to correct rectocele, urethrocystocele with or without stress incontinence, and procidentia becomes negligible.

ULTRASONOGRAPHY

Ultrasonography is utilized in obstetrics in at least four main areas: (1) early pregnancy, for diagnosis and complications; (2) fetal cephalometry with vertex and breech presentation; (3) placental localization; and (4) multiple pregnancy.

A gestational sac may be visualized at six weeks' menstrual age and persists to approximately 10 weeks when the decidua capsularis probably fuses with the decidua vera and the sac is obscured. During this interval, clinical suspicion of impending spontaneous abortion may be confirmed by an ultrasonogram showing a poorly defined sac or one that is implanted low in the endometrial cavity. Hydatidiform mole can be diagnosed by absence of fetal structures and by a generalized intrauterine stippling pattern which represents echoes from multiple dilated villi. These multiple echoes disappear at low-gain setting, revealing what appears to be an empty uterus.

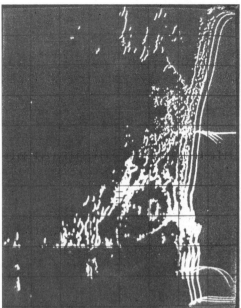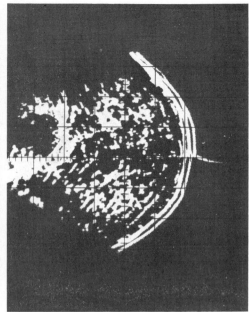

Figure 24. Ultrasonography in early pregnancy. A, Longitudinal view; normal gestational sac in uterus at 6 weeks from last menstrual period. The symphysis (bladder beneath) and the umbilicus are artificially marked on the anterior abdominal wall. B, Hydatidiform mole. (Courtesy of Dr. Kenneth I. Scheer.)

After 12 weeks' gestation, the fetal head begins to appear on sonogram and at 16 weeks the characteristic midline echo from the falx cerebri may be visualized. From this point on, ultrasonic cephalometry is most useful in serial determinations of normal growth, or more particularly for detection of intrauterine growth retardation. There is a fairly good linear correlation between fetal biparietal diameter growth and gestational age. It is less satisfactory although still useful for dating pregnancies with unknown menstrual history or for resolving size-date discrepancy.

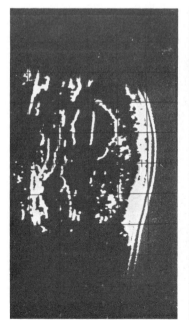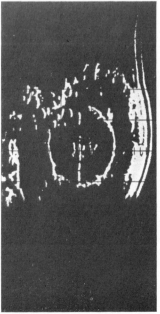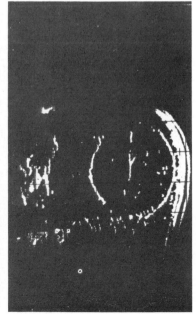

Figure 25. Ultrasonography in cephalometry: Fetal head showing biparietal diameter with characteristic midline echo at 22, 28, and 36 weeks' gestation. (Courtesy of Dr. Kenneth I. Scheer.)

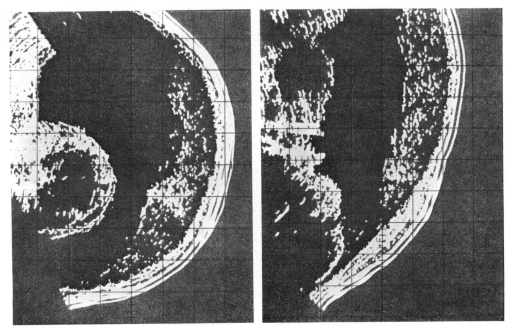

Figure 26. Placental localization by ultrasonography: Placenta implanted on anterior wall, transverse and longitudinal views (also demonstrating polyhydramnios). (Courtesy of Dr. Kenneth I. Scheer.)

In cases of second- and third-trimester bleeding, placental localization by ultrasound is at least as reliable as any other diagnostic mode (97 per cent success rate) and avoids the hazards of radiation. When the placenta is implanted on the anterior wall it can easily be mapped out so that amniocentesis in cases of erythroblastosis may avoid "bloody taps" and possible exacerbation of Rh sensitization.

There is no increased incidence of congenital anomalies or evidence of tissue damage due to sound energy in infants delivered of mothers who have undergone sonography at any stage of gestation.

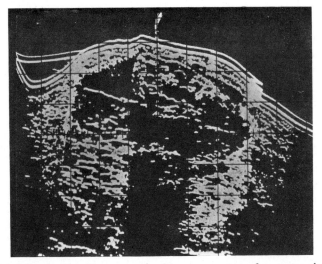

Figure 27. Placental localization by ultrasonography: Transverse view of posterior placenta praevia, taken at level just above symphysis. The nearly solid straight line represents echoes from the chorionic plate. The dark area beneath represents intervillous space, and the ovoid mass above the chorionic plate represents the fetal body. (Courtesy of Dr. Kenneth I. Scheer.)

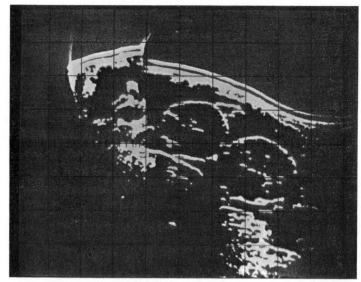

Figure 28. Ultrasonogram in multiple pregnancy: Twinning is definite; interestingly, this is the fourth set of twins for this patient. (Courtesy of Dr. Kenneth I. Scheer.)

BIBLIOGRAPHY

Asherman, J. G.: The myth of tubal and endometrial transplantation. J. Obstet. Gynaec. Brit. Emp., 67: 228, 1960.

Baird, D.: Influence of social and economic factors on stillbirths and neonatal deaths. J. Obstet. Gynaec. Brit. Emp., 52:217, 229, 1945.

Barton, J. J.: Evaluation of the Doppler shift principle as a diagnostic aid in obstetrics. Amer. J. Obstet. Gynec., 102:563, 1968.

Bishop, E. H., and Corson, S.: Estimation of fetal maturity by cytologic examination of amniotic fluid. Amer. J. Obstet. Gynec., 102:654, 1968.

Bourke, G. J., and Whitty, R. J.: Smallpox vaccination in pregnancy: A prospective study. Brit. Med. J., 1:1544, 1964.

Brown, A. D. G., and Robertson, J. G.: The ultrasonic cardioscope in obstetrics. J. Obstet. Gynaec. Brit. Comm., 75:92, 1968.

Burke, B. S., Harding, V. V., and Stuart, H. C.: Nutrition studies during pregnancy; IV. Relation of protein content of mother's diet during pregnancy to birth length, birth weight, and condition of infant at birth. J. Pediat., 23:506, 1943.

Burke, B. S., Stevenson, S. S., Worcester, J., and Stuart, H. C.: Nutrition studies during pregnancy: Relation of maternal nutrition to condition of infant at birth; study of siblings. J. Nutr., 38:453, 1949.

Burnett, C. W. F.: The value of antenatal exercises. J. Obstet. Gynaec. Brit. Emp., 63:40, 1956.

Chanarin, I., Rothman, B., and Berry, V.: Iron deficiency and its relation to folic-acid status in pregnancy: Results of a clinical trial. Brit. Med. J., 1:480, 1965.

Dieckmann, W. J., Turner, D. F., and Ruby, B. A.: Diet regulation and controlled weight in pregnancy. Amer. J. Obstet. Gynec., 50:701, 1945.

Donald, I.: Sonar study of prenatal development. J. Pediat., 75:326, 1969.

Donald, I., and Abdulla, U.: Placentography by sonar. J. Obstet. Gynaec. Brit. Comm., 75:993, 1968.

Gray, M. J.: Use and abuse of thiazides in pregnancy. Clin. Obstet. Gynec., 11:568, 1968.

Haddon, W., Nesbitt, R. E. L., and Garcia, R.: Smoking and pregnancy: Carbon monoxide in blood during gestation and at term. Obstet. Gynec., 18:262, 1961.

Hardy, J. B.: Virus and the fetus. Postgrad. Med., 43:156, 1968.

Horowitz, H. S., and Heifetz, S. B.: Effects of prenatal exposure to fluoridation on dental caries. Public Health Rep., 82:297, 1967.

Jacobson, H. N., Burke, B. S., Smith, C. A., and Reid, D. E.: Effect of weight reduction in pregnant obese women on pregnancy, labor and delivery, and on the condition of the infant at birth. Amer. J. Obstet. Gynec., 83:1609, 1962.

Jeffcoate, T. N. A.: Amenorrhoea. Brit. Med. J., 2:383, 1965.

Jones, W. E.: Traumatic intrauterine adhesions. A report of 8 cases with emphasis on therapy. Amer. J. Obstet. Gynec., 89:304, 1964.

Kerr, M. G.: The problem of the overweight patient in pregnancy. J. Obstet. Gynaec. Brit. Comm., 69:988, 1962.

Knapp, E. L., and Stearns, G.: Factors influencing urinary excretion of calcium; II. Pregnancy and lactation. Amer. J. Obstet. Gynec., 60:741, 1950.

Kraus, G. W., Marchese, J. R., and Yen, S. S. C.: Prophylactic use of hydrochlorothiazide in pregnancy. J.A.M.A., 198:128, 1966.

Lenz, W.: Malformations caused by drugs in pregnancy. Amer. J. Dis. Child., 112:99, 1966.

Low, J. A., Johnston, E. E., McBride, R. L., and Tuffnell, P. G.: The significance of asymptomatic bacteriuria in the normal obstetric patient. Amer. J. Obstet. Gynec., 90:897, 1964.

Macy, I. G., and Hunscher, H. A.: Evaluation of maternal nitrogen and mineral needs during embryonic and infant development. Amer. J. Obstet. Gynec., 27:878, 1934.

Mandelbaum, B., LaCroix, G. C., and Robinson, A. R.: Determination of fetal maturity by spectrophotometric analysis of amniotic fluid. Obstet. Gynec., 29:471, 1967.

Nelson, M. M.: Production of congenital anomalies in mammals by maternal dietary deficiencies. Pediatrics, 19:764, 1957.

Perl, G.: Metronidazole treatment of trichomoniasis in pregnancy. Obstet. Gynec., 25:273, 1965.

Read, G. D.: Correlation of physical and emotional phenomena of natural labour. J. Obstet. Gynaec. Brit. Emp., 53:55, 1946.

Singer, J. E., Westphal, M., and Niswander, K.: Relationship of weight gain during pregnancy to birth weight and infant growth and development in the first year of life. Obstet. Gynec., 31:417, 1968.

Smith, C. A.: Effects of maternal undernutrition upon newborn infant in Holland (1944–1945). J. Pediat., 30:229, 1947.

Smith, C. A., Worcester, J., and Burke, B. S.: Maternal-fetal nutritional relationships; effect of maternal diet on size and content of fetal liver. Obstet. Gynec., 1:46, 1953.

Speert, H., Graff, S., and Graff, A. M.: Nutrition and premature labor. Amer. J. Obstet. Gynec., 62:1009, 1951.

Thoms, H., and Karlovsky, E. D.: Two thousand deliveries under a training for childbirth program. Amer. J. Obstet. Gynec., 68:279, 1954.

Tompkins, W. T., and Wiehl, D. G.: Nutritional deficiencies as a causal factor in toxemia and premature labor. Amer. J. Obstet. Gynec., 62:898, 1951.

Underwood, P., Hester, L. L., Laffitte, T., Jr., and Gregg, K. V.: The relationship of smoking to the outcome of pregnancy. Amer. J. Obstet. Gynec., 91:270, 1965.

Warkany, J.: Congenital malformations induced by maternal nutritional deficiency. J. Pediat., 25:476, 1944.

Willocks, J., Donald, I., Campbell, S., and Dunsmore, I. R.: Intrauterine growth assessed by ultrasonic foetal cephalometry. J. Obstet. Gynaec. Brit. Comm., 74:639, 1967.

Yerushalmy, J.: Mother's cigarette smoking and survival of infant. Amer. J. Obstet. Gynec., 88:505, 1964.

Zabriskie, J. R.: Effect of cigaret smoking during pregnancy. Study of 2000 cases. Obstet. Gynec., 21:405, 1963.

Chapter 24

The Normal and the Abnormal Obstetric Pelvis

The proper conduct of a normal labor or of one requiring operative or instrumental delivery is predicated on a knowledge of the anatomic landmarks and major planes of the bony pelvis. Accordingly, the clinician must be familiar with the overall pelvic architecture and with the various regions or zones within the birth canal that are utilized by the fetus during parturition.

To understand the mechanism of labor and delivery and to comprehend the significance of pathologic labor, one should begin with an inquiry into the extent to which the anatomy of the human pelvis is modified in the female to make it especially suitable for the birth process. As a corollary to this, it is equally necessary to assess those features of the human female pelvis which might act as deterrents to labor and delivery.

Physicians have long appreciated the fact that the male and the female bony pelvis differ in certain anatomic respects. They were not aware, however, as were the anatomists and the anthropologists, of the normal variations in the female pelvis. The transformation of this knowledge into obstetric practice found its inception in the epochal work of Caldwell, Moloy, and D'Esopo, and in the classic contributions of Thoms and Greulich. Through the medium of accurate and practical methods of x-ray pelvimetry developed and introduced by these workers, it became possible to examine, measure, and describe at will the pelvis of the living subject. As a result of this facility, the normal variation in the bony architecture of the female pelvis was more clearly defined. These workers corroborated the finding of skeletal differences between the male and the female pelvis previously recorded by the anatomist and the anthropologist. In addition, their observations established the fact that the female pelvis is subject to considerable deviation in its normal architecture, frequently exhibiting some of the features characteristic of the male pelvis.

Further, these investigations demonstrated that for obstetric purposes it is preferable to classify the different pelvic types according to morphologic characteristics, in contrast to previous classifications in which variations in pelvic types were attributed to pathologic changes occurring congenitally or acquired through disease and malnutrition. Through this medium it was possible to record accurately the mechanism of labor in the normal and in the abnormal pelvis, through serial stereo-roentgenograms taken during the passage of the fetus through the birth canal.

From these studies in pelvimetry, the physical examination of the obstetric pelvis has acquired more meaning. By learning to identify the anatomic landmarks that these roentgenographic studies have revealed are significant, the clinician can train himself to recognize by physical examination the deviations from normal, and thereby classify a pelvis according to its morphologic characteristics. Being aware of the pelvic contour, and the size and shape of the various planes of the pelvis, from either his examination or roentgenographic study, he is in a position to offer a reasonably accurate prognosis as to the outcome of labor. Any discussion of the architecture of the obstetric pelvis and the process and mechanism of labor must acknowledge and evaluate the concepts which have evolved from the studies of Caldwell and Thoms and their associates. Such an evaluation is facilitated by a consideration of some of the special characteristics of the human pelvis, the differences that exist in the pelves of the two sexes, and the normal variations of the female pelvis and how these may affect parturition.

ANATOMIC CHARACTERISTICS OF THE HUMAN PELVIS

The anthropologists, although they may differ in opinion regarding the immediate predecessor of man, agree that few parts of the human body have undergone more profound evolutional changes than has the bony pelvis. These changes in position, shape, and proportions are due chiefly to the special mechanical requirements brought about through man's attainment of the upright posture. The human pelvis has thus acquired bony landmarks which are distinctive and characteristic. These changes deserve consideration in order to acquaint one with those anatomic features which may either favor or impede labor and parturition in the human female.

With assumption of the erect position of the body, the pelvic cylinder has become modified, for now, in conjunction with the lower extremities, it must support the weight of the major portion of the body. In man the symphysis is inclined at about 45 degrees from the vertical axis of the body. This is in contrast to other primates, in which the symphysis is almost parallel to the trunk. Also, in man the lumbosacral curve overhangs the pelvic cavity. To provide for the attachment of muscles that cause lateral flexion, the ilium is enlarged and extends laterally. It is a distinctly human attribute that the internal face of the ilium is directed upward and in this position supports a portion of the weight of the internal organs. These anatomic modifications serve to locate the viscera more over the symphysis and ilium and less over the pelvic outlet. Were it not for this arrangement, prolapse of the female reproductive organs undoubtedly would occur with greater frequency.

Changes in the sacrum, ischia, and pubes are also related to an erect attitude and bipedal progression. The acetabulum is larger and more centrally located in the human innominate bone than in that of other primates (Fig. 1), while man in the upright position has acquired a heavy sacrum with a large articulation. In the human pelvis, the caudal end of the sacrum lies far below the symphysis, but in the lower primates there is no fixed bony structure opposite the pubic bones (Fig. 2). In the subhuman primates, therefore, only at the inlet can the sacrum interfere with the passage of the fetus. The ischial spines, which serve as sites of insertion of the great sacrosciatic ligaments, are

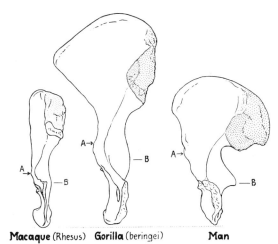

Figure 1. Comparison of innominate bone of macaque, gorilla, and man. A, Acetabulum; B, ischial spines. (From Schultz, A. H., Quart. Rev. Biol., 11:259, and 425, 1936.)

greatly developed in the human pelvis, compared with that of subhuman primates.

In the evolution of the human pelvis, the last lumbar segment is sometimes incorporated into the sacrum (sacralization), mark-

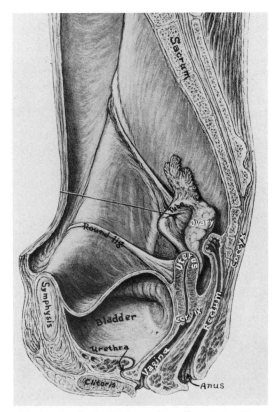

Figure 2. Sagittal view of gorilla pelvis. (From Wislocki, G. B., Contrib. Embryol., 23:163, 1932.)

ing a further attempt to increase the size of the sacroiliac articulation and provide a stronger joint. Routine roentgen-ray examination of the female pelvis will reveal this modification of the sacrum in a certain number of pelves, the incidence having been variably reported between 5 and 20 per cent. In obstetrics, when the sacrum contains six segments, the term "high assimilation" has been proposed to designate the resultant pelvis. Considerable importance was once given to this finding, particularly as it related to a funneling effect on the pelvis. Except for a lengthening of the anteroposterior diameter of the inlet, which increases the tendency for the fetal vertex to assume an occipitoposterior position, for clinical purposes this type of pelvis need not be considered abnormal. A "low assimilation pelvis," in which the sacrum has only four segments (lumbarization), is shallow, but neither has this any special clinical significance.

It can be concluded that the principal change taking place in the human pelvis since the appearance of the giant primates is a shortening of the lumbar spine by one segment, with enlargement of the sacrum to knit the pelvis more firmly to the spine, resulting in a pelvic girdle that is broader and more shallow. The iliac crest is thickened and strengthened, and the ilium has acquired an increased width. In all other primates except man, the sacrum articulates with the ilium at a point far above the acetabulum. The human pelvis has ischial spines that are often enlarged, while the sacrum ends caudally well below the level of the symphysis pubis and opposite the pubic rami, a condition nonexistent in primates other than man.

In considering natural phenomena, it is perhaps well to emphasize those features of the human pelvis capable of causing dystocia or difficult labor that are not present in the pelvis of other primates. The human sacrum, unlike that of other primates, continues downward and normally ends well below the inlet. The ischial spines, if prominent, may interfere with the passage of the fetus through the midpelvic and outlet planes. Also, the human female must deliver a fetus through a pelvic outlet that is confined by a pubic arch that permits only the posterior component of the perineum to distend and allow delivery. To offset these apparent defects, the human pelvis is more shallow and the pelvic inlet has a more generous aperture.

It is evident, however, that, through the process of evolution, the pelvis has acquired anatomic features capable of causing a higher incidence of dystocia, with a greater likelihood of harm to the fetus during labor and delivery than probably occurs in the subhuman primate. Labor under these circumstances could be expected to cause some degree of damage to the soft tissues of the pelvis, especially to the perineum and the fascial supports of the bladder and rectum.

SEX CHARACTERS OF THE MALE AND THE FEMALE PELVIS

Although there are anatomic differences between the male and the female bony pelvis, designated sex characters, the pelvis of the individual may have anatomic features distinctive of the opposite sex. In any collection of dried female pelves, specimens will be found that may resemble or be difficult to distinguish from the male pelvis. Consequently, to determine whether the pelvis is male or female when the sex is unknown, the anthropologist must consider the pelvis as a whole, for he dare not rely on the appearance of one plane or anatomic landmark as a distinguishing feature. Obstetrically, this is important for at least two reasons: the diagnosis of pelvic type should be made on the overall architecture and not on the appearance of the inlet alone; the evaluation of the various etiologic factors that determine the ultimate shape of the pelvis must be based on their possible effect on the pelvis as a whole and not be restricted to the inlet. This latter point is the subject of some controversy, and will be considered further in a discussion of the factors that contribute to the shaping of the adult pelvis.

In general, the inlet of the female pelvis is round to slightly ovoid; by comparison, the inlet of the male pelvis tends to have a wedge-shaped outline (Fig. 3). In the male the posterior segment of the inlet, i.e., the portion of the superior strait situated posterior to the transverse diameter, has a flattened appearance. Consequently, the posterior segment is shallow and the posterior sagittal diameter is shortened. The anterior segment of the pelvic inlet characteristically is narrower in the male, and the retropubic angle is described as being convergent. In the female, the retropubic angle is wide and both segments of the inlet are rounded in appearance.

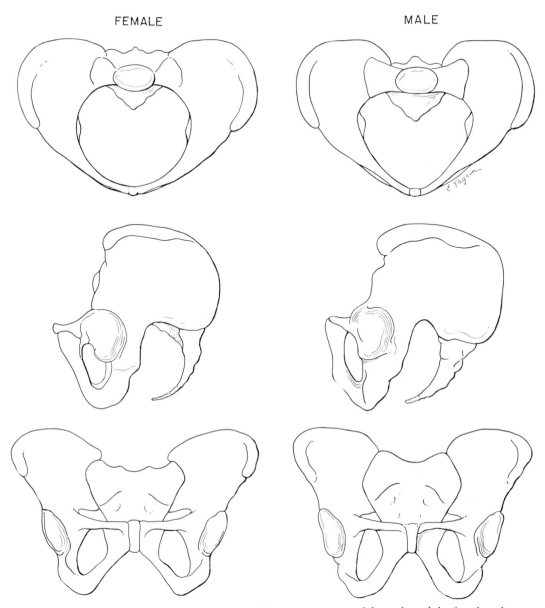

Figure 3. Drawings illustrating comparison of the various aspects of the male and the female pelvis.

The lateral view of the pelvis of the two sexes presents striking differences in both the size and shape of the sacrosciatic notch. In the female, the apex of the notch is wide and the posterior border passes almost directly backward to merge into the sacrum. The sacrosciatic notch in the male is long and narrow, and the ilium extends downward to form a portion of the posterior boundary of the notch. This narrowing effect is accentuated in the male by a forward inclination of the sacrum, which causes a shortening of the posterior sagittal diameters of the midpelvic and pelvic outlet planes. The capacity of the midpelvic com-partment, especially the posterior segment, is greater in the female than in the male, for in the female the sacrum is placed more posteriorly and the side walls of the pelvis are either straight or slightly divergent. In the male, because of the narrowing of the side walls, the pelvis from the midplane downward tends to converge, causing a reduction in the length of the bispinous and bi-ischial diameters. These features, combined with a forward encroachment of the sacrum, give the pelvis a funnel effect. Because of the narrowing of the pubic rami, the subpubic angle is small and the pubic arch in the male has a Gothic-arch outline.

The rami of the pubes in the female are well curved and the contours have a rounded Roman-arch appearance. Finally, the male pelvis has a greater height and depth than that of the female.

The presence of certain male characters in the pelvis of the obstetric patient may offer hazards to successful pelvic delivery. These are summarized as follows:

1. Posterior displacement of the transverse diameter of the inlet toward the sacral promontory

2. Narrowing of the retropubic angle with convergence of the forepelvis

3. Decrease in the capacity of the posterior pelvis by a forward position of the sacrum, associated with a narrow sacrosciatic notch

4. Constriction of the capacity of the midpelvis and lower pelvis by convergence of the side walls

5. Decrease in the transverse diameter of the outlet by narrowing of the subpubic angle

It must be emphasized that, although the obstetric patient may have a pelvis with an inlet characteristic for the female, there may be evidence of maleness elsewhere. Before the pelvis can be completely classified and a diagnosis appended, all of its various areas and landmarks must be taken into account and the pelvis studied as a whole.

Conversion of the Pelvis to the Adult Form

The pelvis of the newborn infant is characteristically funnel-shaped, and until the child attempts to stand upright the vertebral column is straight. As the child begins to walk, changes in the shape of the pelvis appear. To appreciate fully these changes, it is necessary to recall that there are certain fixed supporting structures within the pelvis. These are the sacroiliac, sacrosciatic, and pubic ligaments, and the acetabular articulation. In the upright position, a downward thrust of weight-bearing is brought against the sacrum, with the maximum force directed slightly anterior to the sacral promontory. The latter moves forward and encroaches into the pelvic cavity, while the body of the sacrum assumes a more posterior position. Resistance is offered at two points, the strong posterior sacroiliac and equally strong sacrosciatic ligaments. Hence, with pressure from above on these

fixed points, the sacrum loses its straightness and becomes concave.

A certain degree of anterior bowing of the vertebral column occurs in the lumbosacral region. The ilia of the innominate bones tend to flare lateralward. Prior to and coincident with puberty, there is a rapid growth of the sacrum and a lengthening of the pubic portion of the innominate bone. Although the mechanical factor of weight-bearing in the upright position accounts for the conversion of the pelvis to the adult form, being common to both sexes it cannot account for the apparent anatomic differences that normally exist between the male and the female pelvis. There must be genetic and environmental factors that influence the final shape of the pelvis.

Factors Influencing Anatomic Variation in the Female Pelvis

The difference in the incidence of the various pelvic types, when analyzed, introduces the possibility that there are genetic as well as environmental factors operating in determining the shape of the pelvis.

The anatomist and the anthropologist have long been interested in whether sex differences could be identified in the pelvis of the fetus. The earliest study regarding the question of sex determinants, made on a limited number of cases, revealed anatomic differences in the pelves of fetuses of the two sexes. These observations found additional support when a much larger series was studied, and it was concluded that the fetus possesses a pelvis that is morphologically characteristic of its sex. The extent of the anatomic differences recorded, however, did not warrant the conclusion that pelvic types are entirely predetermined.

In fact, more recent observations tend to show that the pelvic inlet in the male and in the female do not differ appreciably in contour during early life. Only at or near puberty do the major differences which characterize the pelvis of each sex appear. In one radiographic study of the pelves of young girls between the ages of 5 and 15 years, over 80 per cent were dolichopellic or anthropoid in type, an incidence that changes perceptibly with puberty. In another study of boys and girls ranging in ages from 5 to 15 years, the pelvis in nearly every instance had an anteroposterior diameter larger than the transverse diameter. In the males, with the approach of puberty, the transverse diameter of the inlet assumed a position closer to the sacral promontory, indicating a beginning tendency to form a pelvis characteristic for this sex (android). The change seen in the female was a significant flattening of the anteroposterior diameter, with the emergence of a characteristic oval type (gynecoid). These normal changes in pelvic contour peculiar to the two sexes following puberty are attributed to environmental effects of endocrine origin. That a genetic factor is operating, however, is suggested by the fact that the pelvis of the female apparently is endowed with a greater potential of lateral growth. In both sexes at birth the body of the first sacral vertebra is twice as broad as the alae. This ratio tends to remain stationary in the male; the difference disappears in the female, by virtue of a greater growth of the sacral alae, resulting in a greater width of the pelvic inlet.

That the pelvic type is genetically determined and modified by endocrine and nutritional factors gains additional support from a roentgenographic study of the pelvic architecture of a series of male and female patients with hypogonadal states of various etiologies. The pelves retained the contour of the appropriate sex, although the secondary sex characteristics were absent or deficient.

Of the environmental or acquired factors, disease may cause pelvic abnormality directly, as in osteomalacia and rickets, or indirectly from diseases of the spine and lower extremities should they develop in childhood when the pelvis is malleable. Trauma in this age of technology plays an increasing role in the etiology of the abnormal pelvis.

The nutritional status of the patient during childhood and adolescence is believed by many to be the most important factor concerned with shaping of the pelvis. The remolding of the pelvic inlet from infancy to adulthood has been ascribed to possible derangement in calcium and vitamin D metabolism, with the tendency of the pelvis to change from a dolichopellic or a mesatipellic toward a platypelloid form. In nearly every instance, however, this change is arrested midway between the round and flat types, for most females have an oval or brachypellic or gynecoid type, and rarely is the stage of flattening reached. Accordingly, the concept is formulated that the contour and shape of the adult pelvis is determined by the proportionate rate of growth of the various bones comprising the pelvis just preceding and following puberty. If growth is symmetric, the pelvis will retain the dolichopellic appearance of childhood, but usually the growth rate is less in the anteroposterior than in the transverse diameter, with the tendency for the pelvis to broaden.

This is an elaboration of an older study wherein the ultimate contour of the pelvic inlet was thought to be due not so much to mechanical factors of the upright position as to the comparative rate of prepubertal bone growth of the sacral, iliac, and pubic portions of the innominate bones. It was further contended that in rickets the pubic bone grows at the normal rate, but in the iliac and sacral areas growth is retarded, causing a flattening of the inlet.

In keeping with these observations that the normal female pelvis is round and that tendency to the oval shape or flattening of the pelvic brim is a nutritional effect, the problem has been subjected to intensive study from a socioeconomic point of view. The patients studied were divided into five classes, ranging from the professional and well-to-do to unskilled workers. Social gradients based on food, housing, and education were considered important criteria. In general, women in the privileged socioeconomic group were usually taller. These women had long or mostly round pelves, whereas the flat type of pelvis was more commonly found in the shorter persons. Presumably, with a poor diet in youth, the individual's growth may be impaired, with a greater possibility that the pelvis will become contracted.

In an attempt to assess any possible relationship between body build and pelvic type, it had been shown that women with long oval pelves are taller and the width of the pelvis is smaller in proportion to the shoulders. The women with a transversely elongated pelvis are the shortest in stature, with hips and pelvis proportionately larger than their shoulders. It was concluded, however, that the external body measurements varied so much that it would be extremely hazardous to predict the pelvic type on the basis of these body dimensions.

A major difficulty in interpreting the studies concerned with the etiology of the various types of female pelves is the fact that different criteria have been used for purposes of classification. The proponents of the nutritional theory employ the pelvic index of the inlet in classifying pelves. Those who favor endocrine influence as a possible genetic expression emphasize that

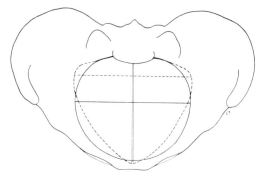

Figure 4. Drawing illustrating the identical value of the pelvic indexes in a gynecoid and an android inlet (the latter represented by the broken line).

what they have designated the android pelvis is distinguishable not by the pelvic index but rather by its shape and outline (Fig. 4). Furthermore, those who consider nutrition the paramount factor sometimes fail to mention that male characters can be present in other parts of the pelvis, even when the pelvic inlet is not android in configuration. Although the nutritional status of the individual during the periods of growth and development undoubtedly influences the pelvic contour, the genetic factor cannot be ignored and, indeed, needs to be explored further. A determination of the pelvic types of near relatives of individual patients might yield interesting information on this question.

It may be concluded that genetic and acquired or environmental factors intermingle in the formation of the adult female pelvis. Anatomic sex differences may be present at birth, but these are not detectable by roentgenographic examination. Generally speaking, both males and females start life with an identical type of pelvis (dolichopellic). At puberty the various types emerge through a transition from the long, oval type (dolichopellic or anthropoid), influenced by endocrine and nutritional factors. The pelvis may be further modified by disease and trauma at any time during the life of the individual. Until there is additional information on total families, however, the comparative roles which the environment and genetic or sex determinants play in the formation of various pelvic types must remain an open question.

PLANES OF THE PELVIS

The true pelvis is divided into several planes or areas for the purpose of relating

the pelvic architecture and the part it plays in the mechanism of normal and abnormal labor. These areas are referred to as the superior plane, or pelvic inlet; the midpelvic plane; and the inferior plane, or pelvic outlet.

The superior plane (the pelvic or obstetric inlet), which in the female is normally an oval area, is bounded posteriorly by the promontory of the sacrum, laterally by the iliopectineal line, and arteriorly by the rami of the pubic bones and the upper margin of the symphysis pubis (Fig. 5A). The midpelvic plane is bounded posteriorly by the sacrum near the junction of the third and fourth sacral vertebrae, laterally by the ischial spines, and anteriorly by the inferior and inner aspect of the symphysis (Fig. 5B).

The inferior plane (the pelvic or obstetric outlet) is not a single geometric plane, but is made up of two components (Fig. 5C). These are triangular in outline, with a common base represented by a line connecting the two ischial tuberosities (bi-ischial diameter). The posterior component is bounded behind by the sacrococcygeal joint, laterally by the sacrotuberous ligaments, and anteriorly by the common base. The anterior component extends from the common base or bi-ischial diameter upward and forward to the inferior margin of the symphysis. The lateral limits of this area are the inner margin of the pubic arch. The floor of the pelvic outlet is composed of the soft tissue of the perineum and the urogenital diaphragm.

Certain subordinate planes have been described. The first of these is the plane of greatest pelvic dimension (Fig. 5D). It lies approximately midway between the superior and midpelvic planes. This area is bounded posteriorly by the sacrum near the junction of the second and third sacral vertebrae, laterally by the ischium, and anteriorly by the midportion of the inner surface of the symphysis. The inferior strait, which is not to be confused with the inferior plane or pelvic outlet, is an area bounded posteriorly by the tip of the sacrum, laterally by the sacrotuberous ligament, and anteriorly by the lower and inner margin of the symphysis. Advantage may be taken of the plane of greatest pelvic dimension in forceps operations involving rotation of the vertex. Otherwise, these two planes are of little obstetric significance, for problems concerned with cephalopelvic relationships are influenced principally by the size and

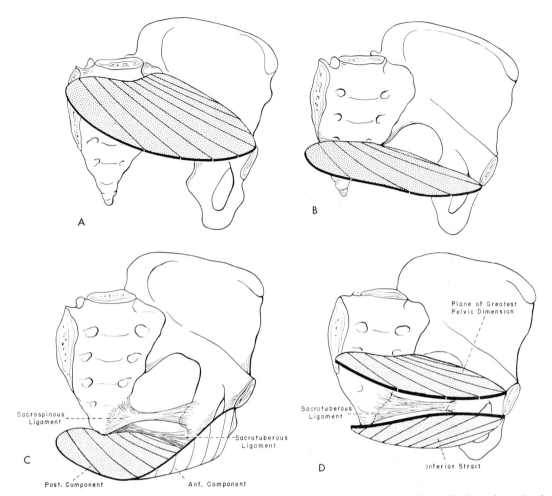

Figure 5. Planes of the pelvis. A, Superior plane of the pelvis: obstetric inlet. B, The midpelvic plane. C, The inferior pelvic plane: obstetric outlet. D, Subordinate planes of the pelvis.

contour of the superior, midpelvic, and inferior planes.

DIAMETERS OF THE PELVIS

Each of the three major pelvic planes has an anteroposterior and a transverse diameter. The anteroposterior diameter of each plane is then subdivided, by its intersection with the transverse diameter, into an anterior and a posterior sagittal diameter. In the superior plane, or pelvic inlet, the anterior and posterior sagittal diameters measure approximately 6.5 and 4.5 cm., respectively (Fig. 6A).

Several diameters have been proposed to describe the anteroposterior dimension of the inlet, and these extend from various points on the inner or inferior and superior surfaces of the symphysis to the sacral promontory (Fig. 6B). The first of these is the true conjugate diameter, normally measuring 11.0 cm. or more, which extends from the superior border of the symphysis to the sacral promontory. The length of this diameter is derived indirectly by subtracting 1.5 cm. from the diagonal conjugate. A second anteroposterior diameter of the superior plane is the obstetric conjugate, which extends from the point of maximum convexity of the symphysis to the sacral promontory. Owing to the curvature of the surface of the symphysis, this diameter is slightly less than the true conjugate, but for clinical purposes they may be considered identical. Neither of these diameters can be determined by direct physical examination. They can be estimated with reasonable accuracy from the length of the diagonal conjugate as measured on vaginal examination. (See Chapter 23.)

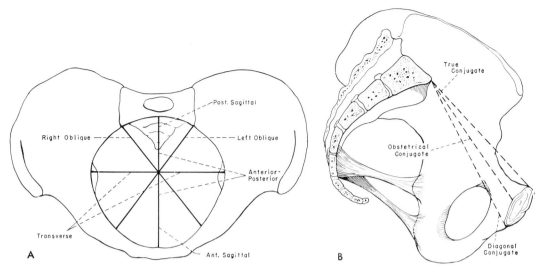

Figure 6. Diameters of the pelvis. A, Diameters of the superior plane, or inlet of the pelvis. B, Conjugate diameters of the superior plane of the pelvis.

If recourse is made to roentgenographic mensuration, in addition to identification of the true and obstetric conjugates, a third anteroposterior diameter of the inlet can be determined, the x-ray conjugate. The latter is defined as the shortest diameter of the inlet, and in the normal pelvis is identical in length to the obstetric conjugate. If, however, the lower border of the first sacral vertebra projects into the pelvic inlet, the x-ray conjugate may be shorter than either the obstetric or the true conjugate.

The transverse diameter of the superior plane is represented by an imaginary line connecting the most lateral aspect of the iliopectineal line on either side. This measures approximately 13.0 cm., or 1 or 2 cm. greater than the anteroposterior diameter of the inlet. Of nearly equal length, and peculiar to the superior plane, are the two oblique diameters, extending from the region of each sacroiliac synchrondrosis to the opposite iliopectineal eminence located on the superior ramus of the pubis, and designated "right" or "left," depending on the sacroiliac joint from which they originate. These diameters measure approximately 12.0 to 13.0 cm.

The anteroposterior diameter of the midpelvic plane is slightly longer than the corresponding diameter of the inlet. It extends from the inferior border of the symphysis, intersecting the bispinous diameter, to end on the anterior surface of the sacrum, most often at the junction of the third and fourth

sacral segments (Fig. 7). The anterior and posterior sagittal diameters of the midpelvic plane, although slightly longer than their counterparts of the superior plane, have the same relative ratio, the anterior being longer than the posterior. The transverse diameter of the midpelvic plane, represented by an imaginary line connecting the ischial spines, is referred to as the bispinous diameter. Its length in the normal pelvis is 10.0 to 10.5 cm.

The anterior sagittal diameter of the inferior plane extends from the inferior border of the symphysis to the midpoint of the transverse or bi-ischial diameter and measures about 5.5 cm. The posterior

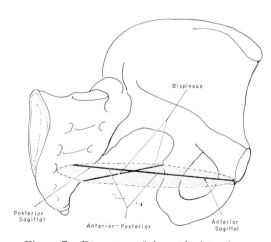

Figure 7. Diameters of the midpelvic plane.

sagittal diameter continues from the midpoint of the transverse diameter to the sacrococcygeal joint and measures 6.5 cm. (Fig. 8). The transverse or bi-ischial diameter of the pelvic outlet extends between the two ischial tuberosities and normally measures 10.0 to 11.0 cm.

The anteroposterior diameter of the outlet is often erroneously stated to be the distance from the inferior border of the symphysis to the tip of the sacrum. This actually is the length of the anteroposterior diameter of the inferior strait and, as stated previously, is not relevant to obstetrics. This diameter is not a true measure of the size of the pelvic outlet or available space, as indicated in Table 1. It will be noted that there is no difference in the length of this diameter in the pelves of the two sexes, but there is a marked difference in the size of the inferior pelvic plane in the male and in the female. This difference is readily demonstrable by measurement of the bi-ischial and posterior sagittal diameters and an assessment of the contour of the pubic arch. Again, the inferior strait must not be regarded as synonymous with the inferior pelvic plane. If careful attention is given to the measurements of the inferior pelvic plane, one need not resort to x-ray examination of this area. This brief description of the pelvic planes and diameters will be amplified in the discussions devoted to roentgenographic examination of the pelvis.

The Pelvic Axis

The pelvic axis has been defined for the purpose of describing the direction through which the fetal head traverses the pelvic

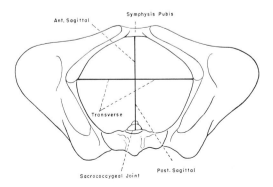

Figure 8. Diameters of the inferior plane, or outlet of the pelvis.

TABLE 1. Comparison of the Mean Values of the Principal Characters Shown Radiographically in a Series of 500 Female and 50 Male Pelves[*]

Pelvic Characters	Mean Values Females	Males
Obstetric true conjugate diameter	11.8 cm.	11.5 cm.
Anatomical true conjugate diameter	12.2 cm.	12.0 cm.
Greatest transverse diameter at brim	13.1 cm.	12.1 cm.
Pelvic brim index		
(1) with obstetric conjugate	90.8	95.3
(2) with anatomical conjugate	93.9	99.2
Approximate area of pelvic inlet		
(1) with obstetric conjugate	121.6 sq. cm.	109.5 sq. cm.
(2) with anatomical conjugate	126.8 sq. cm.	113.4 sq. cm.
Anteroposterior diameter at pelvic outlet	11.9 cm.	11.9 cm.
Interspinous diameter	9.9 cm.	8.3 cm.
Intertuberous diameter	10.1 cm.	9.3 cm.
Approximate area of pelvic outlet	93.7 sq. cm.	78.0 sq. cm.
Subpubic angle	93.5°	75.8°

[*]Young, M., and Ince, J. G. H., J. Anat., 74:374, 1940.

cylinder during labor. Conventionally, it has been described as an imaginary line that passes downward from the inlet to the outlet, bisecting the anteroposterior diameter of the major pelvic planes en route (Fig. 9). The portion above the midplane is called the superior axis, and that below this point, the inferior axis. The superior axis is approximately straight, while the inferior portion curves forward to emerge at the midline of the perineum in the region of the transverse perineal muscles.

Serial stereoroentgenograms taken for the purpose of delineating the normal mechanism of labor, however, show that the course followed by the vertex differs from that described above. Consequently, Caldwell and his associates have proposed that the superior and inferior axes are not continuous, but rather are separate entities. The superior axis originates at the intersection of the transverse and anteroposterior diameters of the inlet and descends downward parallel to the sacrum, ending at the sacrococcygeal area, or what Caldwell aptly chooses to call the "sacrococcygeal platform." The inferior axis of the forepelvis begins at the center of the anterior sagittal diameter of the inlet and descends parallel to the posterior surface of the symphysis, emerging at or slightly anterior to the center of the bi-ischial or transverse diameter of the outlet. However, only the portion that

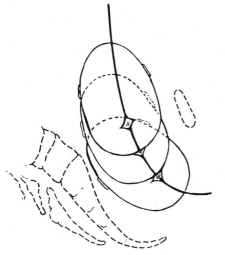

Figure 9. Drawing illustrating the older concept of the direction and location of the pelvic axis.

descends parallel to the sacrum through the superior axis, thereby avoiding the bony resistance of the fore-pelvis, the upper pubic arch, and the ischial spines. As it moves below the midpelvic plane, the vertex meets bony resistance at the sacrococcygeal platform, which causes it to move forward into the area of the inferior axis. Rather than sweeping forward and anteriorly in accordance with the conventional description of the pelvic axis, the vertex continues downward in the direction of the inferior pelvic axis as described. This is consonant with the belief that the vertex should be maintained in flexion and should not be allowed to extend during delivery until such time as the biparietal diameter of the vertex has reached the transverse diameter of the outlet, which means that the occiput is about to bypass the inferior border of the symphysis (see Mechanism of Labor in Chapter 25). It is suggested, therefore, that whatever tendency the vertex has to extend is not by preference but rather because of the resistance offered by the pubococcygeus muscle

lies at or below the level of the ischial spines is utilized by the fetal vertex (Fig. 10).

According to this concept of the location and direction of the pelvic axes, the vertex in its course through the upper pelvis

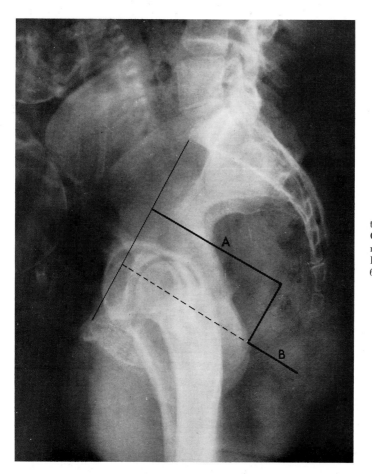

Figure 10. The location and direction of the pelvic axes, according to Caldwell, Moloy, and D'Esopo. A, Superior axis; B, inferior axis. (From Reid, D. E., J. Obstet. Gynaec. Brit. Emp., 66:709, 1959.)

and the transverse perineal muscles. If extension occurs, the larger occipitofrontal diameter of the fetal vertex must pass through the inferior pelvic plane, rather than the smaller suboccipitobregmatic diameter, which passes through this plane when the head is well flexed. The extension that occurs during the course of normal labor is at the expense of distention and ofttimes disruption of the structures within the perineum and the endopelvic fascia beneath and supporting the bladder. To prevent this, an episiotomy is performed to allow the rectum to fall away from the oncoming flexed head. The routine use of this operation is in keeping with modern obstetrics, in which the objectives are to avoid undue pressure on the fetal vertex by the perineum and to avoid damage to the perineum and fascial supports of the bladder that might necessitate gynecologic surgery at some later date. This is in contrast to the natural way with its subsequent disabling consequences.

THE PARALLEL AND CORONAL PLANES OF THE PELVIS

The pelvis has long been conventionally subdivided into four parallel planes, in order to describe more accurately the mechanism of labor as it relates to the direction of descent, the level of rotation, and the possible arrest of the presenting part. Since the introduction of x-ray pelvimetry, the location of these planes has been slightly modified and another plane, the coronal plane, has been added. The latter coincides with an imaginary line that passes downward through the transverse diameter of the inlet and the bispinous diameter of the midpelvis and divides the pelvis into an anterior and a posterior segment.

It has been suggested that the parallel planes be located at right angles to the coronal plane. From the lateral film of Thoms' method of x-ray pelvimetry, the following planes are drawn, parallel to each other and at right angles to the coronal plane:

1st plane — at the level slightly below the superior strait;
2nd plane — at the level of the ischial spines;
3rd plane — at the level of the tip of the sacrum;
4th plane — at the level of the ischial tuberosities.

According to this method of placement of the parallel planes, the distances between the planes may differ somewhat, depending on the depth of the pelvis and the level at which the sacrum ends. For example, the third plane which is drawn from the tip of the sacrum usually is located above the ischial tuberosity (Fig. 11). In some instances the third and fourth planes may nearly coincide, and, when the sacrum is long and ends low in the pelvis, their respective locations may actually be reversed. As will be seen, the ease of labor and delivery is related to these variations in location of the pelvic planes. In problems concerned with contracture of the midpelvis and pelvic outlet, the relationship of the third plane to the second and fourth planes is especially important.

CLASSIFICATION OF THE NORMAL AND THE ABNORMAL PELVIS

Prior to the 18th century when Hendrik van Deventer first made measurements of the pelvis in the living subject and recorded the differences, little attention had been given to the atypical or abnormal pelvis and its possible effect on labor. Following this, William Smellie verified these observations and found that the pelvic inlet could be contracted in the anteroposterior diameter alone or in all of its dimensions.

Throughout the 19th century the obstetric pelvis was exhaustively studied, especially by the French and German schools. Various forms of pelvic contracture were recognized, including many kinds of congenital defects, and from these observations several classifications were proposed. Modifications of the pelvis by congenital defects and diseases other than rickets were described in the most minute detail. When the pelvis was small throughout and no obvious cause was apparent, familial or racial influences were held responsible. However, many of the pelves included in these classifications are extremely rare, and prior to the use of roentgen rays those reported were found in dissected bodies rather than in the living patient.

In general, when the pelvic brim was contracted in all its dimensions, it was called a "generally contracted" or a "justo-minor" type. The term "flat" was used to describe the pelvis when the anteroposterior diam-

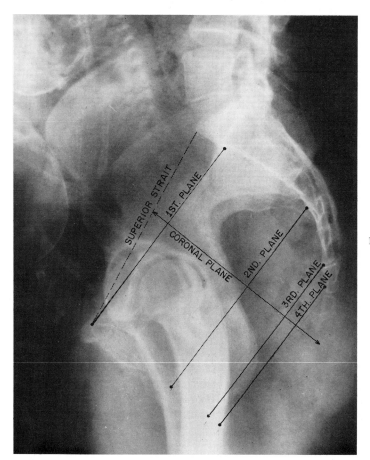

Figure 11. The coronal and parallel planes of the pelvis.

eter of the inlet was appreciably reduced. If both forms of contracture were believed present, the pelvis was termed "generally contracted flat." When rachitic changes were observed in these three parent types, the terminology was modified accordingly, that is, generally contracted rachitic pelvis, and so forth.

The idea that the outlet of the pelvis could be abnormally contracted emerged from investigations conducted mostly in the early part of the present century. This type of contracture was designated a funnel pelvis and was considered due either to a sacralization of the last lumbar vertebra (high assimilation pelvis) or to a generally contracted state of the pelvis. Perhaps not appreciated at the time, the discovery of this funneling effect associated with a contracted outlet was a forerunner of the obstetric concept that the female pelvis could embody male sex characters.

Since the introduction of the newer concepts of Caldwell, Moloy, and D'Esopo, and of Thoms, there has been a tendency to disregard previous terminology and to use and

teach the classifications proposed by these authorities. For the student and clinician this is a fortunate turn of affairs, for over the years the pelvic nomenclature was frequently modified, and consequently the classifications of the abnormal obstetric pelves became unnecessarily complex and without uniformity.

Modern systems of classification still suffer from a lack of universality of terms. It will be noted that in some instances the nomenclature as used by the anatomist and anthropologist conveys different meanings when applied to the obstetric classification of the pelvis. In order to reconcile these classifications and to inquire into the appropriateness of the terms used, some consideration must be given to the anthropologic and anatomic classifications from which the nomenclature was derived. Table 2 lists some of the more important classifications proposed by the anatomists and anthropologists, based on the appearance of the pelvic inlet.

When applied to the present-day classification of the obstetric pelvis, the wedge-

TABLE 2. COMPARATIVE TERMINOLOGY OF
PELVIC TYPES

Weber	von Stein	Turner
1) oval	truncated-cordate	–
2) round	round	mesatipellic
3) four-sided	elliptical-longitudinal	dolichopellic
4) wedge-shaped	elliptical-transverse	platypellic

shaped type of inlet presumably represents maleness, the elliptical-longitudinal would be similar to the anthropoid or dolichopellic pelvis, and the elliptical-transverse would denote the platypellic form. Turner's classification of pelvic type was derived and expressed by the pelvic index, while Weber and Stein used terms to denote only the outline of the inlet. Turner made no provision in his classification for the female pelvis, since his chief purpose was to relate racial effects on the male pelvis.

The obstetric pelvis is segregated into four parent types in the Greulich and Thoms classification, whereas the Caldwell-Moloy-D'Esopo classification, in addition to the parent types, recognizes a number of intermediate types. In each classification there is a relatively small number of pelves that cannot be classified by these methods. These are the pelves that are modified by disease, trauma, or congenital influences.

The Thoms classification, an elaboration of the Turner method, groups pelves according to the pelvic index of the inlet. The pelvic index is the relationship between the anteroposterior and transverse diameters of the inlet as expressed in the equation,

$$\frac{\text{anteroposterior diameter} \times 100}{\text{transverse diameter}} = \text{pelvic index.}$$

The extremes of the pelvic index are represented by the dolichopellic pelvis, with a value of 95 or more, and the platypellic type, with a value of 90 or less. Falling between these extremes are the indexes representing the mesatipellic and brachypellic types. As a result of applying this method in the study of a large number of pelves, Greulich and Thoms classified the inlet as follows:

1. Dolichopellic, or elongated type (i.e., the anteroposterior diameter exceeds the transverse diameter).

2. Mesatipellic, or round type (i.e., the anteroposterior and transverse diameters are of equal length, or the latter exceeds the anteroposterior diameter by not more than 1 cm.).

3. Brachypellic, or oval type (i.e., the transverse diameter exceeds the anteroposterior diameter by more than 1 cm. and less than 3 cm.).

4. Platypellic, or flat type (i.e., the transverse diameter exceeds the anteroposterior diameter by 3 cm. or more).

This classification recognizes the possible overlap in sex characters, and, if any evidence of maleness is present, it is included in the description of the pelvis. Such evidence may appear in the shape and size of the sacrosciatic notch and in the pubic arch and the contour of the anterior segment of the inlet.

Caldwell, Moloy, and D'Esopo base their nomenclature on the size and shape of the inlet and sex characters without regard to the pelvic index. Accordingly, the parent types of pelves are classified as follows:

1. *The anthropoid pelvis*, characterized by a long anteroposterior diameter of the inlet that equals or exceeds the length of the transverse diameter. The angle of the forepelvis of the superior strait may be long and narrow and average in size. The transverse diameter is located well in advance of the sacral promontory, denoted by a relatively long posterior sagittal diameter. The sacrosciatic notch is large, while the subpubic angle is usually wide and the size of the arch is normal (Figs. 12 and 13).

2. *The gynecoid pelvis*, characterized by a round or an oval pelvic inlet. The transverse diameter is placed well ahead of the promontory, and the sacrosciatic notch is large. The sacrum slopes backward, causing divergence of the pelvic bore. The subpubic angle is wide and the rami diverge to form a large Roman-type arch (Figs. 14 and 15).

3. *The android pelvis*, characterized by a wedge-shaped inlet with a narrow forepelvis. The transverse diameter is situated close to the sacrum, resulting in an extremely short posterior sagittal diameter of the inlet, i.e., *less than 3 cm.* The sacrosciatic notch is small, with the sacrum inclined forward toward the ischial spines, and the splay of the pelvis is convergent. The subpubic angle is more acute, with a narrow Gothic-type arch. It is recognized that the convergence of the side walls and

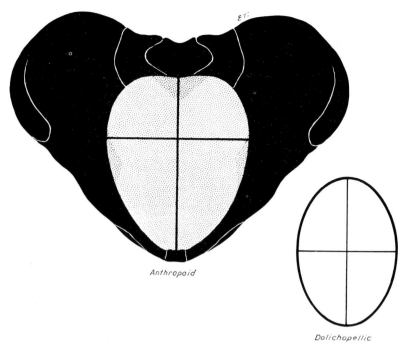

Anthropoid

Dolichopellic

Figure 12. Anteroposterior and transverse diameters of anthropoid pelvis, compared with dolichopellic pelvis.

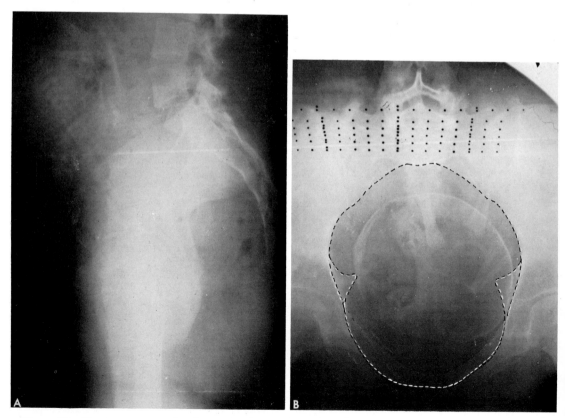

Figure 13. Roentgenograms of anthropoid pelvis. A, Lateral, and B, anteroposterior view. (Thoms' method of x-ray pelvimetry.)

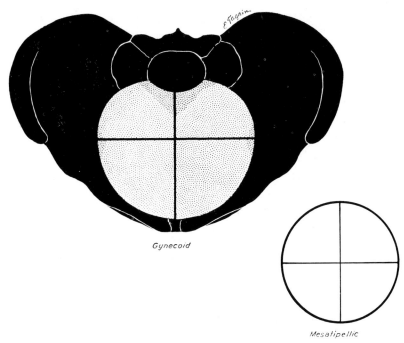

Gynecoid

Mesatipellic

Figure 14. Anteroposterior and transverse diameters of gynecoid pelvis, compared with mesatipellic pelvis.

the narrow subpubic arch represent masculine characteristics which may occur in other types of pelves (Figs. 16 and 17).

4. *The platypelloid pelvis*, characterized by flattening of the pelvic inlet with a short anteroposterior and a wide transverse diameter. With the exception of rachitic changes and resultant bony exostoses on the anterior surface, the sacrum has a normal curve. The sacrosciatic notch is large,

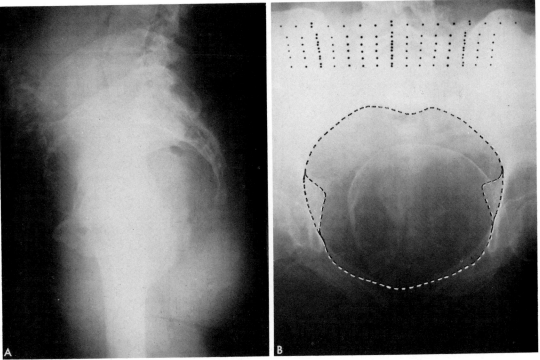

Figure 15. Roentgenograms of gynecoid pelvis. A, Lateral, and B, anteroposterior view.

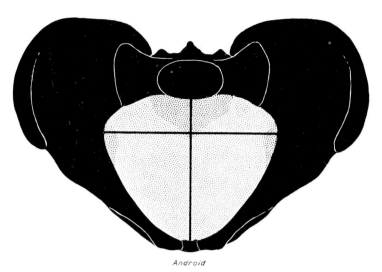

Android

Figure 16.   Anteroposterior and transverse diameters of android pelvis.

the pelvic bore divergent, and the pubic arch is wide (Figs. 18 and 19).

Except for the gynecoid type, the parent types listed above are relatively uncommon. An intermediary type of pelvis is one in which the inlet is composed of an anterior and a posterior segment of different parent types. The shape of the posterior segment, i.e., the area of the inlet posterior to the transverse diameter, determines the type; that of the anterior segment determines the tendency. For example, if the posterior segment of a pelvis has android characteristics and the forepelvis is gynecoid in outline, it would be classified as an "android pelvis with a gynecoid forepelvis."

For each parent type, therefore, the following intermediary types are possible:

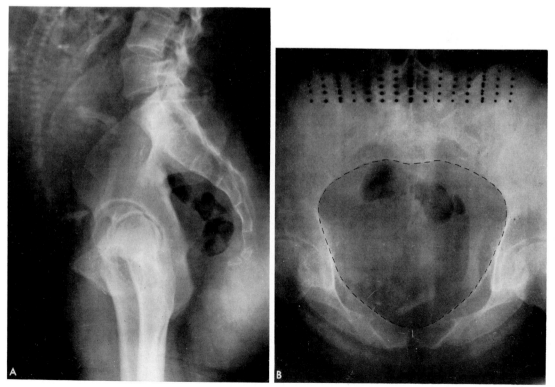

Figure 17.   Roentgenograms of android pelvis. A, Lateral, and B, anteroposterior view.

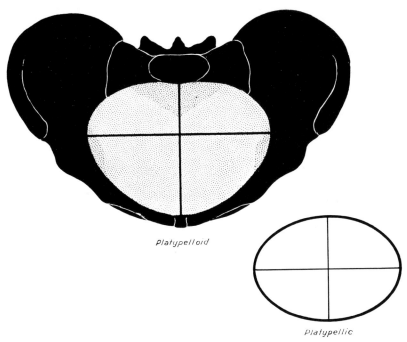

Platypelloid

Platypellic

Figure 18. Anteroposterior and transverse diameters of platypelloid pelvis, compared with platypellic pelvis.

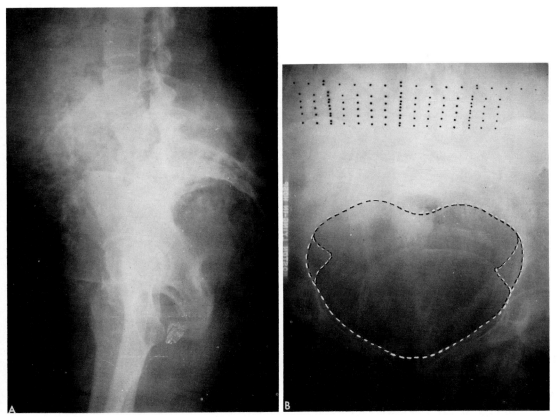

Figure 19. Roentgenograms of platypelloid pelvis. A, Lateral, and B, anteroposterior view.

1. Gynecoid
   (*a*) with anthropoid tendency;
   (*b*) with platypelloid tendency;
   (*c*) with android tendency.
2. Android
   (*a*) with anthropoid tendency;
   (*b*) with gynecoid tendency;
   (*c*) with platypelloid tendency.
3. Anthropoid
   (*a*) with gynecoid tendency;
   (*b*) with android tendency.
4. Platypelloid
   (*a*) with gynecoid tendency;
   (*b*) with android tendency.

These terms used to describe pelvic types are not completely acceptable to the anthropologists and anatomists, who use the term *gynecoid* to describe female sex characters in the male pelvis and *android* to denote male sex characters in the female pelvis. The term *anthropoid* (manlike) seems inappropriate, for the term *pithecoid* (apelike) would be more nearly correct in describing an elongated type of pelvis. The nomenclature of the Caldwell classification seems preferable despite the fact that it may lack the anthropologic correctness of the Thoms classification. Caldwell and his associates rightly believe that the shape of the forepelvis and the location of the transverse diameter of the inlet have great obstetric import, and these cannot be delineated by a classification that utilizes the pelvic index (see Fig. 4). This applies more especially to the android pelvis in which the forepelvis is narrow and the transverse diameter is located in close proximity to the sacral promontory.

INCIDENCE OF THE DIFFERENT PELVIC TYPES

Where the pelves have been routinely examined radiologically during the antepartum period, the incidence of the various types of pelves reported varies from series to series, depending upon the ethnic and racial groups studied and possible differences in their economic and nutritional status. In the original study of Caldwell et al., the pure gynecoid type of pelvis was observed in 40 per cent of the patients examined, while the pure android and anthropoid types of pelves each occurred in 12 per cent. The platypelloid pelvis was observed in approximately 1 per cent, leaving about 35 per cent of the intermediate forms (Table 3.).

TABLE 3.   INCIDENCE OF THE OCCURRENCE OF THE VARIOUS PELVIC TYPES

Classification	Incidence, Per Cent
True gynecoid type	40
Gynecoid type with android tendency	12
Gynecoid type with anthropoid tendency	4
Gynecoid type with platypelloid tendency	3
True android type	12
Android type with gynecoid tendency	5
Android type with anthropoid tendency	3
Android type with platypelloid tendency	2
True anthropoid type	12
Anthropoid type with gynecoid tendency	6
True platypelloid type	1
	100

*From Caldwell, W. E., Moloy, H. C., and D'Esopo, D. A., Amer. J. Obstet. Gynec., 28:482, 1934.

In other series the incidence of platypelloid pelvis has been reported to be as high as 3 per cent, while an incidence of 30 per cent or more has been reported for the anthropoid and android types. The incidence of anthropoid pelvis is said to be higher in black women than in white women, with the white women having a much higher incidence of android pelves.

MODIFICATION OF THE PELVIS BY DISEASE, CONGENITAL DEFECTS, OR TRAUMA

Mention must be made of the rachitic pelvis, for it has been the subject of much study and elaborate description and has always been regarded as a classic example of the effect of nutrition and disease on the pelvis. According to the usual description, the rachitic pelvis characteristically shows marked flattening in the anteroposterior diameter, causing the ilia to flare outward. The sacrum encroaches into the pelvic excavation, and in the presence of a flattish contour in the extreme gives the inlet a kidney-bean shape as viewed from above. There is a marked flare to the pelvic arch, with the ischial tuberosities situated wide apart. The sacral promontory, as indeed the entire sacrum, shows marked changes. The surface of the first sacral vertebra is flattened, and near the inferior border a false promontory may extend into the superior strait. Through bony exostoses over the anterior surface the sacrum loses its normal curvature and becomes straight (Fig. 20). In some instances, near the junc-

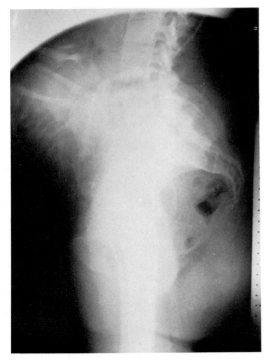

Figure 20. Lateral roentgenogram of a pelvis with the sacrum showing presumably marked rachitic changes.

tion of the bodies of the third and fourth sacral vertebrae, it may angulate forward acutely. It is now appreciated that rachitic changes may occur in any type of pelvis. The condition may be suspected when stigmata of the disease are apparent on physical examination.

The pelvis may be obliquely contracted owing to either congenital or acquired causes. This type of pelvic contracture may develop from a defect in the sacral ala, either from a congenital absence (Naegele's pelvis) or from destruction by an infectious process. Unilateral lameness or scoliosis of the spine, if present before puberty, may also cause the pelvis to be obliquely contracted. Although this type of pelvic deformity may be suspected from the history and pelvic examination, verification of the diagnosis depends on x-ray examination. In Naegele's pelvis there is a general cave-in of the wall of the pelvis on the affected side and the resultant contracture is accentuated from inlet to outlet. On pelvic examination the wall of the pelvis is easily palpated on the side involved (Fig. 21).

Transverse contracture of the pelvis, due to the absence of both sacral alae, known as a Robert pelvis, is sometimes referred to as a double Naegele pelvis. Again, the trans-

versely contracted pelvis is believed to be due either to congenital absence of the sacral alae or to their destruction by infection. As one might anticipate, the marked narrowing of the pelvis is readily recognized on pelvic examination.

The kyphotic pelvis develops secondary to diseases of the spine. Severe kyphosis may be present, however, especially above the lumbar region, without affecting the shape of the pelvis. Characteristically the kyphotic pelvis shows enlargement of the inlet and contracture of the lower portion of the pelvis. When the kyphosis is located in the lumbar region, the outward displacement of the involved vertebrae pulls the sacrum backward, causing the innominate bones to rotate outward. This outward rotation tends to bring the ischial spines and tuberosities and lower portion of the pelvis closer together, causing a contracture of the midpelvic and inferior pelvic planes.

The pelvis of osteomalacia has a characteristic appearance. The sacral promontory moves forward and downward into the excavation of the pelvic cavity, and with the upward thrust of the femur there is marked constriction of the midpelvis with characteristic narrowing of the pubic arch, which in the extreme brings the pubic rami very

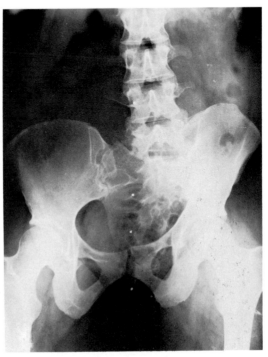

Figure 21. Anteroposterior roentgenogram of Naegele pelvis.

nearly in apposition to each other. From above downward the pelvis presents a triangular shape, and in extreme cases the inlet may be nearly obliterated. (See discussion of Osteomalacia in Chapter 30.)

In dwarfism not only is the pelvis small, but there is a disproportionate decrease in the anteroposterior diameter, causing a flattening of the inlet (Fig. 22).

Spondylolisthetic pelvis is the result of a pathologic displacement of the last lumbar vertebra, which in the extreme may cause inlet contracture. The initial symptoms may develop during pregnancy, owing to increased weight-bearing and relaxation of the pelvic ligaments. In the more severe cases the lumbar vertebra may be readily palpated on pelvic examination as it encroaches over the pelvic inlet. Diagnosis of the more frequent and milder forms of the condition is dependent on x-ray rather than on pelvic examination. Rarely is the displacement of the vertebra of such magnitude, however, that the presenting part of the fetus is unable to enter the superior strait.

PELVIC CONTRACTURE

From the exhaustive studies of the obstetric pelvis beginning in the 18th century, values were established for the true conjugate for the purpose of defining a contracted pelvis. Today, these standards, when translated into modern nomenclature, continue to have obstetric meaning. It was believed that a true or obstetric conjugate of 10.0 and 9.5 cm. characterized the generally contracted (small gynecoid) and the flat (platypelloid) pelvis, respectively. The degree of pelvic contracture was graded from borderline to absolute, the latter indicating an inlet with a true conjugate of 5.5 cm. It was appreciated that the large transverse diameter of the platypelloid pelvis could compensate for a significant degree of anteroposterior shortening.

The definition of pelvic contracture, therefore, must be somewhat arbitrary, for the type of the pelvis in which contracture occurs is of equal significance. As has been stated, an enlargement in one diameter may compensate for contracture in another, and permit pelvic delivery. By contrast, the diameters of the pelvis may be of normal length, but so arranged, as in the android pelvis, that they cannot be utilized effectively by the fetal vertex, and pelvic delivery may thus fail.

Although the original definition of a contracted pelvis was derived from the size of the pelvic inlet, it later became apparent that all three of the major planes might be

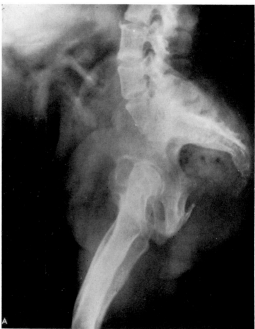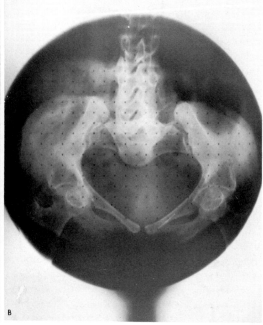

Figure 22.   Roentgenograms of the pelvis of an achondroplastic dwarf. A, Lateral, and B, anteroposterior view.

contracted, either singly or in combination. Therefore, a pelvis in which any major plane is reduced below normal size is considered a contracted pelvis. Classification of the contracture is based on the pelvic type, the planes involved, and the calculated capacity. For example, a contracted pelvis might be designated an "android pelvis" with possible "inlet, midpelvic, or outlet contracture" and with a "pelvic capacity" of a certain percentage of normal.

Pelvic contracture at the inlet must be suspected when the anteroposterior diameter is reduced below 11.0 cm. Some degree of midpelvic contracture is present when the bispinous diameter is less than 9.5 cm. and the posterior sagittal diameter of the midpelvic plane is less than 5.0 cm. The latter measurement is consistent with a sacrum that curves forward and reduces the size of the sacrosciatic notch. Equally important and not sufficiently emphasized is the fact that the sacrum may end *at* or *above* the level of the ischial tuberosities and near the level of the ischial spines. Such a condition prevents the presenting fetal part from descending sufficiently low in the pelvis to take full advantage of the bi-ischial diameter of the outlet. To offset this disadvantage, the sacrum must be situated well posterior, as indicated by a long posterior sagittal diameter or by a large sacrosciatic notch. Conversely, although the sacrum may curve forward and decrease the size of the sacrosciatic notch, this need not necessarily cause midpelvic contracture and thereby impede labor, provided the sacral tip as determined by the third plane is situated at or below the level of the ischial tuberosities. This concept is a departure from the conventional and will be considered further in the discussion of the abnormal pelvis.

Outlet contracture may be defined as a condition in which the sum of the bi-ischial and posterior sagittal diameters of the inferior plane is less than 15.0 cm. Normally, the bi-ischial diameter is 11.0 cm., and the posterior sagittal diameter is 7.0 to 9.0 cm. A bi-ischial diameter of 8.5 cm. or less is consistent with a contracted outlet and will not allow delivery from below unless the infant is small or there is compensatory space in the posterior segment of the outlet, as indicated by a posterior sagittal diameter longer than normal.

Opinion differs on how best to define and detect outlet contracture. It has been proposed that the anteroposterior diameter of the outlet (inferior strait), as measured from the inferior or lower border of the symphysis to the tip of the sacrum, is the most reliable index of the size of the outlet. It has been shown that the length of this diameter of the outlet does not differ in the two sexes. The same study, however, revealed a marked difference in the area or usable space of the pelvic outlet in the male and the female pelvis, being 78.0 sq.cm. and 93.7 sq.cm., respectively (see Table 1). The average bi-ischial (intertuberous) diameter was 10.1 cm. in the female and 9.3 in the male, while the subpubic angle was 93.5 degrees in the female and 75.8 degrees in the male. It is suggested that the adequacy of the outlet is determined by what has been here defined as the inferior pelvic plane, as assessed by the flare of the arch and the length of the bi-ischial and posterior sagittal diameters, rather than by the length of the anteroposterior diameter of the inferior strait.

Although the pelvic planes are described separately, it is important to emphasize that the midpelvis and outlet should always be considered together in evaluating the adequacy of the lower pelvis. Outlet contracture without midpelvic contracture can occur and should be recognized, but is infrequent. Five anatomic features are involved in midpelvic and outlet problems:

1. The length of the bispinous diameter
2. The sacral inclination as indicated by the size of the sacrosciatic notch
3. The location of the sacral tip in relation to the second and fourth pelvic planes
4. The shape of the pubic arch and size of the subpubic angle
5. The length of the bi-ischial and posterior sagittal diameters

Except for the bispinous diameter, which can be accurately measured only by x-ray pelvimetry, physical examination of the pelvis should enable one to evaluate the remainder adequately for clinical purposes. If all of these features are unfavorable, pelvic delivery may be impossible unless the infant is small. A wide pubic arch, however, can compensate to a degree for a shortened bispinous diameter and a forward sacrum. Likewise, marked shortening of the bi-ischial distance and a Gothic-type arch may still allow pelvic delivery if the spines are widely spaced and the sacrum has a normal curve and ends well below the ischial spines, all of which means that the posterior sagittal diameter of the outlet is ample.

The incidence of pelvic contracture associated with specific pelvic types has not been reported in any sizable series. Because the gynecoid pelvis occurs with greater frequency, it may be expected that the greatest number of contracted pelves are of this type. The pelvis is contracted proportionately in all dimensions, and, therefore, all of the three major planes are involved. A pelvis so contracted is often referred to as a "small gynecoid" type. The clinical problem is usually one of inlet disproportion, but the descent of the presenting part into the pelvis does not exclude the possibility of the presence of midpelvic outlet contracture. Pelvic contracture is seemingly next most frequently encountered in the android variety. This type of pelvis is associated with midpelvic and outlet contracture, although all of the pelvic planes may be involved. Pelvic contracture is less commonly seen in the anthropoid type, and only when the bispinous diameter is decreased significantly by virtue of the narrowing of the side walls. Because of its low incidence, pelvic contracture associated with a platypelloid pelvis is comparatively rare, although the frequency of this type of pelvis differs appreciably, depending on the locale. The clinical problem is principally that of the superior strait, for the lower pelvis is not contracted with the possible exception of marked deformity of the lower sacrum from rickets.

X-RAY PELVIMETRY

After the introduction of roentgenology, sporadic attempts were made to visualize the pelvis, but not until the invention of the moving grid by Potter in 1921 was there sustained interest in the problem. Since then many methods and techniques of x-ray pelvimetry have been developed, and some of these are concerned with fetometry, the chief purpose of which is to determine the size and maturity of the fetus.

The objectives of any method of pelvioroentgenography are:

1. To provide a description of the general architecture of the obstetric pelvis
2. To ascertain the length of the diameters of the significant pelvic planes
3. To compute the pelvic capacity

4. To outline the cephalopelvic relationship
5. To determine progress in labor by means of serial roentgenograms

All methods of x-ray pelvimetry suffer from the fact that the roentgen rays diverge as they originate from the x-ray tube, with resultant distortion of the image of the pelvis on the x-ray film. In some techniques corrections must be made for oblique as well as for divergent distortion.

The following outline lists the divisions and subtypes of the techniques of x-ray pelvimetry which have been developed.

   I. Position Methods
      A. Isometric scales
      B. Proportional scales
      C. Triangular proportion
         1. Direct application of equations
         2. Graphs of equations
         3. Slide rules
  II. Parallax Methods
      A. Stereoscopic
         1. Direct parallax
         2. Measurement of virtual image
         3. Geometric construction
            a. Plane
            b. Solid
      B. Nonstereoscopic
         1. Single film
         2. Multiple films
            Cartesian coordinates
 III. 90-Degree Triangulation
      A. Empiric
      B. Geometric construction
         1. Plane
         2. Cartesian coordinates
 IV. Orthometric Reproduction
      A. Pantographic
      B. Orthoscopic
      C. Geometric

Only a few of these techniques are considered here, and only one is discussed in detail.

Position methods involve arrangement of the patient to the x-ray tube so that the part to be examined bears a known relationship to the film. For example, the obstetric conjugate is measured on a lateral roentgenogram because of the accepted belief that it lies in a plane which is parallel to the sagittal plane of the body. Similarly, the true conjugate of the inlet can be measured on the anteroposterior film because of the assumption that it lies in the superior plane of the pelvis. In the position method, isometric rulers, proportional scales, slide rules, and specially prepared charts are used to correct distortion.

The second large division includes the parallax methods, which are based on the apparent displacement of an object as viewed from two different points. The effect is demonstrable, for example, by the perceivable movement of an object when it is viewed alternately by one eye and then the other. A comparable effect is produced by substituting the x-ray tube for the eyes. Two films are exposed, with the x-ray tube shifted a measured distance between exposures. When these films are superimposed, the amount of displacement or parallax between the images of the parts may be measured. This method may disregard the relation of the anatomic parts to body surfaces or to the film, or their distance from the x-ray tube. When the maternal or fetal part lies parallel to the plane of the film, a direct measurement can be made from the latter without further equipment. If the pelvis or fetal part is not parallel to the film, the two films or stereoroentgenograms must be viewed through a measuring stereoscope to correct the oblique distortion. Geometric reconstruction, in which a true geometric model is made of the object portrayed in the roentgenogram, has also been used to interpret stereoroentgenograms.

Another commonly used technique has been referred to as the 90 degree triangulation method. This technique specifies pelvic dimensions, capacity, and the volumetric mensuration of the fetal head by the use of anteroposterior and lateral-view roentgenograms of the pelvis. Linear and volumetric magnification or distortion of the pelvis and fetal head may be corrected by an instrument known as the pelvocephalometer and a specially prepared chart. When the fetal cranium and pelvic diameters have been measured in units of volume and volume capacity, respectively, a definite fetal cranium–pelvic diameter ratio is evolved.

The fourth division comprises methods of true scale drawings made of the various sections of the pelvis. These orthometric reproductions obtained from x-rays permit a complete and permanent record of the pelvis without subsequent reference to the films.

When measurements of the pelvis obtained by the various methods outlined were compared, it was found that there was less than 1.0 cm. deviation in all measurements made. All of these techniques evidently give accurate results, provided the procedure is carefully performed. One should seek, therefore, a method that provides: (1) simplicity of performance, (2) clear recognition of the pelvic architecture, (3) ready measurement of the pelvic diameters, (4) an index of the fetopelvic relationship, and (5) ease of x-ray interpretation. It is proposed that these criteria are best fulfilled by the method developed by Thoms.

The Thoms Technique

The Thoms technique is a position method. The distortion is corrected by the use of a radiopaque ruler and grid. These appurtenances, being subjected to the same distortion as the pelvis, may be regarded as isometric scales for the diameters to be measured.

The technique employs two views of the pelvis: the first, an anteroposterior view of the inlet, and the second, a lateral view. For the anteroposterior film, the patient is arranged on the x-ray table in a semi-reclining position with a back rest placed at about a 35- to 40-degree angle in relation to the table (Fig. 23A). With the patient in a reclining position, the gonads of a fetus in vertex presentation are protected from exposure to irradiation.

By so placing the patient, the superior plane is nearly parallel to the x-ray film. Two measurements are required to provide this relationship: the first is taken from 1.0 cm. below the superior margin of the symphysis to the x-ray table (line A); the second is taken posteriorly from the junction of the fourth and fifth lumbar vertebrae to the table top (line B). A satisfactory silhouette of the inlet is obtained when these measurements are nearly identical. By adjustment of the back rest, the patient's pelvis is tilted forward or backward slightly to equalize these distances. The x-ray tube is centered about 5 cm. superior to the patient's symphysis and 32 inches from the x-ray film.

After the film has been exposed, the patient is removed from the table. A lead plate or grid containing rows of perforations along one margin is placed on the x-ray table over the area previously occupied by the patient. From the measurements used above to align the pelvic inlet the grid is adjusted to coincide with the superior plane. A flash exposure is then made, projecting the several rows of perforations onto the top edge of the x-ray film. In the first row

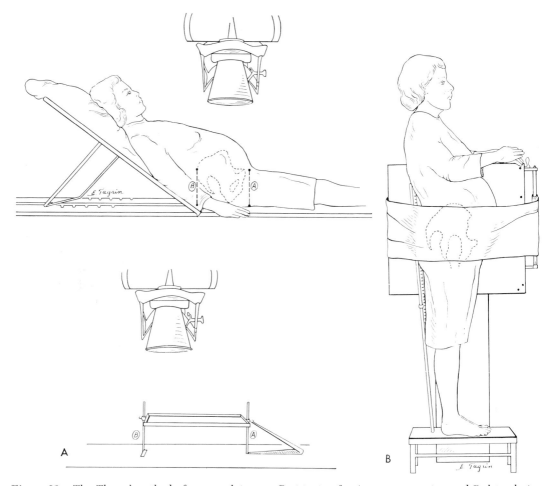

Figure 23. The Thoms' method of x-ray pelvimetry. Positioning for A, anteroposterior, and B, lateral view.

the area between each perforation represents a centimeter with respect to any measurement taken on or about the superior plane of the pelvis. The area between each perforation of the other five successive rows represents a centimeter distance of any measurement taken at 5, 6, 7, 8, and 9 cm. below the pelvic inlet, respectively. From the finished film of the anteroposterior exposure, the conjugata vera and the posterior and anterior sagittal, transverse, and oblique diameters of the inlet can be readily demonstrated and measured directly.

A lateral view of the pelvis is obtained by placing the patient in a standing position with her side against the Bucky diaphragm (Fig. 23B). The x-ray tube is centered at a distance of 5 feet. A movable stand with a calibrated notched rod which can be raised or lowered conveniently is placed between the buttocks of the patient. The rod is notched at 1.0-cm. intervals, and this isometric scale is superimposed on the lateral portion of the film at the time of exposure. This provides a scale to correct distortion. The lateral film affords a view of five diameters, which are directly measurable and which are clinically significant:

1. The obstetric conjugate—from the innermost area on the posterior surface of the symphysis to the sacrum

2. The true conjugate—from the upper border of the symphysis to the sacral promontory

3. The anteroposterior diameter of the midpelvic plane—from the inferior margin of the symphysis to near the lower border of the fourth sacral vertebra

4. The posterior sagittal diameter of the midpelvic plane—from the visible ischial spine to the near border of the fourth sacral

vertebra. It is this diameter which best serves as an index to the size of the sacrosciatic notch

5. The posterior sagittal diameter of the inferior plane—from the ischial tuberosity to the end of the sacrum

Strictly speaking, the posterior sagittal diameters of the midpelvic and inferior planes should be measured from the points where they bisect the bispinous and bi-ischial diameters, but this is impossible. The distortion is negligible, however, and may be disregarded. In order to measure the bispinous diameter, both inlet and lateral films must be utilized. A line is first drawn on the lateral film from the superior border of the symphysis to the sacral promontory. From this line, at the point where the transverse diameter and conjugata vera intersect, a perpendicular line is dropped to the ischial spine. The length of this perpendicular line is the distance from the inlet to the bispinous diameter of the midpelvic plane. A direct measurement is now taken of the bispinous diameter from the inlet film. The measurement obtained is placed on the appropriate row of perforations required to correct distortion of the bispinous diameter. For example, if the bispinous diameter is 7 cm. below the pelvic inlet according to the perpendicular line on the lateral film, the fourth row of calibrations as seen on the inlet film is used to provide an isometric reading of the correct length of the bispinous diameter.

The method of Thoms has been modified somewhat, especially in regard to positioning of the patient to bring out certain pelvic and fetal details, or by improving the isometric scale for the correction of distortion. In essence, the principles of pelvimetry are the same, and the differences in technique are concerned primarily with detail.

Some clinics advocate and prefer a combination of a position method similar to the Thoms technique and a parallax method utilizing a precision stereoscope. In the classification of normal and abnormal pelves and a more precise description of the mechanism of labor, Caldwell, Moloy, and D'Esopo found the stereoroentgenograms indispensable. Undoubtedly, this combined method of x-ray examination affords a more complete view of the birth canal. Not only does it provide measurements of the various diameters, but it allows the examiner to observe the relationship of the fetal head to the planes of the pelvis. But, again,

the size and location of the pelvic diameters, which are easily discernible in the Thoms method, are the important factors in governing the outcome of labor.

In the simplest technique for measuring the pelvic outlet, the patient is seated at the end of the x-ray table and is asked to bend as far forward as her condition will permit. The tube is centered over the lower sacrum posterior, and the film is exposed. In such a position the bi-ischial tuberosities and the pubic arch can be visualized, and the bi-ischial diameter measured. The value of x-ray examination of the outlet must be questioned, however, for the information gained may indeed be misleading. The bi-ischial diameter may not reflect the size or shape of the pelvic arch. Moreover, this is the one plane of the pelvis that can be accurately evaluated by pelvic examination and measured by external pelvimetry, thereby eliminating the necessity of an x-ray examination. On the rare occasion when the examiner may still be in doubt as to the size of the lower pelvis, an examination with the patient anesthetized will dispel this uncertainty. If required, this is most informative in the early hours of labor when fetal size can also be evaluated.

The interpretation of the Thoms roentgenograms includes the measurements of the various diameters of the major pelvic planes, a description of the pelvis, a calculation of the pelvic capacity, a statement regarding the cephalopelvic relationship, and, if pelvic contracture is thought to exist, determination of the pelvic planes involved. In addition to the diagnosis of pelvic type, a prognosis is offered as to the outcome of labor. As previously noted, the pelvic type is determined from the inlet film, but the final diagnosis is dependent also upon the appearance of the pelvis as observed in the lateral film.

The shape of the superior plane or inlet is described in toto and according to the configuration of the anterior and posterior segments. Depending on the relative size of the retropubic angle, the shape of the anterior segment is described as oval or convergent. The outline of the posterior segment is reported as shallow or deep, as it relates to the distance between the sacral promontory and the position of the transverse diameter of the inlet. The size and shape of the sacrosciatic notch are recorded and, in addition to the measurement of the bispinous diameter, some notation is made of the prominence of the ischial spines. The bore of the pelvis is described as being straight, divergent, or convergent, according to the position and appearance of the sacrum. Normal divergence is dependent on a sacrum that is located posteriorly and is normally concave. The position of the sacrum is perhaps more accurately described by determining the size of the angle formed where it meets the superior plane. This value can readily be obtained by lines drawn from the upper margin of the symphysis to the sacral promontory and from the promontory to the tip of the sacrum. Normally the angle so formed is 90 degrees or more. Some convergence may exist if the angle is less than 90 degrees, particularly when it measures less than 70 to 80 degrees. Convergence may be produced if the sacrum is straight rather than concave. Should the sacrum be straight, the areas involved should be carefully and accurately described. The sacrum may be straight throughout, or only in its upper portion. These differences should be accurately noted because of their relationship to the contracture of the various major planes of the pelvis.

The location of the sacral tip as it relates to the ischial spines and tuberosities, or its possible encroachment on the lower portion of the sacrosciatic notch, should be mentioned. This relationship may be best established by drawing the parallel planes on the lateral film as previously described (see Fig. 11). The height at which the sacrum terminates should be interpreted also because of the way it may influence the length of the posterior sagittal diameter of the outlet. When the sacrum ends high, this diameter, although it may be normal or longer than normal, may give a false impression that the posterior segment of the midpelvic and inferior planes is spacious. Finally, when taken in the latter weeks of pregnancy or during labor, the lateral film can aid in establishing whether the fetopelvic relationship is normal as it pertains to engagement of the presenting part or whether any disproportion exists at the superior and midpelvic planes.

MEASUREMENT OF PELVIC CAPACITY

The capacity of the pelvis has been measured by a variety of x-ray methods, many of which are so complicated that they hardly lend themselves to routine usage. Recently, simpler methods have been presented for estimating the pelvic capacity.

One method calculates the surface area of the superior plane by introducing the x-ray measurements of the anteroposterior (A) and transverse (B) diameters of the inlet in the following formula: $\pi \times \frac{1}{2} A \times \frac{1}{2} B$. Should the inlet area be 110 sq.cm. or more, it is stated that the baby's head will invariably enter the pelvis. The level of uncertainty is reached when the area is reduced to 90 sq.cm.; if the inlet is less than 80 sq.cm. it is said that the term-size fetal head will enter the pelvis in only one of five cases.

A second method calculates the surface areas of the inlet and midpelvic planes from appropriate radiographs, and the values are expressed in terms of pelvic capacity. This method can be applied to roentgenograms taken by the Thoms technique. Being the product of the true or obstetric conjugate (11 cm.) and the transverse diameter (13 cm.), the normal surface area of the pelvic inlet or capacity is approximately 145 sq.cm. The normal surface area of the midpelvic plane is similarly calculated from the anteroposterior diameter (12 cm.) and the bispinous diameter (10.5 cm.), which gives a value of 125 sq.cm. Dystocia is anticipated if the surface areas of the inlet and midpelvic planes are less than 85 per cent of the calculated normal. Therefore, pelvic capacity is believed to be restricted when the inlet and midpelvic planes, respectively, are approximately 123 sq.cm. and 107 sq.cm., or less.

More important than methods of estimating capacity is the question whether pelvic volume or pelvic diameters are more significant in determining the outcome of labor. Pelvic capacity is undoubtedly meaningful when all of the major diameters are contracted, as in the small gynecoid type of pelvis. In the platypelloid pelvis, however, the capacity of the inlet may be reduced below the norm because of the unusually short anteroposterior diameter, but the fetal vertex may pass through the superior strait by taking advantage of the longer transverse diameter. By contrast, engagement may fail to occur in the android pelvis, even when the capacity of the superior plane is normal. Under these circumstances the fetus may be unable to avail itself of the adequate transverse diameter because of the proximity of this diameter to the sacral promontory. Accordingly, it is proposed that the outcome of labor depends more on the length and location of the pelvic diameters than on pelvic capacity. *The success with which the fetal head negotiates the birth canal is dependent principally on a diameter of adequate length, properly located within each of the major planes of the pelvis.*

FETAL CEPHALOMETRY

Fetal cephalometry, the purpose of which is to estimate the maturity and size of the fetus, has been performed with a number of x-ray techniques. This information would be useful clinically when premature termination of pregnancy is contemplated or the fetopelvic relationship is uncertain. Until recently, cephalometry received little acceptance in clinical obstetrics, for the techniques are complicated and only chance positioning of the fetal head in utero will allow accurate x-ray visualization of the desired diameters of the fetal skull. With ultrasound, it now appears possible to measure the biparietal diameter of the fetus from the 28th week onward with an accuracy of 3 mm. The technique is applicable in cases of cephalopelvic disproportion and breech presentation. As indicated previously, the method is extremely useful in determining fetal development and growth, since it is said that from the 28th week onward the biparietal diameter normally increases 1.8 mm. a week.

IRRADIATION HAZARDS IN PREGNANCY, WITH SPECIAL REFERENCE TO X-RAY PELVIMETRY

With the arrival of the nuclear age, the potential hazards of ionizing radiation on biologic processes has assumed greater significance and caused rightful concern. This is particularly pertinent to the biology of pregnancy.

Many of the effects of irradiation have long been known, but more recently emphasis has been placed on its remote effects as they relate to the etiology of malignant disease, more particularly leukemia, and the influence on the mutation rate. Both of these must receive the serious attention of those responsible for the care of pregnant women. The literature on this subject has reached voluminous proportions, and the student must seek the current thoughts on this subject elsewhere. Only a few aspects of the principles as they apply to clinical obstetrics will be discussed here.

Although no sharp division is possible, the problem of the term fetus involves principally the overall irradiation effect. As previously stated, by proper positioning of the mother on the x-ray table, the Thoms method can be and has been modified so that in vertex presentations the fetal gonads are not exposed. Consequently, in this circumstance the main concern with the fetus is the possible relationship of irradiation to malignant conditions in later life. By contrast, the hazard to the mother is chiefly gonadal or genetic.

Progress in the evolutionary process, although due to mutation, is made at the expense of a number of resultant environmental misfits. Therefore, most mutations are detrimental, with a tendency to reduce normal survival time. However, it has been pointed out by many that, as medical science is able to save and prolong life with greater frequency, more individuals with congenital defects will survive and reproduce. In other words, in an individual whose life has been saved by medical care, a set of genes persists which otherwise might have been eliminated by natural selection. This is a further sobering thought when irradiation is being used in the presence of a fetus.

It has been recommended by the National Academy of Sciences that efforts be made to ensure that members of the general population receive no more than 10 roentgens (R) to the reproductive cells before the age of 30; during this time background and cosmic radiation contribute approximately 4.3 to 5.5 R. Further, no person should receive more than a total accumulated dose of 50 R up to that age, and no more than an additional 50 R before the age of 40. The relationship between mutation rate and irradiation dosage is apparently a linear one, and it has been stated that to equal or thereby double the spontaneous mutation would require 100 R. There is ample evidence, however, to indicate that a comparable mutation rate can be produced with less irradiation in mammals than in lower forms of life. The clinician is forced into the position that, in terms of future generations, there is no "safe" dose of irradiation.

Radiation can reach the reproductive organs either from the direct beam during investigation of the pelvic region or through scatter during investigation in other parts of the body. The dosage can be measured directly in males, but in females it must be computed indirectly. Skin dosage must be converted to ovarian dosage. Using water phantoms and cadavers, into which an ionization chamber has been deposited, attempts have been made to determine the skin-to-ovary dosage ratio, taking into consideration the thickness of the patient and the distance of the ovary from the source of the radiation. These values are regarded within the range of 50 per cent of absolute accuracy. On this basis, a fragment of the available data relating to irradiation dosage at x-ray examinations commonly used for the obstetric patient is presented in Table 4. The data on x-ray pelvimetry are calculated for the modified Thoms method. The dosages to the two ovaries differ substantially in the lateral exposure.

The small amount of radiation expended seems not to preclude placentography or x-ray examination for fetal position, both of which are extremely useful in patient management. The overall irradiation to the fetus and maternal gonads in the course of pelvi-

metry represents the greatest obstetric hazard. The dosage presumably is reducible to 1 or 2 R. The factors that influence dosage should be constantly scrutinized—namely, positioning of the patient, beam filtration, skin distance to field and target, type of screen and film used, and the kilovoltage. Further, in pyelography in pregnancy only one or possibly two films need be taken rather than the conventional four.

On sound indication, roentgen examination is permissible in pregnancy, but, if possible, the procedure should never be repeated. Certainly opinions vary as to which method of x-ray pelvimetry is the most valuable. It follows that the profession must decide not only what types of x-ray examination can be safely done during pregnancy, but also what technique should be used. Finally, if x-ray pelvimetry is to be performed, it should be postponed until the last weeks of pregnancy when, except in event of breech presentation, irradiation to the fetal gonads can be largely avoided.

INDICATIONS FOR POSSIBLE X-RAY EXAMINATION

The possibility of performing x-ray examination should be considered
(1) when the history reveals:
  (a) previous obstetric difficulties associated with labor and delivery,
  (b) unexplained stillbirth or neonatal death,
  (c) longstanding infertility,
  (d) previous cesarean section and pelvic delivery is contemplated;
(2) when pelvic examination reveals:
  (a) inlet contracture, with the diagonal conjugate less than 12.5 to 12.0 cm.,
  (b) mid-pelvic contracture, as suggested by
    (i)   estimated small bispinous diameter,
    (ii) small sacrosciatic notch,
    (iii) a straight sacrum with a forward inclination,
    (iv) converging pelvic side walls, or
    (v)   small clinical measurements of the outlet;
(3) in test of labor without progress;
(4) in an elderly primipara;
(5) in patients who require therapeutic induction of labor, as in pregnancy tox-

TABLE 4. AMOUNT OF IRRADIATION IN X-RAY PROCEDURES USED IN OBSTETRIC MANAGEMENT

	(Source°)	Fetal Gonads	Center of Fetus	Maternal Gonads
Placentography	(1)	0.1	0.16	0.45–0.02
Lateral pelvis	(1)		0.9	1.75–0.05
	(3)		1.0	2.7 –0.12
Inlet	(1)	3.0	1.1	1.4 each
	(2)		0.47	0.44
	(3)		1.0	1.4
Outlet	(1)		0.2	0.2
	(3)		0.1	0.02
I.V. pyelogram	(3)			0.4 (2 films)
Photofluorogram of the chest				0.0053†
Regular chest film				0.00025†

°Compiled from:
(1) Clayton, et al: Brit. J. Radiol., 30:291, 1957 (Thoms' method);
(2) Moir, J.: Lancet, 2:99, 1956;
(3) Modified Thoms' method of x-ray pelvimetry.
†Estimated values.

emia, diabetes mellitus, and other medical conditions, and when the size of the pelvis is in doubt; and

6) in case of abnormal presentations: breech, brow, face, and transverse position.

The physical examination of the pelvis should not give way to reliance on the x-ray examination to identify deviations in the pelvic architecture. It is entirely possible for the clinician to become so proficient in pelvic examination as to be able to render a prognosis relative to subsequent labor and delivery with an accuracy approaching that based on x-ray pelvimetry.

The intent of these remarks is not to minimize the value of x-ray pelvimetry, but rather to attempt to place the examination in its proper perspective. Similar to x-ray examination of other parts of the body, radiographic pelvimetry finds its greatest usefulness when it is correlated with the physical examination. *It is essential that the obstetrician interpret the x-ray films himself, for only in this manner can pelvimetry be properly related to the obstetric problem at hand.*

RÉSUMÉ

This chapter attempts to discuss the subject of the obstetric pelvis within the context of the physical attributes of the human pelvis and the effect these anatomic characteristics may have on parturition and its consequences. The writer has the impression that most students, like himself, did not have the wit or the opportunity to take a course in physical anthropology. The acquisition of the upright position in the human has brought about changes in the pelvic architecture that distinguish man from the other primates and that have relevance to the problems associated with the birth process and those gynecologic problems and complaints which may arise later through a disturbance of the supporting structures of the pelvic organs—more precisely, the urinary bladder, uterus, and rectum.

The location and contour of the sacrum and the prominence of the ischial spines are anatomic characteristics of the human pelvis that can influence parturition markedly. In primates other than the human the pubic arch flares widely like outstretched arms and is nearly parallel to the symphysis. We must be reminded that the term perineum applies to the soft tissues incorporated within the area of the symphysis, the pubic arch, and the coccyx, and not simply the tissue between the posterior fourchette of the vagina and rectum. Hence, in the subhuman primate, the entire perineum can dilate in the process of birth but not so in the human. In the human, it is the perineal body and surrounding structures that are subject to the greatest amount of pressure from the presenting part of the fetus in the course of delivery.

Attempt has been made to distill the older literature and relate some of the previous terms used to describe the pelvis in accordance with the more modern terminology, and by so doing, discard the cumbersome pelvic nomenclatures of the past. Actually, many of the older classifications are hard to compare one with another. There are wide discrepancies in the literature of the 18th and 19th centuries of what constitutes normal and abnormal pelvic measurements. In fact, the unit used to express the pelvic diameter differed from one section of the European continent to the other and between the French, German, and English schools.

From the writings of the present century, paradoxes and controversy continue over the relative influence of the genetic and environmental factors in the shaping of the pelvis. Because of reluctance to use x-ray except when needed diagnostically, it is doubtful that additional information will be forthcoming, for such studies would require serial and periodic roentgen examination of female siblings during childhood and through puberty and of the pelvic architecture of the mother, with an evaluation in accordance with the ethnic and socioeconomic environment of the family.

But the greatest exception taken to the past is the introduction of the writer's concepts of the location of the pelvic axis, the four important planes of the pelvis, as he interprets the writings of Caldwell, Moloy, and D'Esopo. The location of the pelvic axis has relevance to the direction in which the fetal vertex traverses the birth canal, and the level in the pelvis where rotation and extension of the fetal vertex occurs. Moreover, adherence to the anatomic principles of the direction, pelvic axis, and the location of the pelvic planes, as herein defined, is basic to gentle, atraumatic forceps delivery.

With the lower two planes and their relation to the vital triangle of the ischial spines, tip of the sacrum, and ischial tuberosities in mind, the diagnosis of lower and midpelvic contracture is easily made on pelvic examination. Although rare, the failure to diagnose midpelvic and outlet contractures is the greatest of all obstetric mistakes in the conduct of trial labor. X-ray examination adds little and is not required for diagnosis. Its greatest value resides in identifying inlet contracture, the contour of the inlet, and the cephalopelvic relationship.

Also, adherence to the direction of the pelvic axis, as outlined here, when performing a forceps delivery will avoid trauma (of any form) to the anterior portion of the vagina, urethra, and clitoris and will preserve the integrity of the endopelvic fascia supporting the bladder. This presupposes that the vertex is maintained in a state of flexion until its biparietal diameter is in line with bi-ischial diameter, in accordance with Caldwell. This means that before extension of the vertex is permitted, the fetal occiput is well beyond the inferior border of the maternal symphysis and away from the crucial area of the structures about the bladder neck. To extend the vertex by using the symphysis as a fulcrum is to invite trauma, both fetal and maternal—sometimes of serious proportions. Traumatic pelvic delivery has no place in modern obstetrics, and should it happen, is an admission of faulty judgment or technique.

BIBLIOGRAPHY

Baird, D.: The cause and prevention of difficult labor. Amer. J. Obstet. Gynec., 63:1200, 1952.

Ball, R. P.: Roentgen pelvimetry and fetal cephalometry. Surg. Gynec. Obstet., 62:798, 1936.

Caldwell, W. E., and Moloy, H. C.: Anatomical variations in the female pelvis and their effect in labor with a suggested classification. Amer. J. Obstet. Gynec., 26:479, 1933.

Caldwell, W. E., Moloy, H. C., and D'Esopo, D. A.: Further studies on the pelvic architecture. Amer. J. Obstet. Gynec., 28:482, 1934.

Caldwell, W. E., Moloy, H. C., and D'Esopo, D. A.: Roentgenologic study of the mechanism of engagement of the fetal head. Amer. J. Obstet. Gynec., 28:824, 1934.

Caldwell, W. E., Moloy, H. C., and D'Esopo, D. A.: Further studies on mechanism of labor. Amer. J. Obstet. Gynec., 30:763, 1935.

Caldwell, W. E., Moloy, H. C., and D'Esopo, D. A.: Studies on pelvic arrests. Amer. J. Obstet. Gynec. 36:928, 1938.

Caldwell, W. E., Moloy, H. C., and Swenson, P. C.: Use of the roentgen ray in obstetrics; I. Roentgen pelvimetry and cephalometry; technique of pelvioroentgenography. Amer. J. Roentgen., 41:305 1939.

Caldwell, W. E., Moloy, H. C., and Swenson, P. C.: Use of the roentgen ray in obstetrics; II. Anatomical variations in the female pelvis and their classification according to morphology. Amer. J. Roentgen. 41:505, 1939.

Caldwell, W. E., Moloy, H. C., and Swenson, P. C.: Use of the roentgen ray in obstetrics; III. Mechanism of labor. Amer. J. Roentgen., 41:719, 1939.

Clifford, S. H.: Stereoroentgenometric method of fetometry and pelvimetry with its obstetrical application. W. Virginia Med. J., 31:3, 1935.

Colcher, A. E., and Sussman, W.: Practical technique for roentgen pelvimetry with a new positioning Amer. J. Roentgen., 51:207, 1944.

D'Esopo, D. A.: The occipitoposterior position. Amer J. Obstet. Gynec., 42:937, 1941.

Elftman, H. O.: Evolution of the pelvic floor of the primates. Amer. J. Anat., 51:307, 1932.

Eller, W. C., and Mengert, W. F.: Recognition of midpelvic contraction. Amer. J. Obstet. Gynec., 53:252, 1947.

Fehling, H.: Die Form des Beckens beim Foetus u. Neugeborenen. Arch. Gynäk., 1876. (The relation of the pelvis of the fetus and newborn to the adult.) From Thomson, A.: The sexual differences of the foetal pelvis. J. Anat. Physiol., 33:359, 1899.

Greulich, W. W., and Thoms, H.: Study of pelvic type and its relationship to body build in white women J.A.M.A., 112:485, 1939.

Greulich, W. W., and Thoms, H.: Growth and development of the pelvis of individual girls before, during and after puberty. Yale J. Biol. Med., 17:91, 1944

Hooten, E.: Up from the Ape. Macmillan Co., New York, 1949.

Kaltreider, D. F.: The contracted outlet. J.A.M.A. 154:824, 1954.

Mengert, W. F.: Estimation of pelvic capacity. J.A.M.A. 138:169, 1948.

Moloy, H. C.: Clinical and Roentgenologic Evaluation of the Pelvis in Obstetrics. W. B. Saunders Co. Philadelphia, 1951.

Morton, D. G., and Gordon, G.: Observations upon the role of the sex hormones in the development of bony pelvic conformation. Amer. J. Obstet. Gynec. 64:292, 1952.

Morton, D. G., and Hayden, C. T.: Comparative study of male and female pelves in children with a consideration of the etiology of pelvic conformation. Amer. J. Obstet. Gynec., 41:485, 1941.

Muller, H. J.: Damage to posterity caused by irradiation of the gonads. Amer. J. Obstet. Gynec., 67:467, 1954.

Nicholson, C.: Interpretation of radiological pelvimetry. J. Obstet. Gynaec. Brit. Emp. 45:950, 1938.

Reynolds, E.: Evolution of the human pelvis in relation to the mechanics of the erect posture. Papers Peabody Mus. Amer. Arch. Ethnol., 11:255, 1931

Reynolds, E. L.: The bony pelvic girdle in early infancy; A roentgenometric study. Amer. J. Phys Anthrop., 3:44, 1945.

Robert F.: Beschreibung eines in höchsten Grade

querverengten Beckens u.s.w. Karlsruhe u. Frieburg, 1842. (Description of contracted pelvis of extreme degree.)

Schultz, A. H.: Characters common to higher primates and characters specific for man. Quart. Rev. Biol., 11:259, 425, 1936.

Steele, K. B., and Javert, C. T.: Roentgenography of the obstetric pelvis; a combined isometric and stereoscopic technique. Amer. J. Obstet. Gynec., 43:600, 1942.

Taylor, E. S., Holmes, J. H., Thompson, H. E., and Gottesfeld, K. R.: Ultrasound diagnostic techniques in obstetrics and gynecology. Amer. J. Obstet. Gynec., 90:655, 1964.

Thoms, H.: Newer aspects of pelvimetry. Amer. J. Surg., 35:372, 1937.

Thoms, H.: The Naegele pelvis. Yale J. Biol. Med., 10:513, 1938.

Thoms, H.: Clinical application of roentgen pelvimetry and a study of the results in 1,100 women. Amer. J. Obstet. Gynec., 42:957, 1941.

Thoms, H.: The role of nutrition in pelvic variation. Amer. J. Obstet. Gynec., 54:62, 1947.

Thoms, H., and Greulich, W. W.: Comparative study of male and female pelves. Amer. J. Obstet. Gynec., 39:56, 1940.

Thoms, H., and Wilson, H. M.: Roentgenological survey of the pelvis. Yale J. Biol. Med., 13:831, 1941.

Thomson, A.: Sexual differences of the foetal pelvis. J. Anat. Physiol., 33:359, 1899.

Turner, W.: Index of the pelvic brim as a basis of classifications. J. Anat. Physiol., 20:125, 1886.

von Stein, —.: Ueber die Meinung von Raçenverschiedenheit der Becken. Neue Z. Geburtsh., 15:41, 1844.

Washburn, S. L.: Sex differences in the pubic bone. Amer. J. Phys. Anthrop., 6:199, 1948.

Weber, M. J.: Die Lehre von den Ur- und Rassenformen der Schadel und Becken des Menschen. Düsseldorf, 1830. From Turner, W.: The index of the pelvic brim. J. Anat. Physiol., 20:125, 1886.

Weinberg, A., and Scadron, S. J.: The value and limitations of pelvioradiography in the management of dystocia, with special reference to midpelvic capacity. Amer. J. Obstet. Gynec., 52:255, 1946.

Williams, J. W.: The funnel pelvis. Amer. J. Obstet., 64:106, 1911.

Young, M., and Ince, J. G. H.: Transmutation of vertebrae in the lumbosacral region of the human spine. J. Anat., 74:369, 1940.

Young, M., and Ince, J. G. H.: Radiographic comparison of the male and female pelvis. J. Anat., 74:374, 1940.

Chapter 25

Physiology and Mechanism of Labor in Parent Types of Pelves

THE PHYSIOLOGY OF LABOR

DEFINITION AND STAGES OF LABOR

Labor is the process by which the products of conception are expelled from the uterus and vagina into the external environment. It is divided into four stages. The *first stage* of labor is the interval from its onset until the cervical os becomes completely or fully dilated. In normal labor this stage is characterized by the development of synchronized myometrial contractions of the upper segment of the uterus or the uterine corpus, which increase in frequency and force, causing the cervix to efface and dilate.

The *second stage* of labor is the period between attainment of full dilatation of the cervical os and expulsion of the fetus from the birth canal. Since the upper vagina surrounding the cervix expands in equal measure with dilation of the cervical os during the first stage, the forces of labor on the presenting part during the second stage serve to dilate the lower vagina and to allow passage of the fetus from the birth canal.

The *third stage* of labor begins with the delivery of the fetus and ends with the delivery of the placenta, thus concluding the active process of labor.

The *fourth stage* denotes the hour or two after delivery, when uterine tone is established. If there is neither undue bleeding nor other complications at the end of this period, it may be assumed that labor is safely completed.

THE ETIOLOGY OF LABOR

The cause of labor remains a mystery. Presumably the control of the reproductive cycle is a carefully integrated neuroendocrine process. Certain observations may be recorded but their relationship one to each other is a matter of speculation.

During the female's reproductive life the uterus is never completely quiescent, although, as has been noted previously, the degree of motility varies with the different phases of the menstrual cycle. The uterus also contracts throughout pregnancy, and as term approaches, these contractions increase in frequency and at times in intensity. Thus, the etiology of labor may depend on factors that deter the uterus from expelling the fetus until it has attained sufficient maturity to survive in an extrauterine environment, rather than on factors that evoke uterine contractions. The presence of a fetus is not a requisite for either the continuation or the termination of pregnancy, at least in the subhuman primate. In the macaque, when the fetus was removed by abdominal hysterotomy and the placenta was left in situ during a period comparable to the fourth to eighth month of human pregnancy, the placenta was retained and not expelled until term, following an episode of labor. A somewhat similar circumstance is observed in human pregnancy when labor is occasionally postponed for several weeks or even months after fetal death in utero.

Whether there is a true prelabor decrease

480

of estrogens is debated, but there is agreement that the free form of estriol rises. The effect of progesterone on myometrial activity in the rabbit has been emphasized in the "progesterone block theory." Supposedly, under the influence of progesterone there is a reported increase in intracellular sodium and a diminution of potassium. This decrease in the intracellular potassium-sodium ratio is postulated to favor a quiescent muscle. Thus, the degree of uterine motility will depend on whether the myometrium is under estrogen or progesterone domination. In human material, although intracellular myometrial sodium increases during pregnancy without potassium loss, there is no discernible change in values of these electrolytes in association with labor. Further, blood progesterone levels do not change significantly until the placenta is expelled, when there is a prompt fall.

Because of its therapeutic importance, perhaps, oxytocin is assigned a prominent role in the etiology of labor. The response of the uterus to the oxytocic factor appears to increase as pregnancy progresses. Extensive studies have been made during various periods of pregnancy and under a variety of obstetric circumstances, using dilutions of standardized natural and synthetic oxytocin, in which 10 units of oxytocin (10,000 milliunits) is added to a liter of glucose solution. Patients who are "favorable," "ready," or about to enter labor, respond to minimum doses of 1 to 8 milliunits (2 to 12 drops) per minute or a maximum of 32 milliunits. These values have relevance whenever oxytocin is used therapeutically, as in the treatment of desultory labor. Conventionally 5 units of oxytocin placed in a liter of glucose solution permits the administration of the hormone in the amount to cause physiologic myometrial contractions.

Direct measurements of oxytocin in blood have proved to be formidable procedures and require further refinement. Evidence of oxytocin activity in maternal blood is indirectly deduced from the behavior of the myoepithelial cells of the human mammary gland when the gland pressure is measured by a polyethylene tube introduced into the duct.

The mammary gland pressure response is directly related to the dose of oxytocin administered and is observed to rise spontaneously in labor. The letdown or milk-ejecting factor of oxytocin may also be demonstrable by the above method. This is consistent with the observation that the nipple of the breast opposite to the one being suckled will ofttimes ooze milk—a sort of "sympathetic suckling" effect. The so-called "after-pains" from contraction of the uterus experienced by the patient in the early days of the puerperium are usually maximal when the infant is nursing.

As assayed with the milk-injection technique in the lactating rabbit, the jugular vein blood from women in labor is stated to be four to nine times more potent for oxytocin than venous blood taken simultaneously from the peripheral circulation.

Finally, alcohol has been administered to patients in premature labor to suppress the release of the antidiuretic hormone and presumably indirectly oxytocin. There is little doubt that when alcohol is given to patients in labor myometrial activity appears to diminish, usually to reappear as the alcohol is discontinued.

One must list the catecholamines as possible factors in the etiology of labor. In brief, epinephrine is released almost exclusively by the adrenal medulla and affects both alpha (excitatory) and beta (inhibitory) receptors. Norepinephrine, stored and released peripherally, affects alpha receptors only.

The catecholamines have taken on added interest in human reproduction because of the recent attempts to prevent premature labor through substances that influence alpha and beta receptors. Epinephrine derivatives such as isoxsuprine and isoproterenol are being studied intensively. These agents will decrease uterine motility in both normal labor and induced oxytocin contractions, supposedly through beta receptor stimulation, but they have adverse side effects on the cardiovascular system, resulting in tachycardia and hypotension. This inhibitory effect will continue but apparently to a lesser degree when a beta-blocking agent (propranolol) is administered simultaneously, and the cardiovascular responses of hypotension and tachycardia are somewhat diminished. By contrast, norepinephrine will activate the uterine myometrium, presumably by stimulation of alpha receptors. Hence, a beta-blocking agent might enhance labor by removing the inhibitory beta effect of epinephrine, or perhaps by the unopposed action of norepinephrine. Theoretically, myometrial activity could be reduced by a beta stimulator (isoxsuprine) or an alpha blocker (phentolamine). It has been authoritatively stated, however, that none of the agents mentioned are capable of permanently eliminating labor, and their side effects are substantial.

Investigation of prostaglandin has uncovered some interesting effects on myometrial activity. In a small series of patients at term, uterine contractions have been observed following infusion of prostaglandin F_{2a}. Labor continued when the infusion was stopped with the cervix 5 to 6 cm. dilated. The same fraction of prostaglandin has been isolated from the blood of women in labor but it is absent at other times in pregnancy. Prostaglandin is found in amniotic fluid, and the decidua is stated to be rich in the substance. (See Chapter 1.)

In summary, the control of pregnancy and parturition is difficult to assign to a single factor. Instead of being directly related in initiating labor, perhaps the function of the sex steroids is to maintain a favorable milieu for the fetus. The placental-fetal unit is becoming a more viable concept. As stated by Barcroft, there comes a time when the fetus must escape or perish. It would be pleasing to believe that the fetus has some control over his destiny. Certainly he will find it difficult to do so once born. What, then, is the trigger mechanism in the etiology of labor? Once committed to labor, the uterus can and will respond to oxytocin, catecholamines, and a host of related substances.

UTERINE TOCOGRAPHY

Human tocography, or the graphic study of the contractions of the human uterus, has been attempted by various methods. The instrument used to record the pattern of myometrial contractions is known as a tokodynamometer (TKD), of which there are both internal and external types.

In the earlier studies a small balloon was introduced through the cervix and placed between the fetal membranes and uterine wall, that is, in an extraovular location. By means of a catheter inserted through the cervix, a polyethylene tube was introduced into the uterus, bypassing the presenting part to enter the amniotic sac. This prevented any escape of amniotic fluid, and valid readings of uterine motility were

obtained through measurements of changes in the intrauterine or amniotic fluid pressure. Direct measurements of the amniotic fluid pressure have been obtained by the transabdominal insertion of a No. 15 needle into the amniotic cavity (Fig. 1).

It has long been appreciated that the presence of a foreign body will stimulate the uterus. To reduce this effect, a method has been developed whereby microballoons are placed transabdominally into the wall of the uterus through a proper-sized needle. After the needle is introduced under local anesthesia, a fine polyethylene catheter with a microballoon attached is threaded through the needle into the myometrium. The catheter connects the microballoon with an electromanometer, which records the intramuscular pressure from various areas of the uterus.

To eliminate totally the stimulating effect of a foreign body, attempts have been made to record uterine contractions by external tocography. Until recent times these methods were restricted to observations from a single location on the abdomen. From these early observations, it was demonstrated that the uterus contracts throughout pregnancy and becomes more irritable as term approaches. These studies have been extended by use of a multi-channel type of tokodynamometer, providing simultaneous observations of myometrial activity at various areas of the uterus. The success of this instrument depends on a receptor contain-

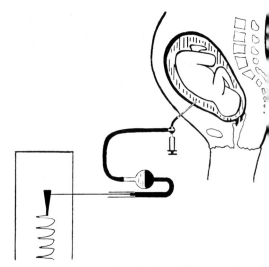

Figure 1. Internal method used for recording the contractility of the whole uterus: the amniotic fluid pressure is recorded with a mercury manometer. (From Caldeyro-Barcia, R., Alvarez, H., and Reynolds, S. R. M., Surg., Gynec. Obstet., 91:641, 1950.)

ing a strain gauge, which transmits to a recording manometer the frequency and intensity of the uterine contractions. Six of these outlets are placed, three on each side, over the abdomen in areas representing the right and left fundus, midzone, and lower uterine segment. From use of this method has come a better understanding of the pattern of the uterine contractions associated with normal and abnormal or nonproductive labor. Other studies have employed the multi-channel tokodynamometer in conjunction with the transabdominal needle method of internal tocography, with the objective of determining how uterine contractions affect amniotic fluid pressure. From these observations it has been deduced that effective labor is associated with the synchronization of overall uterine motility and a rise in amniotic fluid pressure to 40 to 50 mm. Hg with a return to a normal resting level of 10 mm. Hg (Fig. 2).

SIGNIFICANCE OF AMNIOTIC FLUID AND INTRAUTERINE PRESSURE IN PREGNANCY AND LABOR

In the discussion on intervillous blood flow (Chapter 7), reference was made to the possible relationship of intrauterine pressure and how it could influence rate of flow. Here, the interest is how intrauterine pressure may relate to uterine motility and the character of myometrial contractions under normal and abnormal conditions; that is, the status of the intrauterine pressure in early and late pregnancy, during the different stages of labor, and in so-called desultory labor or functional dystocia.

Amniotic fluid or intrauterine pressure has come to be regarded as an index of uterine tonus and of the intensity of the uterine contractions. Uterine tonus is de-

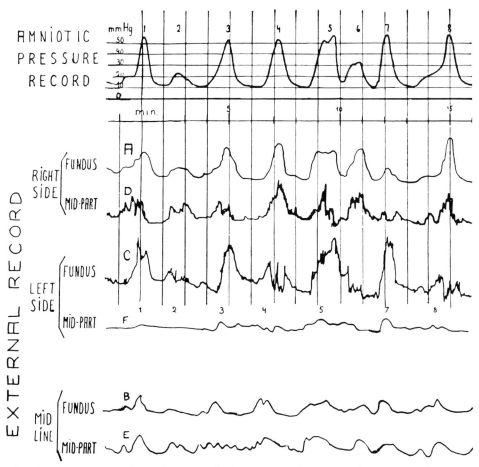

Figure 2. Simultaneous recording of amniotic fluid pressure and intensity of contractions from various areas of the uterus in normal labor. (From Caldeyro-Barcia, R., Alvarez, H., and Reynolds, S. R. M., Surg., Gynec., Obstet., 91:641, 1950.)

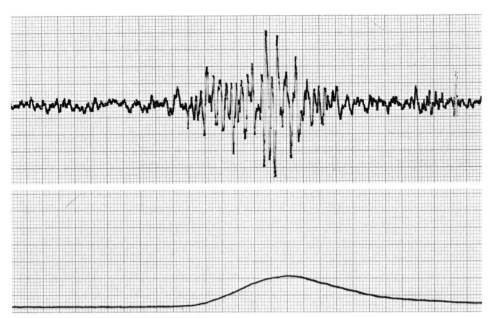

Figure 3. A uterine contraction of 60 seconds' duration as recorded by an electronic monitor on the patient's abdomen (top) with a rise of 30 mm. Hg of amniotic fluid pressure via an intrauterine catheter (bottom). (Courtesy of Dr. Jess B. Weiss.)

fined as the intrauterine pressure between contractions, or during the resting phase.

The intrauterine resting pressure in the early weeks of pregnancy is sometimes barely perceptible, but values between 3 and 8 mm. Hg have been recorded when measured by the transabdominal method. The resting pressure, or normal uterine tonus, gradually rises, and near term it is between 8 and 12 mm. Hg. Uterine contractions of early pregnancy will raise the pressure to levels of 18 to 20 mm. Hg or more, whereas with prelabor or so-called Braxton Hicks contractions the amniotic fluid pressure may occasionally rise to 30 to 35 mm. Hg.

Some recent observations by the associates of the writer indicate that the uterine contraction begins sometime before there is any measurable increase in amniotic fluid pressure (Fig. 3). This response is consistent with the onset of pain arising from a uterine contraction. By placing one's hand over the anterior surface of the uterus, one can readily perceive that the uterus is contracting several seconds before the patient is aware of pain. In fact, it is this phenomenon that permits effective pain relief with intermittent administration of nitrous oxide. (See Pain Relief in Chapter 26.)

By the transabdominal catheterization method the amniotic fluid pressure in normal labor ranged between 20 and 50 mm.

Hg, and at these values the cervix was found to dilate readily. As the patient entered the second stage of labor, the superimposed expulsive efforts raised the intrauterine pressure to approximately 70 mm Hg. The intrauterine pressure in the third stage of labor was determined from measurements taken through a needle in the umbilical vein, after the cord had been clamped and with the placenta presumably still in situ and not separated. Under these conditions, the umbilical vein pressure was recorded to be between 35 and 40 mm. Hg.

In cases of functional dystocia or desultory labor, the myometrium may develop an exaggerated tonus. In contrast to normal labor, in functional dystocia the intrauterine or amniotic fluid pressure remains elevated at 15 to 20 mm. Hg during the basal or resting phase, indicating a high sustained myometrial tonus. Further, in functional dystocia the amniotic fluid pressure during the height of a contraction increases only slightly over the resting pressure, rarely exceeding a value of 2 mm. Hg. However, with the catheterization technique, no increase in the basal intrauterine pressure was found. These observations lend some support to the clinician's impression that effective labor is associated with forceful, frequent, and regular uterine contractions, between which the uterus is relaxed and soft in consistency. In cases of prolonged labor arising from functional dystocia, as labor continues the uterus fails to contract and relax in a normal pattern.

THE UTERINE THRUST ON THE FETUS

When the intrauterine pressure and the area of the fetal head exposed to the pressure are known, a calculation can be made of the pressure being supported by the fetal head, or the total uterine thrust on the fetal head in various intrauterine states. Table 1 has been prepared from several sources of the earlier literature, but the values contained therein are substantiated by the more recent observations.

The force required to cause the fetal membranes to rupture varies greatly, a fact that is borne out by clinical experience. They may rupture before or early in the first stage of labor, or, despite the increased uterine thrust, may fail to rupture in the second stage. Under this circumstance, progress in labor may be enhanced by amniotomy.

It is evident that the total uterine thrust of second-stage labor is markedly increased after administration of oxytocin. The values listed for the force required to extract the fetus by forceps are those for low and mid-forceps operations and do not pertain to outlet forceps. In fact, the force involved in outlet forceps delivery may be less, or little more, than the thrust of second-stage labor.

TABLE 1. TOTAL THRUST TRANSMITTED TO FETUS, SUMMARY OF ESTIMATIONS BY DIFFERENT METHODS°

INTRAUTERINE BAG METHOD

(a) Resting tension plus uterine contractions (average) — 14 lb.

(b) Resting tension plus uterine contractions plus secondary expulsive powers (average) — 25 lb.

(c) As in (b), but after injection of pituitary extract — 32 lb.

FETAL CORD METHOD

Resting tension plus uterine contractions — 24 lb.

BURSTING STRAIN OF FETAL MEMBRANES

Average measurement — 16 lb.

Greatest measurement — 38 lb.

TRACTION ON OBSTETRIC FORCEPS

Average traction (for primigravidae) — 35 lb.

°Modified slightly from Moir, C.: Lancet, 1:417, 1936.

Delivery by outlet forceps properly performed can exert less force on the fetal vertex than a normal delivery in the presence of expulsive labor following a prolonged second stage.

CHARACTER AND PATTERN OF UTERINE CONTRACTIONS IN STAGES OF NORMAL LABOR

At the beginning of labor, uterine contractions generally occur at 15- to 20-minute intervals; however, labor may start abruptly, especially in the multiparous patient, with contractions occurring frequently and with great intensity. Usually two to three hours after the onset, the contractions, which have been somewhat sporadic, become more regular. From this time on, they increase in frequency and intensity until the patient is experiencing contractions every two or three minutes, and they continue at that interval through the remainder of the first and second stages of labor. When the presenting part contacts the perineum, the patient has a reflex urge to expel the fetus. As the uterus contracts, the patient holds her breath and bears down in this expulsive effort. During this phase, the pain of labor is accentuated by the pressure of the presenting part on the tissues of the vagina and the perineum.

The uterus may remain quiescent for several minutes following delivery, after which the contractions are resumed. The uterus will respond to abdominal massage and will react to administration of oxytocic substances, particularly when given intravenously, by contracting vigorously. After several contractions the placenta is extruded, and the contractions tend to become less frequent. Although they are for the most part painless, the contractions may continue to cause the patient some discomfort in the early puerperium, and this is commonly referred to as "after-pain." The latter usually disappears within 48 hours, except under the stimulation of suckling, when the contractions may again be of sufficient strength to produce discomfort.

From studies in the macaque, the uterine contractions were thought to initiate simultaneously from pacemakers located near the insertion of each fallopian tube. Flowing in a concentric fashion, the contractions were observed to spread over the uterine fundus and merge at the midline before moving downward toward the lower uterine segment and cervix. The exact origin of uterine contractions in the human has been the subject of some controversy, and even those who believe that the uterus contains pacemakers differ in their interpretation as to how they may operate.

Although there is some difference of opinion regarding whether the lower uterine segment contracts, there is general agreement that the contractions of the fundal portion of the uterus are much stronger and last much longer than those of the midzone area. These comparative differences in the intensity of the contractions at different locations in the uterus are referred to by many terms, such as fundal dominance, uterine polarity, or gradient of activity. Tocographic studies and measurements of differences in electrical activity of the various areas of the uterus support the concept that there is a decrease in the gradient of uterine activity from the fundus of the uterus downward toward the cervix. Attention has been called to the probability that abnormal myometrial contractions, as interpreted from external measurements, can be effected by factors other than a disturbance in uterine physiology. A distended bladder or an unengaged head may produce a pattern consistent with lower zone preponderance and reverse dominance. More-

over, it has been suggested that the resistance offered by the cervix and other soft tissues has more bearing on the progress in labor than the character of the recorded contractions.

OBSTETRICALLY SIGNIFICANT LANDMARKS AND DIAMETERS OF FETAL SKULL

The obstetrically significant landmarks of the fetal skull include the anterior and the posterior fontanelle, the occipital, the parietal, and the frontal bones and their connecting sutures, and the fetal ear. The frontal, or anterior, fontanelle is identified by the joining of four sutures: the two coronal, or lateral, sutures, the sagittal suture (posteriorly, and the frontal suture anteriorly; Fig. 4). The occipital, or posterior, fontanelle is recognized by the joining of three sutures, the two lambdoid sutures posterolaterally, and the sagittal suture anteriorly. The sagittal suture occupies a position between the anterior and posterior fontanelles. It has clinical importance in the management of labor, for its location indicates the parallel relationship of the planes of the fetal vertex to the various planes of the pelvis (synclitism). The location of the posterior fontanelle denotes the pelvic position of the fetal

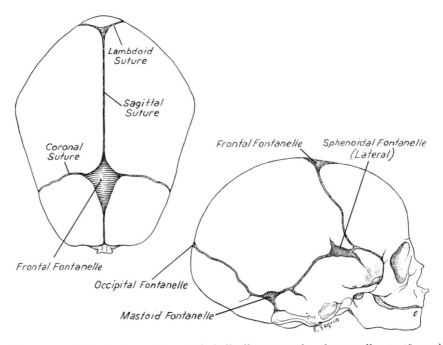

Figure 4. Superior and lateral views of the fetal skull, illustrating the obstetrically significant landmarks.

occiput. Besides being important in locating the posterior fontanelle, the lambdoid sutures are significant obstetric landmarks in the performance of forceps operations.

The fetal ear can be helpful in establishing the position, especially in the case of a markedly molded head with an edematous scalp (caput succedaneum). This condition is more frequently seen in prolonged labor, and, when present, makes difficult the accurate palpation of the sutures and fontanelles. The pinna of the ear is the most reliable landmark, for it is invariably directed toward the occiput. If reliance is placed on the position of the ear lobe, a mistake in diagnosis is possible, for the ear may be folded forward with the lobe pointing away from rather than toward the occiput.

The obstetrically significant diameters of the fetal skull include the biparietal (9.5 cm.) (Fig. 5), and the suboccipitobregmatic (9.5 cm.), occipitofrontal (11.5 cm.), and occipitomental (12.5 cm.) (Fig. 6). The biparietal diameter is the greatest distance from the lateral surface of one parietal boss to the other. The suboccipitobregmatic diameter is the distance from the point where the posterior margin of the anterior

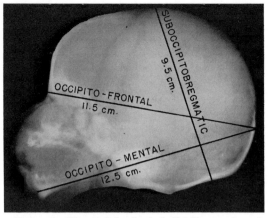

Figure 6. X-ray of the fetal skull following breech delivery, showing no evidence of molding. The important anteroposterior diameters are shown, with their respective values.

fontanelle and the sagittal suture join, designated the bregma, to the inferior edge of the occipital bone. The suboccipitobregmatic and biparietal diameters, of equal length (9.5 cm.), are concerned with the mechanism of labor in the normally flexed vertex presentation. The occipitofrontal and occipitomental diameters are related to the problems surrounding deflection of the vertex, namely in brow and face presentations.

MOLDING OF FETAL SKULL

As the vertex accommodates to the birth canal in the course of labor, some degree of molding usually occurs. The process is evident when a comparison is made of the contour of the vertex of an infant born by the breech and that of one born by the vertex. In fact, in vertex presentation molding may occur before the onset of labor, for x-ray pelvimetry in the last weeks of pregnancy sometimes reveals overlapping of the skull bones in what at birth proves to be a normal infant. This should be kept in mind also as it relates to the question of fetal death in utero when, in the absence of labor, overlapping of the skull bones is regarded as an important diagnostic sign.

In the course of extreme molding (Fig. 7), the coronal and lambdoid sutures tend to close, and the margin of the parietal bone in the region of the anterior fontanelle slides beneath the posterior edge of the frontal bone. Posteriorly, however, the parietal bone overlaps the occipital bone.

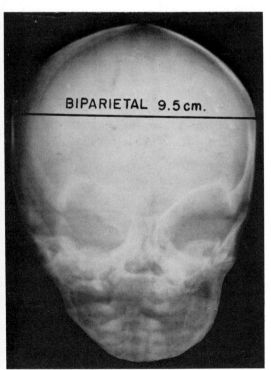

Figure 5. X-ray of the fetal skull, showing the important transverse diameter, that is, the biparietal diameter.

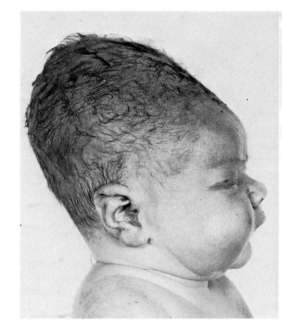

Figure 7. Marked molding of the fetal skull.

It has been said that the angle formed by the sphenoid-petrous bones at the base of the skull decreases, supposedly preventing unusual tension on the tentorium cerebelli, which might otherwise rupture from elevation of the vault of the skull, the result of molding. Thus, both the base and the vertex participate in the molding of the fetal skull. Whether lacerations of the sinuses and veins occur about the base of the brain as the result of molding has been the subject of considerable interest. Actually, cerebral hemorrhage, when associated with marked molding, is probably the result of a difficult or ineptly performed forceps operation or intrauterine asphyxia attendant upon prolonged labor rather than of the molding per se.

MECHANISM OF LABOR IN THE PARENT TYPES OF PELVES

The pelvic architecture has been described, and the pelvic axes, the parallel planes of the pelvis, the presentation and position of the fetus, and the landmarks and diameters of the fetal skull have been defined. The mechanism of labor will now be considered in the three positions of vertex presentation in the parent types of pelves.

The mechanism of labor may be defined as the accommodation of the fetal ovoid to the birth canal brought about by the coordination of the expulsive forces of the uterine contractions, which are reinforced in the second stage by the voluntary contractions of the abdominal muscles. As a result, the fetus undergoes certain important changes in habitus or posture during labor, imposed by the interplay of the forces of expulsion and counterforces of resistance offered by the surrounding tissues and bones of the birth canal.

Before the mechanism of labor is discussed further, however, it is necessary to define what is meant by engagement, synclitism, asynclitism, and positioning of the uterus and fetus, and to describe the soft tissue changes in the reproductive tract during labor.

ENGAGEMENT

Engagement of the vertex is sometimes described as the state that exists when the largest diameter of the fetal vertex has passed through the superior strait or inlet. Before this condition can be attained, however, the presenting part must be on or near the pelvic floor, a situation which may not occur until the second stage of labor. A preferable definition is: *engagement has occurred when the biparietal diameter of the flexed vertex has passed through and is below the superior strait or inlet of the pelvis.* By this definition, the cephalopelvic relationship at the superior strait can be established at a much earlier period, an important consideration in the conduct of both normal and abnormal labor.

This should not be construed to mean that engagement is postponed until after the onset of labor. As stated previously, the antepartum examination some two to six weeks before term, particularly in the primigravida, may reveal that the fetal head is already engaged. In fact, an unengaged vertex in the primigravida at term should be viewed with some concern. By contrast, more often than not in the multiparous patient, abdominal palpation and rectal or vaginal examination at the onset of labor will reveal the vertex in the pelvic brim, or unengaged. This difference is assigned to the tonicity of the abdominal muscles, which, in the case of the primigravida, forces the lower pole of the fetus into the pelvis.

The clinical discernment of engagement is considered in Conduct of Normal Labor in Chapter 26. Suffice it to say that, with engagement of the vertex, labor and delivery in most instances are relatively normal. Exceptions occur, however, as in functional dystocia, failure of anterior rotation of the vertex, and the comparatively rare instances of midpelvic and outlet contracture.

SYNCLITISM AND ASYNCLITISM

By definition, *synclitism* denotes a state of parallelism. In obstetrics this means a parallel relationship between a designated plane of the fetal head and one of the parallel planes of the pelvis. Under normal conditions, with the vertex flexed, the fetal plane of reference is a circular area wherein the suboccipitobregmatic and the biparietal diameters intersect each other. When the vertex is incompletely flexed, the fetal plane might lie within an area where the occipitofrontal and the biparietal diameters intersect each other. Regardless, the point of reference is the sagittal suture, and, when it abuts on the parallel plane in question, the head is designated as being synclitic.

The term *asynclitism* denotes a lack of parallelism of the fetal and the pelvic planes, and in this situation the sagittal suture fails to rest on the parallel pelvic plane in contact with the presenting vertex. When the sagittal suture is anterior to the parallel plane, that is, nearer the symphysis, it is referred to as posterior asynclitism, or posterior parietal bone presentation (Litzmann's obliquity). When the sagittal suture is posterior to the parallel or pelvic plane, that is, near the sacral promontory, the condition is known as anterior asynclitism, or anterior parietal bone presentation (Naegele's obliquity). In the normal mechanism, the unengaged vertex is often moderately asynclitic prior to the onset of labor. With engagement the vertex levels off, so to speak, in the upper pelvis and becomes synclitic. During descent through the upper pelvis the sagittal suture is located near the coronal plane and the superior axis, and in the lower pelvis the sagittal suture is midway between the inferior border of the symphysis and sacrum and somewhat posterior to the inferior axis of the pelvis.

In a platypelloid or flat pelvis, the vertex may impinge against the sacral promontory, causing the anterior parietal bone to present. In an android pelvis with a narrow anterior segment or forepelvis, bony resistance may be met at the symphysis. In consequence, the posterior parietal bone will present. In either case, if asynclitism persists in the course of engagement, it must be regarded as a pathologic state and is indicative of cephalopelvic disproportion.

POSITIONING IN LABOR

In early labor the uterus moves forward in the abdomen so that its long axis comes to point directly downward at right angles to the superior strait. Simultaneously, the fetal body loses its posterior curvature, and its vertebral column tends to straighten, depending to a degree on the amount of forewaters present. When the membranes are ruptured and there are no forewaters, the vertebral column is more likely to be straight. This forward movement of the uterus and the change in the fetal posture enable the force produced by the uterine contractions to be transmitted with maximal effectiveness against the cervix. It is doubtful that positioning of the mother has any special influence on the eventual outcome of labor.

CHANGES IN SOFT TISSUES OF REPRODUCTIVE TRACT PRIOR TO AND DURING LABOR

In discussion of the normal changes in pregnancy, it was stated that the lower segment of the uterus is formed largely from the uterine isthmus, and, near term, or with the onset of labor, the upper portion of the cervix also becomes incorporated into the lower segment (Fig. 8A). This process, known as the "taking up," or effacement, of the cervix, may occur to a degree before the onset of labor. The length of the cervical canal varies greatly in the latter weeks of pregnancy; hence, at the onset of labor the cervix may vary between 1 and 2 cm. in thickness. A shorter labor, particularly in the primigravida, is anticipated when the cervix is effaced at the onset. Many hours of labor may be spent before the cervix becomes effaced and dilation begins.

At the beginning of labor the intact fetal membranes egress into the upper cervix and serve as a hydrostatic dilator. With each uterine contraction the pressure of the membranes causes the cervix to dilate (Fig. 8B). As it becomes fully dilated, the cervix comes to lie in contact with the surrounding vaginal wall. Should the membranes rupture before the onset of labor or during the first stage, the presenting part must act as the dilator. It serves as effectively as the intact membranes in dilating the cervix, except in cases of cephalopelvic disproportion or malposition of the fetus, when the presenting part may be unable to fit tightly against the cervix.

To the uterine muscle is attributed the faculty of shortening without losing its ability to contract, a phenomenon known as retraction or brachystasis. By this action, the upper segment becomes shorter and thicker as labor progresses. In turn, the lower segment becomes stretched and distended, with the muscle fibers manifesting the same tension at a greater length, a process known as mecystasis. Consequently, during the course of labor, the cervix dilates by a dual mechanism: through the effect of retraction, and by the force of the uterine contractions transmitted through the presenting part of the fetus or the amniotic fluid when the fetal membranes are intact.

COURSE OF LABOR

In recent times normal and abnormal labor has been described in graphic form by plotting cervical dilatation against time. The earlier hours of labor are devoted to effacement and dilatation of the cervix up to 3 cm. and is referred to as the latent

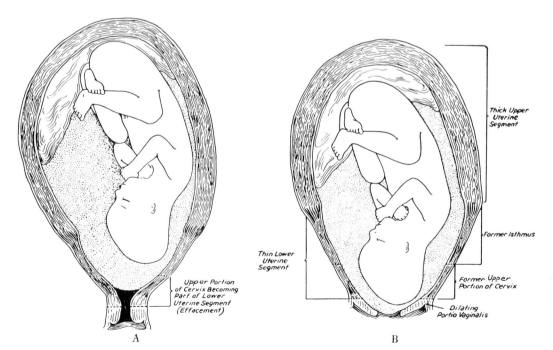

Figure 8. The anatomic status of the pregnant uterus. A, In late pregnancy. B, In labor with effacement and dilatation.

phase. This may represent more than half the total length of labor. From that point on, cervical dilatation is more rapid, the process being completed in three to four hours followed by a second stage of an hour on the average (Fig. 9). The hours in each phase vary from patient to patient but it is proposed that the relative time in each phase permits the characteristic sigmoid curve to apply to the individual patient.

However, the cervix in the latter weeks of pregnancy is usually partially if not totally effaced, and often dilated to 1 to 2 cm. or more prior to the onset of labor. It is this phenomenon that allows for elective induction of labor that is commonly practiced, and for most of these patients the time from the onset of labor to its completion is usually less than eight hours. If this were not so, there would be no advantage to such procedure, for its possible hazard must be recognized (see Elective Induction of Labor in Chapter 29). Indeed, the primiparous patient who enters labor with an uneffaced and closed cervix should be suspect as a possible candidate for prolonged labor. It has been stated that one of the advantages in recording cervical dilatation against hours is to anticipate dysfunctional or desultory labor, and it follows that the latter when identified should be actively treated and the hazards of prolonged labor avoided. Indeed, it is here that depicting labor graph-ically may have its greatest clinical useful-ness.

MOVEMENTS IN THE MECHANISM OF LABOR

The major movements in accommodation of the fetal ovoid to the birth canal in labor are the following: (1) *descent* and *flexion* of the vertex; (2) *internal rotation* of the vertex; (3) *extension* of the vertex with birth; (4) *restitution* of the vertex wherein the occiput assumes the position which it oc-cupied at the time of engagement; (5) *internal rotation* of the shoulders; and (6) *delivery* of the shoulders and body.

The mechanism of labor in the parent and mixed types of pelves has been determined by serial roentgenograms taken during labor and interpreted by the use of the precision stereoscope. It is apparent that the pelvic type may influence the ultimate position the fetus assumes at term and prior to labor. For example, in the platypelloid type, the fetus invariably and indeed must engage in the transverse position.

The narrow forepelvis of the android type is undoubtedly a contributory factor in in-creasing the incidence of malrotation of the occiput, whereas the anthropoid or longitu-dinal pelvis favors engagement in an an-terior or a posterior position in preference

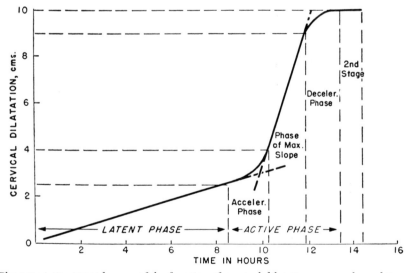

Figure 9. Characteristic sigmoid curve of the function of cervical dilatation versus elapsed time in labor, mean pattern for labor in nulliparas depicted, subdivided into phases for both theoretical statistical and practical clinical value. (From Friedman, E. A., in Reid, D. E., and Barton, T. C.: Controversy in Obstetrics and Gynecology. W. B. Saunders Co., Philadelphia, 1969.)

to the transverse. In the gynecoid pelvis, the unengaged fetal head at the onset of labor is often observed to be in a transverse position (L.O.T. or R.O.T.).

Gynecoid Pelvis: Transverse Position of Vertex

In early labor, the anterior parietal bone slips behind the symphysis under the impact of the downward thrust of the uterine contractions. The sagittal suture of the vertex moves backward toward the sacral promontory to take up a position slightly anterior to the superior axis of the pelvis (Fig. 10).

Flexion of the vertex occurs simultaneously with descent and is conventionally described as a lever-like action, the fulcrum being located near the fetal foramen magnum and the long arm represented by the sagittal suture, whereby the infant's chin is brought in approximation to its upper chest.

Flexion facilitates the accommodation of the fetal head to the birth canal by substituting the smaller suboccipitobregmatic diameter (9.5 cm.) for the larger occipitofrontal diameter (11.5 cm.). Consequently, the flexed fetal vertex enters the birth canal as a slightly oval to round object, presenting the biparietal and the suboccipitobregmatic diameters, the values of which are regarded as identical (9.5 cm). With flexion, the leading point of the vertex is the area slightly anterior to the posterior fontanelle. The process of flexion is attributed to the uniform resistance offered to the head by the normal tonicity of the lower uterine segment. It is said that the anterior portion of the lower uterine segment is more firmly fixed by its fascial and ligamentous attachments. This may account for the cervix moving anteriorly from its frequent location in the posterior fornix, a feature commonly observed in early labor coincidental with effacement and beginning dilation.

Attention has been drawn to the fact, however, that the above description does not provide an explanation for failure of complete flexion, which is sometimes seen in labors when the vertex is in an occiput posterior position, or in those cases of brow or face presentation that occur in the presence of a normal pelvis and without any obvious cause. Accordingly, flexion or deflection is dependent on the length of the lever arm, which is determined by the direction of the line of force transmitted to the vertex through the fetal spine. If the fetal spine is straight, the line of force would fall presumably through the foramen magnum to emerge slightly anterior to the posterior fontanelle, causing flexion. Should the fetal spine be curved backward, the line of force would be directed nearer the anterior fontanelle, which would favor deflection.

The second major movement in the mechanism of labor is *internal rotation* of the vertex, with the occiput usually occupying an anterior position. The cause for internal rotation has been the subject of much discussion, and a number of theories have been advanced. The more obvious anatomic relationships would seem to provide an acceptable explanation. In essence, the pelvic diaphragm is inclined downward and forward, favoring spiraling in accordance with the lines of least resistance, and this condition, together with the comparative difference in space available in the anterior and posterior pelvic segments, accounts for rotation. Consequently, whatever portion of the vertex reaches the pelvic diaphragm first will be the part that will tend to rotate anteriorly. Further, with descent, the vertex meets resistance of the ischial spines and, more particularly, the sacrococcygeal platform, and moves forward to take up its position in relation to the inferior axis. The normal forepelvis at this lower level is more spacious than the posterior segment. This favors the probability that the larger occipital and parietal portions of the vertex rotate anteriorly, allowing the smaller frontal and sincipital areas to occupy the relatively less expansive posterior segment of the pelvis. In summary, rotation occurs as the result of the inclination of the levator ani muscles of the pelvic diaphragm, together with the accommodation of the vertex to the space available. With rotation there is further descent accompanied by flexion, until the vertex rests firmly against the perineum.

Whether the vertex rotates, and the direction in which it will rotate, depends on the difference in size of the anterior and posterior segments of the lower pelvis and the status of flexion, and this in turn will determine the area of the vertex that first contacts the pelvic diaphragm. Posterior occiput rotation is more frequently encountered in anthropoid and android pelves in which the anterior segment is small in comparison with that of the gynecoid pelvis,

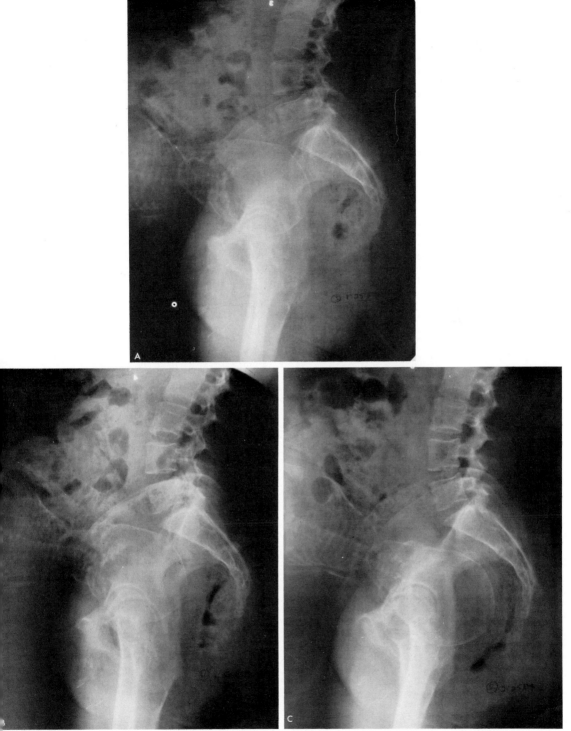

Figure 10.   Roentgenograms showing progress in normal labor. Taken with the patient standing, hence the absence of lateral flexion. (From Reid, D. E., J. Obstet. Gynaec. Brit. Emp., 66:709, 1959.) A, Biparietal diameter of the fetus passing through the superior strait (engagement). B, Vertex engaged, parallel to the sacrum. Leading point of the vertex is slightly anterior to the superior axis of the pelvis. C, Further descent of the vertex. Leading point is below the ischial spines; the vertex is nearing the sacrococcygeal platform, about to move forward, and the occiput about to rotate.

and there is an inclination toward deflection of the vertex. By contrast, there is a tendency toward anterior rotation in brow and face presentation, a mechanism that favors spontaneous delivery and indeed is a requirement for successful forceps delivery.

The third major movement is *extension* of the vertex, brought about by the slope of the levator ani muscles of the perineum and the resistance offered by these and the deep transverse perineal muscles. The older literature describes extension as the process whereby the occiput impinges against the inferior border of the symphysis, thus acting as a fulcrum, with the forces of labor causing the vertex to extend. As the perineum distends, the brow emerges, followed in turn by the face and the chin. Thus the occipitofrontal diameter (11.5 cm.) is presented to the inferior plane or outlet.

According to the concept proposed by Caldwell, however, extension occurs only after the biparietal diameter of the vertex and the occiput have passed the bi-ischial diameter and the inferior margin of the symphysis, respectively. In other words, before extension begins, the head is virtually free of the confines of the bony pelvis. This delay in extension causes the smaller biparietal and suboccipital fetal diameters (9.5 cm.) to present to the outlet. It is evident that the perineum must distend appreciably before extension occurs. This indicates that maintaining the vertex in a state of flexion during delivery and performing a perineotomy or episiotomy at the proper time, together, will cause less pressure by the occiput against the anterior vaginal wall and will preserve the surrounding perineal tissues and the supporting structures of the bladder.

The fourth major movement in the mechanism of labor is *external restitution* of the vertex, whereby the occiput returns to the position which it had assumed at the beginning of labor. In the case of a transverse presentation, the occiput points to the mother's inner thigh, either left or right, depending on the original position of the vertex.

The mechanism now finds the shoulders undergoing *internal rotation*. After delivery of the head, the bisacromial diameter of the shoulders engages in the pelvis in the oblique diameter of the inlet opposite that traversed by the occiput and meets the resistance of the pelvic floor. The shoulder that lies in the anterior segment of the pelvic cavity meets this resistance before its fellow, and is guided forward to lie behind the symphysis, at the same time the posterior shoulder rotates to the sacrum. Thus, the bisacromial diameter now lies directly within the anteroposterior diameter of the midpelvic and the outlet planes. While this movement of internal rotation of the shoulders is taking place within the birth canal, the born head maintains its sagittal suture in alignment at a right angle to the shoulders. After internal rotation has occurred, the continuing force of uterine contractions delivers the posterior shoulder over the perineum. Following this movement, the anterior shoulder is released from behind the symphysis and delivered beneath the pubic arch. In many cases the reverse sequence occurs, and the anterior shoulder is delivered first beneath the arch, followed by extrusion of the posterior shoulder. The infant's body follows, born by lateral flexion.

Gynecoid Pelvis: Anterior and Posterior Positions of Vertex

Labor in the anterior position begins with the occiput engaging in either of the two anterior quadrants of the pelvis (R.O.A. or L.O.A.), utilizing one or the other of the oblique diameters (Figs. 11 and 12). In any pelvis with a large anteroposterior diameter, as in the anthropoid, the vertex may engage directly anterior (O.A.), but this is of little consequence and has no adverse effect on the course of labor. The mechanism of labor in an anterior position is similar to that in a transverse with only a few minor differences. Obviously, the degree of internal rotation is less, being 45 degrees, and the leading point of the well flexed head descends downward anterior to the coronal plane.

The mechanism of labor in an occiput posterior position finds the vertex entering either of the posterior quadrants of the pelvis, utilizing one of the oblique diameters (R.O.P. or L.O.P.). The occiput occupies a position near the sacroiliac synchondrosis, and, except when rotation fails to occur, the mechanism of labor is similar to that of other vertex presentations. There is descent with flexion, internal rotation of 135 degrees, and birth by extension, followed by external restitution (Fig. 13).

On occasion the occiput fails to rotate

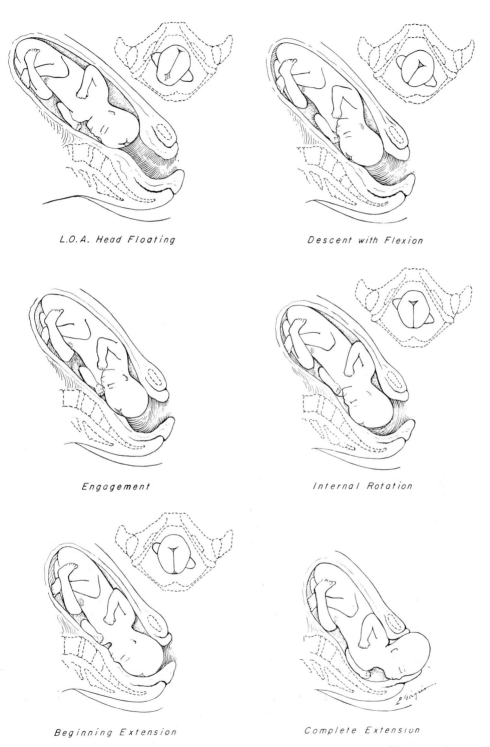

L.O.A. Head Floating

Descent with Flexion

Engagement

Internal Rotation

Beginning Extension

Complete Extension

Figure 11.   Mechanism of labor in left occiput anterior position of fetus.

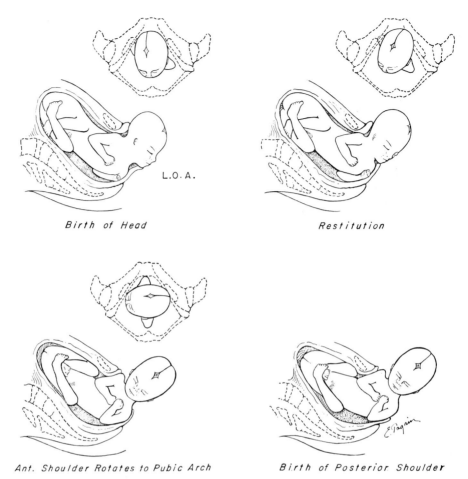

L.O.A.

Birth of Head   *Restitution*

Ant. Shoulder Rotates to Pubic Arch   *Birth of Posterior Shoulder*

Figure 12.   Final movements of mechanism of labor in left occiput anterior position of fetus.

anteriorly, or rotates directly posteriorly (see Chapter 27). When the pelvis is normal, failure of the occiput to rotate anteriorly is attributed to incomplete flexion. If the bregma is the area of the vertex that first encounters the pelvic diaphragm, this would favor anterior rotation of the sinciput. As previously stated, a less spacious forepelvis would foster lack of anterior rotation and favor a persistent occiput posterior position (Fig. 14). In some instances this condition is aggravated by an abnormally short bispinous diameter, owing to narrowing of the pelvic side walls and unusually prominent ischial spines.

A feature of the mechanism of labor of an occiput posterior position is the tendency for the vertex to extend or fail to remain completely flexed. The opinion has been expressed that whatever extension occurs takes place early in labor at the time the head enters the pelvis. The occiput meets with resistance from the posterior lower uterine segment and, perhaps to a minor degree, the sacral promontory, which, combined, causes some degree of extension. It is visualized that the force of the uterine contractions is transmitted forward along the occipitofrontal diameter near the region of the bregma. The fact that a brow or face presentation fails to develop is due to resistance of the forepelvis encountered by the sinciput at the inlet. Accordingly, with descent into the lower pelvis, the head again becomes flexed.

From personal experience, extension more likely occurs at a time when the occiput enters the lower pelvis and encounters the resistance of the ischial spines and the sacrococcygeal platform. Failing to rotate, the head may extend. This is indicated by finding the anterior fontanelle located near the lower margin of the symphysis, either to the right or to the left of the midline, depending on whether the occiput is right or left. The posterior fontanelle, which is normally near the axis of the pelvis in a well flexed vertex, is now located

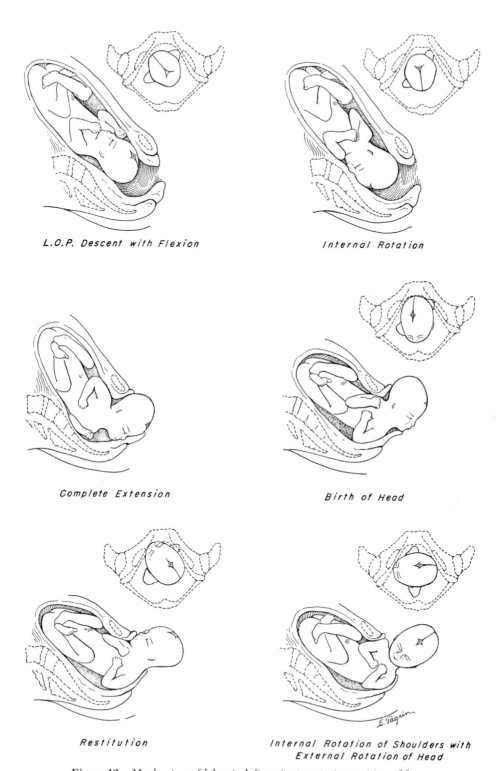

L.O.P. Descent with Flexion

Internal Rotation

Complete Extension

Birth of Head

Restitution

Internal Rotation of Shoulders with
External Rotation of Head

Figure 13. Mechanism of labor in left occiput posterior position of fetus.

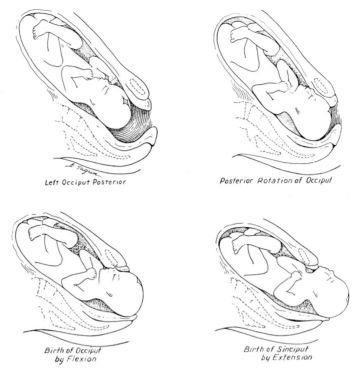

Left Occiput Posterior

Posterior Rotation of Occiput

Birth of Occiput
by Flexion

Birth of Sinciput
by Extension

Figure 14. Spontaneous birth in persistent occiput posterior position of fetus.

near the respective ischial spine. Whatever the mechanism, incomplete flexion is a major factor in lack of progress in labor in occiput posterior position and must be dealt with in its management.

A fetus in posterior face presentation is incapable of being born unless it is extremely small or the pelvis large, for it is impossible for the head and neck to pass through the pelvis at the same time (Fig. 15A). Thus, in the case of a face posterior presentation, the normal mechanism of labor involves spontaneous rotation to an anterior position, as the chin is the portion of the presenting part that first contacts the pelvic floor. With descent the anterior face tends to extend, but birth is by flexion (Fig. 15B). The chin rotates about the symphysis and the vertex is born over the perineum, after which the chin restitutes to its original position. The shoulders rotate in a transverse position following the direction of

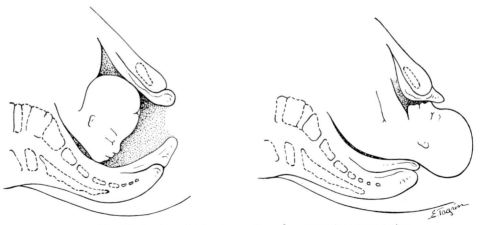

Figure 15. Mechanism of labor in mento or face posterior presentation.

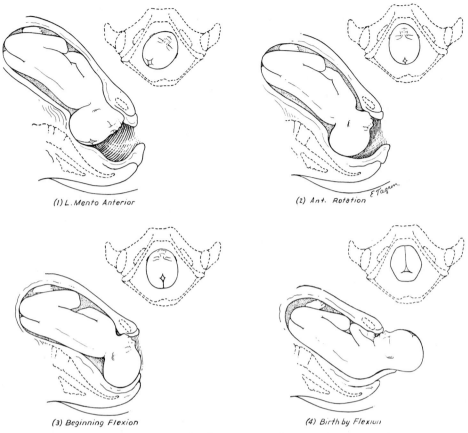

(1) L. Mento Anterior

(2) Ant. Rotation

(3) Beginning Flexion

(4) Birth by Flexion

Figure 16. Spontaneous birth in mento or face anterior presentation.

the chin, with the anterior shoulder impinging beneath the symphysis. The mechanism of labor in a mento or face anterior presentation is depicted in Figure 16. The face may become markedly edematous and the cranium somewhat flattened by molding. From the effects of prolonged extension, the baby may hold its head in a state of opisthotonos for several hours after birth.

A brow presentation may become flexed in the course of early labor, or it may extend into a face presentation or remain a brow. As such, it is a most unfavorable presentation; the diameters of the pelvis are confronted with the occipitomental diameter of 12 to 13 cm. If descent is possible, the brow contacts the pelvic floor and rotates anteriorly, as in a face presentation, and the brow, the bregma, and the occiput are born by flexion. The occiput then recedes posteriorly and the face and chin are born by extension. The remainder of delivery is similar to that in a vertex presentation. The vertex shows a characteristic molding with an extremely high forehead or sinciput and some flattening of the cranium.

Android, Platypelloid, and Anthropoid Pelves

It is envisioned that the mechanism of labor in the android type of pelvis begins with the unengaged head in a posterior parietal bone presentation (posterior asynclitism). With effective labor, the anterior parietal bone descends with greater rapidity and, with engagement, the vertex follows downward along the superior axis parallel to the sacrum. Accordingly, the sagittal suture must pass through the superior strait forward to the transverse diameter, for it must be recalled that the latter is a comparatively short distance from the sacral promontory as indicated by the length of the posterior sagittal diameter (3.5 cm. or less), a characteristic of the android pelvis. Consequently, for the term fetus to engage in the pure android pelvis, it is evident that the forepelvis must be sufficiently large to enable the vertex to move far enough anterior to the transverse diameter of the inlet to permit it to pass the sacral promontory. It is stated that only when the forepelvis is long and narrow, that is, in the so-called "android-anthropoid" pelvis, can the head enter the inlet through the oblique diameters of the pelvis.

By comparison with the gynecoid pelvis, rotation must occur at a lower level, at or below the third parallel plane, for, until the head is low in the pelvis, the temporal region of the vertex meets the lateral surface of the sacral alae which, owing to their proximity in the android pelvis, prevents rotation. The head moves forward into the forepelvis by anterior lateral flexion, and, with further descent, the brow passes beneath the sacral promontory, allowing for anterior rotation. The remainder of the mechanism of labor is similar to that in the gynecoid pelvis.

Provided the inlet admits the fetal head, labor and delivery in the platypelloid pelvis are usually normal. The vertex enters the pelvis in the transverse position, sometimes in marked anterior asynclitism with the anterior parietal bone presenting, the result of meeting obstruction in the region of the sacral promontory, near which the sagittal suture is now located. Under the impact of labor the posterior parietal bone bypasses the sacral promontory and the vertex becomes engaged. At the same time, the vertex becomes synclitic, and the sagittal suture is found slightly anterior to the superior axis of the pelvis. In the large platypelloid pelvis the vertex passes through the superior strait in a state of synclitism. In each instance, however, the normal mechanism prevails throughout the remainder of labor, with the vertex remaining in a transverse position until it comes into contact with the pelvic floor. Dystocia in the lower pelvis rarely occurs unless there are rachitic changes of the sacrum, for the bore of the pelvis is divergent and the arch is ample. Except for the occasional transverse arrest and the extremely rare occiput posterior position, whatever difficulty is encountered occurs at the pelvic inlet.

Labor in the anthropoid pelvis follows the normal mechanism, although in some instances anterior rotation fails to occur. As might be expected, the vertex engages with a greater frequency in the anteroposterior diameter of the inlet, it being longer than the transverse diameter; hence, the vertex often enters the pelvis in an anterior or a posterior position. When the vertex engages in the occiput posterior position, it may or may not rotate to an anterior position. In

fact, the occiput may rotate directly posterior into the excavation of the sacrum, particularly when the distance between the pelvic side walls is short or the bispinous diameter is abnormally decreased. The pubic arch as a rule is normal and, indeed, may be large, and thus with an ample outlet the vertex may be delivered spontaneously in the occiput posterior position by flexion followed by extension. According to this mechanism, the brow impinges beneath the symphysis, the occiput is born over the perineum, and the brow and face are delivered by extension. When the vertex delivers in an anterior position following normal anterior rotation, the occiput restitutes to a posterior position. Except for the fact that the anterior shoulder must rotate an extra few degrees, the shoulders and body are born according to the normal mechanism.

THE THIRD, OR PLACENTAL, STAGE OF LABOR

The placenta begins to separate through the spongiosa layer of the decidua, usually immediately following the delivery of the fetus, and is extruded from the vagina within a matter of minutes thereafter. Placental separation is noted by the fact that the uterus rises upward out of the pelvis and changes from a discoid to a globular shape. Some bleeding occurs, and advancement of the umbilical cord follows, indicating that the placenta has been extruded from the corpus into the lower uterine segment or the upper vagina. In the rare event that the placental stage continues beyond 30 to 60 minutes and there is no bleeding, preparations should be made to remove the placenta manually.

The placenta separates by a dual mechanism: through a decrease in the size of the placental site and the formation of a retroplacental hematoma. Following delivery the uterus continues to contract and relax. The decidual veins close and the marginal sinus decreases in size, occluding venous return from the intervillous space. The spiral arterioles remain patent and bleed into the intervillous space when the uterus relaxes. The resultant hematoma detaches the placenta by dissecting through the spongiosa or central zone of the decidua basalis. This requires that the margins of the placenta remain intact until separation

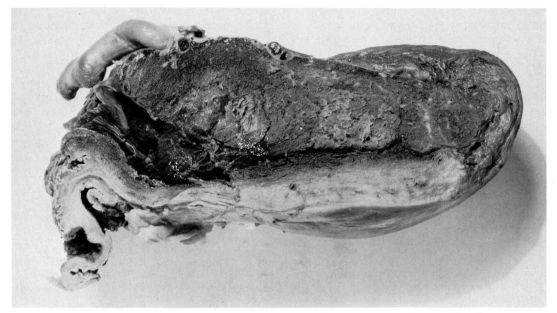

Figure 17.   Section of placenta, showing separation through spongiosa layer of decidua.

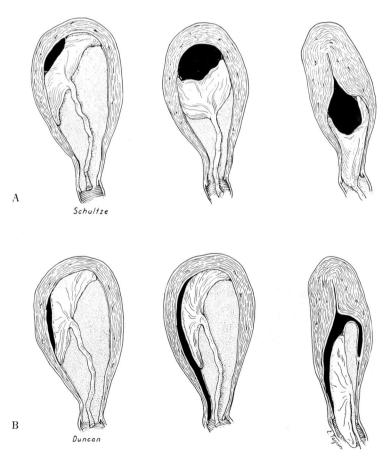

Figure 18.   Mechanisms of placental separation: A, Schultze method. B, Duncan method.

has occurred; otherwise, the bleeding will be external and the physiologic effect of retroplacental hematoma formation will not be produced (Fig. 17). In normal separation, external bleeding is delayed until the placenta is actually expelled from the uterus. By this mechanism (Schultze method, Fig. 18A), which is considered the normal, the placenta appears at the vulva as a glistening organ with the fetal chorionic surface presenting.

Should a portion of the placental margin become detached with the birth of the infant, bleeding from the placental site is largely external. In this event the placental separation depends principally on a decrease in the size of the placental site, for the physiologic effect of hematoma formation is lost. The placenta slides away from the uterine wall into the vagina and is expelled over the perineum with the dull reddish maternal surface exposed (Duncan method, Fig. 18B). In such cases incomplete separation and placental retention are frequent and the risk of postpartum hemorrhage is increased. This type of placental separation is often brought about by unwarranted abdominal uterine massage to hasten completion of the third stage of labor.

THE FOURTH STAGE OF LABOR

The hour or two immediately after delivery must be considered a part of labor, for during this period the parturient's vital signs should become stabilized. The patient must be under constant nursing supervision in accordance with the technique of the modern recovery room.

During this time effective uterine hemostasis is established by the contraction of the muscle bundles surrounding the myometrial blood vessels and thrombosis of the decidual blood vessels. As in control of bleeding from any body surface, hemostasis of the placental site is attained by ligature and thrombosis of the involved blood vessels. In this instance the ligature effect is created by the contraction of the entwining myometrial muscle bundles, while thrombi form in the distal decidual blood vessels (Fig. 19). Normally thrombus formation is never observed in the blood vessels of the myometrium, a fine arrangement on the part of nature. Were it otherwise, the contraction and relaxation of the uterus in the early days of the puerperium would favor the release of thrombi from the myometrial veins into the systemic circulation. Evidence that the blood must clot in the decidual blood vessels for complete hemostasis is derived from observations on delivered patients who have received excessive amounts of heparin or Dicumarol or those patients in whom a hypofibrinogenemia develops. In the absence of uterine atony, serious uterine hemorrhage has been encountered that has been controlled only after the clotting mechanism was restored to normal, that is, after clotting or thrombosis formation has occurred in the decidual vessels.

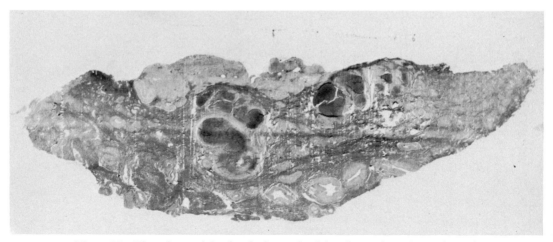

Figure 19.   Thrombosis of the decidual vessels of the placental site (sagittal view).

BIBLIOGRAPHY

Alvarez, H., and Caldeyro-Barcia, R.: Contractility of the human uterus recorded by new methods. Surg. Gynec. Obstet., 91:1, 1950.

Alvarez, H., and Caldeyro-Barcia, R.: The normal and abnormal contractile waves of the uterus during labour. Gynaecologia, 138:190, 1954.

Barden, T. P., and Stander, R. W.: Effects of adrenergic blocking agents and catecholamines in human pregnancy. Amer. J. Obstet. Gynec., 102:226, 1968.

Caldeyro-Barcia, R., Alvarez, H., and Reynolds, S. R. M.: A better understanding of uterine contractility through simultaneous recording with an internal and a seven-channel external method. Surg. Gynec. Obstet., 91:641, 1950.

Caldeyro-Barcia, R., Sica-Blanco y Poseiro, J. J., Gonzalez-Panizza, V., Mendez-Bauer, C., Fielitz, C., Alvarez, H., Pose, S. V., and Hendricks, C. H.: A quantitative study of synthetic oxytocin on the pregnant human uterus. J. Pharmacol. Exp. Ther., 121:18, 1957.

Caldwell, W. E., Moloy, H. C., and D'Esopo, D. A.: A roentgenologic study of the mechanism of engagement of the fetal head. Amer. J. Obstet. Gynec., 28:824, 1934.

Caldwell, W. E., Moloy, H. C., and Swenson, P. C.: The use of the roentgen ray in obstetrics; the mechanism of labor. Amer. J. Roentgen., 41:719, 1939.

Csapo, A.: Progesterone "block." Amer. J. Anat., 98:273, 1956.

Danforth, D. N., and Ivy, A. C.: The lower uterine segment; its derivation and physiologic behavior. Amer. J. Obstet. Gynec., 57:831, 1949.

D'Esopo, D. A.: The occipitoposterior position. Amer. J. Obstet. Gynec., 42:937, 1941.

Embrey, M. P.: External tocography in the study of uterine motility. A critical examination of the method. J. Obstet. Gynaec. Brit. Emp., 65:200, 1958.

Friedman, E. A.: Primigravid labor: A graphicostatistical analysis. Obstet. Gynec., 6:567, 1955.

Fuchs, F., Fuchs, A., Poblete, V. F., and Risk, A.: Effect of alcohol on threatened premature labor. Amer. J. Obstet. Gynec., 99:627, 1967.

Hellman, L. M., Harris, J. S., and Reynolds, S. R. M.: Characteristics of the gradients of uterine contractility during the first stage of true labor. Bull. Johns Hopkins Hosp., 86:234, 1950.

Hendricks, C. H.: Dysfunctional labor. In Reid, D. E., and Barton, T. C., eds.: Controversy in Obstetrics and Gynecology. W. B. Saunders Co., Philadelphia, 1969, p. 168.

Horvath, B.: Ovarian hormones and the ionic balance of uterine muscle. Proc. Nat. Acad. Sci., 40:515, 1954.

Ivy, A. C.: The functional anatomy of labor, with special reference to the human being. Amer. J. Obstet. Gynec., 44:952, 1942.

Ivy, A. C., Hartman, D. G., and Koff, A.: The contractions of the monkey uterus at term. Amer. J. Obstet. Gynec., 22:388, 1931.

Karim, S. M. M.: Appearance of prostaglandin F_{2a} in human blood during labour. Brit. Med. J., 4:618, 1968.

Karim, S. M. M., Trussell, R. R., Patel, R. C., and Hillier, K.: Response of pregnant human uterus to prostaglandin-F_{2a}-induction of labour. Brit. Med. J., 4:621, 1968.

Little, A. B., Smith, O. W., Jessiman, A. G., Selenkow, H. A., van't Hoff, W., Eglin, J., and Moore, F. D.: Hypophysectomy during pregnancy in a patient with cancer of the breast; case report with hormone studies. J. Clin. Endocr., 18:425, 1958.

Lurie, A. O., Reid, D. E., and Villee, C. A.: The role of the fetus and placenta in maintenance of plasma progesterone. Amer. J. Obstet. Gynec., 96:670, 1966.

Marshall, J. M., and Burnett, W. M., eds.: Initiation of Labor. Proceedings of Interdisciplinary Conference on the Initiation of Labor. National Institute of Child Health and Human Development, Bethesda, Md., 1963, p. 50.

Moir, J. C.: The expulsive force of the uterus during labor. Lancet, 1:414, 1936.

Moloy, H. C.: Studies on head molding during labor. Amer. J. Obstet. Gynec., 44:3, 1942.

Reynolds, S. R. M., Harris, J. S., and Kaiser, I. H.: Clinical Measurement of Uterine Forces in Pregnancy and Labor. Charles C Thomas, Springfield, Ill., 1954.

Reynolds, S. R. M., Heard, O. O., Bruns, P., and Hellman, L. M.: A multi-channel strain-gauge tokodynamometer; an instrument for studying the patterns of uterine contractions in pregnant women. Bull. Johns Hopkins Hosp., 82:466, 1949.

Schaffner, F., and Schanzer, S. N.: Cervical dilatation in the early third trimester. Obstet. Gynec., 27:130, 1966.

Smith, P. E.: The nonessentiality of the posterior hypophysis in parturition. Amer. J. Physiol., 99:345, 1932.

Stander, R. W.: Phenethanolamines and inhibition of human myometrium. Amer. J. Obstet. Gynec., 94:749, 1966.

Stolte, L., Eskes, T., Seelen, J., Moed, H. D., and Vogelsang, C.: Epinephrine derivates and the activity of the human uterus. Amer. J. Obstet. Gynec., 92:865, 1965.

van Wagenen, G., and Newton, W. H.: Pregnancy in the monkey after removal of the fetus. Surg. Gynec. Obstet., 77:539, 1943.

Williams, E. A., and Stallworthy, J. A.: A simple method of internal tocography. Lancet, 1:330, 1952.

Chapter 26

Conduct of Normal Labor and the Puerperium

The patient, having been instructed regarding the signs of imminent labor, should immediately enter the hospital with the appearance of "show," with rupture of the fetal membranes, or as soon as the uterine contractions become regular and occur every 10 to 12 minutes. By preference, the patient should enter the hospital at the beginning of the first stage of labor, which will permit those in attendance to prepare her properly for labor.

Occasionally, from their onset, the contractions may occur every 2 or 3 minutes and the patient may arrive at the hospital in or near second stage labor. Under such circumstances she must be taken directly to the delivery or case room, and the enema that is routinely given is omitted because it may not be completely expelled, and it only adds to the risk of contamination and infection. After a cursory history is taken and a general physical examination is made, the fetal heart tones and the presentation and position of the fetus are established. A rectal examination is made to determine the station of the presenting part and the dilatation of the cervix, and thus to ascertain whether delivery is imminent or if the patient is still in the first stage of labor. She is then managed accordingly.

It is emphasized that all who come in contact with the parturient from the time of her entrance until her discharge from the hospital must protect her from any possibility of infection. Thus, the technique of patient management must be faultless, and only persons free of infection can be permitted to come in contact with the maternity patient or her infant. Masks should be worn by all who approach the mother's bedside. Hand washing is mandatory before and after each examination. The wearing of gowns, scrub suits, and clean conduc-

tion shoes in the labor and delivery rooms is basic in the prevention of infection. In short, the adherence to the principles of aseptic technique are essential in defending the maternity patient from infection.

ADMISSION OF THE PATIENT

Every obstetric patient should be weighed on admission and her pulse, temperature, respiratory rate, and blood pressure should be taken and recorded. The physician in charge, on seeing the patient, writes the admission orders. These orders will include permission for the nurse to administer a cleansing enema and perform a perineal shave.

Admission History and Physical Examination

The physician reviews the patient's prenatal record and refreshes his memory regarding her past medical, surgical, and obstetric history. Special attention should be given to the interval since the last prenatal visit, particularly in relation to pregnancy toxemia or vaginal bleeding. The history should note any recent respiratory infection, the onset and character of the uterine contractions, whether the membranes are intact or ruptured, and the time when the patient last took food or fluids.

The physical examination should include a reexamination of the throat, heart, and lungs. If the patient has fever, steps should be taken immediately to determine the possible source of infection and whether the patient should be removed from the so-called "clean" area of the labor and delivery floor and cared for under isolation precautions. Cultures of the urine, and of material from the throat, the vagina, and the cervix may be indicated, depending on the signs, symptoms, and circumstances of the case. Any elevation of the blood pressure demands an explanation, particularly if it persists after mild sedation.

The Obstetric Examination

On admission, the obstetric examination is preceded by a review of the obstetric findings at the last prenatal visit and of the recorded description of the pelvis. By observing and palpating the uterus during several contractions, together with performing a rectal examination, the physician should ascertain if the patient is in labor and determine the character of the labor. For emphasis, *the patient is considered to be in labor only when the uterine contractions cause changes in the cervix, that is, effacement, dilatation or both.* This is the definition of labor.

The examiner next turns his attention to confirming the presentation, position, and estimation of the size of the fetus. By auscultation the location, rate, and quality of the fetal heart tones are determined. If the fetal size seems smaller than would be indicated by the gestational dates, there is the possibility of prematurity, in which event the conduct of labor will have to be modified. If by chance the uterus appears unduly large, polyhydramnios with its connotations or a multiple pregnancy must be considered.

Any question about the cephalopelvic relationship or the type of fetal presentation must be decided unequivocally, if necessary by vaginal or x-ray examination. Also,

in order to distinguish a normal cephalopelvic relationship and possible cephalopelvic disproportion or dystocia from an abnormal presentation, special attention should be given to two features of abdominal palpation. These are *whether the vertex is well flexed, and if there is any overriding of the mother's symphysis by the fetal vertex.* Flexion indicates that the vertex is so positioned that the biparietal and the suboccipitobregmatic diameters (both 9.5 cm.) present at the superior strait. The sinciput is more prominent than the occiput when the head is well flexed, and the reverse relationship exists when a brow or a face presents (see Malpresentation, Chapter 28).

Deflection of the vertex in the patient in labor leads to dystocia in some instances. Actually, in the primiparous patient at term, it should be considered indicative of cephalopelvic disproportion until proved otherwise by x-ray pelvimetry or vaginal examination, with the patient anesthetized if necessary. The early diagnosis of extension of the vertex is dependent on abdominal examination, for the cervix must be dilated by one third or more before the physician is usually aware on rectal examination that, because of the irregularity of the presenting part, he may be dealing with a brow or a face presentation. Because it is not unusual in deflection attitudes for the membranes to rupture before the onset of labor, it is readily conceivable that a long interval may pass after spontaneous rupture before labor begins and reaches the stage at which the cervix is dilated sufficiently for the diagnosis to be made on rectal ex-

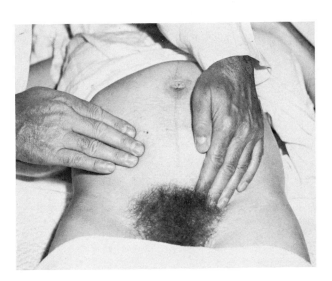

Figure. 1. Abdominal findings in a left vertex presentation, consistent with an occiput posterior with the vertex well flexed. The examiner's right hand is on the fetal sinciput; the left hand is on the occiput. Characteristically, the sinciput is more prominent and a greater distance from the midline of the mother's abdomen.

amination. If cephalopelvic disproportion exists, cesarean section is the treatment. Thus it can be seen why early diagnosis of deflection attitudes is so important, particularly if the fetal membranes are ruptured, for then uterine infection becomes a threat. For emphasis, the early diagnosis of deflection attitudes is dependent on abdominal examination, verified by x-ray examination of the abdomen.

Overriding, a term used when the anterior parietal bone of the fetus rises above the superior border of the mother's symphysis (Fig. 2), when present, raises the question of cephalopelvic disproportion. Prior to or in the early hours of labor, such a finding may be due to a thick lower uterine segment rather than to a contracted pelvis (Fig. 3A), in which event, after a few hours of labor, the lower segment becomes thinner, and what at first appeared to be overriding no longer exists. (Fig. 3B). If it persists during the course of labor, however, it must be regarded as strong evidence of cephalopelvic disproportion at the pelvic inlet (Fig. 3C). Since molding of the vertex may permit pelvic delivery in some cases, the extent of the overriding and the type of pelvis in which it occurs become important in determining the eventual outcome of a test of labor. In other words, some degree of overriding in a platypelloid pelvis is less serious than it is in an android or a small gynecoid pelvis.

Also, on abdominal palpation an impression may be gained that the vertex is engaged, that is, that the vertex is deep in the pelvis. Engagement is determined, however, by rectal examination or, when this does not provide the necessary information, by vaginal examination. Again for emphasis, *engagement has occurred when the biparietal diameter of the flexed vertex has passed through and is below the superior*

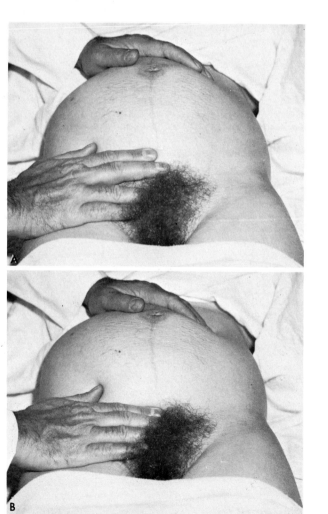

Figure 2. Examination for overriding. The findings are negative in B, positive in A. Note the difference in the spread of fingers when placed on the symphysis and the upper surface of the vertex.

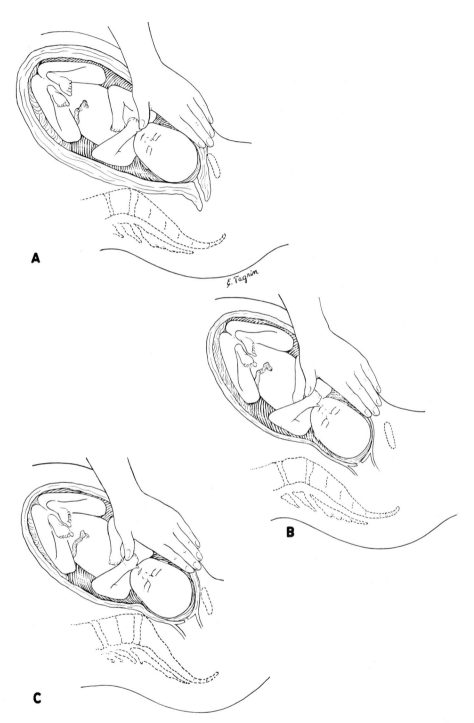

Figure 3. Findings of overriding, apparent and real. A, Apparent overriding, the result of a thick lower uterine segment in a normal pelvis. B, Finding eliminated by thinning of the lower segment in the course of labor. C, True overriding in the presence of cephalopelvic disproportion.

strait or inlet of the pelvis. This is considered to have occurred when the leading point of the vertex is at or below the level of the ischial spines, and the angle formed by the descending vertex with the inner surface and lower border of the symphysis pubis is obliterated or nearly so (Fig. 4). If the vertex is markedly molded (Fig. 5A) or the head is extended (Fig. 5B), both of these criteria can be fulfilled and the vertex not be engaged.

A rectal examination is next performed, but before it is done it is well to palpate the pubic arch and the symphysis to be reassured that the outlet is of ample size. The rectal examination should determine the degree of effacement and dilatation of the cervix. Even for the experienced, this examination may be difficult to perform accurately when the cervix is not dilated, or the vertex is unengaged. In fact, it may be almost impossible if the presenting part is floating or the cervix is in an extreme posterior position. If there is doubt as to the findings, a sterile vaginal examination is indicated.

The station of the presenting part is next determined in relation to the bispinous diameter or line and that is designated zero. When the presenting part is above this line, it is described as being minus

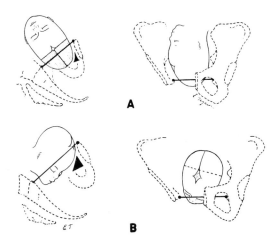

Figure 5. Conditions creating a false impression of vertex engagement. A, Marked molding of the fetal vertex. The biparietal diameter is above the inlet, the head is unengaged, and disproportion is more than a possibility. B, An extended head. The biparietal diameter (broken line) is well above the inlet, the head is not engaged, and disproportion is more than likely.

1, 2, 3, or 4, depending on its distance in centimeters above the line. Minus 4 is consistent with totally unengaged or floating presentation. When the presenting part is below the bispinous diameter, it is recorded as plus 1, 2, 3, or 4. Plus 4 means that the presenting part is on the perineum.

As part of this examination, the physician must confirm whether the vertex is well flexed. Otherwise, in the case of deflection, that is, a brow or face presentation, the examiner may falsely assume that the vertex is engaged because the leading point of the presenting part is at or below the interspinous line (Fig. 5B). An attempt should therefore be made to locate the posterior fontanelle, which is near the pelvic axis when the vertex is well flexed. Also, its location in the pelvic quadrants will designate the position of the occiput, that is, O.P., O.A., or O.T., the three cardinal positions of the fetus in a vertex presentation. Unless the lower uterine segment is extremely thin, however, or until the cervix is dilated 3 cm. or more, it may not be possible by rectal examination to identify the fontanelles and suture lines. If there is doubt, a vaginal examination may be necessary, for the examining fingers can invade the cervix and lower uterine segment and thus locate these landmarks of the fetal vertex, or, if the presentation is a breech, the position of the fetal sacrum. Most labors, however, can be

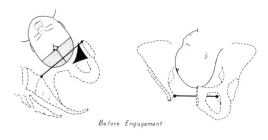

Before Engagement

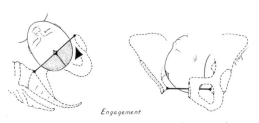

Engagement

Figure 4. Engagement is indicated by the descent of the leading point of the flexed vertex to the level of the intraspinous line, tending to obliterate the angle formed by the vertex and the symphysis, as shown in black. The junction of the stippled and clear area of the vertex indicates the position of the biparietal diameter of the fetal vertex.

followed entirely satisfactorily with abdominal palpation and rectal examination.

When searching for the various pelvic and fetal landmarks, it may prove helpful after the examining finger has passed the rectal sphincter to turn the finger so that its palmar surface is toward the sacrum. The coccyx and the tip of the sacrum are now located, and the lateral border of the sacrum is followed upward about 2 cm. Here, the examining finger will encounter a semilunar bandlike structure, which is the sacroiliac ligament. Following this lateralward some 2 to 4 cm. will bring the examining finger to the iliac spine. After turning his hand anteriorly, the examiner can then relate the station of the vertex to this structure and, by sweeping the finger to the midline, usually locate the cervix.

In summary, a rectal or vaginal examination in a vertex presentation should elicit whether the head is engaged, its station in the pelvis, the position of the occiput, flexion or evidence of deflection, the degree of effacement and dilatation of the cervix, and its consistency, that is, whether it is soft and pliable or firm and unelastic (Fig. 6).

Status of the Fetal Membranes

Whether the fetal membranes are ruptured or intact at the time of the patient's admission is a question that is asked because of its important clinical implications. If the membranes have apparently ruptured prior to hospital entrance, the time at which the event occurred should be recorded. The patient's story may be difficult to evaluate, for vaginal and cervical secretions increase in normal pregnancy, and the patient may not be able to differentiate between this, mild urinary incontinence, and a slight loss of amniotic fluid. More often, however, the patient is able to state that at a precise time there was a sudden gush of fluid from the vagina with a subsequent continuing loss of fluid sufficient to necessitate the wearing of a perineal pad. Despite the fact that patients have been instructed that it is important to enter the

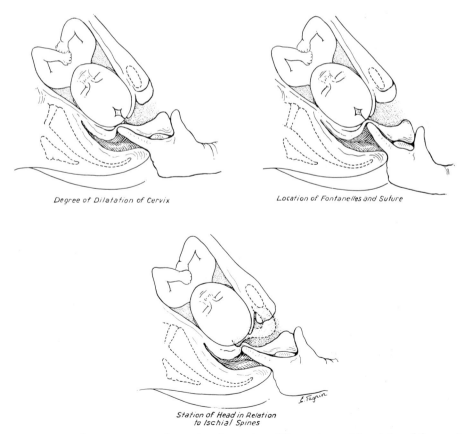

Degree of Dilatation of Cervix

Location of Fontanelles and Suture

Station of Head in Relation to Ischial Spines

Figure 6. Rectal examination to determine the station of the vertex and the status of the cervix.

hospital immediately when the membranes rupture, some fail to do so. It is disturbing to have a patient who may require a cesarean section enter the hospital many hours after rupture of the membranes, sometimes even a day or more.

There are several good reasons why the patient whose membranes have ruptured should enter the hospital immediately even though she is not experiencing uterine contractions. The fetal membranes are the main barrier in preventing intrauterine infection, an important consideration should cesarean section become necessary. In addition, the fetus may become infected secondary to intrauterine infection. With loss of fluid the uterus contracts about the fetus, adding to the risk of fetal distress with the advent of labor. Finally, a tightly contracted uterus limits obstetric manipulation should it be required to accomplish delivery. When labor is prolonged, early rupture of the membranes permits a contraction ring (Bandl's ring) to develop sooner and, although infrequent, this is an additional risk to the existing dystocia problem. The point is that if the patient were in the hospital and near term, to prevent the above possibilities, it would seem sound to stimulate the uterus by oxytocin drip in the hope of initiating labor. Hence, the patient should be under careful nursing surveillance after the membranes have ruptured to detect the earliest signs of infection or any evidence of fetal distress.

Usually there is no problem in establishing whether or not the fetal membranes are ruptured. A fluid containing whitish flecks of vernix caseosa is seen over the vulva or escaping from the introitus. On rectal examination, the presenting part may be gently displaced upward and away from the lower uterine segment, permitting fluid to be released from the uterus. In patients in whom the outcome of labor and the method of delivery are in question, that is, in patients who are to have a trial labor in the presence of borderline disproportion, it may be wise to perform a gentle sterile vaginal examination to determine with certainty the status of the fetal membranes, for the findings may influence the immediate method of management. Again, displacement of the presenting part upward by pressure of the examining fingers against the lower segment will allow fluid to come away if the membranes are ruptured. When the cervix is dilated at least 1 or 2 cm., the finding of forewaters confirms the fact that the membranes are intact, except when there is a rupture somewhere high in the corpus of the uterus. In the latter the threat of infection is notably less than when the membranes rupture in the region of the cervix.

Indicators have been used to determine the reaction of the vaginal secretions and thus attempt to detect whether or not the fetal membranes have ruptured. Their usefulness is based on the fact that normally the vagina is acid, with a pH value of about 4 to 4.5, and the pH of the amniotic fluid is nearly that of the body fluids, 7 to 7.5. The nitrazine test is commonly used and consists of a mixture of dyes that turn blue at a pH of 6 to 6.5. Bromthymol blue has also been used as an indicator; it reacts at the same pH. The presence of blood or cervical secretions will give a positive test with either indicator. Thus, such tests are of limited value, and when there is doubt a vaginal examination as described may be necessary to obtain the desired information.

ASSESSMENT OF THE CONDITION OF THE FETUS DURING LABOR

The obstetrician is concerned at all times during the course of labor with the status of the fetus. Assessment of the condition of the fetus in labor is dependent largely on auscultation of the fetal heart tones and the fetal blood pH. There is abundant recent literature on these subjects, and one of the problems is to reconcile several investigators' results and how these can be applied to patient management.

It is recognized that auscultation of the fetal heart tones is rather perfunctory and what is needed and is on the horizon is a constant external monitoring device that provides a permanent written record. However, with methods to measure amniotic fluid pressure, the influence of uterine contractions on fetal heart rate patterns has been extensively studied. Certain generalizations appear possible.

1. The fetal heart rate remains remarkably unchanged in many labors but it may accelerate and decelerate during a normal contraction.

2. The fetal heart rate of 140 beats per minute has a normal range of between 120

and 160 beats per minute. Indeed, the range might be extended to 110 to 170.

3. The deceleration that begins almost simultaneously with the start of the uterine contraction and recovers rapidly within 20 seconds from the peak of contraction is regarded as not pathologic and within the range of normal.

4. Deceleration is regarded as pathologic when it occurs later in the cycle of the uterine contraction, in some instances near the end, and when the recovery period is delayed beyond 20 seconds.

5. By interpretation, the former is related to cord compression and the latter to uteroplacental insufficiency.

It is apparent that the status of fetal heart rate is more significant in the latter part of a uterine contraction or the period immediately following it. It is the writer's opinion that deceleration with pathologic implication is commonly preceded by a period of acceleration (160 beats or more per minute), i.e., tachycardia followed by bradycardia. Also, the impression is gained that in some instances there is momentary flurry of fetal activity at the onset of acute fetal distress.

Sampling of fetal blood obtained by means of an endoscope introduced through the cervix and applied to the fetal scalp is now a means of assessing the status of the fetus in labor. From the results of many studies, it is safe to conclude that blood pH (normally 7.30 to 7.40) is a more reliable index of fetal homeostasis than blood oxygen levels. There appears to be slight fall in fetal blood pH in normal labor, more especially in the second stage of labor. This buttresses the concept long expressed that even normal labor contains an asphyxial element (see Fetal Distress in Chapter 27). Also, it would support the view that once the second stage of labor has been reached, the patient should be delivered at a time consistent with safe obstetric practice. That is to say, allowing a prolonged second stage to continue simply to obtain a spontaneous delivery may not be in the best interest of the fetus. Deviations in fetal heart rate are common during contractions when the vertex is arrested on the maternal perineum.

The relationship of the fetal blood pH to the conventional signs of fetal distress—tachycardia, bradycardia and the presence of meconium in the amniotic fluid—has received much attention but has not been entirely resolved. However, there appears to be growing agreement that a blood pH of 7.20 is crucial. Below this value, the fetus may well be in serious trouble and suffering from severe asphyxia.

Perhaps the greatest value of blood sampling is to reassure the clinican that the fetus is not facing impending doom, regardless of the status of the fetal heart, when the blood sample reveals a pH well above 7.20. To deliver the patient by some means, usually cesarean section, when bradycardia develops, is an easy answer to a rather common obstetric problem. Whether the operation is justified or necessary is the question. It is hoped that fewer rather than a greater number of cesarean sections will be performed for what is regarded as fetal distress if blood sampling is available for routine use. If this is to be meaningful, it must be recognized that serial blood sampling must be done in perhaps 10 per cent or more of patients. Moreover, time is of the essence when there is evidence of fetal distress and the necessary treatment must be promptly instituted (see Fetal Distress in Chapter 27).

Undoubtedly the most important result of determining blood pH will be that the values obtained can be correlated with deviations in fetal heart rate so that monitoring of the fetal heart tones will be more meaningful in identifying the fetus in distress.

In summary, the rate and rhythm of the fetal heart beat continues to be the most reliable practical gauge of the condition of the fetus in utero. Fetal blood sampling is far from a routine procedure. Deviations in the rate and regularity of the fetal heart beat can occur in the course of normal labor. The question is, when do changes in the fetal heart tones denote fetal distress in which survival is threatened or irreversible damage to the central nervous system may occur? Under what circumstance should or must the obstetrician intervene? (See Fetal Distress in Chapter 27).

ASSESSMENT OF THE INFANT AT BIRTH

A number of physiologic and clinical observations have been suggested for the evaluation of the physical state of the infant at birth. Such an evaluation may have several purposes, including assessment of the various methods of resuscitation. The main purpose, however, is to try to relate the condition of the infant at birth with its subsequent growth and development.

Considerable significance has been attributed to the oxygen content of the cord blood obtained at birth, with comparisons being made between the values obtained in normal and abnormal states. A body of such data is available, but definite limitations are imposed by the techniques of collection so that a degree of caution must be exercised in interpretation. (See Fetal Physiology in Chapter 31.) Rather than being based on separate samples obtained simultaneously from the umbilical vein and artery, the results of several of the oft-quoted studies are based on a pooled sample or a sample from one or the other vessel.

Although umbilical blood with a normal oxygen saturation (50 to 70 per cent) at birth undoubtedly means that the tissues of the newborn have an adequate oxygen content, in many instances the infant is vigorous and not depressed when the umbilical arterial blood has an oxygen saturation of 10 per cent or less. Although it was concluded that the oxygen values of blood from the umbilical artery more nearly reflect the oxygen content of the fetal tissues, these values alone are not a reliable index of the clinical state of the infant at birth.

Much has been made of the observation that the oxygen content of the cord blood is often low in babies born of mothers with pregnancy toxemia, prolonged labor, and postmaturity. Despite the low values, when blood from both the umbilical artery and vein of these infants is available for analysis, the oxygen difference often falls within the normal range of 4 to 5 volumes per cent. Thus, the oxygen difference between arterial and venous blood, rather than the oxygen levels from a pooled sample or from a single vessel, is perhaps a more precise reflection of the status of the oxygen content of the fetal tissues. Also, if the oxygen content of the cord blood is meaningful, the rate of umbilical blood flow should also be known, and this information is obtainable only under special circumstances when the cord can be exposed with the conceptus in situ, such as at the time of cesarean section.

It is evident that determinations of oxygen saturation and capacity, pCO_2 and pH, of scalp blood during labor and of cord blood at delivery are beyond the reach of routine clinical practicability as a method of assessing the physical state of the infant at birth. Rather, the clinician must continue to depend on certain physical signs and symptoms that the newborn exhibits at delivery.

During the last three or four decades several ways of evaluating the physical status of the infant at birth have been proposed. In recent times the scoring system of Apgar has gained wide popularity (Table 1). With 2 assigned for an optimum, 1 for an average, and 0 for an absent response, the infant is scored against five items, including a heart rate of less or more than 100 beats per minute, respiratory effort together with the character of the cry, muscle tone, reflex irritability, and color. The baby is first assessed at the end of the first minute and, when the first score is low, is scored periodically thereafter. According to this scheme, the heart rate and respiratory effort are more important than the muscle tone and reflex irritability, and the infant's color is least important of all. Deterioration of the infant is accompanied by a fall in heart rate. Scores below 6 at five minutes are unacceptable, and the obvious is to strive for a perfect score of 10.

TABLE 1.   EVALUATION OF NEWBORN INFANT[*]

Sign	0	1	2
Heart rate	absent	slow (below 100)	over 100
Respiratory effort	absent	slow, irregular	good; crying
Muscle tone	limp	some flexion of extremities	active motion
Response to catheter in nostril (tested after oropharynx is clear)	no response	grimace	cough or sneeze
Color	blue, pale	body pink, extremities blue	completely pink

*From Apgar, V., Holaday, D. A., James, L. S., Prince, C. E., Weisbrot, J. M., and Weiss, I.: J.A.M.A., 165:2155, 1957.

A large number of infants thus scored are being followed with periodic neurologic examinations and pertinent psychometric tests to determine whether this method of assessing the baby at birth can offer an accurate prognosis as to its future growth and neuromuscular development. Certainly uniformity of description of infant status at birth, by these or other methods, would appear necessary to the validity of any study concerned with the possible effects of the events surrounding pregnancy, labor, and delivery on the development of cerebral palsy and other neurologic deficits, including disturbance in the learning process.

THE LABOR AND DELIVERY RECORD

A careful recording of the events of labor is essential for use both immediately and later as it may relate to circumstances surrounding delivery and the puerperium and their consequences to the fetus and newborn. The following might be regarded as the minimal requirements.

The fetal heart beat during the first stage of labor is recorded at least every 15 minutes. A method of constant electronic monitoring is the ideal. During the second stage of labor the fetal heart tones are observed after each contraction and recorded every five minutes. Unfortunately, the constant elicitation of the rate of the fetal heart beat once the patient is prepared and draped for delivery is difficult. This applies especially in cases of cesarean section, when a period of some 15 minutes or more may elapse between the time of abdominal preparation and draping, and delivery of the infant. In the interim, particularly if there is a drop in blood pressure, the fetal heart rate may vary considerably without being detected.

The blood pressure is taken and recorded hourly, and the temperature at least every four hours. The maternal pulse is recorded every 15 to 30 minutes, together with other vital signs, including respiratory rate. In the course of labor frequent notation is made of the duration, the interval, and the strength of the uterine contractions, the latter as determined by the firmness of the uterus at the height of the contraction. If the membranes are intact at the onset of labor, the time of rupture is recorded, and some nota-tion should be made as to whether the amniotic fluid is normal in appearance or is meconium-stained. Although the fetal heart rate may be normal, meconium-stained amniotic fluid in a vertex presentation has been accepted as evidence of fetal distress prior to or during labor.

For patients who are sedated a record should be kept of their reaction to medication, that is, whether they are quiet or agitated with contractions, and the general status of their sensorium. All medications, their dosage and route, and all procedures must be recorded. Also included in the nurse's notes is the time when the patient enters the second stage of labor.

The vital information on the delivery record, besides a résumé of the events of labor and a description of the delivery by the physician, must include the time of birth, the method of delivery, and the infant's sex in terms of boy or girl, rather than male or (fe)male. The record must also state the type of anesthesia, the time and method of delivery of the placenta, whether an episiotomy was performed (and its type), an estimation of blood loss (normally 50 to 200 ml.), and any complication or deviation from normal.

CONDUCT OF THE VARIOUS STAGES OF NORMAL LABOR

It is assumed that the parturient has been well instructed about the events of labor and delivery, and that the method of pain relief has been discussed with her.

Ideally the patient should be in a single room with a nurse in attendance. Until she is medicated, the husband, properly gowned and masked, can be present, and the patient should be aware that he will be nearby until she is delivered and will be with her again when she is returned to her room. No patient who has received any drugs for pain relief is to be left alone until she is completely awake following delivery. In fact, no patient in labor should ever be left alone, a principle that is respected in the most primitive societies.

The medical support of the patient in labor involves the provision of good nursing care, adequate means of pain relief, maintenance of fluid balance, and care of the bladder. The nursing care consists of careful observation of labor, as well as offering encouragement to the patient. The nurse should report immediately any vaginal bleeding beyond that acceptable as excessive "show," a deviation in the rate and quality of the fetal heart tones, the appearance of meconium in a vertex presentation, or any variation in the vital signs of the mother.

As the patient becomes uncomfortable, medication for pain relief is administered, as ordered by her physician. For many patients this will become necessary only when the cervix is effaced and dilated 2 to 3 cm. Others may complain before this, and meperidine, 50 mg., or its equivalent, may be sufficient; it may be repeated in two to four hours until such time as the cervix has reached the state described. By this time the patient is usually in what is commonly referred to as "good labor"; the contractions are two to four minutes apart and last 40 to 60 seconds. From this time on it is anticipated that the patient will make satisfactory progress in labor, and the regular regimen for pain relief is instituted.

Intravenous administration of fluids is not required unless the patient has experienced a waiting period, as in the case of ruptured membranes without labor, or when duration of labor exceeds 8 to 10 hours.

The bladder is checked frequently, and in a few instances catheterization may be needed. When the presenting part is above the pelvic inlet, a full bladder may prevent engagement. Once the presenting part becomes engaged, however, the bladder and its contents are no longer a factor in the progress of labor. In fact, when it contains any appreciable amount of urine, the bladder moves up out of the pelvis and becomes an abdominal organ. Once the vertex or

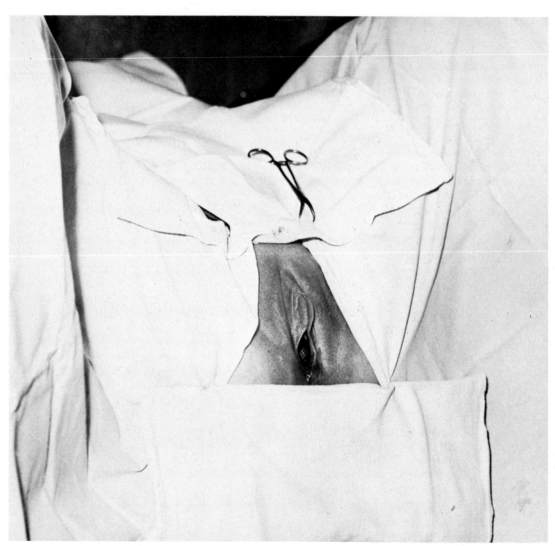

Figure 7.   Patient draped for delivery. Vertex beginning to crown.

presenting part is deeply situated in the pelvis, the patient need not be catheterized unless labor is prolonged several hours and the bladder becomes markedly distended. Further, catheterization at delivery is unnecessary, regardless of whether the delivery is normal or by forceps. In fact, damage to the bladder is less likely to occur if the bladder is an abdominal rather than a pelvic organ. The incidence of postpartum catheterization is not increased and most patients void spontaneously post partum. The few who require catheterization are usually those who have had a rather difficult operative delivery.

When the patient enters the second stage of labor the pains are more frequent and sustained, and she usually becomes more restless. Often the patient feels nauseated and may vomit. She exhibits the desire to bear down and expel the fetus, as indicated by holding her breath with the contractions, thus fixing her diaphragm, and at the same time tensing her abdominal muscles. When these signs become evident, the presenting part is usually at or near the perineum. If the membranes are intact, they may at this point impede progress. At the time of the rectal examination, with the vulva prepared with an antiseptic and the labia separated by sterile pledgets, a hemostat may be introduced into the vagina and directed, by the rectal finger, to the membranes, which can be grasped by the instrument and ruptured. This may hasten the completion of the second stage of labor and prepare the patient for delivery. Occasionally, with intact membranes, the cervix may become fully dilated and the presenting part unengaged. In this event it is wise to prepare the patient for a sterile pelvic examination and amniotomy. With the fingers or hand in the vagina it is possible to allow the amniotic fluid to escape slowly. Otherwise, spontaneous rupture of the membranes under these circumstances, with the sudden release of fluid, may result in prolapse of the cord. With the second stage, the patient is moved to the case room and, as the presenting part is seen at the introitus, she is placed on the delivery table. The patient is administered either a pudendal, a conduction,

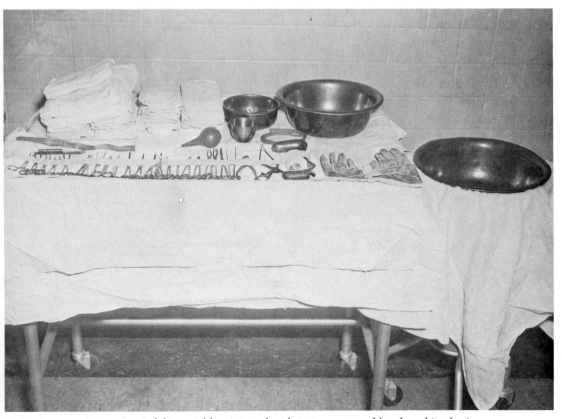

Figure 8. A delivery table equipped with instruments and hand-washing basin.

or a general anesthetic, in accordance with the indications. She is prepared and draped for delivery (Figs. 7 and 8).

DELIVERY

In accomplishing spontaneous and controlled delivery, one of two methods can be used. With the first, three fingers of the hand are spread over the fetal occiput as the vertex begins to crown and emerge from beneath the symphysis. Covered by a towel, the tips of three fingers of the other hand are placed at the midline between the sacrum and the anus. Immediately after each contraction the fetal brow is advanced over the perineum by an upward pressure of the lower hand. Both hands are kept immobile during contractions. The above technique is repeated until the chin is delivered. The vertex is thus delivered by extension, with the larger occipitofrontal diameter presenting at the outlet. In practice, extension of the head, even with an episiotomy, and certainly if episiotomy is not performed, causes lacerations about the urethra and clitoris and disruption of the endopelvic fascia supporting the urethra and bladder through accentuating the pressure of the occiput against these structures. This maneuver, modified or otherwise, demands that the head be born by extension rather than in a state of flexion.

According to the second and preferred technique of delivery, the vertex is maintained in a state of flexion until the occiput has bypassed the symphysis and the brow has been born over the perineum. Thus, the smaller suboccipitobregmatic diameter, rather than the larger occipitofrontal diameter, passes through the outlet. With contractions and following an episiotomy (Fig. 9A) the flexed vertex is guided over the perineum with the fingers of one hand on the occiput and the fingers of the second hand supporting the sinciput (Fig. 9B). With the patient anesthetized, the vertex is guided through the outlet in a similar manner with forceps. It is appreciated that the views expressed here may be at variance with statements in other texts.

With the birth of the head the neck region is explored for cord entanglements, for commonly the cord may encircle the neck once or twice or several times. If there is a single encirclement, the cord should be loosened and slipped over either the head or shoulders. Otherwise, it may be necessary to clamp and cut the cord in order to release it. One has the impression that the infant breathes and responds better when the cord does not have to be severed early.

To aid in the delivery of the anterior shoulder the fingers of one hand are inserted behind the infant's back and along the posterior shoulder, sweeping it into the hollow of the sacrum (Fig. 9C). This causes the anterior shoulder to rotate to the arch. For example, in an anterior occiput position, the anterior shoulder will be found rotated into the right upper quadrant of the pelvis. By the maneuver described above, the anterior shoulder rotates to the left to impinge beneath the arch, and is more easily delivered, with little or no traction being necessary.

As the vertex restitutes and the anterior shoulder is born, it is well to milk the infant's trachea to bring any secretions into the nasopharynx where they can easily be removed by suction (Fig. 9D). In fact, slow delivery of the shoulders and chest will result in compression of the chest, and commonly large amounts of amniotic fluid are seen to exude from the mouth and the nose. This physiologic effect may be one of the reasons why it is more beneficial for the infant to be born pelvically than by cesarean section, for in cesarean section compression of the chest during delivery is not a special feature. Consequently, there is a considerable amount of amniotic fluid in the respiratory tract at the first breath, which may or may not be detrimental, depending mostly on the presence or absence of infection in the amniotic fluid.

With birth of the anterior shoulder the posterior shoulder is then born (Fig. 10A). On occasion the posterior shoulder will deliver itself before the anterior shoulder. Traction on the neck, with its possible injury to the brachial plexus, must be avoided at all times.

With the birth of the shoulders and chest the infant is rotated with its abdomen upward. The back lies along the obstetrician's forearm and the baby is balanced by the other hand (Fig. 10B). The hand of the arm on which the newborn is resting searches for the infant's feet as the buttocks and thighs are born (Fig. 10C). The baby is then grasped by its feet and suspended, to encourage drainage of secretions from the trachea, and the mucus is aspirated with a bulb

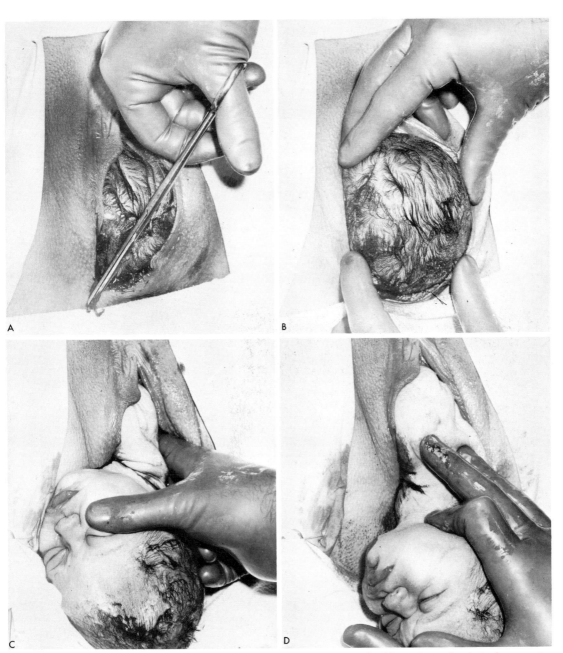

Figure 9. Technique of delivery. A, Right mediolateral episiotomy, preferably performed early in the crowning of the vertex. B, The sinciput is born over the incised perineum; the occiput has bypassed the inferior border of the symphysis. C, The infant's left shoulder is rotated manually into the hollow of the sacrum to cause the anterior shoulder to impinge under the pubes, to avoid any need for traction on the neck. D, Anterior shoulder being born. The trachea should be milked at this point.

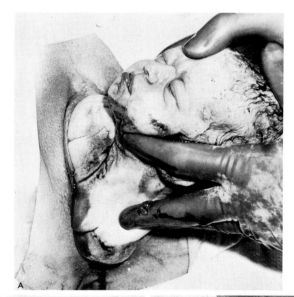

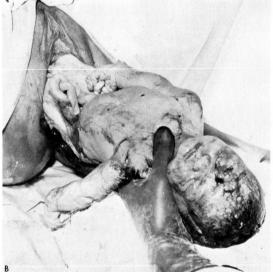

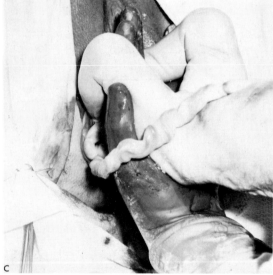

Figure 10.   Technique of delivery (continued). A, Delivery of the posterior shoulder. B, The baby's abdomen is turned anteriorly. Towels over the rectum have been removed to demonstrate the position of the operator's left hand. The baby now rests on the operator's forearm. C, The operator seeks the baby's feet, passing one or two fingers between. With the thumb meeting the fingers, the baby is securely locked and can be readily suspended.

syringe (Fig. 11). Or with the infant's head lowered the trachea is again stripped toward the nasopharynx, and the latter is emptied of mucus (Fig. 12). For a time the bassinet should be tilted so that the infant's head is lower than its body. This will promote drainage and prevent aspiration. The nasopharynx should be periodically suctioned for excessive mucus.

Resuscitation of the Newborn

Resuscitative measures for the newborn are rarely necessary beyond the stage of

bulb suction. With the infant suspended, gentle tapping of the chest encourages drainage from the bronchioles and bronchi. The infant should be suspended until the airway seems clear, aided on occasion by one or two coughs on the part of the infant. Before the infant is placed on the table, it is well to make certain that the airway is clear, rather than to chance aspiration in the supine position. At the same time, if the infant is not breathing normally, there should be no great delay in pursuing more definitive treatment.

More active resuscitation of the infant at

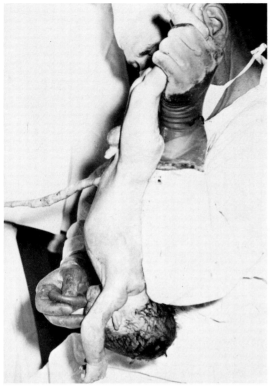

Figure 11. Baby suspended. Note locking of the physician's fingers about the baby's ankles. The upper airway is being aspirated, the procedure being facilitated by the operator flexing his forearm, permitting the extension of the infant's neck.

birth should be a rare event and restricted in the main to patients with high-risk pregnancies, in which one should anticipate the possibility that the fetus may be depressed at birth. On occasion, however, asphyxia neonatorum may occur in a supposedly

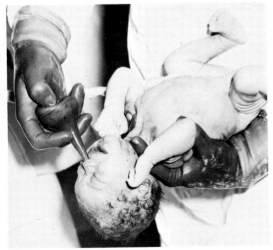

Figure 12. Alternate method of aspirating the infant's upper airway.

full-term normal labor and for an indiscernible cause (see Fetal Distress in Chapter 27).

The vast majority of infants will breathe promptly with an immediate Apgar score of 7 to 10. However, if at birth the fetus fails to breathe promptly and appears to lack normal tone, no time should be lost over considering a plan of action. Some infants will require only pharyngeal suction and administration of oxygen by mask. But those of concern are those who fail to respond after the above measures. Within 30 to 60 seconds, more active methods must be considered; time is of the essence. The cord should be clamped and cut and the infant removed to an adjacent room especially equipped with both personnel and facilities for coping with the resuscitative problem. The room should be temperature-regulated to preserve the infant's body heat. The medical team should be especially knowledgeable and adept in methods of resuscitation. The following are basic objectives:

1. A clear airway should be immediately established. At the beginning this may be a mouth airway with administration of oxygen.

2. If this proves insufficient and no respiratory response occurs, intubation should be performed by one skilled in the use of the laryngoscope. If after tracheal aspiration the infant fails to breathe from the stimulus, gentle pressure breathing (a modification of mouth-to-mouth resuscitation) will assist in expanding the lungs.

3. External cardiac massage by gentle compression of the lower third of the sternum may assist the emptying and filling of the heart.

4. Rapid correction of the low blood pH favors recovery, and glucose and bicarbonate solutions should be administered via umbilical vein as soon as is feasible.

In summary, avoidance of the need for resuscitation of the newborn is the objective of every delivery. Careful obstetric management, especially in patients with high-risk pregnancies, includes the elimination of as much of the second stage of labor as is consistent with safe delivery. This applies especially to the fragile premature infants, who make up the bulk of those requiring resuscitation.

No delay should be permitted when there is evidence of asphyxia. Evidence can be marshaled to indicate that placental transfusion might be detrimental to a depressed infant and is not essential for any infant. Hence, the cord should be promptly cut and the baby given to a medical team that includes an anesthesiologist and pediatrician, as well as an obstetrician, all of whom are versed in the methods of resuscitation.

The umbilical cord is eventually clamped and cut; the time after birth at which this should be done has been the subject of controversy. There is no doubt that the newborn infant can recover 50 ml. or more of blood from the placenta if clamping of the cord is delayed until it ceases to pulsate. Although placental transfusion is without danger to the normal infant, this procedure may prove detrimental in infants with anomalies of the cardiovascular system, or with asphyxia, circulatory failure, maternal-fetal blood group incompatibility, and possibly intracranial hemorrhage. Regardless of controversy, if there is any doubt about the newborn's respiratory function, the cord should be clamped and cut and whatever resuscitative measures seem indicated should be started immediately. The same procedure applies when the mother requires immediate attention. If one chooses, however, clamping of the cord may be postponed until it ceases to pulsate, which is ordinarily a minute or so after birth.

THIRD STAGE OF LABOR

With the birth of the infant, oxytocic drugs are administered to initiate effective uterine contractions for the purpose of expelling the placenta and to prevent uterine atony. There are those who prefer ergonovine (Ergotrate), or a synthetic product, methylergonovine (Methergine), to be given either intravenously or intramuscularly. When the drug is given intravenously, the uterus contracts more promptly but, owing to the hypertensive effect, this method is sometimes contraindicated in patients under regional anesthesia. One technique has been to administer the drug with birth of the infant's shoulder, but the uterus contracts to the extent that the placenta may become trapped and require manual removal.

Some believe that intravenous ergonovine causes the uterus to contract more effectively than any of the oxytocic substances but, in the writer's opinion, if given intravenously, oxytocin causes the uterus

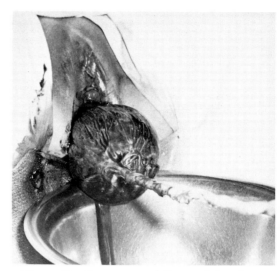

Figure 13. Spontaneous delivery of the placenta (Schultze mechanism). When necessary, as in this instance, the membranes are released from the uterus by placing the hand palm upward between the symphysis and the anteriorly flexed uterus. With upward pressure, the anterior flexion is overcome and the membranes are released and delivered (Brandt maneuver).

to contract almost instantaneously and in a more physiologic fashion; that is, the uterus contracts and relaxes at frequent intervals.

One method preferred by the writer is to administer intravenously 2 ml. of a mixture of one-half an ampule (0.5 ml.) of Pitocin, or its synthetic equivalent, diluted in 4.5 ml. of saline solution. This relatively small dose (equal to 2 to 3 units of oxytocin) can be used with any form of anesthesia without any side effects. After the placenta is delivered, ergonovine, 0.2 mg., is then administered intramuscularly.

In most instances, following the intravenous administration of oxytocin, the placenta is spontaneously extruded into the vagina within three to five minutes after delivery (Fig. 13). If this fails to occur, the placenta may be expelled by gently compressing the uterus with the hand on the abdomen (Credé maneuver), combined with pressure to lift the uterus upward and backward out of the pelvis (Brandt maneuver).

EXAMINATION OF THE PLACENTA

The inspection of the placenta is a routine procedure in every delivery, to make certain that none of the placental and fetal membranes have been retained in the uterus and to identify any gross changes of pathologic significance. The inspection may begin with the chorionic surface by noting the site of insertion of the umbilical cord. If it inserts on the membranes, this is termed membranous or velamentous insertion of the cord. It is important to note the status of the large fetal vessels of the cord, for because of their location they are easily traumatized. Further, if these vessels are disrupted, the baby will have bled, and can be near exsanguination at birth. Care must be taken to see whether or not the chorionic vessels near the margin are intact or disrupted, disruption meaning that there may still be some placental tissue in the uterus in the form of a succenturiate lobe.

The cut end of the umbilical cord should be inspected, and it should be recorded whether three or only two blood vessels are seen. Infants with only one rather than two umbilical arteries have a much greater incidence of malformation, often recognized at birth but sometimes not until later in life. Whoever is responsible for the medical care of the baby should be aware of this anomalous finding in the cord and thus be forewarned.

After the fetal surface is examined, the maternal surface is examined more closely. First, notation is made of the absence or presence of coagula, particularly old clots which may be attached to the placenta. Such clots may be indicative of old or recent abruptio placentae. The margin of the placenta should be closely examined to detect marginal sinus thromboses.

When one examines the maternal surface, attention should be given to the fissures that normally divide the cotyledons (Fig. 14), noting whether the cotyledons are all present and intact, as an indication that there is no missing or retained placental tissue. At times the placenta is grossly torn and it is difficult to piece the cotyledons together. Because retained placental tissue is often the cause of subinvolution and postpartum hemorrhage, when cotyledons are missing the uterus should be explored immediately and any retained placental tissue removed.

Although some favor routine exploration of the uterus after expulsion of the placenta, if the membranes appear intact, the placenta is complete, and the patient is not bleeding, this seems unnecessary. One cannot deny, however, that when routine exploration has been the policy of the management of the

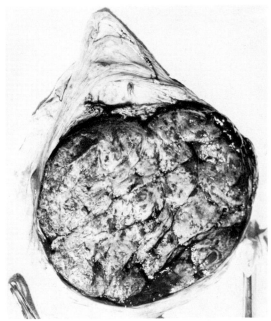

Figure 14. A normal placenta with the usual fissuring and distribution of cotyledons.

third stage, experienced clinicians have recovered placental tissue and membranes in a percentage of cases (1 to 4 per cent). Despite antibiotics and chemotherapy, invasion of the uterus must be regarded as carrying some risk. However, if there is doubt as to whether the placenta is intact or there is possibility of trauma, the uterus certainly should be explored.

CARE OF THE MOTHER

After tagging and placing the baby in the bassinet, the physician changes his gloves, which may possibly have become contaminated during delivery, and turns his attention to the mother, who is redraped for the episiotomy repair (Fig. 15). In operative deliveries, it is good practice to inspect the vaginal vaults and the cervix and to explore the uterus. Otherwise, if the patient bleeds following episiotomy repair, this inspection may have to be carried out with resultant marked tension on the recently placed sutures and damage to the episiotomy wound.

The incision is closed with 0 and 00 chromic catgut. In principle, the closure of the vaginal mucous membrane is postponed so that the interrupted sutures in the levator ani muscles can be placed under

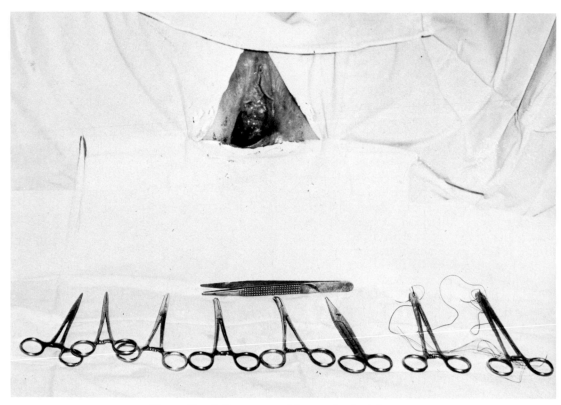

Figure 15. Patient prepared for repair of episiotomy.

direct vision. This permits the suture to include the endopelvic fascia surrounding the rectum and closes the wound from its base outward. If the vaginal mucous membrane is closed first, the sutures in the levator ani muscles must be placed by touch; in an effort to avoid the rectum, the physician may fail to place the sutures deep enough to restore normal perineal support. The end-result is a poor repair, devoid of normal amounts of muscle and fascia, and made up mostly of skin and vaginal mucous membrane. In order to facilitate subsequent closure of the vaginal mucous membrane, the deep sutures are not tied until this has been accomplished (Fig. 16).

The hymenal ring is a useful landmark to aid in restoring previous anatomic relationships and provide proper closure of the vaginal mucous membrane. As demonstrated, the continuous vaginal suture dips beneath it to emerge on the perineal side. At this point, the wound is wiped dry before each deep suture is tied, for a dry field promotes healing by first intention, prevents edema formation, and consequently reduces patient discomfort. The continuous suture next closes the deep fascia of the perineum and the skin (Fig. 17).

In the mediolateral type of episiotomy it must be appreciated that there is considerable distortion of the anatomic relationships, resulting from upward and downward retraction of fascia containing the pubococcygeus muscle. To restore the perineum and achieve a correct repair, the tissues of the lower perineal incision must be brought anteriorly and approximated to the vaginal portion of the tissue of the upper incision. To suture together the opposing tissues will result in a repair with poor perineal support. Another point of difference is that the skin is closed by interrupted sutures because the tissue tension does not permit the use of the subcuticular type of sutures, which serve for closing a median episiotomy (Fig. 18).

Any complications arising in a normal birth are more apt to occur in the first hour or two after delivery. To emphasize its importance in terms of patient care, this period is designated or referred to as the *fourth stage of labor*. Laryngospasm, which may lead to vomiting and its attending risks, is also a possibility as the patient emerges from the anesthesia. The patient should be carefully watched during this period and should not be moved from the recovery room to her own room. In the interim, all

(Text continued on page 526)

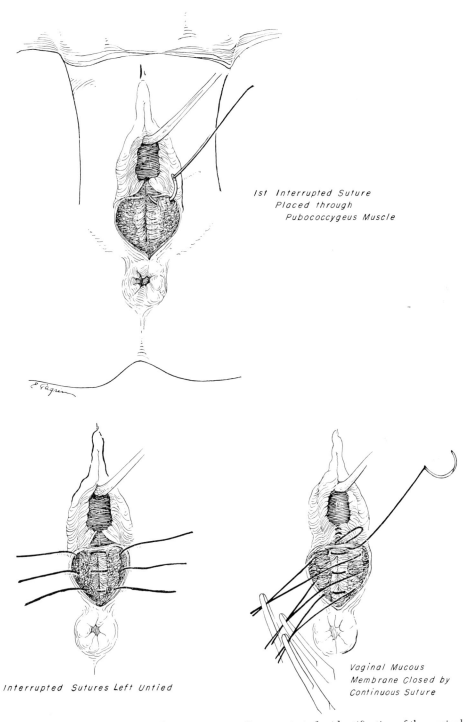

1st Interrupted Suture
Placed through
Pubococcygeus Muscle

Interrupted Sutures Left Untied

Vaginal Mucous
Membrane Closed by
Continuous Suture

Figure 16. First steps in repair of median episiotomy. Gauze strip is for identification of the vaginal tampon.

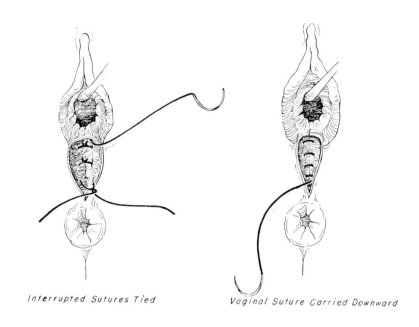

Interrupted Sutures Tied   *Vaginal Suture Carried Downward*

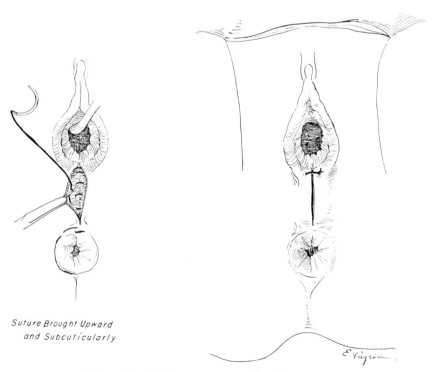

*Suture Brought Upward
and Subcuticularly*

Figure 17.   Final steps in repair of median episiotomy.

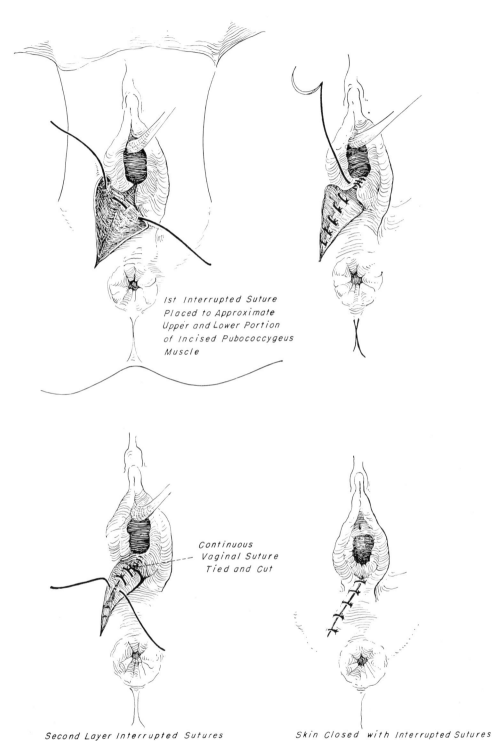

1st Interrupted Suture
Placed to Approximate
Upper and Lower Portion
of Incised Pubococcygeus
Muscle

Continuous
Vaginal Suture
Tied and Cut

Second Layer Interrupted Sutures   Skin Closed with Interrupted Sutures

Figure 18.   Steps in repair of right mediolateral episiotomy.

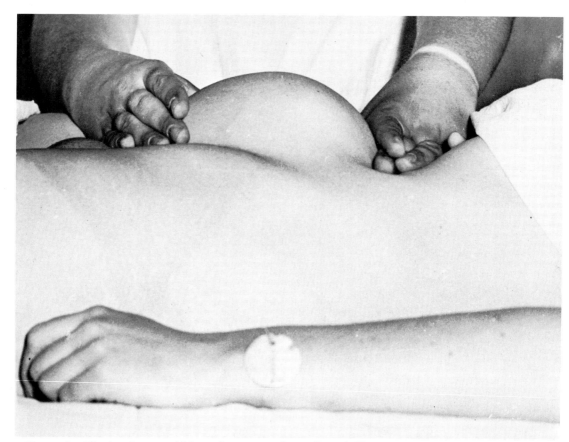

Figure 19. The fourth stage of labor. The uterus is being "guarded" to prevent uterine atony, or to detect it early.

of the vital signs should be observed and recorded. A nurse should guard the uterine corpus (Fig. 19) for a minimum of 45 minutes from the time of delivery. By so doing, she will detect at once any tendency to atony. Also, she will be able to assist the patient who has postanesthesia nausea and give general nursing care.

CARE OF THE NEWBORN

The newborn should be ushered into a temperature environment not too different from the one he departed. Although the newborn contains increased amounts of brown adipose tissue, which plays a role in both heat conservation and heat production, he responds rapidly to environmental temperature change. In fact, he may respond more rapidly than at any other time of his life. The thermoregulation range bears a reciprocal relation to body size; hence the range is comparatively less for the newborn, whose body surface is greater per mass of

generating tissue than the adult's. This applies to a greater degree in the premature or dysmature infant. Despite the concept that a state of hypothermia might be useful in reducing energy requirements, for purposes of the care of the newborn the oxygen consumption is said to be minimal when the skin temperature as measured on the abdomen is 36 to 37° C. Also, improved survival in birth asphyxia is associated with the lowest energy costs. Conservation of energy will be enhanced by an environment that will maintain the skin temperature at the value mentioned above. In short, it is essential to keep the infant warm in its sojourn in the delivery room as well as the nursery.

Definite means of identifying the baby should be affixed by a physician in the delivery room. A variety of methods are used in different hospitals, including metal discs with numbers, lettered beads, or tapes bearing the identification data. A print of the walking surface of the infant's foot, similar to a fingerprint, is frequently made.

To prevent ophthalmia neonatorum of

neisserian origin, the infant's eyes are treated with 1 per cent silver nitrate solution. The technique is to clean the eyelids with cotton pledgets moistened with sterile distilled water, and to turn the infant's head from one side to the other and gently irrigate each conjunctival sac with an ear syringe. One drop of silver nitrate solution is instilled near the outer canthus of each eye. After two minutes, the conjunctival sacs are again irrigated with sterile water, and a small amount of 1 per cent yellow oxide of mercury ointment is applied along each eyelid.

A usual routine is to give vitamin K to the newborn in a dosage of 2.5 mg. or less, intramuscularly (see Fetal Growth and Physiology, Chapter 31). Because it is possible to produce icterus experimentally by the administration of vitamin K, the question has been raised whether the drug should be used, and, if so, in what dosage. Regardless of its therapeutic value, which is still debated, the amounts given are well within the range of safety in comparison with the rather huge amounts that must be used to produce icterus in the experimental animal.

The infant is examined by the obstetrician at the end of delivery. The head should be palpated for any evidence of trauma, and the mouth inspected for abnormalities of the jaws and the hard and soft palate. The examiner must be satisfied that the lungs are well aerated and the heart sounds are normal. The abdomen should contain no masses, nor should there be any enlargement of the liver or spleen. The anus should be patent and the external genitalia normal. In a male, the testes should be in the scrotum. It should be realized that hypospadias, usually mild, is not uncommon.

PAIN RELIEF IN LABOR AND DELIVERY

The adoption of measures to relieve pain in the parturient marked a milestone in the history of both anesthesia and obstetrics. As an anesthetic, chloroform was introduced into clinical medicine by Dr. James Y. Simpson, of Edinburgh, who first anesthetized an obstetric patient on January 19, 1847, using this agent. There were sharp differences of opinion regarding both the moral and the medical justification for the use of agents for relief of pain during labor and delivery; only after Dr. John Snow successfully administered chloroform to Queen Victoria at the birth of Prince Leopold, on April 7, 1853, was anesthesia accepted by the medical profession and the lay public as a helpful adjunct to obstetric practice.

Since that time, particularly in the past 25 years, many investigations have added materially to the knowledge and techniques of the control of pain during labor. The indications and contraindications have been established for the different methods and techniques. Thus, the practice of pain relief has now benefited several generations of women. The aura of fear and expectation of agonizing pain that were once associated with childbirth have, as a result, been substantially dispelled. It is of considerable consolation to the parturient that effective and safe methods of pain relief are available for her if the need arises.

Although it is argued that analgesics can inhibit uterine contractions, progress in labor can be improved by the use of these agents by allaying pain and also the anxiety that often develops in the patient in the course of labor.

However, the use of agents for pain relief requires that the obstetrician be familiar with the indications and the limitations of the different analgesic and anesthetic agents if he is to use them with safety and benefit to his patient. Working closely with the anesthesiologist, the obstetrician must be aware that there is a preferred method of pain relief, depending on the circumstances in each case. Both must appreciate the physiologic changes that occur in pregnancy and how these may influence the cardiorespiratory and renal systems.

Certainly no obstetric patient may properly be regarded as a "routine case," and the safety and welfare of the mother and her fetus are poorly served when the administration of anesthesia is placed in the hands of persons who are not competent in all of the types and phases of anesthetic management. This means the presence at all times of a highly competent anesthesiologist who acknowledges that obstetric anesthesia has certain features peculiar to it. He must appreciate that the obstetric patient is often not as well prepared to receive an anesthetic as are patients for elective surgery.

SOURCE AND DEGREE OF PAIN IN LABOR

It is assumed that the pain of labor is due not to the contractions of the body of the uterus, but to the effect of the forces initiated by these contractions. In cesarean section performed under local block of the anterior abdominal wall, incision of the uterus is not painful but the extraction of the infant is, at the least, most uncomfortable. The latter is probably the result of stretching of the utero-sacral ligaments at the time the baby is extracted from the uterus. Thus, it would appear that the pain of labor arises from tension on the supporting ligaments of the uterus and pressure of the uterine contents produced through the forces of labor against the lower uterine segment and cervix. The pain is transmitted through the 11th and 12th thoracic and the 4th and 5th sacral segments by way of the ganglia located in and about the uterus.

The problem of determining the presence and estimating the amount of pain accurately and quantitatively is a difficult one. Awareness of pain and the degree to which it is felt are both subjective experiences. If a standardized technique of questioning and recording answers is used for determining whether or not a patient experiences pain, there is probably nothing more reliable than the patient's own statement. An attempt has been made to estimate the amount of pain experienced during labor by use of the thermal radiation apparatus. The patient's awareness of the intensity of pain during labor was compared with her response to a known, quantitatively graded, painful stimulus from this apparatus. In a limited number of unmedicated patients during the first, second, and third stages of labor, pain began from a threshold value of 2 dols* in intensity, and increased as labor progressed. During the second stage, pain intensity was reported as 10 dols, the latter being ceiling pain, the most intense pain which can be experienced. The authors further observed that the intensity of pain

in the first stage of labor was roughly proportional to the extent of cervical dilatation and inversely proportional to the duration of the interval between uterine contractions.

It is concluded that the labor contractions are painful, and the pain can be as intense as any encountered in medical practice. Many factors, however, may tend to minimize or aggravate the amount of discomfort and pain that a patient experiences.

CONTROL OF PAIN IN LABOR

The pharmacologic agents commonly used to control pain during labor are the barbiturates and the phenanthrene alkaloids. These may be supplemented by scopolamine for amnesia and those agents with a tranquilizing effect. Intermittent inhalation of trilene and nitrous oxide during painful uterine contractions may be used, and also sensory nerve block including the paracervical and epidural methods. The use of hypnosis completes the list of methods of pain relief during labor.

Barbiturates

The barbiturates, of which there are many, produce sedation and hypnosis, but are not analgesics, for they do not produce insensibility to pain. The rationale for their use in labor lies in the fact that a patient adequately medicated will sleep between uterine contractions. The barbiturates are not without effect on the fetus, as they cross the placenta readily, but satisfactory sedation can be obtained with doses that will not cause respiratory depression of the newborn, provided the total dose is restricted to 0.3 to 0.4 gram. When the dosage has been so restricted, these drugs have been scarcely detected in the cord blood.

The potency, toxicity, duration of action, and hypnotic effect of these drugs vary. Administered orally, the short-acting barbiturates are secobarbital (Seconal) and pentobarbital (Nembutal), and the intermediate-acting one is amobarbital (Amytal). Other short-acting barbiturates in the form of vinbarbital (Delvinal), and thiopental (Pentothal), often administered intravenously, have their advocates. These agents come into equilibrium in the fetal and maternal blood within a few minutes after they are given.

---

*The *dol* is a unit of pain, with a value of approximately one tenth the intensity of maximal pain.

The shorter-acting barbiturates are detoxified in the tissues, particularly in the liver, and the longer-acting (barbital and phenobarbital) are eliminated in the kidney, so that caution must also be exercised in the use of these drugs when there is liver or renal impairment, as in pregnancy toxemia. Untoward reactions to the barbiturate drugs are readily avoided by careful history-taking, accurate evaluation of the physical and emotional status of the patient, and proper administration of these agents.

Phenanthrene Alkaloids

The phenanthrene alkaloids, of which morphine is a principal member, have been widely used in obstetrics as analgesic agents. These drugs have a selective action by depressing pain sensibility without necessarily producing sedation. Morphine, as well as the synthetic preparations with similar action, finds its chief usefulness in the relief of discomfort of early labor. These drugs, moreover, may be used to differentiate so-called true from false labor. In false labor, the uterus will become quiescent, and the patient's discomfort will disappear after administration of a small amount of morphine (10 mg.) or a comparable dose of a morphine-like drug. In the event that the patient is in labor, uterine contractions will continue.

The depressant action of the alkaloids on the fetus, especially the premature fetus, or the fetus at risk for any other reason, contraindicates their use near the end of the first and during the second stage of labor and in many obstetric complications. Typically, the term infant whose mother has mistakenly received morphine within a period of one or two hours before delivery, although born with excellent tone and color, is likely after a few breaths to become apneic and flaccid. Because of depressed reflexes, the newborn finds it difficult to handle the collection of mucus in the nasopharynx that is often normally present in the early hours of life. Frequent suctioning is necessary to maintain a clear airway for some hours after delivery. The nursing personnel should be forewarned and instructed to stimulate the infant to cry, and to clear the air passages of mucus periodically; they should also keep the baby under constant surveillance for at least 12 hours after delivery.

The newer synthetic alkaloids have largely supplanted morphine. A derivative of pyridine, referred to as meperidine or pethidine (Demerol), has been used extensively as an analgesic agent in labor. In substance, this drug combines a worthwhile weak atropine-like property with the analgesic effect of morphine. Caution must be exercised in the intravenous administration of the drug, for the average dose may cause a significant fall in blood pressure, tachycardia, and respiratory and cerebral depression. Rarely, a profound peripheral vascular collapse has been known to occur when this drug was given intravenously, and maternal death has been attributed to this form of administration. Also, like morphine, the use of meperidine should be restricted to early labor. In fact, when the drug is given intramuscularly in the commonly advocated dosage of 100 mg. every two to four hours in the course of labor, fetal depression is a distinct hazard, particularly if inhalation rather than conduction anesthesia is used at delivery. Recent work has shown that significant levels of meperidine are found in infants when delivered from one to two hours after administration of the drug to the mother.

A synthetic derivative of morphine, dihydromorphinone (Dilaudid) has 10 times the analgesic potency of morphine, and is effective in pain relief when large doses of morphine fail. The drug may be safely administered intravenously when restricted to a dose of no more than 0.3 mg. (gr. 1/200). As with morphine, however, this drug is best not given when delivery is imminent. The impression is gained that, as a postoperative or postpartum agent for pain relief, it surpasses morphine. Other synthetic analgesic agents are available, some less potent than morphine, such as alphaprodine (Nisentil), and others, such as methadone, that are several times as potent. Nisentil is commonly used in early labor, in 20 to 40 mg. dosage. Equi-analgesic dosage appears to range from 6 to 10 mg. for morphine, 50 to 100 mg. for meperidine, and 30 to 60 mg. for alphaprodine.

N-allyl-normorphine and levallorphan counteract the respiratory depressant action of morphine and morphine-like substances. They reach the fetus when administered intravenously to the mother a few minutes prior to delivery. The dosage of N-allyl-normorphine is 5 to 10 mg.; that of levallorphan, 1 to 2 mg. The venous (umbilical vein) administration of N-allyl-normorphine (0.5 to 2.0 mg.) or levallorphan (0.1 to 0.2 mg.) to the newborn will immediately improve respiration that has been depressed through the injudicious use of morphine and its derivatives.

Scopolamine, or hyoscine, is frequently used to supplement the action of the hypnotics and analgesics. Although the drug has some sedative action, its chief use in obstetric medication is to produce amnesia. In general, the patient who has received hypnotics or analgesics in the correct amounts with scopolamine will move about, indicating pain during a uterine contraction, but the memory of this in most cases is erased.

Scopolamine, like atropine, is a parasympatheticolytic drug, and therefore has the property of preventing or eliminating the vagal type of carotid sinus syndrome characterized by bradycardia and hypotension, with its associated low pulse pressure. The drug, when introduced into obstetrics, was used in conjunction with morphine, a combination designated "twilight sleep." Because of the depressant action of morphine on the fetus, this form of medication in labor has long been discarded.

The drug has no apparent ill effect on the fetus or upon uterine motility and is reputed to have a wider margin of safety than atropine. Reducing the secretions of the respiratory tract, the drug will also combat vagal stimulation and prevent laryngospasm and bronchospasm. Thus, scopolamine helps to counteract the vomiting, laryngospasm, and stridor occasionally seen in the second or expulsive stage of labor or during an operative pelvic delivery. It may be given intravenously with equal safety and will afford a therapeutic effect within 20 minutes after administration.

Scopolamine has the distinct disadvantage of causing restlessness and excitement in approximately 5 to 10 per cent of patients in labor. The pupils become dilated, and flushing and dryness of the skin are characteristic reactions. More recently, chlorpromazine and other tranquilizing drugs have been shown to reduce the incidence of hyperexcitability from scopolamine.

The recently introduced drugs noted for their tranquilizing effect have constituted a welcome addition in the programs of medication for pain relief in labor. The introduction of chlorpromazine has been followed by a long list of tranquilizers. These include promethazine (Phenergan), proma-

zine (Sparine) and other drugs such as diazepam (Valium). These agents have little or minimal effect on the fetus. These drugs have an additive effect on other obstetric analgesic agents and have reduced perceptibly the amount of such drugs necessary to control the discomfort of labor. For example, 50 mg. of meperidine (Demerol) together with 25 mg. of promethazine (Phenergan) is a popular combination.

Trichloroethylene, commercially available as Trilene, is used alone as an analgesic agent during labor and as a supplement to other forms of anesthesia. Because of rapid decomposition to dichloroacetylene and other highly noxious agents, particularly in the presence of an alkali, Trilene must never be used as an anesthetic with carbon dioxide absorption techniques. Also, the patient who has received Trilene for its analgesic effect during labor should not be given another form of inhalation anesthesia at delivery. Conceivably, the amount of Trilene absorbed and expired during the course of the anesthesia might be sufficient to lead to toxic manifestations from the resultant degradation products. When Trilene is used as an anesthetic, cardiac arrhythmias are not infrequent, and cardiac deaths have been reported. The drug has some of the virtues as well as the hazards of chloroform.

For self-administration, a special canister has been devised, with an appropriate facepiece, which the patient places over her face as she anticipates a contraction. Inhaling deeply several times, the patient absorbs sufficient Trilene to relieve pain in the course of the uterine contraction. The facepiece inevitably falls away should the patient reach a stage of beginning unconsciousness. The drug can be self-administered for long periods, apparently without any significant ill effects. However, this method abuses the principle that patient medication in hospital should always be administered by medical or nursing personnel; and the self-administration of a potent drug in hospital practice is difficult to condone. Hence, Trilene administration should be carried out by the anesthesia service or by the physician in charge. When analgesic drugs are contraindicated, or it is reasonably expected that they will not afford appreciable relief, patients may benefit greatly by the careful, intermittent administration of nitrous oxide analgesia as a 50-50 mixture of the gas and oxygen. With practice, the physician will readily be able to anticipate the patient's needs, and the desired objective is to relieve pain without loss of consciousness. Since the uterus begins to contract a few seconds before the patient is aware of pain, the administration of nitrous oxide analgesia should start at the beginning of each contraction, as determined by palpation of the uterus. As the pain subsides, the anesthetic mask is removed, to be replaced when the next contraction begins. This type of analgesia should always be administered by a physician who is familiar with the method and the possible complications. Breath-holding, nausea, and vomiting may be precipitated or associated with the second stage of labor.

Paracervical block anesthesia is used to afford pain relief in the first stage of labor. Besides relieving pain, this technique has been used to treat cervical dystocia with reported success. The cervix is said to dilate rapidly following paracervical block. The technique differs only in the area injected and the anesthetic solutions used. By using radiopaque material, it has been shown that the anesthetic agent, regardless of where it is deposited in the paracervical region, will diffuse anteriorly and posteriorly into the tissues surrounding the cervix.

With the patient in the lithotomy position, the vagina is prepared with an aqueous antiseptic solution. A 19 to 21 gauge needle, 18 to 20 cm. long, surrounded by a metal sheath except for the distal 2 cm., is used for the injection. To avoid the uterine vessels, some prefer that the point of entry be slightly above the insertion of the uterosacral ligaments and posterior to the descending branch of the uterine artery. The needle is never inserted beyond 2 cm. Preferably the injection is made when the cervix is 3 or 4 cm. dilated and the vertex is 0 to plus 2 station. The solution used is determined largely by personal preference, the choice depending somewhat on the length of action of the particular drug. Lidocaine, 1 to 2 per cent solution, is commonly used, 10 ml. being injected into each of the right and left parametrial areas. The duration of the anesthesia is 60 to 90 minutes; a Teflon catheter-in-situ can permit repeated injections (Fig. 20). Epinephrine added to the anesthetic solution to prolong its action is contraindicated, for it may disturb uterine motility to the point of cessation of labor, and possibly cause

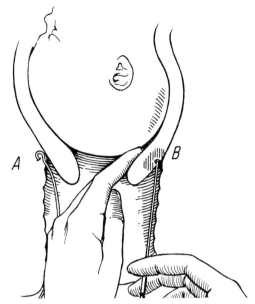

Figure 20. Techniques of paracervical anesthesia. A, Placement of a Teflon catheter in the region of the broad ligament for continuous paracervical anesthesia. B, Placement of the needle at the junction of the cervix and vagina for single-injection paracervical (intracervical) anesthesia. (From Flowers, C. E., Jr.: Obstetric Anesthesia and Analgesia. Paul B. Hoeber Div., Harper & Row, New York, 1967.)

vasoconstriction of uterine arteries and their branches, thereby decreasing uterine blood flow. It is perhaps on the basis of the latter that fetal brachycardia has been encountered. An additional complication is maternal vasomotor collapse, which is understandable in view of the fact that the anesthetic agent is injected into an area where the blood vessels are abundant and there could be rapid absorption of the anesthetic agent.

On the basis of recent work quantitating the transplacental passage of regional blocking agents used with paracervical block, as well as the fetal hypoxia, acidosis, and bradycardia that frequently is associated with the technique, certain precautions must be taken with the use of this method.

1. Direct injection into maternal circulation or fetal tissues must be avoided at all times.

2. The technique should not be used in cases in which the fetus may already be hypoxic and acidotic, as in maternal toxemia, diabetes, and postmaturity.

3. Prior fetal heart irregularity or the presence of meconium should contraindicate its use.

4. Constant fetal heart monitoring should

be mandatory in all cases in which the block is used.

In fact, a review of the recent investigations that have been done to quantitate the transplacental transmission of local anesthetic agents establishes the fact that the widely used regional blocking agents, such as procaine, lidocaine, tetracaine (Pontocaine), mepivacaine, and prilocaine, are rapidly absorbed into maternal circulation with all of the commonly used blocking techniques, and that this is followed by equally rapid passage of these drugs to the fetus.

It is now well known that these drugs may intoxicate the fetus in the event of overdosage, to produce apnea and vascular collapse from medullary depression, bradycardia because of the quinine-like effect on the myocardium, and convulsions due to cortical excitation. Like all forms of medication for pain relief, regional anesthetic technique and agents must be constantly under appraisal. In this regard, it should be mentioned that one fourth the initial dose is required for spinal anesthesia when compared with the initial dose for the epidural form.

Caudal analgesia and anesthesia as a form of extradural block in obstetrics has now come to mean a continuous or multiple injection technique, rather than a single dose as when it was first introduced into clinical medicine. It is administered with the patient in the lateral decubitus position, the lower limb extended, and the upper thigh flexed on the abdomen. The skin of the sacrococcygeal area is properly prepared with an appropriate antiseptic, and the patient is draped. The sacral hiatus is located beneath the upper margin of the intergluteal cleft, 2 to 3 inches above the tip of the coccyx. A skin wheal is raised, and a needle is introduced 1 to 2 inches into the epidural space (Fig. 21). This is easily done because, in almost every instance, the dural sac terminates considerably above the point of the needle, that is, superior to the second sacral spine. In some patients, however, anatomic differences make the sacral hiatus difficult to locate, and it is impossible to introduce the needle into the epidural space. Should spinal fluid be obtained, it is evident that the needle has pierced the dura mater and entered the subarachnoid space, so that administration of the total amount of drug necessary for an effective caudal anesthesia would produce a wide-

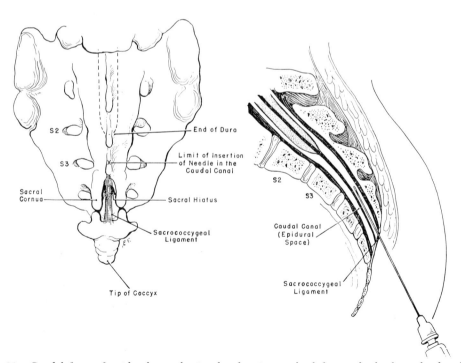

Figure 21. Caudal form of epidural anesthesia; the drawing at the left reveals the bony landmarks in the region of the sacral hiatus. (From Hershenson, B.: Obstetrical Anesthesia. Charles C Thomas, Springfield, Ill., 1955.)

spread, rapidly ascending spinal anesthesia with serious consequences. To avoid the hazard of the needle entering the subarachnoid space without the usual appearance of spinal fluid, a test dose of some 5 to 8 ml. of the anesthetic solution is first injected and the patient is observed for a brief period to rule out the possibility of a spinal anesthetic. The needle can then be replaced by a catheter, which is more adaptable to prolonged administration. Besides the risk of depositing the anesthetic agent within the subarachnoid space, there is possibility of contamination of the area where the needle or catheter is introduced, and the danger of introducing infection into the peridural space is real.

Pain is relieved soon after injection. Additional injections are made at determined intervals, depending on whether a long- or short-acting drug is used. A tilting downward of the patient's head (Trendelenburg position) will cause the anesthetic effect to move cephalad. It is anticipated that during labor and pelvic delivery anesthesia will result in the areas served by the coccygeal, hemorrhoidal, perineal, pudendal, ilioinguinal, and iliohypogastric nerves. For cesarean section the 11th and 12th thoracic or slightly higher, as well as the sacral nerves, must be blocked.

As in continuous lumbar epidural block, the anesthetic is started only when the patient is definitely committed to productive labor. It may be continued for several hours, to include delivery. The patient is at all times awake and comfortable, and, except for a tightening sensation of the abdomen created by the uterine contractions, is unaware of labor. As when lumbar epidural anesthesia is employed, the patient rarely experiences the desire, and, in fact, is unable, to utilize fully her abdominal muscles to push in the second stage of labor. The patient must be coached in this maneuver. As the nurse detects the uterine contraction, she should instruct the patient to take a deep breath, hold it, and push downward.

Epidural analgesia with a lumbar approach has at least two advantages over the caudal form. First, there is no problem of cleanliness, as in the sacral region. Second, because of the absence of variations of bony structure encountered in the sacral region, lumbar epidural block rarely fails.

The patient is placed in a lateral position as for spinal anesthesia, and a generous area of the back is prepared with tincture of Zephiran. The anesthetist infiltrates the skin and deeper tissues at the chosen site of the epidural tap, usually the L4 to L5 intervertebral space, with 0.8 to 1.2 per cent lidocaine (Xylocaine). He then introduces a No. 16 or No. 17 Tuohy needle through the skin and into or close to the interspinous ligament of the chosen interspace (Fig. 22). The stylet of the needle is then removed, and a drop of fluid is placed in the hub, or, alternatively, a small syringe containing fluid and a bubble of air is attached to the hub. The needle is then advanced in a very slow and carefully controlled fashion until the fluid in the hub of the needle is "sucked in" because of the negative pressure existing in the epidural space. A 5-ml. syringe filled with air is then attached to the needle, and the plunger is tapped; the air should enter the space freely and without resistance. The purposes of the last maneuver are two: first, it serves as an additional check that the needle is in the epidural space; second, it tends to expand the epidural space, which is only a potential space between the dura mater and vertebral periosteum.

A disposable catheter with a minute bore, with an obturator of No. 25 stainless steel wire, is then introduced through the needle, and the obturator is pulled back by an assistant so that its end is always visible to the operator. The catheter is first advanced slowly until it meets a definite resistance, indicating that it has reached the bevel of the needle. It is then advanced for a distance of 2 to 3 cm. with such firm pressure as may be required. *Under no circumstances should an attempt be made to withdraw the catheter without also withdrawing the needle,* lest the end of the catheter be cut off at the bevel and remain as a foreign body in the epidural space. When the catheter has been advanced the appropriate distance, it is stabilized with one hand while the needle is slowly withdrawn with the other hand. The catheter is thus kept in place while the needle is removed. The same method is applicable to continuous spinal anesthesia (see inset, Fig. 22).

The site of the catheter insertion is then supported by sponges and taped, the catheter is taped up the back to the shoulder, and a No. 24 needle is introduced into the distal end. A test dose of 3 to 5 ml. of 0.8 per cent lidocaine with 1:200,000 epinephrine is then given through the catheter.

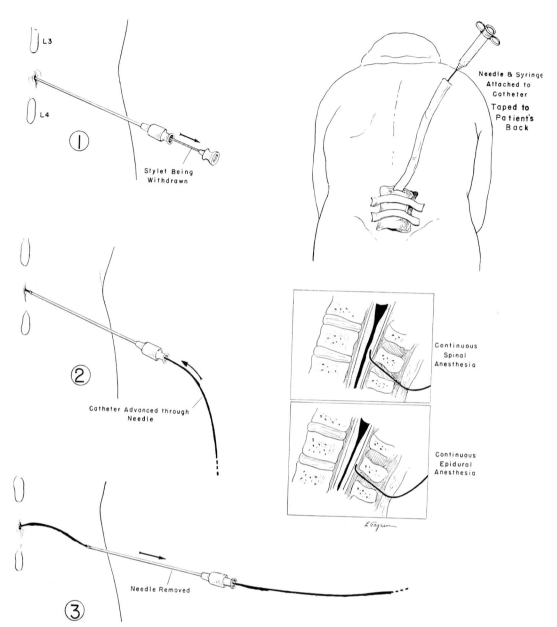

Figure 22. Continuous spinal block with catheter technique and the epidural approach. (From Hershenson, B.: Obstetrical Anesthesia. Charles C Thomas, Springfield, Ill., 1955.)

Some effect will usually be apparent to the patient five to eight minutes after the test dose. The anesthesia is then supplemented by repeated doses of the agent (with 5-ml. increments), as may be required in the judgment of the anesthetist; the position of the patient is altered from time to time to assure spread of the solution downward and equally to both sides of the body. Occasionally the 0.8 per cent concentration of lidocaine will prove insufficient. In such event 1.0 per cent or 1.2 per cent solution may be used.

The impression is held that, compared with spinal anesthesia, there is less likelihood of a drop in blood pressure with continuous epidural anesthesia, but this must be questioned when the level of anesthesia must rise to T12 to T11 or above. It eliminates the hazard of arachnoiditis and chemical meningitis. Also, in a patient so anesthetized, if fetal distress or some other complication arises in the course of labor, no further anesthesia is required for delivery even if cesarean section is indicated.

In summary, besides its near-routine use

in labor, extradural analgesia and anesthesia is particularly advantageous in patients with metabolic disease, such as diabetes mellitus, those with lung and heart disease, some patients with pregnancy toxemia, and those in whom a test of labor is anticipated, or if there is special concern for the fetus for any reason.

Hypnosis has been explored as a method of control of pain during labor and delivery, and the literature contains many and some rather complete articles on the subject. It is stressed that no physician should use hypnosis for purposes that are beyond the range of his competence. Further, the technique should not be used as a routine procedure but only on a selective basis, for harmful results have been noted with the appearance of psychotic reactions following this form of therapy.

There is little doubt that patients, perhaps 25 per cent or more, depending on those selected and the ability of the therapist, may be managed through labor and delivery under hypnosis with apparently little or no discomfort, sometimes with pudendal block at the time of delivery. The failure rate can be substantial, however, with patients requiring medication for pain relief. The biochemical status of the infant at birth is comparable to that noted in infants delivered under conduction anesthesia.

PAIN RELIEF AT DELIVERY

Inhalation and Intravenous Methods

Chloroform is more of historical interest and, although rarely used today, has certain advantages as an obstetric anesthetic. It is a nonexplosive agent, and anesthesia is quickly induced. It is also nonirritating and easy to inhale, which simplifies its administration to the patient who has received little premedication. Being nonirritating, it causes little respiratory secretion, and has therefore been the anesthetic of choice in some patients with mild respiratory infection. Overdosage is a hazard, toxic concentrations of the drug being readily reached, as manifested by cardiac irregularities. Because of its potency and hepatotoxicity, chloroform should never be used except on strict indication and by an anesthesiologist.

Being nonexplosive, unless combined with other gases that are explosive, nitrous oxide when used properly has a wide field of usefulness in obstetrics.

Because its action is comparatively weak, when used as an anesthetic nitrous oxide must be supplemented by other agents. Nitrous oxide concentration above 70 per cent is capable of causing both maternal and fetal hypoxia; concentrations in the 90 per cent range are decidedly dangerous.

Ether continues to be a useful anesthetic to assist in the management of many of the more serious obstetric complications; it is probably the safest for the cardiac patient. Ether crosses the placenta readily, however, and, if it is not used solely as a supplement and if the delivery demands a deep anesthetic over a period of time, it may easily be detected on the infant's breath for some hours after delivery. Used in conjunction with other anesthetics, ether effects good muscle relaxation. In the average forceps delivery, it can be used as an adjunct with nitrous oxide during the period of induction and while the forceps are being applied. At this point, the patient is controlled sufficiently that in the next 10 to 15 minutes, during extraction of the fetus, the ether can be discontinued and the mother permitted to breathe 100 per cent oxygen. With proper timing, which is easily attained when the anesthesiologist and the obstetrician are working together as a team, the patient experiences pain relief and the fetus is free of the anesthetic agent and breathes spontaneously at birth. After the cord is clamped, nitrous oxide – ether may be resumed and the third stage of labor completed, including episiotomy repair. This technique applies to other inhalation anesthetics as well, and with experience the anesthesiologist can anticipate the obstetric needs for the proper conduct of delivery, at the same time preventing the absorption of any quantity of anesthetic agent by the fetus.

Ethylene possesses more potent anesthetic qualities than nitrous oxide, for analgesia is accomplished with mixtures of less than 50 per cent ethylene and oxygen, and surgical anesthesia is obtained with a concentration of about 80 per cent.

The danger of explosion with this anesthetic must not be minimized. In surgery, where all of the necessary safeguards can be enforced, this hazard is almost nil; in obstetrics, however, the precautions are more difficult to maintain. Imminent delivery creates a sense of urgency. Moving the patient into the case room and transferring her to the delivery table in the presence of anesthetic agents with explosive potential is not consistent with absolute safety.

Cyclopropane is an extremely potent agent, capable of producing analgesia in 3 to 4 per cent concentration. Anesthesia is maintained with a mixture of 10 to 20 per cent cyclopropane with oxygen, which is nonirritating and easy for the patient to inhale. Further, induction is rapid. The greatest usefulness of cyclopropane in obstetrics is in the patient with active antepartum bleeding in an amount that shock is a distinct threat and definitive obstetric treatment is urgent.

Because of its use with a high oxygen concentration, cyclopropane anesthesia would appear to be ideal for obstetric use, but, despite this, it has certain definite drawbacks. It has a high degree of toxicity, and cardiac irregularities are more likely to occur with it than with other agents. It also carries a high explosion hazard. Despite the high oxygen concentration of the anesthetic mixture, the oxygen content of the fetal blood fails to reflect this supposed advantage. One may notice at cesarean section that the uterus is in a state of contraction and is rather blanched in appearance. This would suggest that the rate of intervillous blood flow might actually be reduced, with the fetus failing to receive its full quota of oxygen.

Halothane (Fluothane) is a potent, nonexplosive, halogenated hydrocarbon that has become very popular in surgical anesthesia since its introduction. Besides its noninflammability and nonexplosiveness, its advantages include rapid induction, ease in variation of depth of narcosis, quick recovery with minimal nausea and vomiting, and minimal stimulation of salivary secretions. Moreover, halothane is said not to influence the vasomotor system, in that it does not prompt the usual sympathoadrenal responses produced by other anesthetic agents.

It has been shown, however, that halothane results in a reduction of the cardiac output and stroke volume, due primarily to myocardial depression. It has been observed that unless halothane is administered in low concentrations that are rigidly controlled, an unusually high incidence of uterine flaccidity with concomitant serious uterine bleeding can result. It is evident the advantage of this agent is dependent on its skilled administration.

Pentothal sodium has been used as an anesthetic at the time of delivery. This agent passes readily across the placenta and reaches a maximum concentration in the fetal blood within five minutes after injection. It may readily cause respiratory depression in the infant. The slow rate of detoxification of Pentothal sodium is an added hazard. Even in small amounts, the drug can cause laryngospasm, which a preliminary dose of scopolamine or atropine will tend to diminish.

Pentothal sodium can be used to abolish the momentary pain that accompanies spontaneous birth. The perineal area should be aseptically prepared and the patient draped before the anesthetic is administered. After the infant is delivered and the cord is clamped and cut, the patient can then be taken through the remainder of her delivery and perineal repair with additional amounts of the drug.

When muscle relaxation is the objective, the amount of Pentothal required is capable of producing maternal respiratory and circulatory depression. In doses of 100 to 200 mg., Pentothal sodium has proved useful to facilitate induction of inhalation anesthesia, but as an anesthetic alone for prolonged forceps operation or cesarean section it is contraindicated.

Drugs causing muscle relaxation have their place in obstetrics in the hands of the trained anesthesiologist. Succinyl choline appears to be the drug of choice, with a lesser if any fetal effect. In the case of inhalation anesthesia, Pentothal sodium (100 to 200 mg.) and 30 to 60 mg. of succinyl choline will facilitate endotracheal intubation and inflation of the cuff. This so-called balanced form of anesthesia has its advocates and the patient may thus be carried on nitrous oxide and oxygen.

Regional Anesthesia

Local block anesthesia for cesarean section has become less of a necessity than in former years with the general progress in the field of anesthesia. However, this form of anesthesia does have a place in cases in which there is great concern about the welfare of the fetus. At the same time, local block anesthesia requires a courageous mother and a surgeon who will take ample time to inject the tissues and has the temperament to wait for the anesthetic agent to take full effect.

The success of this type of anesthesia depends on complete cooperation between the patient and the surgeon. This is best gained through the patient having a clear understanding of the procedure and the steps to be taken in the technique of local block. Through detailed explanation, the patient should appreciate the fact that she will experience a sense of pressure and some degree of dull discomfort. She should be told that when the fetus is extracted as gently as possible from the uterus the re-

sultant tension on the uterosacral ligaments may cause extreme backache. If the patient is aware of this and is prepared for this momentary experience, it should be bearable. Except for preoperative atropine, no other medication should be given when local block is to be used for abdominal delivery, at least until the baby is born. Barbiturates or other sedatives may cause the patient to be confused and prevent her cooperation, which is so essential to the success of this type of anesthesia.

The block can be attained by injecting the anesthetic solution some 2 or more

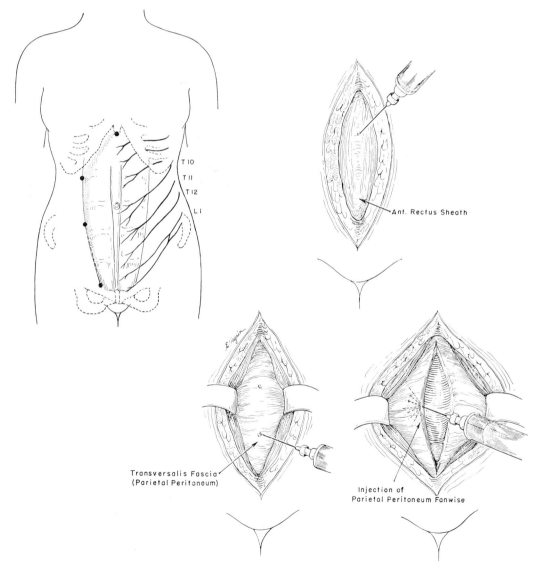

Figure 23. Areas of abdominal field block for abdominal hysterotomy. (From Hershenson, B.: Obstetrical Anesthesia. Charles C Thomas, Springfield, Ill., 1955.)

inches away from the midline of the abdomen. The skin is first injected, and then a second injection deposits the anesthetic solution beneath the anterior rectus sheath (Fig. 23).

If the area is to be effectively anesthetized, the upper and the lower angles of the field, in approximation to the umbilicus and the symphysis pubis, should be carefully injected. At least five minutes should elapse after the second injection to permit the anesthetic agent to act fully before the skin is incised. As the peritoneum is approached, a third injection may be necessary to prevent pain. Once the abdomen is open, gentle retraction is permitted. Because of discomfort, gauze packs cannot be used. Spillage of amniotic fluid and blood into the peritoneal cavity may be minimized, however, by having an assistant place his hands parallel along the abdominal incision and pressing the anterior abdominal wall against the unopened uterus. A suture placed deep in the myometrium near the upper angle of the abdominal incision will permit upward traction and help to keep the uterus in apposition to the abdominal wall. Incision of the uterus is painless, but, as stated previously, extraction of the fetus can cause considerable discomfort. In most cases it should be possible to conduct the operation totally without supplementary anesthesia. Unless there is some maternal contraindication, however, once the fetus is removed, Pentothal sodium (200 mg.), together with nitrous oxide or some other appropriate inhalation anesthesia, may be given for the remainder of the procedure.

Pudendal block anesthesia for pelvic deliveries is used in many clinics. Although the technique is not difficult, it may fail to afford adequate pain relief, and this is true particularly when the vertex must be rotated or any amount of traction is required to extract the fetus.

The anesthetic solution, to which epinephrine is added to prolong duration of the anesthesia, is deposited in the region of the ischial spines where lies the pudendal nerve, as well as medial to the ischial tuberosities as the nerve emerges from Alcock's canal to distribute itself over the perineum (Fig. 24). The patient should be prepared in the same general way as for any other anesthetic. Blood pressure, pulse, and respirations should be recorded. The patient should have received some barbiturate medication to prevent or counteract the stimulating effects of the regional anesthetic agent on the central nervous system, and atropine to dry the secretions

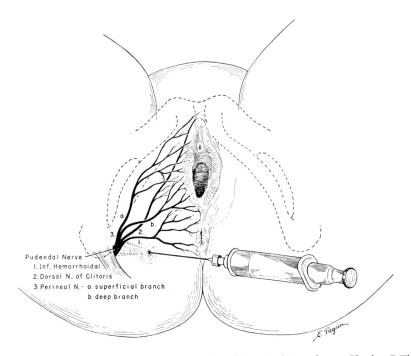

Pudendal Nerve
1. Inf. Hemorrhoidal
2. Dorsal N. of Clitoris
3. Perineal N. - a. superficial branch
                b. deep branch

Figure 24. Pudendal nerve block. (From Hershenson, B.: Obstetrical Anesthesia. Charles C Thomas, Springfield, Ill., 1955.)

of the respiratory tract in the event that general anesthesia is needed.

The patient is prepared and draped, and after the skin wheal is raised a No. 20 spinal needle is then introduced and guided, by the fingers placed in the vagina, until its tip comes to lodge 1 cm. posterior and inferior to the ischial spine. The needle traverses the ischiorectal space well lateral to the rectal wall. Some 5 to 10 ml. of 1 per cent lidocaine, to which is added 1:200,000 epinephrine solution, is deposited in this region. As the needle is withdrawn, it is redirected toward and just medial to the ischial tuberosity and additional solution is injected here. It is a common practice also to infiltrate the skin and underlying muscle ½ to 1 inch away from the projected episiotomy incision. Some also inject the ilioinguinal and iliohypogastric nerves in the region of the symphysis, hoping to block the nerve fibers that supply the anterior third of the vagina, thereby eliminating the pain aroused by pressure of the presenting part on the anterior vagina and contained structures. The total maximal safe dose of lidocaine is about 4 mg. per pound of body weight, or about 40 to 50 ml. of 1 per cent solution in the average-sized woman.

Spinal anesthesia or subarachnoid block for pelvic delivery is in the form of a so-called saddle block or a low spinal. A saddle block confines its anesthetic effect to the sacral nerves and possibly L5. In practice, however, the block is frequently not so restricted, including L4, 3, 2, and possibly 1, and, in essence, is a low spinal. The term saddle block is more acceptable to patients than "low spinal," for some patients have certain reservations about spinal anesthesia in any form and, in fact, definitely request that it not be employed unless there are substantial indications, particularly fetal, for its use.

For a low spinal sufficient for pelvic delivery the patient is placed on her side and a generous area of skin is prepared with tincture of Zephiran. The L3 to L4 or L4 to L5 intervertebral space is chosen for lumbar puncture (Fig. 25). A skin wheal is raised by injection of the local anesthetic, both for comfort and for possible identification of allergy to the agent used. A reddened wheal or itching should arouse suspicion of sensitivity to the drug. A 1 to 1½-inch No. 20 needle is used as an introducer, and a No. 26 spinal needle is passed through it for the actual tap; clear fluid must be seen before the anesthetic solution is introduced. This small-bore needle virtually eliminates postspinal headaches. If it is not immediately apparent, the needle is aspirated with an empty 2-ml. syringe to demonstrate clear spinal fluid. The solution is injected slowly with the bevel of

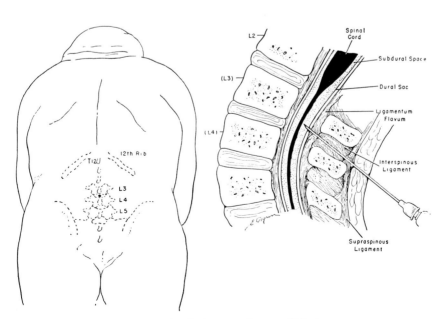

Figure 25. Technique of a spinal block.

the needle directed downward. Following injection, the patient is immediately placed in lithotomy position, and the head and shoulders are raised on a double pillow. The drugs and doses of spinal anesthetic agents vary for pelvic delivery, but 1 per cent tetracaine (Pontocaine) 0.3 to 0.5 ml., in 10 per cent dextrose solution, 0.5 to 0.8 ml., or 5 per cent Xylocaine in 7.5 per cent dextrose solution, 0.8 to 1 ml., is commonly used. The level of anesthesia sought is between the 11th or 12th and 7th thoracic dermatome.

The technique of spinal anesthesia for abdominal hysterotomy varies to the extent that (1) the dose of Pontocaine is increased in a dose range of 6 to 8 mg. in 10 per cent dextrose. Lidocaine (Xylocaine) and mepivacaine (Carbocaine) may be used in a dose range of 50 to 75 mg. in 7.5 per cent dextrose made up to a 5 per cent solution; (2) prophylactic administration of a pressor drug and local infiltration with procaine at the lumbar puncture site are used; and (3) following injection the patient is placed in slight Trendelenburg rather than lithotomy position. Anesthesia should ascend to the 6th or 7th thoracic dermatome.

Any blood pressure fall is not necessarily due to a sudden or unpredictable rise in the level of spinal anesthesia but, rather, to obstruction of the venous return from the lower extremities and pelvic viscera by the gravid uterus, with a pooling of blood in the occluded area at the expense of the general circulation. The hypotension can usually be partially corrected by raising the patient's legs and turning her on one side. As indicated, the prophylactic use of vasopressor drugs and lactated Ringer's solution may avoid a hypotensive episode.

The intravenous use of oxytocin in small doses with spinal anesthesia is a safe procedure; but intravenous injection of ergonovine or methylergonovine may cause a startling and dangerous rise in blood pressure, frequently accompanied by severe headache and other central nervous system symptoms.

The summation of current experience of authorities in the field of obstetric anesthesia tends to support the view that fetal mortality and morbidity are less when conduction anesthesia is used. Account must be taken, however, of the obstetric circumstances surrounding the cases analyzed. If the patients are individualized and no one form of anesthesia is used routinely, it may be found that the less complicated cases are delivered under spinal anesthesia, and the more complicated cases, under inhalation type. An example is the patient with serious bleeding from a placenta praevia or abruptio placentae. The fetal mortality and morbidity may be higher in cesarean section under cyclopropane anesthesia than under spinal anesthesia, but the former is used because of the urgency of the situation and the adverse effects of unpredictable blood loss. Such variables deserve careful assessment in reviewing anesthetic results, both maternal and fetal.

DEATHS AND MATERNAL COMPLICATIONS FROM OBSTETRIC ANESTHESIA

With the overall decrease in maternal mortality in recent times, the percentage of maternal deaths from anesthesia may have increased. Actually, there are today fewer deaths from this cause, but these deaths must nevertheless be considered preventable.

It might be reasonable to estimate that obstetric anesthesia is responsible for some 5 per cent of maternal deaths. However, it is difficult to determine with accuracy the number of maternal deaths and complications that occur with the various forms of obstetric analgesia and anesthesia. Unless there is autopsy proof, unexpected death during delivery is too often assigned to causes other than the anesthetic. This applies especially to conduction forms of anesthesia when death usually occurs suddenly and without signs of impending disaster, in contrast to death from inhalation anesthesia when the provoking factors are readily evident.

Factors that contribute to anesthesia deaths include failure to employ all means to avoid allergic or toxic drug reactions; the selection of improper anesthesia for the particular case; dereliction in correcting an existing anemia; misunderstanding of drug action; poor technique in administration of the anesthetic; human error with excessive amounts of anesthetic agent being given; and delay in instituting supportive therapy, for example, failure to transfuse immediately when appreciable blood loss has been experienced.

Deaths from spinal anesthesia are more specifically the result of overdosage causing either vasomotor collapse or respiratory paralysis. The effects and implications of various levels of spinal anesthesia are shown in Figure 26.

Sequelae of spinal anesthesia in obstetrics are not easily acceptable, if for no other reason than that the patients are young and the situation might have been met by the use of some other form of anesthesia. With the advances in this form of anesthesia and with skilled technique, neurologic sequelae occur in less than 1 in 10,000 patients. In the writer's institution no serious neurologic complication has occurred in over 60,000 patients who had spinal anesthesia in a 12-year period. However, it must be kept in mind that complications from inhalation anesthesia are a hospital affair, whereas the delayed effects of spinal anesthesia are sometimes not recognized until after hospital discharge and hence never appear in the overall statistical results.

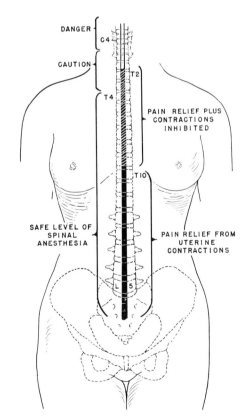

Figure 26. Various levels of spinal anesthesia as they pertain to pain relief and the patient's safety. (From Hershenson, B.: Obstetrical Anesthesia. Charles C Thomas, Springfield, Ill., 1955.)

Albeit extremely rare, cauda equina paralysis is a devastating consequence in which recovery is slow and tedious and not always complete. It becomes immediately obvious, with failure to recover function. A more serious complication is a progressive arachnoiditis, wherein the cord is compressed and finally destroyed.

The incidence of postspinal headache, which is assumed to be due to a leakage of spinal fluid through the hole in the dura mater caused by the needle, has been reduced to a minimum (now less than 1 per cent) by employing the smallest spinal needle possible. Despite this, these headaches seem to occur with a greater frequency in the obstetric than in the surgical patient. This may be due to failure to adhere to the rule of introducing the spinal needle and the anesthetic agent only between contractions when the patient is quiet and not straining. Characteristically, the headaches appear on the second postpartum day, or shortly thereafter. The patient is relatively comfortable when recumbent, but the headache develops immediately when the patient is in the upright position. The pain can be severe and disabling, and the headache may last for several weeks. No treatment has been altogether successful.

Deaths from inhalation anesthesia may follow aspiration due to cardiac arrest or pulmonary complications. Aspiration of the stomach content is especially threatening to obstetric patients, for they are often unprepared to accept an inhalation anesthesia as when, without previous warning, the onset of labor follows a recent meal. Despite the fact that it is difficult to demonstrate a delay in the emptying time, brownish, highly acid material tends to collect in the stomach in the course of labor, particularly when labor is prolonged. The material is extremely irritating to the respiratory tract, setting in motion a rapidly spreading chemical pneumonitis referred to as Mendelson's syndrome (Fig. 27). Aspiration can occur during labor as well as during induction of anesthesia for delivery. It is most likely to be precipitated during second stage labor through the sacrocerebral parasympathetic reflex, initiated by pressure of the presenting part on the perineum. Whenever difficulty of induction is encountered in inhalation anesthesia, it is wise to stop the anesthesia and evaluate the situation, and perhaps change to a conduction type.

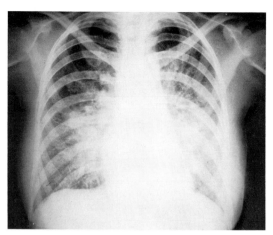

Figure 27. A diffuse chemical pneumonitis, as shown by x-ray 6 hours after aspiration at the time of emergence from anesthesia; bronchoscopy considered at 12 hours post partum and rejected. The patient died, 36 hours after delivery, of respiratory failure. Autopsy confirmed the diagnosis of a diffuse chemical pneumonitis.

When aspiration is obvious, increased pulse rate, cyanosis, and respiratory embarrassment appear simultaneously. Tracheal aspiration should be instituted promptly. "Silent" or unsuspected aspiration of the irritating stomach content can occur, in which event the first and most important sign is elevation of the pulse rate to 100 or more beats per minute; the increased respiratory rate and cyanosis may appear later. In fact, a pulse rate of 110 to 120 beats per minute in an uneventful delivery without blood loss should arouse suspicion of an aspiration. The clinician should realize that tachycardia may precede the onset of respiratory symptoms by an hour or more. A chest x-ray should be considered. Delay in diagnosis is to be avoided at all cost.

The writer holds the conviction that, although tracheal suction may suffice, if there is any question as to its effectiveness, bronchoscopy should be performed immediately. In the hands of the expert, this procedure adds little to the risk of this potentially serious situation and may be lifesaving. It permits the removal of gastric secretions from the main bronchi, the deposition of an antacid solution to counteract the irritating effect of this material, and the placement of antibiotics into the involved areas.

It is appreciated that many anesthesiologists may oppose this opinion, believing that in location of the tissue effects of aspiration, bronchoscopy is of little or no value. In fact, these procedures may be considered harmful, and be thought to aggravate the existing chemical trauma. This liquid stomach content seems particularly noxious in the obstetric patient, however, and personal observation would indicate that bronchoscopy, performed at the earliest moment, is of great help in arresting the spread, and consequently the extent and duration, of the process (Fig. 28).

Regardless of controversy, the following measures should nevertheless be undertaken. Laryngoscopy, orotracheal intubation, and tracheal suction should be tried to remove any accessible material. Three or four intratracheal instillations of 5 or 10 ml. of physiologic saline solution containing 1 per cent sodium bicarbonate will tend to dilute or neutralize any acidified material it may reach. Humidified oxygen is admin-

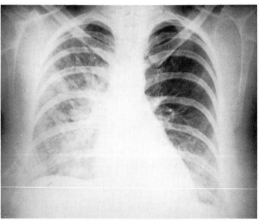
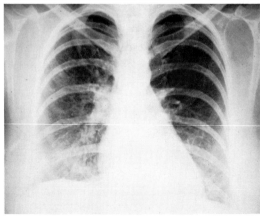

Figure 28. Aspiration with chemical pneumonitis. Immediate x-ray and bronchoscopy, with recovery in 48 hours.

istered by catheter or mask. Antibiotic therapy is also instituted, for some degree of bronchopneumonia is inevitable. The patient should be encouraged to cough and change position frequently. The prognosis in these patients may remain uncertain for days, but complete recovery is the rule.

Cardiac arrest during any form of anesthesia has an element of preventability. Important measures include the correction of anemia prior to administration of the anesthesia, the maintenance of fluid balance in labor, and the avoidance of trauma and blood loss. Further, in the case of inhalation anesthesia in cesarean section, one must not employ extreme Trendelenburg position with its resultant decrease in tidal exchange and respiratory volume, which is contributed to by the large uterus and the marked elevation of the diaphragm, which in this position has a limited excursion.

The disappearance of blood pressure and of palpable pulsations of peripheral and carotid pulses, or of palpable aortic pulse if the abdomen is open, establishes beyond doubt the diagnosis of cardiac arrest. Dilatation of the pupils and blanching or cyanosis of the skin are late signs; gross movement of somatic muscles and gastrointestinal peristalsis may occur for a moment or two after arrest or fibrillation has occurred.

When the condition is suspected, surgery or delivery must stop at once, and the efforts of the entire team must be directed toward establishing the diagnosis unequivocally and undertaking immediate resuscitative measures. One or two ampules of epinephrine should be added to the intravenous glucose solution and the rate of infusion should be increased. External cardiac massage should be started promptly. With the patient in a supine position, the operator places the heel of one hand over the lower sternum, with the second hand over the first, and exerts his weight over the area. The pressure is maintained for 30 seconds, alternating with release, with the sternum showing an excursion of 3 to 5 cm. Mouth-to-mouth ventilation is applied until the anesthesiologist is able to apply assisted breathing with the insertion of an endotracheal tube. Trendelenburg position is instituted to avoid aspiration and to improve cerebral blood flow.

It has been cautioned that minimal force be used in external massage to avoid rib fractures and soft tissue injury. The effectiveness of therapy is gauged by the volume of the femoral pulse and the status of the pupils. In obstetric patients, who are usually free of underlying disease, this method should prove comparatively successful in maintaining circulation and, it is hoped, recovery. At least it may maintain the circulation until electrodes can be applied either externally or directly to the heart. The electrodes when applied externally are placed at the apex and over the sternal notch.

If the abdomen has been opened, the surgeon should palpate and massage the heart through the diaphragm. When the diagnosis is cardiac standstill, he should inject 0.2 mg. of epinephrine, diluted to 4 to 5 ml., directly into the left ventricle. If these measures do not produce a palpable peripheral pulse in the following 30 to 60 seconds, thoracotomy should be done without delay, even without sterile precautions. Asepsis, of course, is preferable, but the delay in skin preparation could cost the patient's life.

In patients who are in the Trendelenburg position, particularly pregnant patients, one must be aware that the heart is displaced upward and laterally because of the elevation of the diaphragm by the enlarged uterus. If the standard approach for cardiac thoracotomy through the fourth or fifth intercostal space in the midclavicular line is used, there is danger of incising the heart. The safest area for the incision in these circumstances is through the third or fourth intercostal space, near the midaxillary line.

If the heart is flaccid, and massage does not improve myocardial tone within 30 seconds, injection into the left ventricle of 0.2 to 0.3 mg. of epinephrine (diluted to 5 ml. with saline) is suggested. This will usually improve the myocardial tone and make the surgeon's compression of the heart effective, whether the situation is arrest or asystole. When epinephrine is not effective and the myocardium remains flaccid, several doses of calcium chloride, 100 to 300 mg., may be given intracardially at 5- to 10-minute intervals. Sodium bicarbonate solution should be started to combat the mounting acidosis.

Once effective massage is maintained for one minute, the exact cardiac status should be determined by direct observation. If the operator does not feel that he is accomplishing effective massage through the intact pericardium, he should incise it without delay or hesitation. The establishment of effective massage, with use of epinephrine, calcium, and pericardiotomy in that sequence, if necessary, is the first requisite of adequate treatment.

If a diagnosis of ventricular fibrillation is now established, defibrillation should be undertaken by electrical countershock, using the defibrillator, regardless of whether or not massage has been considered effective at the end of the third minute. After application of repetitive countershock for 10 to 15 seconds, massage must be resumed. The intracardial injection of 200 to 500 mg. of procaine or of potassium chloride following another brief period of massage may contribute to the success of the subsequent attempts at electrical defibrillation.

If myocardial tone can be maintained while ventilation is adequate, and there is improvement in peripheral color or tone, there is hope of recovery. The mechanical stimuli applied by massage, injections, and so forth may result in the prompt resumption of a spontaneous and effective heart beat. If a spontaneous beat does not return under these circumstances, the defibrillator (440 volts for 0.25 seconds), or the pacemaker, with application of the "hot" electrode near the area of the sinoatrial node, is used.

Initial dependence on the use of the external electrodes for defibrillation and pacemaking may result in lapse of too much time, so that the battle is lost before definitive therapy (thoracotomy and massage) has been instituted. It is worth reiterating that there is no time for discussion or temporization once the question of cardiac arrest has been raised. Diagnosis and treatment should take immediate precedence over all other activities.

PROGRAMS OF PAIN RELIEF

It is the responsibility of the physician in charge to be sufficiently familiar with the patient's history, and to inform the anesthesiologist of any condition that may reasonably influence the choice of analgesia and anesthesia, regardless of his own or the patient's preference.

Uncomplicated Labor, with Vaginal Delivery Expected

With the onset of regular contractions producing changes in the cervix, that is, either effacement or dilatation, or both, secobarbital (Seconal), 200 mg., or Vistaril, 100 mg., may be administered. Some 20 to 40 minutes later, with continuing labor causing pain and discomfort, promazine (Sparine), 25 mg., is administered intramuscularly. At two-hour, or longer, intervals thereafter, promazine, 25 mg., may be given intramuscularly, depending on the patient's progress and need for medication, as evaluated by the physician.

As an alternative to promazine in this circumstance, meperidine, 50 mg., may be given intramuscularly. Narcotics are avoided if delivery is imminent, regardless of circumstances. Intermittent nitrous oxide is preferred to alleviate discomfort in the last hour or minutes of the second stage.

The writer's preference is to administer Nisentil, 20 to 30 mg., every one to two hours of early labor. Usually within three to four hours or when the cervix is 3 to 4 cm. dilated and labor is well established with the patient becoming uncomfortable and restless, a lumbar epidural form of conduction anesthesia is administered with the expectation that the second stage will be attained within three or four hours. The patient can be delivered under this form of pain relief, usually by outlet forceps, and the episiotomy readily repaired. The patient is totally comfortable and awake at delivery; the infant breathes and cries immediately, and altogether the patient, the baby, and the physician find it a highly satisfactory method of management.

Modification of Medication Schedule According to Maternal and Fetal Complications

MEDICAL COMPLICATIONS. Patients with active asthma or a history of the condition should not receive barbiturates, for an acute attack may follow their administration. Initial medication with 50 to 100 mg. of meperidine or Nisentil, 30 mg., is permissible, followed by lumbar epidural analgesia. If the patient has a complicated history of allergies, conduction anesthetic techniques are perhaps preferable for delivery, although nitrous oxide — oxygen — ether anesthesia is not contraindicated.

In pulmonary complications (such as pneumonia, bronchiectasis, tuberculosis, emphysema, or a history of thoracic surgery), when the pulmonary function is not seriously impaired, the patient is dealt with as an uncomplicated case. If pulmonary function is moderately impaired, medication should be held to a reasonable minimum. When pulmonary function is severely impaired, continuous lumbar epidural analgesia is used for pain relief in labor, and suffices also for delivery.

The cardiac patient is medicated moderately during labor, and certain other reservations are imposed. Early in labor she may be given 100 mg. of meperidine initially, followed by 50 mg. doses at two- to four-hour intervals as required. As the time of delivery approaches, promazine in 25 mg. doses may be used instead of meperidine to avoid the risk of fetal depression. Atropine sulfate, 0.4 mg., is given intramuscularly about 30 minutes before delivery. The anesthesia can be spinal, or nitrous oxide and oxygen with local or pudendal block. Skillfully administered, ether–oxygen is a time-honored form of anesthesia for cardiac patients.

In renal disease, when renal function is only mildly to moderately impaired, the medication for pain relief in labor is decreased to one half to three fourths of the normal dose. When there is advanced renal impairment, medication is reduced drastically (one fourth to one half the usual dose). If such medication proves inadequate, continuous lumbar epidural anesthesia may be instituted.

In patients with central nervous system complications, including poliomyelitis, meningitis, tumors, multiple sclerosis, central nervous system trauma or vertebral surgery, the medication is individualized, but in general it follows the pattern for uncomplicated cases. Spinal and epidural anesthesia are contraindicated; thus, general anesthesia is used, but pudendal block may be acceptable when general anesthesia appears to be a risk.

Whether the patient with epilepsy or a history of convulsions is or is not on anticonvulsant therapy does not influence the situation greatly except that, if she has been on medication, this should be continued during labor and her hospital stay.

It should be recognized that the tolerance of both mother and baby to sedatives is likely to be high if the mother has been on anticonvulsants. The doses of barbiturates may be increased with discretion according to apparent requirements, but the patient must be carefully watched. Narcotics are contraindicated in epileptics. A single dose of atropine is given about 30 minutes before delivery, and the method of choice is inhalation anesthesia.

Of the metabolic disturbances, the most common in most pregnancy clinics is diabetes mellitus. Because it is associated with a high incidence of fetal difficulties of all types, the policy is to withhold medication to the greatest extent possible. Meperidine, 50 to 75 mg., may be given at three-hour intervals during early labor, but not within four hours of expected delivery. When the cervix begins to dilate (3 cm. or more) and labor is progressing well, continuous lumbar epidural analgesia is highly satisfactory.

OBSTETRIC COMPLICATIONS. The patients who deserve special attention are those whose examination necessitates a "double set-up" preparation to establish the diagnosis and permit the appropriate method of delivery because of antepartum bleeding, premature labor, fetal distress from any cause, difficult forceps delivery, breech extraction, test of labor, and pregnancy toxemia.

In patients who enter the hospital with moderate to severe bleeding requiring immediate treatment, cyclopropane, with tracheal intubation, is chosen because of its rapid action, spinal anesthesia being contraindicated in patients who may be in or on the verge of shock. There is no contraindication to conduction anesthesia for patients who are stabilized and not bleeding actively.

It is accepted that the premature fetus tolerates medication less well than does a term fetus. In such cases medication is held to a minimum. One or two doses of secobarbital, 100 mg., may be given early in labor (not within three hours of expected delivery). As the time of delivery approaches, other methods of analgesia may be sought. Continuous lumbar epidural anesthesia is ideal. In vertex presentations forceps delivery is favored; the "splinting" effect of forceps will reduce the chance of intracranial damage in the immature infant.

In all cases of prematurity, some form of

conduction anesthesia, barring any contra-indication, should be selected for delivery. Spinal anesthesia is preferable to local or pudendal block, because it immediately affords better relaxation of the maternal soft tissues, thus diminishing the risk of fetal trauma.

In the presence of developing fetal distress, further medication is withheld and, as soon as obstetric conditions permit, delivery is accomplished under conduction anesthesia. However, when circumstances require intrauterine manipulation, general anesthesia with rapid induction and tracheal intubation must be considered. This may be superimposed on lumbar epidural analgesia to obtain uterine relaxation. This likewise applies to difficult forceps and breech extraction.

In test-of-labor cases, the patient is medicated conservatively. Continuous lumbar epidural anesthesia may be added to the régime, and is especially useful when oxytocin infusion is being given, for it permits the patient to be completely comfortable while remaining awake, quiet, and cooperative.

In the toxemias of pregnancy, medication during labor should be minimal since the threat of liver damage and of oliguria is always present. Furthermore, in the therapy of the disease the patient is often under some degree of sedation before the onset of labor. In fact, the prescribed treatment of the disease will usually provide adequate sedation. The epidural method is not contraindicated, but if pelvic delivery can be accomplished under pudendal block, especially in severe toxemia, this is also a desirable method. The choice must be individualized, however, and either general or spinal anesthesia is not entirely excluded.

SUMMARY

An attempt has been made to present the medical issues concerned with medication for pain relief in labor. A brief résumé is given of the more pertinent features of the drugs and methods used, with emphasis on the dangers as well as on the value of each. If any drug or method has been omitted, it is done so deliberately, primarily because it is of questionable worth, at least in obstetric practice. Not that they occur, except rarely, in a well conducted anesthesia service, but the complications are discussed in some detail, for the obstetrician must be prepared to meet them and to aid the anesthesiologist in their treatment. Further, if a fair appraisal is to be made of the pros and cons of the different methods and techniques used for pain relief, it is necessary to be familiar with the anesthetic complications that can occur and the eventual extent of such complications. Such an assessment applies to anesthesia generally, but certain differences exist in obstetrics, including the unique situation that two lives are simultaneously at stake. One of the greatest single services any hospital can offer the parturient is anesthesia of the highest quality—a goal that is difficult to achieve and maintain.

In an era of regional planning of hospitals and medical facilities, there is perhaps no single type of service more important than obstetric anesthesia to illustrate what could be achieved by such planning. If standards of care are to be met in a time when medical manpower shortages are mounting, the question is posed whether only the hospitals that are able to provide round-the-clock quality anesthesia service should be permitted to maintain an obstetric service.

THE PUERPERIUM

POSTPARTUM CARE

The postpartum bedside chart should include pulse, temperature, blood pressure, and respiratory rate recorded every four to six hours for 48 hours. A careful intake and output chart is kept for three days after delivery. Ambulation and bathroom pri-vileges are permitted 12 hours after delivery. In the normal case, a house diet is permissible from the beginning.

The parturient represents a patient with an open wound, that is, the placental site, and her care must be planned and governed accordingly. The nurse and all in attendance, and the patient herself, must treat the perineal area as a surgical field. The avoidance of contamination and cross-contamination is a basic consideration, for puerperal infection is rarely the result of delivery; rather, epidemics may result from cross-infection in the early days of the puerperium. Proper masking and proper hand care are fundamental requirements in the postpartum care of the patient. With early ambulation, a safe technique for perineal care can be taught to patients, which they are able to use beginning on the second postpartum day.

Urine retention complicating the puerperium may occur in the patient with a normal delivery, but is more likely following a difficult forceps procedure. The patient should be given every opportunity to void before catheterization is resorted to. At the same time, postpartum diuresis usually begins with delivery, and several hundred milliliters of urine may collect in the bladder every two to three hours for at least the first day of the puerperium. Amounts of 500 milliliters or more invite bladder atonicity, causing a delay in spontaneous voiding. Hence catheterization may be required for several days before the bladder will regain its tone. The constant desire to void, with urination of only small amounts, usually means urine retention or an overflow bladder. Also, characteristically, the full bladder displaces the uterus out of the pelvis; abdominal palpation will reveal the uterus away from the midline and in extreme situations its fundus may reach nearly to the costal margin. In the patients who are not voiding in average amounts, the abdomen should be palpated every two hours for evidence of urine retention. If there is any doubt as to whether the patient is emptying her bladder, or if she complains of bladder discomfort, she should be catheterized at least once. Intermittent catheterization is thought to be less of an infectious hazard than use of an indwelling catheter. This means, however, that the nurse in charge must be fully aware that, because of normal postpartum diuresis, the patient may require catheterization as frequently as every two to four hours instead of the customary six to eight hours.

In their preparation for childbirth, patients should be made to realize that some emotional letdown is often experienced on the third to the fifth postpartum day, so that when this happens it comes as no surprise. Patients and their husbands should both be aware of this, and it might be regarded as a normal part of the postpartum course. Tears without obvious cause is a prominent symptom, and the patient is quick to state that she can find no reason for her behavior and tends to be apologetic. One might speculate that this is a state of emotional exhaustion following the successful completion of a new medical experience, but it happens to multipara and primipara alike.

Reassuring the patient that she is no different from the majority of her recently pregnant contemporaries is usually sufficient. In some instances, however, this is not enough. Most important is to make certain that the patient does not feel somewhat inadequate as a future mother, a state of mind sometimes fostered by her mother. The patient should be told with emphasis that her husband and her new family take precedence over all other considerations. She should realize that she must manage her parents and others with a degree of emotional detachment, out of respect and affection, but not from any feeling of loyalty. Perhaps she and her husband should reread and be familiar with the literal interpretation of and practice the precepts contained in Genesis 2:24, and, in some instances, they might bring this reference to the attention of their respective parents.

BREAST FEEDING

Successful breast feeding begins with the antepartum preparation of the patient. She should be familiar with the advantages to the infant, and at the same time be aware that 7 to 10 days must elapse after delivery before the baby is nursing satisfactorily. Breast feeding should be supervised by the obstetrician who, after all, is the mother's physician, and because the infant belongs to her, by simple deduction, he is the infant's physician. The management of breast feeding is a responsibility that is difficult to share with the pediatrician, lest the patient become confused by conflicting advice.

The patient should realize that the baby will show little interest in nursing until the third day post partum, tending to sleep when at breast. Further, it should be made apparent to the patient that engorgement and milk production are not synonymous. Characteristically, on the second and third days the breasts become engorged, heavy, and generally uncomfortable. About the fourth or fifth day the breasts begin to soften and produce significant amounts of milk, and the infant begins to nurse with some vigor. For the average-sized infant, the usual schedule calls for nursing every four hours. Provided the infant shows an adequate weight gain, the 2 A.M. feeding may be omitted, affording the mother an opportunity for needed hours of rest. If the baby is small, or excessively large, and the extra feeding is thought necessary, or if it is thought that the breasts need stimulation to meet the demands of the infant, the 2 A.M. feeding is included. More frequent nursing, or demand feeding, in conjunction with the infant rooming in with the mother is undoubtedly an aid to successful breast feeding. Before each feeding the nipples are cleansed with an antiseptic, and to minimize the risk of a breast infection it is now the practice to scrub the entire breast area three or four times daily with a detergent containing hexachlorophene. It is customary to have the infant nurse 7 to 10 minutes at each breast.

If the baby is not receiving an adequate amount of milk, as indicated by failure to gain, two possibilities exist: either the mother, at least at the moment, has insufficient milk, or the baby is failing to obtain it, perhaps because the breasts are engorged, or the nipples are flat or inverted. Nipple shields may be tried, but pumping each breast at low pressure (3 to 5 lb.) with a breast pump for five minutes softens the breasts and tends to draw out the nipples.

To settle the issue of whether the mother has sufficient milk or the baby is failing to obtain it, the baby is weighed both before (AC) and after feeding (PC). If the weight after feeding exceeds that before by 2 oz. or more, it is concluded that the mother has enough milk and the baby will soon begin to gain. If the weight is approximately the same, the breasts are pumped to see whether the mother is producing any milk or if it is simply that the baby is not able to obtain it. If the baby appears discontented on breast feedings, the mother should be reassured that it is not due to the quality of the milk. There is no reason to expect formula feeding to rectify the situation. Rather, greater attention should be given to the technique of nursing to make certain that the infant is not swallowing abnormal amounts of air. The patient should be expected to breast feed the baby for several months. Only when the milk supply dwindles or there is evidence of breast infection should the infant be placed on formula feedings. The breasts go through a cycle of production that usually covers a three- to six-month period, with their gradual involution. To interrupt the process is to invite failure of normal involution, which may contribute to chronic cystic disease of the breast. Some weeks or months after birth the milk output may not satisfy the demands of the infant. The common procedure is to omit one or more breast feedings and substitute a formula feeding, and in about two to four weeks the baby will be weaned completely from the breast.

In women who do not choose to breast feed, or during the course of weaning the baby, endocrine substances, of which there are a great number, are commonly used and advocated to suppress lactation. Without doubt these substances will prevent some engorgement with its associated discomfort, which reaches its peak on the third postpartum day. Both patients and nurses will testify, however, that the breasts become engorged when the medication is discontinued, which often means when the patient is at home and nursing care is not at hand. The time-honored method of the breast binder, ice caps to the breasts, and administration of adequate analgesics is effective. The breasts are held upward and to the midline by the binder. A mistake is to bind the breasts tightly to the chest wall, which causes passive congestion and produces additional discomfort. Ice bags, three in all, one between the breasts and one lateral to each breast, are applied for an hour or two and then omitted for an equal length of time. To prevent the possibility of an "ice burn," the breasts should be covered with petrolatum or muslin. Mild analgesics may be given in liberal amounts. Usually within 24 to 72 hours the breasts become softer and the discomfort disappears. The patient should be aware that the nipples will frequently discharge a milky to almost clear fluid for at least two or three months after the return of the menses.

Besides lymphangitis and breast abscess, which are discussed in Chapter 21, there are three common complications of breast feeding. The patient may produce excessive milk (polygalactia), and for a week or more comfort may necessitate pumping of the breasts after alternate feedings. In time supply and demand will become regulated. Insufficient milk (agalactia) is common, and this may be corrected by breast stimulation through more frequent nursings. Fissures of the nipples, which of course provide an entry of infection, are of two types, circular and radial. Although the infant should be removed from the affected breast, to do so for more than 24 to 48 hours will invite agalactia. At the same time, this is frequently insufficient time for the fissure to heal, particularly the circular type which develops at the base of the nipple. Local application of antibiotic creams is commonly recommended to avoid infection and promote healing. The patient should be carefully observed, however, to detect any evidence of a lymphangitis. In the interim, pumping of the breast at low pressure or nipple shields may stimulate the breasts to some extent. After 24 to 48 hours the infant is usually returned to the breast.

POSTPARTUM DISCHARGE AND PATIENT INSTRUCTIONS

Some physicians advocate that a gentle vaginal examination be performed prior to the patient's hospital discharge. The only possible advantage is to be assured that a sponge has not been inadvertently left in the vagina, which need not occur if the vagina is inspected at the end of delivery. Otherwise, there are a number of disadvantages, including the possibility of introducing infection and of traumatizing the episiotomy wound; in addition, the examination is obviously uncomfortable to the patient at this time.

Patients should be instructed to obtain three or four hours of rest each day and to climb stairs no more than once daily for at least one or two weeks. Although patients are ambulatory from the second day after delivery, they should realize that such a period is required before they regain their strength sufficiently to take over their household duties. It must be emphasized that the emotional and physical strain of caring for a new baby, particularly in the first three months, is considerable.

Douches may be advisable if a brownish or yellowish vaginal discharge persists some two weeks after the patient has left the hospital. The patient should realize that douches are of limited value, however, and need not be continued for more than a week.

Furthermore, the normal healthy woman should not require douches for any reason. Many otherwise normal women believe that in order to be "clean" and not have a repugnant odor it is necessary to take douches almost daily. Such self-criticism is entirely unwarranted and deserves further questioning to determine the basis for such an attitude. If the vaginal discharge continues in abnormal amounts or is irritating in character, the patient should return for an early postpartum checkup, which may reveal a cause for this state of affairs.

Exercises to restore the tone of the abdominal muscles are advocated, but they should be postponed for approximately four weeks post partum. In fact, the impression is gained that the abdominal muscles regain their tone more readily after the menses have returned and the pregnancy is truly completed. Many forms of exercise have been recommended to strengthen the abdominal muscles. An effective method is for the patient to lie on the floor with her arms at her sides. The thighs and legs are elevated together to approximately a 70-degree angle from the floor. The limbs are rotated together clockwise and counterclockwise three or four times. Before the legs and thighs are returned to the floor, they are raised and lowered a few times. The last time they are lowered, they are held as long as possible without actually touching the heels to the floor. At first this is an exhausting exercise, but with practice it will be possible to rotate the lower extremities a number of times. If the exercises are performed three or four times daily for a period of 5 to 10 minutes, the abdominal muscles will regain much of their tone.

The patient should be told that ovulation and the menstrual periods usually recur within 6 to 10 weeks post partum unless she is breast feeding, in which case amenorrhea may continue. In the non-nursing mother, however, it is possible for the catamenia to be delayed some five or six months. (See Figure 26 in Chapter 4.)

The flow at the initial menstrual period is likely to be somewhat profuse, and the passage of small clots is not unusual. It is wise for the patient to rest for a few hours in the hope that the flow will subside. Rarely will the bleeding be of such a degree that hospitalization is necessary. (See Subinvolution of the Placental Site in Chapter 16.) The patient should realize that it is possible to become pregnant before the menses reappear. Sexual intercourse is best postponed until after the postpartum check-up, which is customarily performed at the sixth to eighth postpartum week. However, contraceptive advice and methods are discussed and steps taken for conception control.

POSTPARTUM EXAMINATION

The postpartum examination should include a history covering the interval from the patient's discharge from the hospital. The patient should be weighed, her blood pressure taken, and the hemoglobin determined. The breasts should be examined, and the patient instructed concerning self-examination of the breasts.

Before proceeding with the vaginal and rectal examinations the cervix is first inspected and on occasion the cytologic smear may be repeated. The cervix often appears eroded at the first postpartum visit; however, it may look quite normal following one or more periods.

After the speculum is removed, vaginal and rectal examinations are performed as previously described. In addition, the bimanual examination determines the muscular support of the perineum and the status of the episiotomy site. Family planning is reviewed and contraceptive methods individualized.

If an erosion persists, and a smear is negative, the cervix may then be cauterized. It is not necessary to see the patient for 8 to 10 weeks after cauterization, for it will take at least that long for the cervix to heal. The patient should be told that a vaginal discharge will develop, usually brown or yellow in color, and will persist for two or three weeks. For the sake of cleanliness, a warm water douche may be taken daily. At the next visit, a uterine sound should be passed through the cervical canal to prevent stenosis.

Return visits will depend on the patient's general condition, but two or more postpartum examinations are necessary before the patient is discharged. The patient should be instructed to return for periodic checkups, the frequency depending somewhat on her age. Before the age of 35, the patient should return every two years; after that age she should return annually. On these visits an interval history is taken, and a general physical examination, including a pelvic and rectal examination, is performed. Besides routine blood and urine studies, a vaginal smear is taken for cytologic study and the cervix is stained by the Schiller method. Women who plan to have more children should be told that a preconceptional examination is advisable.

BIBLIOGRAPHY

Albert, C. A., Anderson, G., Wallace, W., Henley, C. E., Winshel, A. W., and Albert, S. N.: Fluothane for obstetric anesthesia. Obstet. Gynec., 13:282, 1959.

Apgar, V., Holaday, D. A., James, L. S., Prince, C. E., Weisbrot, I. M., and Weiss, I.: Comparison of regional and general anesthesia in obstetrics; with special reference to transmission of cyclopropane across the placenta. J.A.M.A., 165:2155, 1957.

Apgar, V., Holaday, D. A., James, L. S., Weisbrot, I. M., and Berrien, C.: Evaluation of the newborn infant—second report. J.A.M.A., 168:1985, 1958.

Apgar, V., and Papper, E. M.: Transmission of drugs across the placenta. Anesth. Analg., 31:309, 1952.

Bieniarz, J., Fernandez-Sepulveda, R., and Caldeyro-Barcia, R.: Effects of maternal hypotension on the human fetus; 1. Fetal heart rate during normal labor. Amer. J. Obstet. Gynec., 92:821, 1965.

Bonica, J. J.: Principles and Practice of Obstetric Analgesia and Anesthesia. Philadelphia, F. A. Davis Co., Vol. 1, 1967, Vol. 2, 1969.

Briscoe, C. C.: Routine exploration of the uterus for retained secundines. Obstet. Gynec., 4:375, 1954.

Bromage, P. R., and Robson, J. G.: Concentrations of lignocaine in the blood after intravenous, intramuscular, epidural and endotracheal administration. Anaesthesia, 16:461, 1961.

Busby, T.: Local anesthesia for cesarean section. Amer. J. Obstet. Gynec., 87:399, 1963.

Douglas, R. G., Bonsnes, R. W., and du Vigneaud, V.: Natural and synthetic oxytocin; preliminary report on the use of both for the induction and stimulation of labor. Obstet. Gynec., 6:254, 1955.

Flowers, C. E.: Trilene; an adjunct to obstetrical anesthesia and analgesia. Amer. J. Obstet. Gynec., 65:1027, 1953.

Gainey, H. L.: Postpartum observation of pelvic tissue damage; further studies. Amer. J. Obstet. Gynec., 70:800, 1955.

Gordon, H. R.: Fetal bradycardia after paracervical block: Correlation with fetal and maternal blood levels of local anesthetic (mepivacaine). New Eng. J. Med., 279:910, 1968.

Hardy, J. D., and Javert, C. T.: Studies on pain; measurements of pain intensity in childbirth. J. Clin. Invest., 28:153, 1949.

Hardy, J. D., Wolff, H. G., and Goodell, H.: Studies on pain; an investigation of some quantitative aspects of the dol scale of pain intensity. J. Clin. Invest., 27:380, 1948.

Hershenson, B. B., Isaac, S. J., Romney, S. L., and Reid, D. E.: A new sedative (antipsychomotor) drug useful in labor. New Eng. J. Med., 251:216, 1954.

Hon, E. H.: Observations on "pathologic" fetal bradycardia. Amer. J. Obstet. Gynec., 77:1084, 1959.

Jacobson, E.: Relaxation methods in labor. Amer. J. Obstet. Gynec., 67:1035, 1954.

James, L. S., and Adamsons, K., Jr.: Respiratory physiology of the fetus and newborn. New Eng. J. Med., 271:1352, 1403, 1964.

James, L. S., Weisbrot, I. M., Prince, C. E., Holaday, D. A., and Apgar, V.: The acid base status of human infants in relation to birth asphyxia and the onset of respiration. J. Pediat., 52:379, 1958.

Javert, C. T., and Hardy, J. D.: Influences of analgesics on pain intensity during labor. Anesthesiology, 12:189, 1951.

Johnson, L. D.: The role of the obstetrician in the prevention of cervical cancer. New Eng. J. Med., 262:1297, 1960.

Kennedy, F., Effron, A. S., and Perry, G.: The grave spinal cord paralyses caused by spinal anesthesia. Surg. Gynec. Obstet., 91:385, 1950.

Klink, E. W.: Perineal nerve block; an anatomic and clinical study in the female. Obstet. Gynec., 1:137, 1953.

Kobak, A. J., and Sadove, M. S.: Combined paracervical and pudendal nerve blocks—a simple form of transvaginal regional anesthesia. Amer. J. Obstet. Gynec., 81:72, 1961.

Lurie, A. O., and Weiss, J. B.: Blood concentration of mepivacaine and lidocaine in mother and baby after epidural anesthesia. Amer. J. Obstet. Gynec., 106:850–856, 1970.

Marx, G. F.: Placental transfer and drugs used in anesthesia. Anesthesiology, 22:294, 1961.

Mathews, D. D., and Loeffler, F. E.: The effect of abdominal decompression on fetal oxygenation during pregnancy and early labour. J. Obstet. Gynaec. Brit. Comm., 75:268, 1968.

Morris, E. D., and Beard, R. W.: The rationale and technique of foetal blood sampling and amnioscopy. J. Obstet. Gynec. Brit. Comm., 72:489, 1965.

Moya, F., and James, L. S.: Medical hypnosis for obstetrics. J.A.M.A., 174:2026, 1960.

Moya, F., and Kvisselgaard, N.: The placental transmission of succinylcholine. Anesthesiology, 22:1, 1961.

Moya, F., and Smith, B. E.: Uptake, distribution and placental transport of drugs and anesthetics. Anesthesiology, 26:465, 1965.

Paul, W. M., Gare, D. J., and Whetham, J. C.: Assessment of fetal scalp sampling in labor. Amer. J. Obstet. Gynec., 99:745, 1967.

Phillips, O. C., and Frazier, T. N.: Obstetric anesthesia care in the United States. Obstet. Gynec., 19:796, 1962.

Phillips, O. C., et al.: The role of anesthesia in obstetric mortality. Anesth. Analg. 40:557, 1961.

Ranney, B.: Paracervical block for first-stage pain in primigravidas. Obstet. Gynec., 27:757, 1966.

Russell, J. T.: Halothane and caesarian section. Anaesthesia, 13:241, 1958.

Shnider, S. M., and Moya, F.: Effect of meperidine on newborn infant. Amer. J. Obstet. Gynec., 89:1009, 1965.

Silverman, W. A., and Sinclair, J. C.: Temperature regulation in the newborn infant. New Eng. J. Med., 247:92, 146, 1966.

Stenger, V., et al.: Extradural anesthesia for cesarean section: Physiologic and biochemical observations. Obstet. Gynec., 25:802, 1965.

Taylor, P. M., Bright, N. H., and Birchard, E. L.: Effect of early versus delayed clamping of the umbilical cord on the clinical condition of the newborn infant. Amer. J. Obstet. Gynec., 86:893, 1963.

Telford, J., and Keats, A. S.: Narcotic—narcotic antagonist mixtures. Anesthesiology, 22:465, 1961.

Vandam, L. D.: Local anesthetics. Clin. Pharmacol. Ther., 3:131, 1962.

Weiss, J. B.: Obstetric analgesia and anesthesia. *In* Cyclopedia of Medicine, Surgery, Specialties. Philadelphia, F. A. Davis Co., in press.

Weiss, J. B., Kagey, K. S., and Frink, R. D.: Fetal heart rate monitoring in clinical practice. Obstet. Gynec., to be published.

Chapter 27

Conduct of Abnormal Labor and Its Complications

ETIOLOGY

Dystocia, or difficult labor, may be either mechanical or functional in etiology, and in some cases there is an element of both. Mechanical dystocia is more commonly due to maternal obstacles, the most frequent of these being a contracted pelvis, and rarely an obstructive tumor, either of the ovary or a uterine fibromyoma. The fetal causes include failure of the vertex to rotate, as in occiput posterior and occiput transverse position; malpresentations; malformation of the fetus, as in hydrocephalus; and excessive size of the infant. Mechanical dystocia in the form of cephalopelvic disproportion occurs most often at the inlet, but may result from midpelvic and outlet contracture. In fact, contracture below the inlet is more treacherous, for its presence may not be appreciated until late in labor or when attempt is made to deliver the patient pelvically.

Functional dystocia or dysfunctional labor is a term used to describe conditions in which uterine contractions are regarded as deviating from the normal. The contractions from their very onset may be extremely forceful and lead to rapid and damaging labor resulting in a precipitous delivery, but more frequently labor is attended by ineffectual uterine contractions. Certain recognized contributing conditions are: (1) anomalous conditions of the uterus; (2) overdistention of the uterus associated with multiple pregnancy or polyhydramnios; (3) delayed labor, or postmaturity; (4) multiple fibromyomata, which may disrupt the normal pattern of uterine contractions; (5) scar-tissue formation in and about the cervix from a previous delivery or from ill advised and improperly selected gynecologic procedures; and (6) miscellaneous factors, such as a debilitating disease or

a pendulous abdomen with redundancy of the uterus. Statistically speaking, in the majority of patients who fail to have effective or productive labor there is no apparent cause. Thus, the cumbersome term "idiopathic functional dystocia" perhaps more correctly describes the syndrome. These patients contribute the majority of instances of prolonged or desultory labor.

Admittedly, one is confronted with a variety of paradoxes when attempting to assess the etiologic factors and the clinical aspects of functional dystocia. Certainly clinical experience supports the idea that cervical resistance (cervical dystocia) is involved in the etiology of functional dystocia, for with rare exceptions the syndrome is restricted to first labors. This suggests that once the cervix has dilated it no longer offers any appreciable resistance in a subsequent labor.

Idiopathic functional dystocia has come to mean a failure of complete synchronization of myometrial activity. These aberrations in uterine contractility have been classified in several ways and are subject to various interpretations. From tocographic studies it has been found that the uterine contractions may remain localized instead of involving the entire uterus. The contractions may be stronger in the lower than in the upper segment; in fact, they are sometimes said to become reversed and propagate upward rather than downward, and the uterus loses its fundal dominance or normal polarity. Uterine fibrillation and high uterine tonus are synonymous with failure of the cervix to dilate. As interesting and important as these observations are, it still remains a question why the uterus behaves in such a manner. If the etiology of functional dystocia resides in the uterine corpus and not in the cervix, one might expect the syndrome to recur in subsequent labors, *but, as stated above, such is not the case.* Regardless of theoretical considerations in idiopathic functional dystocia, it is the failure of the cervix to dilate that bothers both the patient and the obstetrician.

Considerable weight has also been placed on whether the uterus in functional dystocia is in a hypotonic or a hypertonic state. Hypertonicity is believed to be associated with reversal or loss of uterine polarity or an inversion of the normal gradient of myometrial activity. The opinion has been expressed that if the uterus is flaccid and hypotonic, labor of an indefinite length can be permitted, and will not be accompanied by any significant increase in fetal morbidity and mortality. Although labor may last for several days, time and supportive therapy will eventually result in a nontraumatic pelvic delivery. By contrast, if the uterus is hypertonic and contracts in a so-called colicky fashion, the prospect is for a much less favorable outcome for the infant, and more active measures of management are indicated in conformity with those outlined in the treatment of prolonged labor. Further, the uterus is less likely to respond favorably to oxytocin stimulation. In other words, the fetal morbidity and mortality are determined more by the tonicity of the uterus than by the hours of labor per se.

Appealing as this distinction may be, the tonicity of the uterus in idiopathic functional dystocia may be related more to the effect of labor than to any specific type of uterine dysrhythmia. That is to say, the uterus may be in a state of hypotonicity at the beginning of labor, but becomes hypertonic as labor continues and as the cervix fails to dilate. Accordingly, hypertonicity of the uterus is the result and not the cause of functional dystocia.

Further, it has become customary to divide the uterine inertia of functional dystocia into a *primary* and a *secondary* type. Primary uterine inertia is considered when there is lack of progress from the very onset of labor, in contradistinction to secondary uterine inertia, which develops after labor has been established. It may be questioned whether this is a necessary or a useful division. Actually, what the clinician often chooses to call primary inertia is, in fact, false labor, in which case the total length of labor and the incidence of protracted or desultory labor are incorrectly computed and reported. Further, in contradistinction to secondary uterine inertia, in so-called primary inertia the use of oxytocic drugs is contraindicated. Rather, the treatment should be one of watchful expectancy, including adequate sedation and attention to fluid balance. It is recommended, therefore, that the terms "primary" and "secondary" be discarded and that the term "uterine inertia" be used only to denote the failure of effective uterine contractions to develop after the onset of labor.

In summary, much of the literature bearing on the subject of idiopathic functional dystocia supports the belief that the difficulty resides principally in the corpus and not in the cervix, and that ineffectual labor is due initially to a disturbance in uterine motility. Whether the latter represents cause or effect is open to question, but in either event the cause of the syndrome remains unknown. Although it may be associated with what some may choose to call uncoordinated uterine contractions, these can be coordinated apparently by therapy, for to assume otherwise is at variance with the observation that in most instances labor can be completed by stimulation with oxytocic drugs provided treatment is not postponed until the uterus reaches a state of hypertonicity. Whether the condition is or is not the result of uterine dysrhythmia, the clinical fact remains that with few exceptions cervical resistance can be overcome by uterine stimulation.

The concept is put forward here that ineffective uterine contractions reflect soft-tissue resistance or a disparity between the strength of the uterine contractions and the resistance offered by the cervix, comparable on occasion to that seen when the presenting part encounters bony resistance. Composed principally of fibrous tissue which, in order to dilate, must stretch, the cervix could be expected to offer considerably more resistance in the first than in subsequent labors. The comparative amounts of muscle, with its ability to contract, and connective tissue may differ from patient to patient, but any causal relationship of these proportions to functional dystocia has never been precisely determined. Again, once the cervical tissue is stretched by the initial labor, it could be expected that subsequent labors might be less prolonged. Further, could it not be that functional dystocia develops when the cervix is not properly prepared for labor? Certainly when this syndrome does occur, the cervix at the onset of labor is often uneffaced and closed.

A patient with idiopathic functional dystocia presents certain characteristic clinical features. At the onset, the contractions are of short duration and limited intensity. As the patient enters a state of prolonged labor, of 20 hours or beyond, the uterine tone increases and the uterus often takes on an hourglass outline. The physiologic retraction or constriction ring may at first be palpable above the symphysis, and as the hours of labor go by the ring rises toward the region of the umbilicus. Whether the constriction reaches pathologic proportions, that is, becomes a Bandl's ring, and contracts about the infant, making pelvic delivery hazardous, will depend on whether, because of cervical resistance, labor is permitted to continue indefinitely. In the extreme, the patient will show signs of exhaustion, and the strain of unproductive labor on the fetus may be revealed by disturbances in the rhythm and rate of the fetal heart tones or by the passage of meconium-stained amniotic fluid.

The patient, realizing the lack of progress, becomes anxious and apprehensive and may lose her morale. If fluid balance is not maintained, tachycardia and fever appear, and there is acetonuria. Perhaps through a disturbance of the sympathetic nervous system, ileus is commonly seen. In fact, for 48 to 72 hours after delivery is accomplished, abdominal distention is usually present; it may be rather marked at times, but no special treatment is indicated. This is the clinical picture after 30 or more hours of unproductive labor. It is here that the fetal morbidity and mortality begin to rise (Table 1).

The reported perinatal mortality in prolonged labor is totally unacceptable in current obstetric practice (Table 1). Furthermore, the fetal damage caused by intrauterine hypoxia is not entirely reflected in the stillbirth or neonatal death rates. The number of infants lost in utero or in the neonatal period as the result of prolonged labor undoubtedly is matched by an equal number of infants who survive but, because they have experienced hypoxia, show residual central nervous system damage. The ultimate effect on the fetus is a matter of great concern and it is imperative that delivery not be delayed indefinitely.

TABLE 1. INCIDENCE OF PROLONGED LABOR AND PERINATAL MORTALITY REPORTED BY VARIOUS AUTHORS

Author	Time Factor (Hours)	Per Cent Prolonged Labor	Per Cent Perinatal Mortality
Cosgrove (1940)	36	6.0	7.0
Douglas and Stander (1943)	30	9.0	–
Mac Rae (1944)	48	3.2	11.47
Reid (1946)	20	5.4	11.7
Odell et al. (1947)	30	2.7	10.4
Eastman (1947)	24	8.4	5.0
Schmitz et al. (1947)	24	4.0	7.4
Willson and Alesbury (1951)	24	1.8	4.23
Daro and Gollin (1951)	18	3.9	4.5
Starr (1952)	24	5.0	7.4
Evans (1955)	24	5.3	4.67
Keettel and Pettis (1956)	30	3.2	11.2
Winterringer (1957)	25	2.1	10.0
Fields et al. (1959)	24	3.7	–
Goodwin and Reid (1963)	20	1.4	5.4

It is proposed that the term prolonged labor and all it denotes be discarded and desultory labor be substituted for such cases with the proviso that labor be completed within 18 to 20 hours, the extreme period for normal labor. Hence, desultory labor will be the term used for cases in which progress is not sustained in the course of labor. Accordingly, if one believes that the welfare of both the mother and the infant can be seriously jeopardized by unproductive labor, and active measures are instituted to improve labor whenever it becomes desultory, thereby effecting earlier delivery, the incidence of prolonged labor will be substantially reduced and, it is hoped, eliminated.

A TRIAL OR TEST OF LABOR

A trial or test of labor is the amount and length of labor permitted prior to delivery in cases of mechanical and functional dystocia. What constitutes a test of labor has been defined in a variety of ways, but in practical terms *it is the length of labor, designated in hours, during which time the clinician concludes that the patient can be safely delivered pelvically, or that recourse must be made to abdominal delivery.* It must never be a test of endurance for either the fetus or the mother, and the length of time of a test of labor will depend to a degree on whether the dystocia is mechanical or functional.

In patients with cephalopelvic disproportion, only rarely is the disproportion absolute (Fig. 1), permitting a cesarean section without a test of labor. In fact, when a pelvic delivery seems unlikely, as determined by obstetric and x-ray examination, surprisingly the patient may have a comparatively uneventful labor and pelvic delivery. Also, if a patient with mechanical dystocia is permitted to enter labor, the clinician is assured that the pregnancy has continued as long as it will and that cesarean section, if necessary, is not performed prematurely.

In cases of "borderline" mechanical dystocia, labor is rarely allowed to progress beyond 6 to 12 hours, for at the end of this period it should be evident whether pelvic delivery is possible. In inlet disproportion the question may be settled much sooner, and, in fact, if the uterus is contracting vigorously, harm may come to the fetus if labor extends beyond four to six hours.

In patients with functional dystocia, a test of labor involves additional hours, but the length of time is subject to individual experience and judgment. Opinions differ much more in the management of these patients than in that of patients with mechanical dystocia. Admittedly, these are the most trying cases, for they generally occur in primiparous women in whom the clinician wishes to avoid a reproductive career requiring cesarean section with its possible additional hazards and complications. At the same time, there is good reason to believe that a test of labor beyond 18 to 20 hours is not in the best interests of the fetus.

PRECIPITATE LABOR

A labor of two hours or less in duration must be considered abnormal. In such a rapid labor the uterus may contract with sufficient frequency and violence to cause both fetal and maternal trauma.

From the very onset the uterine con-

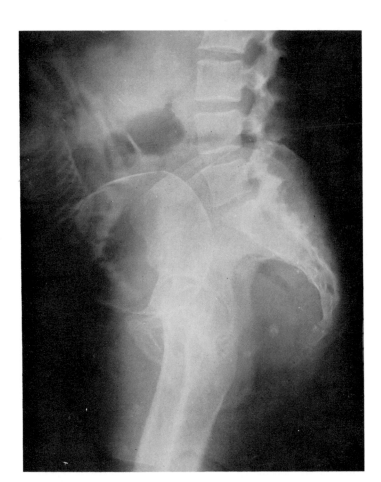

Figure 1. Absolute cephalopelvic disproportion.

tractions are often tumultuous, and the uterus relaxes for only a moment between contractions. Consequently, the intervillous blood flow may be impaired with a resultant hypoxic effect on the fetus. The rapid propulsion of the fetal head through the birth canal, caused by the violent action of the uterus, may result in gross intracranial hemorrhage. Because of the precipitate nature of the labor, delivery may be unattended, the baby may not receive the benefit of immediate resuscitation, and the mother may experience severe lacerations of the birth canal. Such labors form the background for some cases of rupture of the lower uterine segment and severe cervical and vaginal vault lacerations. In most instances, however, the lacerations are restricted to the perineum, labia minora, and the area about the urethra and clitoris. Precipitate labor is especially hazardous when the vagina or the cervix has been lacerated during a previous labor or delivery. Also, amniotic fluid embolism has been related to this type of labor.

Clinical experience recalls the rare patient who has lost one or more babies from intracranial hemorrhage as a result of rapid and precipitate labor. These patients deserve special attention, and, to forestall a recurrence, consideration must be given to elective induction and control of labor. With the onset of labor following amniotomy, the character and the type of uterine contractions should be carefully observed by continuous abdominal palpation and monitoring. If the contractions become excessively strong, the patient should receive some form of anesthesia for the purpose of decreasing the strength of the contractions. Controlling the contractions should maintain a normal rate of intervillous blood flow and adequate oxygenation of the fetus, as well as prevent fetal and maternal trauma.

DESULTORY LABOR

Desultory labor may become evident within six to eight hours after the onset of labor, and with few exceptions it is the result of an idiopathic functional dystocia. Among the exceptions, distention and distortion of the myometrium may contribute to a deficiency in uterine contractility, with polyhydramnios, multiple pregnancy, and fibromyomata being the conditions most commonly encountered. At times, and despite the fact that the fetuses are small, a patient with multiple pregnancy may experience very desultory labor with ineffective uterine contractions, and, what is more, the uterus may not respond to carefully administered oxytocin stimulation. A so-called "dry birth," in which the membranes have ruptured before the onset of labor and the amniotic fluid is lost, is no longer regarded as a cause of desultory labor. In some cases reducing the amount of amniotic fluid may improve uterine motility by allowing the myometrium to contract more effectively. It is stated that labor is more prolonged in certain fetal presentations and positions, more specifically breech presentation and occiput posterior position, but the mean average of length of labor, shortened perhaps by operative delivery, falls within the normal range. The same conclusion applies to those cases in which the pelvis is borderline in size.

A primipara who is 35 years or older, frequently referred to as "elderly" in the reproductive sense, is generally regarded as a possible candidate for desultory labor and, although statistically this appears to be true, these patients often experience normal labor. Consequently, age alone is no contraindication to a trial labor in a primiparous patient. The multipara who has not borne a child for several years sometimes worries about pregnancy, labor, and delivery, and also wonders whether because of her increasing age parturition may be hazardous. She should be reassured that labor will not be protracted provided she is otherwise obstetrically normal.

As stated previously, desultory labor due to functional dystocia with rare exception is a syndrome of primiparity. Therefore, a woman with normal pelvis who experiences desultory labor in the first pregnancy will have a normal labor in subsequent pregnancies, and such patients should be reassured of this fact for they are naturally apprehensive with respect to future pregnancies.

The same considerations which are important in primiparas are also highly important in the management of the multiparous patient whose labor becomes desultory. Here again, the obstetric history should be reviewed, the patient's status re-evaluated, and a careful search made to explain the lack of progress in labor. The patient may possibly have a contracted pelvis which has previously gone unrecognized; the fetus may be larger than her previous infants, or it may be presenting abnormally. Another possible cause is an undiagnosed obstructing tumor of the pelvis, such as a fibromyoma on the posterior surface of the lower uterine segment, which reasonably may not have been detected. Also, scar-tissue formation in the cervix may prevent dilatation and impede labor. All of these must be excluded before it can be assumed that the multiparous patient has functional dystocia as the cause for the desultory labor.

Treatment of Desultory Labor

Basic in the management of desultory labor is the belief that once true labor has started, progress should be definite and sustained until the patient has been successfully delivered within the period of time defined for normal labor, i.e., within 20 hours. Treatment is predicated on the concept that the patient is given the usual supportive measures and that uterine inertia, as defined, is treated by uterine stimulants. It is presumed that the pelvis is normal and that functional dystocia is the problem. Whether a shorter labor brought about by oxytocin stimulation is less harmful than a desultory labor of considerably greater length may be debated. However, there is no doubt that a definite time limit is necessary, for when labor exceeds a certain number of hours there is a resultant increase in the fetal morbidity and mortality. There is ample literature to attest to this conclusion.

In patients with desultory labor who are candidates for prolonged labor, a decision must eventually be made regarding the length of labor that is to be allowed and the steps to be taken to effect delivery.

To complete labor within the time limit and without immediate recourse to cesarean section, an attempt is made to stimulate and improve the quality of the labor. The efficacy of amniotomy to improve labor must be considered. On occasion such a procedure is followed immediately by excellent progress in labor, but at times no change is noted. Moreover, there is introduced an increase in the fetal and maternal risk, and in general one is committed to an earlier delivery.

A subject of continuing controversy, oxytocin, in some form to stimulate and im-prove the character of the uterine contractions, is now accepted therapy. Since its reintroduction nearly three decades ago, which was permissible with the advent of x-ray pelvimetry to afford the clinician an accurate means of determining the cephalopelvic relationship, oxytocin has been administered for the prevention and definitive treatment of functional dystocia.

Oxytocin is given primarily for two reasons: (1) to produce uterine contractions sufficiently strong to increase the dilatation of the cervix, and (2) to demonstrate over a comparatively short period of time whether the uterus will contract effectively to complete at least the first stage of labor, that is, overcome cervical resistance. If progress in labor is reestablished by oxytocin infusion, the cervix should be dilated completely within three to four hours from the time of the initial medication. Pelvic delivery can then be accomplished either normally or by low forceps. If appreciable progress has not been made at the end of that time, however, it is fair to assume that additional doses of the drug will not produce the desired results. Actually, continuation of oxytocin therapy and indefinite delay in delivery may increase the risk of irreversible hypoxic damage to the fetus.

For continuous intravenous administration, 5 International units of oxytocin is added to 1000 ml. of 5 per cent glucose in buffered water. Beginning with 10 drops of this solution, the rate is increased to 20, 40, or 60 drops or more per minute, depending on the uterine response. The use of specialized pumps for administration is a refinement that does not eliminate the hazard of this form of therapy or add to its efficacy.

Because it has certain advantages, intravenous drip administration of oxytocin has become more popular than the intramuscular method. There is little doubt that uterine contractions will ensue from minute doses of oxytocin administered intravenously. In addition, the drug can be titrated more accurately by this method to produce the type of labor desired, and in this sense it is more readily controlled. Also, once myometrial contractions are reestablished and desultory labor disappears, the oxytocin therapy on occasion may be discontinued. Pain relief adds to the success rate and this is quickly and satisfactorily attained by lumbar epidural form of analgesia.

The physician in charge should be in constant attendance during oxytocin therapy to make careful observations on the contraction and relaxation of the uterus. Tetanic contractions of the uterus are rare but, should they occur, usually appear immediately when oxytocin drip is started. Transient slowing of the fetal heart rate below 100 beats per minute may occur during a matter of minutes when the physiologic dosage of oxytocin is being determined.

Although adverse effects have been recorded after administration of oxytocin, particularly when it was first introduced into obstetrics in the second decade of the present century, whatever complications have arisen in the first and second stages of labor have usually been caused by its improper use in cases in which there were definite contraindications. Because the syndrome of desultory labor is seen mainly in primiparous women, it is hereby recommended that oxytocin not be given to the multiparous woman with uterine inertia except under the *most strict* supervision and consultation. In fact, a perusal of reports of rupture of the uterus associated with uterine stimulation by oxytocin indicates that almost invariably the patient was a multipara. If oxytocin therapy fails to produce some progress within three or four hours, it is usually abandoned in this clinic for fear that its continuation will contribute to fetal morbidity. Moreover, the fetal risk prohibits resting such a patient and then administering the drug for a second period of time. The efficacy of the therapy should be evident with the initial administration.

When oxytocin fails—this should be obvious in four hours or less, and it may occur in perhaps 5 per cent of patients— the decision regarding the type of delivery depends on two factors, namely, the degree of cervical dilatation, and the station of the presenting part. If the cervix is more than half dilated, the presenting part nearing the pelvic floor, and the outlet ample, pelvic delivery with the aid of Dührssen's incisions is warranted. If these criteria are not fulfilled, abdominal hysterotomy is less traumatic and a far safer procedure.

Use of the ventouse or vacuum extractor has been applied to a longstanding concept that traction on the presenting part might enhance labor. As with the use of scalp forceps, the results have not been impressive. Actually, evulsion of the cervix may occur without furthering dilatation.

FAILURE OF ANTERIOR ROTATION OF THE VERTEX AND ITS MANAGEMENT

Lack of anterior rotation of the occiput is a common cause of arrested labor. "Persistent occiput posterior" and "persistent or deep transverse arrest of the vertex" are clinical terms conventionally used when the occiput fails to move into an anterior position in accordance with the mechanism of internal rotation. Although this failure to rotate anteriorly may occur in the gynecoid pelvis, it is more prevalent in the other parent types of pelves.

Hence when the occiput assumes a posterior position and fails to rotate, there may be certain anatomic reasons for this malposition. These include an anteroposterior diameter of the inlet which exceeds the length of the transverse diameter, a narrowing of the *forepelvis*, or a significant decrease in the interspinous diameter. In the first instance, characteristic of the anthropoid pelvis, the occiput often engages in the posterior position. Together with a narrow forepelvis and a short interspinous diameter, an occiput posterior position may develop from a primary transverse position, which is more typical in the android pelvis but is seen in rare instances in the platypelloid pelvis.

For the vertex to engage in the android pelvis the forepelvis must be of sufficient size to accept the bulk of the vertex, allowing it to move forward and avoid the sacral promontory. If this is to occur, the oblique diameters of the inlet must be, and indeed they are, longer than the anteroposterior diameter. Further, it can be assumed that, if the vertex becomes engaged, the oblique diameters are located a greater distance from the side walls of the pelvic inlet than is the transverse diameter from the sacral promontory (Fig. 2). That is to say, this distance is greater than the length of the posterior sagittal diameter of the inlet. This suggests that to correct either a transverse arrest or a persistent occiput posterior position in the android pelvis it is perhaps best to displace the vertex upward or, if need be, to disengage it, and rotate it above the inlet, utilizing the longer oblique diameters, a method preferred by the writer, rather than to attempt to bring the vertex to the pelvic floor and rotate it, with the possibility of causing considerable trauma to the maternal soft parts.

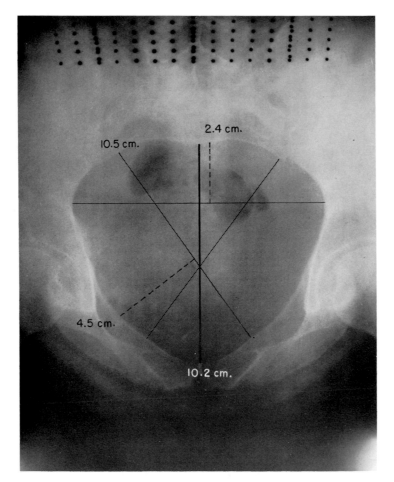

Figure 2. Diameters of the inlet in an android pelvis, indicating the value of the oblique diameters if one chooses to rotate to an anterior position, a "transverse arrest" or a "persistent occiput posterior" above the inlet.

In persistent occiput posterior position, there are two important features of labor that have a bearing on each other. The head, as it meets resistance at the sacrococcygeal platform and the ischial spines, tends to become deflexed. If the patient is examined rectally at the height of the uterine contractions, one gains the impression that the vertex is advancing. What is actually happening is that there is some extension of the vertex with a temporary descent of the sinciput, or brow, in which case the anterior fontanelle may be easily palpated. This unfavorable mechanical situation of partial deflection tends to prevent complete descent and the head arrests somewhere between the spines and the perineum. Secondly, in the case of a partially deflexed head, the cervix may fail to dilate completely, and in some instances becomes passively congested and edematous from being incarcerated between the presenting vertex and the symphysis. Labor

in a persistent occiput posterior position may thus reach an impasse, and further delay may make the delivery more difficult. If there is no question of midpelvic or outlet contracture and progress has ceased for the reason mentioned above, delivery should not be postponed more than an hour after the condition is recognized, for the vertex will become further extended and the cervix more edematous, which will only add to the dystocia problem.

To improve progress in labor in an occiput posterior position, it has been recommended that some effort be made to flex the head by introducing the hand vaginally and exerting pressure against the sinciput during contractions. This maneuver is uncomfortable to the patient, however, and usually does not permanently correct the deflection. Turning the shoulders through 180 degrees has also been advocated (Pomeroy maneuver) to bring the baby's back to an anterior position and thereby cause the occiput to rotate, but such a procedure requires a deep inhalation anesthesia and a cervix dilated some 8 cm. to permit the operator to pass his hand beneath the baby's posterior shoulder for the purpose of turning. This means that the vertex must be displaced out of the pelvis, thus creating the danger of a prolapse of the cord at a time when the cervix is completely dilated. The occiput, moreover, frequently reverts to a posterior position once the patient has recovered from her anesthesia and uterine contractions are reestablished. During labor, therefore, the management of an occiput posterior position is that of watchful expectancy until such time as no further progress is anticipated.

When operative interference is needed, there is less risk of soft tissue damage if the vertex can be rotated and delivered in an anterior position, rather than from a persistent occiput posterior position. Otherwise, the sinciput must first be brought well below the inferior border of the symphysis and the vertex delivered by flexion. This means that the larger occipitofrontal diameter (11.5 cm. or more) of the vertex is presented to the outlet, causing marked distention of the perineum with separation of the underlying endopelvic fascia, despite extensive episiotomy.

There are exceptions, however. Delivery without rotation can be considered when the outlet is large, which applies more often in the anthropoid pelvis. Also, although persistent occiput posterior is rare in a flat platypelloid pelvis, it is unsatisfactory to try to rotate the occiput at any level, and delivery is best accomplished in the occiput posterior position. Although the head may be rotated above the inlet in a platypelloid pelvis, personal experience has shown that the occiput will return to a posterior position as traction is applied at the time of forceps extraction. Rather, after a mediolateral episiotomy, the vertex is best delivered in a posterior position, although it is at some expense to the integrity of the endopelvic fascia and there is a greater likelihood of residual rectocele and urethrocystocele.

It is stated that the amount of force necessary to extract the child is lessened by some three times if the occiput is rotated into an anterior position before the fetus is extracted. Thus, with the exceptions listed above, the vertex, whether it is occiput posterior or transverse, is disengaged from the station of its arrest and rotated either manually or by forceps in the pelvic plane of the greatest dimension or, if need be, above the inlet.

Scanzoni Maneuver versus Manual Rotation

The belief is generally expressed and taught that in the management of an occiput posterior position manual rotation is preferred to the double application of forceps (Scanzoni maneuver), principally because it is stated that there is less danger of traumatizing the soft tissues of the pelvis. Those who follow this precept contrast the higher incidence of vaginal lacerations that accompanies the Scanzoni operation with their near absence when manual rotation is employed. Such a comparison may not be entirely valid, however, if account is taken of the type of case involved, and provided also that important principles and a careful technique of forceps operation are followed.

There is no doubt that in most cases the occiput can be manually rotated anteriorly (Fig. 3). When this is impossible, either the baby must be extracted from the original position as a persistent occiput posterior, or the vertex must be rotated by forceps. If one subscribes to the concept that there is less chance of causing maternal and fetal trauma when the occiput is rotated to an anterior position before the fetus is extracted, except for the rare occurrence of occiput posterior in a platypelloid pelvis or an anthropoid pelvis that is characterized by a large outlet, rotation must be accomplished by forceps when manual rotation fails. Consequently, the results are hardly comparable if this means that the Scanzoni operation is performed on the most difficult cases, and manual rotation on the least difficult.

Perhaps the success of manual rotation is due in part to the fact that during the procedure the vertex is displaced upward into the pelvic plane of the greatest dimension or on occasion above the pelvic inlet. Simply placing the hand in the vagina automatically displaces the vertex upward and away from the station of arrest. This supports the contention that the key to success in performing the Scanzoni maneuver is to displace the vertex upward to a plane where it rotates easily.

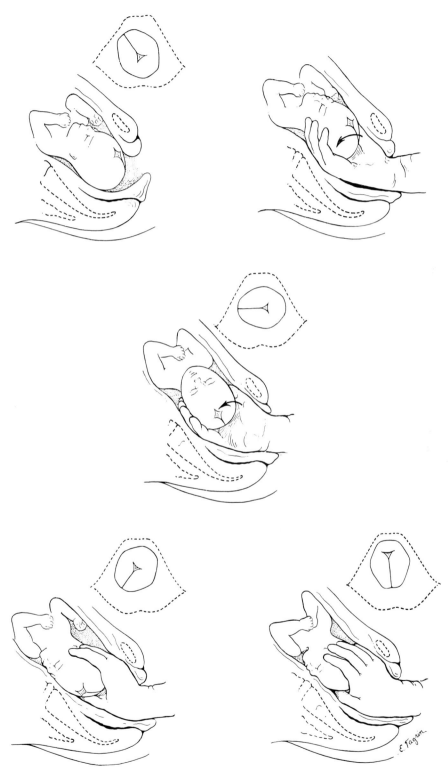

Figure 3. Manual rotation of persistent occiput posterior.

Application of the forceps in a case of left occiput posterior (L.O.P.) is illustrated in Figures 4 to 6. The forceps are applied as to right occiput anterior (R.O.A.) (Fig. 4). The vertex is now displaced upward to a level in the pelvis where it appears to rotate easily. This may be in the plane of greatest pelvic dimensions, approximately midway between the inlet and midpelvic plane, thus avoiding the impediment of the ischial spine; or it may mean that the vertex is displaced upward above the pelvic inlet and rotated. As depicted, the occiput is overcorrected into an R.O.A. position (Fig. 4D). This is to prevent the occiput from rotating backward to its original position during the reapplication of the forceps. To aid the vertex in maintaining its new position, mild suprafundic pressure is exerted by an assistant. The forceps, which are now upside down, are brought into normal relationship (Figs. 5 and 6). This consists

of removing what will be the right blade (Fig. 5B) and sweeping the left blade over the baby's face, which will tend to prevent the occiput from rotating back to an L.O.P. position. The right blade is reintroduced, both blades are adjusted as to an L.O.A. position (Fig. 6C), and the infant is extracted. (See Forceps Deliveries in Chapter 29.)

In summary, if the Scanzoni maneuver is used routinely in the management of occiput posterior position, the results compare favorably with manual rotation. The latter is not always successful, however. In fact, the space the forceps occupy in the vagina is less than that occupied by the operator's hand, and altogether the Scanzoni maneuver is preferred by some to manual rotation. The skillful performance of a Scanzoni maneuver, like that of any operation, depends on the operator's technical familiarity and experience with the procedure.

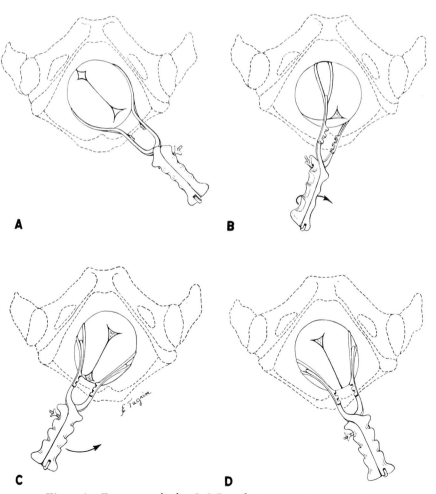

A　　　　　　　　**B**

C　　　　　　　　**D**

Figure 4.　Forceps applied to L.O.P. and rotation to R.O.A. position.

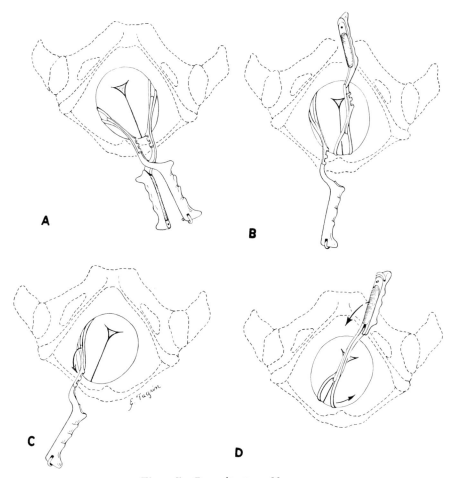

Figure 5. Reapplication of forceps.

PERSISTENT TRANSVERSE POSITION OF THE OCCIPUT

Until recent times, a so-called "transverse arrest" of the vertex had been regarded as a variant of an occiput posterior position in which only partial rotation had occurred. From observations of labor as depicted by stereoroentgenograms, it became evident that in the majority of cases a transverse arrest was a failure of rotation in a primary occiput transverse position. A transverse arrest of the occiput, should it occur in the gynecoid pelvis, rarely presents any special problem. Rotation is easily accomplished, and forceps extraction is not difficult. In the platypelloid or the android pelvis, however, delivery can be a formidable procedure, requiring experienced judgment and skillful operative technique. Certainly in the android pelvis there is always the possibility of midpelvic and outlet contracture. Consequently, the pelvis must be carefully

reevaluated at the time of delivery, because cesarean section is preferable to damage to the infant or serious injury to the maternal soft parts, the consequence of a difficult and ill advised forceps delivery.

It has been said authoritatively that to rotate a transverse arrest of the vertex to an occiput anterior position is advantageous, but only if the shape of the upper pelvis will allow it. It is implied that rotation must on occasion be performed low, especially in the android pelvis in which, at the inlet, there is a narrowing of the forepelvis. Moreover, when a transverse arrest occurs in this type of pelvis, it has been recommended that, to avoid the resistance to anterior rotation imposed by the midpelvis through its characteristic shallow posterior pelvic segment and prominent ischial spines, the vertex may be laterally flexed anteriorly toward the symphysis and by traction brought to the pelvic floor and rotated, utilizing the Barton forceps. This

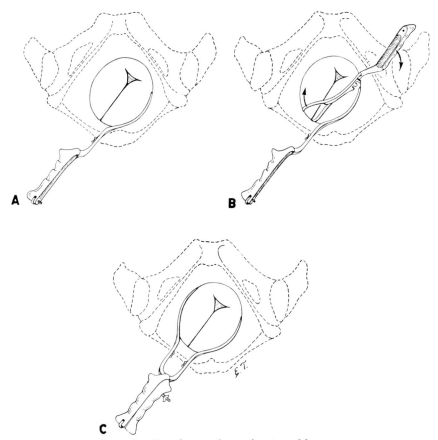

Figure 6.   Completion of reapplication of forceps.

method of management has tended to produce vault and lateral sulcus lacerations of the vagina, and these are compounded when anterior spiral rotation is attempted, as is sometimes advocated. *Rotation of the vertex at the time of traction can be very traumatic to the maternal soft parts under any circumstance.* In other words, first rotate, then exert traction, but never combine the two procedures. In principle, except in the platypelloid pelvis, the vertex is no longer rotated at or below the level of arrest, but rather at a higher station and, if need be, above the pelvic inlet. The fact that the vertex is engaged is adequate evidence that the anterior segment of the inlet is of sufficient size for the fetus, for otherwise engagement would not have occurred. In a discussion of labor in the parent types of pelves, it was suggested that the oblique diameters offer an index of the adequacy of the anterior segment of the pelvic inlet. Further, their distance from the pelvic side walls, as shown in Figure 2, would permit rotation above the ischial spines or

inlet, thus lessening the hazard of maternal trauma.

After rotation, the vertex is slowly brought into the pelvis through one of the oblique diameters. Through axis traction downward, in accordance with the direction of the pelvic axes, the head becomes flexed, and a point slightly anterior to the posterior fontanelle again becomes the leading point of the vertex. After the vertex has reached the lower pelvis and moved forward from the ischial spines, the occiput is gently rotated from the oblique to a direct anterior position. The head is then carefully and slowly extracted, being kept well flexed until the occiput is beyond the inferior border of the symphysis.

Perhaps the most important factor in the management of a transverse arrest in an android pelvis is not the exact method of delivery but rather that the physician appreciates the fact that the android pelvis is prone to midpelvic and outlet contracture. Also, despite different points of view, there is general agreement that, whether the occiput is posterior or transverse, no attempt should be made in the android pelvis to rotate the vertex in the midpelvis lest severe trauma ensue. In the platypelloid pelvis, however, the divergent bore and ample outlet permit anterior rotation at a low level; in fact, with an adequate episiotomy done prior to rotation, the lower it is performed, the better.

The delivery of an arrested transverse position demands a careful assessment of the pelvis to determine the safest method of management. Even when pelvic delivery has been anticipated, it is sometimes better judgment to consider abdominal delivery. (See Avoidance of Birth Trauma.) When pelvic delivery is elected, this is perhaps the one situation in which more than one type of forceps may be needed. Should the arch be Gothic in outline and the symphysis wide, owing to the deep cephalic curve of the Simpson type of forceps the operator may encounter difficulty in sweeping the anterior blade over the infant's face and bringing it in close apposition to the lambdoidal suture (Fig. 7). The forceps handle must be depressed posteriorly, and even then the broad symphysis may prevent movement of the anterior blade into its proper position. Forcing the forceps blade may traumatize the vaginal wall or cause the occiput to move posteriorly so that a satisfactory application is difficult to achieve. Further, the vertex may be asynclitic and molded in accordance with a posterior parietal bone presentation, and even at best the inferior margin of the anterior blade may be a bit forward, near the outer canthus of the baby's eye. This location is permissible for purposes of rotation, but the forceps must always be adjusted to a perfect application before extraction is attempted.

To surmount these difficulties, the Barton (Fig. 8) or Kjelland type of forceps is often used. It is recommended that, once the head is rotated, the Barton or Kjelland type of forceps should be replaced by axis-traction forceps for the extraction. The shallow cephalic curve of the Kjelland forceps permits the anterior blade to be introduced between the vertex and the symphysis with its cephalic curve uppermost (Fig. 9). With the blade so placed, it is rotated, and its superior margin comes to within a fingerbreadth of the upper lambdoidal suture. The posterior blade is applied, the handles approximated, and the vertex rotated in the manner described. Because of the shallow cephalic and pelvic curves, it is also possible to rotate the anterior blade of the Kjelland forceps around the occiput, as well as the face, and obtain a proper application.

At the beginning of the extraction after rotation, the lambdoidal sutures and the posterior fontanelle are barely palpable, being situated behind the symphysis, a finding consistent with some degree of extension. With traction downward in accordance with the directions of the superior and the inferior axis, the head will tend to flex and the posterior fontanelle is more readily palpated. After the vertex has reached the lower pelvis and has moved forward to the ischial spines, the occiput is rotated from the anterior oblique to a direct anterior position. The vertex is extracted in accordance with the technique of low forceps in an occiput anterior position. (See Forceps Deliveries in Chapter 29.)

AVOIDANCE OF BIRTH TRAUMA

The management of any dystocia problem revolves about the avoidance of trauma to either the baby or the mother. Difficult forceps operations with their hazard of both maternal and fetal trauma are performed less frequently than heretofore, and rightly so. Cesarean section has been made a safer procedure by improved anesthesia and the availability of antibiotics and chemotherapeutic drugs. Furthermore, x-ray studies of the pelvic architecture have made the forceps operation a more scientific procedure. The anatomic variations in the bony pelvis that can impede labor and possibly cause trauma at the time of delivery are now well understood.

At least four anatomic features of the human female pelvis deserve emphasis in the avoidance of traumatic pelvic delivery. These include the position and direction of the pelvic axes, the influence of the position of the sacrococcygeal platform, the location of the tip of the sacrum as it may influence the available space in the midpelvic and outlet planes, and, finally, whether the inferior strait or the inferior plane more nearly reflects the size of the pelvic outlet.

First, and briefly, the pelvic axis is not a continuous affair, but rather is a composite of two separate entities in both location and direction, an important consideration in

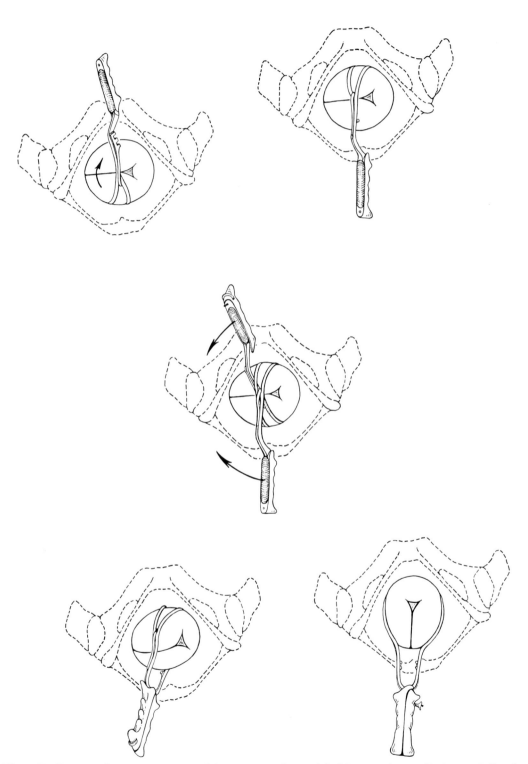

Figure 7. Rotation of a transverse arrest of the occiput with a modified Simpson forceps (Irving type). Note how the forceps handle of the anterior blade must be depressed to facilitate sweeping the blade into proper position. Vertex is displaced upward prior to rotation.

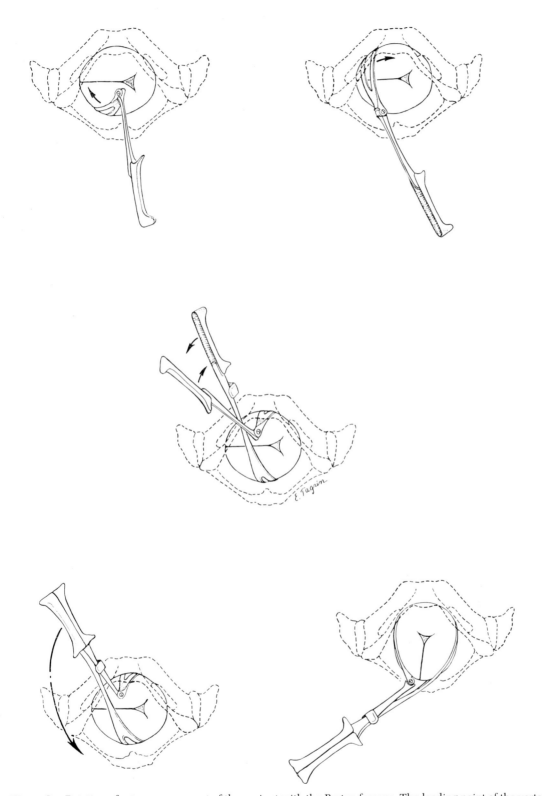

Figure 8. Rotation of a transverse arrest of the occiput with the Barton forceps. The leading point of the vertex is deliberately depicted midway between the ischial spines and the perineum to emphasize the difficulty of placing the anterior blade of the forceps in the proper position. Following rotation, the Barton forceps is removed and a Simpson type forceps is applied for extraction of the fetus.

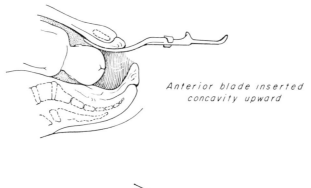

*Anterior blade inserted
concavity upward*

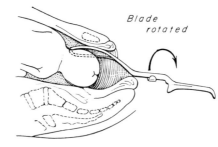

*Blade
rotated*

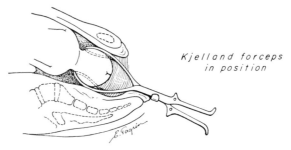

*Kjelland forceps
in position*

Figure 9.

directing the presenting part through the birth canal in the course of operative delivery.

Second, in a normal pelvis, the sacrococcygeal platform or lower third or fourth of the sacrum, including the coccyx, is well posterior, as indicated by an angle of 90 degrees or more formed by a line drawn from the inferior edge of the symphysis to the sacral promontory and from the latter to the tip of the sacrum. An angle of less than 90 degrees (Fig. 10) means a convergent bore; this, however, may be readily offset in its implication by a sacrum that normally ends low in the pelvis, that is, at or below the ischial tuberosities (Fig. 11).

Third, if the sacrum ends high, that is, well above the ischial tuberosities, midpelvic or outlet contracture, or both, is likely to be encountered (Fig. 12). A sac-

rum that ends high, however, may be offset by a divergent pelvic bore (Fig. 13).

The location of the pelvic planes, as drawn in the lateral Thoms x-ray film, can reflect the relationship between the position of the end of the sacrum and the ischial spines and tuberosities, which in turn are concerned with the problems surrounding midpelvic or outlet contracture and the ease or difficulty of labor and delivery. The cases are presented to illustrate these anatomic features and relationships as they may affect the course of labor and delivery. Even if the sacrum is set forward, that is, at an angle of less than 90 degrees, the fact that it is long and ends at or below the ischial spines will permit the vertex to descend to the perineum and permit it to take full advantage of the space available at the outlet. By contrast, if the sacrum ends

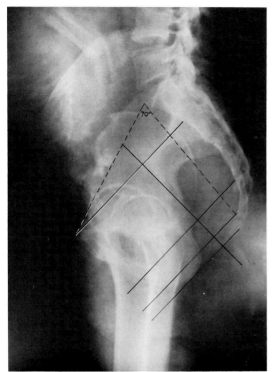

Figure 10. Android pelvis (77 per cent midpelvic capacity—Mengert). (Parallel lines represent parallel planes of the pelvis as described in Chapter 24.) Convergent bore. Sacrum ends well above the ischial tuberosities. Short first stage of labor; prolonged second stage. Firm low midforceps—infant 7 lb. No sequelae. Future delivery: prognosis guarded. (From Reid, D. E., J. Obst. & Gynaec. Brit. Emp., 66:709, 1959.)

well above the ischial tuberosities, the vertex will fail to bypass the sacrococcygeal platform and descend to the perineum (Fig. 12). Bringing the vertex downward to the perineum (by axis-traction forceps) may require considerable force, particularly if the sacrum is forward, with the possibility of severe trauma to the mother and the fetus.

As the fourth feature deserving emphasis, it is concluded that the adequacy of the outlet is determined by the flare of the arch and the length of the bi-ischial and the posterior sagittal diameter as the latter relates to the level of the sacral tip, rather than by the length of the anteroposterior diameter of the inferior strait. Further, all of these relationships and landmarks are discernible clinically, and x-ray examination of the outlet is unnecessary despite the insistence of some.

Regardless of the fact that the pelvis is thought to be normal on antepartal examination, in some cases the method of delivery will remain in doubt even after many hours

of labor. These include the few patients with a borderline pelvis or functional dystocia, or both, who it is anticipated can be delivered pelvically but who fail to make the progress expected in the latter hours of labor. Reexamination of the midpelvis and outlet, and an estimation of the size of the fetal vertex by pelvic examination with the patient anesthetized will afford the information necessary for the clinician to choose the correct procedure. The question to be answered is simply: What is the safest method of delivery for the mother and her infant? In the extreme, the choice can be between a midforceps procedure, with or without forceps rotation or Dührssen's incisions, in the presence of borderline midpelvic or outlet contracture, and a cesarean section on a patient who has experienced a long labor and may be potentially infected. This infrequent but extremely important group includes those in whom the fetus is more likely to be damaged by ill-advised forceps delivery through previous failure to identify midpelvic and outlet contracture. Examination should be conducted in the operating room, which has been made ready for either pelvic or abdominal delivery and the anesthesia planned accordingly. In this clinic this preparation is

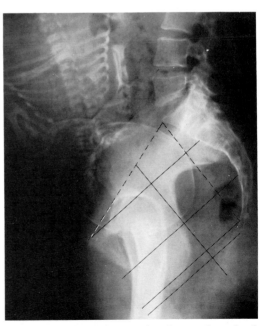

Figure 11. Small gynecoid pelvis with android forepelvis (84 per cent midpelvic capacity—Mengert). Sacrum ends low, at the ischial tuberosities. Hence, easy low forceps—8 lb. 2 oz. infant. (From Reid, D. E., J. Obst. & Gynaec. Brit. Emp., 66:709, 1959.)

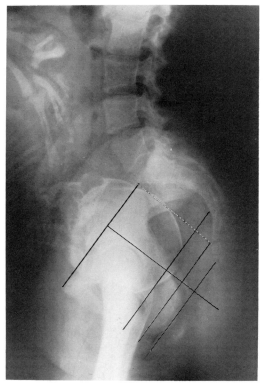

Figure 12. Small gynecoid pelvis. Obstetric conjugate 10.2 cm. (100 per cent midpelvic capacity— Mengert). Regarded originally as an inlet problem, but because the *sacrum ends extremely high* the problem is that of midpelvic contracture. Roman type arch. Twenty-three hours' labor with Pitocin stimulation; "double set-up" examination; vertex +1–2 station; extraperitoneal cesarean section—9 lb. infant. (From Reid, D. E., J. Obst. & Gynaec. Brit. Emp., 66:709, 1959.)

referred to as a "double set-up" procedure. A trial forceps is sometimes attempted; if forceps delivery seems contraindicated after careful reassessment of the pelvis, abdominal delivery can be performed forthwith. When these preparations are not made and the patient is managed in the case room, there is the tendency to deliver the patient pelvically, even when it is unwise to do so.

FETAL DISTRESS

The term "fetal distress" is synonymous with fetal hypoxia, a condition that is associated with a variety of obstetric complications. It is an illusive, all-encompassing term, filled at the clinical level with innumerable paradoxical situations.

In discussing the assessment of the infant at birth, it was implied that a precise definition of what constitutes intrauterine as-

phyxia of the newborn is still to be formulated. Every obstetrician has had the experience on more than a single occasion of performing a cesarean section for fetal distress and having the baby scream lustily as soon as it was extracted from the uterus, when prior to or during labor the fetal heart rate without demonstrable cause had dropped below 100 beats per minute and the amniotic fluid was heavily stained with meconium. In other cases, under almost identical conditions, the infant at delivery has shown severe asphyxia pallida, was limp and pale, and failed to respond to the usual stimuli. These preliminary remarks are made to familiarize the student with the vagaries of fetal distress, and to give some indication of how difficult it is for the clinician to decide on the proper method of management. Without question, subjecting a mother to the risk of an operative delivery for an infant who has received irreversible central nervous system damage is a most remorseful experience.

Deliberateness but not procrastination

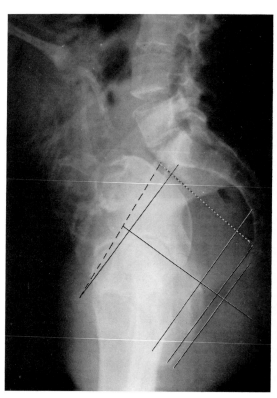

Figure 13. Anthropoid pelvis. A divergent bore, as indicated by the large sacrosciatic notch which compensates for a sacrum ending at a rather high level, as seen by the third pelvic plane located well above the ischial tuberosities. Low forceps delivery—8 lb. 2 oz. infant.

might well be the rule for the clinical management of fetal distress.

As a guide to clinical treatment, intrauterine asphyxia might usefully be classified into either acute or chronic forms. In the latter there would be such conditions as pregnancy toxemia, diabetes mellitus, Rh incompatibility, and postmaturity or dysmaturity with placental dysfunction. The acute form of asphyxia occurs in cases of late pregnancy bleeding or it develops in the course of labor and delivery, especially with compression of the cord and a decrease of intervillous blood flow.

In the conditions listed under the chronic form, there is literally a race between fetal medical maturity and death in utero from intrauterine asphyxia. Here the clinician is constantly confronted with the question of whether premature birth gives the fetus a better chance for survival than remaining in utero (see Assessment of the Fetus in Utero in Chapter 23).

The patient often volunteers the information that the baby seemed unusually active for a period, and then became rather quiet. Granted, this is purely a subjective symptom, but it is deserving of attention, particularly in the conditions listed under the causes of chronic asphyxia. Also, in the course of routinely checking the fetal heart tones, a bradycardia or irregularity is a chance finding that may portend fetal disaster.

If, after an evaluation of the estimated fetal size in relation to the gestational age and of the obstetric and medical factors surrounding the case, the decision is reached to deliver the patient, this should be done immediately. Cases can be recalled in which the fetal heart tones disappeared some hours after delivery had been decided on but the procedure had been postponed until the following day for reasons of operating room time or convenience.

Turning now to the question of acute fetal distress encountered in labor, it is recalled that the fetal heart rate often increases by 10 to 30 beats over the normal range of 130 to 150 beats per minute in the course of a normal uterine contraction. (See Chapter 26, Conduct of Normal Labor.) As the head enters the pelvis, it is not uncommon for the fetal heart rate to misbehave for a time, particularly in an occiput posterior position, presumably from pressure on the occiput as it bypasses the sacral promontory. Once the vertex negotiates the inlet, the fetal heart rate will become steady and return to normal rate. In an occasional case, however, the fetal heart rate will become truly pathologic as the vertex descends deeper into the pelvis, perhaps as a result of tightening of the umbilical cord about the neck or shoulder, or because of its prolapse, or as a result of a state of insufficiency of intervillous blood flow.

From the extensive studies on fetal heart rates, there should be general agreement that fetal distress exists when the fetal heart rate falls below 100 beats per minute and certainly when it drops into the low range of the 60s late in the course of the uterine contraction and the bradycardia persists for a half minute or more. Marked tachycardia of 180 beats or more per minute also is undoubtedly an ominous finding.

Placing the patient on her side and in the Trendelenburg position may improve the fetal heart rate, presumably by removing pressure on the inferior vena cava. Administration of oxygen (6 L. per minute) to the mother is conventional treatment. If oxytocin therapy is being used, this should be stopped. If the contractions are prolonged and are tetanic in character, some form of inhalation anesthesia should be considered.

Preferably the patient should be in the operating room, which is in readiness for an immediate cesarean section.

If the fetal heart rate fails to return to a normal range, the patient should be quickly anesthetized and rapidly prepared and draped, and a vaginal examination should be performed to determine if there is any obvious cause for the fetal distress. If the cervix is 4 cm. or more dilated, the examining hand can enter the lower uterine segment and ascertain whether or not the umbilical cord is by chance alongside the vertex, a so-called occult prolapse, in contrast to a frank prolapse, where the cord is found in the vagina. If the degree of cervical dilatation permits, the hand may explore upward to see if the cord is coiled about the fetal neck. During the examination, auscultation of the fetal heart tones should be continuous to determine if they have responded favorably to oxygen administration and upward displacement of the presenting part. If there is no evidence of prolapse or entanglement of the umbilical cord, it must be decided whether to permit the patient to awaken and allow labor to resume or to perform an immediate cesarean section. The decision rests primarily on the degree of cervical dilatation and the parity of the patient.

If a conservative policy is elected, it is envisioned that after one or two hours of labor the patient will reach the second stage and can be delivered pelvically with comparative ease. This usually means that the patient is a multipara with an uneventful past obstetric history, and that the cervix is at least half dilated at the time of the vaginal examination. The patient is kept in the operating room throughout the remainder of her labor, with constant observation and frequent auscultation of the fetal heart tones. Oxygen administration is continued with the patient in mild Trendelenburg position. In a few instances, if the fetal distress is mounting, it may be reasonable to deliver the patient with forceps, with the aid of Dührssen's incisions, before the second stage is reached. If the fetal heart fails to return to an acceptable rate, or if it continues to fall below 100 beats per minute with each contraction, and the patient does not make the anticipated progress in labor, the physician is justified in performing a cesarean section. He must accept the fact that all too often a reason for the fetal distress will not be found.

An additional word is needed concerning the treatment of a patient with prolapse of the cord. This accident occurs with a frequency of about 1 in 200 deliveries, being more common when the presentation is other than a vertex, or when the vertex is unengaged. The prolapse is more likely to occur in conjunction with rupture of the fetal membranes, although the cord may be found between the vertex and the intact membranes. The immediate management is the same as that outlined above for fetal distress. When cervical dilatation is insufficient to permit pelvic delivery, and the fetus is regarded to be in reasonably good condition, immediate transperitoneal lower segment cesarean section is indicated. In the multiparous patient, with the cervix 6 to 8 cm. dilated, the use of Dührssen's incisions and forceps delivery is permissible. Attempt to replace the cord is of questionable worth.

IMPACTION OF THE SHOULDERS

Having delivered the vertex, usually by forceps, the physician is confronted suddenly with the problem of impacted shoulders. This can be a dangerous complication to the mother as well as to the infant. The mother must never be placed in jeopardy in an attempt to deliver the infant alive, for when the mother is subjected to serious trauma the fetus rarely escapes unscathed. Mothers have been lost by frantic attempts to deliver the child alive. Excessive abdominal uterine and suprasymphyseal pressure may cause rupture of the lower uterine segment. Undue traction on the infant's neck can result in permanent damage to the brachial plexuses (Erb's palsy) or dislocation of the cervical vertebrae leading to spinal cord damage and sometimes death. Once an airway is established for the infant, at least 10 to 15 minutes is available for completion of the delivery without great danger to the infant.

Reference was made in Chapter 26, Conduct of Normal Labor, to the fact that delivery of the shoulders is facilitated by placing the hand against the posterior shoulder and rotating it directly posterior, causing the anterior shoulder to impinge beneath the symphysis. If the shoulders then assume an anterior-posterior position, gentle traction on the vertex and moderate suprafundic pressure should result in birth of the anterior shoulder. If this fails, the hand is passed beyond the vertex, and the posterior arm and hand are identified. The hand and arm are swept over the infant's chest in a wide arc and delivered, thereby releasing and permitting delivery of the posterior shoulder. There is some risk that the humerus may be fractured by this maneuver, but such injury can be readily treated. If one is unable to deliver the posterior arm and shoulder, cutting of the anterior clavicle should be considered. This procedure may be lifesaving, assuming that the subclavian vessels escape damage. Cleidotomy markedly reduces the size of the shoulder girdle, thus relieving the impaction. The clavicle heals readily without deformity. In fact, in the course of normal delivery spontaneous fracture of the clavicle occurs more frequently than is probably appreciated, with no residual disability even when it is undetected and untreated.

The difficulty encountered in the delivery of a large infant is usually with the shoulders and not with the vertex, for with the vertex the question is one of cephalopelvic relationship, generally at the inlet, and the case is managed accordingly. Excessively large infants are proudly reported when they are delivered successfully, but actually the fetal morbidity and mortality are significantly increased in pelvic delivery when the weight of the fetus exceeds 4500 grams.

AMNIOTIC FLUID EMBOLISM

Maternal death during labor occurs infrequently when compared with the number of deaths during pregnancy, delivery, and the puerperium. Of the few deaths that do occur in labor, however, amniotic fluid embolism is a major cause. The chief clinical signs are sudden dyspnea and cyanosis, and whenever these appear in a patient in labor the diagnosis should be suspected. The predisposing factors in the causation of this syndrome are tetanic uterine contractions and multiparity, often associated with an exceedingly large infant. Patients may die undelivered, with the classic signs and symptoms of embolism, and those who survive the initial shock may succumb from postpartum hemorrhage. When there is vaginal bleeding it is attributed to atony of the uterus secondary to shock, but this can be an erroneous assumption.

Widespread embolization of the pulmonary arterioles and capillaries by particulate matter contained in amniotic fluid is believed responsible for the essential pathologic lesions. When fatal cases are reviewed, however, two observations demand explanation. One is that in most instances the amount of mechanical blockage of the pulmonary vessels by amniotic debris is hardly sufficient to be the cause of death. The other is the finding that the blood is liquid at postmortem examination, and clotting of any degree in the large vessels is rarely seen. One must hasten to add that such a finding may be observed in cases of sudden death, regardless of its cause. It appears, therefore, that death in this syndrome cannot always be explained by the effects of embolism alone. Should the patient survive her original vascular insult, she may develop a hemorrhagic diathesis.

Uncontaminated amniotic fluid contains a substance that behaves like thromboplastin. The fluid has the ability to reduce the clotting time of hemophilic blood. Thus, death in this syndrome may result from extensive intravascular clotting and subsequent postpartum hemorrhage. Clot forma-

tion is deficient at the uteroplacental site, more specifically in the decidual arterioles, and a lethal postpartum hemorrhage can eventuate. (See discussion of Coagulation Defects in Chapter 18.)

The fact that in most instances the syndrome occurs near the end of the first stage of labor suggests that a certain set of circumstances must exist for its development, including both an available portal of escape and the forceful ejection of amniotic fluid from the uterus. Two avenues of entrance of amniotic fluid into the maternal circulation may be postulated.

The commonly accepted route involves rupture of the membranes somewhere in the upper segment of the uterus, with eventual escape of fluid through the uteroplacental site. Amniotic fluid has been identified between the amnion and the chorion, in the placental margin, the decidual sinusoids, and the myometrial veins. Following rupture of the fetal membranes, the amniotic fluid may accumulate between the membranes and the uterine wall, and may reach the placental margin to enter the venous sinusoids and the systemic circulation. The process is apparently expedited by vigorous uterine contractions. The escape of the fluid from the uterus is enhanced by those conditions in which the myometrial veins or sinuses are exposed, as in marginal separation of the placenta, rupture of the uterus, and hysterotomy, especially of the lower segment type.

The second mode of escape of amniotic fluid is through the endocervical veins. These blood channels become lacerated during normal labor and account for the appearance of "bloody show." Since the upper portion of the cervix becomes completely incorporated within the lower uterine segment during labor, some of the endocervical veins are also included in it. When the fetal membranes rupture the endocervical veins may become exposed, allowing the amniotic fluid to come in contact with them. Were the fetal vertex to tamponade the cervix, intrauterine pressure as the result of labor might increase sufficiently to permit the trapped fluid to enter the exposed endocervical veins of the lower uterine segment.

The most significant contributing factor would appear to be tumultuous and exceedingly rapid labor. The improper administration of oxytocin preparations may contribute to the production of amniotic fluid

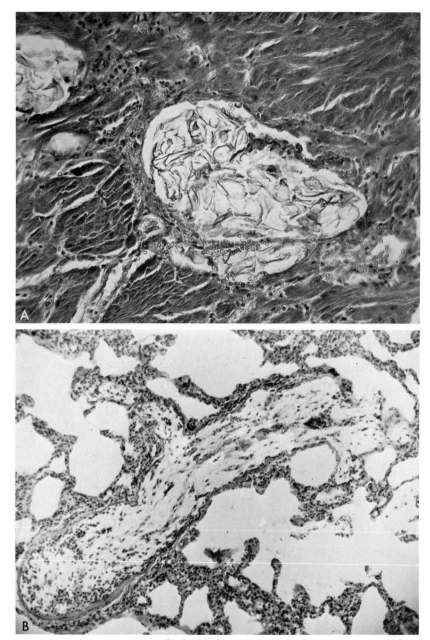

Figure 14. Pathologic findings in amniotic fluid embolism. A, Squames in uterine vein. B, Squames in lungs.

infusion through the medium of vigorous labor.

The treatment of amniotic fluid embolism is preventive, supportive, and definitive. Turbulent labor, whether originating spontaneously or stimulated by oxytocin, may be counteracted by administration of ether to near-anesthetic levels.

The belief that amniotic fluid embolism is invariably fatal would indicate that any treatment is futile. It is true that in the event of a large infusion of amniotic fluid death

often follows within half an hour from the onset of symptoms. Although some patients with this condition will die, prompt and energetic treatment will enable others to survive. Initially, the treatment is directed toward the relief of respiratory distress. Even when the case is apparently hopeless, the patient occasionally rallies, and further treatment may be rewarding. In these patients, the therapy must be directed toward prevention of death from a coagulation defect. In the interim, the fetus is in grave jeopardy, and an immediate sterile vaginal examination should be performed. The cervix will often be found completely or nearly completely dilated, and a forceps operation may salvage the fetus and reduce the mother's respiratory obligations. The vagina and the uterus should be quickly explored to exclude any possibility of lacerations or uterine rupture as cause of the bleeding.

Recovery will depend ultimately on maintenance of the normal blood volume. In addition to adequate blood replacement, the treatment must include, without undue delay, the restoration of the clotting mechanism to normal. (See Coagulation Defects in Chapter 18.)

PATHOLOGIC RETRACTION RING (BANDL'S RING)

A pathologic retraction ring is infrequent in current obstetric practice, for it means that there has been some negligence in the conduct of labor, and the patient has been exposed to an excessively prolonged labor from either functional or mechanical dystocia.

The considerable controversy surrounding the topic is concerned primarily with whether a muscular ring can develop in any area other than at the junction of the upper and the lower uterine segment, and, if so, whether it has the same clinical significance. Review of the pertinent literature, however, discloses that there is only one type of pathologic uterine ring and this always develops at the anatomic internal os. The student must be aware that this conclusion is at variance with some that are expressed, and that the confusion has been compounded by differences in nomenclature.

A retraction ring is more likely to occur in neglected cases of cephalopelvic disproportion; it can also be encountered in functional dystocia with extremely long labor, especially if the membranes have been ruptured for any great length of time. In either event, when a retraction ring is suspected the uterus may be in danger of imminent rupture, and the patient shows anxiety and signs of exhaustion. Palpation of the abdomen reveals what is obviously an attenuated lower uterine segment, which is often quite tender. As the examining hand moves upward over the uterus, it may or may not encounter a transverse bandlike structure. Whether the baby is alive or dead, the patient has reached a state where she should be delivered by the safest means.

When question of a retraction ring arises, the patient should be managed in the operating room with preparations for either pelvic or abdominal delivery. The anesthesia chosen must provide maximal relaxation of the uterus. After the patient is properly prepared, diagnosis can be established by passing the examining hand well into the uterus to the junction of the upper and the lower segment. If a retraction ring is present, a ridge of tissue will be found tightly encompassing the fetus. Its location will be gauged by the station of the presenting part, but it is usually found about the fetal neck.

Various pharmacologic agents have been suggested as a means of relaxing the ring, but all are of questionable value. Abdominal delivery is less hazardous than pelvic delivery unless the fetus is dead and the cervix is near full dilatation to permit embryotomy. At cesarean section, the ring must be incised before the fetus is extracted, lest uterine rupture occur. This demands a vertical incision, for when the band is incised it immediately disappears. The likelihood of uterine infection from prolonged rupture of the fetal membranes also must be given consideration in patient management.

RUPTURE OF THE UTERUS

Rupture of the uterus is one of the most serious accidents encountered in obstetric practice. The complication may develop during pregnancy or in labor; it may be spontaneous or traumatic; it may occur in an intact uterus, or in one that has previously been subjected to incision, either cesarean section or, in very rare instances, myomectomy.

In the past two decades the overall incidence has remained fairly constant, but there has been a relative change in the percentage of ruptures attributed to particular causes. Rupture of the uterus due to obstetric trauma has shown a marked decrease. This is the result of the policy of not permitting unproductive labor to continue indefinitely, the use of x-ray pelvimetry to verify the clinical impression of cephalopelvic disproportion, the elimination of hazardous obstetric maneuvers, such as manual dilatation of the cervix or ill advised internal podalic version, and the more frequent use of abdominal hysterotomy when difficult pelvic delivery is anticipated. The resultant increase in the incidence of cesarean section, however, accounts for failure of the overall incidence of uterine rupture to decrease significantly. In other words, the major cause of uterine rupture currently is a previous cesarean section scar.

Rupture of the intact uterus during pregnancy is extremely rare. It may occur in the rudimentary horn of a double uterus because of failure to adapt to the growth and distention necessary to contain the developing fetus. Cases have also been encountered in which adenomyosis has caused pathologic thinning of the uterine wall. The most frequent cause of spontaneous rupture of the intact uterus is labor, especially when obstructed. Besides cephalopelvic disproportion and abnormal presentation, excessive cervical scar tissue resulting from a previous labor and delivery may cause rupture of the cervix extending into the lower uterine segment, particularly when the labor is tumultuous. Oxytocin stimulation may also cause rupture of the uterus by precipitating violent uterine contractions. Excluding those occurring in cesarean section scars, spontaneous ruptures begin in the lower uterine segment and commonly extend into the corpus (Fig. 15). When rupture occurs in a cesarean section scar, the type of the operation will determine the location and direction of the laceration.

Spontaneous rupture of a previous cesarean section scar may be either overt or si-

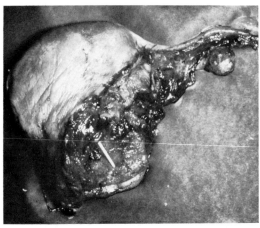

Figure 15. Spontaneous rupture of the uterus in labor, beginning in the lower segment and extending upward along the side of the uterus. At operation baby and placenta were found extruded into the abdomen.

lent, silent rupture being referred to as dehiscence and being discovered incidentally at repeat cesarean section. (See Cesarean Section in Chapter 29.) Overt rupture is nearly always associated with the so-called classic type of cesarean section. The onset is usually sudden and without warning, with a clinical picture of sudden abdominal pain and shock from intraperitoneal hemorrhage, with or without some vaginal bleeding. Rupture may occur at any time during pregnancy, but is rarely observed before the third trimester.

The silent rupture, or dehiscence, is found at repeat cesarean section, becoming visible after the bladder has been displaced downward, exposing the lower uterine segment. The chorion sac and its contents are readily seen through the defect. The involved area of disruption may vary from 2 to 3 cm. long to a length that will allow delivery of the presenting part without further incision of the lower uterine segment.

Impending rupture may be suspected when in prolonged or obstructive labor there is increasing tenderness over the lower uterine segment. The uterine contractions are prolonged and tetanic in character, and the uterus fails to relax appreciably between contractions. Rupture itself is signaled by a sharp stabbing pain over the lower uterus, with a sensation of something giving way. This is followed by a cessation of contractions and the disappearance of pain. The fetal heart tones are soon lost, and the patient exhibits signs of shock. The fetus may be extruded from the uterus and become palpable. Vaginal bleeding may be considerable or comparatively slight.

Traumatic rupture of the intact uterus can occur when an ill timed or an inappropriate operation is attempted to effect delivery. Application of forceps and extraction of the fetal vertex or of a breech before the cervical os has dilated completely can result in uterine rupture. If delivery is mandatory, it is much wiser and safer to incise the cervix (Dührssen's incisions). The performance of an internal podalic version after the fetal membranes have been ruptured for a period of time, with loss of the amniotic fluid permitting the uterus to contract tightly about the fetus, is an invitation to uterine rupture. In addition, a vigorous attempt to deliver the head of a hydrocephalic infant without first decompressing it by intraventricular tap or some other means may result in uterine rupture. Finally, excessive suprafundic pressure in a desperate attempt to deliver impacted shoulders may cause the uterus to rupture. In the course of intrauterine or intracervical manipulation, the operator may feel the uterus give way. Otherwise, the signs and symptoms of traumatic rupture at delivery may not be immediately apparent. As in spontaneous rupture, the patient soon shows the clinical signs of shock and blood loss, and evidence of intra-abdominal hemorrhage.

The maternal prognosis is guarded, especially in uterine rupture of traumatic origin. Even with present-day treatment, the mortality is in the neighborhood of 5 to 10 per cent, but this is a far cry from the mortality of 25 per cent or more of only a few decades ago. The prognosis for the fetus is grave, for it often dies of asphyxia prior to delivery, or suffers permanent damage from the effects of hypoxia.

The treatment begins with the prevention of spontaneous rupture of the uterus, which can be accomplished largely by accurate evaluation of the maternal pelvis and the fetal position before labor, and the avoidance of prolonged labor. After rupture has occurred, whether it be spontaneous or traumatic, the treatment is immediate abdominal hysterectomy. One or two venous cut-downs are invaluable for ensuring that adequate amounts of blood may be delivered to the patient. The patient's condition may be temporarily precarious, and a supracervical rather than a complete hysterectomy may be the better choice. The basic objective is to obtain complete hemostasis at the earliest moment by the easiest and quickest means. Even if the cervix is lacerated, it can be sutured abdominally in the course of a supracervical hysterectomy. (See Cesarean Hysterectomy in Chapter 29.) Difficulty in identifying the uterine vessels is not unusual, particularly in a transverse rupture. If the uterine vessels are disrupted, they tend to retract deeply into the broad ligament. The presence of a hematoma may compound the problem. Ligation of the hypogastric arteries should be considered, even preliminary to hysterectomy.

ANNULAR DETACHMENT OF THE CERVIX

Because patients are no longer subjected to prolonged tests of labor as in previous eras, annular detachment of the cervix is indeed rare today. Seldom is the detachment complete, but rather the cervix is usually found to be 3 or 4 cm. dilated, with a portion still attached at the cervicovaginal junction. The detachment supposedly occurs through ischemic necrosis produced by pressure of the presenting part against the walls of the pelvis. So insidious is its development that the physician is not forewarned by bleeding from the detached area. In fact, very little bleeding occurs when the remainder of the cervix is excised, and a few mattress sutures will suffice to control whatever ooze there may be. Delivery can be completed, assuming that the pelvis is normal; however, in some cases cephalopelvic disproportion necessitates cesarean section.

The patient's outlook for future childbearing contains an element of uncertainty, because she has in essence a high amputation of the cervix. Abortion and premature labor are a threat. Although patients have been successfully delivered pelvically in subsequent pregnancies, cesarean section to avoid rupture of the lower uterine segment would seem a more prudent procedure, particularly when one considers that the patient has been fortunate to retain the fetus until it reaches a stage of medical viability.

THE RETAINED PLACENTA

The problem of retained placenta affords a situation that serves to illustrate what is meant by the necessity of providing maximal safeguards for the parturient. Retention of the placenta must be regarded as a complication of delivery with a risk that has been only partially removed through the chemotherapeutic control of infection, the latter being a possibility whenever the uterus is invaded. Obviously, in the presence of an alarming hemorrhage from partial separation of the placenta during the third stage of labor, manual removal must be performed immediately. When the placenta fails to separate spontaneously, and the degree of bleeding is such that the patient is not in immediate danger from hemorrhage, one should consider a more deliberate and planned method of management.

Although the bleeding may be only slight, indefinite delay in the hope that the placenta will eventually deliver itself is accompanied by a rise in the morbidity rate. Thus,

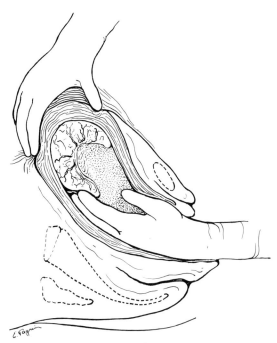

Figure 16. Schematic drawing showing manual removal of the placenta.

PLACENTA ACCRETA

Placenta accreta is the union of the placenta and the myometrium through a lack of the normal amount or a complete absence of the decidua (Fig. 17). The condition is encountered more often when implantation occurs in the lower uterine segment or in the region of the cornua where the decidua is normally less luxuriant. Previous manual removal of the placenta, abortion, curettage, and endometritis are predisposing factors in the etiology of placenta accreta, presumably through interference with normal decidua formation. In many cases, however, the reproductive history is entirely normal.

The placenta may be only contiguous to the myometrium or it may actually invade it. Further, all or portions of the maternal surface of the placenta may be attached to the myometrium. Thus, placenta accreta may be classified according to the amount of the maternal surface of the placenta that is involved and, if the placental tissue invades the myometrium, the depth to which

within 30 to 60 minutes after delivery of the infant preparations should be made to remove the placenta in the operating room under the so-called "double set-up" procedure, with the realization that laparotomy will rarely be necessary. Hindsight in most instances would indicate that these tedious details could be dispensed with, but they are more than justified in the rare case of placenta accreta in which the control of hemorrhage depends on immediate hysterectomy.

After the patient is anesthetized, before exploration the uterus should be compressed (Credé maneuver) in an attempt to dislodge the placenta. If this fails, the placenta should be removed by placing the hand into the uterus and establishing a line of cleavage through the spongiosa layer of the decidua. *The outside hand should compress the uterus into the pelvis*, for one must be prepared to reach the top of the fundus and the cornua, which is where the placenta is commonly located when it fails to separate. A line of cleavage being established, it is usually not difficult to free the placenta (Fig. 16). Once the placenta is extracted, the uterus is reexplored to make certain that no placental tissue remains.

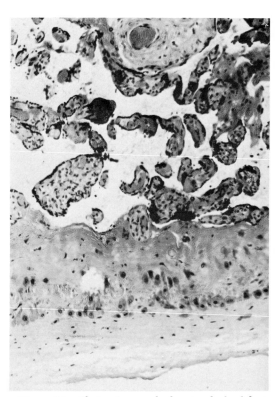

Figure 17. Photomicrograph showing lack of decidua in placenta accreta in the lower uterine segment in a patient with placenta praevia, who died because hysterectomy was not performed immediately.

invasion occurs. A complete placenta accreta involves the entire maternal surface. This type is extremely rare. More common are the partial type, which includes several cotyledons, and the focal type, which involves one cotyledon only. When the placental tissue invades the myometrium it is referred to as a "placenta increta." In "placenta percreta" the invasion extends to the covering serosa (Fig. 18A); this is seen more often when implantation occurs over the site of a previous cesarean section incision and, in fact, contributes to uterine rupture by weakening the scar.

The wide variation in incidence of the condition is due perhaps to the fact that only the complete and the partial types are considered; or, if it is the policy of the particular clinic to treat the partial or the focal type by removing the placental tissue piecemeal by placental forceps, these cases may be diagnosed as "adherent" placenta rather than as placenta accreta.

The diagnosis of placenta accreta is made when a line of cleavage cannot be established between the uterine wall and the placenta in the course of manual removal, and it is verified by subsequent histologic examination (see Fig. 17). Although some obstetricians try to preserve the uterus in the partial or the focal type, the treatment is immediate supracervical hysterectomy, regardless of the type. One must ask whether the occasional maternal death from postpartum hemorrhage and shock associated with manual removal was, in reality, due to a partial or a focal placenta accreta (Fig. 18B). Certainly furious hemorrhage may ensue when the placental tissue is forcefully removed, with fragmentation and exposure of the adjacent myometrial sinusoids. Further, many late postpartum hemorrhages, attributed to what is referred to as a "placental polyp," are in fact due to a previously unrecognized partial or focal type of placenta accreta. Here, again, attempts to dislodge this tissue by curettage or placental forceps may be met by a hemorrhage of such serious proportions that it can be controlled only by immediate abdominal hysterectomy. The bleeding that brings the patient to the hospital may be due to subinvolution of the placental site created by presence of a focal accreta or placental polyp (Fig. 18B). This is in contradistinction to the hemorrhage that may ensue when the polyp is forcefully removed.

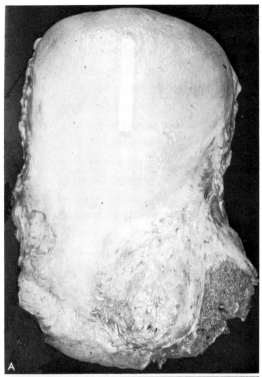

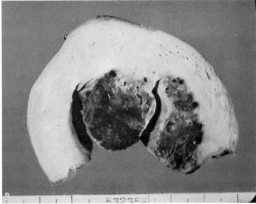

Figure 18. Types of placenta accreta. A, Uterus reveals placenta percreta. B, Cross-section of uterus, showing focal placenta accreta (? placental polyp). Note large caliber of blood vessels at base of the accreta. On right, subinvolution of the placental site with no placental tissue present on histologic examination. Hysterectomy five weeks post partum. (Courtesy of Dr. William Ober and Dr. Hugh Grady.)

INVERSION OF THE UTERUS

Inversion of the uterus is a rare but serious complication of the third stage of labor and the puerperium. It is generally taught that mismanagement of the third stage of labor is an important etiologic factor. Many cases of puerperal inversion of the uterus, however, occur when the placental stage has been entirely normal. Consequently, it has been suggested that routine vaginal examination should follow delivery if uterine inversion is to be detected early. Since this is not included in the prescribed techniques for the conduct of delivery, a certain number of cases are not recognized until some hours or days later.

Inversion of the uterus may be suspected when shock suddenly appears without appreciable blood loss. Shock is apparently precipitated by irritation of the serosal surface of the uterus resulting from the inversion. The definitive diagnosis is made on abdominal palpation and vaginal examination. One is unable to outline the uterine corpus abdominally, and, in the extreme, there may actually be a dimpling effect identified at the junction of the upper and lower uterine segment. With proper exposure the inverted uterus can be visualized vaginally.

It seems evident that no one method of management can suffice. These cases can be classified as follows: (1) an *acute inversion* is discovered before there is cervical ring formation, that is, in the course of the third and fourth stages of labor; (2) *subacute inversion* is diagnosed after the cervical ring has formed; and (3) *chronic inversion* includes all those neglected cases that have passed through the subacute stage.

Manual replacement is generally successful when the inversion is recognized at the time it occurs. Pressure is exerted by the operator's fingers about the periphery of the cervical ring, which means that the portion of the corpus that prolapsed last is reduced first. There should be no special concern about reinversion, either immediately or in subsequent pregnancies, and packing of the uterus is unnecessary, although an oxytocin drip will ensure that the uterus remains well contracted.

If recognition of the inversion is delayed, attempts at vaginal replacement may fail. Through marked passive congestion and edema formation (Fig. 19), the corpus may enlarge to fill completely and distend the vagina. Under this circumstance, if the operator fails to reduce the uterus, the patient may be lost from hemorrhagic shock. By the time the inversion has reached the subacute stage, therefore, abdominal reduction seems preferable. With adequate blood replacement, the patient is anesthetized, and the abdomen is prepared and draped and opened through a lower midline incision. The cervical ring is identified, the round ligaments and the anterior and posterior uterine wall are grasped with appropriate hemostats, and with traction the corpus is quickly reinverted. If this attempt is unsuccessful because the cervical ring is firmly contracted, incising the ring posteriorly will cause its release and permit the uterus to be quickly reinverted (Fig. 20). The uterine incision that must now be

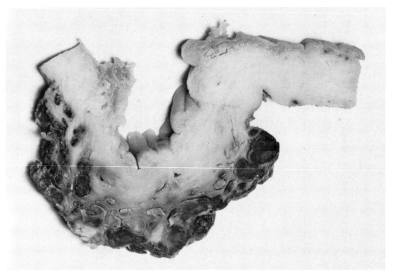

Figure 19. Section of inverted uterus, showing edema and marked dilatation and thrombosis of venous sinusoids. No placental tissue present.

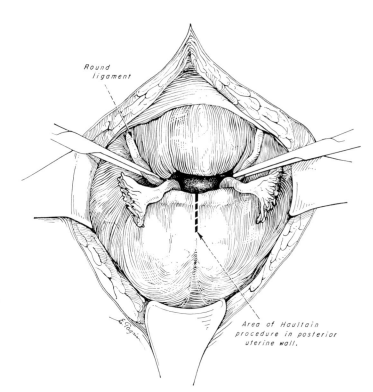

Round
ligament

Area of Haultain
procedure in posterior
uterine wall.

Figure 20. Haultain procedure for correction of inversion of the uterus.

closed is similar to that observed in the classic type of abdominal hysterotomy, except that in this instance it is located in the posterior uterine wall. This can be quickly closed by continuous and interrupted sutures. Altogether it is a procedure that requires little time, and is predictable and nontraumatic, all of these features being so necessary in preventing additional shock.

Chronic inversion finds the uterus completely involuted and returned to its nonpregnant size. Although this condition can occur in the nonpregnant, undoubtedly most of the cases of chronic inversion are the result of the inversion not being recognized at the time of delivery and the patient failing to return for a postpartum examination. Reinversion can be brought about by the Spinelli operation, which, in principle, is similar to the procedure just described but is performed vaginally.

PERINEAL LACERATIONS

Lacerations of the perineum and tissues about the introitus are more likely to occur when episiotomy is not performed. Perineal lacerations are classified into four categories, with the belief that the category of third-degree laceration, which often is defined as a laceration of the rectal sphincter with or without involvement of the rectal mucosa, should be classified. Only when the rectal mucosa is torn or severely traumatized is a perineal or a rectovaginal fistula likely to develop. No disability through failure of rectal control should occur when the rectal sphincter is lacerated, provided it is recognized and repaired. Accordingly, the following classification of perineal lacerations is offered:

First degree. The laceration involves the vaginal mucous membrane and the skin of the perineum in the region of the posterior fourchette.

Second degree. The laceration involves the endopelvic fascia, the levator ani muscles, and the perineal body.

Third degree. The laceration involves the entire perineum and the external sphincter of the rectum, either partially or completely.

Fourth degree. The laceration is complete, involving the entire perineum and the rectal sphincter, and to some degree the mucous membrane of the rectum.

The repair of first- and second-degree lacerations is similar to that of a median episiotomy, as, indeed, is that of the third-degree, except that one or two mattress sutures are added to ensure approximation of the rectal sphincter. No special nursing care is needed.

A fourth-degree laceration, or complete perineal tear, requires a careful step-by-step repair (Figs. 21 and 22). The apex of the rent in the rectal mucosa is identified, and the edge of the rectal mucosa is inverted into the bowel lumen by a Connell suture that is continued slightly beyond the mucocutaneous junction. This suture is reinforced by several interrupted sutures in the surrounding endopelvic fascia. Next, three or more interrupted sutures are placed in the levator ani muscles but are not tied until later. The ends of the sphincter are next identified. The torn ends of the sphincter are not obvious, for they tend to retract lateralward and posteriorly, disappearing within the fascial sheath where the sphincter is encased. A slight dimpling, seen lateral to the anus, will indicate their location. With each grasped by an Allis forceps they are brought to the midline and approximated with mattress sutures. The remainder of the repair is similar in all respects to that of a median episiotomy, with the exception that further treatment is required for the rectal mucosa. After the perineum is repaired, including closure of the skin, the anterior rectal mucosa is gently pulled down, everted, and approximated to the adjacent skin by three or four interrupted

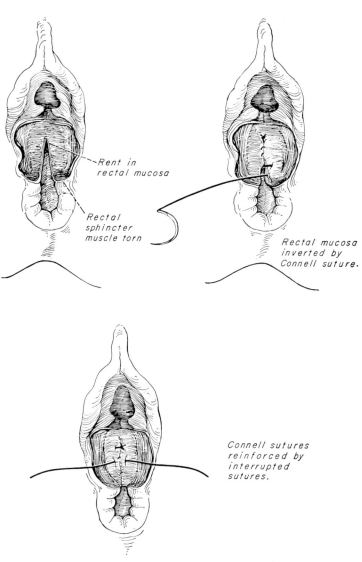

Rent in rectal mucosa

Rectal sphincter muscle torn

Rectal mucosa inverted by Connell suture.

Connell sutures reinforced by interrupted sutures.

Figure 21.　First steps in repair of perineal lacerations.

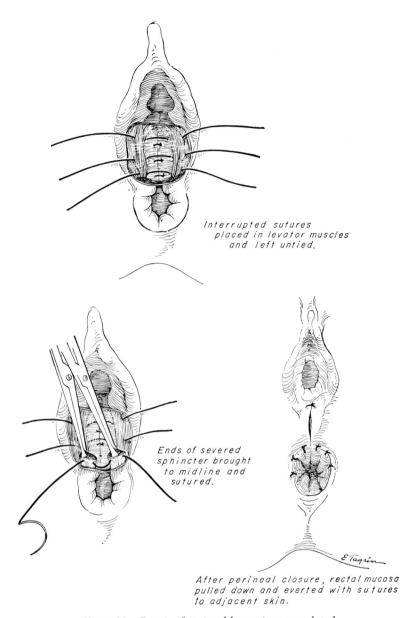

Interrupted sutures
placed in levator muscles
and left untied.

Ends of severed
sphincter brought
to midline and
sutured.

After perineal closure, rectal mucosa
pulled down and everted with sutures
to adjacent skin.

Figure 22. Repair of perineal lacerations completed.

sutures. The rectal mucosa, as it heals, tends to retract upward, so that if there is any leakage at the mucocutaneous junction a fistula may result. The above technique reduces the risk of rectoperineal or rectovaginal fistula, or both.

The patient is placed on a low-residue diet, and, beginning on the second postdelivery day, mineral oil is ordered. At about the sixth day, in the absence of a spontaneous bowel movement, an oil retention enema should be administered by an experienced nurse; if the bowels then fail to move, a soapsuds enema is given. Pelvic delivery in a subsequent pregnancy is not contraindicated provided the outlet is ample. Common sense dictates that a mediolateral type of episiotomy be performed.

PELVIC HEMATOMA

Hematoma of the reproductive tract is extremely rare *during* pregnancy, but cases of spontaneous rupture of the tubo-ovarian veins have been reported. Even in the presence of large vulvar varicosities, hematoma of the perineum is unusual. Broad-ligament or vaginal hematoma, however, may develop in the course of labor or as the result of operative pelvic delivery. Vaginal hematoma may develop because of faulty hemostasis in an episiotomy repair. A hematoma beneath the bladder may occur as a complication of a transperitoneal lower segment cesarean section.

A broad-ligament hematoma incidental to labor and delivery, besides being potentially serious, also contains an element of uncertainty as to its origin. A hematoma in this region may arise from spontaneous rupture of a broad-ligament vein or be one of the presenting signs in rupture of the lower uterine segment.

The development of pain lateral to the uterus within a few hours after delivery, together with exquisite tenderness and spasm on palpation, is strongly suggestive of a broad-ligament hematoma. Tenderness may appear in the flank and, in the extreme, extend up to the lower pole of the kidney as a result of retroperitoneal extension of the hematoma. The upper border of the distended broad ligament may be felt as a ridgelike structure above the brim of the pelvis, extending laterally to the abdominal wall. Abdominal distention is not unusual. A rectal examination may reveal tenderness and a sense of fullness high in the cul-de-sac and to the side. In the absence of external bleeding, which is an important sign in differentiating uterine rupture and spontaneous hematoma, surgical intervention will be influenced by an hour-to-hour evaluation of the condition of the patient, including frequent hematocrit determinations. If there is doubt as to the integrity of the uterus, the latter should be explored, but only in the operating room, for if there is a rupture the examination may intensify the bleeding by further disrupting the exposed uterine vessels. In the absence of uterine rupture, conservative management with adequate blood replacement is usually sufficient and certainly is to be preferred. It is anticipated that the bleeding will cease, and the process will show no evidence of extending. Should laparotomy and exploration be required, one should be prepared to meet the effects of unpredictable blood loss. After opening the broad ligament and removing the hematoma, one may experience difficulty in recognizing the offending vein or veins. To control the bleeding, hysterectomy and a bilateral oophorectomy may be necessary with ligation of the hypogastric vessels.

If a hematoma develops in conjunction with an episiotomy, the episiotomy wound should be reopened, and in reclosing it greater care should be given to proper hemostasis. When a hematoma develops in the vulvar area, a compression bandage may suffice, or the hematoma may be opened and the cavity packed with gauze, to be removed in 24 to 48 hours.

In the extreme a hematoma may dissect upward into the area of the broad ligament and fill the ischiorectal space and encroach across the midline of the vagina. It may take several weeks or months for the blood to be absorbed and the hematoma to disappear. The question arises whether the hematoma should be surgically treated or left alone. Aspiration of the hematoma always introduces the risk of infection, but slow absorption is an annoyance to the patient and may cause considerable discomfort. In the early stages it is possible that the hematoma may reach such proportions that shock intervenes. After the blood volume is restored to normal, consideration should be given to opening and evacuating the hematoma and ligating the bleeding vessels. Packing of the cavity created by the hematoma may be necessary, but it delays recovery.

Spontaneous rupture of a utero-ovarian vein must be thought of when in the latter half of pregnancy or during labor a patient suddenly complains of diffuse abdominal pain followed by signs consistent with hemoperitoneum of some magnitude. The cases of this complication appear to be about equally divided between those that develop in the prenatal period and those arising during labor. Considering the great distention of these veins in normal pregnancy, the marvel is that they do not rupture more often. The resultant bleeding may be intra-abdominal, retroperitoneal, or both. As rapidly as preparations permit, laparotomy with ligation of the offending vessels is indicated.

BIBLIOGRAPHY

Aaberg, M. E., and Reid, D. E.: Manual removal of placenta; policy of treatment. Amer. J. Obstet. Gynec., 49:368, 1945.

Alvarez, H., and Caldeyro-Barcia, R.: The normal and abnormal contractile waves of the uterus during labor. Gynaecologia, 138:190, 1954.

Caldwell, W. E., Moloy, H. C., and D'Esopo, D. A.: Studies on pelvic arrests. Amer. J. Obstet. Gynec., 36:928, 1938.

Chung, F., and Hon, E. H.: The electronic evaluation of fetal heart rate; I. With pressure on the fetal skull. Obstet. Gynec., 13:633, 1959.

Cope, I.: Amniotic fluid embolism. Report of a case with survival of mother and child. J. Obstet. Gynaec. Brit. Comm., 71:112, 1964.

D'Esopo, D. A.: The occipitoposterior position. Amer. J. Obstet. Gynec., 42:937, 1941.

Douglas, L. H., and Kaltreider, D. F.: Trial forceps. Amer. J. Obstet. Gynec., 65:889, 1953.

Easterday, C. L., and Reid, D. E.: Inversion of the puerperal uterus managed by the Haultain technique. Amer. J. Obstet. Gynec., 78:1224, 1959.

Eller, W. C., and Mengert, W. F.: Recognition of midpelvic contraction. Amer. J. Obstet. Gynec., 53:252, 1947.

Evans, T. N., and Stander, R. W.: Cervical incisions in obstetrics. Amer. J. Obstet. Gynec., 67:322, 1954.

Fara, F., Steward, M., Jr., and Standard, J. V.: Occiput transverse position; a modified technique for the application of the Kjelland forceps. Obstet. Gynec., 6:633, 1955.

Fenton, A. N., and D'Esopo, D. A.: Prolapse of the cord during labor. Amer. J. Obstet. Gynec., 62:52, 1951.

Ferguson, R. K., and Reid, D. E.: Rupture of the uterus: A twenty-year report from the Boston Lying-in Hospital. Amer. J. Obstet. Gynec., 76:172, 1958.

Friedman, E. A., and Sachtleben, M. R.: Dysfunctional labor; II. Protracted active phase dilatation in the nullipara. Obstet. Gynec., 17:566, 1961.

Friedman, E. A., and Sachtleben, M. R.: Dysfunctional Labor; III. Secondary arrest of dilatation in the nullipara. Obstet. Gynec., 19:576, 1962.

Friedman, E. A., and Sachtleben, M. R.: Amniotomy and the course of labor. Obstet. Gynec., 22:755, 1963.

Garnet, J. D.: Uterine rupture during pregnancy—an analysis of 133 patients. Obstet. Gynec., 23:898, 1964.

Goodwin, J. W., and Reid, D. E.: The risk to the fetus in prolonged and trial labor. Amer. J. Obstet. Gynec., 85:209, 1963.

Hellman, L. M., Kohl, S. G., and Schechter, H. R.: Pitocin—1955. Amer. J. Obstet. Gynec., 73:507, 1957.

Hendricks, C. H.: Dysfunctional labor. In Reid, D. E., and Barton, T. C., eds.: Controversy in Obstetrics and Gynecology. W. B. Saunders Co., Philadelphia, 1969, p. 165.

Hodgkinson, C. P., and Christensen, R. C.: Hemorrhage from ruptured utero-ovarian veins during pregnancy; report of three cases and review of the literature. Amer. J. Obstet. Gynec., 59:1112, 1950.

Huntingford, P. J.: The vacuum extractor in the treatment of delay in the first stage of labor. Lancet, 2:1054, 1961.

Huntington, J. L., Irving, F. C., and Kellogg, F. S.: Abdominal reposition in acute inversion of the puerperal uterus. Amer. J. Obstet. Gynec., 15:34, 1928.

Jeffcoate, T. N. A.: Prolonged labour. Lancet, 2:7193, 1961.

Jeffcoate, T. N. A., and Lister, U. M.: Annular detachment of the cervix. J. Obstet. Gynaec. Brit. Emp., 59:327, 1952.

Landing, B. H.: Pathogenesis of amniotic fluid embolism; uterine factors. New Eng. J. Med., 243:590, 1950.

Leary, O. C., Jr., and Hertig, A. T.: Pathogenesis of amniotic fluid embolism; possible placental factors—aberrant squamous cells in placentas. New Eng. J. Med., 243:588, 1950.

McCain, J. R., Anderson, C. L., Lester, W. M., and Pilkington, J. W.: Prolonged labor: clinical evaluation. J.A.M.A., 153:695, 1953.

McElin, T. W., Bowers, V. M., Jr., and Paalman, R. J.: Puerperal hematomas; report of 73 cases and review of the literature. Amer. J. Obstet. Gynec., 67:356, 1954.

Munsick, R. A.: The pharmacology and clinical application of various oxytocic drugs. Amer. J. Obstet. Gynec., 93:442, 1965.

Ranney, B.: Relative atony of myometrium underlying the placental site secondary to high cornual implantation—a major cause of retained placentas. Amer. J. Obstet. Gynec., 71:1049, 1956.

Reid, D. E.: The treatment of prolonged labor with posterior pituitary extract. Amer. J. Obstet. Gynec., 52:719, 1946.

Reid, D. E.: Remote effects of obstetrical hazards on the development of the child. J. Obstet. Gynaec. Brit. Emp., 77:709, 1959.

Reid, D. E., Weiner, A. E., and Roby, C. C.: Intravascular clotting and afibrinogenemia, the presumptive lethal factors in the syndrome of amniotic fluid embolism. Amer. J. Obstet. Gynec., 66:465, 1953.

Ritson, E. B.: An investigation of the psychological factors underlying prolonged labor. J. Obstet. Gynaec. Brit. Comm., 73:215, 1966.

Sluder, H. M., and Lock, F. R.: Sudden maternal death associated with amniotic fluid embolism. Amer. J. Obstet. Gynec., 64:118, 1952.

Steiner, P. E., and Lushbaugh, C. C.: Maternal pulmonary embolism by amniotic fluid. J.A.M.A., 117:1245, 1340, 1941.

Theobald, G. W., Kelsey, H. A., and Muirhead, J. M. B.: The Pitocin drip. J. Obstet. Gynaec. Brit. Emp., 63:641, 1956.

Chapter 28

Malpresentations

BREECH PRESENTATION

DEFINITION

On the basis that vertex presentation is normal since it accounts for nearly 95 per cent of all births, breech presentation, the extended vertex presentation, and transverse lie will be regarded as deviations from the normal.

Breech presentation is that variety of longitudinal presentation in which the cephalic pole of the fetus occupies the fundal segment while the caudal or podalic pole lies in the lower segment of the uterine cavity. The frequency of breech births is listed to be 4 per cent.

Since the fetus does not necessarily assume its final presentation and position within the uterine cavity until the final weeks of pregnancy, breech presentation occurs more often in premature labor than at term.

ETIOLOGY

Among the most frequently cited causes for breech presentation are prematurity, placenta praevia, fetal hydrocephalus, multiparity, multiple pregnancy, hydramnios, contracture of the maternal pelvis, congenital uterine anomalies, and tumors of the pelvic organs. Some of the conditions mentioned occur so rarely as to represent coincidence rather than cause-and-effect relationship. However, in premature delivery breech birth is more likely because of the occurrence of labor before the "law of accommodation" has become operative.

Multiple pregnancy and breech presentation are frequently associated. Here two factors account for the breech presentation: excessive distention of the uterine cavity which interferes with development of normal uterine polarity, and the presence of another fetus to interfere with the normal occurrence of cephalic polarity.

Hydramnios is said to be associated with a somewhat increased incidence of breech presentation. The great distention prevents development of uterine polarity and the fetus tends to assume a random presentation. Gross fetal deformities, chiefly anencephaly and hydrocephaly, influence the incidence of breech presentation through a reversal of the polarity of the fetal ovoid. In addition, many of these cases are associated with hydramnios to a greater or lesser degree.

It has been considered that placenta praevia may cause breech presentation. This is inferred because placenta praevia is associated with transverse presentation so frequently as to suggest an important etiologic relationship of the former to the latter. The much lower frequency of placenta praevia observed in association with breech presentation does not permit drawing the same conclusion.

Congenital uterine anomalies may be an important cause of abnormal presentations, including breech, and so may pelvic tumors.

VARIETIES

Breech presentation may be observed in several varieties (Fig. 1). The *frank breech* (Fig. 1A) is characterized by flexion of the thighs on the abdomen with extension of the legs in such a way that the feet lie at the level of the fetal thorax or shoulders while the rounded caudal pole alone occupies the lower uterine segment. In the *complete* or *full breech* (Fig. 1B) the thighs are flexed on the abdomen and the legs on the thighs, an attitude that disposes the feet to lie in the birth canal at approximately the same level as the caudal pole of the fetus. In some cases the habitus of one lower extremity may correspond to that of a frank, the other to that of a complete, breech. In some instances (Fig. 1C), a thigh and leg may be extended, the foot maintaining a level in the birth canal considerably in advance of the breech proper. This variety

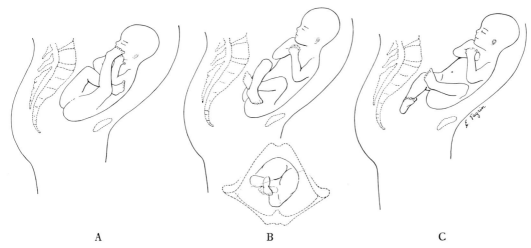

Figure 1. Varieties of breech presentation. A, Frank breech. B, Complete breech. C, Single footling breech.

is designated as a *footling*, with the extremity occupying either the anterior or posterior segment of the birth canal in the characteristic extended attitude. If both extremities are thus extended a *double footling* results. Very occasionally one or both thighs may become extended while the legs remain flexed, resulting in presentation of *one or both knees*. Knee presentation is so rare as to be an obstetric curiosity.

The majority of the several varieties of presentation are the frank breech, followed by double and single footling and full breech in that order.

PRIMARY POSITIONS OF THE BREECH

Regardless of the variety of breech presentation the primary position of the breech

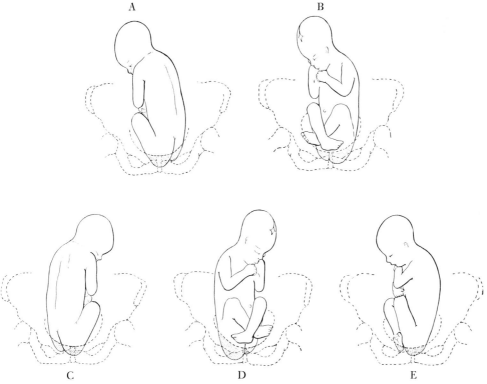

Figure 2. Primary positions of breech presentation. A, Left sacroanterior (L.S.A.). B, Left sacroposterior (L.S.P.). C, Right sacroanterior (R.S.A.). D, Right sacroposterior (R.S.P.). E, Left sacrotransverse (L.S.T.).

results from the orientation of the back with respect to one of the quadrants of the maternal pelvis. For descriptive purposes the fetal sacrum is used as the point of reference. If this landmark is oriented to an anterior quadrant of the pelvis, a left or right sacroanterior position results—L.S.A. or R.S.A.; if it lies in the transverse plane of the pelvic brim the position is left or right sacrotransverse—L.S.T. or R.S.T.; if the sacrum is inclined toward a posterior quadrant the position is left or right sacroposterior—L.S.P. or R.S.P. These are shown in Figure 2.

DIAGNOSIS

Diagnosis of breech presentation is usually made by abdominal palpation in the later weeks of pregnancy, complemented by vaginal examination and verified by roentgenogram (Fig. 3). In most cases palpation alone suffices for accurate diagnosis, but vaginal examination is often necessary to determine whether the presentation is frank, complete, or footling.

The first three maneuvers of palpation that are employed for diagnosis of cephalic presentation are used to diagnose breech presentation. If a breech presents, the first maneuver reveals the rounded mass of the

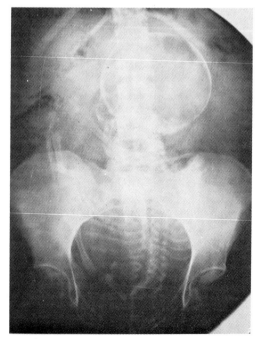

Figure 3.   Flat x-ray film showing breech presentation.

fetal head occupying the fundus of the uterus. The second maneuver shows the right or left side of the uterus subtended by the smooth contour of the fetal back, which may occupy a position somewhat anterior to, in alignment with, or somewhat posterior to the midaxillary plane of the maternal body, corresponding to anterior, transverse, and posterior positions of the sacrum, respectively. Conversely, the fetal small parts are found on the side opposite that occupied by the back and are more distinctly identifiable with sacroposterior than with sacroanterior presentations. The third maneuver reveals the irregular contours of the caudal pole of the fetus, usually well above the pelvic brim, but occasionally fixed in the inlet. The fourth maneuver is noncontributory with a breech presentation for obvious reasons.

The fetal heart tones, when the breech presents, are often heard above the level of the maternal umbilicus. Otherwise they are usually transmitted through the fetal back to the left side of the abdomen in left sacral positions and to the right side in right sacral. However, their location should never be considered sufficient evidence to controvert a diagnosis otherwise adequately assured by palpation.

Vaginal examination when the breech presents gives results that vary considerably according to circumstances, such as whether the examination is done before the onset of labor, in early labor, or late in labor; whether the breech is frank, complete, or footling; and whether the amniotic sac is intact or ruptured.

In labor, as in the late antepartum examination, much depends on the station of the presenting part, the variety of presentation, and the degree of effacement and dilatation of the cervix. Occasionally, especially when there is an excess of amniotic fluid, the caudal pole is so high in the birth canal that it can barely be reached, and its contour cannot be defined. More often, however, the presenting part is more easily palpable, and the examining fingers are able to trace the outline of the caudal pole through the lower uterine segment. If the breech is of the frank variety it fills out the vaginal vault on all sides to a considerable degree, but not as uniformly as does the head when the vertex presents; furthermore, the breech does not reveal the regular rotundity of the presenting vertex. At this particular time the anatomic landmarks characteristic of the breech cannot be defined. If the breech is of the complete variety the irregularity palpated in the vaginal vault is much more marked. The breech proper tends to occupy one side of the vault; on the other side one or more smaller masses may be felt, which correspond to one or both feet alongside the breech. Occasionally a frank breech may have descended well into the pelvis by the time of prelabor examination, and, if the amniotic fluid is scanty, may be very difficult to differentiate from a head. In this case the dilemma is usually resolved by reference to the first maneuver of palpation, which has already revealed the head in the fundus. If the status is still in doubt, an x-ray examination may be made.

During labor, after the cervical os has undergone a moderate degree of dilation, especially if the membranes have ruptured, the landmarks of the breech become distinguishable and the variety of the presentation is established with relative facility by vaginal examination. The entire fetal pole is irregular in contour. The gluteal cleft and anus are identified, with the two fetal ischial tuberosities palpable one on either side of the anus. The direction in which the finger traces the gluteal cleft is indicative to a certain degree of the position of the breech, but this cannot be established definitely until the finger can trace the sacrum and its spinous processes at one end of the cleft. If the breech is of the complete variety, one or both feet may be felt; if the examination is made after a foot has prolapsed through the dilating os it may be identified as right or left by locating the great toe. Certain diagnostic mistakes should be guarded against. Occasionally a frank breech that has descended well into the pelvis may be diagnosed as a face, especially if preceding abdominal palpation has not made the differentiation plain. In this event the gluteal cleft may be mistaken for the mouth and the ischial tuberosities for the malar bones. This error can be avoided if one reflects that the cleft separates the two tuberosities, whereas the mouth runs parallel to a line between the two malar bones. Finally, even though the examiner feels certain that he knows the sex of the unborn child at this time, he will be well advised to avoid predicting, since the differentiation between male and female genitalia may be obscured by compression and by edema.

Rectal examination is useful primarily to indicate the station of the breech as it descends through the pelvis during labor. It does not yield information concerning the fetal landmarks or degree of cervical dilatation with more than a fraction of the accuracy of that obtained by vaginal examination, however, and should never be relied on to determine the type or position of a breech presentation.

In rare instances the diagnosis of breech presentation can be established only by x-ray examination. Palpation of the abdomen of an extremely sensitive and apprehensive primigravida may be inadequate for accurate diagnosis, and in the same circumstances vaginal examination may not succeed in differentiating the presenting part as either a head or a breech. Palpation may also be of little value in the obese patient, or when there is an excessive amount of amniotic fluid; furthermore, hydramnios, as described before, may make vaginal examination inconclusive.

MECHANISM OF LABOR IN BREECH PRESENTATION

Breech birth takes place in three successive phases. The fetal hips are the first to engage in the birth canal and to be delivered, the shoulders are next, and the aftercoming head, last. Each phase is concerned with adaptation of certain diameters and circumferences of the fetus to the diameters and circumferences of the various planes through which the fetus must pass. Whether the breech is of the complete or of the frank variety, its greatest presenting diameter is the bitrochanteric, which is usually 9 cm. in length. The circumference of the shoulders is somewhat greater, the bisacromial diameter being 12 cm.; this is also somewhat reducible by compression and by the range of mobility of the shoulder girdle. The aftercoming head, when flexed, presents a plane subtended by the suboccipitobregmatic and biparietal diameters. These diameters can be reduced little if at all by compression save by a long process of molding that is impossible in a breech presentation.

X-ray studies in recent years have added much to the understanding of cephalic labor, especially with regard to the mechanism of engagement, descent, and rotation of the head. Similar studies of breech labor have yielded comparatively little information other than demonstration of variations in attitude that may be assumed by the arms and head within the uterus and confirmation of facts already known concerning descent and rotation of the hips.

It is a matter of general observation that engagement, or passage of the hips through the inlet, usually occurs in one of its oblique diameters. When the primary position is L.S.A. or R.S.P. the left oblique diameter is traversed; when it is R.S.A. or L.S.P., the right oblique. However, because the bitrochanteric diameter of the hips measures 9 cm., adequate space is available for engagement to take place through the true conjugate, resulting in a primary position of either L.S.T. or R.S.T.

In contradistinction to engagement of the vertex presentation, which so frequently occurs several weeks before term, the breech ofttimes fails to enter the pelvis until labor has begun. Nor is this finding prior to labor necessarily suggestive of disproportion between the presenting part and the maternal pelvis.

The mechanism of the first phase of breech labor, accommodation of the hips, follows a pattern that is approximately uniform in the frank and complete varieties of the presentation. With the onset of labor the longitudinal axis of the contracting uterus becomes sufficiently aligned with that of the superior strait to force the hips down through the inlet (Fig. 4A). Descent

continues in this axis to the floor of the pelvis in a direction that is inclined somewhat posterior to a perpendicular dropped from the plane of the inlet (Fig. 4B). Because the bitrochanteric diameter of the breech maintains a right angle with its axis of descent, the breech is inclined in such a way that the hip that lies in the anterior segment of the pelvis reaches the pelvic floor sooner than does the hip that lies posterior (Fig. 4B).

Whenever labor starts with the breech in primary sacroanterior or sacroposterior position the second movement of the hips commences when the anterior, or leading, hip impinges on the pelvic floor. The movement comprises simultaneous internal rotation of the anterior hip through an arc of 45 degrees to the symphysis and of the posterior hip through an equal arc in the opposite direction to the concavity of the sacrum.

The anterior hip is guided in the direction of least resistance by the elastic contour of the pelvic musculature. The direction of least resistance is toward the space between the portion of the two levator ani muscles beneath the pubic bones; consequently the anterior hip rotates forward. The net effect of internal rotation is thus to bring the bitrochanteric diameter into the anteroposterior diameter of the pelvic outlet and to adapt the elliptical contour of the breech as a whole to the elliptical space developing in the outlet of the pelvis (Fig. 5).

The third movement of the breech begins

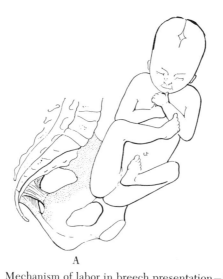

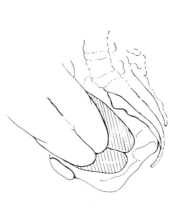

A   B

Figure 4.   Mechanism of labor in breech presentation—first phase. A, Breech entering pelvic brim. Bitrochanteric diameter in posterior asynclitism. Leading hip is posterior. B, Breech descending through pelvis. Posterior asynclitism becomes anterior as descent proceeds. Anterior hip becomes leading point.

with the anterior hip rotated to the pubic arch and lying at a level slightly below that of the lower border of the symphysis (Fig. 6A). The posterior hip is now forced downward, overcomes the slight resistance offered by the coccyx, and comes to rest on the perineum. The fetal body flexes laterally toward the symphysis on the fulcrum provided by the anterior hip at the level of either the trochanter or the iliac crest (Fig. 6B). The posterior hip passes over the perineum and the bitrochanteric diameter becomes disengaged from the birth canal,

thus completing birth of the hips (Fig. 6C). In frank breech the movement of lateral flexion may be delayed somewhat by the resistance offered by the extended legs, and operative assistance is more often required at this point than when a complete or footling breech presents. Usually, however, after the bitrochanteric diameter has cleared the outlet the body is rapidly extruded to the umbilicus, the legs slipping out of the birth canal spontaneously but sometimes requiring manual assistance (Fig. 6D).

Immediately after disengagement of the breech and legs the fetal sacrum normally rotates 45 degrees or more anteriorly. This movement is in no sense a restitution of the presenting part, such as occurs in vertex labor, and has been termed "overrotation." Forward rotation of the back after delivery of the hips is unquestionably a movement that is favorable to simultaneous forward rotation of the interscapular region of the shoulders prior to or at the time of engagement of the latter in the pelvic inlet. In like manner it undoubtedly is equally favorable to forward rotation of the occiput of the aftercoming head.

In single footling presentation, when the prolapsed leg is attached to the anterior hip, the mechanism is the same as that in the double footling, in that the anterior hip rotates 45 degrees to the pubis, either above or at the pelvic floor, after which lateral flexion proceeds in the usual way (Fig. 7).

In the case of prolapse of the leg attached to the posterior hip, however, the leg extends across the long arc of the posterior segment of the birth canal and is deflected forward at an angle that diverges considerably from the line of the pelvic axis. So long as this leg remains posterior the direction of force imposed by the uterine contractions causes the anterior half-breech to impinge upon and straddle the brim of the bony pelvis anteriorly. Progress in labor is therefore delayed until either a natural mechanism or assistance by the physician causes the posterior hip to rotate to the arch and become anterior.

Each phase of breech labor exerts some degree of influence on the next succeeding phase. By the time the hips have been delivered the second phase—delivery of the shoulders—has already begun. Although the shoulders, as will be described, are normally born with their widest diameter, the bisacromial, passing through the an-

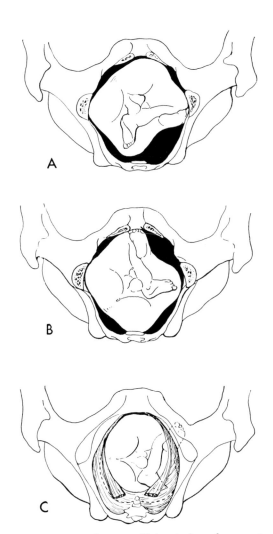

Figure 5. Mechanism of labor in breech presentation. A, Right sacroanterior before rotation. Effect of rotation will be to change the position to right sacrotransverse. B, Right sacroposterior before rotation. Effect of rotation will be to change the position to right sacrotransverse. C, Right sacrotransverse. This figure may represent a position originally sacrotransverse or the effect of internal rotation upon a position originally either right sacroanterior or right sacroposterior.

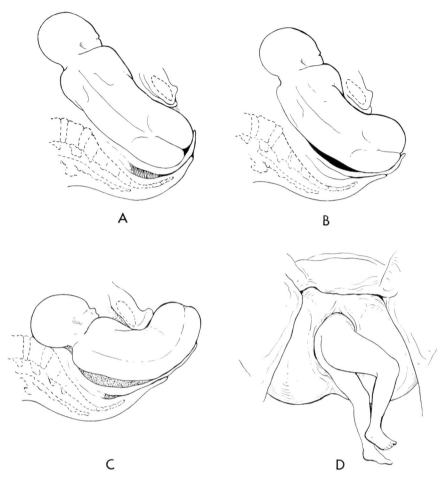

Figure 6. Mechanism of third movement in breech labor. A, Breech has descended to pelvic outlet. Anterior hip rotated to symphysis, posterior to sacrum and coccyx. Little or no lateral flexion of trunk. B, Anterior hip has descended well below symphysis. Posterior hip has passed by coccyx and is supported only by the soft tissues of the perineum. Lateral flexion of the trunk has begun. C, Bitrochanteric diameter of breech distending perineum. Lateral flexion of trunk is marked. D, Breech is born. Lower extremities disengaged from birth canal. Characteristic anterior rotation of fetal sacrum has taken place regardless of originally anterior, transverse, or posterior orientation of sacrum at beginning of labor.

teroposterior plane of the pelvic outlet by a movement of lateral flexion, the manner in which they engage in and pass through the pelvis is described differently by various authorities.

The extent to which successive internal and external rotation of the hips is accompanied by simultaneous and similar rotation of the shoulders within the birth canal is not definitely known. It seems probable that the sequential internal and external rotations of the hips impose immediate or almost immediate coordinate rotation of the shoulders within the birth canal. Such coordination would support the observations of many authorities who describe the shoulders as engaging in dorsoanterior rotation regardless of the original position

of the breech, whether sacroanterior or sacroposterior.

After the shoulders have passed the pelvic brim they descend to the pelvic floor, at which point they undergo internal rotation in a manner similar to that which has previously been described for the hips. The anterior shoulder rotates forward to lie behind the symphysis, while the posterior shoulder rotates backward to lie in the concavity of the sacrum. The bisacromial diameter now occupies the anteroposterior diameter of the lower birth canal. In strictly unassisted delivery the weight of the legs, hips, and trunk, now freed from the birth canal, causes the anterior shoulder to descend further and appear beneath the pubic arch (Fig. 8). The next few uterine contractions cause the

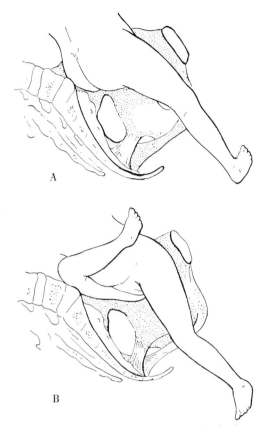

Figure 7. Mechanism of labor in single footling breech—anterior foot and leg presenting. A, Right sacroposterior position. Anterior hip will rotate 45 degrees to symphysis. B, Left sacroanterior position. Anterior hip will rotate 45 degrees to symphysis.

posterior shoulder to pass over the perineum and the second phase of breech birth is completed. So long as the arms of the fetus remain flexed on the chest they are born alongside the thorax as it emerges.

The arms, however, do not necessarily maintain a flexed position on the fetal chest throughout labor. One or both may become extended to lie at or above the level of the shoulder girdle or even to lie alongside the aftercoming head. In this event delay may occur in delivery of the shoulders and manual assistance by the physician may be required to correct the malposition; otherwise the fetus, subjected at this time to rapidly increasing hypoxia from compression of the umbilical cord after the umbilicus has passed the vulvar outlet, incurs a grave risk of perishing before delivery is complete.

Extension of the arms may be due to one or to several causes, chief among which are minor degrees of contraction at any of the

pelvic planes through which the shoulder girdle must pass. It is also possible that in any breech delivery the degree of cervical dilatation that permits unobstructed passage of the hips may still offer sufficient resistance to passage of the shoulder girdle, because of its slightly greater circumference, to cause the arms to become extended upward. It follows, therefore, that one or both arms may be found extended in any breech delivery even though the hips and legs have been extruded spontaneously. Under these circumstances, the physician must be fully prepared to disengage the arms without delay, so that no time need be lost in correcting the abnormality as soon as it is discovered.

Occasionally in breech labor an arm may be found not only extended but also inclined so far backward in relation to the frontal plane of the thorax that the elbow and forearm lie across the nape of the neck, giving rise to a *nuchal position*. In very rare instances both arms have been observed in this position. Either condition is a serious complication of labor since further descent of the shoulders is prevented by impaction of the arm or arms between the occiput of the aftercoming head and the inner surface of the maternal pubis. Unless such nuchal position is recognized promptly during the course of delivery of the fetal trunk, and unless the condition is promptly corrected by the maneuvers described later in connection with breech extraction, the risk to the fetus of perishing from anoxia or of undergoing traumatic damage from im-

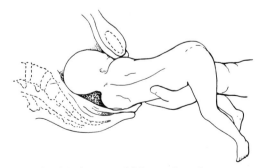

Figure 8. Mechanism of labor in breech presentation—second phase. Shoulders have rotated on pelvic floor. Bisacromial diameter in anteroposterior diameter of pelvic outlet; anterior shoulder beneath symphysis. Lateral flexion of body will sweep posterior shoulder over the perineum.

proper application of traction becomes enormous.

During delivery of shoulders and arms in completion of the second phase of breech birth, the third phase is already beginning as the aftercoming head passes through the pelvic brim. Because in the normal intrauterine position of the head prior to labor its sagittal plane is assumed to maintain a right angle to the bisacromial diameter, it has been generally believed and taught that the head follows the shoulders through the pelvic brim with its sagittal plane engaging in a diameter at a 90-degree angle to that previously traversed by the bisacromial diameter. If this is the case, the head engages with its occiput obliquely anterior or obliquely posterior to correspond to the preceding dorsoanterior or dorsoposterior engagement of the shoulders. Although this may be applicable to the three phases of breech labor when the original position is sacroanterior, the evidence is against it when the primary position is sacroposterior. In the latter the shoulders have normally undergone sufficient rotation within the birth canal prior to engagement to change their orientation through an arc of 90 degrees from dorsoposterior to dorsoanterior, with the corollary that the head also, prior to engagement, changes from occiput posterior to occiput anterior orientation. From this it follows that normal engagement of the aftercoming head takes place with the occiput directed toward one of the anterior quadrants of the pelvis, a circumstance that applies to practically all breech mechanisms.

Regardless of any degree of deflection or extension of the head within the uterus during pregnancy, a movement of flexion normally results during the first stage of labor. Coming into direct contact with the head, the uterine fundus exerts equal pressure on occiput and sinciput. Inasmuch as the head, in its longitudinal dimension, is divided into two unequal segments by the fulcrum represented by the occipital condyles, because the segment from condyles to sinciput is longer than that from condyles to occiput, the mechanical result of pressure brings about some flexion of the head, usually in advance of engagement. On occasion the head will be found to be markedly deflexed, as verified by roentgenography. Cesarean sections have been unnecessarily performed because of fear that the head would not or could not be flexed.

The suboccipitobregmatic diameter of the head thus enters the pelvic brim with the suboccipital region obliquely anterior. Descent then occurs until the suboccipital region impinges on an anterior quadrant of the pelvic floor, where the former turns to the pubic arch, a movement accounted for by the guidance exerted by the levator ani muscle. The cervical spine, which now is the region of maximal flexibility, is brought into the concavity of the curve of the lower birth canal in the pelvic outlet.

With anterior rotation completed, the head lies with its sagittal plane in alignment with the anteroposterior diameter of the outlet. The suboccipital region now acts as a fulcrum around which the chin, mouth, face, vertex, and finally the occiput of the fetus are successively extruded over the perineum, and thus the third and final phase of breech birth is completed (Fig. 9). During this final movement a descrip-

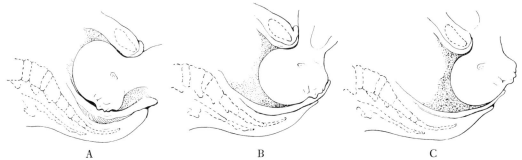

A   B   C

Figure 9.   Mechanism of labor in breech presentation—third phase. A, Head has entered pelvis and occiput has rotated anteriorly. Face in hollow of sacrum. B, Suboccipital region of head pivots around lower border of symphysis as fulcrum. Beginning flexion of head has caused face to descend from hollow of sacrum to perineum. C, Continued flexion of head on suboccipital region around lower border of symphysis has resulted in disengagement of chin, mouth, and nose from the vulvar outlet. Birth of head will be completed by continued flexion.

tive paradox appears. The head, although already flexed, is born by increased flexion on its cervical spine, a movement that becomes graphically apparent if, as is the usual procedure, the legs and body of the fetus are raised by the attending physician to a level above the horizontal.

PROGNOSIS OF BREECH PRESENTATION

For several reasons the mechanism of labor is more hazardous to the fetus when it presents as a breech than when it presents as a vertex. In breech labor the breech, whether or not it is augmented by the bulk of the lower extremities, does not fill the lower segment as completely as in vertex presentation, thereby affording a greater opportunity for the cord to prolapse when the membranes rupture. When the vertex presents, a degree of cephalopelvic disproportion that has not been demonstrable before the onset of labor may become evident early enough that the decision to deliver the patient by cesarean section in the interest of the fetus does not expose the mother to an additional risk. However, when the breech presents, a degree of cephalopelvic disproportion not demonstrable prior to labor may become apparent only after delivery of the hips and shoulders, leaving the aftercoming head obstructed within the birth canal. Under such circumstances attempt to extract the head is practically certain to cause crippling or lethal trauma to the fetus, whereas cesarean section exposes the mother to grave risk of death from infection and at the same time offers little hope of saving the fetus from the effects of the hypoxia which always occurs cumulatively after the hips and shoulders have been released from the birth canal.

Aside from the contingencies of prolapse of the cord and cephalopelvic disproportion, certain factors that are intrinsic in the mechanism of breech labor, but that do not occur in vertex labor, predispose to development of fetal hypoxia. These are listed in Table 1.

The principal causes of neonatal mortal-

TABLE 1. FACTORS PREDISPOSING TO FETAL HYPOXIA IN BREECH LABOR THAT ARE NOT PRESENT IN VERTEX

Vertex Labor	Breech Labor
1. The fetal umbilicus and adjacent cord are not subjected to pressure until they enter the pelvis. This does not occur until *after* birth of the head and at a time when pulmonary respiration becomes available to the newborn infant.	1. The fetal umbilicus and adjacent cord may become subjected to pressure in the first stage of labor after the breech engages, are usually subjected to pressure after birth of the breech, and are practically always subjected to pressure after disengagement of the shoulders.
2. During the second stage of labor and prior to birth of the head, the greater bulk of the fetus remains within the uterine cavity. Retraction of the placental site proceeds very slowly until the fetus is completely born. Consequently, oxygenation of the fetus through placenta and cord is but little diminished until birth of the head allows institution of pulmonary respiration.	2. During the second stage of labor, after birth of the breech, the greater bulk of the fetus is usually expelled suddenly from the uterine cavity. This predisposes to rapid retraction of the placental site or even to complete separation of the placenta at a time when the aftercoming head is still undelivered. Consequently a critical delay is apt to occur from the instant when the fetal circulation becomes impaired or cut off until birth of the head permits pulmonary respiration to start.
3. Full dilatation of the cervical os with respect to passage of the forecoming head indicates that the shoulders and hips will not be resisted by the cervix during the second stage of labor. The head, ordinarily of a circumference equal to that of the shoulders and greater than that of the hips, is less compressible than the latter two levels of the fetal cylinder.	3. Full dilatation of the cervical os with respect to passage of the breech does not guarantee that the shoulders or aftercoming head will not meet resistance from the cervix. The circumference of the hips is smaller than that of the shoulders, although both are reducible by compression. The circumference of the aftercoming head, though it is equal to that of the shoulders, is less reducible by compression than the latter, and is in any case greater than that of the hips.

ity associated with uncomplicated breech birth at full term, aside from such unpredictable conditions as antepartum intrauterine death and congenital malformations, include anoxia, intracranial damage from rupture of the tentorium with or without associated hemorrhage from the vein of Galen, and traumatic injury of the spinal cord. In addition, the factors mentioned, if they are not fatal to the newborn infant, may cause mental retardation from cerebral hypoxia, paralyses of various types from intracranial or spinal damage, peripheral paralysis of the upper extremities from injury to the brachial plexus, and fractures of the clavicle or extremities.

MANAGEMENT OF BREECH PRESENTATION

Aside from the management of breech delivery, the only treatment for breech presentation as such consists in converting it into a cephalic presentation by performance of external cephalic version. In view of the increased fetal risk associated with breech birth, previously discussed, external version is entitled to a definite place as a prophylactic measure.

Successful performance of external version depends on a number of circumstances that should be carefully assessed before the operation is attempted. Of these, accurate diagnosis of presentation and position is an essential preliminary. The uterus should not be irritable, inasmuch as external version is seldom successful when the uterus is in a phase of increased contractility. The amniotic sac should contain sufficient fluid to allow the fetus to be turned within the uterine cavity. The breech should be unengaged or at most only lightly engaged in the superior strait. Finally, for the practical reason to be discussed, the rate and rhythm of the fetal heart tones should be carefully determined before the operation is begun.

If the situation is favorable in respect to the foregoing factors, external version may well reward the attempt to perform it. The technique is simple. The patient is instructed to empty her bladder, after which she is placed on a bed or on an examining table. She lies in the dorsal recumbent position with her legs extended and her abdomen bared. A mild degree of Trendelenburg position may be used if the breech is found to be lightly engaged. The fetal heart tones are auscultated and recorded. In order to disengage the breech from the pelvic inlet to facilitate turning, the obstetrician displaces the breech upward (Fig. 10A). He then grasps the caudal pole of the fetus in the lower uterine segment through the abdominal wall with one hand and the cephalic pole in the fundus with the other, and guides the breech upward and outward to the side occupied by the fetal back, simultaneously pressing the head downward and outward to the side occupied by the fetal small parts (Fig. 10B); in this way he gradually turns the fetus end for end to a transverse lie and finally brings the caudal pole into the fundus and the head into the lower uterine segment (Fig. 10C). Moreover, turning the fetus toward the side of the back favors maintaining the vertex in flexion, which may contribute to successful version.

When version has been accomplished in the manner described the rate and rhythm of the fetal heart tones should again be carefully determined, since the reversed fetal habitus may have resulted in tension on the cord or in compression of the cord between the fetus and the uterine wall. If the heart tones become and continue to be slow and irregular, the fetus should be reconverted without any delay to a breech and further operative attempts given up. It is not too unusual for the rate of the fetal heart to be momentarily slowed, but in a minute or two the rate should return to normal. The manipulations described must be applied slowly, methodically, and intermittently, being halted temporarily when the uterus contracts and recommenced when relaxation occurs.

Although it is a subject of some controversy, except for a situation to be mentioned subsequently, it is questionable whether anesthesia should be used for the procedure. The amount of force that can be tolerated by the unanesthetized patient, and that at the same time suffices to turn the fetus, entails little or no danger of rupturing the amniotic sac or of detaching the placenta. The exception is the young primipara with a borderline pelvis whose infant, if the vertex presented, most likely

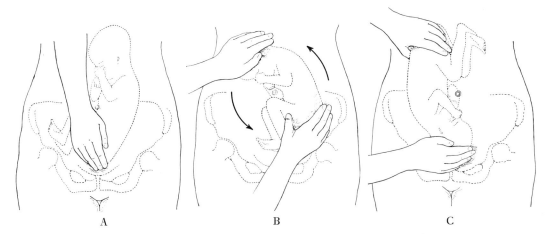

Figure 10. Technique of external version in breech presentation. See text.

would be born without risk. Successful external version could avoid the necessity for a cesarean section in this and future pregnancies. Here, anesthesia appears justified, if the operator keeps in mind the fact that only moderate force should be used.

The optimal time to perform external version is between the 34th and the 35th week, when the fetus can usually be turned with a minimum amount of force and with less likelihood of its reconverting to a breech. Furthermore, if an accident should occur, such as premature rupture of the membranes, the baby is sufficiently mature to survive. At this time the fetus is small in bulk in relation to the mass of amniotic fluid within the sac; the breech is seldom if ever engaged; the maternal abdomen is relatively undistended by the uterus and its contents, and the abdominal wall is comparatively relaxed; also, the uterus is less irritable than in the final weeks of gestation. Nevertheless, reversion to a breech presentation may take place, and in some cases the operation must be repeated before a permanent cephalic presentation is obtained.

The likelihood of successful performance of external version diminishes steadily with the passage of time. This is especially true in the primigravida. Although successful versions have been done after labor has commenced, most of these have been in multiparas with relaxed abdominal walls and with coincident large amounts of amniotic fluid.

The statistical results of external version when applied to a series of breech presentations are very difficult to calculate.

In discussing the etiology of breech presentation, the frequency with which spontaneous cephalic version takes place in the later weeks of gestation has been mentioned. It is a matter of observation that spontaneous version often takes place before labor in cases in which external version has been attempted without success, and also that such version may on rare occasion occur during labor. It seems at least probable that some of the breech presentations that are successfully changed by external version would have undergone the change spontaneously without the operation. At the same time, careful palpation and recognition of the breech make it possible to reduce breech delivery to 1 per cent or less.

MANAGEMENT OF BREECH DELIVERY

This relatively simple-sounding subject covers a wide variety of circumstances. It entails, for example, the management of premature labor which takes place at a time when the fetus presents as a breech. It concerns the question of delivering by cesarean section, at full term, the patient whose pelvis is significantly contracted and whose fetus lies in breech presentation. It involves decision concerning the administration or withholding of analgesic drugs during labor. It requires careful consideration of the type of anesthesia, if any, to be employed for delivery or extraction. For this reason it seems advisable to discuss the broad subject under several categories, the first dealing with breech labor at full term conducted in anticipation of pelvic delivery, the second with breech labor and delivery that occurs prior to the 36th week of gestation, and the third with the cases in which cesarean section, in preference to birth through the pelvis, is indicated in the interests of the fetus.

Breech labor is notorious for the rapidity with which normal progress may be punctuated by sudden and unpredictable complications that jeopardize the unborn infant and that require prompt delivery if they are to be properly dealt with. *This fact imposes on the obstetrician in charge of the case the obligation to present himself at the patient's bedside without delay once the onset of labor is established and to remain in constant attendance until delivery has been completed.* Finally, no obstetrician should undertake single-handed the management of breech labor and delivery. An assistant and an anesthesiologist should be immediately available for any contingency, and both should be in attendance in the delivery room at all times during the second and third stages of labor, until delivery is completed.

In breech presentation at full term the first stage of labor should be conducted in much the same way as if the vertex were presenting. Periodic rectal examinations should enable the operator to follow the progress of cervical dilation and descent and rotation of the breech, and in any case in which the information thus obtained is equivocal, vaginal examination should be performed. Close attention should be paid to the rate and rhythm of the fetal heart tones, which should be unfailingly checked, especially when the membranes are observed to rupture. Diagnosis of fetal distress at this time may call for immediate termination of labor—by extraction if the second stage has begun or by cesarean section if the cervical os is not completely dilated. Medication for pain relief may be used during the first stage according to indication exactly as it is in vertex presentations.

The most crucial phase of breech labor, from the standpoint of fetal prognosis, coincides with the second stage and ends only with completion of delivery. During this phase several factors that are intrinsic in the mechanism of labor and inseparable from it may occur singly, or in combination, to bring about varying degrees of fetal hypoxia before pulmonary respiration can become established.

Some compression of the umbilical cord becomes inevitable as the fetus passes through the lower birth canal. Although this is not usually significant until the hips have been born, it becomes more significant during delivery of the thorax and shoulder girdle, and thereafter increases markedly as the cord unavoidably becomes subjected to pressure between the aftercoming head and the walls of the maternal pelvis. As a rule, therefore, in the interval between the successive extrusion of shoulders and head the fetal circulation and hence the supply of oxygen to the fetus frequently become reduced to a critical level.

Coincidentally with cord compression, at this time the uterus, the cavity of which has been emptied of the greater bulk of its contents, may suddenly shrink down, causing rapid retraction of the placental site and placental separation, thus adding another factor that favors the development of fetal hypoxia.

To compound the potentially serious effects of the two factors mentioned, delay in the progress of disengagement of the fetus from the birth canal may occur between birth of the hips and delivery of the shoulders and again while only the head remains undelivered. Because such delays occur at the exact times when hypoxia is most likely to take place, they add appreciably to the fetal risk associated with breech birth.

In view of the foregoing considerations it follows that constant and unremitting vigilance is essential to successful conduct of breech labor, particularly during the second stage. As soon as this stage has begun the patient should be placed on the delivery table. The obstetrician, capped, masked, and gowned, should be prepared to assist the delivery should the need arise. The anesthetist should be present in the delivery room at all times. Only in this way can prompt and effective countermeasures be provided against the hypoxic complications that so often occur.

With these precautions the obstetrician is now prepared to conduct the second stage under conditions that can be effectively controlled. The fetal heart tones should be constantly monitored. If the uterine contractions, combined with the characteristic reflex contractions of the patient's diaphragm and abdominal muscles, are adequate to bring about consistent descent of the fetus through the lower birth canal, and if at the same time no slowing in the rate or irregularity in the rhythm of the fetal heart tones betokens development of fetal distress, it is sometimes possible to achieve a completely spontaneous delivery by the characteristic mechanism of breech birth. On the other hand, it is never possible to predict if or when delay will occur or fetal embarrassment develop. Consequently, it sometimes becomes necessary to deliver the fetus by breech extraction. More often it becomes necessary to extract the shoulders and head after the hips have been born spontaneously, and very frequently delay in completion of delivery after spontaneous birth of breech and shoulders requires that the head be flexed over the perineum manually or by means of forceps.

In general there are three recognized policies or methods for management of the second stage of breech delivery. These will be discussed in the following order: (1) spontaneous or assisted delivery; (2) extraction of shoulders and aftercoming head; and (3) total breech extraction.

Spontaneous Breech Delivery

In spontaneous breech delivery the breech, body, shoulders, and aftercoming head of the fetus are extruded successively from the birth canal by the force of uterine contractions, aided, when possible, by the conscious expulsive efforts exerted by the patient. No traction is applied at any time, and the obstetrician simply supports the infant as it is born. In this way, it is claimed by some, extension of the arms does not occur and there should be no obstruction to birth of the shoulders as a result. Assistance is given to facilitate flexion of the head through the pelvic outlet by performing a preliminary mediolateral episiotomy under pudendal block, by raising the fetal body upward over the maternal pubis, and by insertion of a finger into the fetal mouth to guide the latter into the vulvar opening.

Spontaneous delivery by this method may be successful in many cases, especially if the fetus is of less than average size (i.e., 3000 grams) and if the maternal pelvis is of ample dimensions. On the other hand, any thought of achieving spontaneous delivery must be abandoned promptly in favor of partial extraction at any time if evidences of fetal distress appear or if progress in delivery is not continuous.

Extraction of Shoulders and Aftercoming Head

Since delay in birth of the shoulders frequently necessitates resort to partial extraction, the second method available for delivery of the breech is to allow spontaneous birth of the hips, to extract the shoulders and arms under anesthesia, and finally to complete the delivery by extracting the head. This method of management is advocated and practiced by many obstetricians. It permits free employment of analgesic medication in early labor since the conscious cooperation of the patient in the second stage is largely unnecessary. Anesthesia may be planned in advance and methodically administered. Inhalation anesthesia is most effective in quieting the patient and relaxing the maternal soft tissues, and for the latter purpose is preferable to local and regional forms.

Total Breech Extraction

Total or complete extraction is a method of delivery that frequently becomes necessary if fetal distress or delay in the progress of labor occurs in the second stage prior to birth of the hips. The absolute indications for its performance include prolapse of the cord, hypoxia resulting from compression of the cord, and intrapartum separation of the placenta. Delay in the progress of labor unassociated with fetal distress is a relative indication and results most frequently from the splinting action of the legs of a frank breech which inhibits lateral flexion of the trunk or from failure of anterior rotation of the posterior hip when the breech is of the single footling variety with the posterior leg prolapsed.

For total extraction the patient should be under complete surgical anesthesia before the operation is begun. The first step in total breech extraction is delivery of the breech itself by freeing the hips. The technique for this purpose depends primarily on the disposition or habitus of the lower extremities and secondarily upon the station of the breech in the birth canal.

If the presentation is that of a double footling it is ordinarily simple to disengage the hips by making traction first on the feet and subsequently on the legs as the lower extremities are drawn upon. Extraction of the complete or full breech is begun in the same way.

In frank breech presentation application of traction becomes more complicated. Three methods are available: (1) to secure the feet, disengage the lower extremities, and proceed as described for extraction of a double footling; (2) to deliver the breech by means of fingers inserted into the fetal groins; or (3) to achieve the same results by application of forceps to the breech, one blade over each hip.

Of the three methods the first is most commonly used. It may be utilized regardless of the station of the breech, and is the only method that is successful when the breech occupies a station at or above midpelvis when the operation is commenced. It should be done after a preliminary mediolateral episiotomy has been performed. To perform the maneuver, the obstetrician uses the hand that, if held in semipronation, will present its palmar surface toward the ventral surface of the fetus after insertion through the vagina into the uterus—the right hand for right sacral positions, the left hand for left. After a mediolateral episiotomy to facilitate delivery, the hand is then carried upward as far as may be necessary and the operator carefully palpates the ventral surface of the fetus, identifying the thighs and legs and their relationships to the respective hips which lie in the anterior and posterior quadrants of the birth canal. The legs may be found widely separated or, conversely, they may be crossed. If they are separated, the operator identifies the anterior leg, and makes pressure in its popliteal space (Pinard's maneuver), thus causing shortening of the hamstring muscles and bringing the foot down against his fingers. He next relaxes his pressure, grasps the foot between his fingers, and draws it down past the breech in an arc across the infant's body. Having thus converted the presentation to a single footling, he proceeds in the same way to release the posterior foot and leg, again by sweeping it across the infant's abdomen, as a result of which the presentation becomes a double footling (Fig. 11).

If the infant's legs are crossed it may become necessary to release the lower leg first, regardless of whether it is anterior or posterior; in this event the operator should determine carefully which is the lower leg and should, especially if it proves to be posterior, be sure to bring down the other leg as well before continuing the extraction.

It is highly desirable to spend the time necessary to bring down both feet and both legs before proceeding further. By so doing the operation is facilitated in that the force required to draw the breech down through the vagina is transmitted through the ankle, knee, and hip joints of two legs rather than of one. Although it is possible to extract the fetus by grasping the anterior leg, the necessary force must be transmitted through the joints of this leg only, and may result in epiphyseal damage, especially if the fetus is large. Extraction by the posterior leg alone should be avoided whenever possible. It is quite liable to result in injury to one or more of the joints, since not only traction but also rotation must be applied to the extremity in order to bring about anterior rotation of the corresponding hip. Otherwise traction, if applied alone, will cause the anterior half-breech to straddle the ischiopubic ramus of the maternal pelvis toward which it is oriented, thus obstructing further progress until corrective measures have been taken.

When a frank breech has reached the pelvic outlet and the anterior hip has rotated to lie behind and below the maternal symphysis by the time extraction is begun, it often proves possible, especially if the patient is a multipara with a relaxed perineum, to start delivery of the hips by means of an index finger hooked into the anterior fetal groin. Lateral flexion of the trunk induced by this maneuver permits insertion of the other index finger into the posterior groin, in this way completing disengagement of the hips. This method of delivery is entirely safe for the fetus, since the force that can be exerted by the flexed fingers does not endanger either the femur or the femoral vessels and nerves. The traction thus applied, however, may not be adequate to disengage the breech when the fetus is large or in a primipara despite a preliminary mediolateral episiotomy. Use of a blunt hook to effect extraction is permissible only when the fetus is known to be dead, for, if used when the fetus is alive, it may inflict irremediable trauma to the femoral vessels

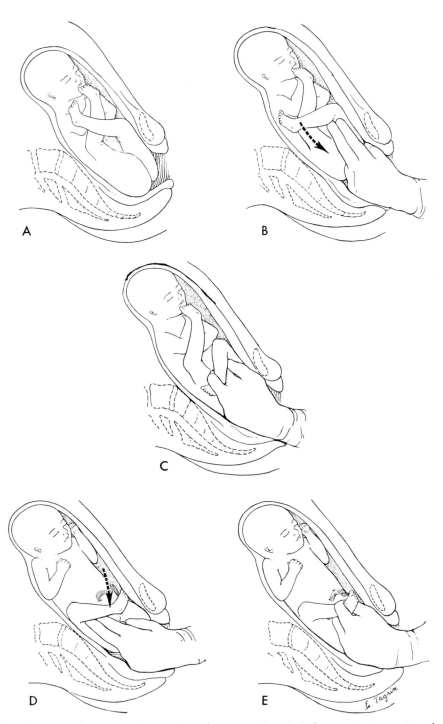

Figure 11. Technique of extraction in frank breech presentation. A, Left sacroanterior position, legs crossed. B, Pressure exerted in the popliteal space of the anterior (left) leg of the fetus brings the foot down against the operator's fingers. C, Foot is grasped and brought down in an arc across the infant's body. D and E, Second leg is brought down in similar fashion before extraction is continued.

and nerves and even fracture the femur.

Whenever finger traction does not suffice to deliver the frank breech as such from a low station at the outlet there should be no hesitancy about pushing the fetus upward in the birth canal, disengaging the feet and legs, and performing a breech extraction as described. It is in this situation particularly that inhalation anesthesia shows its greatest value in securing the necessary relaxation of the uterus and pelvic soft parts.

In a single footling presentation, the method to be employed for extracting the hips depends chiefly on whether the prolapsed foot lies anterior or posterior. If by the time extraction is begun the entire anterior leg is already extruded from the vagina and the anterior hip is deeply impinged behind and beneath the symphysis, it is ordinarily simple to free the posterior buttock and deliver the breech by drawing the prolapsed extremity first slightly downward, then forward, and finally slightly upward, allowing the posterior leg to emerge after the hips have been disengaged (Fig. 12). However, in cases in which the anterior leg is prolapsed but not extruded, and in all cases in which the posterior leg presents, the retained foot should be sought, grasped, and brought down by the technique described for management of the frank breech, before extraction of the hips is begun.

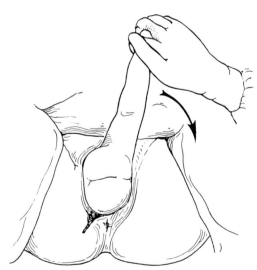

Figure 12. Delivery of single footling breech in which the anterior leg and foot present. Upward traction on the anterior leg after the hip has become disengaged beneath the symphysis causes birth of the posterior hip over the perineum. The posterior leg will be freed spontaneously during the further course of the extraction.

Except in those cases in which a frank breech is delivered as such in one of the ways already described, every total breech extraction begins when the feet have been grasped (Fig. 13). The hips are now extracted in the following manner. Gentle and even traction is applied to the two feet in such a way as to make pressure on the fourchette. As the breech emerges over the perineum the heels and posterior aspects of the legs will tend to rotate transversely to the pelvic outlet, corresponding to internal rotation of the hips to a sacrotransverse position. If time is a factor owing to a prolapse of the cord, or if it proves impossible to secure and deliver the anterior leg readily, the posterior leg can usually be easily converted into an anterior by rotating the infant 180 degrees. Rotation – counterclockwise if the position is right, and clockwise if the position is left – is quickly accomplished by sweeping the leg with slight traction in a wide arc. The procedure tends to sweep the infant's arms away from the anterior chest, increasing the possibility of the complication of a nuchal arm, but this is readily correctable in the extraction of the shoulders. The legs and soon the thighs are grasped through a sterile towel and gradually lifted upward, with stronger traction applied to the posterior thigh. The posterior hip appears over the perineum and disengagement of the breech is completed.

The next step after birth of the hips should be to grasp the pelvic girdle through a sterile towel and gently rotate the sacrum and buttocks forward until the bitrochanteric diameter of the hips lies transversely across the pelvic outlet (Fig. 14A and B). This step ensures simultaneous orientation of the interscapular region of the shoulders and of the occiput of the aftercoming head to the anterior segment of the birth canal. Downward traction is now applied to the hips, depressing the incised perineum. As the umbilicus is drawn over the perineum the obstetrician draws down the umbilical cord in order to secure as much slack as possible and to avoid tension on it during the balance of the operation. If no slack is available the findings may betoken either that the cord is congenitally short or that it is wrapped around the neck or an upper extremity of the fetus. In such event it may be necessary to clamp, cut, and release the cord.

Traction is now continued, keeping the back upward (Fig. 14C and D) until the lower portion of one or both scapulae may

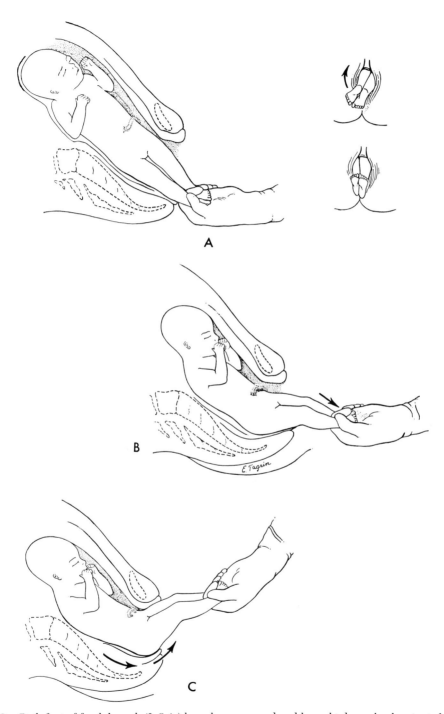

Figure 13. Both feet of frank breech (L.S.A.) have been secured and brought down, heels oriented toward the left and anterior.

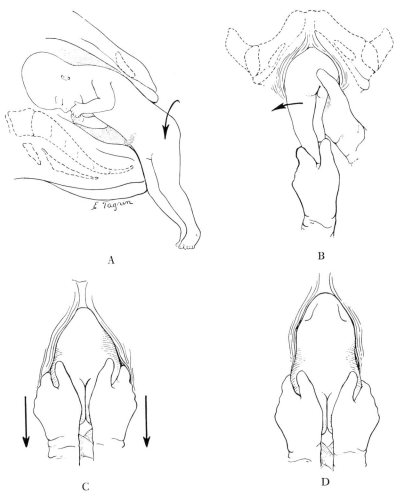

Figure 14. Succeeding steps after birth of hips. A, Hips have been freed by downward traction applied to feet, legs, and thighs, successively. Note spontaneous anterior rotation of fetal sacrum and lower back after birth of breech. B, Operator completes anterior rotation of hips so as to bring fetal back directly anterior. C, Downward traction continued, with back maintained forward (uppermost). (Sterile towel not shown.) D, Angles of scapulae appearing below pubic arch as downward traction is continued.

be seen, or outlined by digital palpation, below the ischiopubic rami. The shoulder girdle and arms are now ready for delivery (Fig. 15). The operator shifts the grasp of his hands to the sides of the fetal thorax, still using a sterile towel to assure his grip. He rotates the torso on its long axis toward the shoulder that originally lay anterior in the birth canal until the shoulder in question lies directly beneath the symphysis (Fig. 15A).

While the shoulder is undergoing rotation in the pelvic outlet, the corresponding arm, held back somewhat by the constriction of the lower birth canal, lags behind, and usually drops downward behind the ischiopubic ramus with the humerus flexed on the thorax and the forearm flexed at the

elbow. Slight pressure applied to the axillary border of the scapula in the direction of the vertebral column may be helpful in facilitating this movement. The entire arm is now freed from the birth canal by passing two fingers over the shoulder, and using these fingers to splint the humerus, while pressure in the bend of the elbow sweeps the forearm downward and outward along the lateral wall of the thorax (Fig. 15B).

As soon as the anterior arm has been freed, the operator rotates the entire delivered torso through an arc of 180 degrees, in such a way that the fetal back is carried uppermost beneath the pubic arch in transit, until the shoulder that had previously been posterior is brought beneath the symphysis. The corresponding arm lags behind

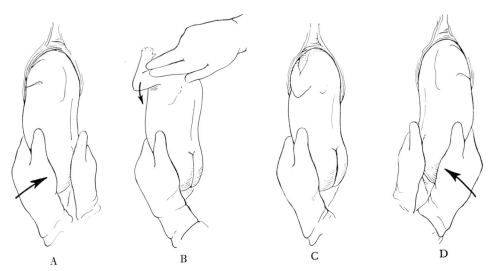

Figure 15. Birth of shoulder girdle and arms. A, Shoulder originally anterior in L.S.A. position has been brought beneath the symphysis by rotation of the fetal body toward the shoulder in question—in this case, clockwise. B, The arm is found flexed and is swept down and out. C, Elbow delivered; forearm and hand will follow. D, The shoulder originally posterior—in this case the right—has been made anterior by rotating the fetal body through an arc of 180 degrees in a direction which causes the back to turn beneath the pubic arch—in this case, counterclockwise. The right arm is now ready for delivery.

the shoulder while rotation is being carried out, and practically without exception is found to lie alongside the thorax as had been the case with the first arm. It is then easily delivered by the same maneuver that was used previously to free its fellow (Fig. 15D).

If extension of the arms has resulted in one or both of them assuming a nuchal position, the arm(s) will be found lying behind the neck. If digital pressure is applied to secure flexion, it becomes a practical certainty that the humerus, clavicle, or both will be fractured. No attempt, therefore, should be made to deliver an anterior extended arm first; instead, the fetal torso should be rotated 180 degrees away from the nuchal arm, thus making anterior the shoulder that was originally posterior. Since the arm lags behind, it will be found flexed and becomes easy to release. If the other arm is in nuchal position, the torso is rerotated 180 degrees in the opposite direction to bring the posterior shoulder beneath the symphysis, at which point it will be found that it too has been freed from its abnormal or nuchal posture and can be delivered easily.

Delivery of the aftercoming head is the final step in total as well as in partial breech extraction. As mentioned before, in discussing extraction of the body following birth of the hips, maintenance of the back for-

ward (or uppermost) until disengagement of the shoulders is begun causes the head to enter the pelvis with its occiput directed anteriorly regardless of its original orientation prior to labor. When the fetal body is rotated outside the birth canal to effect delivery of the shoulders and arms, the occiput may change position somewhat within the pelvic cavity. However, provided external rotation is properly applied in such a way as to maintain the fetal back uppermost in transit from side to side, any corresponding movement transmitted to the head must keep the occiput in the anterior segment of the pelvis and prevent it from turning backward into the hollow of the sacrum. Accordingly, as soon as the shoulders and arms have been delivered, the operator drops the towel previously used to facilitate traction, and places the body of the fetal abdomen downward astride either his right or left forearm (Fig. 16). He then inserts two fingers of the corresponding hand into the vagina and seeks the fetal mouth within the birth canal. Having found this orifice, and having guided it into the midline of the pelvic axis when necessary, he proceeds to extract the head by flexion (Mauriceau's maneuver).

In some cases, especially in a multipara with a yielding and relaxed perineum, or in a primigravida who has been prepared for extraction by a preliminary mediolateral

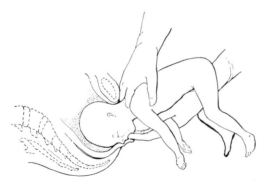

Figure 16. Extraction of aftercoming head. The fetus is placed belly downward on the forearm of the operator, who inserts the index and middle fingers of the corresponding hand into the fetal mouth. He forms a fork of the index and middle fingers of the other hand and grasps the shoulders *for guidance only but not for traction.*

episiotomy, it is possible for the operator, by making pressure about the symphysis with his free hand, to flex the head sufficiently to bring the chin, mouth, face, and crown over the perineum and thus complete the extraction unaided. To distribute the force over the larger area, he should use the entire palmar surface of the hand to exert suprapubic pressure. If the force thus available does not free the head from the pelvic cavity, application of forceps to the head should be resorted to without delay (Fig. 17), with due regard to the possibility that some of the resistance to passage of the circumference of the aftercoming head is offered by the cervical rim. A Simpson forceps or its modification is sufficient for this purpose. No attempt should ever be made to apply forceps to the aftercoming head if it is not completely engaged in the pelvis. If the aftercoming head cannot be brought into the pelvis by manual manipulation, to do so with forceps will potentially cause great harm to the mother and cause irreversible cerebral damage in the infant. If the head refuses to enter the pelvis, a further attempt should be made to flex the head and try to maneuver the occiput into either the larger oblique or transverse diameter. Should the infant succumb, craniotomy will permit completion of the delivery without serious trauma to the mother.

Rotation of the aftercoming head with its occiput in the hollow of the sacrum in properly conducted breech delivery or breech extraction is a rarity. On recognition of the abnormal rotation the operator should

insert his hand between the fetal neck and the symphysis, spread his third and fourth fingers widely apart, and by applying the fork thus formed on either side of the chin, rotate the face 180 degrees into the sacral concavity, and complete the delivery of the head in the usual way. If this maneuver is tried and proves unsuccessful, the entire fetal body should be carried downward and backward so as practically to be suspended by its neck. In this way the chin, face, and forehead may become disengaged successively from behind the symphysis and delivery thus completed. It is possible that gentle forceps rotation could succeed; the forceps is removed after rotation and the head is delivered by flexion.

Routine or elective total extraction for pelvic breech delivery at or near full term is advocated and practiced by many experienced obstetricians, who believe that termination of the second stage of labor by extraction under full surgical anesthesia not only avoids the hazards of delay and fetal hypoxia inherent in the more conservative methods of management, but also permits a more deliberate and more skillfully applied technique to be used than when partial extraction suddenly becomes neces-

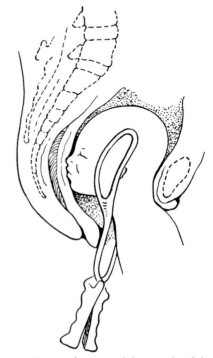

Figure 17. Application of forceps for delivery of aftercoming head.

sary. In assessing neonatal results, account must be taken of the value of x-ray pelvimetry, of the decrease in the incidence of contracted pelvis, and of the quality of anesthesia, all factors in reducing the fetal mortality and morbidity. It is possible, therefore, that a policy of performing elective partial extraction after spontaneous delivery of the hips can, under meticulous guidance and supervision, give comparably good results.

Cesarean Section for Delivery

When the breech presents, disproportion may be suspected because of pelvic contracture at any level, because the fetus is larger than average size, or because of the existence of both factors. Accurate clinical measurement of the pelvis is essential before every breech labor and should be supplemented by x-ray study and measurement whenever doubt of pelvic adequacy exists. A trial labor, which is often useful to confirm or rule out disproportion when the vertex presents, is less reliable in breech presentation. Thus valid indication for cesarean section in breech presentation is when disproportion is predictable or anticipated. Here ultrasound is of immeasurable assistance, for the biparietal diameter of the fetus may be determined with accuracy at the onset of labor. If ultrasonography is used together with x-ray pelvimetry, the cephalopelvic relationship may be established.

Summary of Management of Breech Labor

In all instances in which the fetopelvic relationship is normal the conduct of labor in breech presentation is little different from that in vertex presentation, except that it must be recognized that conditions in breech presentation cause additional hazards to the fetus. Consequently the patient in breech labor must be under constant surveillance by the obstetrician in charge. In the absence of fetal distress and, with continuous progress, the patient should be allowed to labor without interference. Breech presentation per se is not a contraindication to oxytocin stimulation of labor if uterine inertia develops in the first stage of labor.

It is a sound policy to await spontaneous delivery with assisted breech extraction as long as the patient makes progress in the second stage of labor. Breech extraction is indicated when the obstetrician is convinced that progress in the second stage of labor has virtually ceased. It must be understood that a breech extraction in a patient at full term, especially if she is a primigravida, can be as difficult as an internal podalic version. For reasons already mentioned, more infants are lost or damaged as a result of hypoxia in the second stage of labor in breech than in vertex presentation. Breech birth therefore demands supervision by one skilled and experienced in the operation of breech extraction if the fetal mortality and morbidity are to approach those in vertex presentation.

BROW AND FACE PRESENTATION

These abnormal presentations are considered together, although it is granted that the management of the two conditions differs in certain respects. In the main they have the same etiology and are diagnosed by the same methods. Considerable attention has already been given to the diagnosis of an extended vertex in the section on obstetric examination, and the concern here is more with its management. The potential fetal mortality and morbidity are substantially higher in face and brow than in the normal vertex presentation, owing principally to failure to recognize the condition until many hours of labor have elapsed.

The early diagnosis of an extended vertex, as previously emphasized, depends primarily on abdominal palpation. *A brow or face presentation should be suspected when the most prominent portion of the vertex appears to be on the side of the fetal back.* This is obviously a correct statement, but it may lead to a faulty diagnosis for the reason that characteristically the chest is also extended and can be mistaken for the fetal back. This would lead to the erroneous belief that the back is on the side opposite the area it actually occupies, which would be consistent with a well flexed vertex. To avoid this mistake, the following definition is suggested: *when on abdominal palpation the most prominent portion of the vertex is opposite the fetal small parts, the diagnosis is that of an extended head* (Fig. 18A). Confirmation of a brow or face presentation will depend largely on an anteroposterior x-ray of the abdomen (Fig. 18B) or vaginal examination, or both.

Besides pelvic contracture, there are other factors, such as fetal abnormalities, which contribute to an extended vertex, but in some instances there is no demonstrable cause. In fact, with the maternal pelvis large, apparently the vertex can become extended and remain so, with the baby being born by a brow or a face mechanism.

Several avenues are open in the management of labor and delivery. First, provided the pelvis is normal and the membranes are intact, watchful expectancy seems indicated in most multiparous patients and in many primiparas because spontaneous conversion can occur. Second, if the membranes remain unruptured until the patient enters the second stage of labor, internal podalic version is a possible procedure but is not without hazard. Third, if the cervix dilates readily, an attempt may be made to flex the vertex, but extension frequently recurs once the patient emerges from her anesthesia, presumably because of the established opisthotonos state of the fetus, and prolapse of the cord is more than a possibility. If this procedure is to be tried, the cervix must be dilated 6 to 8 cm. With the patient under deep inhalation anesthesia, the operator passes his hand behind the fetal occiput

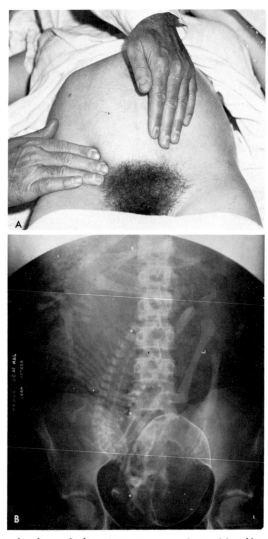

Figure 18.   Abdominal and x-ray findings in a mentoposterior position. Note the extended chest.

in an attempt to flex the vertex and simultaneously "reduces" the infant's chest by pressure imposed by his external hand over the corresponding area of the mother's abdomen. The case is then left to the influence of the natural powers of labor. This procedure is mentioned but not recommended. Fourth, if the cervix becomes fully dilated and the pelvis is normal, a brow presentation may be converted to a face presentation by traction with the operator's finger in the baby's mouth. The face is rotated anteriorly, either manually or by forceps, and delivery is accomplished by forceps through the mechanism of flexion. Rarely is a brow or a posterior face delivered unaided, but when in the latter the face rotates anteriorly the fetus may be delivered spontaneously, or by forceps. Whenever the membranes rupture early, or progress in labor is unsatisfactory, cesarean section must be seriously considered, and, in fact, must be used liberally if the fetal mortality and morbidity are to be kept low.

TRANSVERSE PRESENTATION

Many of the factors involved in production of face and brow presentation apply also to a transverse presentation. These factors include pelvic contracture, obstructing tumors of the pelvis, leiomyomata with uterine distortion, and fetal anomalies. It is also reemphasized that in many cases of placenta praevia the fetus is in a transverse position. In addition, women who have borne many children, and in whom the uterus is relaxed as the result of several pregnancies, are more likely to have a transverse lie of the fetus.

External version is usually attempted to convert either one of the poles of the fetus to the inlet, but the fetus often reverts to its original position. Placental localization, especially if the patient is in the last month of pregnancy, even in the absence of bleeding, is indicated in an attempt to exclude or establish the diagnosis of placenta praevia.

Whether to await the onset of labor or to attempt to correct the position of the fetus and induce labor is the question. If the fetal membranes rupture at home, the patient may arrive at the hospital with a prolapsed cord and a dead or compromised fetus. Or, if the membranes rupture and the amniotic fluid drains away, attempts to manipulate the fetus and correct the presentation are rarely successful. In fact, even if the patient enters labor some hours after rupture of the membranes and the cervix becomes fully or almost fully dilated, which would be unusual under these circumstances, internal podalic version could be fraught with danger. It is possible, however, that as the patient enters the second stage of labor, despite the fact that the membranes are ruptured, one or the other of the fetal poles might enter the pelvis and the patient be delivered rather uneventfully.

Instead of awaiting the onset of labor, at least in the multipara with a normal pelvis who has reached term with the cervix favorable for induction, an attempt can be made with the patient anesthetized to entice the vertex over the inlet. If the attempt is successful, the membranes are then ruptured, and in order to avoid prolapse of the cord the amniotic fluid should be permitted to drain slowly with the operator's hand in the vagina. The vertex can then be guided into the pelvis and maintained in this position by a scalp forceps (Willett forceps). This method of management may prevent the fetal accidents referred to and, in some instances, eliminate the necessity for delivery by cesarean section.

If the patient with a transverse position enters labor spontaneously and the membranes remain intact until the second stage of labor, internal podalic version under deep inhalation anesthesia is a satisfactory procedure. If in a transverse presentation the fetal back lies against the uterine fundus (Fig. 19A), the baby is easily turned, for the feet and legs can be readily grasped. If the fetal back is down and the fetal small parts are in the fundus (Fig. 19B), the operation of turning is more difficult, for it means that the operator's hand must bypass the fetal back and grasp the fetal foot, preferably the distal or posterior foot, and, with traction, bring the thigh over the fetal abdomen, thus rotating the fetal pelvis. By further traction on the foot, the breech is brought over the inlet and the fetus delivered in conformity with a breech extraction.

SUMMARY

The literature on the subject of brow, face, and transverse presentations deplores the fact that these conditions are too often diag-

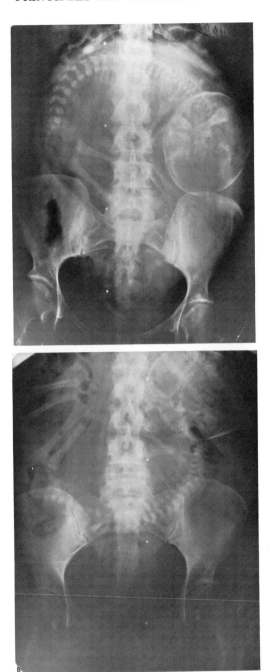

Figure 19. X-ray findings in transverse presentation. A, Fetal small parts are over the inlet. B, Fetal back is over the inlet.

nosed late in labor. To avoid the risk of abdominal delivery long after the membranes have ruptured, or after prolonged labor, pelvic delivery is sometimes attempted unwisely. For example, internal podalic version is an accepted method of delivery but, when performed on a term fetus under the conditions just alluded to, the outcome may be disastrous for the fetus and the mother, with the risk of uterine rupture.

There are many variables surrounding a case of brow, face, or transverse presentation, such as the estimated weight and maturity of the fetus, as well as the size of the pelvis, so that each patient must be managed on her own merits. On the assumption that the pelvis is normal, the most important factors are the status of the fetal membranes and whether the labor is normal as gauged by the progress of cervical dilation. If the cervix reaches full dilatation with the membranes intact or recently ruptured, pelvic delivery can be anticipated in the multipara and occasionally in the primipara.

Corrective manipulation during labor is generally unsatisfactory, and might be classified as meddlesome obstetric practice. If there is any question about the size of the pelvis, possible fetal macrosomia, premature rupture of the membranes with or without labor, or unsatisfactory progress in labor, cesarean section is the safest for both the mother and the infant.

BIBLIOGRAPHY

1. Friedlander, D.: External cephalic version in the management of breech presentation. Amer. J. Obstet. Gynec., 95:906, 1966.
2. Goethals, T. R.: Management of breech delivery. Surg., Gynec. Obstet., 70:620, 1940.
3. Goethals, T. R.: Cesarean section as method of choice in management of breech delivery. Amer. J. Obstet. Gynec., 71:536, 1956.
4. Harris, B. A., and Epperson, J. W. W.: An analysis of 131 cases of transverse presentation. Amer. J. Obstet. Gynec., 59:1105, 1950.
5. Meltzer, R. M., Sachtleben, M. R., and Friedman, E. A.: Brow presentation. Amer. J. Obstet. Gynec., 100:255, 1968.
6. Morris, N.: Face and brow presentation. J. Obstet. Gynaec. Brit. Emp., 60:44, 1953.
7. Reddock, J. W.: Face presentation, a study of 160 cases. Amer. J. Obstet. Gynec., 56:86, 1948.
8. Stevenson, C. S.: Principal cause of breech presentation in single term pregnancies. Amer. J. Obstet. Gynec., 60:41, 1950.
9. Vartan, C. K.: Cause of breech presentation. J. Obstet. Gynaec. Brit. Emp. 52:417, 1945.

Chapter 29

Operative Obstetrics

FORCEPS DELIVERIES

The obstetric forceps possesses a potential for the preservation of life greater than that of any other surgical instrument. Also, when used improperly, it is capable of great harm. The favorable consequences of forceps delivery depend not only on the technical capacity of the operator, but also on the presence of the accepted and established obstetric indications and conditions for its performance. Failure to adhere to these principles may result in irreversible damage to the fetus and disability to the mother.

HISTORY

Probably no subject has received more attention in medical history than have the obstetric forceps and the forceps operation. This is understandable, for, like cesarean section, the forceps operation was one of the earliest surgical procedures known. Several historical references are listed in the Bibliography, but only a brief résumé is attempted here.

Instruments to grasp and assist in the delivery of the fetus were used by the ancients, but it is an open question whether prior to the 16th or 17th century the instruments were designed to give consideration to the safety of the unborn child. Authorities on the history of the obstetric forceps appear to agree that the famous, and also somewhat infamous, Chamberlen family, which included several generations (A.D. 1601–1818), perhaps without knowing of its pre-existence, developed an effective instrument for delivery of a living child. As depicted in Figure 1, it seems probable that forceps similar to those introduced by the Chamberlens did exist at a much earlier time.

Regardless, the elevation of the obstetric forceps from a mere instrument for delivery to that of a lifesaving instrument (in the Chamberlen era) marks a period when physicians, rather than midwives whose training had been gained through experience only, began to assume responsibility for the parturient prenatally, during labor and delivery, and post partum. Prior to the 16th century, and certainly before what might be regarded as the Chamberlen era, the services of a physician or surgeon were sought only when the mother, the child, or both were already in grave jeopardy.

Being Huguenots, the Chamberlen family, because of their religious beliefs, felt obliged to leave Paris and settle in England in the year 1569. The family at the time comprised the father William, a physician, the mother, and three children—one named Peter, who became known as the "elder," because another son, born in England, was also named Peter, and became known as the "younger." This Peter's son Peter is credited by some with the development of the "modern" obstetric forceps, although there are authorities who believe he inherited the instrument from the two previous Peter(s) Chamberlen, i.e., his uncle and father. This controversial and provocative family, who were vitally interested and involved in correcting the social injustices of their times, have to their discredit the fact that the instrument they devised was a family secret, kept from the profession for almost a century. The introduction and acceptance of forceps procedures into general medical practice began in the early part of the 18th century, but the question of responsibility for this is a matter of individual interpretation.

What did the Chamberlens contribute to advancing the design of an instrument that would ensure, if properly used, the delivery of a live, unharmed child? In brief, the blades were disjointed and could be introduced separately into the birth canal. Up to this time it is said that the blades were joined and could only be introduced to-

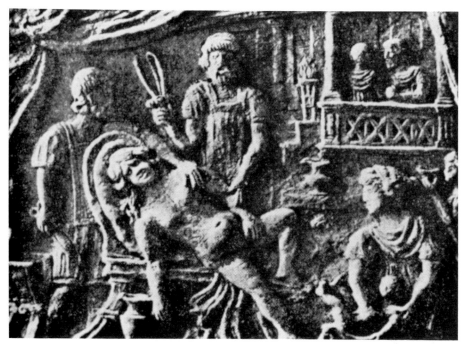

Figure 1. Bas relief mural in marble found near Rome. The dress and surroundings suggest the second or third century. Baby recently born alive; size of uterus suggests that the placenta is still in situ. Forceps not unlike many of the 19th century. (From Baglione, S.: Conoscevano glia antichi l'uso del forcipe? (Did the ancients know the use of forceps?) Societa Laziale de Obstetricia e Ginecologia, Rome, 1937. Fisiologia e Medicina.)

gether, obviously limiting their use. They enlarged and fenestrated the blades. The forceps had a respectable cephalic curve, but no special consideration was given to the need for a pelvic curve, and the articulation might be described as what is referred to as the French type.

Although the necessity of a pelvic curve was appreciated, and forceps had been so designed, Sir James Y. Simpson in 1848 introduced an instrument with a pelvic curve, and its popularity continues but primarily because the cephalic curve of the blades more closely follows the contours of the fetal head. Some 30 years later, Tarnier introduced the principle of axis traction, whereby traction could be exerted along the pelvic axes. Owing to the mobility of the handles, from which the force is applied, the vertex is free to follow the direction of the birth canal, permitting the head to accommodate to the pelvic bore as in natural labor. In more recent times, together with other modifications, Irving applied the Tarnier axis-traction device to the Simpson forceps. In the present century, other forceps have also been designed to deal with special situations, such as a persistent occiput posterior,

a transverse arrest of the occiput, and delivery of the aftercoming head in a breech birth. These are considered in the following section, under the heading The Instrument and the Purpose of Special Design. Since the time of the Chamberlens, hundreds of forceps have been devised. Das, in a classic book on the subject, described 550 up to 1929. Since then it is estimated that 100 or more models, new or modified, have been added to the list, which indicates the scope of the subject. At the risk of not mentioning many sound instruments that a number of clinicians prefer, the writer is concerned here with the principles or the objectives sought in forceps design.

THE INSTRUMENT AND THE PURPOSE OF SPECIAL DESIGN

The obstetric forceps consists of handles, a lock upon which the forceps articulates, blades, and a shank situated between the handles and the blades. The lock may be one of three types, an over-and-under design held together by a screw (French type, i.e., Tarnier's), a mortised lock (English type, i.e., Simpson's), or a sliding lock, as in

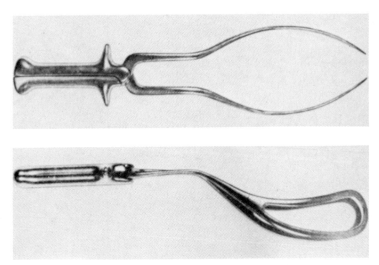

Figure 2.   Hawks-Dennen forceps.

the Kjelland forceps. The shanks may be short or long, and some are narrower than others. The blades are either solid (Tucker-McLean type; Fig. 3A and C), or fenestrated (Simpson and others). The instrument has two curves—the cephalic curve, which in use is in apposition to the fetal vertex, and the pelvic curve—and the extent of these curves varies in the different types of forceps. Certain forceps may be provided with an axis-traction apparatus, or posterior traction is accomplished without these appurtenances, the shank being curved to avoid the perineum, as in the Hawks-Dennen forceps (Fig. 2).

It has been suggested that there should be some universality of forceps design in order to afford the greatest safety for the mother and infant, for certainly forceps of bad design may apply unwarranted stress to the fetal head. The measurements recommended for the ideal obstetric forceps include the following:

(1) tips of blades at least 3 cm. apart;
(2) maximal width of blades, 9 cm.;
(3) length of blades, 16 cm.;
(4) radius of pelvic curve, 17.5 cm.;
)5) radius of cephalic curve, 16 cm.;
(6) length of shank, 6.25 cm., with its greatest width, 2.5 cm.

These values are listed simply as a point of reference for use in comparing one forceps with another. All of the features listed differ to a degree in the various types of instrument. The Irving forceps qualifies in the measurements listed above. Forceps that have been arbitrarily selected on the basis that they represent certain principles

and objectives in forceps design are illustrated in Figures 2 to 7.

The Tarnier axis-traction forceps (Fig. 3B and D), a commonly used instrument, is rather heavy in design, and the cephalic curve is shallow compared with the deeper curve of the Simpson forceps. The Irving modification of the Simpson forceps (Fig. 4), besides the axis-traction appliance, has a slightly greater cephalic curve. The ad-

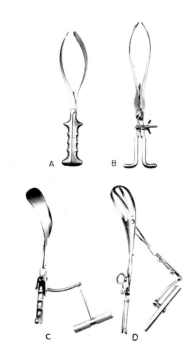

Figure 3.   Representative types of obstetric forceps. A and C, Tucker-McLean type; B and D, Tarnier type.

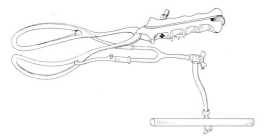

Figure 4. Irving forceps.

vantage is that, once applied, the forceps never moves from its original position during the course of traction. However, the exaggerated cephalic curve, unless one is familiar with use of the instrument, makes it a bit more difficult to apply, especially to a transverse arrest of the vertex (L.O.T. and R.O.T.). The shank is rather wide, requiring early episiotomy to release pressure on the perineum. The traction rods, like those of the Tarnier forceps, have a generous perineal arm, permitting the force to be exerted along the posterior line of traction consistent with bringing the vertex to the perineal floor in accordance with the direction of the pelvic axes. Like other axis-traction instruments, the traction rods are attached after the forceps is in place and are held in a mortised joint by a sliding sleeve or collar. A set screw is located at the end of the handles to keep them apart, thus preventing undue pressure of the forceps blades on the fetal vertex. It is appreciated that there are some who believe that the forceps blades, in order to avoid pressure on the fetal vertex, should move away from and toward each other in a parallel relationship, and there are forceps so constructed.

The Kjelland forceps (Fig. 5) was designed to assist in the delivery of a deep transverse arrest of the vertex, but it has become more popular for the correction or delivery of an occiput posterior as well as a transverse position. This instrument has a shallow cephalic curve, little or no pelvic curve, and a sliding lock. Two small metal knobs, which are essential in the presence of a sliding lock, are located on the anterior surface of the handles. These tell the operator the position of the blades, and when they oppose each other the blades are in the conventional relationship. Also these knobs are used to indicate the direction in which rotation of each branch of the forceps is to take place. It is said that the sliding lock permits the blades to adjust to an asynclitic head when the occiput is in a transverse position, but this feature is not entirely appealing, for the blades may slide beyond one or the other malar eminence and cause serious compression of the vertex.

The Barton forceps (Fig. 6) was designed specifically to cope with a transverse arrest of the vertex. For ease of application, the hinged blade permits a reduction in the cephalic curve. An axis-traction apparatus is also available for the extraction, but this involves certain obvious mechanical disadvantages, and it is recommended that another type of forceps be used once the occiput is rotated to an anterior position.

An instrument designed specifically to assist in the delivery of the aftercoming head in a breech presentation or following internal podalic version is the Piper forceps (Fig. 7). This has a fenestrated, mildly curved cephalic blade and a long, posteriorly curved shank. Certain of the advantages assigned to this forceps, however, may also be regarded as disadvantages. Owing to the long shanks and thin construction of

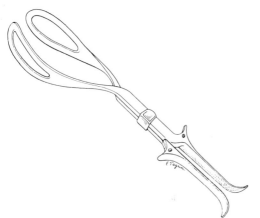

Figure 5. Kjelland forceps.

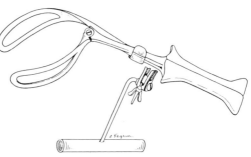

Figure 6. Barton forceps.

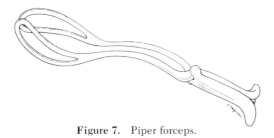

Figure 7.   Piper forceps.

the blades, the latter possess an unusual amount of flexibility or resiliency, which is said to prevent compression of the vertex. This may be true, but this virtue may be detrimental at times when a considerable amount of traction is required. Because of their flexibility, the blades may slip, and whenever this accident occurs in any forceps operation the resultant sudden release of pressure may be as damaging to the blood channels of the fetal brain as undue compression.

The length of the shank of the Piper forceps is said to be an aid in application of the forceps when the aftercoming head is high in the pelvis. It must be emphasized, however, that no forceps of any design should ever be applied to the aftercoming head until it is well engaged, for great harm may otherwise come to both the mother and her child. Engagement must be accomplished by manipulation, with use of forceps reserved when necessary for extraction after the vertex has entered the pelvis.

There is no doubt that certain situations demand specially designed forceps to accomplish a safe, nontraumatic delivery, and in some instances more than one instrument is necessary. In the final analysis, a familiarity with one good forceps is of far greater importance to successful forceps operations than the particular instrument used. Equally significant is knowledge of the indications and contraindications for a forceps procedure.

CLASSIFICATION OF FORCEPS OPERATIONS

Forceps operations are classified into various types, for several reasons: (1) to serve in describing the clinical situation existing at the time of performance of the operation; (2) to provide an accurate reference to the events surrounding the delivery should the infant reveal evidence, either immediately

or remotely, of damage to its central nervous system or other vital structures; and (3) to relate the type of delivery to any obstetric or gynecologic sequelae, and to serve as a guide in the conduct of the patient's subsequent deliveries.

No method of classification of the type of forceps procedure tells the complete story of any forceps operation. Regardless of how it is classified, qualifying terms are necessary if one is to have an accurate account of whether the forceps operation was easy or difficult. Included are such terms as "the occiput was rotated from position X," the rotation was "easy" or "difficult," and the traction required was either "minimal," "moderate," or "extreme." Even such a phrase as "a firm forceps extraction was required" has some clinical meaning. Undoubtedly the effect of the forceps delivery on the fetus could be more accurately described if one could measure the amount of traction needed to advance the fetal head and the amount of compression imposed on it by the forceps. The data are limited, and the results are rather widely divergent. The maximal traction recorded by different methods ranged between 33 and 75 lb., and the average compression, between 3 and 5 lb. These values hardly apply in an outlet forceps, where no significant amount of traction is required in most cases.

The types of forceps are classified according to the arrest of the station of the vertex, not according to where the presenting part may be after the malrotation is corrected. That is to say, the vertex may arrest low but be at midstation after rotation. Many classifications have been proposed. A long-time student of forceps and forceps procedures, Dennen, has proposed the following classification:

(1) **High forceps**—the biparietal diameter of the fetal vertex is in the inlet and the leading point of the vertex is barely above the ischial spines. Anything higher is referred to as forceps application to an unengaged head. (In either event, it would appear that disproportion is likely at the inlet; the procedure would be extremely hazardous and is contraindicated totally.)

(2) **Midforceps**—the leading bony part of the vertex is at or just below the ischial spines, with the biparietal diameter below the superior strait.

(3) **Low midforceps**—the biparietal diameter is at or below the level of the ischial spines, with the leading bony part within a

fingerbreadth above the perineum between contractions.

(4) **Low forceps** — the bony vertex is on the perineum between contractions and is visible during a contraction. The biparietal diameter is judged to be below the plane of the ischial spines with the sagittal suture in or nearly coinciding with the anteroposterior diameter of the outlet.

Any classification is open to criticism, and, as previously suggested, one cannot describe by type alone the total events associated with a forceps procedure. Most obstetricians, however, consider that, besides high forceps (which is no longer acceptable in obstetric practice and could therefore be deleted from any classification), three categories are necessary in describing forceps delivery of the engaged vertex.

Pelvic landmarks obviously must be taken into account in any classification, but because the pelvic planes are described in a variety of ways it is difficult to use these interchangeably in recording the station of the vertex. It seems logical, and is therefore suggested, that the type of forceps be designated according to the scheme of denoting the station of the vertex in the conduct of labor, qualified by indicating the necessity for rotation and the degree of traction required. That is to say, the station of the leading bony part of the vertex should be designated as *minus* 1 to 4 cm. when it is above the interspinous line, which is zero, and *plus* 1 to 4 cm. when it is below the interspinous line.

Thus, a *minus* value would mean a high forceps; in fact, minus 4 would indicate a floating vertex. A *midforceps* would mean that the bony part of the vertex is zero to plus 1 cm. below the interspinous diameter, that is, the biparietal diameter is slightly below the inlet and the vertex is engaged. A *low forceps* would indicate position of the vertex as plus 2 or 3 cm., with the leading point nearing the perineum. An *outlet forceps* would indicate the bony vertex at plus 4 cm., meaning that it is visible and distending the perineum, and the biparietal diameter is near the bi-ischial diameter. As can be seen, this does not differ appreciably from the Dennen classification, but attempts to be more definitive.

A second category would designate the degree of rotation, if needed. Third, and finally, the amount of traction required would be stated as *minimal, moderate,* or *maximal.* Thus, for example, a final diagnosis of a forceps operation might be: (1) *a low forceps;* (2) *manual rotation from L.O.P. position,* and (3) *moderate degree of traction.*

Whatever scheme is used, forceps operations can be mistakenly classified as the result of molding and caput formation of the vertex. Also, the clinician may classify the procedure somewhat arbitrarily, for the natural instinct is to minimize any difficulties encountered in a forceps delivery. Admittedly, when outlet contracture exists, a low forceps as here defined can be a reasonably formidable procedure even for the experienced. But outlet contracture alone is rare, and most authorities agree that, when it occurs, it is associated with midpelvic contracture. It is these cases that are of the greatest concern, for it is in this group that mistakes are made and that, in midforceps operations, the fetal morbidity and mortality reside. In retrospect, cesarean section in some instances would appear to have been preferable. If the diagnosis of midforceps is to be applied to all cases other than outlet forceps, the frequency of the operation will be comparatively high, and the fetal morbidity and mortality should be low. By comparison, midforceps as here defined has been known to be accompanied by a comparatively high fetal morbidity and mortality. In view of all these considerations, it seems desirable to include three types of forceps for delivery of the engaged head if the fetal morbidity and mortality are to be factually portrayed and a critical review is to be made of the results in any one clinic.

Outlet forceps as defined accounts for nearly all forceps operations. Although performed for a specific indication, the procedure is generally used to reduce the length of the second stage of labor. The operation is thus used as a preventive measure, that is, to remove the possibility of fetal distress and intracranial damage through a prolonged perineal arrest. The value of decreasing fetal mortality and morbidity through eliminating a prolonged second stage of labor by masterful interference with forceps was appreciated long ago, and, encompassing the idea of prevention, the term "prophylactic forceps" was introduced.

In general, in an outlet forceps procedure the occiput is found in an anterior position, and the need for traction following an episiotomy is slight. At the same time, the occiput may have rotated directly posterior and, if it is not corrected, the amount of traction required can be considerable. This is mentioned to emphasize the necessity for classifying the forceps operation otherwise than according to type.

A low forceps procedure can be either easy or moderately difficult, depending on the need for correction of malrotation and whether the pelvic outlet is ample. The same may be said of a midforceps, but generally the procedure is more difficult. In fact, both low and midforceps, as here defined, require skill and experience if fetal and maternal trauma are to be avoided.

In summary, forceps delivery should be categorized as belonging to one of four types, however one chooses to define them, besides being characterized on the basis of two or possibly three additional categories, including (1) the correction of malrotation, (2) the amount of traction required, and (3) whether the procedure was easy or difficult.

TRIAL FORCEPS AND FAILED FORCEPS

Trial forceps is an accepted obstetric practice; failed forceps must be regarded as the result of the use of forceps when the operation is contraindicated, and it is therefore not acceptable. Failed forceps denotes inability to deliver the patient because of failure either to recognize cephalopelvic disproportion or a pathologic retraction ring, or to diagnose the fetal position correctly; it may also result from technical error, that is, from improper application of the forceps. If failure is the result of cephalopelvic disproportion or a contraction ring, there are two alternatives of management. One is to consider a destructive operation if the fetus is presumably already severely damaged or dead; the other is to deliver the patient by abdominal hysterotomy. The baby, if living, is usually suffering from hypoxia or is traumatized as a result of prolonged manipulation, and the mother is potentially if not actually infected. Fortunately, failed forceps is rarely seen in current obstetric practice.

A trial forceps is permissible with the "double set-up" preparation as discussed under Avoidance of Birth Trauma in Chapter 27. Being experienced in forceps procedures, the operator is aware that the cephalopelvic relationship is borderline; he is certain of his diagnosis, and realizes that a forceps operation must be carefully performed if fetal and maternal trauma are to be avoided. He is not committed unreservedly to pelvic delivery. Rather, he proposes to apply the forceps and correct any malrotation if this can be accomplished with relative ease, after which he will apply traction, and, depending on the progress obtained, decide whether the patient can or cannot be delivered safely by the pelvic route. When trial traction results in little or no progress, the operator desists from any further attempt before the condition of the mother or fetus has in any way been compromised, and proceeds with abdominal delivery. It is evident that there is a clear distinction between "trial" and "failed" forceps.

INDICATIONS FOR AND INCIDENCE OF VARIOUS TYPES OF FORCEPS OPERATIONS

The myth may still prevail in the minds of patients and others that a forceps delivery is all too frequently associated with fetal trauma. Suffice to say, intracranial damage from trauma should not occur in current obstetric practice, primarily because of the more liberal use of cesarean section in cases in which the midpelvic and outlet pelvic capacity may be in question. There should be agreement that a difficult midforceps operation must be avoided in such cases.

Studies of the forces of traction and compression by means of strain gauges applied to the handles and blades of the forceps reveal the compression force of the maternal tissue on the fetal head to be substantially greater than the compression force from the forceps blades on the zygomatic arches of the fetal head. Moreover, the forces generated by uterine contractions and the maternal resistance that cause the head to mold may well exceed the forces engendered by forceps per se. Hence, whenever intracranial damage occurs, it may be due to forces of labor rather than those required for delivery itself.

Forceps operation should be regarded as a procedure performed as a preventive measure. Certainly fetal distress from whatever cause with its accompanying hypoxia is readily treatable by a properly performed forceps delivery. The splinting effect of the forceps can protect the fetal brain from maternal compression, especially important in the fragile premature infant. The ill effects of maternal compression of a prolonged second stage of labor may be eliminated by episiotomy and easy outlet forceps operation.

Most forceps operations are performed to reduce the length of the second stage of labor, and nearly all of these procedures are of the outlet variety. A slowing of the fetal heart rate and the passage of meconium indicate fetal distress, which occurs most frequently when the vertex is arrested on the perineum. In other specific situations a prolonged second stage may be detrimental to the mother, as when she has cardiac or a metabolic disease, or when she has previously undergone cesarean section or myomectomy. In current obstetric practice maternal exhaustion alone should not be an indication for forceps delivery.

The second most common indication for forceps delivery is to overcome dystocia, whether idiopathic functional dystocia, or dystocia due to malrotation of the vertex, brow and face presentations, macrosomia, contracture of the midpelvic and outlet planes bordering on disproportion, and, finally, the resistance of the perineum.

Third, forceps delivery is indicated for fetal distress of a specific cause, such as occult or frank prolapse of the cord or premature separation of the placenta, provided the patient is in or nearing the second stage of labor.

Exactly how long a patient should be permitted to remain in second-stage labor depends largely on whether or not she is making progress. As a general policy, the vertex should not be allowed to remain on the perineum much beyond an hour, and during this period the fetal heart tones should be constantly auscultated and recorded. The patient should be delivered promptly in the event of any evidence of fetal distress. In the multiparous patient who has had her previous babies easily, however, a second stage of longer than an hour, regardless of the station of the vertex, should be viewed with some suspicion; in fact, a prolonged second stage in the multipara is to be deplored. One should perform a vaginal examination in search for a cause of the apparent dystocia. In contrast, no harm comes to the primiparous patient or her fetus in a second stage lasting more than one or two hours provided the vertex is off the perineum, the patient is making progress, and her general condition is satisfactory. For example, the primiparous patient who enters the second stage of labor with the bony point of the vertex at or slightly below the interspinous line and whose pelvis is believed to be of sufficient size to permit pelvic delivery may be given two to three hours of labor if the vertex continues to advance, for a low forceps is preferable to a midforceps procedure. Naturally the patient must be closely supervised and delivery expedited if there are any untoward developments.

The incidence of various types of forceps deliveries will depend on the policies regarding the indications for these procedures, more particularly in relation to the length of time allowed for second-stage labor without progress and the definition and classification of the various types of forceps. With oxytocin infusion to stimulate desultory labor, and the gradual decrease in the incidence of contracted pelvis, the need for midforceps and, indeed, for low forceps has diminished, but the incidence of outlet forceps probably will not be decreased, at least when the procedure is used to avoid the hazards of a prolonged second-stage labor.

In summary, the need for forceps delivery in the absence of fetal distress is determined by the resistance of the perineal tissue, the efficiency of the forces of labor, the size of the fetus, the position of the vertex, and the size and type of the pelvis. In present-day obstetrics, the most frequent indication for forceps delivery is prevention of fetal hypoxia and fetal brain damage from pressure effect of prolonged second-stage labor offered by resistance of the perineal tissues. The elimination of prolonged perineal arrest of the vertex, which as a rule requires only an outlet forceps operation, is consistent with sound obstetrics based on the clinical observation that under these circumstances, during the course of a contraction, the fetal heart tones frequently become slow in rate and irregular in rhythm. This is interpreted to mean that the fetus may be in some distress, presumably from oxygen lack, although it is recognized that pressure on the fetal vertex will cause a diminution in fetal heart rate. Prolonged perineal arrest also leads to disruption of the supporting structures of the bladder and rectum, with resultant gynecologic lesions.

THE REQUIREMENTS FOR FORCEPS DELIVERY

The forceps operation requires fulfillment of at least five conditions: (1) the cervix must be completely dilated; (2) the membranes must be ruptured; (3) the cephalopelvic relationship at the major pelvic planes must be normal or must not preclude pelvic delivery; (4) the vertex must be engaged; and (5) the fetal position must be correctly diagnosed. These requirements having been listed, some deserve qualification.

Emphasis is placed on the errors in determining engagement, and these result principally from three features: caput succedaneum, or edema formation of the scalp, which may be mistaken for the bony vertex; extreme molding; and faulty attitudes. All of these may be interpreted as indicative of engagement when the biparietal diameter of the vertex is above the superior strait with the leading point at or below the bispinous diameter. The vertex is not engaged, however, although cephalopelvic disproportion may not necessarily exist (Fig. 8).

In some cases of prolonged labor, pelvic

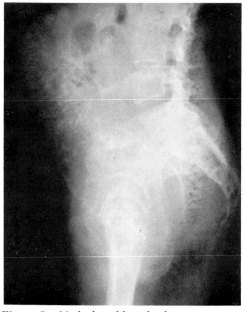

Figure 8. Marked molding leading to erroneous determination of engagement. Note overriding of the parietal bones in the area of the sagittal suture. Biparietal diameter at the inlet; leading point at spines. Sacrum ends well below ischial tuberosities. Eventual safe pelvic delivery.

delivery may be brought about by incising the cervix when it is not completely dilated (see Dührssen's Incisions, later in this chapter). The conditions and circumstances under which this procedure is permissible must be fulfilled. The same management is indicated if fetal distress suddenly develops when the patient is near the end of the second stage of labor, provided the cephalopelvic relationship is normal.

TECHNIQUE OF FORCEPS DELIVERY

In this discussion it is the writer's desire not to become involved in minutiae that have little bearing on the end-results, but rather to dwell on those principles of technique of application and extraction that pertain equally to all forceps operations, of whatever type, whether outlet, low, or midforceps. The choice of the instrument is not so important as the judgment, dexterity, and gentleness of the operator.

The patient is anesthetized, prepared, and draped for the forceps operation. The bladder is not necessarily catheterized, for it is less likely to interfere with the forceps procedure when it is an abdominal rather than a pelvic organ. Injury to the point of defect in the bladder is not related to failure to catheterize the patient, but is rather the result of faulty technique in performing a forceps delivery or of utilizing the operation when it is contraindicated, as in the presence of midpelvic contracture.

Besides a correct diagnosis of fetal position and proper application of the forceps, several details of forceps operations are vital to prevention of fetal and maternal trauma (Figs. 9 to 13). When there is marked molding of the fetal vertex, or edema of the scalp or caput succedaneum, the diagnosis of position may at first be uncertain. Under these circumstances, rather than relying on fontanelles and suture lines to establish the fetal position, it is well to locate the fetal ear and ascertain its point of direction. (See Obstetrically Significant Landmarks and Diameters of the Fetal Skull in Chapter 25.) Furthermore, locating the fetal ear can be an aid in placing the forceps in the proper position if, because of edema of the scalp, one cannot be certain of the location of the lambdoidal sutures. If the fetal ear rests in the fenestra of the forceps blade, the operator may be assured that he has a proper application, that is, that the anterior edge of the blades near the shank is within a fingerbreadth or two of the lambdoidal suture. To accomplish this, the operator places the index finger of the hand in the vagina in the fenestra of the left blade to guide the blade upward and along the side of the vertex until it overlies the ear.

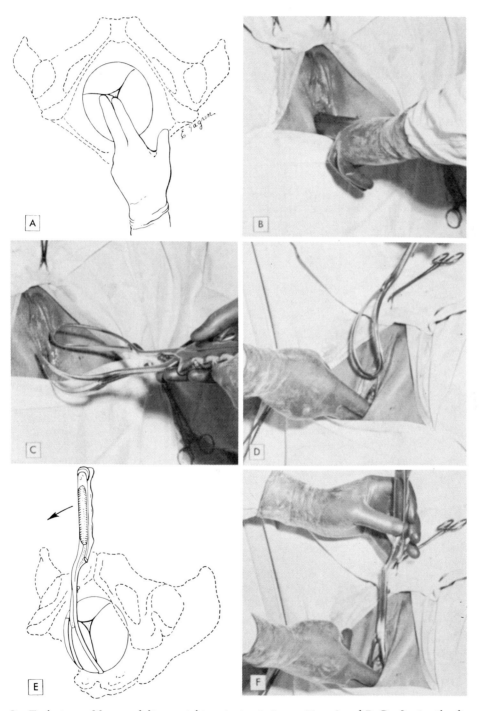

Figure 9. Technique of forceps delivery, right occiput anterior position. A and B, Confirming the diagnosis of position. The examining fingers detect the posterior fontanelle and the lambdoidal and sagittal sutures. C, Orienting the forceps to the position of the vertex. D, About to insert the left blade in the vagina. E and F, Inserting the left blade into the vagina along the curve of the sacrum.

With an assistant steadying the forceps handle so that the blade will not wander, the right blade is next applied. This technique is especially helpful when it is essential to apply the instrument with great accuracy, as in a low forceps or midforceps procedure. In an outlet forceps, slight deviations in application can occur without producing any harmful effects on the fetus, but this is not true in the more formidable types of forceps operation.

To begin, after confirming the diagnosis of position, the operator holds the instrument in position to orient himself as to how he must apply it (Fig. 9C). The middle and index fingers of the guiding hand are introduced into the vagina over the anterior surface of the lower sacrum (Fig. 9D). The left blade is then inserted into the vagina over the palmar surface of the fingers of the guiding hand (Fig. 9F). Remembering that there is ample room in the hollow of the sacrum beneath the vertex, the operator

thus introduces the blade into the midline of the vagina (Fig. 10B). Often the blades are depicted as being inserted along the side of the vertex, but this method only invites abrasion of the infant's cheek or of the vaginal mucous membrane. If the forceps handle is held as one would a pencil, the weight of the handle will be sufficient to cause the blade to drop into the hollow of the sacrum. The blade is now swept into place near the lambdoidal suture by the guiding hand. There is little necessity to exert appreciable force on the handles; rather, the hand in the vagina should be the more responsible for application of any force necessary. The shank and anterior edge of the blade is brought to approximately 2 cm. from the lambdoidal suture (Fig. 10C). This places the forceps blade in a position where it will not cause pressure on the infant's facial nerve, for the tip of the blade rests on the malar eminence, from which position traction may be ap-

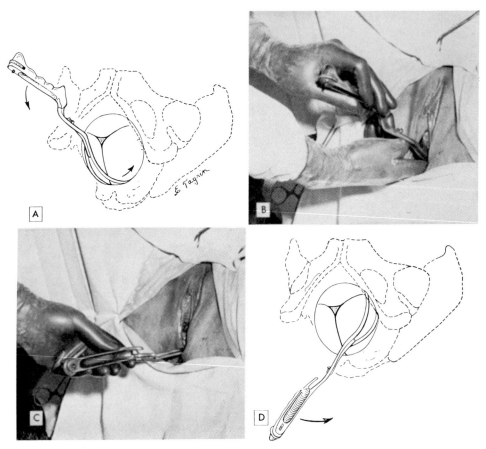

Figure 10.   Technique of forceps delivery, R.O.A. (*continued*). A and B, Left blade properly inserted into the vagina. C and D, Left blade correctly placed over the infant's ear and about 2 cm. from the lambdoidal suture.

plied without harm. The right blade is similarly applied, each blade being the same distance from its respective lambdoidal suture (Fig. 11).

The handles are now gently brought together; if resistance is met, an attempt should be made to see how far apart the handles must be to avoid encountering this sensation, and they are then kept at that distance. This means that the handles are separated sufficiently to ensure the operator that the blades will not cause fetal compression. The handles should be held in this position for the extraction. If, when the position of the forceps is checked, the shanks are not equally distant from the lambdoidal sutures, the handles should be unlocked and the forceps adjusted to a near

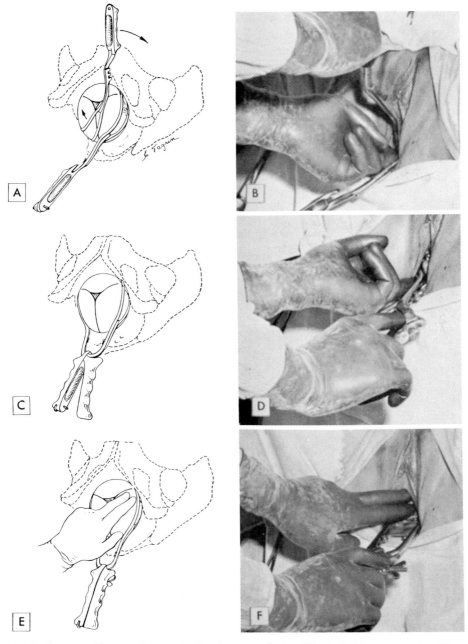

Figure 11. Technique of forceps delivery, R.O.A. (*continued*). A and B, Right blade inserted and being placed in correct position. C and D, Forceps in place, handles unlocked. E and F, Rechecking the diagnosis and the position of the forceps.

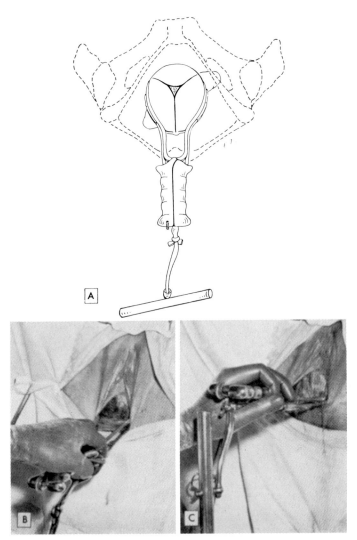

Figure 12. Technique of forceps delivery, R.O.A. (*continued*). A, Forceps in position. Occiput rotated directly anterior. Traction rod in place. B, Beginning of the extraction. Traction by right hand not visible. C, Handles and traction rods held together preliminary to performing the episiotomy.

perfect application. When required, the occiput is first rotated to an anterior position prior to extraction.

Next, the axis-traction apparatus is applied and the extraction is begun (Fig. 12). To appreciate the direction of traction, one must envision the direction of the pelvic axes with the patient in the lithotomy position. The traction should be exerted along the line of the pelvic axis (Fig. 14) and hence must be directed posteriorly and downward.

Both interesting and important, Tarnier believed that the line of traction must be directed well posterior, in fact, from the midpelvis toward the tip of the sacrum (Fig. 15). In many publications on the subject, as

noted by the illustrations used, the view has been expressed that the direction of traction advocated by Tarnier was extreme (Fig. 16), but Tarnier's ideas appear to be more in keeping with the modern concept of how the vertex traverses the birth canal, as demonstrated by Caldwell, Moloy, and D'Esopo. In the drawing of the lateral view of the pelvis showing Tarnier's idea of direction of traction (Fig. 15), the curve of the sacrum is more like the normal. The sacrum in Figure 16 is comparatively straight, however, and hence what is stated as the proper line of traction hardly applies to the normal pelvis.

There is a great tendency to direct the traction anterior to the inferior axis, which

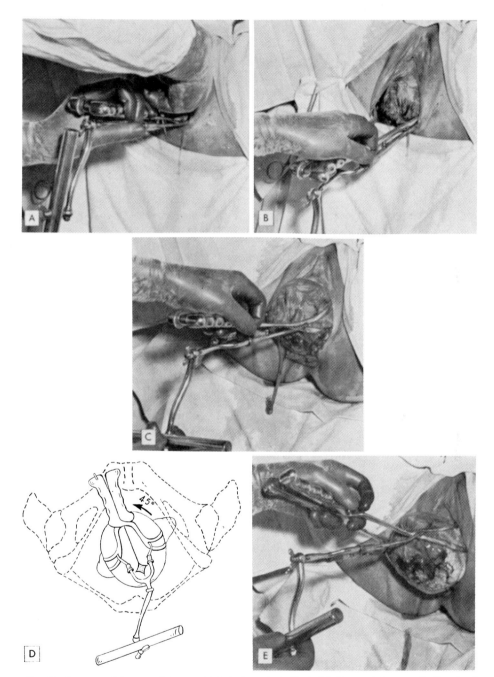

Figure 13. Technique of forceps delivery, R.O.A. (*concluded*). A, Median episiotomy. B, Continuing extraction after episiotomy. C, Extraction of vertex nearly complete. Perineal towel deliberately removed for exposure purposes. Forceps handles elevated. D, Forceps in situ, vertex delivered, shoulder rotating 45 degrees counterclockwise. E, Vertex delivered, forceps in situ.

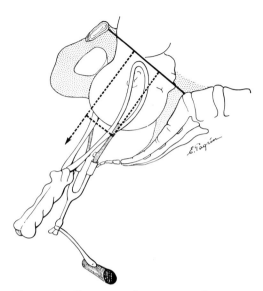

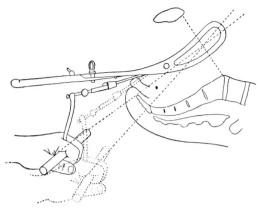

Figure 16. Ribemont-Dessaignes axis traction. Upper hand regarded as representing proper line of traction, which may be true for this rather straight sacrum. Lower hand represents the line of traction favored by Tarnier when the sacrum is normal. (From Ribemont-Dessaignes, A., and LePage, G.: Traité d'obstétrique. Masson et Cie, Paris, 1914, p. 1176.)

Figure 14. Direction of traction in the superior axis of the pelvis.

is permissible only after the occiput has bypassed the symphysis. Thus the direction of the line of traction advocated by Tarnier, which may seem exaggerated, should be followed, for it eliminates any possibility of the occiput exerting pressure on the anterior vaginal wall and bladder. The vertex is therefore brought to the perineum, and only after the biparietal diameter is at the level of the ischial tuberosities is the vertex permitted to extend, simulating in detail the normal mechanism of labor.

Directing the vertex along the pelvic axis *without* axis traction is not without its dangers. Hence it is not illustrated, and is only briefly described. With the forceps

in place, one hand exerts downward pressure over the shanks of the forceps and the other hand furnishes traction backward and downward (Saxtorph-Pajot maneuver). By this maneuver an attempt is made to bring the vertex into the posterior segment of the pelvis, but the forceps blades tend to traumatize the lateral fornices of the vagina, the pressure of the occiput against the symphysis favors disruption of the pubo-cervical fascia, and the skin covering the infant's malar eminences may become abraded. These happenings are readily prevented by the routine use of axis-traction forceps.

The duration of traction should simulate that of normal labor contractions; that is, traction is exerted for 30 to 35 seconds followed by the release of the forceps, including separation of the handles, for some 30 to 60 seconds. The first traction might be designated *trial traction* whereby the operator should demonstrate advancement of the vertex. After trial traction, he should recheck his diagnosis of the position, as determined by the posterior fontanelle, making certain that the forceps are correctly placed and have not moved from their original position on the fetal head. If progress fails to occur, the operator may even wish to remove the forceps to check his diagnosis more accurately, and to reassess the midpelvis and lower pelvis, making certain that no cephalopelvic disproportion exists.

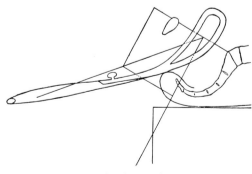

Figure 15. Tarnier's idea of direction of traction. Note curve of sacrum which is more in keeping with the normal pelvis in Figure 14, compared with the relatively straight sacrum in Figure 16.

Traction is applied periodically, remembering that there is no need for haste, and that gentleness is the watchword. Constant checking of the fetal heart with the fetoscope is a nicety, but pressure over the skin of the scalp can keep the operator informed as to the infant's condition. Finger pressure will cause the skin of the fetal scalp to blanch; with release, the blanching will immediately disappear, indicating that the capillary circulation is intact and the infant's condition is satisfactory. Further, the rate of the fetal heart tones may decrease with traction, presumably owing to some compression, causing the inexperienced operator undue worry, but this is no reason to reduce the operating time, for more harm will come to the baby through haste than otherwise.

Slow, steady progress is the desired objective, and 15 or more minutes should be required for low and midforceps extraction. As noted, traction is directed posteriorly until the occiput has bypassed the symphysis. An episiotomy is performed early, that is, when the vertex reaches the perineum and is barely seen at the introitus. The vertex is guided through the outlet by forceps. Following the delivery of the vertex, the mechanism is similar to that of spontaneous delivery. In case the forceps is to be removed prior to delivery, the blade last applied is swept posteriorly to the hollow of the sacrum and removed first, and the blade initially applied is then removed in similar fashion. The ischial spines may be an impediment, but raising the handle anteriorly will release the blade.

VACUUM EXTRACTOR VERSUS FORCEPS DELIVERY

A vacuum extractor has been reintroduced into obstetrics to be used in place of forceps as a method of delivery. It is also used in the treatment of functional dystocia to bring the presenting part against the partially dilated cervix, reputedly to enhance labor.

In principle, the device consists of a steel cup with an attached rubber suction tube containing a traction chain. The cup is applied to the scalp of the leading point of the infant's vertex, and is held in place by a regulated vacuum created by an appropriate pump. Internal traction is applied to the chain and the fetus is delivered. It is said that the instrument is capable of accomplishing delivery in cases comparable to those in which the midforceps operation is used. Also, a malrotated or arrested vertex (O.T. or O.P.) is reported to rotate into an occiput anterior position with traction on the chain. With the negative pressure that is applied during placement of the cup, the scalp beneath becomes markedly edematous, protruding several centimeters, and exceeding the largest caput succedaneum. This swelling of the scalp following delivery with the vacuum extractor persists for at least 24 to 48 hours, and should create some anxiety in most mothers. One may wonder whether such traction might in some way damage the blood vessels covering the brain, especially when considerable traction is required. With the station of the vertex above the perineum, traction cannot readily be applied in the proper pelvic axis.

There is of course no splinting effect with the vacuum extractor as with forceps. The distortion of the fetal skull—a tenting effect that can occur with traction of the vacuum extractor—is quite different from normal molding. The tenting may give rise to rupture of the sagittal sinus and falx.

As this instrument has been used and evaluated by more clinics, it has become apparent that it has definite limitations. After a trial experience, the writer abandoned its use, being convinced that it did not possess any advantage over forceps but rather definite disadvantages. Damage to the fetus has been alluded to and these results would be totally unacceptable in forceps procedures.

The instrument is not regarded as appropriate for the premature infant, for certainly there is the loss of the splinting effect of forceps which is believed necessary to protect the fragile brain of the premature. Also, it takes at least 5 to 10 minutes to create the vacuum necessary to hold the extractor, which would be most undesirable in the delivery of an infant with fetal distress when time is of some importance.

Varying results have been reported when the vacuum extractor is applied through the partially dilated cervix to improve desultory labor. The principle has been applied by other methods, i.e., traction to the fetal scalp, and the results were unsatisfactory. Prolonged traction can be damaging to the infant, and the admonition that the cervix should be inspected after delivery suggests that lacerations can occur. Moreover, oxytocin stimulation is highly effective in the treatment of this syndrome.

A failure rate of 10 per cent to effect delivery has been recorded. Altogether,

to suggest that delivery by the vacuum extractor should be regarded as an alternative to a forceps procedure seems inconsistent with safe obstetric practice.

CESAREAN SECTION

HISTORY AND SURGICAL OBJECTIVES OF VARIOUS TYPES

Cesarean section and abdominal hysterotomy are terms used interchangeably to designate the operation by which a child is delivered abdominally through a surgical opening of the uterus. The literature concerning the operation and its history is voluminous, and numerous books and monographs are readily available on the subject. Only a brief résumé as it relates to the development of the various types of operation and the objectives sought will be attempted here.

The operation was known to the ancients and became a recognized procedure under the Roman Law. The name of the operation is derived from the Latin verb *caedere* (to cut) and lex caesarea is included in the codification of the Roman Law (715 B.C.). As in antiquity, the purpose of the Roman Law was twofold: namely, to salvage a living fetus should the mother die undelivered or, under these tragic circumstances, to provide the child a separate burial. The preservation of the life of a viable fetus after death of the mother is still regarded as one of the indications for the operation. Undoubtedly only a percentage of the total number of cases has reached the literature. As might be expected, the fetal mortality is quite high, for the operation is performed after the mother has expired but when the fetal heart tones are believed to be still present. A careful follow-up is needed of the children so delivered; the risk of irreparable damage to the central nervous system from intrauterine hypoxia obviously is substantial.

The first authentic report of a cesarean section performed on a living woman was by Trautmann of Wittenberg in 1610. The gravid uterus was contained in a large ventral hernia, and pelvic delivery was deemed impossible. Although the infant survived,

the mother died some 25 days postoperatively, presumably from protracted uterine and generalized sepsis. In the absence of aseptic technique and failure to close the uterine incision the mortality was 85 per cent.

From that time until late in the 19th century, it was vigorously debated whether cesarean section was ever justified as opposed to a destructive operation, that is, craniotomy and embryotomy, when pelvic contracture precluded safe vaginal delivery and the fetus was still alive. Those who advocated craniotomy on a living child to preserve the life of the mother were condemned by some medical as well as religious groups.

The appalling mortality continued until 1876 when Porro advocated the extirpation of the uterine corpus and ovaries at the time of cesarean section. It was his hope that such a procedure would prevent death from hemorrhage or peritonitis resulting from contamination of the peritoneal cavity. In the original operation, after removal of the corpus, the cervix was mobilized upward out of the pelvis and sutured into the abdominal incision. In the operation today, the ovaries are generally not removed, and the cervix is removed or if left in situ is covered with the uterovesical fold of peritoneum.

The operation that bears Porro's name had been contemplated from the early 1800's. Actually, the removal of a gravid uterus at term was probably first performed by Storer of Boston in 1869. The procedure was born of necessity as a desperate measure to control hemorrhage at the time of cesarean section. The indication for cesarean section was a large degenerating uterine fibroid that completely obstructed the birth canal. The patient died on her third postoperative day. In the early years after its introduction, the Porro operation had a mortality rate of approximately 15 per cent. Obviously this operation marked a significant milestone in increasing the safety of abdominal delivery.

In 1882, Sänger of Leipzig recommended suturing and coaptation of the uterine wound; this brought the operation of cesarean section to the stage of development where it warranted acceptance as a surgical procedure. Prior to that time, with few exceptions, reliance was placed on the contraction of the myometrium to control hemorrhage, and the uterine incision was not sutured. Although closure of the uterus had been attempted previously, notably by American surgeons, the methods were less well conceived and consisted simply of placing a few silver wire sutures through the uterine wall. In his technique, Sänger employed two layers of sutures, and the closure was so complete that previous attempts to suture the uterus were hardly comparable. The first suture was continuous and included the entire thickness of the myometrium but avoided the decidua and the visceral peritoneum. Interrupted sutures were used for the second row in an effort to invert the edges of the incision and bring the peritoneum into close apposition about the uterine wound.

Even with the notable improvement in operative mortality following Sänger's contribution, a significant death rate from infection continued in patients following prolonged labor and earlier failure of operative pelvic delivery. Before that time, and subsequently during the 19th and the early part of the present century, two other important contributions were made in the technique of cesarean section. The first was an attempt to expose and enter the uterus extraperitoneally; the other was the placement of the incision in the lower uterine segment. The purpose of both was to decrease the hazard of peritoneal infection.

In the early part of the 19th century, Ritgen devised an operation whereby he was able to enter the uterus extraperitoneally. This resulted in many complications, however, and deaths from hemorrhage were frequent, which is understandable in view of the extreme vascularity of the region selected for the operation, namely, the lowermost portion of the uterus and the upper part of the vagina. Through a semilunar skin incision above the right inguinal ligament, the peritoneum was visualized and displaced upward; the uterus and vagina were then incised and the infant extracted. Although the operation (gastroelytrotomy) was used sporadically for the next century in this country and elsewhere, it was eventually discarded, for blood loss was unpredictable and wound sepsis was the rule.

Physick, the renowned Philadelphia surgeon, in 1824 stated that in his opinion the lower uterine segment could be approached extraperitoneally if the visceral peritoneum overlying the upper portion of the urinary bladder were dissected and displaced upward. Nearly a century later, in 1908, Sellheim demonstrated that this approach was possible, and thereby performed an extraperitoneal type of cesarean section. After a Pfannenstiel incision, the bladder was distended with fluid. The dissection, begun at the lateral border of the bladder caudad to or below the peritoneal reflection, was carried toward the midline, allowing the peritoneum with the prevesical fascia to be displaced upward. The lateral border of the bladder on the opposite side was treated in a similar fashion, and when the dissection met at the midline the peritoneum and the bladder were freed from each other. The bladder was then displaced downward, and the peritoneal fold was displaced upward, exposing the lower uterine segment, which was excised longitudinally. Apparently Sellheim's first case was his most successful, for in his subsequent papers he favored an operation that excluded the lower segment from the peritoneal cavity. After recognizing Frank's contribution (1906), Sellheim proceeded to describe an operation that included incising the parietal peritoneum near the fundus of the bladder and suturing it to the visceral peritoneum of the uterus. The fetus was then delivered through an incision in the lower uterine segment. The extraperitoneal operation he chose to call Sellheim I, and the peritoneal exclusion procedure, Sellheim II.

Latzko, in 1909, advocated an extraperitoneal type of operation in which the dissection was restricted to one side of the lower uterine segment. The bladder was displaced to the midline, and the lower uterine segment was exposed sufficiently to permit a vertical incision long enough to allow extraction of the fetus.

Waters, in 1940, proposed an extraperitoneal type of cesarean section, utilizing more closely the dissection as recommended by Physick, with an approach to the lower uterine segment and surgical treatment of the peritoneum overlying the bladder similar to that advocated by Sellheim.

The development of the peritoneal exclusion types of cesarean section began with the present century. The first of these operations was proposed by Frank in 1906 and, as previously noted, was followed closely by a similar operation introduced by Sellheim. According to Frank's technique, the abdomen was opened through a transverse suprapubic incision of the Pfannenstiel type. The peritoneum over the upper portion of the lower uterine segment was incised close to the bladder and sutured to the parietal peritoneum, excluding the peritoneal cavity. The uterus was opened transversely through the area now devoid of peritoneum. To accomplish greater exposure of the lower uterine segment and place the uterine incision at a lower level, this procedure has been modified by Smith.

Kehrer of Heidelburg in 1882 was the first to devise a procedure that approached the lower uterine segment transperitoneally. He believed that the poor results following classic cesarean section were due to leakage of lochia through the uterine wound into the peritoneal cavity, with subsequent peritonitis. To obviate this situation, he proposed an operation in which the lower uterine segment was opened transversely through the uterovesical fold of peritoneum, with care taken not to disturb the bladder. The uterus was closed by two lines of interrupted sutures, the first including the entire myometrium, and the second approximating the uterovesical fold of peritoneum.

Krönig, in 1912, reiterated the beliefs of Kehrer, and also stated that any favorable results encountered in the extraperitoneal or exclusion type of operation were due mainly to placement of the incision in the lower uterine segment. To support his position he called attention to the fact that the lower uterine segment is relatively quiescent and less likely to extrude lochia into the peritoneal cavity through the incision. Further, he contended that the peritoneal cavity should be protected from subsequent infection by covering the lower uterine incision with uterovesical peritoneum. The risk of sepsis being diminished, a longer test of labor was permissible and thereby a lesser need for cesarean section. Krönig also believed that postoperative convalescence would be improved when compared to the classic type of procedure. Extending the procedure of Kehrer, Krönig dissected the upper bladder free of the lower uterine segment, thereby exposing the latter, which he opened with a *longitudinal* incision. He replaced the bladder following uterine closure.

Beck modified the operation by covering the closed uterine wound with peritoneum that had been previously dissected from the nearby upper uterine segment. The uterovesical fold of peritoneum, or bladder flap, was subsequently sutured above the upper peritoneal fold, making the uterine incision both retrovesical and retroperitoneal. The operation was somewhat inaccurately designated a transperitoneal cesarean section with an extraperitoneal closure. DeLee became an exponent of this type of cesarean section, and suggested the term laparotrachelotomy to describe the procedure.

An operation similar to that devised by Kehrer was advocated and popularized later, in 1926, by Kerr, who also found adequate space at the uterovesical fold to open the uterus *transversely* without displacing the bladder. It was Phaneuf who, following the ideas propounded by Krönig, first placed a *transverse* incision in the lower uterine segment in an area beneath the bladder after it had been dissected free and displaced downward, the most popular technique in current practice.

With all these developments, the transperitoneal lower segment cesarean section soon began to displace the classic operation, and today many clinics perform only the former.

So far as the records reveal, the first successful cesarean section in America was performed in 1794 by Dr. Jesse Bennett upon his own wife in the backwoods country of Virginia. Following a consultation after an unsuccessful attempt at pelvic delivery by forceps in the presence of a contracted pelvis, it was decided that two courses were open: cesarean section or craniotomy. The decision was influenced in no small measure by the patient, who, thinking that she would die anyway, insisted that the child be saved if possible. Although it was decided to perform a cesarean operation, the consultant refused to do the procedure but did consent to assist Dr. Bennett. The mother survived and lived for another 25 years, while the baby girl, unharmed, lived to the impressive age of 77 years. The records are authentic, although Dr. Bennett refused to report the case, for he believed his critics would question his veracity and asserted that "no doctor with any feeling of delicacy would report an operation he had done on his own wife."

INCIDENCE AND RISK OF CESAREAN SECTION

The concomitant advances in surgical technique and improvement in anesthesia, the increased availability of blood for transfusion, and the use of antibiotics and chemotherapy have resulted in material reduction of the mortality associated with cesarean section, and have permitted broadening of the obstetric indications for abdominal delivery. There has been a trend to substitute cesarean section for difficult midforceps operations or internal podalic version as a method of delivery. The avoidance of traumatic pelvic delivery, with its associated high fetal morbidity and mortality, is a desirable goal. The gratifying decrease in the incidence of cerebral hemorrhage of the newborn attests to the soundness of such a policy.

The incidence of both primary and secondary, or repeat, cesarean section will be influenced by the frequency of contracted pelvis and of medical and obstetric complications. A *primary* cesarean section rate of 2 or 3 per cent and a total incidence of 5 to 6 per cent is an acceptable rate in present-day practice. The latter incidence is influenced by a number of factors—one being the desire to have a concomitant tubal sterilization at the time of repeat cesarean section, not always acceptable in some hospitals.

The modern literature contains several reports of large series of cases, some of which are without a single maternal death. Although a study of maternal mortality statistics reveals a high percentage of deaths associated with cesarean section, it is not the operation itself, but other factors—medical and obstetric complications—that contribute mostly to the mortality. Regardless of the decrease in cesarean section risk, it is well to be reminded that deaths following uncomplicated labor and delivery have likewise been markedly reduced. These differences in relative risk are more pertinent to the question of the advisability of performing the primary cesarean section than to the choice between a repeat cesar-

ean section or pelvic delivery. The mortality from the operation per se is 0.5 to 0.1 per cent.

ONCE A CESAREAN SECTION ALWAYS A CESAREAN?

Since the operation has been used for conditions other than cephalopelvic disproportion, the proper method of delivery to be used after a previous abdominal hysterotomy continues to be debated. In view of the improvement in cesarean section mortality, the question of vaginal delivery after an antecedent abdominal hysterotomy has become even more controversial. When the conditions that impelled the primary cesarean section are permanent or recurring, the decision is obvious. If the indication for the initial abdominal delivery was temporary and the conditions in the current pregnancy appear favorable for pelvic delivery, the choice of attempting pelvic delivery rather than performing a repeat cesarean section becomes a matter of clinical judgment. The data reported from many clinics testify to the fact that results in selected cases justify vaginal delivery as the preferred method of management.

The facts to be considered in determining the method of delivery to be employed after previous cesarean section include the type of section that was performed and whether the postoperative course was afebrile or febrile, indicative presumably of primary healing of the uterine scar although this has probably been overstressed; the presentation of the fetus; the station of the presenting part; and the status of the cervix and the membranes at the onset of labor. Finally, the presence of pain and tenderness about the region of the previous uterine incision is generally held to reflect the possibility of impending or beginning rupture of the uterine wound.

The condition of the cesarean section uterine scar is obviously the most important consideration from the standpoint of labor. Much has been written about the method of the healing of these uterine incisions. The earliest contention was that the uterus heals by the regeneration of muscle fibers. Others believe that the eventual integrity of the wound depends on the extent to which the incision is bridged by fibroblastic tissue growth. In the presence of serum or exudate, healing of the uterine wound would require extensive fibroblastic proliferation. Under these circumstances approximation of the muscle fibers could not occur, and the uterine incision would be composed entirely of connective tissue. Should the exudative process be marked, effective bridging would fail to occur. It would appear that the tensile strength of the uterine scar depends on the amount of the cut surface of uterine wall involved in the repair rather than on the nature of the tissue taking part in the repair.

An index to the success or failure of the healing of the uterine incision is said to be the presence or absence of infection as measured by postoperative fever. If the convalescence following the previous cesarean section was marked by a febrile response, many clinicians assume that there may be defective healing of the uterine wound, and subsequent pelvic delivery is contraindicated. Although infection will prevent healing by first intention, the tensile strength of the resultant scar tissue may well be sufficient to withstand the forces of labor. Conversely, and equally significant, the absence of postoperative fever is no assurance that primary union occurred and that firm uterine scar is present. Attempts to ascertain the integrity of the uterine scar before pregnancy by hysterography have been sporadically made, but it remains to be shown whether this has clinical value.

Pain and tenderness to palpation in the region of the cesarean section scar in a subsequent pregnancy must be taken to suggest possible disruption. The absence of pain does not exclude the possibility of threatened uterine rupture, for pain and tenderness are by no means invariable precursors of the event. These symptoms, however, find their chief value in calling to the physician's attention the possibility of uterine rupture; but many times the uterine scar will be barely perceptible at repeat cesarean section. Should these symptoms appear in a patient prior to term, clinical judgment must dictate whether to delay or perform a cesarean section immediately. If the procedure is postponed for the purpose of securing greater fetal maturity, the patient should be in the hospital under close observation until she is delivered.

Some clinicians hold that an equally important factor in determining the soundness of a cesarean section scar is the part of the uterus in which the incision is placed. It is commonly thought that scars of incisions in the body of the uterus rupture with much greater frequency than those in the lower segment. Several reasons are given for the decreased incidence of rupture following the lower segment operation. Exponents of this operation emphasize that the various tissue layers composing this area of the uterus can be brought into better approximation than is possible in the upper segment procedure. The lower segment is in a greater state of rest than is the corpus post partum, and this is presumed to promote and encourage better healing.

These reasons appear to be conjecture and are difficult to accept completely. Regardless of whether, as stated, the lower segment is less active than the upper segment during the healing period, extensive involution must occur in the lower segment of the uterus in order that it may regain its nonpregnant isthmic dimension of approximately 1 cm. in length. In reality, precise approximation of the various tissue layers of the lower segment is difficult and, except for the overlying endopelvic fascia, the tissue borders are not easy to delineate, especially when the lower segment is thin. Undoubtedly the future integrity of the wound in the lower uterine segment depends chiefly on the coaptation of the endopelvic fascia.

The incidence of rupture of the uterine scar in a subsequent pregnancy following the classic type of cesarean section is reported as between 1 and 3 per cent; following the lower segment type, less than 1 per cent. It must be noted that many of the lower segment operations are performed for a permanent indication, and the classic type is usually performed for a more temporary indication.

Silent ruptures found at the time of repeat operation are reported infrequently. Hence, these silent ruptures discovered at repeat cesarean section rarely reach the record rooms of hospitals or the literature. Until occult or incomplete dehiscences are accepted as uterine ruptures and so reported, the true incidence of uterine disruption in the various types of cesarean section will remain uncertain. For when account is taken of the dehiscence of the lower segment incision at subsequent cesarean section, the incidence of uterine disruption differs little from that following the classic type. This is mentioned to emphasize what may happen in the course of labor in the lower segment type.

Before the subject of uterine rupture in a previous cesarean section scar is dismissed, one must ask the reason for the discrepancy between the rather high frequency of dehiscence of the lower uterine segment reportedly seen at repeat cesarean section and the infrequent rupture at subsequent pelvic delivery. A partial answer, at least, may be found in the fact that such a separation occurs or may be present at the time of labor without producing symptoms as long as the uterovesical peritoneum remains intact. This is interesting, for the cessation of labor is a classic sign of uterine rupture. In any event, a normal puerperium has been reported in patients in whom routine exploration of the uterus immediately following pelvic delivery revealed a defect in a transverse incision of a previous cesarean section, and in whom, because the uterovesical peritoneum was intact, nothing more was done. This is not cited to indicate, however, that when a silent uterine rupture is found a hysterectomy is unnecessary or future deliveries can be managed pelvically. Indeed, with respect to future pregnancies, abdominal delivery would seem to be the safer procedure.

The behavior of the upper and of the lower segment scars differs with respect to pregnancy and labor. Rupture of an upper segment scar tends to occur in the seventh or eighth month of pregnancy when the uterus is accommodating itself to the rapidly growing fetus. Moreover, the rupture is dramatic and complete and usually happens without warning to either the patient or the physician.

By contrast, rupture of the lower segment scar is more insidious and tends to occur near term or during labor when this portion of the uterus becomes attenuated. This suggests that a patient with a classic type of incision who reaches term is a safer candidate for labor and pelvic delivery than a patient with a previous lower segment type of cesarean section. This is not always the case, for rupture of the classic scar has occurred during labor. By virtue of the vertical incision located in the upper segment, the operative management of rupture of a classic scar is much less difficult and is associated with fewer problems than that of rupture of the lower segment. When the lower segment uterine scar ruptures in a complete rather than an incomplete fashion, particularly if it is a transverse incision, the uterine vessels may be torn, and recognition of these vessels can be difficult and uncertain. An added complication of this type of uterine scar rupture is that the bladder, being incorporated in the old uterine incision, has been known to rupture concomitantly.

The decision to remove the uterus should it rupture will be governed by the parity of the patient and the extent and location of the rupture. On occasion the wound edges may be freshened and the uterus closed. However, uterine rupture can recur in a subsequent pregnancy. Also, despite the fact that the patient was successfully delivered pelvically after a cesarean section, there is no assurance that the uterus may not rupture in a later pregnancy and labor.

The risk of uterine rupture re-emphasizes the fact that the all-important decision in patient management is whether the primary cesarean section is entirely necessary or justified, not whether the patient should be delivered by a repeat cesarean section. Future pregnancies will pose the risk of subsequent uterine rupture to these patients, regardless of the type of cesarean section performed, the antibiotics administered to prevent or control infection, or any special skill or technique that the surgeon may possess.

If pelvic delivery is to be considered for a patient previously delivered by cesarean section, the presentation must be normal, the pelvis adequate, the cervix partially effaced and somewhat dilated, and the membranes preferably intact.

Despite the fact that a certain number of cesarean sections are performed for temporary indications, as in late pregnancy bleeding, it is difficult to be dogmatic as to the method of delivery in a subsequent pregnancy. The decision will be tempered somewhat by the hospital environment, which means that assistants should be immediately available and the operating room in constant readiness for cesarean section in the event that complications arise in the course of labor.

The conduct of labor is somewhat modified in patients delivered previously by cesarean section. The stronger and expulsive contractions of the second stage should be minimized to relieve undue tension on the cesarean section scar. Forceps delivery is indicated as the patient enters the second stage. Oxytocic drugs should be withheld until after the placenta has been delivered.

Once the placenta has been expelled, the uterus should always be explored. To one who has not palpated a thin scar, the experience may be somewhat startling. In the case of the classic scar, one may encounter a deep furrow, involving one half or more of the uterine wall. Unless the defect extends to the peritoneum, however, the scar should be considered intact and the patient so treated. Administration of oxytocic drugs before such exploration may cause the uterus to be so tightly contracted that a small rupture may go undetected at the time of the examination, and fatal peritonitis has been known to follow when the rupture has occurred in the upper angle of a previous vertical incision that may not have been covered by vesical peritoneum.

INDICATIONS FOR PRIMARY CESAREAN SECTION

The indications for primary cesarean section include late pregnancy bleeding, that is, placenta praevia and abruptio placentae. Absolute cephalopelvic disproportion is rare, but borderline disproportion following a failed test of labor is a major indication for the operation. A relatively few patients may require abdominal delivery following unproductive labor in the presence of a normal cephalopelvic relationship. This condition may be classified under a number of terms, such as dysfunctional labor and cervical dystocia. As previously mentioned, these are patients in whom, despite the use of oxytocin, the cervix fails to dilate sufficiently to permit safe pelvic delivery. Cesarean section is justified when fetal distress develops in the presence of partial dilatation of the cervix. On rare occasions a pelvic tumor may obstruct the birth canal and prevent delivery through the pelvis. Malpresentation, such as a transverse, or a brow or a face presentation, particularly in the primiparous patient, is also a bona fide indication for cesarean section. To prevent fetal injury, cesarean section is not infrequently required in breech presentation.

Patients with severe and progressive pregnancy toxemia, with a sufficiently mature fetus but with the cervix unfavorable for the induction of labor, are often best managed by cesarean section. Women with medical diseases complicating pregnancy may also require cesarean section, particularly patients with diabetes mellitus. In addition, there is a long list of miscellaneous indications, including patients with poor obstetric histories and no living children and certain patients with Rh incompatibility when death in utero is a threat.

TYPE OF CESAREAN SECTION IN ACCORDANCE WITH OBSTETRIC CIRCUMSTANCES

The better policy is not to adhere strictly to any one type of cesarean section, but rather to employ the operation that will most safely deal with the obstetric problem at hand.

Many, if not most, clinics routinely use the transperitoneal lower segment operation. There is no question that, compared to the classic type, the postoperative convalescence following the lower segment operation is more comfortable, and the incidence of postoperative adhesions is less in this type of procedure, with the subsequent risk of intestinal obstruction being thereby diminished. The same may be said for the extraperitoneal type, for, besides the absence of peritoneal signs and symptoms, it assures a smooth convalescence, a fact often not considered or emphasized. The blood loss in the lower segment operation varies, however, and in the absence of labor, when a thick lower segment usually exists, the amount lost may be excessive. Certainly this is true in patients with placenta praevia. It is here that the classic type has a place in patient management. Also, most clinics hold the view that there is little danger of peritonitis following the transperitoneal lower segment operation when antibiotics are used as adjunctive therapy, and therefore the extraperitoneal type is an unnecessary procedure.

With respect to the control of infection, it is difficult, if not impossible, to determine whether the transperitoneal or extraperitoneal cesarean section in combination with antibiotic therapy has the lower mortality and morbidity rate. By comparing the results of some of the larger maternity services in this country, one might be impressed that in the institutions where extraperitoneal cesarean section is employed the incidence of cesarean section following a trial labor tends to be lower than where the lower segment transperitoneal operation is used, indicating that the inherent fear of infection leads to a shorter test of labor.

Moreover, there is no certain way of excluding the possible presence of intrauterine infection prior to cesarean section. It seems logical, therefore, to avoid peritoneal contamination by utilizing the extraperitoneal type (Waters) or the exclusion type (Smith). For if the uterus is infected, and the uterine wound suppurates, it will drain extraperitoneally rather than intraperitoneally. That is not to say that septicemia may not develop after either type of operation, and in some few instances cesarean hysterectomy is unquestionably the safer procedure.

It is here suggested that the extraperitoneal or exclusion type be considered in test-of-labor cases when the membranes have been ruptured for 12 hours, or when labor has exceeded 12 hours. It is readily admitted that the uterine cultures will be negative in most of these cases.

In more recent years, some clinicians have advocated complete removal of the uterus when it has previously been decided that this is the patient's final pregnancy. It is argued that this is preferable to tubal ligation, for, besides accomplishing sterilization, it removes the possible need for a hysterectomy later because of dysfunctional bleeding or pathologic condition of the uterus. There is no question that complete hysterectomy is a formidable procedure in the pregnant patient. In the face of reportedly good results, however, the operation of cesarean section accompanied by complete abdominal hysterectomy would appear to have a place in obstetric operations, but only in the hands of the experienced.

When the reason for removal of the uterus is postpartum hemorrhage, placenta accreta, or uterine rupture, often these patients are not in the best condition, and the simplest procedure, namely, a supracervical or subtotal rather than complete hysterectomy, should be considered. The fear of cancer in the cervical stump is hardly sufficient reason for routinely performing a complete hysterectomy. Moreover, a cervicectomy can be easily performed vaginally some months later after the patient is fully recovered.

The question arises whether normal-appearing ovaries should be removed at the time of cesarean section hysterectomy or at hysterectomy in the nonpregnant patient because of the possibility of subsequent ovarian disease resulting, presumably, from interference in the ovarian blood supply incident to the operation. This leads to a second question—whether the age of the patient is a factor when considering incidental oophorectomy.

Those who consider it proper to remove apparently normal ovaries prior to the age of 40 have in mind that a certain number of patients (about 5 per cent) will require a secondary operation some years later because of ovarian disease.

It is apparent that in women who have had a hysterectomy, regardless of indication, the ovaries function for as long a period of time as those of comparable controls who have not had a hysterectomy, as determined by vaginal cytology and hormone assays. Why, then, should a patient before the age of 40 to 45 be surgically deprived of her ovarian function, provided the ovaries appear healthy at the time of hysterectomy?

TECHNIQUE OF CESAREAN SECTION

In preparation for operation, the patient's hemoglobin and hematocrit are determined and 2 units of properly matched blood should be in readiness for transfusion. In the transperitoneal type, once the abdomen is opened the uterus should be examined to see whether it has rotated. Such rotation, if it occurs, is usually to the right. If this has happened, the uterus is rotated back to its normal position to ensure that in case of a vertical incision it is placed in the midline. Moist gauze packs are placed along the sides of the uterus to reduce spillage of amniotic fluid and blood into the peritoneal cavity. As the uterus is incised, ring forceps are placed along the cut edge to close the large sinuses and to reduce blood loss. The uterus is routinely cultured before the baby is delivered.

As the presenting part is extracted, an oxytocic agent should be given, preferably intravenously, as described for pelvic delivery. Oxytocin may also be administered by the drip method, and continued for an hour or more after operation as insurance against uterine atony. Ample time should be allotted for the placenta to separate. In the lower segment operation, with a transverse incision, the physiologic retraction ring separating the upper and lower segments of the uterus may contract, trapping the placenta in the upper segment and frequently necessitating its manual removal. The uterus is explored to determine that the placenta and membranes are completely removed. During the operation the uterus is palpated frequently to make certain that it is well contracted.

Following uterine closure, the peritoneal cavity should be carefully toileted. The omentum is directed behind the uterus to keep the small bowel away from the uterine incision. It is well to explore the abdomen before it is closed, and the adnexa should always be inspected. It is poor practice to fail to recognize an ovarian cyst or a tumor that will necessitate a later operation.

Although the classic type is briefly described, only the transperitoneal, the extraperitoneal, the peritoneal exclusion types and cesarean hysterectomy are illustrated in the following pages, for they embody all of the surgical and obstetric principles involved.

The **classic method** of cesarean section consists of placing an incision in the uterine corpus, beginning above the uterovesical junction and extending upward 10 to 12 cm. After the baby is extracted and the placenta is expelled, the uterus is closed in three layers. A continuous suture is placed in the myometrium near the uterine cavity but not to include the decidua, followed by a second row of interrupted figure-of-eight sutures to embrace most of the myometrial wall. The serosa is closed with a continuous Connell-type suture.

The **transperitoneal lower segment procedure** (Figs. 17 and 18) involves exposure of the lower uterine segment by incising above the uterovesical fold of the peritoneum (Fig. 17A). With scissors the peritoneum is dissected laterally, with care to remain close to the peritoneum to avoid ooze from the veins overlying the uterus. The bladder is displaced downward, so that the lower uterine segment is exposed (Fig. 17B). The uterus can then be opened either vertically (Krönig, Beck, DeLee) (Fig. 17C and D), or transversely (Phaneuf, Kerr). The baby's head is rotated so that its mouth is in the wound, and the operator's hand is passed behind the occiput. The vertex is then delivered by flexion either manually or by forceps. A specially devised spoonlike instrument (Fig. 19) serves the same purpose as the hand, but is less bulky. The uterus is then closed by three rows of sutures, careful attention being given to approximating the overlying endopelvic fascia. The bladder flap is sutured back to its original relationship, and the abdomen is closed (Fig. 18).

Unless the lower segment of the uterus has considerable width, as seen following a test of labor, it is often impossible to contain the vertical incision completely in this segment. In an attempt to accomplish this by extending the distal portion of the incision, the vagina may be inadvertently entered; although this is disturbing, it is not crucial, provided the accident is recognized. Certainly, one of the advantages of the transverse incision is that it is completely in the lower segment, and it is readily covered with the bladder and its peritoneum. In all types of procedures in which the incision is restricted to the lower segment, if a Bandl ring is encountered the peritoneum covering it should be dissected upward and the ring cut. Personal experience can testify to the fact that forcing the infant's shoulders past the pathologic retraction ring at cesarean section may result in unwarranted uterine rupture. Cutting the ring causes it to disappear dramatically, and the infant can be extracted easily. The T-shaped incision created in the uterus presents no problem in closure.

In the **peritoneal exclusion operation (Smith)** (Figs. 20–24), the abdomen can be opened by either a vertical lower midline or a Pfannenstiel incision (Fig. 20). The uterovesical fold is identified (Fig. 21), and the visceral peritoneum is incised from the dome downward along the lateral border of the bladder (Fig. 22). The upper edge of the visceral peritoneum is sutured to the parietal peritoneum, and the abdominal cavity is excluded (Fig. 23). The bladder is displaced downward, and the lower uterine segment uncovered. The fetus is delivered through a transverse incision (Fig. 24). After the uterus is closed the bladder is restored

(*Text continues on page 642.*)

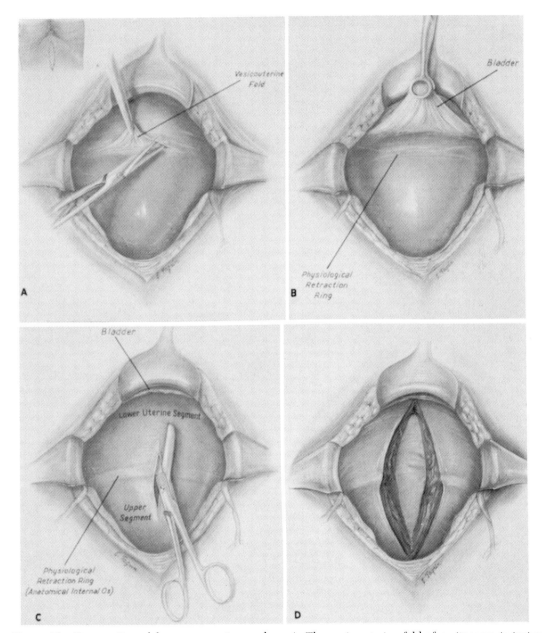

Figure 17. Transperitoneal lower segment procedure. A, The vesico-uterine fold of peritoneum is incised. B, The incision in the vesico-uterine peritoneum has been extended laterally and the bladder is dissected off the lower uterine segment. C, The incision in the lower uterine segment is extended downward. In this instance the incision involves a portion of the upper segment. D, Incision of the uterus is now complete. The baby's face is visible. After the membranes are ruptured, the operator places his finger in the infant's mouth and rotates the face into the wound. The vertex is then extracted by flexion.

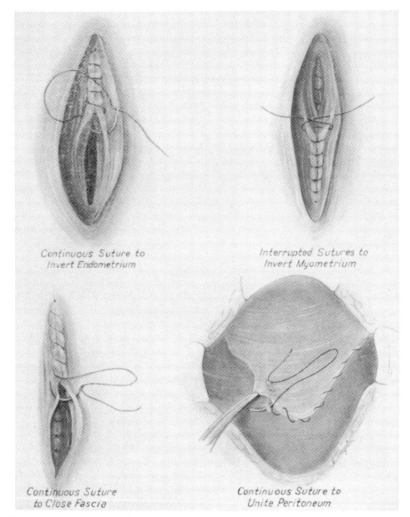

Continuous Suture to
Invert Endometrium

Interrupted Sutures to
Invert Myometrium

Continuous Suture
to Close Fascia

Continuous Suture to
Unite Peritoneum

Figure 18. Closure of the uterus in the transperitoneal lower segment procedure. The bladder is restored, so that it covers the uterine incision.

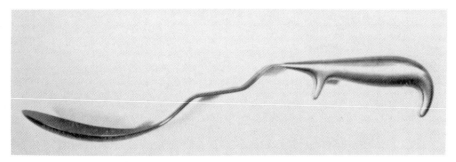

Figure 19. The instrument used to aid in delivery of the vertex at cesarean section. After the face is rotated into the uterine wound, the spoon is passed behind the occiput, and, with upward lift, the vertex is delivered.

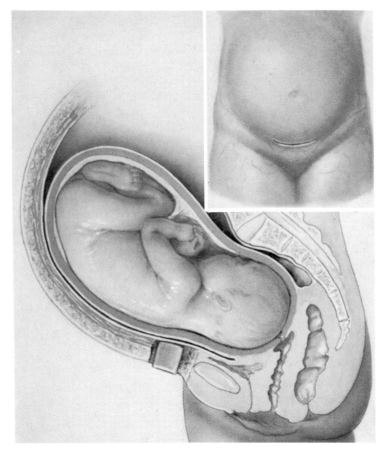

Figure 20. A vertical lower midline incision, as well as the Pfannenstiel incision depicted here, provides sufficient exposure. (Courtesy of Dr. E. F. Smith.)

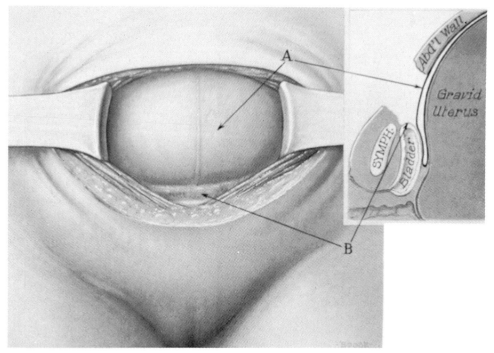

Figure 21. The rectus muscles retracted laterally allow the parietal peritoneum (*A*) and bladder (*B*) to balloon up, with the urachus glistening in the midline. Rarely is this structure as prominent as shown here. (Courtesy of Dr. E. F. Smith.)

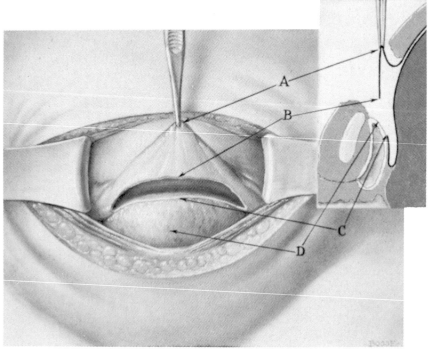

Figure 22. The parietal peritoneum (*A*) is opened (*B, C*) just over the bladder (*D*). The parietal peritoneum may be opened more cephalad and the visceral peritoneum incised along the bladder margin, much in the manner of the conventional transperitoneal lower segment procedure. There will be adequate visceral peritoneum for suturing without tension to the parietal peritoneum. (Courtesy of Dr. E. F. Smith.)

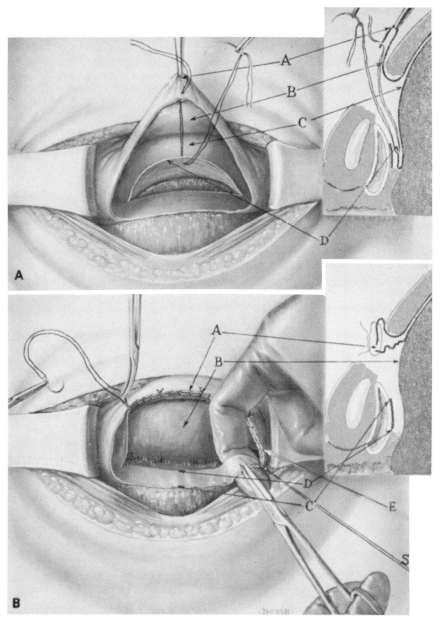

Figure 23. The abdominal cavity is excluded by suture of the cut edges of the visceral and parietal peritoneum. A, The vesico-uterine fold of peritoneum (*D*) is opened transversely (as in the low flap operation) and sutured to the superior parietal peritoneum (*A*) to exclude peritoneal cavity (*BC*). It is helpful to extend the incision of the visceral peritoneum along the bladder to its inferior lateral border, thus ensuring closure of the peritoneum without tension. B, The visceral peritoneal bridge, which varies in width (*CD*) in different patients, being cut at the closed apex (*S*) of suture after complete stitching of parietovisceral peritoneal layers (*AE*), which then excludes bilaterally and entirely the peritoneal cavity from the lower uterine segment (*B*). Incision of the peritoneum along the lateral borders of the bladder eliminates the incising of the visceral peritoneum shown here. (Courtesy of Dr. E. F. Smith.)

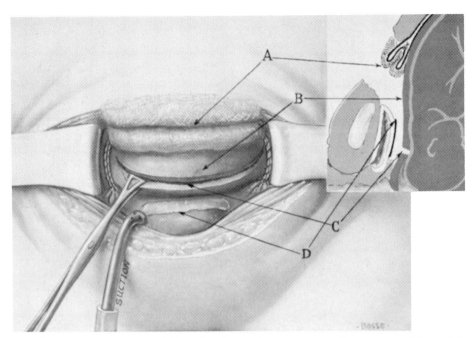

Figure 24. The protective gauze strip (*A*) is placed over the parietovisceral peritoneum. The mobilized bladder (*D*) is shown just before the retractor hides it under the symphysis. The incision (*C*) in the lower uterine segment (*B*) curves upward. (Courtesy of Dr. E. F. Smith.)

to its original relationship by several interrupted sutures. A drain is placed beneath the bladder, and the muscle, fascia, and skin are approximated. The catheter may be removed the following day, and the drain completely removed on the fourth or fifth day if the wound is not infected. When preservation of the uterus is desirable in a patient with an obvious or suspected uterine infection, this type of procedure is useful in that it affords an added barrier against peritonitis. The operation moves along in a predictable manner, and is generally easier to perform than the extraperitoneal type, unless the operator has had a reasonable amount of experience with the latter.

As stated previously, the **extraperitoneal type of operation (Waters)** (Figs. 25 and 26) requires exposure of the lower uterine segment without opening the peritoneal cavity. After abdominal preparation, a left rectus incision is made through the skin and the fascia, and the left rectus muscle is retracted laterally. To facilitate dissection, the bladder is moderately distended with saline. The prevesical fascia is incised transversely in the region of the junction of the middle and upper thirds of the distended bladder. Near the lateral margins of the bladder the incision is directed inferiorly toward the

inguinal region to avoid opening the peritoneum (Fig. 25A). The prevesical fascia above the incision is dissected upward and away from the dome of the bladder (Fig. 25B). The urachus is identified and incised.

The lower uterine segment is approached through a small triangular area near the margin of the bladder. The triangle is bounded medially by the bladder, above by the peritoneum, and laterally and inferiorly by the broad ligament (Fig. 25C). The blunt scissors dissection is made slightly toward the midline through several layers of loose areolar tissue to expose the endopelvic fascia of the lower uterine segment with its characteristic glistening, smooth, gray appearance (Fig. 25D). When this incision is in the proper line of cleavage, between the two layers of endopelvic fascia covering the posterior wall of the bladder and the lower uterine segment, respectively, the operator's index finger, inserted through it, can pass readily and easily beneath the bladder to the opposite side (Fig. 26A). Next, the operator's finger is swept upward to the dome of the bladder between the fused endopelvic fascia of the anterior and the posterior bladder wall and the overlying peritoneum. As an aid in the dissection, it is helpful at this point to drain

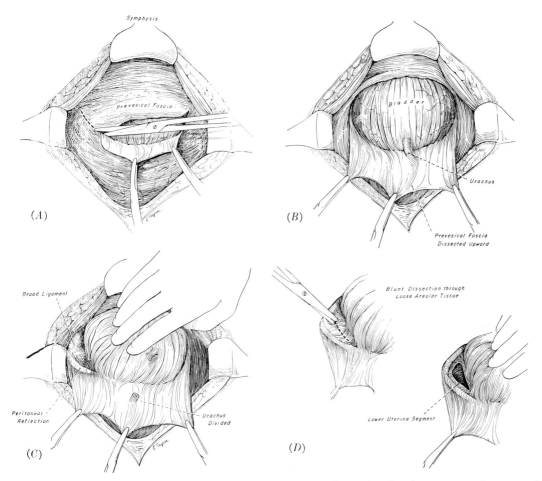

Figure 25.   Extraperitoneal lower segment procedure. A, Prevesical or endopelvic fascia is incised transversely after the bladder is inflated. Note downward direction of the incision to avoid opening the peritoneum as it is reflected off the lateral border of the bladder. B, The prevesical fascia is dissected off the bladder. Extending the dissection over the dome of the bladder and onto its posterior wall will be of great aid later in the operation when attempt is made to identify the peritoneal reflection. C, The vital triangle, gateway to the lower uterine segment. The structures are deliberately exaggerated by the artist to emphasize the anatomic relationships. D, Opening the angle and exposing the lower uterine segment.

the bladder. The prevesical or endopelvic fascia at the angle of the bladder must be carefully incised to avoid opening the peritoneum (Fig. 26B). When this is done the peritoneal fold will be readily seen extending over the dome of the bladder to the opposite side. The distance between the peritoneum and the bladder varies considerably in different patients, ranging from a few millimeters to a centimeter or more. The incision of the fused layers of the prevesical fascia is continued close to the margin of the bladder, and, when it is completed, the peritoneum is free of its bladder attachment and retracts upward (Fig. 26C). The bladder is displaced below

the symphysis, and the lower uterine segment is widely exposed (Fig. 26D). The baby and placenta are delivered through a transverse incision, after which the lower uterine segment is closed in three layers. A continuous suture includes the myometrium, followed by a row of interrupted sutures in the endopelvic fascia. The third suture is continuous and approximates the edges of the endopelvic fascia. The bladder is replaced and sutured to the prevesical fascia attached to the peritoneum. A drain is placed between the bladder and the lower uterine segment; this is removed in two to five days, depending on the clinical course of the patient.

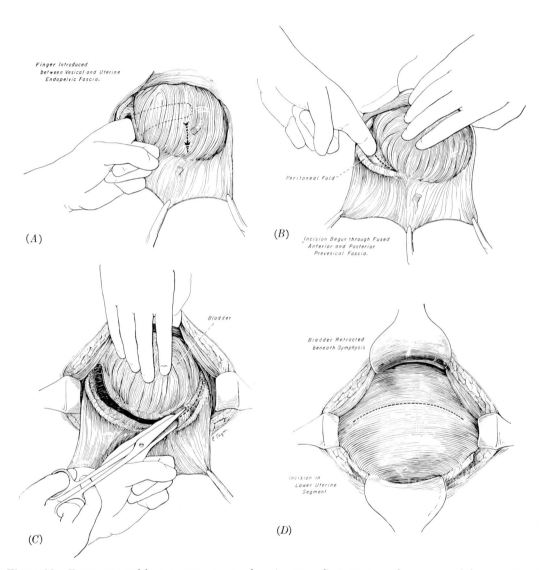

Figure 26. Extraperitoneal lower segment procedure (*continued*). A, Basic to the success of the operation is identification of the layers of endopelvic fascia covering the bladder and lower uterine segment. B, The most important area where careful dissection of the fascia is necessary to avoid opening into the peritoneal cavity. C, The prevesical or endopelvic fascia is incised along the bladder border, and the peritoneum retracts cephalad; the bladder is displaced beneath the symphysis. D, The bladder is retracted beneath the symphysis. A transverse incision, as in the transperitoneal cesarean section, is made in the lower uterine segment, and ample room is available for extraction of even the largest infant.

CESAREAN HYSTERECTOMY

The technique of **cesarean hysterectomy** is depicted in Figures 27 to 32. This procedure obviously will differ somewhat, depending on the type and location of the uterine incision, which in the technique illustrated is the classic type. It must be appreciated that in the recently pregnant uterus the ovarian vessels are hypertrophied, increasing the risk of ineffective hemostasis. Hence these vessels and the round ligament are clamped, cut, and sutured separately and should never be sutured together, as is sometimes practiced in the nonpregnant uterus. For when the round ligament is included in the ovarian pedicle, there is some tension on the ovarian ligaments, because the round ligament retracts downward, and the ovarian pedicle retracts upward and laterally, which may cause displacement of the suture ligature,

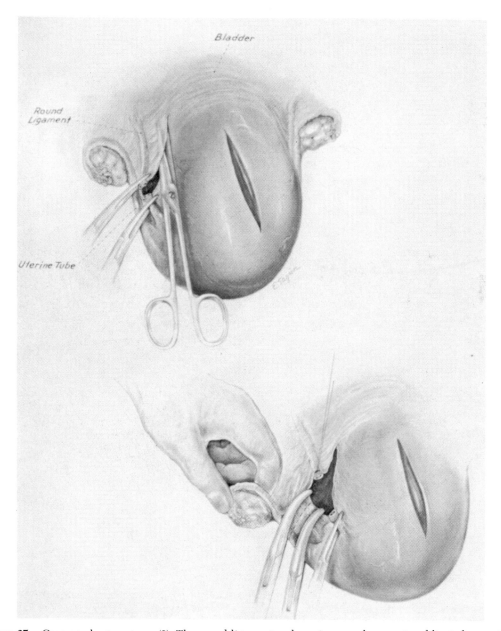

Figure 27. Cesarean hysterectomy (I). The round ligament and ovarian vessels are cut and ligated separately.

resulting in bleeding from the ovarian vessels. In a hysterectomy performed in association with pregnancy, both the ovarian and the uterine vessels are doubly ligated.

After the round ligaments are divided and sutured, the ovarian vessels are clamped, incised, and ligated (Fig. 27). The posterior sheath of the broad ligament is incised near the uterus, to expose the uterine vessels and to provide adequate tissue for later peritonealization (Fig. 28). The uterovesical fold of peritoneum is developed, and the bladder is displaced downward, exposing the cervix. The ascending branches of the uterine vessels are clamped, cut, and doubly ligated, or, as in this instance,

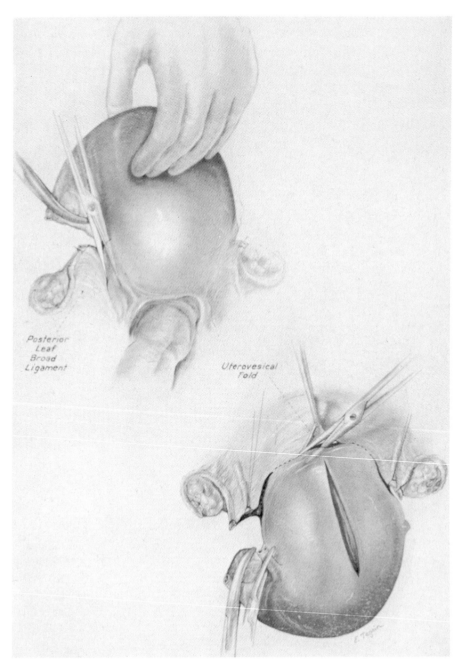

Figure 28.   Cesarean hysterectomy (II). The posterior sheath of the broad ligament is incised, and the neighboring areolar tissue between the leaves of the broad ligament is dissected down to the uterine vessels. The uterovesical peritoneum is incised. (Note the uterosacral ligaments posteriorly.)

clamped and cut, to be ligated later by suture, after the corpus is amputated, a procedure sometimes followed if the patient is bleeding actively from the uterus (Fig. 29). After the corpus is removed, the cervix is closed. To invert the overlying endopelvic fascia and to ensure complete hemostasis, figure-of-eight sutures are used. As will be noted, the needle first passes shallow through the posterior wall of the cervix. The needle is reversed and the suture is placed deep into the anterior and posterior cervical tissues. Again the needle is reversed and passes shallow through the anterior wall of the cervix (Fig. 29). A continuous suture completes the closure. Although the round ligament is illustrated as being sutured to the cervix, this is unneces-

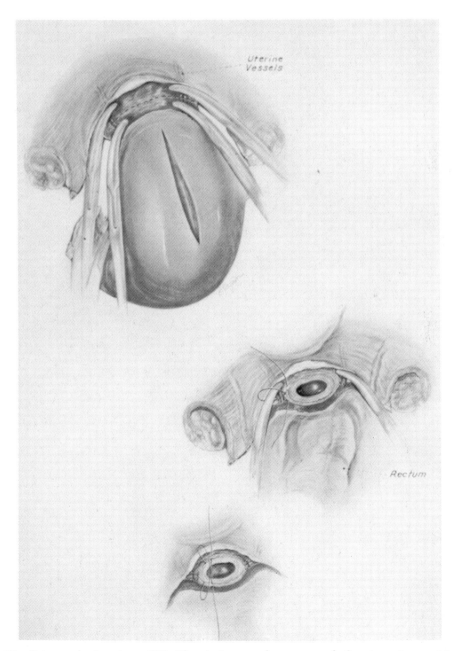

Figure 29. Cesarean hysterectomy (III). The uterine vessels are secured; the uterus is amputated and the cervix is closed.

sary, for it adds little support to the cervix. The ovarian pedicles and cervix are covered by uterovesical and broad ligament peritoneum (Fig. 30).

Complete cesarean hysterectomy is merely an extension of the supracervical type. The bladder is displaced to or slightly below the cervicovaginal junction (Fig. 31). The descending branches of the uterine vessels are clamped, cut, and ligated as the cervix is dissected free. It is reemphasized that the vaginal artery, which encircles the cervix at the cervicovaginal junction, is of considerable size during pregnancy. Thus, it is well to extend the dissection slightly below the cervicovaginal junction and to clamp, cut, and ligate the vaginal artery before proceeding further, to prevent bleed-

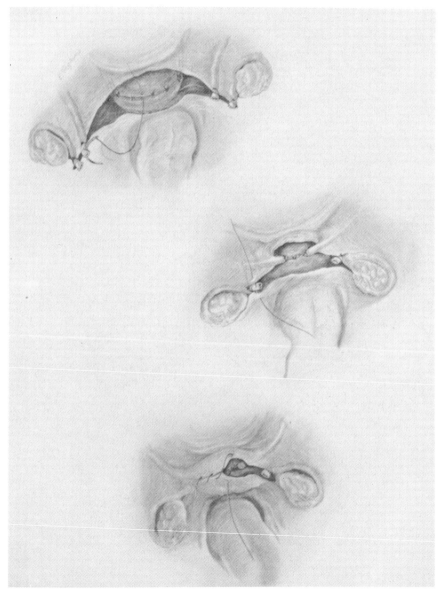

Figure 30. Cesarean hysterectomy (IV). The operative field is covered with peritoneum by closure of the broad ligament and utilizing the uterovesical peritoneum, so that the round ligaments and ovarian pedicles are enclosed. Care is taken to pass the continuous closing suture always distal to the ovarian pedicle suture ligature.

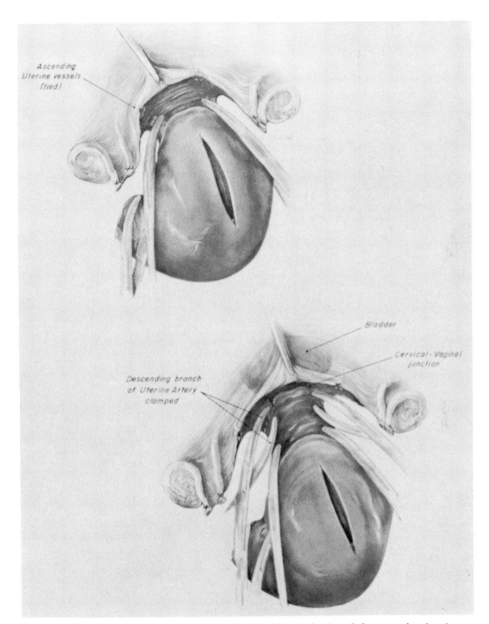

Figure 31. Complete cesarean hysterectomy (I). The bladder is displaced downward either by scissors dissection or by blunt dissection with gauze over the finger, with care to remain between the layers of endopelvic fascia covering the posterior bladder and the anterior cervix. To avoid unpleasant ooze from broad ligament veins, dissection should be restricted to the area of the cervix.

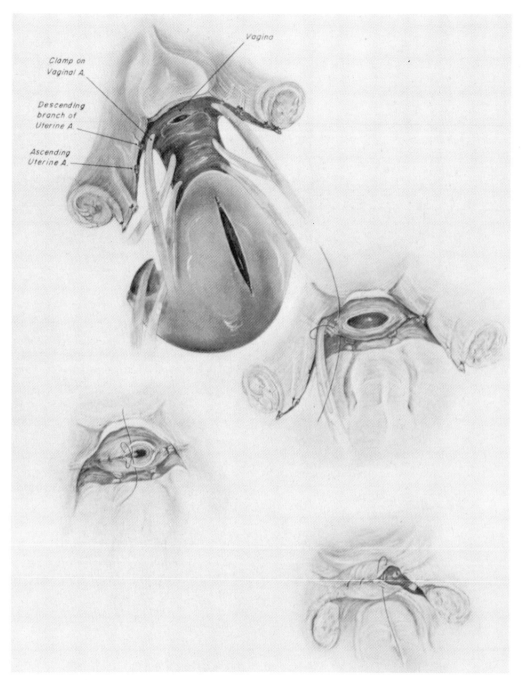

Figure 32. Complete cesarean hysterectomy (II). The cervix is removed, the vagina closed, and the operative field covered with peritoneum.

ing from the vaginal cuff with removal of the cervix. The vagina is opened and incised close to the cervix, thus permitting removal of the uterus (Fig. 32). No special attention is given to the uterosacral ligaments until just before the vagina is opened, when they are cut and ligated. They are incorporated into the vaginal cuff at closure by interrupted figure-of-eight sutures. A continuous suture is used to approximate the endopelvic fascia of the vagina more closely and to ensure complete hemostasis. The operative field is peritonealized (Fig. 32).

POSTOPERATIVE CARE

As in a pelvic delivery, the postoperative care of the patient delivered by cesarean section includes attending the uterus for any evidence of atony; this is especially important after cesarean section performed for complications such as late pregnancy bleeding or prolonged labor, when the uterus is more likely to relax. The uterus, therefore, should be carefully observed for a minimum of two or three hours after the operation, to make certain that it is well contracted and not unduly enlarged, and that there is no unusual vaginal bleeding.

The patient's vital signs should include pulse and blood pressure readings taken at 15-minute intervals for the first two hours postoperatively, and then every 30 minutes for the next four hours. The pulse, temperature, respiration, and blood pressure should be recorded every four hours for at least four days, or until they are normal. The spillage of blood and amniotic fluid into the abdominal cavity invites distention, which is commonplace also in patients who are long in labor. Until the bowel begins to regain its tone, or until the third day, it is best to postpone oral feedings, except for tepid water. During this interval 2000 ml. of a solution of glucose in buffered water is administered daily by intravenous infusion. A progressive diet is started on the 3rd or 4th postoperative day. An oil retention enema is administered on the fourth evening and, if necessary, a cleansing soapsuds enema is given on the following morning.

The patient is taken off catheter drainage after 24 hours. Elastic stockings are used routinely for the first week in the hope of aiding in the prevention of embolism, and early ambulation is encouraged. Attention must be given to the character of the lochia, and the uterus is watched to determine if it is undergoing normal involution. The abdominal sutures are generally removed on the seventh day, and the patient may be discharged from the hospital on the 8th to the 10th day.

In the case of the extraperitoneal type of cesarean section, the catheter remains in place for three to five days. The drain between the bladder and the lower uterine segment is removed gradually, but is completely removed by the fourth or fifth day. Because the peritoneal cavity has not been insulted in the extraperitoneal type of operation, the patient is free of distention. The postoperative reaction resembles more closely that following pelvic delivery, and a regular diet can be ordered on the first postoperative day. When hysterectomy has been performed, the postoperative care of the patient is similar to that following cesarean section.

In summary, whether or not the lower segment type of cesarean section should be performed in all cases is dictated largely by the hospital facilities, the professional personnel available, and the experience of the operator. Despite this rather adamant policy, the classic type has a place in the management of patients with late pregnancy bleeding. Also, the extraperitoneal type affords an additional barrier against infection and is applicable to test-of-labor patients, especially if the fetal membranes have been ruptured for a considerable period prior to operation. Patients so delivered have a postoperative course not unlike that of a pelvic delivery, being devoid of abdominal symptoms or signs.

For the general surgeon whose only contact with obstetrics is to deliver patients who require a cesarean section, the peritoneal exclusion type may prove useful. It is envisioned that when the surgeon is consulted the patient may have been long in labor and is potentially if not actually infected. To preserve the uterus and avoid the risk of peritonitis, this type of procedure may afford the protection of the extraperitoneal type and is no more difficult to perform than a transperitoneal type of cesarean section. If the patient is grossly infected, cesarean hysterectomy may be the more prudent choice of operation regardless of the patient's parity.

As to cesarean hysterectomy, it is being used more frequently in patients who are undergoing their last cesarean section to accomplish sterilization and to avoid dysfunctional bleeding of the menopause and risk of uterine malignancy. The presence of uterine myomata is a more definitive indication for cesarean hysterectomy.

Not unlike the extraperitoneal and peritoneal exclusion types of cesarean section, elective cesarean hysterectomy usually provides a smoother postoperative course with less distention and fewer abdominal signs than transperitoneal cesarean section. In general, the relative risk of removing the uterus electively at the time of cesarean section is certainly greater than that of removal some months later in the nonpregnant state.

Also, when the uterus must be removed in the face of serious blood loss, i.e., uterine atony, placenta accreta, and so forth, a subtotal rather than a total hysterectomy is a more predictable procedure with a shorter operating time, and hence may be the more appropriate procedure. Thus, as in other surgical situations, the operation should be tailored to serve the patient's needs, with her total safety being uppermost in the decision-making.

INDUCTION OF LABOR

Termination of pregnancy is required in obstetric practice for many reasons and at varying times in pregnancy. Whenever possible, it is preferable to accomplish this objective without recourse to abdominal hysterotomy which, besides the immediate risk, places certain compromises on future childbearing, i.e., rarely ruptured uterus, the likelihood of repeat cesarean sections as a method of delivery, and other states such as postoperative adhesions.

Reference has been made to termination of pregnancy in the earlier months of pregnancy, including saline induction. Induction of labor in the latter half of pregnancy must take into consideration both fetal and maternal welfare, especially in the last 8 to 10 weeks of pregnancy.

Labor is induced by either the use of oxytocin or artificial rupture of the fetal membranes, or a combination of the two. Other methods based largely on causing stimulation of the myometrium by mechanical means, with bougies and the like, have been discarded and are of historical interest only. Recently prostaglandin has been introduced, but preliminary results suggest that the agent is no more virtuous than oxytocin.

Controversy exists as to whether oxytocin will suffice in the induction of labor and should be used initially alone or whether the fetal membranes should first be ruptured, with oxytocin stimulation added if labor fails to occur almost immediately thereafter. The time between membrane rupture and the beginning of labor is referred to as the latent period. It should not exceed four hours and when it extends beyond 12 to 18 hours there is reason for concern, for both maternal and fetal welfare. With the fetal membranes ruptured, intrauterine infection is a threat, and the loss of amniotic fluid may give rise to hyperton-

icity of the uterus after a prolonged latent period, with the added risk of fetal distress from hypoxia once labor begins. Moreover, the possible presence of intrauterine infection must be taken into account should abdominal delivery be required. From these remarks it would appear evident that the induction of labor is not without risk and certainly will remain empiric until the factor(s) responsible for labor are known.

The success and failure rate of induction of labor is determined largely by how near to term the patient is. The failure rate mounts rapidly prior to 35th to 36th week; near-total success is encountered if the patient is within one or two weeks of term. Clearly, it is important that the gestational date be accurately known when considering induction of labor for whatever indication and especially when it is performed electively. Also, the multiparous patient, having demonstrated her reproductive capacity, is a more favorable candidate for induction of labor (unless she is in the high gravid group) than is the primiparous patient. When termination of pregnancy is indicated and in the presence of a viable fetus, the appropriate method of delivery must be carefully weighed, that is to say, induction of labor versus cesarean section.

To give reasonable assurance that induction of labor will be successful, certain criteria are regarded as mandatory:

1. The cephalopelvic relationship must be normal.

2. The vertex should be engaged.

3. There should be a singleton fetus.

4. The condition of the cervix must be amenable for induction, i.e., partially effaced and 1 to 2 cm. or more dilated.

The major obstetric indications are: (1) certain cases of late pregnancy bleeding, more especially abruptio placentae or marginal sinus rupture; (2) hypertensive pregnancy in its various forms; (3) fetal conditions—erythroblastosis fetalis, dysmaturity, and postmaturity. Of the various medical conditions, probably the most outstanding example is diabetes mellitus, in which delivery a few weeks before term is indicated to improve the fetal salvage.

Induction of labor, in the presence of sound indications, may be extended to breech presentation when the pelvic capacity is ample. Multiple pregnancy is not altogether a contraindication to induction of labor, but in the overdistended uterus, from whatever cause, inductive labor may fail to occur.

In determining whether the cervix is "ripe" to permit induction, the status of its upper margin, the internal os, is important. If, instead of feeling like a rigid rim-like structure to the examining finger, the internal os has a loose consistency or is not detectable, having been incorporated into the lower uterine segment, this can be taken as useful evidence that induction of labor is feasible. Thus, if the internal os has seemingly disappeared even though the cervix is not appreciably effaced or dilated beyond a fingerbreadth, the condition may be considered favorable for induction of labor.

When termination of the pregnancy is strongly indicated and the cervix is not favorable for induction of labor, i.e., it is uneffaced and undilated, it has been questioned whether the cervix can be "ripened" through oxytocin stimulation to cause it to become effaced and 1 to 2 cm. dilated before the fetal membranes are ruptured. Or better still, the patient will enter labor with continuous oxytocin administration regardless of the status of the cervix and without artificial rupture of the fetal membranes. This approach may be successful on occasion but is by no means universally so. The patient may be subjected to oxytocin infusion over a period of several hours, and the infusion repeated on successive days. During this period some thought must be given to the fetal condition. On occasion time becomes a factor, for example, in a patient with severe toxemia in whom prolonged induction may be contraindicated. Although uterine contractions occur with a frequency and character that mimic spontaneous labor they may cause little if any effect on the cervix. Failure to respond favorably in the presence of the annoying discomfort of the uterine contractions over a period of six to eight hours, and especially on repeated days, is highly disturbing emotionally to most patients. Again, one must question the fetal effects of such a régime.

In the drip method, one ampule containing 10 units of natural or synthetic oxytocin in 1 ml. solution is added to 1000 ml. of 5 per cent glucose in buffered water. The infusion is started at a rate of 5 to 10 drops (3 to 5 milliunits) per minute, and, if need be, is increased up to 40 drops per minute, depending on the uterine response. If the first attempt is unsuccessful after a trial period of three to four hours, it is common practice to make a second attempt to induce labor by the same means some 24 hours later. The failure rate of induction of labor with oxytocin infusion was lowest when the cervix was judged favorable (7 per cent), and was high (63 per cent) when the threshold of the uterine response was high, that is, the uterus was insensitive. Successful induction of labor by oxytocin infusion is related to a "ripe" cervix.

With the criteria fulfilled to permit induction and the patient prepared for labor, including withholding of food and fluids for 8 to 12 hours, a Pitocin infusion may be started or the fetal membranes may be artificially ruptured under sterile precautions. The latter may be followed immediately by an oxytocin infusion to avoid the latent period, or two to three hours later if labor fails to ensue after the fetal membranes have been ruptured. The first method, Pitocin infusion alone, has the clear advantage of avoiding the risk of intrauterine infection by leaving the fetal membranes intact. Also, there is no absolute commitment in hours of time to pelvic delivery in order to avoid intrauterine infection. However, the failure rate of induction appears to be higher by this method than when the fetal membranes are artificially ruptured, to be followed if need be with Pitocin infusion. Those who favor artificial rupture of the membranes hope that the patient will enter labor spontaneously and in most cases will not require Pitocin stimulation. For however carefully administered, adverse reactions to Pitocin infusion occur. Uterine hypertonicity and fetal bradycardia and irregular fetal heart tones may require that the infusion be discontinued, at least for a time. It may be reinstituted, at a cautious rate. Obviously these patients must be carefully monitored at all times by experienced personnel.

The dangers and limitations of the oxytocin methods of induction of labor must not be minimized. This agent may cause tumultuous labor, the precursor of amniotic fluid embolism and uterine rupture. A tetanic contraction may develop, in which the uterus may go into spasm and fail to relax for 5 to 10 minutes, or longer. The fetal heart tones frequently fall to a rate well below 100 per minute and at times are barely perceptible. This response of the fetus is presumably from the hypoxia produced through a decrease in intervillous blood flow brought about by constriction of the endomyometrial blood vessels.

Other complications are those of labor generally—prolapse of the cord, fetal distress, premature separation of the placenta. But more important, a prolonged latent period following artificial rupture of the membranes is to be deplored. Hence, Pitocin infusion should be started soon after the fetal membranes have been ruptured but may be discontinued once labor is established. Should such measures fail and productive labor not occur within 12 to 18 hours after artificial rupture of the membranes, reassessment of the case is mandatory. When all factors are reviewed, that is, age, parity, the reason for induction, and the general status of the patient and the fetus, abdominal delivery may well be the appropriate method of management. In the patient whose childbearing is being completed, cesarean hysterectomy may be warranted and certainly is if intrauterine infection is more than a possibility.

Rarely in current practice will induction fail when the criteria to permit the procedure are met. Oxytocin infusion has added immeasurably to the efficiency of the procedure, so that the success rate of induction of labor for bona-fide indications should be 90 per cent or higher. When the procedure is performed electively, it must be 100 per cent successful.

In résumé, the method or combination of methods used to induce labor depends somewhat on the stage of pregnancy and the circumstances surrounding the case. In patients near term, and with the cervix "ripe" or favorable for induction, labor is initiated either by artificial rupture of the membranes or by the controlled administration of oxytocic drugs, or by a combination of the two. Clinicians hold firm opinions regarding their preference and the writer favors the combined method.

When the fetus is sufficiently mature to have a fair chance of survival, that is, after the 32nd week of pregnancy, and delivery is mandatory but the cervix is uneffaced, closed, and unsuitable for induction by rupture of the membranes, one of two courses is open: either cesarean section on the basis that any delay will increase the maternal or fetal risk, or oxytocin infusion, which may possibly induce labor without the need for artificial rupture of the membranes or may cause the cervix to efface and dilate adequately to permit the membranes to be safely and effectively ruptured. The use of oxytocin drip to prepare the unfavorable cervix for induction can be disappointing.

Technique of Saline Infusion

In the delivery room or operating room, the patient's abdomen is appropriately prepared and draped. Under local anesthesia a 15-cm. No. 15 Tuohy needle is introduced into the amniotic cavity. Following proper placement of the needle, a polyethylene catheter is fed into the amniotic cavity for a distance of some 12 inches. An attempt is made to withdraw approximately 150 ml. of amniotic fluid, which is then replaced with approximately 175 cc. of 20 per cent hypertonic saline solution.

Throughout instillation of the hypertonic solution, aspiration is carried out to ascertain free flow. If in the process of removing the amniotic fluid the sac is inadvertently emptied, normal saline can be used to reestablish flow and assure proper placement of the catheter. This is especially important when the amniotic fluid is meager in amount, as in the "dead-baby syndrome." Radiopaque material is also useful in establishment of proper placement of the catheter. A critical concentration of amniotic fluid sodium appears to be necessary for labor to ensue, usually beginning within 24 to 36 hours. The risk of this method must not be minimized and it should not be considered an outpatient procedure. Whether or not prostaglandin will replace this method is to be determined.

ELECTIVE INDUCTION OF LABOR

In recent years it has become common practice to induce labor at an appointed time, supposedly for the convenience of either the patient or her physician. The reported results of so-called "elective induction of labor" would indicate that the procedure is safe. But these have been compiled from patients selected on the basis of negative past obstetric history and a relatively normal current pregnancy by clinicians capable of meeting any emergency that might arise.

When labor is electively induced, the physician must accept complete responsibility for its outcome. Accidents to either the mother or child may occur in the course of spontaneous labor; should they by chance occur following elective induction of labor, the physician, in conscience and perhaps legally also, must justify the procedure.

In fairness to the controversy, however, it must be stated that elective induction of labor is practiced for reasons other than convenience. The most substantial reason for elective induction is that the patient can be prepared for anesthesia, an important consideration if the inhalation type is preferred. The procedure appears acceptable also in patients who have precipitate labors and deliveries.

The practice of elective induction of labor provides that, if the criteria listed are fulfilled, the patient enters the hospital at term as determined by gestational age and fetal size. After a night's rest, during which time food and fluids are withheld, and following a perineal preparation and a cleansing enema, labor is induced by either oxytocin infusion, artificial rupture of the membranes, or a combination of the two methods. In any event, a short latent period is anticipated, and labor and delivery occur in nearly every instance within a few hours. Programs for pain relief may be started during the latent period or withheld until the patient requests such therapy.

In summary, elective induction of labor is predicated on the belief that labor will promptly ensue, that it will be normal, and that the delivery will not be complicated. It is generally agreed that to permit elective induction the patient must be at or very near term, the presenting part must be the vertex and it must be engaged, and the cervix must be effaced and beginning to dilate. If these criteria are met the perinatal mortality and morbidity in patients induced electively should be substantially lower than the general average for the obstetric service.

Available evidence indicates that mistakes are made by inducing labor when in fact the patient is not at term and the fetus is lost from prematurity. For each of these cases there will be others in which surviving infants may sustain central nervous system damage from the hazards of prematurity. It is apparent that the results of elective induction must be examined in detail when the indications for the procedure lean heavily on convenience for the patient or her physician.

OTHER OBSTETRIC OPERATIONS

INTERNAL PODALIC VERSION

This procedure is used infrequently in current obstetric practice, and consequently the so-called "version artist" no longer exists, which is probably for the best. Actually, this operation is relatively easy to perform, and, if difficult, it is more than a possibility that the procedure has been poorly chosen. A primiparous breech extraction can be more difficult, and familiarity with this type of delivery should afford the physician confidence to perform an internal podalic version should the occasion arise.

In the main, the operation is performed on the second of twins and in the event of fetal distress, as in prolapse of the cord, but the conditions must be present that assure safety to the procedure, that is, a cervix completely or nearly completely dilated, with the membranes intact or only recently ruptured, and the cephalopelvic relationship normal. Further, the operation requires a relaxed uterus, so that the choice and administration of the anesthesia is an important consideration.

Two situations contribute to the ease of the operation: (1) it must be possible (and indeed this is imperative) to displace the vertex into one or the other of the lower quadrants of the uterus before an attempt is made to turn the fetus; and (2) in the event of a transverse presentation when the back is caudad, success depends on turning the fetal pelvis on itself in bringing the breech over the inlet. Whether the operator passes his hand anteriorly over the infant's body and searches for the posterior thigh and foot, or beneath the fetus to grasp the anterior foot, is immaterial except as it may pertain to the location and possible dislodgment of the placenta.

Once the patient is anesthetized, the vertex is displaced by the operator's hand into one of the lower quadrants of the uterus and away from the inlet (Fig. 33). The operator grasps the feet and, by traction, brings them through the completely dilated cervix and delivers them; at the same time the vertex is pushed upward by the outside hand into the area of the fundus. The remainder of the operation is similar in every respect to a breech extraction. In summary, the greatest difficulty with any version is not the turning, but rather the securing of uterine relaxation sufficient to permit displacement of the vertex away

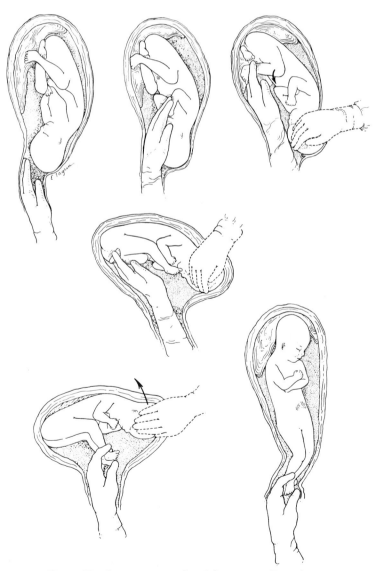

Figure 33. Steps in internal podalic version (Potter).

from the inlet. Attempting to turn the fetus before this is accomplished invites uterine rupture.

BRAXTON HICKS VERSION

Braxton Hicks version by definition is an internal bipolar version performed through a cervix that must be dilated 2 to 3 cm., but is not completely dilated. Once the fetus is turned, its expulsion is left to the uterine forces of labor. Traction is not necessary, but it is often applied to the fetal foot by a fillet to which a kilogram weight is attached. Once the fetus is turned, labor becomes productive, and delivery is usually completed in two to four hours.

The Braxton Hicks version is rarely performed in current practice, although the operation is usually not difficult provided the fetal membranes are intact up to the time of the version. It is fraught with some danger, however, when used in the treatment of placenta praevia, for once the operation is begun some bleeding may ensue until the fetus is successfully turned and converted to a breech. Thus, the procedure must never be considered in a central placenta praevia. Also, the operation becomes difficult when gestation progresses beyond the sixth month, and with a placenta praevia at this stage of pregnancy it can prove to be highly dangerous. Hence, the operation is restricted to cases in which the fetus is medically nonviable and requires judgment and experience in its performance.

DESTRUCTIVE OPERATIONS ON THE FETUS (EMBRYOTOMY)

Embryotomy is the dismembering of the fetus to expedite delivery. These unpleasant procedures are rarely performed in present-day practice, for the infant is less likely to be lost by exposure of the mother to an excessively long labor or obstetric neglect. When the fetus is already dead, regardless of cause, or has a malformation incompatible with extrauterine life, and cannot be delivered spontaneously or by other suitable pelvic procedures, destructive operations must be weighed against delivery by abdominal hysterotomy.

The operations include craniotomy, cleidotomy, evisceration, and decapitation.

Certain basic issues must be considered in determining whether a destructive operation is the indicated procedure. One should be alert to the possibility of a pathologic retraction ring which might defeat any attempt at pelvic delivery, even by embryotomy. Other factors to be weighed are the cephalopelvic relationship, the estimated size of the fetus, the question of uterine infection, and the parity of the patient. Also, these various destructive procedures require that the cervix be at least partially dilated; otherwise the manipulation and necessary instrumentation may result in cervical lacerations which in the extreme may extend into the lower uterine segment and result in uterine rupture. In fact, if the cervix is less than two thirds dilated, abdominal delivery may be the safer procedure. In the infected patient with several children, cesarean hysterectomy must be considered; otherwise an exclusion type or an extraperitoneal type of cesarean section is perhaps the safer form of management.

Craniotomy is rarely performed, except on a hydrocephalic infant when other methods previously described fail. If the cervix reaches near-complete dilatation the cranioclast can be applied to the dead fetus. The anterior fontanelle is first opened, and one branch of the cranioclast is introduced into the skull and placed against the anterior surface. The second branch is placed over the face, and the handles are brought together insofar as is possible so that the cranioclast firmly grasps the fetal head. The instrument should never be applied over the bones comprising the calvaria, for they are so fragile that they will not permit traction. The line of traction is directed in accordance with the pelvic axes, and the amount needed should not be great even in the presence of a contracted pelvis.

A **decapitation** operation has only one indication, that is, in a transverse presentation of a dead fetus when an internal podalic version is contraindicated because of the hazard of maternal trauma. With the neck held firmly by a blunt hook (Fig. 34B) the head can be severed by a long-handled scissors (Fig. 34C). If the cervix is fully dilated, the fetal torso may be extracted immediately; otherwise, a fillet may be

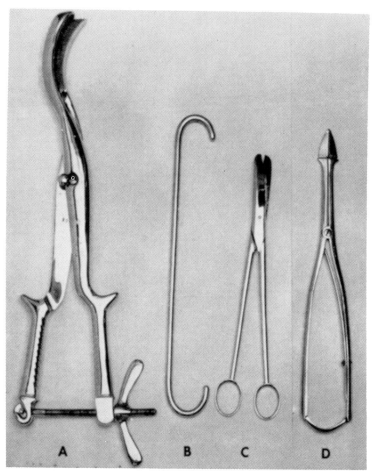

Figure 34. Instruments used for destructive operations: A, cranioclast; B, blunt hook; C, long-handled curved scissors; D, perforator.

applied to the footling presentation and expulsion can be left to the uterine powers. If the vertex is not readily expelled, the base of the skull may be grasped by a tenaculum or the vertex held with a finger in the fetal mouth, and the aftercoming head may be perforated, decompressed, and delivered.

Cleidotomy will facilitate delivery of either a dead or a live fetus when difficulty is encountered with the shoulders. The midpoint of the clavicle of the anterior shoulder is located by the index and middle fingers of the guiding hand. A long-handled scissors is thus directed to the clavicle, which in turn is incised, and this is ordinarily sufficient to release the anterior shoulder which will permit the posterior shoulder to be born. If the shoulders remain impacted, however, a cleidotomy is performed on the posterior shoulder also.

Evisceration may be required in the pres-

ence of an abdominal tumor or polycystic kidney, but perhaps the more common indication is erythroblastosis fetalis with a hydropic fetus. Besides difficulties with delivery of the shoulders, the abdomen may be markedly distended, requiring incision and evacuation of the contents. With the guiding hand along the fetal abdomen, the latter is incised by a long-handled scissors.

The number and types of destructive instruments are many, but those required to meet the various situations are illustrated (Fig. 34). Further, basiotribes and the like are not listed, for even in the hands of the experienced operator these are dangerous instruments capable of causing serious trauma to the mother. The cranioclast is for the compression and delivery of the forecoming head. The blunt hook is used to maintain countertraction when the neck is severed during decapitation. It may be used also to facilitate traction on the groin in a breech presentation, or in the axilla in the delivery of a dead or severely compromised fetus. A long-handled scissors is used for decapitation, cleidotomy, and evisceration. The perforator (Fig. 34D) is used on both the forecoming and the aftercoming head, to reduce its size or as a preliminary to application of the cranioclast.

DÜHRSSEN'S INCISIONS

Incisions of the cervix are preferable to any other management of the situation when immediate delivery is mandatory and failure of complete dilatation is the only obstacle to pelvic delivery. If delivery of the fetus is attempted without first incising the cervix, it will only lacerate, usually at the most vascular areas, namely, on either lateral margin in the region of the descending branch of the uterine artery. When Dührssen's incisions are contemplated, the cervix must be at least 6 to 8 cm. dilated. The operation requires adequate exposure, which is accomplished by applying to the vaginal wall thin, right-angled retractors of a length to permit the operator to see the junction of the cervix and the vagina. When the vertex requires rotation to an anterior position, the question arises whether it is wiser to incise the cervix first, or to apply the forceps, rotate, and then incise the cervix. Personally, the writer prefers the latter method, simply because extraction can be performed immediately after the incisions are made, thereby lessening blood loss. On the other hand, it could be rightfully argued that this method is more likely to traumatize the cervix.

The cervix is handled with a specially designed DeLee cervical tenaculum (Fig. 35) to avoid trauma. Once the cervix is exposed, the incisions are placed in the least vascular areas, at 2 o'clock and 10 o'clock, respectively, and extended nearly to the cervicovaginal junction (Fig. 36). Although these two anterior incisions will usually suffice, a third incision may be placed posteriorly at 6 o'clock. After the fetus is extracted, the uterus is compressed into the pelvis; the incisions are easily exposed, and are closed with appropriate interrupted sutures.

Patients who have had Dührssen's incisions are reputed to deliver without event in a subsequent pregnancy. In other words, the cervix dilates readily and cervical dystocia is not a problem.

VAGINAL HYSTEROTOMY

This procedure could rightfully have been included in the discussion on cesarean section. It is presented here principally because the indications for its use are limited; indeed, some authorities believe it has no place in modern obstetrics. At one time, some three decades ago, it was a rather popular operation, particularly when termination of pregnancy seemed indicated in the middle trimester; and some daring souls performed the operation, apparently with success, in the last trimester of pregnancy.

Vaginal hysterotomy can have a place in the treatment of the occasional patient, but certain rigid conditions must be met to permit complete technical safety in performing the operation. It may be selected only when the operator is certain that he can obtain proper exposure, which is impossible if the pubic arch is narrow or if the

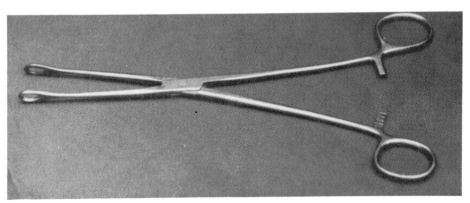

Figure 35. DeLee cervical tenaculum.

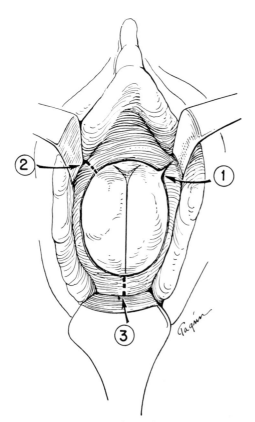

Figure 36. Dührssen's incisions.

cervix cannot be brought nearly to the introitus by traction. The procedure is used when the uterus should be emptied immediately at a stage of pregnancy when induction of labor is tedious and at times unsatisfactory. The gestational period should not exceed five months. The indication conceivably might be the presence of severe renal disease (i.e., chronic glomerulonephritis or pyelonephritis) when the patient is seen for the first time in the fourth or fifth month of pregnancy, and on consultation it is agreed that continuation of the pregnancy would be extremely hazardous. Such patients react adversely medically to abdominal hysterotomy, commonly exhibiting an exacerbation of their renal disease. Thus opening the abdomen is to be avoided when possible, even when there is the general feeling that the uterus should be evacuated promptly.

The operation is not difficult (Fig. 37), if the requirements listed are fulfilled. After the patient is anesthetized, prepared, and draped, the cervix is exposed and grasped with DeLee cervical tenacula,

and an epinephrine solution, 1:200,000, is injected about the lower cervix to reduce bleeding. The vaginal mucosa covering the anterior cervix is incised transversely (Fig. 37). The plane of cleavage between the layers of endopelvic fascia is established between the bladder and the cervix, and the bladder is displaced upward. To facilitate displacing the bladder upward, the so-called pillars of the bladder, that is, the endopelvic fascia at the lateral margins of the cervix, may be cut and sutured. Care should be exercised in retracting the bladder upward away from the cervix, for in pregnancy the nearby veins in the broad ligament are fragile and easily traumatized. A narrow, right-angle retractor with a blade no longer than 4 cm. should be used for this purpose. The cervix must never be permitted to rotate when traction is being applied; rather, the operator must always make certain that he places the incision in its anterior midline lest the veins at the side be cut and cause annoying ooze. Once the bladder is displaced, the operator can feel the anterior cervix in its entirety up to the region of the internal os. The latter is identified by the fact that the cervix is relatively firm and the corpus is extremely soft.

The cervix is incised in its entire length, and with the incision placed in its midline there is surprisingly little bleeding. The uncut cervix barely admits the tip of the finger, but as soon as the internal os is cut the operator will appreciate the fact that the opening into the uterus is 3 cm. or more in diameter. The membranes are now ruptured, with care not to disturb the placenta. The fetus is removed completely, but not always intact, with ovum forceps. The placenta is next removed, and the cervix is closed with interrupted sutures. In fact, as the cervix is cut, the sutures may be placed and carried on a hemostat, and quickly tied after the uterus has been emptied. The vaginal mucosa is reunited and the operation is complete. If by chance the anterior incision fails to permit adequate dilatation, the posterior wall of the cervix can also be incised.

Although it is rare today to encounter a patient who has had a vaginal hysterotomy for what proves to be temporary indications, subsequent labor in these patients, as in those with Dührssen's incisions, is usually normal and unremarkable. There is no reason to deliver the patient by abdominal hysterotomy because of a previous vaginal

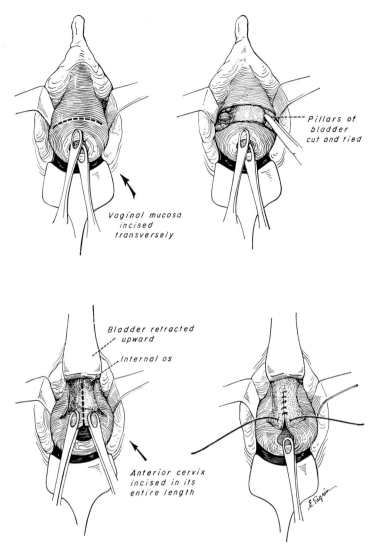

Figure 37. Vaginal hysterotomy.

hysterotomy; she could at least be permitted to enter labor and her progress be observed for a time.

STERILIZATION AT CESAREAN SECTION OR INCIDENTAL TO PELVIC DELIVERY

Comment has been made regarding the procedure required for obtaining permission to perform a sterilization operation, and the medical, surgical, and obstetric indications for the procedure. Here attention is directed to technique.

At least three general methods deal directly with tubal ligation. These include the crushing and ligation of the tube only, using a nonabsorbable ligature (Madlener procedure); the excision of the distal loop of the tube after ligation (Pomeroy procedure, Fig. 38); and placement of the proximal portion of the incised tube in the myometrium (Irving procedure, Fig. 39). The Irving procedure is reputed to have the lowest failure rate. Recanalization of the tube probably occurs in less than 1 per cent with the Pomeroy procedure. The Madlener procedure gives a substantially higher rate of failure (3 to 5 per cent).

Recently tubal sterilization has been accomplished through the use of the laparoscope. Indeed, it is in this area that this instrument may have its greatest usefulness. Also, plastic hoods are being tried for the purpose of temporary sterilization.

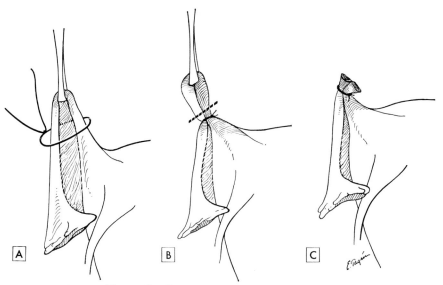

Figure 38.   Pomeroy sterilization procedure.

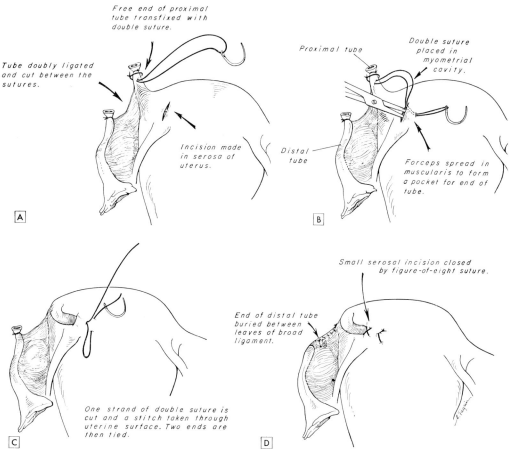

Figure 39.   Irving sterilization procedure.

The hood is sutured in place over the fimbriated portion of the tube. It is envisioned that these can be removed at a later date, if by chance the patient wishes to have another child.

The time at which sterilization should be performed is obvious when it is selected in association with cesarean section. If it is to be performed with pelvic delivery, it may be done coincidentally. This requires, however, that labor and delivery be entirely normal; if there is any question of the patient's condition, sterilization is postponed until some time later, usually several months. Rather than wait for 24 to 72 hours after delivery, there is evidence to support the contention that it is a safer procedure when performed at or almost immediately after delivery. The uterus and the tubes are more likely to be sterile at this time than later in the postpartum period, which lessens the chance of infection. Furthermore, the patient will not have to accept a second anesthetic.

The patient who is to receive a postpartum sterilization is delivered in the operating room with preparation made for laparotomy. After the delivery is completed, with an oxytocin infusion being administered and the uterus well contracted, the abdomen is prepared and draped and opened through a 2- to 3-inch infraumbilical midline incision. The fallopian tubes can be seen nearby. Each in turn is treated according to the Pomeroy or Irving technique, with a total operating time of some 10 to 20 minutes. The patient experiences some postoperative discomfort; to minimize distention, food is withheld for two or three days, and intravenous fluids are given instead. The patient is discharged on the fifth to seventh postpartum day.

The question is occasionally raised concerning a possible disturbance in ovarian physiology in association with sterilization, presumably through some interference with the ovarian blood supply. Whether there is a greater incidence of cystic change in the ovaries, or a higher frequency of premenopausal hypermenorrhea in such patients, is not an easy question to answer, owing to the difficulty in establishing the incidence of these conditions in a group of controls. Certainly there is no convincing evidence that the operation disturbs ovarian or sexual function; in fact, the removal of the fear of pregnancy leads to a more compatible marital state. Thus, patients can be assured that there will be no alteration in their physiology or disturbance in their sexual responses following sterilization.

Articles in popular lay publications have left the impression in the minds of some patients that the uterine tubes, after being incised in the course of a sterilization procedure, can be reunited at some later date should the patient desire another child. This idea should be quickly dispelled from the patient's mind, all of which emphasizes the point that the procedure should be carefully explained to the patient and her husband, and they must realize all of the implications, such as the possibility that the patient might be widowed and wish to remarry and bear other children, or that one or more of their children might be lost from accident or illness. The decision regarding the procedure must not be entered into lightly by either the patient, her husband, or the physician. Also, the procedure is not favored if there is reason to believe that the patient will require some gynecologic surgery in the near future, more precisely, vaginal hysterectomy and plastic repair for the correction of procidentia, urethrocystocele, or rectocele.

BIBLIOGRAPHY

Adams, T. W.: Female sterilization. Amer. J. Obstet. Gynec., 89:395, 1964.

Awon, M. P.: The vacuum extractor—experimental demonstration of distortion of the foetal skull. J. Obstet. Gynaec. Brit. Comm., 71:634, 1964.

Barclay, D. L.: Cesarean hysterectomy. Thirty years' experience. Obstet. Gynec., 35:120, 1970.

Baxter, J.: Vaginal delivery after caesarean section. J. Obstet. Gynaec. Brit. Emp., 65:87, 1958.

Beck, A. C.: The advantages and disadvantages of the two-flap low incision cesarean section, with a report of eighty-three cases done by fifteen operators. Amer. J. Obstet. Gynec., 1:586, 1921.

Bixby, G. H.: Extirpation of the puerperal uterus by abdominal section. J. Gynec. Soc. Boston, 1:223, 1869.

Blakey, D. H., Dewhurst, C. J., and Russell, C. S.: Delivery before full dilatation with special reference to incision of the cervix. J. Obstet. Gynaec. Brit. Emp., 65:644, 1958.

Browne, A. D. H., and McGrath, J.: Vaginal delivery after previous caesarean section. A survey of 800 cases at the Rotunda Hospital, Dublin. J. Obstet. Gynaec. Brit. Comm., 72:557, 1965.

Caldwell, W. E., Moloy, H. C., and D'Esopo, D. A.: Studies on pelvic arrests. Amer. J. Obstet. Gynec., 36:928, 1938.

Cameron, J. M., and Dayan, A. D.: Association of brain damage with therapeutic abortion induced by am-niotic-fluid replacement; report of two cases. Brit. Med. J., 1:1010, 1966.

Chalmers, J. A.: Five years' experience with the vacuum extractor. Brit. Med. J., 1:1216, 1964.

Chamberlain, G.: The vacuum extractor; a possible danger. Lancet, 1:632, 1965.

Choate, J. W., and Lund, C. J.: Emergency cesarean section; an analysis of maternal and fetal results in 177 operations. Amer. J. Obstet. Gynec., 100:703, 1968.

Cooke, W. A. R.: Evaluation of the midforceps operation. Amer. J. Obstet. Gynec., 99:327, 1967.

Crosby, W. M., and Page, E. W.: The clinical observation of an oxytocin infusion. Obstet. Gynec., 18:60, 1961.

Das, K.: Obstetric Forceps; Its History and Evolution. C. V. Mosby Co., St. Louis, 1929.

DeLee, J. B.: The prophylactic forceps operation. Amer. J. Obstet. Gynec., 1:34, 1920.

DeLee, J. B., and Cornell, E. L.: Low cervical cesarean section (laparotrachelotomy). J.A.M.A., 79:109, 1922.

Dennen, E. H.: Forceps Deliveries. In Heaton, C. E., ed.: Obstetrics and Gynecology: A Series of Mono-graphs. F. A. Davis Co., Philadelphia, 1955.

Douglas, R. G., Birnbaum, S. J., and MacDonald, F. A.: Pregnancy and labor following cesarean section. Amer. J. Obstet. Gynec., 86:961, 1963.

Douglas, R. G., and Stromme, W. B.: Operative Ob-stetrics. Appleton-Century-Crofts, Inc., New York, 1957.

Douglass, L. H., and Kaltreider, D. F.: Trial forceps. Amer. J. Obstet. Gynec., 65:889, 1953.

Dunster, E. S.: The use of obstetric forceps in abbrevi-ating the second stage of labor. Trans. Med. Soc. Mich., 7:107, 1877–1880.

Eadie, F. S., and Keettel, W. C.: Trial and failed for-ceps. Obstet. Gynec., 4:241, 1954.

Evans, T. N., and Stander, R. W.: Cervical incisions in obstetrics. Amer. J. Obstet. Gynec., 67:322, 1954.

Ferguson, R. K., and Reid, D. E.: Rupture of the uterus; a twenty-year report from the Boston Lying-in Hospital. Amer. J. Obstet. Gynec., 76:172, 1958.

Fish, S. A.: The Barton obstetric forceps; a history. Amer. J. Obstet. Gynec., 66:1290, 1953.

Fleming, A. R., Brandeberry, K. R., and Pearse, W. H.: Introduction of a metric forceps; preliminary report. Amer. J. Obstet. Gynec., 78:125, 1959.

Frank, F.: Die suprasymphysäre Entbindung und ihr Verhältniss zu den anderen Operationen bie engen Becken. Arch. Gynaek., 81:46, 1907.

Hicks, J. B.: On Combined External and Internal Version. Longman, London, 1864.

Irving, F. C.: The Tarnier axis traction rods applied to the Simpson forceps. Surg. Gynec. Obstet., 20:734, 1915.

Irving, F. C.: A new method of insuring sterility follow-ing cesarean section. Amer. J. Obstet. Gynec., 8:335, 1924.

Kelly, J. V., and Sines, G.: An assessment of the com-pression and traction forces of obstetrical forceps. Amer. J. Obstet. Gynec., 96:521, 1966.

Kehrer, F. A.: Über ein modificirtes Verfahren beim Kaiserschnitte. Arch Gynaek., 19:177, 1882.

Kelly, J. V., and Winston, H. G.: Successful post-mortem cesarean section. Amer. J. Obstet. Gynec., 72:203, 1956.

Kerr, J. M. M., and Hendry, J.: Conservative cesarean section by the lower uterine segment incision. Surg. Gynec. Obstet., 43:85, 1926.

Krönig, B.: Operative Gynäkologie, 3rd ed. Thieme, Leipzig, 1912.

Lane, F. D., and Reid, D. E.: Dehiscence of previous uterine incision at repeat cesarean section. Obstet. Gynec., 2:54, 1953.

Malmström, T.: Vacuum extractor—an obstetrical instrument. Acta Obstet. Gynec. Scand., 33(Suppl. 4):1, 1954.

Mickal, A., Begneaud, W. P., and Hawes, T. P., Jr.: Pitfalls and complications of cesarean section hysterectomy. Clin. Obstet. Gynec., 12:660, 1969.

Miller, J. L.: Cesarean section in Virginia in the pre-aseptic era, 1794–1879. Ann. Med. History, 10:23, 1938.

Nichols, E. E.: Current practices in female steriliza-tion in the United States; incidence and methods. Amer. J. Obstet. Gynec., 101:345, 1968.

Niswander, K. R.: Elective induction of labor. In Reid, D. E., and Barton, T. C., eds.: Controversy in Obstetrics and Gynecology. W. B. Saunders Co., Philadelphia, 1969, p. 121.

O'Leary, J. A., and Steer, C. M.: A 10 year review of cesarean hysterectomy. Amer. J. Obstet. Gynec., 90:227, 1964.

Pearse, W. H.: Electronic recording of forceps delivery. Amer. J. Obstet. Gynec., 86:43, 1963.

Phaneuf, L. K.: The technique of the transverse cer-vical cesarean section. Surg. Gynec. Obstet., 53:202, 1931.

Piper, E. B., and Bachman, C.: The prevention of fetal injuries in breech delivery. J.A.M.A., 92:217, 1929.

Pletsch, T. D., and Sandberg, E. C.: Cesarean hyster-ectomy for sterilization. Amer. J. Obstet. Gynec., 85:254, 1963.

Rhodes, P.: A critical appraisal of the obstetric forceps. J. Obstet. Gynaec. Brit. Emp., 65:353, 1958.

Ribemont-Dessaignes, A., and LePage, G.: Traité d'obstétrique, 8th ed. Masson et Cie, Paris, 1914, p. 1174 (Tarnier's forceps).

Ricci, J. V., and Marr, J. P.: The Physick-Sellheim principle of extraperitoneal cesarean section; eluci-dation of a technique based on 175 cases. Amer. J. Surg., 71:3, 1946.

von Ritgen: Über das Hervorziehen des Uterus aus der Bauchdeckenwunde bei dem Kaiserschnitte, zur Stillung der Blutung der Gebärmutterwunde vermöge kalter Umschläge. N. Z. Geburtsh., 9:212, 1840.

Riva, H. L., and Teich, J. D.: Vaginal delivery after cesarean section. Amer. J. Obstet. Gynec., 81:501, 1961.

Ruiz-Velasco, V., and Gamiz, R.: Prognosis of the cesarean section scar. Amer. J. Obstet. Gynec., 95:1119, 1966.

Sänger, M.: Simplification of the technique of the cesarean section. Amer. J. Obstet., 19:883, 1886.

Schenker, J. G., and Serr, D. M.: Comparative study of delivery by vacuum extractor and forceps. Amer. J. Obstet. Gynec., 98:32, 1967.

Schmitz, H. E., and Gajewski, C.: Vaginal delivery following cesarean section. Amer. J. Obstet. Gynec., 61:1232, 1951.

Schwartz, O. H., Paddock, R., and Bortnick, A. R.: The cesarean scar. Amer. J. Obstet. Gynec., 36:962, 1938.

Sellheim, H.: Weiteres vom extraperitonealen Uterus-schnitt. Zbl. Gynaek., 32:319, 1908.

Simpson, A. R.: The invention and evolution of the midwifery forceps. Scot. Med. Surg. J., 7:465, 1900.

Simpson, J. Y.: On the mode of application of the long forceps. Monthly J. Med. Sci., 9:193, 1848.

Smellie, W.: History of midwifery forceps; theory and practice of midwifery. New Sydenham Soc., 1:77, 1876.

Smith, E. F.: Transcervical cesarean section with peritoneal exclusion and bladder mobilization. Amer. J. Obstet. Gynec., 39:763, 1940.

Tarnier, S.: Description de deux nouveaux forceps. Lauwereyns, Paris, 1877.

Waters, E. G.: Disputed indications and technics for cesarean section. New Eng. J. Med., 234:849, 1946.

Wider, J. A., Erez, S., and Steer, C. M.: An evaluation of the vacuum extractor in a series of 201 cases. Amer. J. Obstet. Gynec., 98:24, 1967.

Young, J. H.: The History of Caesarean Section. H. K. Lewis & Co., Ltd., London, 1944.

Chapter 30

Medical and Surgical Diseases in Pregnancy

With the overall advances in medicine, therapeutic methods and agents have evolved that permit an increasing number of patients with a variety of medical diseases not only to survive childhood and adolescence but, in the case of the female, to consider marriage with the hope that she will be able to fulfill her desire to bear children. Regardless of these advances, there are still some medical conditions in which the risk to the mother and the high fetal mortality contraindicate pregnancy.

Patients who are afflicted with disease or the sequelae of disease, or who are concerned about their genetic background, may seek the counsel of a physician as to the advisability of marriage and subsequent childbearing. The physician may also be asked by his medical colleagues to render an opinion with reference to the desirability of continuation of a pregnancy in the presence of complicating medical disease. His decision will be based on the consideration of many factors, the most important being whether the disease is a greater threat to the patient's life during pregnancy than otherwise, or whether the underlying medical condition will be accelerated or permanently aggravated by pregnancy.

Although the care of a pregnant patient with a medical disease ofttimes demands a team effort, the obstetrician-gynecologist certainly cannot afford to be preoccupied exclusively with the technical aspects of the pregnancy and delegate or relinquish completely the medical responsibility to the internist, for obviously the patient's welfare will not be maximally served.

DISORDERS OF THE REPRODUCTIVE TRACT IN RELATION TO PREGNANCY

LEIOMYOMATA IN PREGNANCY

Patients with leiomyomata, even extensive ones, tend to have uneventful pregnancies and as a rule experience a normal labor and delivery. Actually, patients are seen in early pregnancy with the tumors completely filling the pelvis, and it would be reasonable to expect that pelvic delivery would be impossible; but it is the rule rather than the exception for these tumors to move out of the pelvis, thereby allowing delivery by the pelvic route. It is envisioned that as the uterus enlarges, and particularly as the lower segment forms, the tumors are literally pulled out of the pelvis. Hence, prior to the onset of labor the physician should exercise a degree of caution in expressing an opinion as to how the patient with extensive uterine fibroids will be delivered. In fact, he should convey optimism, for these patients need reassurance as to the possible effect these tumors may have both on the growth and development of the fetus and on the overall outcome of pregnancy. Obviously, if the fibroids remain in the pelvis, and cannot be dislodged, a cesarean section is the only method of delivery.

Leiomyomata tend to enlarge, at times rapidly, in early pregnancy, and recede to their original size after delivery. Perhaps because of a previous upset in blood supply, with degeneration and calcification, tumors that enlarge in one pregnancy may retain more or less their original size in a subsequent pregnancy. Another fact about leiomyomata is that they tend to become pedunculated during pregnancy. That is to say, an intramural leiomyoma or one with a sessile base may actually be pushed or extruded from the uterine wall by the end of pregnancy and become suspended from a pedicle.

The blood supply of leiomyomata occasionally may become compromised during pregnancy, leading to degeneration within the tumor. In fact, an occasional patient may experience recurrent episodes of discomfort in the region of the tumor, presumably as the result of a disturbance in the blood supply as it temporarily enlarges. The tumor becomes tender, and there is generally moderate leukocytosis, but fever, if present, is rarely above 100° F. Surgery is infrequently indicated, for after a day or two of sedation under hospital observation the patient usually becomes free of symptoms. These episodes may recur from time to time during pregnancy, but postponement of surgery until after the patient has finished her childbearing is the ultimate objective. Myomectomy during pregnancy or in the childbearing years is not without risk, and certainly its risk is not to be compared with the low risk of hysterectomy. Thus, conservative management should be sought during pregnancy unless the tumor shows progressive symptoms with evidence of extensive degeneration, or the leiomyoma is believed to contribute to pregnancy failure through distortion of the uterine cavity.

Myomectomy

When myomectomy becomes necessary in pregnancy, even when the tumor is deeply embedded in the uterine wall and the decidua can be seen at the base of the wound after its removal, the pregnancy is likely to continue. If the tumor is located in the broad ligaments or in the lower uterine segment, myomectomy may not be feasible and hysterectomy may be required. The patient and her husband should be fully informed of this possibility.

In removal of the tumor, bleeding is minimal and enucleation is not difficult when the line of cleavage is established between the capsule of the tumor and the myometrium. It is well to place the incision above the base of the tumor and develop a sleeve of serosa that will ensure an adequate amount of tissue for the wound to be closed without tension. To close dead space and to obtain complete hemostasis, figure-of-eight sutures should be placed to

include the base of the myometrial crater. Whether a second layer of interrupted sutures is necessary will depend on the depth of the tumor. The serosal surface is closed by continuous or interrupted sutures. Except perhaps for pedunculated tumors that may become twisted, it is doubtful whether multiple myomectomy is wise at this time, but rather only the tumor or tumors believed to be responsible for the patient's symptoms should be removed.

In patients who have had myomectomies prior to or during pregnancy, the question of management of labor is naturally of some concern. There are surprisingly few documented cases of uterine rupture during pregnancy and labor after myomectomy. Regardless of the size and depth of the uterine wound, these patients can be delivered pelvically unless there are other contraindications. The conduct of labor would consist of all the precautions taken in patients being delivered pelvically after a previous cesarean section.

In summary, patients with leiomyomata do surprisingly well during pregnancy regardless of the size, the location, or the number of tumors present. Rarely do the tumors undergo degeneration during pregnancy to the extent that they require surgical removal. Even when they appear to obstruct the birth canal, at least in early pregnancy, they tend to move up into the abdomen, and labor and delivery may be quite normal.

Thus, in women wishing children, operation for uterine leiomyomata is postponed whenever possible until after childbearing. Some may eventually require hysterectomy, but certainly the presence of the tumor alone does not necessitate surgery. Many women with sizable leiomyomata are entirely asymptomatic. Moreover, these tumors show marked regression with the menopause. Rather, hysterectomy in the nonpregnant is indicated for the following three reasons: if the tumor is growing; if it is submucous in location, causing hypermenorrhea; or if it encroaches on the surrounding structures with pressure symptoms, particularly about the bladder, causing frequency and urgency.

UTERINE PROLAPSE

Pregnancy occurs in the milder forms of uterine prolapse but, of course, never in complete procidentia prior to replacement. According to some, in cases that are reported as prolapse the condition is actually elongation and hypertrophy of the cervix and it should be so designated. It is impossible to distinguish between the two conditions, however, unless the patient has been examined before pregnancy, or is seen in the first trimester when, characteristically, in the case of prolapse the uterine corpus is found resting on the perineum with the cervix protruding from the introitus. If the patient is seen for the first time in the latter weeks of pregnancy, therefore, the precise diagnosis must be postponed until after the patient is delivered. Whichever the condition, the problems are the same, namely, the hazard of uterine infection and the unpredictability of the outcome of labor. Fetal wastage also is increased, by a greater incidence of spontaneous abortion and premature labor.

Treatment consists of use of a properly fitted pessary, which in the first trimester will usually reduce the prolapse and hold the uterus in normal position. Bed rest is recommended, but, as the pregnancy progresses and the uterus becomes an abdominal organ, in some instances the pessary is no longer needed and the patient may be permitted to resume her usual daily activities.

Labor and delivery may be uncomplicated or difficult; the few cases seen by the writer fall into the former category. Actually, during labor the cervix may again protrude from the vagina, and one has the opportunity to observe directly the process of cervical dilatation. The literature, however, bears out the fact that dystocia may be a problem. The cervix may fail to dilate, requiring incision to accomplish delivery, or, in the presence of a dead fetus, craniotomy may be performed.

In women who wish to have more pregnancies, the question arises whether some gynecologic procedure such as the Richardson composite or the Manchester–Fothergill operation should be performed to correct the uterine prolapse. If surgery is done the patient must realize that abdominal delivery will probably be required in any subsequent pregnancy. Instead of surgery, in most cases a pessary can be worn without discomfort, and the patient may be taken through other pregnancies. If possible, gynecologic surgery should

be postponed until the patient has completed her childbearing, when a vaginal hysterectomy will afford complete relief of symptoms.

WOLFFIAN OR GARTNER'S DUCT CYST

Remnants of the wolffian system sometimes fill with fluid and form cysts lateral to the cervix and about the anterior vaginal wall, commonly referred to as Gartner's duct cysts. They often first become evident in pregnancy, increasing in size during its course, and have been regarded as a possible cause of dystocia. Should these cysts become large enough to impede advancement of the presenting part, aspiration will temporarily collapse them and allow pelvic delivery. Certainly their presence is not an indication for abdominal delivery. Further, with the increased vascularity, pregnancy is not the time for their excision, for it is a relatively simple procedure to remove these cysts when the patient is not pregnant.

OVARIAN NEOPLASMS

An ovarian tumor may cause dystocia or become a surgical emergency during pregnancy and the puerperium. Unless the patient is seen in the first trimester, the differential diagnosis between ovarian neoplasm and leiomyoma may at times be uncertain, and once the uterus becomes an abdominal organ it may conceal the presence of the ovarian tumor. At the same time, the ovarian pedicle may become elongated and permit the tumor to move about freely in the upper abdomen, which offers an explanation as to why an ovarian tumor so readily suffers from torsion during pregnancy and requires surgical intervention. With torsion, hemorrhage into the cyst or tumor commonly occurs, and one is often confounded at laparotomy by the marked increase in size of a tumor that had been regarded as rather small.

In the absence of symptoms of torsion the question that arises is whether the tumor should be removed during pregnancy, and if so when. A deciding factor will be the size and consistency of the tumor. When the tumor appears cystic and is no more than 5 cm. in diameter, the patient can reasonably be followed, for certainly a follicle ovarian or a corpus luteum cyst may regress. If the tumor is firm and solid, or actually increases in size, excision of the tumor or oophorectomy is undoubtedly the safer course. Preferably, the removal of an ovarian tumor is delayed until after the second month but not later than the end of the fifth month of pregnancy, in an attempt to avoid early abortion or precipitate premature labor.

Of the solid tumors seen in patients in the childbearing age the majority are dermoids or benign teratomata, and of these, some 25 per cent are bilateral. In the latter situation one ovary is usually less involved, so that it is often possible to enucleate the tumor from one or both ovaries and thus preserve ovarian function. In the diagnosis of a dermoid cyst, skeletal elements can sometimes be visualized by roentgenography, but there is a reluctance to perform roentgenography during pregnancy.

Luteinized tumors of the ovary in the nonpregnant may give rise to a variety of symptoms, from abnormal uterine bleeding to a cushingoid state. When encountered in pregnancy, the question has arisen whether a luteoma is a true tumor or represents hyperactivity of the theca or ovarian stroma from the stimulus of the presence of excessive chorionic gonadotropin. Masculinization in pregnancy has occurred with this rare neoplasm, which has also been encountered bilaterally. The tumor may be 6 to 12 cm. in size, owing in part to hemorrhage, and may be found incidentally at laparotomy. A laparotomy with oophorectomy is usually required because of pain and tenderness. The tumor may go unrecognized and disappear following delivery, more than a theoretical possibility with the disappearance of chorionic gonadotropin. An arrhenoblastoma may be encountered with masculinization appearing in the course of pregnancy.

Dysgerminoma when found in pregnancy brings up the question of how to manage the pregnant patient with a malignant ovarian tumor or one with a malignant potential. Although there are other factors, the decisions are based primarily on the type and gross extent of the tumor and the stage of pregnancy. With dysgerminoma, if it proves to contain only germ cell elements, the prognosis is excellent and nothing further need be done. If the tumor is an admixture of teratocarcinoma or embryonal carcinoma, which occurs in some 20 per cent of dysgerminomata, the survival rate is extremely low irrespective of the type of management. Knowing what her life expectancy may be, the patient may wish to make the choice and decide to continue the pregnancy. Thus, in various forms of malignancy, notably breast cancer when identified initially during pregnancy, the patient's desires must be given consideration.

In the case of a tumor of germinal epithelial origin (carcinoma, papillary cystadenocarcinoma, or adenocarcinoma— all known to be radiosensitive) if the disease is detected early in pregnancy and is restricted to the pelvis and operable, bilateral oophorectomy and complete abdominal hysterectomy should be performed, followed by deep x-ray therapy. If the pregnancy is in the last trimester, however, the procedure might be postponed, with the reasonable anticipation of obtaining a living child. There is no evidence that the survival time will be altered.

Whether the patient should be permitted to enter labor would depend on her general condition at the time and whether the tumor obstructs the birth canal. Even in the absence of such obstruction, conceivably cesarean hysterectomy and bilateral oophorectomy or, when metastases are widespread, cesarean section alone would have to be considered as soon as the fetus has reached medical viability, for certainly one would have some concern regarding its survival under these circumstances.

It is apparent that when ovarian malignancy is at question in pregnancy the patient's treatment must be carefully individualized. If the parametria, the retroperitoneal space, and the lymph nodes are negative to palpation and wedge incision and biopsy of the opposite ovary reveal it to be free of tumor, a conservative procedure of oophorectomy may be considered. The type of tumor will indicate whether a secondary operation will be necessary following delivery. Certainly patients with the pure form of dysgerminoma and other types of ovarian tumor of low-grade malignancy have had successful pregnancies.

CANCER OF THE CERVIX

Of all human cancers, none lends itself more readily to early detection and hence curability than does cervical cancer. It is now conceded that invasive cancer of the cervix is preceded by a preinvasive lesion designated carcinoma in situ or Stage 0.

This lesion is present for months or years before it develops into invasive cancer. The view has been expressed that deaths from cervical cancer could be eradicated if periodic vaginal and cytologic examinations were performed on women from time of puberty.

Certain limitations are imposed on any public health program designed to attain this worthy objective. Perhaps 20 to 30 per cent of women in this country benefit from annual cervical cancer screening. There are many reasons for this, from failure of patient motivation to lack of available screening services. Most disturbing is the fact that cytologic examination is not always included in the physician's pelvic examination. Certainly women between the ages of 30 and 40 years, being usually in good health and many involved in child-rearing, are less likely to visit a physician. It is in this age period when mass screening should be the most rewarding for it is the time when Stage 0 reaches its peak incidence. Also, it is recognized that invasive cancer of the cervix has a higher incidence in the socioeconomically deprived. This raises the difficult question if, when screening is not available for all, the effort should perhaps be directed more toward populations in which the incidence of invasive cancer is highest. All of this implies that the medical manpower is inadequate to perform this prodigious service. Hence, some method other than direct physician participation must be considered, including specially trained paramedical personnel to perform both vaginal and cytologic examinations. Also, it has been shown that examination of irrigation vaginal smears obtained by the patient herself is a suitable method that will uncover an incidence of carcinoma in situ initially of 7 per 1000, and on rescreening, of 4 per 1000, which is comparable to that of more direct methods. However, irrigation specimens require a more tedious search for cells than specimens from a spatula cervical scrape. The method is open to the criticism that the cervix is not inspected and vaginal examination is not performed. In fact, whatever improvement has occurred in reducing incidence of cervical cancer has been due largely to the routine use of the Papanicolaou smear in prenatal care. Thus, pregnancy provides the greatest opportunity for cancer detection through identification of patients with carcinoma in situ and those with dysplasia that in turn may develop, albeit rarely, into a Stage 0 lesion. The dispensing of contraceptives also provides the physician the opportunity to do annual cytologic examinations.

As indicated, the prevalence of carcinoma in situ varies somewhat with the clientele screened and adherence to the strict definition or criteria for the histologic diagnosis of the lesion. For the diagnosis to apply, the entire thickness of the epithelium must be involved, with complete loss of stratification and cellular polarity with atypical mitotic figures throughout and hypochromatic staining of the pleomorphic nuclei (TeLinde) (Fig. 1).

A lesion that fails to fulfill this definition should not be designated carcinoma in situ, but when so defined the incidence of Stage 0 lesion in childbearing women is 4 to 7 per 1000 patients. A lesion with a plethora of terms—atypical epithelium, anaplasia, dysplasia—is more frequently encountered, consisting of an increase in immature cells or abnormal maturation of cells. In the majority of instances of dysplasia the lesion regresses, but when the lesion persists or recurs, carcinoma in situ has been known to develop. The incidence of carcinoma in situ among patients who have dysplasia is approximately 20 times greater than among patients who have negative cytologic smears.

The pathogenesis of Stage 0 lesions has been the subject of many studies and continues to remain an open question. Whether it originates from squamous or endocervical epithelium, the lesion is located in approximation to the squamocolumnar junction. Extension may occur upward into the cervical canal or downward over the vaginal portion of the cervix, and in rare cases, even as far as the vaginal wall. Hence, biopsy of the squamocolumnar junction will include the lesion although it may not outline its extent.

The diagnosis of Stage 0, since it is not a gross lesion, begins with what constitutes an abnormal Papanicolaou smear. Even in preinvasive lesions, the cervical smear technique (aspiration of the endocervical canal and scraping of the vaginal portion of the cervix) should be abnormal

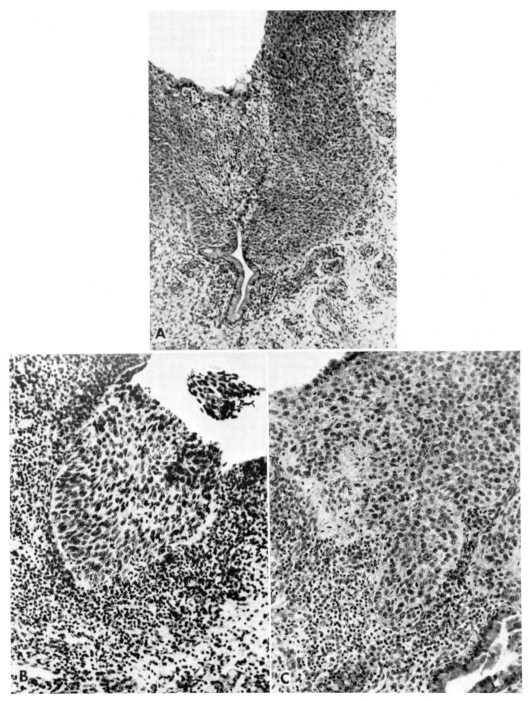

Figure 1. Cervical biopsies demonstrating evolution of invasive cancer. A, At 10 weeks of third pregnancy in a 33 year old patient: metaplasia, negative smears. B, Early in the fourth pregnancy, a year later: positive smear, carcinoma in situ. C, Five months after the fourth pregnancy: question of beginning invasion. Treated by simple complete abdominal hysterectomy, with preservation of the ovaries. Patient living and well five years later.

in 90 per cent of cases. Not unlike the histologic diagnosis, the cytologic smear unfortunately is subject to some individual interpretation and differences of classification.

The following classification is commonly used: Class I—negative cytology in findings; Class II—atypical cytologic smear but no evidence of malignancy; Class III—suggestive of malignancy (dysplasia); Class IV—strongly suggestive of malignancy (carcinoma in situ); Class V—conclusive of malignancy. Class III smears correlate more with dysplasia, and Class IV with carcinoma in situ.

When Classes III, IV, and V smears are found, the examination should be repeated and verified. Patients with Class IV and Class V smears in the absence of a gross lesion will have either severe dysplasia or carcinoma in situ with or without stromal invasion. Roughly a third of the patients with Class III smears will have negative histologic findings in the biopsy and perhaps 15 per cent will prove to have a Stage 0 lesion. The remainder will reveal varying degrees of dysplasia, an entirely and likely reversible lesion disappearing in 50 to 60 per cent of cases so diagnosed.

In the absence of a gross lesion, limitations are placed on establishing a definitive histologic diagnosis. (See the discussion on normal changes in Chapter 11.) The colposcope method is a distinct advance in localizing the lesion after the cervix has been suitably prepared by toluidine blue.

Whether to cone the cervix or rely on multiple punch biopsy continues to be discussed and debated. The complications in conization in pregnancy are certainly greater than in the nonpregnant and substantially higher than with punch biopsy. Although it might be anticipated, there is no evidence to indicate that conization may cause cervical incompetence in a subsequent pregnancy. Despite the added risk of maternal and fetal infection, the likely increase in the rate of abortion and premature labor, and operative hemorrhage to the extent of requiring one or more transfusions, conization continues to be the method more commonly used in securing tissue for histologic diagnosis. This is based on the belief and reported experience that punch biopsy is inadequate in uncovering the lesion. The lesion may be missed by punch biopsy, albeit rarely, but this is true

also for conization in pregnancy, for in order to avoid the risk of serious hemorrhage there is a tendency to limit the extent of the cone, and lesions high in the cervix have been missed. The procedure calls for a cold knife dissection of all the epithelium covering at least the distal two thirds of the cervical canal and the cervical portio to include the eroded areas that fail to take iodine stain, i.e., Schiller positive test. In the pregnant patient the tissue is edematous and more friable and easily fragmented.

Finally, conization in the last trimester is certainly a debatable procedure; rather, if the smears are consistently Class IV or V and the biopsies are inconclusive in a patient first observed at this period of the pregnancy, it might be assumed that the patient may have an invasive lesion. One might strongly consider cesarean section after the 36th week, followed by an immediate postpartum investigation.

It is suggested that because carefully performed punch biopsies will identify 80 to 90 per cent of Stage 0 and dysplasia lesions, conization should be utilized when (1) apparent adequate punch biopsy fails to establish the diagnosis; (2) multiple punch biopsy reveals early stromal invasion; (3) the smears suggest a lesion beyond that accounted for by the histologic findings; and (4) dysplasia is marked.

The procedure of biopsy includes both radial-step and circumferential biopsies, and to obtain these requires a specialized instrument with a rectangular punch that will encompass tissue from the endocervical canal to the portio vaginalis junction. Each piece of tissue is carefully labeled with respect to area of the cervix from which it was obtained.

The management of patients with carcinoma in situ, Stage 0, and dysplasia is to permit the pregnancy to continue and anticipate pelvic delivery, with smears being repeated monthly to make certain they do not reveal progression. In the case of early stromal invasion, the safer treatment may be delivery by cesarean hysterectomy. The patient with Stage 0 without stromal invasion who is desirous of further children may, under careful supervision and with frequent cytologic examination, have one or two additional pregnancies. Conization for the purpose of eradicating the lesion has been recommended. However, abdominal hysterectomy with removal of at least a 1- to 2-cm. cuff of vagina with ovarian preservation will effect a permanent cure.

The question whether dysplasia continues on to carcinoma in situ has been the subject of continuing study. Occasionally this may occur but these cases are the rare exception. The fact that the majority of these lesions regress is a further contraindication to routine conization in the management of the pregnant patient with an abnormal smear. However, patients with dysplasia should be followed in the same way as patients with carcinoma in situ who desire further pregnancies. It would seem self-evident that with her childbearing completed, a patient with persistent and extensive dysplasia, regardless of its ill defined malignant potential, would desire hysterectomy with ovarian preservation.

What has been said about the diagnosis of carcinoma in situ applies also to invasive cervical cancer. Careful inspection of the cervix, with routine prenatal cytologic examination and biopsy, will uncover the rare case. The reported incidence of invasive cancer in pregnancy varies widely, but 1 in 2000 pregnancies is probably a fair figure. Nearly all cases of invasive cancer of the cervix are in multiparous women.

An unfavorable prognosis is often offered for carcinoma of the cervix discovered in pregnancy, but this is more likely due to the failure to make a diagnosis prior to delivery. In those whose disease was identified during pregnancy, the survival rate for the different stages is not appreciably different from that in women who are well away from the event of pregnancy when the condition is discovered. However, when the cancer is found initially in the early puerperium, the outlook is bleak, presumably because the tumor was present in pregnancy, and dilatation of the cervix to permit delivery undoubtedly contributed to its dissemination.

The treatment will be influenced largely by the stage of pregnancy in which the cancer is discovered, and, although it may vary in detail, it follows certain basic principles. There is general agreement that the cervix should be spared the trauma of instrumentation or labor; thus, at least when the cancer is diagnosed in the last half of pregnancy, delivery should be by hysterotomy. The treatment for carcinoma discovered in the first half of pregnancy is irradiation, external as well as intra-cervical radium. Spontaneous abortion usually occurs within two to four weeks; if abortion fails to occur hysterotomy may be required. X-ray exposure precludes the possibility of fetal survival; in fact, this should not be permitted, for extensive irradiation damage to the fetus has been recorded. Successful pregnancy has occurred following irradiation for carcinoma of the cervix, proving, whatever else, that gonadal function is not necessarily destroyed by such therapy.

When the diagnosis is established in the last half of pregnancy, and more especially between the 28th and 34th to 36th weeks, the question is presented whether delivery should be postponed until the 37th week to assure fetal survival. A waiting period of six to eight weeks apparently does not alter the prognosis although this is open to some controversy. Following hysterotomy, irradiation therapy is quickly instituted. At hysterotomy it is well to develop a bladder flap whenever possible to cover the uterine incision, thus decreasing the chance of generalized peritonitis. When there is gross evidence of infection, cesarean section followed by supracervical hysterectomy is possibly the safer procedure. If the uterus is removed, it should be amputated at the junction of the upper and the lower uterine segment. Peritonealization of the area, together with antibiotic therapy, should at least restrict the infection to the pelvis. This probably represents a minority opinion, for many believe it is better to chance infection than to disturb the tumor by supracervical hysterectomy, even when the uterus is amputated well away from the tumor. Regardless, after hysterotomy, irradiation therapy is quickly instituted. From several sources cesarean section combined with radical hysterectomy and pelvic node dissection is being reported in Stage I disease.

OTHER MALIGNANT DISEASES COMPLICATING PREGNANCY

The chief concern of malignant growth as it relates to pregnancy is whether the rate of tumor growth is accelerated by pregnancy and whether pregnancy might invite a recurrence of the disease. In other words, should the patient found to have malignant disease be permitted to continue her pregnancy with the possibility of decreasing her survival time, or should the patient who is apparently cured of a malignant disease ever attempt a pregnancy?

With rare exceptions, the fetus is unharmed directly by malignant disease in the mother. It may be jeopardized secondarily when the malignant process is extensive and causes a severe metabolic upset in the mother. Only melanomata are subject to placental transmission, and then with an extremely low incidence. Metastatic lesions have been noted in the placenta, however, with several types of tumors.

Almost every known malignant tumor has been reported in pregnancy, but because of the overall low incidence of tumors in this age group many papers consist of case reports rather than any cumulative experience. Thus it is difficult to draw any valid conclusions regarding the response to pregnancy of many of these malignant growths.

There is evidence both for and against the contention that pregnancy influences the rate or course of neoplasm of the gastrointestinal tract and its associated organs. Patients effectively treated surgically prior to pregnancy appear to do well, but some require delivery by cesarean section, as in the case of abdominal perineal resection. Despite the young age of many parturients, malignant involvement of the large bowel should be considered in the differential diagnosis of an intestinal obstruction, particularly when the patient has had no previous abdominal surgery.

With the exception of the reproductive system, cancer of the breast is the most frequent malignancy seen in pregnancy. Of the total number of cases of cancer of the breast, 1 in 35 is associated with pregnancy and the puerperium; stated differently, carcinoma of the breast is reported to occur in approximately 1 in 3500 pregnancies. This may actually be a low figure, however, for all too often the diagnosis is missed until months later, and thus the cases that begin in pregnancy are not all reported as such. The normal growth and enlargement of the breasts during pregnancy may mask the presence of a small cancerous lesion.

An inflammatory cancer of the breast has been mistaken for a breast infection. The diagnosis should be suspected when the temperature is normal and there is sudden enlargement of the breast. The involved tissue has a stony hard consistency, and there is a marked redness of the skin. Death often follows within a matter of weeks. Thus, the breasts should be examined periodically during pregnancy and in the postpartum examination; this cannot be stressed too strongly. Suspicious lesions should be investigated as assiduously during pregnancy as at any other time.

At one time breast cancer associated with pregnancy was regarded as hopeless, and pregnancy was placed among the criteria of inoperability of the tumor. It would now appear that patients who, during pregnancy or the puerperium, have a mastectomy for carcinoma of the breast do as well in terms of a five-year cure as do the nonpregnant, provided the axillary nodes are negative for tumor. However, when the lymph nodes are positive the pregnant or recently pregnant patient appears to have a lower five-year survival rate, often as low as 5 to 10 per cent. Some believe that the prognosis is influenced by the state of differentiation of the glandular elements of the tumor. Undoubtedly the prognosis is altered more by the failure to diagnose the disease until it has reached an advanced stage than by the pregnancy per se.

Curiously, in general when the cancer has extended beyond the breast, the disease appears not to be accelerated during pregnancy; but with delivery the tumor often grows rapidly and the patient may run a rapid downhill course and die within weeks or three or four months post partum. Thus, the treatment is directed not toward termination of pregnancy, but rather toward reduction of the growth rate and extension of the tumor by irradiation and other means. In an effort to suppress lactation, large amounts of androgenic substances may be given beginning one or two weeks before the expected time of delivery and continuing indefinitely. Oophorectomy to decrease estrogen stimulation should be considered at the time of delivery. Here the patient is managed in the manner described for postpartum sterilization; that is, she is delivered in the operating room and, immediately afterward, a laparotomy is performed and the ovaries are removed. Hypophysectomy may be considered either prior to or immediately after delivery. Cancer of the breast in pregnancy may be one if not the most notable indication for hypophysectomy as a mode of therapy.

The conduct of pregnancy, labor, and

delivery in a patient with breast cancer is much the same as in the normal patient. If any attempt has been made to suppress the pituitary, or the pituitary has been removed, some thought must be given to increasing the adrenal therapy to meet the stress of labor and delivery. Also, it may be necessary to perform a cesarean section to salvage the infant when the disease is extensive and the mother's life is in the balance.

The termination of pregnancy before the fetus is viable apparently will not influence the rate of growth of breast cancer. If therapeutic termination of pregnancy has a place in patient management, it is only in the very early weeks of gestation. The procedure should be considered in a patient who inadvertently becomes pregnant less than three to five years after her mastectomy, that is, before sufficient time has elapsed to be reasonably assured that the patient is cured. Also, in such an unpredictable disease, the wishes of the patient and her family deserve some consideration. However, there is no clear evidence that termination of the pregnancy after the first trimester will influence favorably cancer of the breast. Accelerated postpartum growth is the rule whether the pregnancy terminates in the first or second half of pregnancy.

Thus, the permissibility of future pregnancy following mastectomy depends on the extent of the tumor at the time of operation. If the lymph nodes were negative, a pregnancy may be attempted four or five years after the breast is removed. Cases are reported in which a successful pregnancy occurred. The writer has had two cases in which the above criteria were fulfilled; each patient had one baby several years after mastectomy, without recurrence of the disease.

ANOMALOUS CONDITIONS OF THE REPRODUCTIVE TRACT

Uterine anomalies occur through incomplete fusion of the müllerian duct system or lack of normal regression of the inner tissue mass as the result of such fusion. Through failure to fuse, there are gradations of a doubling of the uterine corpus and, in the extreme, the cervix as well. Lack of regression may result in varying degrees of septate formation of the uterus and the vagina

(see Embryology in Chapter 5). The vagina may contain a septum, with the cervix and the uterine corpus normal. Certainly vaginal septa are seen when the remainder of the reproductive tract is normal, and, although it is reported that a cervical septum can occur with an otherwise normal uterus and vagina, such a case must be rare indeed.

The multiplicity of classifications proposed to categorize these anomalous conditions suggests that none is entirely acceptable and also contributes to difficulty in comparing therapeutic results. Also, the terms are used interchangeably and rather loosely in relation to specific anomalies. For example, the term *bicornuate* has been used to describe the mildest form of anomaly, the so-called arcuate uterus, with mere dimpling of the corpus, as well as that in which the corpus is nearly double. It would appear desirable to designate the anomalous state in the most appropriate descriptive terms. Thus, a double uterus (uterus didelphys) indicates a complete failure of fusion of the müllerian ducts, which means a duplication of both the uterine corpus and the cervix, with or without vaginal involvement. It has been suggested that, from a functional standpoint, each uterus in this instance is in fact a hemiuterus, the most important feature being restriction of the blood supply to a single uterine artery. An arcuate uterus denotes near-complete fusion, the fundus being relatively flat in contour with slight indentation of its superior surface. Between these two types is the bicornuate uterus with incomplete fusion of the corpus. Septate formation may occur in both the arcuate and the bicornuate uterus. In the former it is usually mild; in the latter it may extend downward through the cervix to the vagina, which may also have a septum.

The diagnosis of anomalous conditions of the reproductive tract is commonly missed, and only after the patient has had pregnancy failures is the condition suspected. It must be recognized also that many forms cannot be diagnosed on pelvic examination, but either hysterography or culdoscopy or both are required. Reference has previously been made to the desirability of exploring the uterus at the time of delivery in patients with repeated pregnancy failures, with the idea that an anomalous condition that could explain the state of infertility might be found. It is true that many of the cases are first identified during manual removal of the placenta or in the course of a curettage.

However one chooses to classify the abnormality, fetal wastage is high when uterine fusion is incomplete or uterine septate formation is extensive. The term hemiuterus to describe a double uterus is undoubtedly useful as the concept pertains to the functional capacity of the uterus. The problem is one of nourishing the conceptus and maintaining the pregnancy at least until the fetus is medically viable. When the anomaly includes the cervix the obstetric difficulties, as might be expected, will be encountered during labor as well.

Depending largely on the extent of the uterine anomaly, then, the fetal wastage from abortion has been cited as between 25 and 50 per cent, and premature labor is reputed to be some three times more frequent than the normal incidence. Because of failed tests of labor and malpresentations, and the special importance of salvaging the fetus in patients in whom the outcome of future pregnancies is in doubt, the cesarean section rate is bound to be high — reportedly 30 to 35 per cent.

Each patient is an individual problem. In the presence of a normal cervix and a mild deformity of the corpus, normal delivery is awaited. A septum of the vagina alone can impede the progress of the presenting part. If the abnormality is recognized prior to pregnancy, resection is in order. When first observed in pregnancy, the septum extending from the base of the urethra cephalad toward the cervix and posterior to the vaginal midline is removed, with mattress sutures used for hemostasis. If at the time of delivery one is unable to displace the septum to one side of the vagina and extract the fetus easily with forceps, the above procedure can be performed safely, although suitable exposure is more difficult.

In the more severe forms of uterine malformation, especially when there has been a series of pregnancy failures, should the patient reach a stage of pregnancy when the fetus is medically viable (35 weeks), cesarean section must be considered as the method of delivery. When the cervix is involved, labor is unpredictable; occasionally one side of a double-barreled cervix will dilate and permit pelvic delivery, but cervical dystocia may necessitate delivery by cesarean section.

When pregnancy failures recur, surgical correction of the anomalous state may be indicated. An authoritative source, with experience in treating such patients surgically, has emphasized that, before surgery is resorted to, these patients should be carefully studied to exclude any metabolic or endocrine disturbance. In a carefully studied series of patients with bicornuate or septate uteri who had an extremely poor reproductive record, it has been demonstrated that correction of endocrine deficiencies can result in successful pregnancy. Surgical correction by the so-called Strassmann operation or its modification (Fig. 2) has a distinct place in the treatment of carefully selected patients, but this should not be attempted until all other methods of management have failed.

When a rudimentary horn has developed from one of the müllerian ducts, pregnancy is a confusing and serious complication. In some 80 per cent of the cases the horn has no connection with the uterus or the vagina. Of these patients, except for those who come to surgery because of a hematometra, those who menstruate from a rudimentary horn must do so into the peritoneal cavity. Not only should this be uncomfortable, but it should also invite endometriosis. One such case has been reported. When pregnancy does occur in these cases, it means transmigration of the sperm, and of the egg also, if the ovary is absent on the affected side. If the rudimentary horn fails to connect with the uterus, rupture will eventually occur. Short of laparotomy, the diagnosis of pregnancy in a rudimentary horn is not easy or certain. The clinical course simulates that of a cornual pregnancy, and, in either case, should rupture occur the resultant hemoperitoneum is usually of considerable magnitude. Further, a nonpregnant rudimentary horn may become incarcerated in the pelvis and obstruct labor.

Superfetation, or the fertilization and implantation of an ovum when the uterus is already occupied by a conceptus, if it ever occurred in the human, would be more likely in the presence of a double uterus. This may offer some explanation for those cases of twin pregnancy in which one infant is delivered several weeks before the second one. Certainly, in a twin pregnancy in a double uterus or in an extreme degree of a bicornuate uterus one may observe

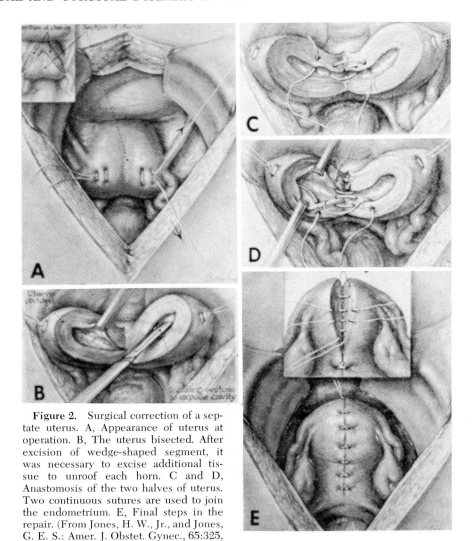

Figure 2. Surgical correction of a septate uterus. A, Appearance of uterus at operation. B, The uterus bisected. After excision of wedge-shaped segment, it was necessary to excise additional tissue to unroof each horn. C and D, Anastomosis of the two halves of uterus. Two continuous sutures are used to join the endometrium. E, Final steps in the repair. (From Jones, H. W., Jr., and Jones, G. E. S.: Amer. J. Obstet. Gynec., 65:325, 1953.)

labor in one uterus and not in the other, an interesting phenomenon to consider when one speculates on the etiology of labor. Also, in a single pregnancy in a double or a bicornuate uterus there may be bleeding from the nonpregnant side or horn throughout gestation, adding to the uncertainty as to normalcy of the pregnancy.

GYNECOLOGIC SURGERY IN CHILDBEARING WOMEN

Ill advised gynecologic surgery may give rise to dystocia, and the presence of successfully repaired gynecologic lesions may necessitate special obstetric management. It is not the purpose here to describe the various gynecologic operations, but rather to consider them in the light of how they may affect the course of pregnancy and its management.

As a principle, gynecologic surgery should be postponed until the patient has completed her childbearing, and there are at least two reasons for this. First, the operative procedure may contribute to infertility or dystocia. When the cervix is appreciably shortened, as, for example, by the Manchester–Fothergill operation for uterine prolapse, miscarriage or abortion and premature labor are distinct possibilities. Further, because of the scar tissue formed incidental to such an operation, the cervix may not dilate in a subsequent labor, thereby necessitating cesarean section. Of the various operations designed to correct cervical lacerations or extensive erosion, the Stürmdorf type of repair is less likely to shorten the cervix. Surgical repair of lacerations of the cervix is rarely required to control an erosion, however, provided the patient is carefully followed and the cervix is cauterized when necessary.

Second, the surgical procedure contemplated may be a compromise to definitive treatment. For example, the patient may have a mild degree of prolapse or mild stress incontinence, neither of which is incapacitating. Rather than being subjected to immediate surgery, the patient should be managed conservatively until she has completed her childbearing, at which time the gynecologic lesions can be properly corrected by a vaginal hysterectomy with plastic repair of the urethrocystocele and rectocele if present. If these lesions are corrected between pregnancies, they can recur as the result of pelvic delivery. Furthermore, it must be appreciated that plastic repair for the correction of urethrocystocele and rectocele as a repeat procedure is never as satisfactory, for the identification of the endopelvic fascia, on which the success of the procedure depends, is never as readily achieved because of the scar tissue created by the first operation. In the case of stress incontinence, a sling type of operation may be needed as a secondary procedure.

There are two situations or exceptions to the above for which gynecologic procedures are acceptable in the treatment of women who desire more children. One is in the relatively young woman who is most miserable from severe stress incontinence and contemplates more than one pregnancy. Here a plastic repair of the urethrocystocele appears warranted. The other is in the patient who in the course of childbearing becomes infertile from an endocervicitis resulting from a severely lacerated or eroded cervix. In this case operative repair of the cervix may occasionally be indicated when cauterization fails to control erosion or endocervicitis.

MANAGEMENT OF LABOR

When a woman in whom a gynecologic procedure has been performed becomes pregnant, certain important principles must be followed in the management of her labor. A successfully repaired vesicovaginal fistula dictates delivery by cesarean section in subsequent pregnancies, for recurrence of the fistula would be tragic. Origin of the fistula frequently can be traced to an ill advised or improperly

executed forceps delivery, or prolonged labor associated with some degree of pelvic contracture.

When the bony pelvis is normal, pelvic delivery is not necessarily contraindicated after operations to correct stress incontinence or to repair a rectovaginal fistula or a complete perineal laceration. Some consideration should be given to the conduct of delivery, however. A relatively extensive mediolateral episiotomy should be performed before the vertex is permitted to crown. With the aid of axis-traction forceps, the fetal occiput is directed posteriorly to avoid any pressure on the urethra and bladder and thus preserve the supporting endopelvic or pubocervical fascia. When attention is given to these details, urethrocystocele with its symptoms will not recur, nor should the perineum again become traumatized.

BARTHOLINITIS AND SKENITIS

Infection of Bartholin's glands may be due to a number of pathogenic organisms, in contrast to infection of Skene's glands, which is usually gonococcal in origin. Skene's glands, when infected, will feel indurated to the examining finger, and pus can be expressed from the duct orifices located lateral to the urethral meatus. Examination of a direct smear of the pus will confirm the diagnosis. A chronic skenitis is rare, and aspiration of the swollen gland may reveal pus from which organisms other than the gonococcus may be cultured.

An infection of Bartholin's gland appears as a swelling located between the posterior fusion of the labia majus and minus and lateral to the posterior fourchette in the substance of the perineum. It may vary in size, at times reaching a diameter of 4 or 5 cm. or more, in which event the medial surface of the gland may impinge against the rectal wall. With the marked induration, the rectal wall has been known to be damaged when the gland is removed in the acute phase, which is one good reason to drain and marsupialize the gland. Bartholinitis fails to respond completely to chemotherapeutic agents. Even if the infection subsides, which it will sometimes do without surgical treatment, or if the inflamed gland goes on to spontaneous rupture, recurrence is the rule, although perhaps not for months or even years later. During the chronic state, removal of the gland is a simple procedure. A small, curved incision is made well outside the hymenal ring over the area occupied by the gland. Rather than indulge in tedious dissection about the gland, it is opened and its base is grasped by two Allis forceps. Traction on the forceps tends to invert the gland and facilitates dissection about its base. The gland is quickly enucleated, hemostasis is established, and the incision is closed without drainage.

During pregnancy conservative treatment would seem indicated. Such treatment consists of the application of heat until the gland is ready for incision, drainage, and marsupialization. Cultures should be taken as a matter of routine.

CONDYLOMATA ACUMINATA

Condylomata acuminata are being encountered with increased frequency in pregnancy. Patients are observed in whom the lesions may extend into the lower vagina as well as the perineum and the surrounding area. If the patient is seen early in pregnancy, the external lesions can be surgically excised or electrocoagulated, for the local application of podophyllin is not altogether successful. A search should be made for associated neisserian infection and syphilis. Cesarean section may be required when the disease is extensive, especially when there is vaginal involvement.

BIBLIOGRAPHY

Asadourian, L. A., and Taylor, H. B.: Dysgerminoma. An analysis of 105 cases. Obstet. Gynec., 33:370, 1969.

Averette, H. E., Nasser, N., Yankow, S. L., and Little, W. A.: Cervical conization in pregnancy. Analysis of 180 operations. Amer. J. Obstet. Gynec., 106:543, 1970.

Bender, S.: Placental metastasis in malignant disease complicated by pregnancy. Brit. Med. J., 1:980, 1950.

Betson, J. R., and Golden, M. L.: Primary carcinoma of of ovary co-existing with pregnancy; report of three cases. Obstet. Gynec., 12:589, 1958.

Brunschwig, A., and Barber, H. R. K.: Cesarean section immediately followed by radical hysterectomy and pelvic node excision. Amer. J. Obstet. Gynec., 76:199, 1958.

Finn, W. .F.: The outcome of pregnancy following vaginal operations. Amer. J. Obstet. Gynec., 56:291, 1948.

Finn, W. F., and Muller, P. F.: Abdominal myomectomy; special reference to subsequent pregnancy and to the reappearance of fibromyomas of the uterus. Amer. J. Obstet. Gynec., 60:109, 1950.

Fisher, J. J.: Effect of amputation of cervix uteri upon subsequent parturition; preliminary report of seven cases. Amer. J. Obstet. Gynec., 62:644, 1951.

Francis, O., and Stevens, R. D.: Pregnancy after primary irradiation for carcinoma of cervix. Medical memoranda. Brit. Med. J., 2:342, 1965.

Gergely, E., and Mason, D. J.: Pregnancy in a non-communicating rudimentary horn; report of a case. Amer. J. Obstet. Gynec., 78:1202, 1959.

Goldman, J. A., and Eckerling, B.: Unusual case of rupture of a pregnant rudimentary horn of a bicornuate uterus. Amer. J. Obstet. Gynec., 78:1205, 1959.

Greene, R. R., Holzwarth, D., and Roddick, J. W., Jr.: "Luteomas" of pregnancy. Amer. J. Obstet. Gynec., 88:1001, 1964.

Haagensen, C. D.: Cancer of the breast in pregnancy and during lactation. Amer. J. Obstet. Gynec., 98:141, 1967.

Holzaepfel, J. H., and Ezell, H. E., Jr.: Evaluation of carcinoma of the cervix associated with pregnancy. Amer. J. Obstet. Gynec., 76:292, 1958.

Israel, S. L., and Weber, L. L.: Prolapse of the uterus complicating pregnancy and labor. Western J. Surg., 58:421, 1950.

Johnson, L. D.: The histopathological approach to early cervical neoplasia. Obstet. Gynec. Survey, 24:735, 1969.

Johnson, L. D., Hertig, A. T., Hinman, C. H., and Easterday, C. L.: Preinvasive cervical lesions in obstetric patients. Obstet. Gynec., 16:133, 1960.

Johnson, L. D., Nickerson, R. J., Easterday, C. L., Stuart, R. S., and Hertig, A. T.: Epidemiologic evidence for the spectrum of change from dysplasia through carcinoma in situ to invasive cancer. Cancer, 22:901, 1968.

Jones, H. W., Delfs, E., and Jones, G. E. S.: Reproductive difficulties in double uterus; the place of plastic reconstruction. Amer. J. Obstet. Gynec., 72:865, 1956.

Jones, W. S.: Obstetric significance of female genital anomalies. Obstet. Gynec., 10:113, 1957.

Keettel, W. C.: Prolapse of uterus during pregnancy. Amer. J. Obstet. Gynec., 42:121, 1941.

Kistner, R. W., Gorbach, A. C., and Smith, G. V.: Cervical cancer in pregnancy; review of literature with presentation of 30 additional cases. Obstet. Gynec., 9:554, 1957.

Little, B., Smith, W. O., Jessiman, A. G., Selenkow, H. A., Van't Hoff, W., Eglin, J. M., and Moore, F. D.: Hypophysectomy during pregnancy in a patient with cancer of the breast; case report with hormone studies. J. Clin. Endocr., 18:425, 1958.

Marchant, D. J.: Hemangioma of the cervix. Obstet. Gynec., 17:191, 1961.

Pack, G., and Scharnagel, I.: The prognosis for malignant melanoma in pregnancy. Cancer, 4:324, 1951.

Piver, M. S., and Spezia, J.: Uterine prolapse during pregnancy. Obstet. Gynec., 32:765, 1968.

Prem, K. A., Makowski, E. L., and McKelvey, J. L.: Carcinoma of the cervix associated with pregnancy. Amer. J. Obstet. Gynec., 95:99, 1966.

Richart, R. M.: Colpomicroscopic studies of the distribution of dysplasia and carcinoma in situ on the exposed portion of the human uterine cervix. Cancer, 18:950, 1965.

Riva, H. L., Hefner, J., and Kawasaki, D.: Carcinoma in situ of the cervix. Obstet. Gynec., 17:525, 1961.

Roberts, D. W. T., and Haines, M.: Conserving ovarian tissue in treatment of ovarian neoplasms. Brit. Med. J., 2:917, 1965.

Robinson, D. W.: Breast carcinoma associated with pregnancy; observation on 1,128 cases of breast carcinoma. Amer. J. Obstet. Gynec., 92:658, 1965.

Rogers, R. S., III, and Williams, J. H.: The impact of the suspicious Papanicolaou smear on pregnancy. Amer. J. Obstet. Gynec., 98:488, 1967.

Shuster, E., and Leake, F. M.: Luteoma of pregnancy. Report of a case. Obstet. Gynec., 32:637, 1968.

Stone, M. L., Weingold, A. B., and Sall, S.: Cervical

carcinoma in pregnancy. Amer. J. Obstet. Gynec., 93:479, 1965.

Strassmann, P.: Die operative Vereinigung eines doppelten Uterus; nebst Bemerkungen über die Korrektur der sogenannten Verdoppelund des Genitalkanales. Z. Gynaek., 31:1322, 1907.

Te Linde, R. W., and Galvin, G.: The minimal histological changes in biopsies to justify a diagnosis of cervical cancer. Amer. J. Obstet. Gynec., 48:774, 1944.

Van Praagh, I. G. L., Harvey, M. H., and Vernon, C. P.: Carcinoma of the cervix associated with pregnancy. J. Obstet. Gynaec. Brit. Comm., 72:75, 1965.

White, T. T., and White, W. C.: Breast cancer and pregnancy; report of 49 cases followed 5 years. Ann. Surg., 144:384, 1956.

Younge, P. A.: Cancer of the uterine cervix; a preventable disease. Obstet. Gynec., 10:469, 1957.

DISORDERS OF THE CARDIOVASCULAR SYSTEM

Disorders of the heart and the blood vessels constitute one of the more important groups of medical complications encountered during pregnancy, perhaps contributing the largest proportion of maternal deaths from medical causes. As a result of the increase in interstitial fluid, blood volume, and cardiac output, pregnancy imposes a temporary burden on the cardiovascular system. Consequently, when the physician is confronted by a pregnant patient with heart disease, he must decide whether she is able to withstand the added circulatory load of pregnancy. In the event that the patient is permitted to continue her pregnancy, he must provide the safeguards to protect her circulatory system against any unnecessary burden.

HEART DISEASE

Incidence of Heart Disease

The incidence and nature of heart disease in the obstetric patient are influenced largely by the frequency of rheumatic fever. The vast majority of pregnant patients with heart disease will have chronic rheumatic heart disease; congenital heart disease is next in frequency, and then a variety of cardiac conditions, such as thyroid heart disease, coronary heart disease, arteriosclerotic heart disease, acute pericarditis, kyphoscoliotic heart disease, and, rarely, syphilitic heart disease. In any group of pregnant cardiac patients with chronic rheumatic heart disease the mitral valve is involved in most cases, with stenosis

being by far the predominant lesion. Next in frequency is mitral regurgitation, followed in turn by aortic regurgitation; aortic stenosis is rare in this age group.

In recent years a decline in incidence of rheumatic heart disease has been noted generally. However, congenital heart disease is seen with increased frequency in the pregnant population, for the advances in management of children with congenital heart disease, especially successful cardiac surgery, have permitted these patients to survive to enter the childbearing age. These patients will seek advice as to marriage and the wisdom of attempting a pregnancy.

Diagnosis of the More Frequent Types of Heart Disease

Pregnancy may afford the first opportunity for recognition of heart disease and for early institution of a therapeutic regimen that may aid in diminishing cardiac disability in later life. Pregnant patients will be encountered who are unaware that they have a damaged heart until their prenatal examination. So important is the diagnosis to the pregnant patient that, even when no cardiac disease is detected at the initial visit, it is good practice to reexamine the heart later in pregnancy to verify the fact that it is normal.

The diagnosis of **valvular heart disease** is dependent on the presence of a diastolic murmur or cardiac enlargement or both. In a large series of patients with heart disease a diastolic murmur was heard in 94 per cent of the cases, and most of these revealed some degree of cardiac enlargement. The diagnosis of heart disease was made in the remaining 6 per cent on the basis of cardiac enlargement alone.

When the heart is definitely enlarged, a diagnosis of heart disease need not be questioned. It should be recalled that in normal pregnancy elevation of the diaphragm may distort the cardiac contour and upset the normal cardiothoracic ratio. During the course of pregnancy, therefore, a few patients will be observed with borderline cardiac enlargement but without pathologic murmurs. A tentative rather than a final diagnosis should be made, and the patient should be treated as a cardiac patient throughout the remainder of pregnancy and labor. Only after delivery will it be possible to determine whether there is definite cardiac enlargement.

Organic murmurs are occasionally difficult to detect in pregnancy when the examination of the heart is conducted with the patient in a supine position. The murmur may be heard only following deep expiration with the patient on her left side, her left arm elevated above the head, and the left breast displaced upward. Auscultation during expiration with the patient sitting up and leaning forward is sometimes helpful in detecting a faint, soft diastolic murmur. Occasionally to subject the patient to mild exercise may accentuate a diastolic murmur and thus facilitate auscultation.

In the diagnosis of **rheumatic heart disease** the diastolic murmur of mitral stenosis, best heard at the apex, is described as a crescendo rumble beginning in early, mid, or late diastole, and ending in a loud first sound. In aortic regurgitation the diastolic murmur is usually high-pitched and is heard close to the left sternal border in the second, third, or fourth interspace. The murmur is not appreciably altered by pregnancy, but because of the frequent presence of a systolic murmur at this time, the diastolic murmur, if faint and of short duration, may be difficult to hear.

In common with the finding in the nonpregnant, a loud Grade II or Grade III apical systolic murmur suggests rheumatic heart disease with mitral insufficiency. In pregnancy, Grade I and soft Grade II apical and pulmonic systolic murmurs, even though transmitted, do not of themselves indicate heart disease. Because of the high incidence of functional murmurs

during pregnancy, therefore, it has been strongly recommended that the final evaluation of both apical and basal systolic murmurs be postponed until after delivery. Such a policy should in no way place the patient in jeopardy, provided the physician is aware of the possibility that a woman with a rather loud systolic murmur may eventually prove to have heart disease and she is treated as a cardiac patient during pregnancy. In these relatively young women, the effects of an erroneous diagnosis of heart disease with its implications of restricted activity could be psychologically and emotionally disastrous.

The diagnosis of **syphilitic heart disease** is tenable, based on the presence of a longstanding history of syphilis, usually positive serologic findings, and aortic insufficiency. For reasons already mentioned, the aortic murmur may not be easy to elicit; hence the diagnosis may be more difficult during pregnancy. The symptoms are variable and depend on the degree of aortitis. In aortitis, the coronary orifices may become partially occluded, causing angina.

The criteria for the identification of the various types of **congenital heart disease** are not altered by the presence of pregnancy, but the development of a functional basal systolic murmur, frequently heard during this period, adds to the uncertainties of accurate diagnosis. A loud, rough systolic murmur, heard along the left sternal border in the third and fourth interspace and associated with a thrill, is consistent with an intraventricular septal defect, as well as with certain other congenital malformations of the heart. If the basal murmur is continuous and extends into diastole with a to-and-fro rhythm, a diagnosis of patent ductus arteriosus is justifiable. In addition to x-ray examination of the heart, cardiac catheterization and other diagnostic procedures may be necessary to determine the exact nature of the abnormality.

Whenever hypertension is found in a pregnant patient, it is well to remember that coarctation of the aorta may be responsible for its presence. Hypotension in the lower extremities, absence of femoral artery pulsations, and an erosion of the lower border of the ribs by dilated intercostal arteries as revealed by x-ray examination are the important diagnostic criteria. A systolic murmur is heard in the middorsal area, sometimes well below the diaphragm. Hypertensive changes may be noted in the retinal vessels.

Diagnosis of the rare types of heart disease in the pregnant patient, including arteriosclerotic or degenerative heart disease, thyroid heart disease, and coronary heart disease, is similar in all respects to that in the nonpregnant person.

Determination of a "Favorable" (Classes I and II) and an "Unfavorable" (Classes III and IV) Cardiac Patient with Respect to Pregnancy

Once the diagnosis of heart disease is established, attention must be directed to an evaluation of the myocardial reserve, although the various tests devised for this purpose are of less value in pregnancy. The fact that a pregnant patient with heart disease may score well in the first trimester with respect to function tests is no assurance that her cardiac reserve is adequate to meet the circulatory burden as pregnancy advances. In addition, the measurement of the vital capacity, the blood volume, and the circulation time, performed in the early weeks of pregnancy, fail to furnish the data needed to permit identification of the cardiac patient who is likely to develop cardiac failure later in pregnancy.

The ability of the cardiac patient to carry out the activities of average daily life is believed to furnish the best index of myocardial reserve. It has been found desirable for clinical purposes to classify patients with heart disease into groups in accordance with their cardiac response to physical activity. The functional classification generally used is that proposed by the New York Heart Association. The classification is as follows:

Class I.   Patients with a cardiac disorder without limitation of physical activity. Ordinary physical activity causes no discomfort.

Class II.   Patients with a cardiac disorder with slight to moderate limitation of physical activity. Ordinary physical activity causes discomfort.

Class III.   Patients with a cardiac disorder with moderate to great limitation of physical activity. Less than ordinary physical activity causes discomfort.

Class IV.   Patients with a cardiac disorder unable to carry on any physical activity without discomfort.

There are certain shortcomings in this functional classification as it pertains to pregnancy, for it assumes that pregnant patients will perform according to expectations when placed on a cardiac regimen that, in the nonpregnant patient, ensures adequate protection to the cardiac reserve. However, the progressive and at times uneven increase in the circulatory load of pregnancy limits the protective features of even the most rigid cardiac regimen. Although the nonpregnant cardiac patient may be able to carry on her normal daily physical activities without circulatory embarrassment, there is no definite assurance that when she is pregnant her myocardial reserve can tolerate the additional circulatory burden. When applied to pregnant patients, the classification also fails to take into account concomitant medical conditions which may prove to be major factors in precipitating cardiac failure during pregnancy. Not included in the classification are certain other features of the cardiac history, specifically, previous episodes of heart failure or a recent attack of rheumatic fever. Finally, the significance of the presence of atrial fibrillation or other dangerous abnormalities of the conduction mechanism of the heart have not been acknowledged, findings that are well known to play an important role in the course of pregnant patients with heart disease.

One classification of heart disease in pregnancy, proposed by Hamilton, recognizes these important features, as well as the patient's ability to perform physical activity. The classification is as follows: Group I includes those patients whose history and cardiac condition indicate that they are "favorable" risks. When the history and cardiac findings reveal that pregnancy will be hazardous, the patient is classified in Group IA, an "unfavorable" cardiac. Group II includes those patients who exhibit questionable cardiac enlargement without any demonstrable organic murmurs. The relatively small number of patients who fall into this class are treated as cardiac patients during pregnancy, labor, and delivery. It is recognized, however, that the apparent cardiac enlargement may in some instances be due to the normal changes of pregnancy. Following parturition, these patients are reclassified into Group I if definite cardiac enlargement persists, or, if the cardiothoracic ratio returns to normal, they are diagnosed as having "no heart disease." Group III comprises patients who have symptoms referable to the vascular system but in whom direct examination fails to reveal any evidence of heart disease. These women may complain of the frequent symptoms of normal pregnancy, such as palpitation, choking sensations, and circulatory instability. Included in this group are those occasional women with anxiety neurosis (neurocirculatory asthenia), whose symptoms are possibly aggravated by pregnancy.

Pregnant patients with heart disease, therefore, fall into one of two major groups, either "favorable" or "unfavorable." The "favorable" or Group I cardiacs of the Hamilton classification would in general include the patients in Classes I and II of the New York Heart Association classification, whereas the "unfavorable" or Group IA cardiac patients as defined in the former would be comparable to those patients in Classes III and IV of the latter classification. In several series, approximately 90 per cent of the cardiac patients fall into the "favorable" group, or Classes I and II of the New York Heart Association classification.

The "favorable" cardiac patients are those who have heart disease as demonstrated by (1) the presence of a diastolic murmur with or without cardiac enlargement; (2) a history that reveals that the patient has never experienced heart failure, either symptomatically or clinically; (3) no significant abnormality of the conduction mechanism of the heart; and (4) freedom from other complicating medical disease.

Other lesser factors may eventually contribute to cardiac difficulties and even to heart failure in a potentially "favorable" cardiac patient, and these must be recognized in addition to the major factors enumerated above. In the rheumatic group the presence of lesions in more than one valve carries a slightly greater incidence of cardiac failure than involvement of a single valve. The incidence of heart failure increases with age, and is significantly higher in cardiac patients past the age of 35.

The development of pre-eclamptic toxemia in the cardiac patient may precipitate heart failure, whereas intercurrent infections during the course of pregnancy add to the hazard. Finally, economic and social factors play a role by not allowing the patient to follow a regimen made necessary by the cardiac condition.

Patients in the "unfavorable" group are those who have heart disease as established by (1) the presence of a diastolic murmur or cardiac enlargement; (2) a history or previous clinical evidence of heart failure in either the pregnant or the nonpregnant state; (3) severe abnormalities of cardiac rhythm; and (4) medical complications other than those of cardiac origin.

The most important single feature of the history in the pregnant cardiac patient is whether she has ever experienced heart failure. Accumulated clinical experience has shown that in approximately 75 per cent of the patients who have had heart failure during pregnancy cardiac failure will recur in a subsequent pregnancy. In some of these patients cardiac failure can be prevented in a repeat pregnancy provided they seek obstetric and cardiac supervision early in pregnancy. Therefore, when the cardiac reserve of the patient who has failed in a previous pregnancy is being evaluated, consideration must be given to the circumstances under which the failure occurred.

Of the abnormalities of cardiac rate and rhythm organically significant in pregnancy, atrial fibrillation is the most frequent, whereas heart block is rarely observed. Because of its association with congestive heart failure, embolism, and, occasionally, sudden death, it has long been appreciated that atrial fibrillation in pregnant patients carries a poor to guarded prognosis. Despite general improvement in the care of obstetric patients with heart disease, the death rate associated with atrial fibrillation has not declined to the same degree as in the nonpregnant.

In addition, the danger of congestive failure is significantly increased if the patient has had rheumatic fever recently. It is recommended, therefore, that pregnancy should be postponed for a year or more after recovery from an attack of rheumatic fever. Finally, pulmonary hypertension, whether or not congenitally acquired, has a guarded prognosis. Indeed, it is one condition in which pregnancy is definitely contraindicated.

The application of these criteria as to

"favorability" and "unfavorability" will allow one to render a reasonably accurate prognosis regarding the response to pregnancy of patients with valvular heart disease, especially if it is of rheumatic origin. In the case of syphilitic valvular heart disease, one is less certain of the outcome, for the recorded experience of the course of syphilitic heart disease in pregnancy is not large. Most pregnant patients with syphilitic heart disease apparently will meet the criteria of the "favorable" category, and a successful pregnancy can be anticipated.

Patients with congenital heart disease, including atrial and ventricular septal defects, and pulmonary and aortic stenosis, appear to do well during pregnancy with careful cardiac management. However, the cardiac failure rate has been reported to be roughly 15 per cent, while the fetal mortality is in the range of 10 to 20 per cent. Patients with cyanotic heart disease also do reasonably well in pregnancy even when the blood oxygen saturation is reduced to 70 to 75 per cent. The patient's hematocrit affords a practical index as to extent of the cardiac disability and the fetal prognosis. There is a high fetal wastage when the hematocrit is 60 or above. If it is below 50 the fetal outlook is comparable to that of a normal pregnancy. The fetus reveals no evidence of hypoxia at birth although there is often a relative increase in the hematocrit with values in the 70s or 80s. Premature labor and small birth weight or intrauterine growth retardation must be anticipated (Fig. 3). In fact, there appears to be a relationship between birth weight and the extent of the maternal polycythemia.

Response of the Cardiac Patient to Pregnancy

As indicated, the course of patients with heart disease in pregnancy is impossible to predict with certainty, for the cardiac status even of those thought to have minimal disease may change. If carefully supervised, most Class I and II (favorable) cardiac patients do well. Even with reasonably good prenatal care, however, some 10 to 20 per cent will require special attention to prevent impending failure or must enter the hospital for active treatment of failure. The fact that a cardiac patient has not had heart failure in a previous pregnancy is no assurance that it will not occur in a subsequent pregnancy. It is well to reemphasize the fact that *any cardiac patient may experience heart failure at any time during pregnancy.*

Heart failure in pregnancy occurs more frequently during the period when the normal circulatory changes of gestation are approaching their maximum (Fig. 4). Hence, cardiac failure is more likely to develop in the sixth, seventh, or eighth lunar month (at 24 to 32 weeks). As has been mentioned, it is of the utmost importance to realize that intercurrent infection, the development of a severe anemia, or a pregnancy toxemia, may impose burdens on the heart and cause it to fail.

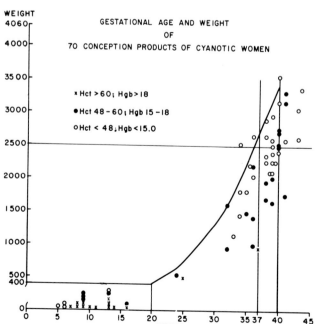

Figure 3. Interrelationship of pregnancy outcome and a maternal polycythemia. (Courtesy of Dr. Helen Taussig.)

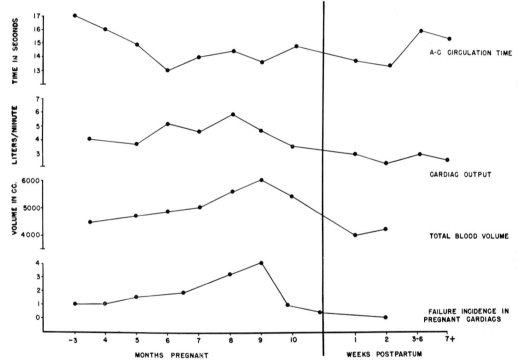

Figure 4. Frequency distribution of cardiac failure as related to hemodynamic changes of normal pregnancy.

Medical Care of the Cardiac Patient in Pregnancy

The patient should be completely familiar with a regimen designed to afford maximal protection to the circulation. This includes instruction to the patient to refrain from shopping tours and excessive physical exercise and to limit her activity to light housework. Cardiac patients should have added hours of rest. Weight control, with restrictions of fluid and salt, must be carried out meticulously. In patients who have developed cardiac failure, a review of their dietary history often reveals that they have neglected to restrict their salt intake as instructed. Supplementary iron is indicated, for any form of anemia is a special hazard to the pregnant cardiac patient. The patient should be instructed to report immediately symptoms associated with cardiac failure, such as dyspnea, orthopnea, and hemoptysis, as well as infections, particularly of the respiratory system.

Pregnant patients with heart disease should be observed weekly throughout the prenatal period. Determination of blood pressure and weight and urine examination are routine, and the obstetric examination should be performed frequently. At each visit the patient should be carefully examined for any evidence of cardiac failure. Persistent rales at the lung bases must be considered due to cardiac failure until proved otherwise. Distended neck veins and liver engorgement with tenderness are late signs of failure. The fact that the vital capacity normally increases in gestation makes this determination useful as part of the weekly examination. A decrease in vital capacity has been observed in pregnant patients with heart disease days or even weeks before there were any outward signs of cardiac failure (Fig. 5).

In the event that heart failure develops, the patient must be hospitalized immediately. Initially, the therapy is purely medical, and the obstetric care assumes secondary importance. The main features of therapy consist of bed rest, fluid and salt restriction, sedation, administration of oxygen if needed, digitalis, and the careful use of diuretics in event of retention of excess extracellular fluid. The development of acute pulmonary edema promptly demands the usual measures, including immediate venesection or the application of multiple tourniquets to the extremities to combat congestive failure. For the purpose of decreasing the hazard of phlebothrombosis and pulmonary embolism, apparently some ambulation is allowed or even encouraged in the nonpregnant cardiac who is being treated for congestive failure. It is doubtful whether such a policy should be followed in the case of the pregnant cardiac. Cardiac failure is less likely to recur if the pregnant cardiac patient is kept at near-complete bed rest. Elastic stockings may aid in the prevention of venous involvement in the cardiac patient at rest.

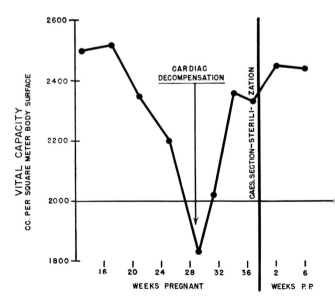

Figure 5. The vital capacity before, during, and after heart failure in a pregnant woman suffering from severe rheumatic heart disease. (From Cohen, M. E., and Thomson, K. J.: J.A.M.A., 112:1556, 1939.)

The signs of cardiac failure often begin to recede within a few hours after the institution of therapy. Even for those patients in whom failure occurs for the first time, however, one or two weeks is usually required before compensation is completely restored and the circulation becomes stabilized. Ideally, before any obstetric procedure is contemplated, the lungs should be consistently free of rales and the pulse rate near normal for several days. The fact that the patient is afebrile while under medical treatment does not exclude a smouldering bacterial endocarditis, and several blood cultures should be taken. Electrocardiograms should be taken periodically to detect changes that might indicate an exacerbation of rheumatic fever.

It is a sound clinical rule never to allow the cardiac patient who has developed congestive failure to leave the hospital until the pregnancy has been completed, even though she has responded well to medical therapy and is fully compensated. Despite good intentions to obtain adequate rest at home, the patient often resumes her ordinary activities, which usually causes a return of congestive failure.

The care of Class III and IV cardiac patients may be concerned more with the wisdom of continuation of pregnancy. Exceptions are encountered, and these will be considered under obstetric management. In the event that the patient wishes the pregnancy to continue regardless of the risk involved, hospitalization is mandatory until after delivery. These patients must receive meticulous medical and nursing care, and every effort should be made to lessen the cardiac burden and forestall further cardiac complications. Open heart surgery during pregnancy has further modified the care of these patients.

Significance of the Less Frequent Cardiac Complications in Pregnancy

Rheumatic fever, bacterial endocarditis, and chorea gravidarum are the cardiac complications that may materially influence the course of an otherwise "favorable" cardiac patient and add to the greater risk already established for the "unfavorable" cardiac.

Recurrent attacks of **rheumatic fever** are infrequently observed during pregnancy, although the cause of this low incidence is not clearly understood. Regardless of its infrequency, a search must always be made for any evidence of an exacerbation of rheumatic fever in the cardiac patient with congestive failure. The leukocytosis and increased sedimentation rate of normal pregnancy limit the value of these tests as diagnostic aids. More definitive evidence is furnished by changes observed in the electrocardiogram, more specifically prolongation of the PR interval.

Although **bacterial endocarditis** may occur at any time during pregnancy, the disease appears most frequently in the puerperium. Hence, in abortion, in premature or full-term pelvic delivery, or in surgical termination of pregnancy, antibiotics should be administered prophylactically to safeguard the patient with chronic rheumatic heart disease against the possibility of this cardiac complication. In the cardiac patient who develops puerperal infection, even though mild, bacterial endocarditis must be regarded as a distinct threat. Furthermore, its possible presence should be investigated in any cardiac patient with fever.

An increasing number of patients successfully treated for bacterial endocarditis have been safely conducted through pregnancy with a uniformly satisfactory clinical course. When the disease has appeared during pregnancy, medical therapy produces results comparing favorably with those obtained in the nonpregnant. On the basis of present-day experience, therefore, therapeutic abortion is no longer indicated in patients in whom bacterial endocarditis develops during pregnancy, or in those who become pregnant following successful treatment of the disease.

The appearance of **chorea** during gestation is regarded as one of the more serious complications of pregnancy. The fact that the condition begins to regress in the puerperium and eventually disappears implies an etiologic relationship to pregnancy and possibly accounts for the origin of the term *chorea gravidarum*. Regardless of terminology, the appearance of this condition has been looked upon by most as a manifestation of rheumatic fever comparable to Sydenham's chorea as it occurs in the nonpregnant cardiac patient. The majority of cases occur in the younger patients, thus accounting for the fact that most of the reported cases have been in primiparas. More than one half of pregnant patients with this disorder give a history of adolescent chorea, and one third state that they have had "rheumatism." The condition usually appears during the first trimester, is characterized by purposeless movements involving the face, arms, and legs, and is associated with muscular weakness. The patient is often unable to take food or to speak articulately. The uncontrolled movements tend to become less violent and often cease during sleep. Hyperthermia is consistently absent in the initial period. Eventually all of the signs of acute rheumatic fever may appear. Death has been known to follow within a few days to several weeks after onset of symptoms.

Divergent views have been presented regarding the value of therapeutic interruption of pregnancy. The present obstetric consensus is that the condition is not influenced one way or the other by the termination of pregnancy. However, cardiologists who are particularly interested in heart disease in pregnancy have expressed the opinion that therapeutic termination of pregnancy will result occasionally in cessation of the chorea and the prevention of complete physical deterioration. Should a trial of medical treatment be unsuccessful, one must consider therapeutic termination of the pregnancy. Moreover, such a procedure must be performed prior to the appearance of hyperthermia, for it is doubtful if any beneficial effect can be derived when the condition has become grave.

Articles appear sporadically raising the question of myocarditis of unknown etiology associated with pregnancy and the puerperium. Indeed, it is sometimes referred to as postpartum heart disease with myocardial degeneration. A wide spectrum of etiologic factors has been suggested, from malnutrition to an autoimmune phenomenon. Viral myocarditis is a distinct possibility.

Obstetric Management of the Cardiac Patient

The obstetric management and care of the cardiac patient should be undertaken with an awareness of the relationship between the occurrence of cardiac failure and the circulatory load of pregnancy. The patient should be treated on an individual basis, but the overall management must take into account certain principles. Although opinion may differ concerning these principles or their relative importance, they do emphasize that the care of the pregnant cardiac patient presents special problems, some of which are obstetric.

As a first principle, obstetric interference must never be undertaken while the patient is in heart failure. One may question the validity of this statement in those patients who are unable to regain their compensation in a reasonable time after the institution of medical therapy. Generally these are patients in the "unfavorable" group, with a prolonged history of severe circulatory disability and little cardiac reserve. Under these circumstances, it is doubtful whether continuation of the pregnancy is any more hazardous than its immediate termination by abdominal hysterotomy or the relief of the heart failure by cardiac surgery. However, two exceptions to the policy of nonintervention in the presence of cardiac failure deserve consideration. The first of these is the cardiac patient who develops paroxysmal dyspnea in the course of pregnancy; the second is the cardiac patient who develops heart failure in association with pregnancy toxemia.

The patients in the first group are relatively free of symptoms in the non-pregnant state, but because of rather severe mitral stenosis, the circulatory changes attendant on pregnancy are apparently sufficient to precipitate attacks of pulmonary edema. The attacks may appear at any time, but they tend to occur more frequently and with greater severity in the last half of pregnancy. The patient may not always respond to medical treatment, and the attacks may continue. The interval between attacks may not allow for complete stabilization of the circulation, and in some instances hemoptysis may become a serious complication. Termination of the pregnancy or emergency valvular surgery must be considered if attacks continue despite medical treatment.

The second exception pertains to the cardiac patient who may develop heart failure in association with pregnancy toxemia. It would appear that the toxemia repreents an additional circulatory burden, and, unless it responds readily to treatment, cardiac compensation will not be restored short of termination of the pregnancy. In fact, worsening of the toxemic condition justifies immediate abdominal hysterotomy, performed with the full realization that the cardiac status at the moment may be precarious. In such cases, one is impressed by the rapid return of cardiac compensation once the pregnancy is terminated.

The second principle of management involves the methods used to terminate the pregnancy in the cardiac patient. In the belief that it involves less risk of infection, a factor of great significance in the cardiac patient, therapeutic abortion by abdominal hysterotomy may be more predictable and safer than by the vaginal route. Also, the induction of labor in the cardiac is avoided whenever possible, for, in addition to infection, these patients may occasionally become somewhat apprehensive and disturbed if labor fails to occur promptly following artificial rupture of the membranes, while oxytocin infusion adds the risk of precipitating cardiac failure. Tranquility is desirable in the cardiac patient. Induction of labor is permissible only when there is an unequivocal indication, as, for example, pregnancy toxemia, and the obstetric conditions favor the prompt onset of labor and a relatively easy delivery. If these criteria cannot be met, and evacuation of the uterus is deemed necessary, abdominal hysterotomy may be the safer procedure.

Therapeutic Termination of Pregnancy

Although pregnancy may not alter the life expectancy of the cardiac patient once she has been safely delivered, this is not the issue. Rather, it is the immediate risk that is of concern. With the general advances in surgical and medical treatment, however, the therapeutic interruption of pregnancy is performed with decreasing frequency. The surgical correction of cardiac disability, the protection of the patient against infection by appropriate antibiotics and chemotherapeutic drugs, and improved anesthesia have all contributed to the increasing numbers of cardiac patients who are able to undertake and to complete their pregnancies successfully. *This assumes, however, that the patient is medi-cally supervised by a cardiologist experienced in the care of pregnant women, working together with an obstetrician who has more than a casual understanding of the patient's cardiac status.* It must also be appreciated that continuation of pregnancy in cardiac patients with limited cardiac reserve requires prolonged periods of hospitalization. Further, the natural history of rheumatic heart disease must be kept in mind when the cardiac patient is being advised concerning further childbearing. That is to say, it must be remembered that the incidence of heart failure is higher in the older than in the younger pregnant cardiac patients.

Whether or not the pregnancy is to be terminated prior to the period of medical viability is decided largely on the recommendations of the cardiologist in consultation with the obstetrician. The final decision must rest with the obstetrician, however, for he is the one who has the ultimate responsibility for the patient during pregnancy, delivery, and the puerperium. Whether a cardiac patient should be permitted to accept the risk of pregnancy will, in the final analysis, *depend on the total cardiac burden which, in some instances, includes the ability of the patient to care for the children whom she has already borne.* The basic principle in estimating the risk involved in pregnancy is to establish the patient's status in the natural course of her heart disease.

When first observed, the Class III or IV cardiac patient is hospitalized immediately for study and treatment. Unless cardiac surgery can place the patient in the "favorable" group as regards risk, therapeutic termination of the pregnancy is considered. An exception is the patient who is seen initially in the last trimester, when her cardiac status should improve with the anticipated decrease in the circulatory load. Following delivery the necessary steps should be taken to protect the patient from the risk of future childbearing.

In the past, termination of pregnancy in the Class I and II cardiac was considered when cardiac failure arose prior to the 25th or 26th week of pregnancy. The plasma volume and the cardiac output are still to reach their maximal values, so that a further circulatory burden can be expected. The advances in cardiac surgery, i.e., open heart surgery, in the past decade have modified this method of management. In the event that failure develops in the last trimester, the pregnancy is allowed to continue, in the realization that the cardiac load will soon begin to lessen. If abdominal hysterotomy is performed, concomitant sterilization is advised unless the cardiac lesion is amenable to surgical correction or the cardiac failure was precipitated by a complicating but correctable medical condition.

Immediate and Long-Term Prognosis of the Childbearing Cardiac Patient

It has long been recognized that the number of deaths in women with heart disease increases during pregnancy, and in the early part of the century the mortality was at least 20 per cent in some maternity clinics. Immediately following the establishment, in and around 1920, of clinics devoted entirely to the care of the pregnant cardiac, the maternal mortality rate decreased some fivefold. Today in this country there is reason to hope that this figure can be reduced to 1 per cent or less.

The immediate prognosis of the pregnant cardiac patient in the various classes is reasonably well established and documented. However, the influence and the ultimate effect of pregnancy on the natural course of heart disease are more difficult to assess. It has been demonstrated that the greatest mortality among persons with rheumatic heart disease occurs during childhood and through puberty, whereas the annual death rate of these patients decreases significantly beginning with the third decade of life. It may be presumed, therefore, that those who attain adulthood have less heart damage. Similarly, the patients with rheumatic heart disease who survive pregnancy might be regarded as having a greater cardiac reserve and, consequently, a longer life expectancy. This is not necessarily true, however, for the annual death rate of cardiac patients who have borne children appears to be somewhat higher than the annual death rate occurring during the third and fourth decades of life in a large series of patients with rheumatic heart disease. What is perhaps more significant is that the mortality rate in the cardiac Classes III and IV is much greater than the overall death rate for cardiac patients surviving

pregnancy. At least 30 per cent or more of the patients in these classes are dead within 10 years from the time they were first classified in pregnancy. For many, the physical activity required for the raising of a family exceeds their cardiac reserve.

Fetal Mortality

Although the overall fetal wastage is higher in the cardiac than in the noncardiac patients, in near-term pregnancies there is very little difference between the fetal mortality rates of the two groups. If perchance the mother develops cardiac failure, concern is often expressed as to the possible hypoxic effect on the fetus. Supposedly, intervillous circulation may be somewhat impaired, but fetal death under these circumstances is rare and these infants react normally at the time of delivery and do well. Any increase in fetal mortality in cardiac patients is due largely to the fact that the pregnancy was terminated therapeutically prior to viability or that labor occurred prematurely.

Relationship of Cardiac Surgery to Pregnancy

The introduction of surgical treatment of cardiovascular disease has given hope to patients who have avoided pregnancy because of severe cardiac disability. This challenges some of the previously held views relative to the obstetric and cardiac management of these patients, and has caused some controversy as to the wisdom of performing cardiac surgery during pregnancy. Today, for the pregnant patient whose cardiac disability from severe mitral stenosis raises the question of whether she should continue her pregnancy, three avenues of treatment are open: (1) Cardiac surgery can be performed and the pregnancy allowed to continue. This would appear to be the ideal solution. (2) The pregnancy can be therapeutically interrupted, with a subsequent operation for correcting the mitral obstruction. (3) The patient can be treated medically, and with hospitalization the pregnancy can be allowed to continue.

Certainly creditable benefits have accrued with mitral valvuloplasty performed during pregnancy. In the earlier periods of cardiac surgery the procedure might have been regarded as successful as far as the mother was concerned, but there was the risk that the conceptus might be permanently damaged by a hypoxic episode. Indeed, congenital defects and mental retardation did occur in association with cardiac surgery in pregnancy when it was first introduced.

Cardiac surgery during pregnancy reached a new dimension when the open heart technique became a reality, for it permitted the cardiac surgeon to design his procedure to meet the lesion encountered without jeopardy to the patient or her fetus. Although the effects of such surgery are yet to be fully appraised, there is reason to believe that congenital anomalies and central nervous system damage will not occur when the flow rate is adequate during the period of bypass circulation. Placement of valve prosthesis during pregnancy is being reported in increasing numbers of cases with a favorable outcome for both the mother and fetus.

To avoid local thrombosis and systemic embolization, long-term anticoagulant therapy is required. Warfarin sodium (Coumadin) with its relatively low molecular weight (1000) crosses the placenta readily, but heparin, with a much greater molecular weight (20,000), does not. The adverse effect on the fetus of warfarin is well documented. Hence, when anticoagulation therapy is required, heparin should be used, at least in the last three to four months of pregnancy.

Despite the reported success in sizable series of patients, the advisability of cardiac surgery during pregnancy must be carefully weighed. Although fetal risk has been reduced, one must still ask whether the patient is not in a more suitable state for cardiac surgery without the presence of pregnancy. Seemingly the patient would be considered better prepared for cardiac surgery if the hemodynamic changes of pregnancy, i.e., increased blood volume and cardiac output, were reduced to a nonpregnant status. Moreover, the risk of pregnancy for the cardiac patient is not removed by valvotomy and valve replacement. The threat of thromboembolism, atrial fibrillation, and cardiac failure remains.

It is well to be reminded that patients with mitral stenosis withstand abdominal hysterotomy with a mortality as low as 1 per cent. Hence, therapeutic termination of the pregnancy by hysterotomy must still be considered, followed by the appropriate cardiac surgery at some later date.

The optimal time for pregnancy to be undertaken is within three years after cardiac surgery. There is no assurance that a patient who has negotiated a pregnancy following valvotomy will do well from a cardiac standpoint in a subsequent pregnancy. Hence, patients who have been recipients of the benefits of cardiac surgery should be carefully assessed and advised prior to each pregnancy.

Conduct of Labor in the Cardiac Patient

The patient with a damaged heart usually withstands normal labor well, and there is no evidence that such an experience increases cardiac disability. Therefore, cesarean section is performed for obstetric reasons, but with some recognition accorded to the possible adverse effect that prolonged and exhausting labor might have on any cardiac patient. Because of the known relationship between beta-hemolytic streptococcus infection and the activation of rheumatic fever, prophylactic penicillin is indicated preoperatively or during labor and should be continued through the early days of the puerperium.

Ideally, both the obstetrician and the cardiologist should be in attendance with the cardiac patient when she is in labor. Periodic auscultation of the chest should be performed to detect the first signs of cardiac failure. During labor most cardiacs find breathing more comfortable when sitting upright; when failure develops, delivery is best performed with the patient in a semi-reclining position.

Patients with heart disease should receive only minimal analgesia and sedation during labor. Scopolamine is contraindicated because of its tendency to produce hyperactivity of the patient. Morphine or morphine-like drugs may be given for pain relief and to assuage apprehension, but, because of their tendency to depress the fetus, their administration must be regulated in relation to the time of delivery. Lumbar epidural anesthesia for pain relief during labor and for delivery in cardiac patients has its advocates.

If labor has any effect on the circulation, it usually becomes evident during the second stage. Brachial artery pressure is increased during this stage of labor with an additional temporary rise with each uterine contraction, presumably resulting from increase in the amount of blood returning to the heart as it is expressed from the uterus. Some thought must be given to the possibility that Pitocin might contribute to myocardial ischemia. The amount of blood returning to the heart may perhaps be increased also by the straining and the bearing-down efforts characteristic of the second stage of labor. Thus, in order to prevent an additional load on the heart, it is advisable to eliminate as much of the second stage of labor as is consistent with safe obstetrics. A short period of second-stage labor—never over an hour—is preferred if by such a policy one can anticipate a low forceps rather than a midforceps delivery.

Should congestive heart failure be present or appear for the first time during labor or delivery, the conventional measures are used in its treatment. Cardiovascular collapse has occurred at the time of delivery in patients with certain congenital cardiac defects. This is attributed to a fall in systemic blood pressure and perhaps a relative increase in right atrial and pulmonary artery pressure, causing a right-to-left shunt through the cardiac defect. The rise in pressure is ascribed to the increased amount of blood entering the systemic circulation from the uterus, the result of its sudden emptying. Prompt steps must be taken to combat the hypotension by increasing peripheral circulatory resistance.

DISEASES OF THE BLOOD VESSELS

Arteries

The diseases of the arteries occurring in association with pregnancy and deserving of mention are Raynaud's disease and dissecting aneurysm of the aorta.

When it occurs in females, Raynaud's disease, characterized by attacks of peripheral cyanosis that involve the hands more commonly than the feet, usually appears sometime between puberty and the menopause. The condition does not seem to be aggravated by pregnancy; it may be temporarily improved during this period.

Dissecting aneurysm of the aorta is uncommon in the young person, but half of the cases reported in women under the age of 40 have been associated with pregnancy or the puerperium. The majority of these catastrophes occurred in the third trimester of pregnancy when the changes in the circulation were maximal. Some cases of dissecting aneurysm in pregnant patients have been associated with coarctation of the aorta, but the initiating cause remains obscure. The onset and course of the disease are dramatic and overwhelming. Death may come quickly, immediately following sudden and severe chest pain, dyspnea, cyanosis, and extreme weakness, or it has been known to be postponed for two weeks following the onset of symptoms, the final cause being cardiac failure, or uremia if the blood flow to the renal arteries is impaired.

Veins

Varicose veins are a frequent manifestation during pregnancy, for the venous return is obstructed by the pregnant uterus and augmented by the large volume of uterine blood that is returning to the caval circulation, causing a further increase in pressure in the femoral vein. Varicose veins are attributed to either an inherent weakness in the venous musculature or a lack of the normal complement of valves, or both. In addition, the increase in the procoagulants and acceleration of the clotting mechanism in pregnancy may predispose to venous thrombosis in the presence of circulatory stasis.

The extent of varicose veins is established by inspection, usually with the patient in a standing position. The saphenous system is visibly prominent, with occasional dilated venous blebs representing localized muscular defects in the venous channels. Interestingly, trophic skin changes, such as eczema or ulcer formation, seen secondary to varicose veins in the nonpregnant, are rarely observed in pregnant patients.

The venous defects coexisting with pregnancy partially regress immediately after delivery. However, when varicosities appear, active therapy during pregnancy is indicated for the following reasons: (1) to relieve symptoms; (2) to reduce the incidence of phlebothrombosis or thrombophlebitis and subsequent embolic disease in the puerperium; (3) to prevent the further spread of venous destruction and the development of permanent varicose veins; and (4) for cosmetic purposes.

The treatment of varicose veins in the pregnant patient is no different basically from that in the nonpregnant. The conventional use of compression bandages, increased rest, and periodic elevation of the affected limbs are beneficial in providing comfort and eliminating symptoms. Should active local treatment in the form of sclerosing solutions be indicated, however, it should not be withheld because of the pregnancy, for the incidence of complications from this form of therapy is rare. The injection of sclerosing agents brings relief of symptoms in 80 to 90 per cent of patients, the best results being obtained when the treatment is initiated early in pregnancy. The operation of vein stripping is restricted to patients whose varicosities are extensive and of long duration, with severe symptoms dating back to the nonpregnant state. In a sense, these patients represent a neglected group who failed to receive adequate treatment when their varicosities first appeared. The extent of vessel involvement in these patients is difficult to determine with accuracy during gestation.

Surgical treatment should be postponed until after delivery. Testing the competence of the valves of the communicating veins is of little aid during pregnancy. For example, since the increased pressure in the femoral veins during pregnancy tends to cause the superficial venous system to fill quickly, giving one the impression that the deep venous system is occluded, the constriction test of Trendelenburg is apt to give falsely positive results. Perthes' test, however, when applied preliminary to injection of the superficial group, will establish the patency of the deep or femoral venous group. Although they tend to subside after pregnancy, vulvar varicosities are particularly annoying. With compression bandages and local injections there is some relief of symptoms.

Contrary to the majority opinion, it is firmly advocated that active treatment of varicose veins should be exercised during pregnancy and the early puerperium, and not postponed until after childbearing. Besides its curative and preventive value, the active treatment of varicose veins in pregnancy also has a cosmetic appeal. If at the onset the involved portion of the vein is injected, the process is less likely to spread. Superficial phlebitis, with its contribution to deep phlebitis, is less probable. When vein stripping is indicated, it is very

successfully performed on the fourth or fifth day of the puerperium, thus removing the need for the patient to return to the hospital at a later date.

In résumé, a plea is made for the prevention of varicose veins by active treatment with sclerosing solutions at the earliest sign of varicosities in pregnancy. If this is done, bandaging and the use of elastic stockings become obsolete and vein stripping will no longer be needed in the otherwise neglected patient.

Thromboembolic disease is recognized in two forms: either as a thrombosis associated with inflammation of the vessel wall (thrombophlebitis), or as a clot formation without vessel involvement (phlebothrombosis). Although such a clot soon attaches itself to the vein wall, in the interim the hazard of embolism is greater than it is in thrombophlebitis.

In the obstetric patient, thromboembolic disease may develop in the deep pelvic veins as well as in the femoral system. When the thrombus originates in the deep pelvic veins, it may propagate into the common iliac vessels proximally or in a retrograde direction into the femoral system. When the femoral system becomes involved, it is designated thrombophlebitis femoris or phlegmasia alba dolens. Although this condition may appear without any obvious provocation, it is more likely to develop secondary to pelvic infection or traumatic pelvic delivery. Similarly, although pelvic thrombophlebitis may appear without any demonstrable precipitating factors, it usually arises secondary to a pelvic cellulitis. When the pelvic infection is controlled, the thrombophlebitis subsides and recanalization of the thrombus begins. In the event that the inflammatory process in the pelvis continues, the thrombus may become infected, necrotic, and purulent. Even with massive antibiotic and anticoagulant therapy, such a suppurative pelvic thrombophlebitis may give rise to septic emboli. A suppurative thrombophlebitis may also occur without any signs or symptoms of femoral thrombosis. Thromboembolic disease develops most often in the immediate puerperium.

Thromboembolic disease may develop silently in the deep veins of the pelvis and, without warning, usually 7 to 10 days after delivery, give rise to an embolism that may be fatal. With the realization that the placental site is a large open wound containing over 400 uteroplacental arterioles with their accompanying veins, all of which have undergone extensive local thrombosis, one might inquire why such embolism does not occur more frequently. Fortunately, however, clot formation is restricted to the decidual vessels, and rarely if ever occurs in the endomyometrial vessels. Thrombosis of the latter can occur in the presence of an abscess or gangrene of the uterine wall. A pelvic thrombophlebitis, therefore, arises from either a lymphatic extension of an endometritis or secondary to a parametritis.

In more recent times, thromboembolic disease of the femoral system is less frequent. The low incidence reflects avoidance of traumatic pelvic delivery, control of pelvic sepsis by chemotherapeutic and antibiotic drugs, and a greater attention to the care of the veins during pregnancy and the puerperium. Early ambulation within 24 hours after delivery also contributes to the reduction in frequency of both thromboembolic disease and superficial phlebitis.

Ovarian vein thrombosis in pregnancy may occur ante partum as well as post partum. When it develops in the right ovarian vein, the symptoms may mimic those of appendicitis with rebound tenderness and mild fever. The diagnosis is most often made at the operating table. The involved portion of the vein is resected and the patient is given heparin for a time.

The diagnosis of thromboembolic disease is never certain in the early stages. An elevation of the pulse rate is often the initial and a very important sign, which may precede other findings, including fever, by several hours. In many instances, a fleeting chest pain is the sole symptom to suggest the presence of thromboembolic disease. Local tenderness of the calf muscles and along the course of the femoral vein, pain on dorsiflexion of the foot (Homan's sign), difference in leg size, fever, and leukocytosis constitute the clinical picture. Reflex vasoconstriction and angiospasm may develop, causing bluish discoloration and mottling of the skin of the involved extremity. The dorsalis pedis artery sometimes can barely be palpated, and the skin temperature may be less than that of the uninvolved limb. The condition may be announced first by the appearance of the signs and symptoms of a pulmonary embolism.

When the process begins in the pelvic veins, as is often the case in pregnancy, the first signs and symptoms may be those denoting involvement of the common femoral or iliac vein. These include engorgement of the superficial veins of the upper thigh and lower abdomen, pain about the hip joint, tenderness in the groin, and a sudden increase (as much as 2 to 4 inches) in the circumference of the thigh. In order to establish the diagnosis of pelvic thrombophlebitis in women, considerable emphasis is placed on the pelvic findings. The involved veins in the broad ligament are said to be tender and cordlike. In view of the induration usually present, and the discomfort of the examination, these findings are difficult to elicit. Hence, pelvic examination is of limited value and, furthermore, may be harmful.

The management and treatment of thromboembolic disease during pregnancy is the subject of some controversy. Majority opinion favors the use of anticoagulants, except when repeated embolic phenomena appear. Certainly if the methods are equally successful, the nonsurgical method is always more appealing, but the dual origin of the disease in the obstetric patient suggests that both forms of therapy are needed.

The proponents of surgical treatment consider that anticoagulant therapy when used in the puerperium has two serious drawbacks. First, it is never certain when anticoagulant therapy can be discontinued without danger of further embolic phenomena. Second, anticoagulant therapy will not remove the hazard of embolism from the unattached portion of a propagating thrombus.

Prothrombin-depressing drugs are avoided prior to delivery because of their adverse effects on the fetus. Heparin therapy can be used without fear of hemorrhagic complications at the time of delivery, for its action is easily controlled by protamine. Warfarin can be used in the puerperium for long-term therapy.

If surgical treatment is employed, it is carried out through the femoral vein just below the origin of the deep femoral branch (Fig. 6). Although the thrombotic process is often restricted to the left side, exploration and ligation should be done bilaterally to protect against a possible silent thrombus on the opposite side. The clot is removed by suction, and its complete removal is indicated by a free backflow of blood. To observe the removal of a large, loosely attached clot from the common iliac vein is a source of relief for those responsible for the patient's care. The femoral vein is

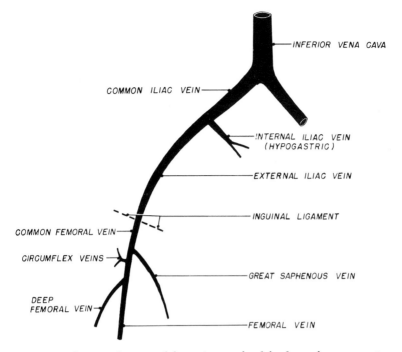

Figure 6. Schematic drawing of the main vessels of the femoral venous system.

then ligated proximally and distally. Ligation of the common femoral vein is condemned, for the sequelae may occasionally lead to severe muscular discomfort, edema of the extremity, and limitation of activity. Since the deep femoral vein is not ligated in this technique, an embolism from this segment of the venous system is a possibility, and therefore anticoagulant therapy should be instituted in the postoperative period. Moreover, because of the probable pelvic source of the thrombosis in the obstetric patient, one is further obligated to administer anticoagulants following surgical exploration. Anticoagulant therapy is also indicated postoperatively to preserve the patency of the distal venous tree and avoid postphlebitic swelling.

Regardless of whether heparin or a prothrombin-depressing drug is used separately or they are used in conjunction with each other, it must be realized that adverse reactions to these drugs may occur in the puerperium as they may after surgery. If these drugs are administered in excess of that necessary to produce their therapeutic effect, bleeding may occur from the placental site, or from the episiotomy or the cesarean section wound. Thus, they must be used with as great care in obstetrics as in any surgical condition. As previously

stated, protamine will promptly counteract a hemorrhagic diathesis from heparin, but such a diathesis is not easily corrected when prothrombin-depressing drugs are used. Vitamin K or K_1 oxide, in a large dosage (72 mg.), should be given intravenously every six hours for as long as necessary to decrease prothrombin time to the nonhemorrhagic level. The response of the patient to vitamin K is somewhat variable, and little or no effect is to be expected until three to five hours after its administration. Multiple transfusions of fresh blood should be given on indication; use of banked blood with reduced prothrombin activity and accelerator substances should be avoided except in emergencies.

Surgical ligation of the inferior vena cava should be considered in patients experiencing recurrent pulmonary infarction caused by emboli arising from suppurative pelvic thrombophlebitis. As the result of a long-standing puerperal infection, these patients often pursue a steady downhill clinical course. Under these circumstances, inferior vena cava ligation is lifesaving. Furthermore, in view of the fact that the ovarian vessels may be involved as frequently as the uterine veins, they, too, should be ligated. When collateral circulation is not completely adequate, residual edema of the lower extremities may be a sequela of venous ligation, but usually it is not crippling. Patients who have been subjected to inferior vena cava ligation have subsequent uneventful pregnancies. Also, inferior vena cava ligation has been performed during pregnancy without sequelae and the pregnancy has continued to term. The prominent collateral veins appear not to be a source of embolism, although this has been questioned.

In summary, if surgery is to be used in the treatment of thromboembolic disease, it is restricted to the early stage of the disease, within 12 to 24 hours after the onset of symptoms. After this time the thrombus has usually become firmly attached to the vein wall, and the likelihood of embolic phenomena is appreciably reduced. Surgical intervention is warranted at any time if, during anticoagulant therapy, one suspects an extension and progression of the disease. When there is evidence that the patient is experiencing showers of septic pulmonary emboli from a deep pelvic thrombophlebitis, ligation of the inferior vena cava and ovarian veins must be considered.

BIBLIOGRAPHY

Becker, F. F., and Taube, H.: Myocarditis of obscure etiology associated with pregnancy. New Eng. J. Med., 266:62, 1962.

Bennett, G. G., and Oakley, C. M.: Pregnancy in a patient with a mitral-valve prosthesis. Lancet, 1:616, 1968.

Benson, R. C., Dotter, C. T., Peterson, C. G., Bristow, J. D., Metcalfe, J., and Kraushaar, O. F.: Congenital arteriovenous fistula and pregnancy: Report of three cases. Amer. J. Obstet. Gynec., 92:672, 1965.

Bland, E. F., and Jones, T. D.: Rheumatic fever and rheumatic heart disease; a twenty year report on 1000 patients followed since childhood. Circulation, 4:836, 1951.

Bunim, J. J., and Appel, S. B.: A principle for determining prognosis of pregnancy in rheumatic heart disease. J.A.M.A., 142:90, 1950.

Burwell, C. S., and Metcalfe, J.: Heart Disease and Pregnancy; Physiology and Management. Little, Brown and Co., Boston, 1958.

Cannell, D. E., and Vernon, C. P.: Congenital heart disease and pregnancy. Amer. J. Obstet. Gynec., 85:744, 1963.

Collins, C. G., Weinstein, B. B., Norton, R. O., and Webster, H. D.: Effects of ligation of inferior vena cava and ovarian vessels on ovulation and pregnancy in the human being. Amer. J. Obstet. Gynec., 63:351, 1952.

Collins, H. A., Daniel, R. A., Jr., and Scott, H. W., Jr.: Cardiac surgery during pregnancy. Ann. Thorac. Surg., 5:300, 1968.

Crane, C.: Deep venous thrombosis and pulmonary embolism; experience with 391 patients treated with heparin and 126 patients treated by venous division, with review of the literature. New Eng. J. Med., 257:147, 1957.

Ellis, J. D.: Pregnancy and delivery after mitral valvotomy. J. Obstet. Gynaec. Brit. Comm., 74:24, 1967.

Genetics of congenital cardiac malformations. Lancet, 1:1349, 1963.

Gilchrist, A. R.: Cardiological problems in younger women: Including those of pregnancy and the puerperium. Brit. Med. J., 1:209, 1963.

Gorenberg, H., and Chesley, L. C.: Rheumatic heart disease in pregnancy; remote prognosis with "functionally severe" disease. Amer. J. Obstet. Gynec., 68:1151, 1954.

Gurewich, V., Thomas, D. P., and Rabinov, K. R.: Pulmonary embolism after ligation of the inferior vena cava. New Eng. J. Med., 274:1350, 1966.

Haig, D. C., and Gilchrist, A. R.: Heart disease complicated by pregnancy. Trans. Edinburgh Obstet. Soc., Edinburgh Med. J., 56:55, 1949.

Hamilton, B. E., and Thomson, K. J.: The Heart in Pregnancy and the Childbearing Age. Williams and Wilkins, Baltimore, 1942.

Harthorne, J. W., Buckley, M. J., Grover, J. W., and Austen, W. G.: Valve replacement during pregnancy. Ann. Intern. Med., 67:1032, 1967.

Jewett, J. F., and Ober, W. B.: Primary pulmonary hypertension as a cause of maternal death. Amer. J. Obstet. Gynec., 71:1335, 1956.

Kinney, T. D., Sylvester, R. E., and Levine, S. A.: Coarctation and acute dissection of aorta associated with pregnancy. Amer. J. Med. Sci., 210:725, 1945.

Lynch, J. K., Sreenivas, V., and Pelliccia, O.: Ovarian-vein thrombophlebitis. New Eng. J. Med., 275:1112, 1966.

MacFarlane, J. R., and Thorbjarnarson, B.: Rupture of splenic artery aneurysm during pregnancy. Amer. J. Obstet. Gynec., 95:1025, 1966.

Meffert, W. G., and Stansel, H. C., Jr.: Open heart surgery during pregnancy. Amer. J. Obstet. Gynec., 102:1116, 1968.

Mowbray, R.: Heart block and pregnancy (a review). J. Obstet. Gynaec. Brit. Emp., 55:432, 1948.

Mullane, D. J.: Varicose veins of pregnancy. Amer. J. Obstet. Gynec., 63:620, 1952.

Novy, M. J., Peterson, E. N., and Metcalfe, J.: Respiratory characteristics of maternal and fetal blood in cyanotic congenital heart disease. Amer. J. Obstet. Gynec., 100:821, 1968.

Pedowitz, P., and Hellman, L. M.: Pregnancy and healed subacute bacterial endocarditis. Amer. J. Obstet. Gynec., 66:294, 1953.

Robinson, M., Newman, N., Creevy, D. C., Katz, J., and Harrison, D. C.: Congenital aortic stenosis in pregnancy; ventricular fibrillation induced by oxytocin. J.A.M.A., 200:378, 1967.

Schenker, J. G., and Polishuk, W. Z.: Pregnancy following mitral valvotomy. Obstet. Gynec., 32:214, 1968.

Schnitker, M. A., and Bayer, C. A.: Dissecting aneurysm of aorta in young individuals, particularly in association with pregnancy, with report of case. Ann. Intern. Med., 20:486, 1944.

Shanahan, W. R., Romney, S. L., and Currens, J. H.: Coarctation of the aorta and pregnancy; report of en cases with twenty-four pregnancies. J.A.M.A., 7:275, 1958.

Stone, S. R., Whalley, P. J., and Pritchard, J. A.: Inferior vena cava and ovarian vein ligation during late pregnancy. Obstet. Gynec., 32:267, 1968.

Szekely, P., and Snaith, L.: The place of cardiac surgery in the management of the pregnant woman with heart disease. J. Obstet. Gynaec. Brit. Comm., 70:69, 1963.

Zegart, K. N., and Schwarz, R. H.: Chorea gravidarum. Obstet. Gynec., 32:4, 1968.

DISORDERS OF THE RESPIRATORY SYSTEM

The acute respiratory disorders encountered in pregnancy that need be mentioned are bacterial and viral infections and pulmonary embolism. To be sure, spontaneous pneumothorax has been reported in pregnancy and other acute respiratory conditions, but the clinical picture and course are not particularly different than in the nonpregnant, granted that the fetus may be temporarily at risk.

Suffice to say, acute infectious diseases of the lung in pregnancy are a less serious complication than they were before the introduction of chemotherapy. However, unless the infection is brought promptly under control, fetal death in utero and premature labor may occur. Also, in influenza epidemics the mortality from this disease has been higher in pregnant than in nonpregnant patients.

Pulmonary embolism, when it occurs in pregnancy, is usually encountered in the puerperium and is considered a complication of thromboembolic disease of the pelvis or lower extremities. However, this need not necessarily be the case when it occurs in the prenatal period when material from the uterus may enter the maternal blood stream. This material may be a foreign substance used to procure an abortion. Also, amniotic fluid may escape from a high rupture of the fetal membranes. In either case, the symptoms and signs are consistent with those of a pulmonary embolism. Angiography and radioisotope lung scan in these latter states may reveal a diffuse rather than a single lesion. Since these methods have become available, the diagnosis of pulmonary embolism, regardless of cause, is being confirmed more frequently in the antepartum period.

Pulmonary embolism all too often is not considered when the symptoms are vague. The diagnosis should be considered in a pregnant patient with unexplained anxiety and palpitation and when the hyperventilation of pregnancy borders on dyspnea. If diagnosed and treated at this stage, a fatality from a large embolus might be averted. The diagnosis is established on the same criteria as in the nonpregnant patient, whether in the prenatal period or during the puerperium. Both in the prenatal and postpartum periods the treatment involves heparin therapy and inferior vena cava ligation as discussed under thromboembolic disease.

The chronic pulmonary disorders may be categorized into three groups. The first includes the infectious conditions, the more important of these being tuberculosis and bronchiectasis. The second group includes those conditions which interfere with alveolar capillary oxygen exchange, an example of which is pulmonary fibrosis. The third category includes diseases that alter ventilatory efficiency by reducing the capacity of the thoracic cage through deformities of the chest (kyphoscoliosis). Present-day medical and sugical therapy has permitted patients with quiescent pulmonary conditions and deviations in the respiratory dynamics to undertake pregnancy.

TUBERCULOSIS

The percentage of maternity patients with pulmonary tuberculosis will depend largely on the prevalence of the disease within the community. Failure to diagnose unsuspected, active tuberculosis in the pregnant patient creates serious public health problems affecting the patient's family and the community. For this reason routine x-ray examination has been recommended in pregnancy. To reduce radiation exposure, the tine test is more desirable for the mass screening of patients for tuberculosis. Only those with a positive test would require x-ray examination of the chest, and in some clinics this might mean only 10 to 20 per cent of the patients. The test does not interfere with other tuberculin tests like the Mantoux test.

Although there may be differences of opinion regarding the effect of pregnancy on the mother's tuberculosis, there is general agreement that maternal tuberculosis seldom affects the fetus. Only after a tuberculoma has formed within the placenta is the tubercle bacillus in a position to attack the fetus. Most present-day opinion favors the view that pregnancy exerts little or no influence on the incidence or course of pulmonary tuberculosis. This belief is based on the assumption that during pregnancy and the puerperium the patient will receive all the benefits of modern therapy for her disease. Regardless of this optimistic viewpoint, patients with pulmonary tuberculosis should be evaluated individually on the basis of the history and the extent and location of the pulmonary lesion. The determining factor seems to be whether or not the lesion is active and how the patient has been reacting to her disease.

The patient whose pulmonary tuberculosis is in the process of becoming stabilized should defer pregnancy for at least two years after the disease has entered the arrested stage, for it should be ascertained whether or not the patient has the resistance to maintain her disease in a quiescent stage. When there is doubt, pregnancy may spell the difference between arrest and reactivation of the infection. Extrapulmonary lesions also are no longer considered a contraindication to pregnancy. In the pregnant patient, as well as in the nonpregnant, the location of the tuberculous lesion is a matter of some importance. In their clinical course basal pulmonary lesions are less predictable than are apical infections. Although the diaphragm is elevated in pregnancy, its excursions are not limited by the presence of an enlarged uterus. In fact, women breathe more deeply during pregnancy. It must not be presumed, therefore, that lesions about the diaphragm will improve with pregnancy, for actually the reverse may occur.

Data are available in the older literature to indicate that some 10 to 15 per cent of patients with tuberculosis react unfavorably to pregnancy, with the condition tending to exacerbate in the early puerperium. As in heart disease, a careful evaluation of the history and physical findings is basic in choosing the safest course for the mother. If the patient is seen in the first trimester of pregnancy, and her history reveals exacerbation of the disease following sufficient periods of sanatorium-like care, continuation of the pregnancy may not be advisable. If, on the other hand, such a patient is seen initially in the last half of gestation, continuation is probably less

hazardous than therapeutic termination of pregnancy.

With sanatorium care and chemotherapy of streptomycin and isoniazid the patient's pulmonary condition can improve remarkably even during pregnancy. The use of streptomycin has been questioned because of its possible deleterious effect on the vestibular and auditory apparatus of the fetus.

Until proved otherwise, fever in the puerperium must be regarded as a possible sign of extension or reactivation of the tuberculous process. If there is doubt concerning the activity of the process, the patient must return for additional sanatorium care for an indefinite period. To protect the newborn, a definitive regimen should be outlined, depending on the status of the mother's tuberculous process. Breast feeding is contraindicated, and the use of BCG vaccine should be considered in the infants of tuberculous mothers.

In some countries, BCG vaccine is given to almost every newborn infant; in the United States, however, it is used primarily for those with an increased risk of exposure to tuberculosis. BCG vaccination is only one step in the prevention of tuberculosis, and it in no way removes the necessity for other routine measures or for the separation of those with active tuberculosis from susceptible persons. Infants must be regarded as being particulary vulnerable to infection.

The infant is vaccinated after the second day of age and before departure from the hospital nursery. The child is isolated from the mother and eight weeks after vaccination is tuberculin tested. The Vollmer patch test is used for a positive reaction; if the result is negative, it is followed by the Mantoux test. The child with a negative tuberculin test, performed 10 to 12 weeks after BCG vaccination, is revaccinated, and isolation is continued for an additional four weeks, when the tuberculin test is repeated. Tuberculin tests and chest x-rays are then repeated at six-month intervals. If the tuberculin test becomes positive following the BCG vaccination, it has obviously lost its value for diagnosing tuberculous infections, and x-rays must be taken at regular intervals to detect early pulmonary tuberculosis. The loss of use of the tuberculin test as a diagnostic aid is a disadvantage of BCG vaccination, but the advantages under these circumstances are thought by some to outweigh this disadvantage.

BRONCHIECTASIS

Bronchiectasis, a severe necrotizing type of bronchitis often occurring early in life, is occasionally encountered in pregnancy. This condition generally results in chronic respiratory difficulties, and emphysema may occur secondary to the process. Intermittent low-grade fever with or without cough and foul sputum are important findings, and when the suppurative process is extensive the patient's health may gradually decline. When the disease process is confined to one lobe, the physical findings may be minimal; when the fibrotic changes are minor, x-ray studies may reveal little. The course of bronchiectasis is not altered by pregnancy, nor is the pregnancy usually affected by the pulmonary changes. The treatment is the same as that followed in the nonpregnant, with postural drainage supplemented by antibiotics to prevent extension of the infection. Patients in whom a lobectomy has been performed, and in whom dyspnea on minimal effort is not marked, may be expected to tolerate pregnancy.

PULMONARY DISORDERS OF DIFFUSION AND ALLIED CONDITIONS

Diffuse involvement of the lung parenchyma has many causes and may follow viral or bacterial infection, but on many occasions etiology is obscure. The characteristic defect in the respiratory physiology is an interference with oxygen diffusion across an impaired alveolar capillary septum, sometimes with a serious reduction in arterial oxygen saturation. Further, there are enlargement of the thoracic cage and diminution of motion which may further embarrass respiration. In contrast to the situation in the cardiac patient, the respiratory discomfort is decreased rather than increased by the supine position.

Pulmonary hypertension and cor pulmonale sometimes evolve in the course of this disease, but only in the more severe state. Any cyanosis, therefore, is usually respiratory and not cardiac in origin. The maximal breathing capacity, or the total minute volume attained under forced ventilation, and the vital capacity may be within normal range. Only when the pathologic changes are so extensive as to reduce lung volume are these respiratory measurements materially diminished. In order to evaluate the respiratory reserve, more elaborate tests are needed to ascertain the status of the alveolar capillary membrane, techniques that are usually available only in cardiopulmonary laboratories.

Although it is rarely seen, two patients with pulmonary fibrosis have been personally observed through three pregnancies. In the first, the patient was orthopneic, her vital capacity was 1400 ml., and the functional residual capacity was at the lower limits of normal (60 per cent). Therapeutic termination of pregnancy was recommended, but the patient elected otherwise. Interestingly, the vital capacity rose to 1800 ml., breathing became more comfortable near term, and dyspnea was experienced only with moderate exertion. Despite the apparent improvement in the patient's condition, a relatively mild respiratory infection in the last trimester caused it to become critical for several days. Except for this episode, the pregnancy was obstetrically uneventful. The second patient, with a disease equally severe, also had two uneventful pregnancies with no new symptoms. Idiopathic pulmonary fibrosis has shown a favorable response to cortisone therapy, and this applies in pregnancy also.

Cystic fibrosis in pregnancy presents two problems—that of the patient herself if she has the disease and that of her offspring. Because of the genetic component, therapeutic abortion and sterilization must be considered. Although the disease may be manageable, the risk of superimposed infection is real and the prognosis must be guarded. Pulmonary hypertension and cor pulmonale may contraindicate pregnancy. The patient's vital capacity may be reduced to less than 50 per cent of normal—indeed less than 1 L.—and the patient survive the pregnancy. At the same time, these patients, like those with other conditions of impairment of the alveolar gaseous exchange, may have misleading vital capacity values. The respiratory reserve should be measured. The disease may illustrate how the fetus can survive apparently without harm when the mother's oxygen saturation may reach the low levels of nearly 60 to 65 per cent.

Patients with bronchial asthma may show a temporary improvement during pregnancy, either from possible cortisone-like effects or for mechanical reasons. Actually, bronchial asthma shows little change during pregnancy; with good medical care it occasionally seems to improve, and only rarely becomes worse. The increased elevation of the diaphragm in normal pregnancy should reduce the residual air and enable these patients to breathe more effectively and with less discomfort.

Other diseases associated with fibrosis and parenchymal infiltration include berylliosis, pneumoconiosis, sarcoidosis, and other granulomatous lesions. The natural course of these diseases is apparently not accelerated by pregnancy, and pregnancy is contraindicated only when the respiratory deficiency is such that the patient's life is endangered as a result of marked alveolar capillary deficiency.

Sarcoidosis is one of the more commonly encountered diseases in this group in childbearing women. There is diffuse organ involvement, especially of the lymph nodes, lungs, liver, and skin. Again, the response to pregnancy is dictated largely by the presence or extent of pulmonary fibrosis and pulmonary hypertension. If these are absent, favorable outcome to pregnancy can be anticipated. In fact, in a comparatively large series of patients with sarcoidosis, it was concluded that pregnancy had a beneficial effect, but, unfortunately, this advantage was often lost after delivery. During pregnancy, cough and shortness of breath improved, and peripheral lymph nodes temporarily decreased in size. Similarly, hilar and mediastinal lymphadenopathy showed a decrease on x-ray examination, with return of enlargement after delivery. These changes were submitted as evidence that the condition was not of tuberculous origin, for in tuberculosis such improvement would not be anticipated in pregnancy. The improvement was attributed to an increased corticoid production during gestation, suggesting that adrenal hormone therapy in the early weeks of the puerperium might prevent serious exacerbation of the disease.

KYPHOSCOLIOSIS

Kyphoscoliosis produces a ventilatory disorder, as the result of a reduction in the lung volume caused by decrease in the capacity of the thorax or interference with its normal mobility. The marked distortion of the chest, resulting from changes in the

cervical and thoracic vertebrae caused by tuberculosis of the spine, rickets, or poliomyelitis, disturbs respiratory function by altering the lung parenchyma and the cardiopulmonary circulation. Because the circulation eventually becomes involved, the condition is often included in circulatory diseases rather than in those of the respiratory system. Dyspnea develops initially from the marked reduction in lung capacity, and later from the cardiac changes as well.

Characteristically, the chest is stunted, with the thoracic cavity shortened so that the total lung capacity or volume is significantly reduced. Compression of the lung on the affected side can cause atelectasis and pulmonary fibrosis. Displacement of the heart may result in some kinking of the pulmonary artery, which, combined with the fibrotic changes in the lung parenchyma, leads to a gradual increase in pulmonary vascular resistance. Pulmonary arterial hypertension with right ventricular hypertrophy or cor pulmonale occurs secondary to these changes. Cyanosis, cardiac arrhythmias, and polycythemia are prominent findings.

The diagnosis of kyphoscoliosis presents no special problem. An evaluation of the underlying cardiac and respiratory alterations, however, necessitates careful medical study. Vital capacity determinations are useful as an approximate index of functioning pulmonary parenchyma, whereas other more elaborate tests must be used to determine functional residual capacity. The thoracic cage may be so fixed, however, that the vital capacity may not rise in pregnancy. Rotation of the spine at the time of x-ray or fluoroscopy of the chest will correct the deformity and aid in restoring the heart to its usual position so that its silhouette can be outlined. Determined in this position, the contour of the heart should be normal, unless anatomic changes have already developed. The electrocardiogram is not thought to be altered significantly by the rotation and displacement of the heart.

The course of pregnancy in women afflicted with kyphoscoliosis will depend primarily on whether cardiac hypertrophy and dilatation are present, and, to a lesser extent, on the degree to which pulmonary volume has been reduced. If the cardiovascular system has not been affected, pregnancy should proceed uneventfully. If signs of cardiac embarrassment are present or develop, however, the prognosis must be guarded. In patients who exhibit inadequate cardiac reserve, termination of pregnancy should be strongly considered.

BIBLIOGRAPHY

Badger, T. L., Breitwieser, E. R., and Muench, H.: Tuberculin tine test. Amer. Rev. Resp. Dis., 87:338, 1963.

Cohen, J. D., Patton, E. A., and Badger, T. L.: The tuberculous mother; 5- to 20-year follow-up of 149 women with 401 full-term pregnancies. Amer. Rev. Tuberc., 65:1, 1952.

Evans, G. L., Dalen, J. E., and Dexter, L.: Pulmonary embolism during pregnancy. J.A.M.A., 206:320, 1968.

Given, F. T., and DiBenedetto, R. L.: Sarcoidosis and pregnancy. Report of 5 cases and 1 maternal death. Obstet. Gynec., 22:355, 1963.

Grand, R. J., Talamo, R. C., Di Sant'Agnese, P. A., and Schwartz, R. H.: Pregnancy in cystic fibrosis of the pancreas. J.A.M.A., 195:993, 1966.

Harvey, R. M., Ferrer, M. I., Richards, D. W., Jr., and Cournand, A.: Influence of chronic pulmonary disease on heart and circulation. Amer. J. Med. 10:719, 1951.

Mayock, R. L., Sullivan, R. D., Greening, R. R., and Jones, R., Jr.: Sarcoidosis and pregnancy. J.A.M.A., 164:158, 1957.

Mendelson, C. L.: Pregnancy and kyphoscoliotic heart disease. Amer. J. Obstet. Gynec., 56:457, 1948.

Novy, M. J., and Edwards, M. J.: Respiratory problems in pregnancy. Amer. J. Obstet. Gynec., 99:1024, 1967.

Novy, M. J., Tyler, J. M., Shwachman, H., Easterday, C. L., and Reid, D. E.: Cystic fibrosis and pregnancy; report of a case, with a study of pulmonary function and arterial blood gases. Obstet. Gynec., 30:530, 1967.

O'Leary, J. A.: A continuing study of sarcoidosis and pregnancy. Amer. J. Obstet. Gynec., 101:610, 1968.

Robinson, G. C., and Cambon, K. G.: Hearing loss in infants of tuberculous mothers treated with streptomycin during pregnancy. New Eng. J. Med., 271:949, 1964.

Rogers, W. N., Wilson, E., and Goodier, T. E. W.: Case of miliary tuberculosis during pregnancy treated by streptomycin. J. Obstet. Gynaec. Brit. Emp., 57:795, 1950.

Schaefer, G., and Silverman, F.: Pregnancy complicated by asthma. Amer. J. Obstet. Gynec., 82:182, 1961.

Swachman, H., Kulczycki, L. L., and Khaw, K. T.: Studies in cystic fibrosis. A report on sixty-five patients over 17 years of age. Pediatrics, 36:689, 1965.

Simpson, G. A., and Long, A. C.: Pregnancy and pulmonary tuberculosis. Amer. J. Obstet. Gynec., 59:505, 1950.

Spellacy, W. N., and Bergquist, J. R.: Hamman-Rich syndrome and pregnancy. Obstet. Gynec., 19:555, 1962.

DISORDERS OF THE ENDOCRINE SYSTEM

DIABETES MELLITUS

Prior to the discovery of insulin, only a few diabetics became pregnant; not only were amenorrhea and infertility common, but even the patient with mild diabetes was forewarned of the hazards of pregnancy. Today, the advances in diabetic therapy and improved obstetric care encourage the attitude that pregnancy is rarely contraindicated in this disease. The advent of insulin therapy has also allowed those with diabetes in childhood to reach the childbearing age. As a result, an increasing number of pregnant patients with juvenile or growth-onset diabetes are being encountered.

Pathogenesis

In the consideration of the natural history of the disease, some and perhaps most authorities believe diabetes is completely genetically determined. The disease is generally inherited as a recessive trait, although some families have been reported in which the condition is a dominant trait.

A variety of terms are used to designate the status of the disease in the course of its life cycle. These are ofttimes used interchangeably, especially in studies on the deviations of carbohydrate metabolism in pregnancy. This applies to the nomenclature of "prediabetes" "chemical diabetes," and other terms such as "suspect" diabetes.

In accordance with the genetic origin of the disease, the term "prediabetes" has been applied to the early period of the offspring of diabetic parents. This state begins with birth or possibly before and terminates when the patient demonstrates an abnormal glucose tolerance test, i.e., "chemical diabetes."

So-called "chemical diabetes" is commonly seen in such conditions as obesity, infection, and pregnancy. There are those who regard these conditions as "stress" situations, which may reveal underlying diabetes. It is recognized, therefore, that a major problem in this field is the difficulty in demonstrating and characterizing the prediabetic state or beginning carbohydrate impairment by what is sometimes referred to as a crude clinical test, i.e., the glucose tolerance test. Hence, it is suggested by many authorities of this disease that "prediabetes" should be used as a research term and not diagnostically, until more sensitive methods are developed for the detection of hormonal, metabolic, and morphologic abnormalities that probably precede measurable impairment of carbohydrate tolerance. This is based, rightly or wrongly, on the belief that diabetes is a hereditary disease, whether or not it is known to the patient involved.

Hence, it would appear preferable to retain the term "chemical diabetes" in pregnancy for those asymptomatic patients with an abnormal glucose tolerance test, in whom regression to normal post partum is the rule rather than the exception. At least the term "chemical diabetes" seems less committal about the future outcome of the patient with regard to overt diabetes.

Classification of Diabetes Mellitus in Pregnancy

In the past and indeed the present, patients are often classified in accordance with their insulin requirements or difficulty of management, for example, the brittle diabetic. Often little attention is given to age at onset and duration of the disease. Actually, the heart of the problem with respect to pregnancy is whether or not maturity-onset diabetes is different from juvenile or growth-onset diabetes, and how the possible difference may affect the course of pregnancy. Thus, for the meaningful assessment of the value of therapy or effectiveness of measures in prenatal care and the time and method of delivery, some attention must be given to categorizing the status of the disease. In so doing, account must be taken of factors other than the extent of the disturbed carbohydrate metabolism, including age of onset and the presence or absence of microvascular disease.

A classification that embodies the criteria alluded to above has proved useful in the care of patients, in assessing the effects of pregnancy on the diabetes, and in evaluating the therapy employed. The following classification has been proposed by Dr. Priscilla White.

Group A. Diabetes on the basis of glucose tolerance test only (chemical diabetes).

Group B. Onset of clinical diabetes after age 20, duration less than 10 years; no demonstrable vascular disease by x-ray, ophthalmologic examinations, and biopsies.

Group C. Onset of clinical diabetes between the ages of 10 and 19, with a duration of from 10 to 19 years; no x-ray evidence of vascular disease.

Group D. Onset of clinical diabetes before the age of 10, or duration of 20 or more years; x-ray evidence of vascular disease in legs (pelvic arteriosclerosis excluded); retinal changes in funduscopy.

Group E. Same as Group D, with the addition of pelvic arteriosclerosis by x-ray examination.

Group F. Vascular disease in the kidneys (Kimmelstiel-Wilson syndrome, or diabetic nephritis).

Group R. Active retinitis proliferans.

Long experience has demonstrated that placing patients in these categories is useful in predicting the course of the disease in pregnancy and the fetal and maternal outcome.

Pregnancy may be thought to aggravate the diabetes, for the insulin requirement increases, changes may be seen in the retinal vessels, and proteinuria (previously not evident or present) may appear. These effects are mostly temporary, however, and except for retinitis proliferans there is no firm evidence that pregnancy accelerates the natural course of the disease. Consequently, the patient may be reassured that changes in her diabetic status during pregnancy are not necessarily permanent and that after delivery her insulin requirement should return to its prepregnancy level. Microvascular disease (Groups D, E, and F) may be encountered in about 10 per cent of pregnant patients with growth-onset diabetes. These patients present special problems and the fetal mortality is high despite expert care of the diabetes and the pregnancy.

Diagnosis of Diabetes Mellitus in Pregnancy

The symptoms and signs of diabetes mellitus, such as excessive thirst, hunger, polyuria, and glycosuria, are not uncommon in pregnancy; hence the diagnosis must be considered rather frequently during this period. Moreover, the normal changes in pregnancy may influence the carbohydrate metabolism and at times simulate chemical diabetes.

The diagnosis of overt diabetes is tenable

when the fasting blood glucose level is elevated above normal, or the abnormal glucose tolerance test is accompanied by the classic symptoms of the disease, and the test remains abnormal after delivery. So far, there is no special controversy. Rather, it is when asymptomatic pregnant women with abnormal glucose tolerance tests are encountered that diagnostic problems arise. Actually the diagnosis may not be clear until after completion of the pregnancy. Moreover, the fact that a chemical diabetic-like state may appear in pregnancy is important not only with respect to both diagnosis and patient management but also in determining whether or not pregnancy truly is "diabetogenic"—that is to say, whether pregnancy initiates the disease or it is acquired during this period. Also, this has relevance as to whether there is an entity that should be referred to as "gestational diabetes" or whether this is simply another term for "chemical diabetes" encountered in pregnancy. Such concepts are excluded by the thesis of predetermined inheritance, but could properly fall into place as expressions of stages of the natural development of the disease.

Regardless, one is confronted with establishing the diagnosis through the glucose tolerance test, and the value of this test in pregnancy must be viewed with some reservation. The oral glucose tolerance test is not universally accepted as authoritative in pregnancy. Besides the possible influence of the endocrine change in pregnancy, misgivings concerning the reliability of the oral glucose tolerance test are further based on the facts that delayed intestinal absorption of carbohydrate occurs during pregnancy and that unusual eating habits may influence carbohydrate tolerance. Certainly the intravenous glucose tolerance test is sometimes normal in pregnant patients in whom the oral test was reported as abnormal. Hence a positive oral glucose tolerance test should be followed by an intravenous one.

What then is the diagnostic value and prognostic significance of an abnormal glucose tolerance test encountered during pregnancy, and what pertinence may it have to immediate patient management? Whatever may be its clinical value in discovering unsuspected or latent diabetes in pregnancy, it must be assessed with respect to two circumstances: (1) mass screening and (2) testing patients selected on the basis of history, to include family history of diabetes, the delivery of babies of excessive size, unexplained stillbirth and neonatal deaths, repeated abortions, obesity, and glycosuria.

With regard to mass screening, besides the several endocrine and physiologic changes in pregnancy that can influence carbohydrate metabolism, the interpretation of a positive glucose tolerance test in asymptomatic patients is further compounded by additional variables, such as the overall incidence of overt diabetes in the population or ethnic group screened, and their general state of health as regards nutrition, obesity, and chronic infection. These factors, together with the variable of the endocrine changes in pregnancy, may account in part at least for the observation that only about 25 to 30 per cent of women with an abnormal glucose tolerance test in pregnancy will show an abnormal curve in a following pregnancy.

When patients are preselected for testing as outlined above, the incidence of abnormal oral tests is quite uniform, ranging from between 11 to 13 per cent. But then, if these patients were considered in relation to the general population from which they were initially selected, the incidence of overt diabetes would appear no higher than in the nonpregnant population. In other words, the incidence of the disease in women of this age group would not differ from those genetically destined to develop diabetes (2 to 3 per cent). Thus, the oral glucose tolerance test in pregnancy finds its greatest usefulness in pregnancy in supplementing a detailed family, medical, and obstetric history in the identification of the patient who may develop diabetes.

Despite the limitations of the test in pregnancy, unquestionably a certain percentage of asymptomatic patients with an abnormal glucose tolerance test in pregnancy, when followed over a period of years, eventually demonstrate overt diabetes. Again, the magic number appears to be some 25 to 30 per cent. Thus, from retesting patients with an abnormal glucose tolerance test in subsequent pregnancies and from follow-up of patients with an abnormal curve it may be concluded that pregnancy is not diabetogenic if this term is meant to imply that pregnancy may cause the disease. However, the term gestational diabetes may be acceptable, recognizing that overt diabetes will develop in only one in four patients.

Furthermore, any diabetogenic effect in pregnancy would be more in keeping with a response to an already existing disease. This is supported by and is consistent with the observations that pregnancy appears not to influence appreciably the life expectancy of the mother with overt diabetes, although certain complications arise in pregnancy that may be detrimental, albeit temporarily. Thus, in the patient who will eventually become diabetic, the disease may first manifest itself in pregnancy, and with it there may be an increased risk, at least to the fetus. As noted above, for each such patient there will be three or more with an abnormal glucose tolerance curve in pregnancy in whom overt diabetes will not develop. With respect to management, the question is, which patient with an abnormal glucose tolerance test initially found in pregnancy is indeed a diabetic?

Hence, until more refined methods are available to determine precisely which of the asymptomatic patients with an abnormal glucose tolerance test in pregnancy actually have or will have diabetes, based on clinical experience it appears that these patients should be treated as diabetics, realizing that perhaps only one in four will develop the disease. This is analogous to other medical states seen in pregnancy, most notably the blood pressure response in the patient in whom essential hypertension is predestined to develop. A parallelism with respect to treatment may be seen in the occasional patient with a question of heart disease in pregnancy, in whom the diagnosis will not be clear until after delivery. In the interim period of pregnancy, it is safer to treat the patient as a cardiac, though realizing that this may not necessarily be the case.

Insulin Needs and Metabolic Response

For most diabetic patients the insulin requirements may double or triple during pregnancy although in a few they may remain unchanged. The percentage of increase in insulin needs for the complete diabetic is less than may be required for patients with milder forms. The needs may change rather suddenly and an insulin reaction may be an ominous sign. If the insulin requirements fall and tend to approach prepregnancy needs it may indicate that the pregnancy is in jeopardy; and if the fetus is of sufficient age to survive, immediate delivery may be warranted and indeed indicated. Furthermore, the insulin needs may fall precipitously (sometimes within two to three hours after delivery) to the prepregnancy level and the patient may show evidence of a hypoglycemic reaction.

In normal pregnancy there is an elevation of plasma insulin, both in the fasting state and after intravenous glucose administration. (See Endocrinology of Human Pregnancy in Chapter 4.) Although the levels are elevated in normal pregnancy, insulin may be more securely protein-bound and, hence, metabolically less active. It is a hallmark of pregnancy that plasma-binding capacity for many substances is increased. One may speculate that such an arrangement could insure a stable, normal maternal blood sugar level in the interest of maintaining fetal homeostasis.

However, this increase in insulin levels may be in response to other hormone changes, including the presence of placental lactogen. Whatever may be the latter's other physiologic properties, it can potentiate the effects of human growth hormone. The effect of placental lactogen separately or together with growth hormone and the fact that insulin is degraded by proteolytic placental enzymes furnish additional reasons why insulin requirements in the pregnant diabetic increase.

It has been generally postulated that human placental lactogen acts to suppress glucose oxidation by insulin and to mobilize maternal fat to provide the needed energy for the mother's daily metabolic requirements, thus conserving carbohydrate and protein for fetal energy and structural demands. This does not appear to be entirely the case. Although there is a rise in free fatty acids, the proportional amount of fat consumed for maternal fuel remains the same or actually decreases. (See Normal Changes in Chapter 11.) Despite these changes, carbohydrate continues to be the major source of maternal energy even under the stress of physical work. The well controlled pregnant diabetic has a pattern similar to the normal, with at least two exceptions, and these have definite clinical implications. The oxygen consumption in the diabetic begins to fall near the 34th to 35th week, in contrast to the normal patient in whom it continues to rise to near term. This is reflected also in an early and parallel fall in the respiratory quotient in the diabetic patient. This is offered as evidence that perhaps, physiologically at least, pregnancy reaches term earlier in the diabetic and provides some rationale to deliver the diabetic patient by at least the 37th week to avoid fetal death in utero.

Complications in Pregnancy in the Diabetic Patient

The diabetic patient is subject to several serious medical and obstetric complications, the more important of these being pregnancy toxemia, diabetic ketoacidosis, progressive retinal changes, and polyhydramnios.

Hypertension and proteinuria are regarded as the most common complications in the pregnant diabetic. It may well be that the occurrence of proteinuria and hypertension is largely governed by the prevalence of complicating vascular or renal disease rather than by any significant increase in specific pregnancy toxemia. Certainly the number of diabetic patients developing initial hypertension or proteinuria in the latter weeks of pregnancy, that is, specific pregnancy toxemia, hardly exceeds the incidence in the nondiabetic group (5 to 8 per cent). At the same time, in the diabetic patient with vascular and renal disease, the hypertension and degree of proteinuria may increase during pregnancy, representing a state of superimposed toxemia rather than a temporary aggravation of the vascular or renal disease. Influenced by the incidence of vascular and renal disease (microvascular disease) including specific toxemia, the frequency of proteinuria and hypertension in pregnant diabetics may approximate 10 to 20 per cent.

Except for their appearance at an earlier age, the vascular changes in the diabetic hardly differ from those seen in the nondiabetic hypertensive patient. Calcification of the pelvic vessels is sometimes demonstrable in the patients who have had diabetes since childhood. Although the finding is not a contraindication to pregnancy, it must be recognized that, regardless of treatment, the fetal mortality is appreciably higher when atherosclerosis of these vessels exists. The renal changes are in the form of nephrosclerosis, acute and chronic pyelonephritis, and intercapillary glomerulosclerosis (Kimmelstiel-Wilson disease).

The ocular lesions, which are frequently present, may progress during the course of pregnancy and lead to sudden impairment of vision. Although authorities fail to agree on the basis for some of these changes, a characteristic anatomic pattern has been defined and accepted by most. The typical finding is small saclike dilatations of the capillaries, or so-called microaneurysms, appearing deep in the substance of the retina (Fig. 7A). Venous stasis, congestion, and sclerosis of the retinal arteries are part of the general picture of diabetic retinopathy. The ocular fundi show pallor

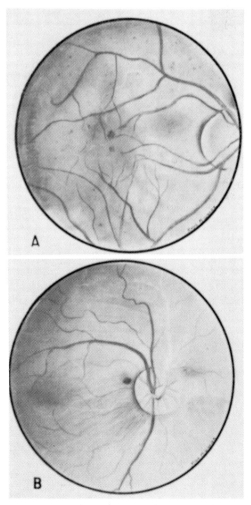

Figure 7. Diabetic retinopathy in pregnancy. A, Characteristic aneurysm. B, Retinitis proliferans. (Courtesy of Dr. William P. Beetham.)

of the retinal arteries, arteriovenous crossing phenomena, and silver-wire appearance, and in advanced stages the arteries may appear white from complete sclerosis. When renal disease is present, "cotton-wool" retinal exudate may be an associated finding.

A rupture of any of the branches of the central vein or capillaries may lead to disturbing hemorrhage. During the process of organization of these small hematomas, minute blood vessels develop to form a network within or over the surface of the retina, and they occasionally extend into the vitreous. This process has been designated retinitis proliferans (Fig. 7B). The condition may progress during pregnancy and cause irreversible damage to vision, sometimes to the point of loss of sight. Because of this fact, ophthalmologic examinations must be performed frequently on all diabetics throughout the course of pregnancy. When diabetic retinopathy is present, the stillbirth rate is increased, undoubtedly reflecting the influence of vascular or renal changes. Actually, retinitis proliferans is the only condition in which pregnancy may be contraindicated.

Ketoacidosis is a constant threat, and in pregnancy it has a dual significance for, in addition to the maternal hazard, it may threaten the life of the fetus. The lowering of the blood bicarbonate, the physiologic lipemia of normal pregnancy, and the slight delay in alimentary glucose absorption, as well as the increment in metabolism, are conducive to the development of ketoacidosis.

Polyhydramnios occurs with greater frequency in diabetic than in normal patients. On occasion, this complication develops with striking rapidity, and within a day or two, or sometimes even within hours, the uterus may become abnormally enlarged and extremely tense from the rapid accumulation of fluid. The use of ammonium chloride and Mercuhydrin has been advocated, and although such therapy decreases the maternal extracellular fluid space, it may have little or no effect on the hydramnios. The excess amniotic fluid may be effectively removed by transabdominal amniotomy. This not only relieves the patient's discomfort, but it may help to maintain normal intervillous blood flow by reducing intrauterine pressure, if elevated, thus restoring the intrauterine environment to normal. The most suitable patients are those who are between the 28th and the 34th weeks of gestation, when continuation of the pregnancy for a few weeks should assure fetal maturity and survival. If the fluid is removed slowly over a period of 12 hours, the risk of precipitating labor is minimal.

Patients with Microvascular Disease

Because they present major problems, these patients deserve special mention. These are patients derived from Classes D, E, F, and R. Even at best, the fetal survival is only about 50 per cent, with the highest fetal loss in the patients with both retinitis proliferans and Kimmelstiel-Wilson disease. Whether patients with retinitis proliferans should attempt a pregnancy is questionable, for the fetal survival rate is low and pregnancy represents a serious risk to vision.

In these patients the blood urea nitrogen may be elevated even in the first trimester, with a further increase in the last trimester. The expected increase in creatinine clearance usually fails to occur and it appears not to deteriorate. Prematurity and fetal respiratory distress syndrome take their toll. The babies of this group of patients show no fetal overgrowth and indeed may show evidences of dysmaturity; nor are congenital anomalies increased over the usual incidence. Changes in the placenta are common, with hyalinization of decidual arterioles and obliteration of small arteries, which undoubtedly contribute to the high fetal loss.

Perinatal Mortality

The perinatal mortality is some five to seven times that of normal pregnancy. At least 15 to 20 per cent of diabetic pregnancies end in failure, with a perinatal mortality of 150 to 200 per 1000, nearly equally divided between fetal and neonatal deaths.

The fetal and infant losses are influenced materially by the severity of the disease and an increased incidence of congenital malformations. The frequency of the latter appears rather uniform for all classes and no correlation can be established with hypoglycemic episodes, ketoacidosis, age, parity, form of therapy, or polyhydramnios.

In many instances the cause of death in utero cannot be established. Ketoacidosis and rarely insulin reactions can be lethal to the fetus, as is the presence of hypertension. The placenta, although characteristically heavier and larger than normal, reveals lesions that may well lead to death in utero. Infarcts are rather common and absence of one umbilical artery occurs with an incidence of 3 to 5 per cent rather than the conventional 1 per cent. Changes in the arterioles of the decidua seen in Classes D, E, and F are observed to a degree in Classes B and C. The changes may eventually obliterate these vessels, and this small artery disease certainly must play a role in the increased stillbirth rate in diabetic pregnancy.

The Fetus and Newborn

Reference has been made to the increased incidence of malformations in the presence of diabetes mellitus and how this may influence the perinatal mortality. The most common cardiac anomaly is a ventricular septal defect. Skeletal deformities are not uncommon and are seen with greater frequency than anomalies of the central nervous and genitourinary systems.

The infants of mothers in Classes A, B, and C may show true gigantism. Except for the brain, the viscera are increased in size. Extramedullary hematopoiesis is commonly observed, and the islets of Langerhans are increased in size and number. The insulin content of the pancreas is increased over that of the infant of the nondiabetic mother. Thrombosis of the renal vein has been observed with relative frequency at autopsy of the infant of the diabetic mother.

The clinician must accept the proposition that the diabetic baby is not endowed with any special safeguards against the ravages of prematurity. The overall incidence of respiratory distress is slightly higher in the infants of diabetic mothers, for even at 37 weeks' gestation it occurs in roughly 15 per cent of the infants. A blood glucose level of less than 20 mg. per 100 ml. is encountered in these infants but rarely observed are the signs and symptoms assigned to hypoglycemia, an important clinical consideration in the management of these infants.

Medical and Obstetric Management of the Pregnant Diabetic

The management and care of the diabetic patient during pregnancy are dependent on a carefully integrated medical and obstetric program. The instability of the insulin requirements of the patient during this period, the ease with which keto-acidosis develops, and the suddenness with which obstetric complications can arise require that the diabetic patient be seen weekly throughout her pregnancy. The diet should consist of at least 200 grams of carbohydrate, 2 grams of protein per kilogram of body weight, and fat in accordance with the patient's nutritional status. The diet in the overweight patient need not provide more than 1200 to 1500 calories.

Protamine insulin alone may effectively control the diabetes, but supplementary crystalline insulin is usually required. Insulin therapy is instituted by the administration of 15 units of protamine insulin daily before breakfast. This is increased by 5 units daily until the preprandial urine tests show blue or light green reduction. If the urine tests before lunch show brown, regular insulin is added by separate injections in doses of 5 to 10 units. Additions are then made slowly until the tests show blue or light green reduction, or until the urine is brought as close to sugar-free as is possible without provoking hypoglycemia. These patients have a tendency toward edema formation. Sodium intake should be curtailed at the first sign of rapid weight gain, and, in some instances, diuretics should be given, together with potassium chloride.

Besides the review of systems and routine obstetric examination, the retinal fundi are examined at each prenatal visit. Postprandial blood sugar determination and examination of the sediment of a clean-voided urine specimen are done, and albumin, sugar, and acetone are determined. At intervals blood urea nitrogen and blood creatinine values are obtained.

The patient should be hospitalized at least a week before delivery is contemplated to provide more careful supervision and early detection of pregnancy toxemia and the various other complications. The timing of delivery is difficult to determine as one attempts to balance the relative risks of death in utero and those from prematurity. The various methods should be brought to bear in the assessment of the status of the fetus, including estriol determination and the ultrasound technique to determine fetal age and size. The total clinical picture must be evaluated daily as it pertains to the development of toxemia and the various complications.

Class A patients should be delivered by the 37th to 38th week for there is a 3 to 5 per cent fetal mortality if the patient is permitted to continue to term. Patients in Classes B and C are delivered by the 36th to 38th week. In those with vascular complications, Classes D and E, the week of delivery must be highly individualized; the same applies for Class F patients. In the presence of vascular and renal changes these patients on occasion must be delivered as early as the 32nd to 34th week.

The method of delivery must take into account macrosomia, prematurity, the avoidance of prolonged labor, and possible difficult pelvic delivery. Induction of labor by amniotomy and Pitocin drip is acceptable in patients in Classes A and B, and possibly in Class C if the criteria to permit this procedure are fulfilled; but this method of management demands that productive labor ensue within four to six hours and delivery be normal or accomplished by outlet forceps. It must be appreciated that fetal gigantism may cause serious shoulder dystocia. Delivery by cesarean section is required when induction of labor is not feasible, labor is unproductive, or there is question of the cephalopelvic relationship.

Preparation of the patient includes withholding breakfast and the administration of one half her prepregnancy dose of insulin. An intravenous infusion of 5 per cent glucose is started. The patient is kept in the delivery room throughout her labor, being carefully monitored. Lumbar epidural anesthesia is ideal for both fetus and mother. Following delivery the remainder of the usual prepregnancy dose of insulin is given. The patient often returns promptly to her nonpregnant diabetic status and her medical management must be planned accordingly.

When delivery is by elective cesarean section no premedication or insulin is given and the operation is performed by pre-ference under conduction anesthesia. Three thousand milliliters of 5 per cent dextrose in water is administered over the first 24 hours and the insulin therapy is again that usually required in the prepregnancy state.

In summary, it is apparent that the treatment and overall patient management must encompass a broad spectrum of a progressive disease from the subclinical form, which in pregnancy may be detected as "chemical diabetes," through the more severe stages to microvascular involvement. In decisions of patient management, account must also be taken of whether the patient has growth-onset or the adult form of diabetes (Table 1).

If a generalization is permissible, it would appear that patients with the juvenile or growth-onset form must have every therapeutic assistance during pregnancy and delivery at the earliest period when it is believed that the fetus is capable of extrauterine survival. This means delivery between the 34th and 37th week and, in most instances, cesarean section will be required as the method of delivery. Meticulous diabetic management is needed, including bed rest in ample amounts from the 20th week onward, with hospitalization by the 30th week. The latter is mandatory for patients with microvascular disease. In this group, anemia is treated vigorously, dietary protein is restricted if the nonprotein nitrogen is elevated, and edema is managed by salt restriction and diuretics, including Mercuhydrin if necessary.

In the case of the adult form of diabetes, obstetrically speaking, the management may be more conservative. Delivery may be postponed until the 37th to 38th week, at which time, it is to be hoped, labor can be induced and pelvic delivery anticipated.

Finally, in the management of "chemical diabetes," insulin comes quickly to mind as the crucial therapy, but it can be shown that control of obesity and dietary management is effective and may in the long run be more beneficial. Certainly, if insulin is indicated, it should be used only when general health rules fail. The patient should be treated as a diabetic during pregnancy, particularly as pertains to fetal survival and with the realization that overt diabetes mellitus will develop in only about 25 to 30 per cent of such patients.

TABLE 1. TRENDS OF COURSE OF PREGNANCY BY CLASS*

Class	A	B	C	D	E	F Nephropathy	R Retinopathy
Spontaneous Abortion Rate	N	N	N	+	++++	++++	++++
Hydramnios Degree	+	++++	+++	++	++	±	±
Excessive Maternal Weight Gain	+	++++	+++	++	++	0	0
Toxemia, i.e., Pre-eclampsia	+	++++	+++	++	++	?	Superimposed ?
Large Placenta	++++	++++	+++	++	+	0	0
Heavy Birth Weight Infant	++++	++++	+++	++	+	0	0
Intrauterine Fetal Loss	+	++	+	+++	++++	++++	++++
Intrapartum Fetal Loss	++++	++++	++	+	+	+	+
Neonatal Fetal Loss	+	++	++	+++	++++	++++	++++
Congenital Anomalies	+	+	+	+	+	+	+
Diabetes Mellitus Intensification	+	++++	+++	+	+	±	+

*Modified from White, P.: Med. Clin. N. Amer., 49:1015, 1965.

DISORDERS OF THE PITUITARY GLAND

Hypofunction of the pars distalis, or anterior lobe, of the hypophysis may arise from the effects of regional tumors, infection, and injury. Sheehan has shown that pituitary insufficiency in the female most frequently follows circulatory collapse from severe obstetric hemorrhage in late pregnancy or during parturition. The adenohypophysis may show varying degrees of damage from local ischemia and, in rare instances, in septic shock and toxemia from thrombosis and infarction. For panhypopituitarism to develop, most of the anterior lobe must be destroyed. The necrosis has been observed to extend to the posterior lobe, and, when this occurs these patients terminally have shown an associated diabetes insipidus. Adenohypophyseal failure resulting from obstetric hemorrhagic shock is now referred to as **Sheehan's syndrome.** This is in contradistinction to pituitary insufficiency from all causes, which is called Simmonds' disease, Simmonds having presented the first cases of panhypopituitarism, including those following complications of pregnancy.

The question arises as to why during pregnancy the adenohypophysis is particularly susceptible to the effects of hemorrhagic shock. Although abundant, the blood supply to the pituitary includes a portal system. From the internal carotid arteries, superior and inferior hypophyseal branches reach the gland and create a sizable plexus around the distal portion of the pituitary stalk. These vessels in turn empty into a secondary plexus located about the anterior lobe or pars distalis. With this type of vascular arrangement and the glandular hypertrophy of pregnancy, the pituitary is especially vulnerable to a reduction in blood supply. The anterior lobe of the pituitary apparently involutes rapidly after delivery, and, when the effects of hemorrhagic shock are superimposed on this rapid involution, the gland may undergo degrees of necrosis. In order for Sheehan's syndrome to occur there must be severe vascular collapse with the patient nearly pulseless for as long as one to three hours. Evidence that the lesion develops in association with the involution is the observation that some 14 hours or more must elapse from the time of the onset of shock before necrosis begins. Patients who succumb from hypovolemic shock immediately or within a few hours after delivery fail to show this destructive lesion at autopsy.

In the more severe cases of Sheehan's

syndrome, the clinical signs and symptoms will be noted immediately after delivery. Colostrum and lactation are absent, and the breasts may involute rapidly; with loss of ovarian function, the menses fail to reappear. In the subsequent weeks, manifestations of thyroid and adrenal insufficiency may develop. There may also be symptoms referable to the gastrointestinal tract, including nausea, vomiting, and abdominal cramps. These patients may show little weight loss, and occasionally may become obese in association with a developing myxedema.

Unless treated, the patient may follow a progressive and steady downhill course after the initial appearance of symptoms. In contrast, the course of the disease may be mild for many years and then suddenly marked panhypopituitarism may appear, with death following rapidly if the diagnosis is not made and substitutional endocrine therapy instituted. There is reason to believe that, if a careful search were made, some women with a history of obstetric hemorrhage or shock would reveal mild forms of hypopituitarism. Patients with milder forms of panhypopituitarism are apathetic and uninterested and may be wrongly judged to have psychiatric illness. This adds to the difficulty of determining the incidence of Sheehan's disease in patients with severe postpartum hemorrhage, for follow-up is unrewarding because of lack of patient response.

Pregnancy may occur in the presence of mild Sheehan's syndrome, and a gratifying and permanent improvement has been noted in the patient's condition, presumably the result of hypertrophy of the residual tissue of the anterior lobe induced by the stimulus of pregnancy. In the event of adrenal hypofunction, the patient may succumb during labor and delivery from an adrenal crisis (Fig. 8). The recognition of adrenocortical insufficiency and the institution of adequate replacement therapy should avert such a catastrophe.

Panhypopituitarism of the Sheehan type is preventable and should not occur when proper obstetric care is given. This reemphasizes the necessity of avoiding traumatic delivery with its attending blood loss, of making provision for the proper care of the patient threatened with late obstetric and postpartum hemorrhage, and of counteracting excessive blood loss promptly and adequately. In a parturient patient who fails to respond completely to the usual measures of treatment of hemorrhagic shock, the diagnosis of Sheehan's syndrome should be considered. Because the condition results from a polyglandular deficiency, replacement therapy must include adrenal and thyroid hormones, as well as testosterone to encourage nitrogen retention and anabolism. In the general supportive measures, attention must be given to water and electrolyte balance. Because both are caused by hemorrhagic shock, Sheehan's syndrome may accompany anuria resulting from acute tubular necrosis.

Tumors of the anterior lobe of the hypophysis will interfere with reproductive function, and amenorrhea is a common and often an early symptom. The more common of these pituitary tumors, the **chromophobe adenoma,** and the occasional craniopharyngioma may lead to pituitary insufficiency. The growing and expanding chromophobe tumor provokes its effect by compression of the neighboring tissue of the anterior lobe of the pituitary. The bodily changes that follow depend on the degree of target gland dysfunction resulting from the decrease in tropic hormone secretion. The gonadotropic hormone activity is usually so greatly reduced that the resulting hypogonadism precludes pregnancy. Craniopharyngioma produces its effect in a similar manner, but, because it may develop before puberty, secondary sex characteristics may fail to appear or be delayed. In either type of tumor, surgical extirpation or shrinkage by roentgen irradiation has restored the menses, and pregnancy has been known to follow. These rare successes, however, have been restricted to patients with the smaller tumors.

Pituitary tumors exhibiting hyperactivity, namely eosinophilic adenoma (causing acromegaly) and possibly basophilic adenoma, eventually inhibit the reproductive function, but in eosinophilic adenoma this need not be an early effect. Similar to the tumors already mentioned, the **eosinophilic adenoma** reduces gonadotropic activity by pressure of the space-occupying lesion. Before the adenoma is large enough to interfere with gonadotropic activity, however, the excessive amounts of growth hormone secreted by the tumor may already have produced the characteristic acromegaloid changes. In other words, hypogonadism may be postponed until after the disease is established clinically, in sharp contrast to

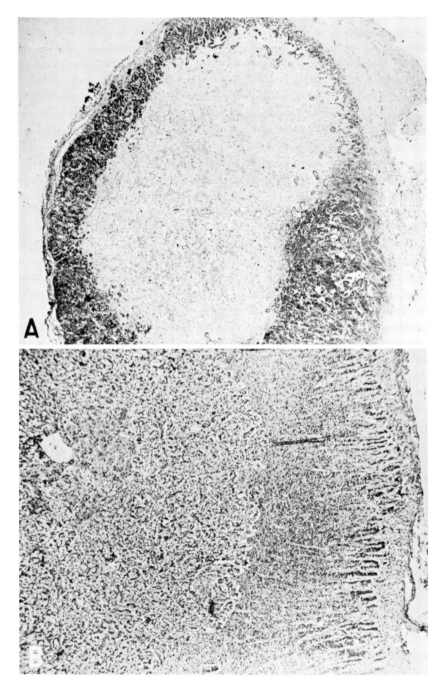

Figure 8. Sheehan's syndrome terminating in death from adrenal crisis in a subsequent pregnancy. A, Massive fibrotic lesion of the anterior lobe of the pituitary. B, Atrophy of zona reticularis and fasciculata with some persistence of the zona glomerulosa of the adrenal. (From Israel, S. L., and Conston, A. S.: J.A.M.A., 148:189, 1952.)

a chromophobe adenoma in which the initial symptom in the female is often amenorrhea. Restoration of the menses and the occurrence of pregnancy have been known to follow palliative x-ray or surgical treatment. The comment has been made that gestation is apt to increase the secretory activity of the tumor, with a recrudescence

of symptoms in the mother and an accentuation of the acromegalic changes. The synergistic action of placental lactogen with pituitary growth hormone may account for the aggravation of the acromegaly.

Basophilic adenoma, a rare pituitary tumor, may be an incidental finding at necropsy, but it is occasionally associated with hyperplasia of the adrenal cortex, a symptom complex that is now known as Cushing's syndrome. Referred to as basophilism, it was thought initially that the characteristic clinical picture was due to the effect of the pituitary adenoma, but this has been seriously questioned.

During pregnancy **diabetes insipidus,** a disorder of the posterior lobe of the pituitary gland, may at times show slight improvement and at others, increase in severity. Despite the possibility that the placenta may contain an antidiuretic hormone–like substance, it is usually more difficult to control urine volume during pregnancy.

Although it is relatively free of oxytocic activity, Pitressin must be used with some caution, particularly in the latter weeks of pregnancy, to avoid precipitating uterine contractions. Labor, delivery, and the puerperium in patients with diabetes insipidus are generally uncomplicated.

Postpartum amenorrhea or the failure of the menstrual periods to return within four or six months after delivery in the nonnursing mother is often a matter of patient concern. Pertinent to patient management is the question as to what constitutes postpartum amenorrhea. It has been suggested that at least a year should elapse after delivery or after weaning of the infant before the amenorrhea is considered abnormal.

Pituitary failure, as in Sheehan's syndrome and chromophobe adenoma, accounts for a few cases. Anorexia nervosa or voluntary starvation may begin following a pregnancy. A condition often discussed as a disturbance in lactation, the so-called Chiari-Frommel sequence, may well be included in postpartum amenorrhea, being characterized by prolonged mammary secretion, galactorrhea, uterine atrophy, and absence of the menses that may continue for a matter of years. The menstrual periods may reappear, and pregnancy ensue, with the entire cycle of events repeating itself. The condition is classified as a hypothalamic disorder (see Chapter 4).

DISORDERS OF THE THYROID GLAND

Thyroid disorders are uncommon complications of pregnancy and the incidence varies from one locale to another. Hyperthyroidism is encountered about once in a thousand pregnancies and hypothyroidism or myxedema is seen even more rarely. Nevertheless, disturbances of the thyroid gland may become aggravated by pregnancy and the mother and the fetus may be jeopardized either by the disorders themselves or by the therapy employed in their treatment.

Evaluation of the thyroid state during pregnancy is at times difficult. The flushed skin, tachycardia, easy fatigability, breathlessness, and increased heat production are suggestive of hyperthyroidism. By contrast, the excessive weight gain, edema, and sometimes pallor, lethargy, and somnolence in pregnancy may give the impression that the patient has myxedema.

Patients with severe **hypothyroidism,** or myxedema, rarely become pregnant, but in the milder form of the disorder, although menstrual disturbances are common, conception may occur. In the event of pregnancy, because of the demands placed on the maternal thyroid, a subclinical hypothyroid state may for the first time become manifest.

In the presence of iodine deficiency and the additional demand for thyroxin, both the mother and the fetus may develop colloid enlargement. In iodine-deficient areas of the world, therefore, endemic goiter in association with pregnancy is not uncommon.

Under these circumstances, the metabolic needs of pregnancy increase the utilization of the limited amount of thyroxin available, and by the reciprocal action of hormones the thyroid-stimulating hormone (TSH), or thyrotropin, is released in greater amounts, causing the acini of the glands to increase in number and the epithelial cells lining them to become columnar in type. With failure of normal thyroxin production through lack of adequate iodine, thyroglobulin or colloid accumulates in the acini, and the thyroid shows a greater increase in size than in normal pregnancy. With delivery and the return to a prepregnancy metabolic state, the secretion of thyrotropin diminishes and the thyroid begins to regress. In many parts of the gland involution is complete, but in other areas hyperplasia and excessive amounts of colloid may persist.

The administration of iodine to pregnant patients with endemic goiter has a two-fold therapeutic purpose. The first of these is to prevent endemic cretinism in the newborn. It must be remembered, however, that cretinism may have a dual etiology, which accounts for the sporadic cases seen in infants of patients with normal thyroid function. Evidently this form of the disease is related to some aberration of the embryonic development of the thyroid gland. Maternal influences have been excluded by the observation that, in dizygotic twins, one was normal and the other had cretinism. Whatever the controversy as to etiology of cretinism in the newborn, endemic cretinism has been reduced when iodine prophylaxis has been given in areas of the world where the water is iodine-deficient.

The second objective of iodine therapy is to promote normal postpartal involution of the thyroid and thereby prevent the development of nodular goiter from which, at some later date, thyrotoxicosis may develop. The latter possibility is increased if areas of hyperplasia persist and normal involution fails to occur. The administration of iodine to the mother with endemic goiter immediately satisfies the needs of the fetus, but the maternal need is fulfilled perhaps more promptly when desiccated thyroid and iodine are given. Thus, from both endogenous and exogenous sources, the serum thyroxin level, as measured by protein-bound iodine, is restored to normal. As the thyrotropic secretion decreases, hyperplasia regresses, colloid production diminishes, and the gland becomes smaller.

Hyperthyroidism is seldom observed during pregnancy, in part because infertility is common in hyperthyroid patients. Menstrual disorders, from amenorrhea to hypermenorrhea, occur in over 80 per cent of thyrotoxic women. When the disease is unrecognized or is inadequately treated, the fetal loss may be high (30 to 50 per cent).

When present prior to pregnancy, the disorder usually remains stationary, but either improvement or accentuation of symptoms may occur. Because of the unpredictable course of hyperthyroidism during pregnancy, it is perhaps better that no generalization be made regarding therapy, and the evaluation and management of the patient should be on an individual basis.

The diagnosis of thyrotoxicosis is never as certain in the pregnant patient as in the nonpregnant. It is evident that the diagnostic criteria must be modified to conform to the altered physiologic effects of pregnancy, including a basal metabolic rate above 20 and a protein-bound iodine of 10 to 12 mg. or more per 100 ml. The serum cholesterol may rise, but not to the level of normal pregnancy; however this value is so variable that, unless it is low, it aids little in establishing the presence of thyrotoxicosis. Perhaps the most useful test is the red blood cell uptake of triiodothyronine. In the nonpregnant female the values range from 11 to 17 per cent. In early pregnancy the values fall to 5 to 10 per cent as protein-binding for thyroid hormones increases. In hyperthyroidism in pregnancy the values rise to range between 17 and 25 per cent.

Hyperthyroidism in pregnancy is associated with two types of anatomic glandular change. The first and most frequent form is diffuse hyperplasia of the gland (Graves' disease); the second most commonly encountered is nodular goiter.

Graves' disease in pregnancy is usually well controlled by medical therapy. Recourse to surgery during the prenatal period is necessary only in the rare patient who fails to respond to medical therapy. However, thyroid surgery is well tolerated during pregnancy and is not contraindicated if the need for it arises. In fact, pregnant patients withstand thyroidectomy as well as nonpregnant persons, and it has no adverse effects on the conceptus. Nodular goiter and associated hyperthyroidism, either pre-existing or recognized initially during pregnancy, may be treated by surgery after adequate medical preparation.

The medical treatment includes the use of iodine or antithyroid drugs, alone or in combination. Although tracer or diagnostic doses of radioactive iodine may be safely given at any time during pregnancy, therapeutic doses should never be considered beyond the first 10 or 12 weeks, and even then they could be dangerous. After the 16th week, the fetal thyroid gland stores iodine, and from that time on there is a definite radiation hazard. Propylthiouracil alone in 100 mg. doses every eight hours has been recommended until the patient is euthyroid for pregnancy, when the dose is reduced to 50 mg.; it may be increased again in the third trimester. Antithyroid drugs have been identified in the milk of mothers who have received such therapy during pregnancy. Although sporadic congenital goiter (Fig. 9) has been observed following administration to the mother of antithyroid substances, in these cases dosage of the drugs was not well controlled, and they were given in excess of the requirements

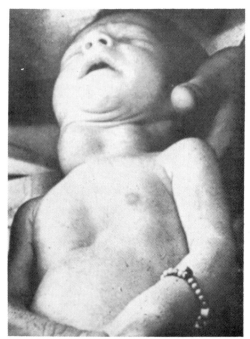

Figure 9. Goiter in a newborn. (Courtesy of Dr. Keith Russell.)

to control the disease. Goitrous hypothyroidism in the fetus and newborn may also be produced by excessive iodine therapy. Actually, the treatment of hyperthyroidism is directed toward the values of normal pregnancy, that is, a protein-bound iodine of 8 mcg. and a basal metabolism rate of plus 20 to 30 per cent. Supplementary thyroid therapy of 180 mg. daily has been advocated to protect the fetus against any adverse effect of antithyroid drugs. However, this has been questioned, for thyroid hormone does not cross the placenta readily and the net gain to the fetus is uncertain.

Despite the controversy regarding the comparative value of radiologic, medical, and surgical management, most pregnant patients with carcinoma of the thyroid have had some surgery. The course of these tumors remains unchanged during pregnancy, which is consistent with the relatively low-grade malignancy of many thyroid tumors. After a free interval period, pregnancy is not contraindicated, the exception being in the patient with the rare anaplastic carcinoma.

DISORDERS OF THE ADRENAL GLAND

With the advances in endocrine therapy, pregnant women with aberrations of the adrenal gland are seen with increasing frequency. The diseases attributable to hyperactivity of the adrenal gland that have obstetric interest are Cushing's syndrome and the adrenogenital syndrome.

Cushing's syndrome is a symptom complex that may arise from either hyperplasia or neoplasia of the adrenal cortex. However, the clinical state stems from excess cortical production. The etiology remains uncertain, and it continues to be debated whether the hyperadrenalism stems from a primary disease of the adrenal cortex or is a secondary effect of stimuli from within the pituitary or the hypothalamic region. When basophilism was first described, it was stated that the basophilic elements of the pituitary adenoma had a highly stimulating effect on the adrenal cortex, causing secondary hyperadrenalism. Supporting this contention has been the amelioration of symptoms occasionally following some forms of therapy directed at the pituitary. It has been speculated in these cases that there is perhaps an aberrant pituitary secretion, a "corticotropin-stimulating" factor. Indeed, in pathologic states elsewhere in the body, notably carcinoma of the lung, ACTH may be secreted in sufficient quantities to result in adrenal cortical hyperplasia, an important diagnostic consideration. Cushing's syndrome is not necessarily associated with basophilic adenoma; in fact, the tumor is found in only about 50 per cent of the cases. It has been stated, moreover, that the latter is found incidentally at autopsy, the patient having exhibited none of the stigmata of basophilism.

Appearing predominantly in women in the childbearing age, Cushing's syndrome is associated with amenorrhea, obesity, hirsutism, prominent purplish striae of the skin, and hypertension. The patient's face is puffy and rounded; the skin is florid, and acne is often present. The obesity is characteristic, involving the head, neck, and entire trunk, and enlargement of the supraclavicular pads causes the neck and shoulders to become prominent (buffalo hump). The striae are found mostly on the skin of the abdomen, hips, breasts, and lower axillae. When the disease is fully developed, the diagnosis is readily made from the patient's general appearance. In the long term there is muscular wasting and weakness, osteoporosis, and arteriosclerotic vascular changes.

The ovaries reveal changes consistent

with lack of gonadotropic stimulation, being devoid of developing graafian follicles and possessing large numbers of atretic follicles. In Cushing's syndrome, hyalinization and vacuolation are commonly seen in the basophilic cells of the anterior lobe of the hypophysis (Crooke's changes). These hypophyseal changes, presumably the result of excessive adrenocortical hormone secretion, undoubtedly alter gonadotropic activity and offer an explanation for the amenorrhea.

Although amenorrhea is a prominent symptom, approximately 20 per cent of the patients have normal menstrual periods, and some have conceived and borne children during the active phase of the disease. It has been commented that the disease is frequently first suspected during or after pregnancy. Whether the condition was present in a mild form during pregnancy and became accelerated following delivery is a matter of speculation.

Adrenal hyperplasia is the more likely finding in Cushing's syndrome, although about a third of the patients have tumors. The treatment is dependent on establishing by appropriate tests the pathologic state of the adrenal and the role of the pituitary. The dexamethasone suppression test, plasma ACTH, and urinary free cortisol values and certain x-ray procedures will differentiate between adrenal hyperplasia and tumor and will to a degree indicate the extent of pituitary involvement. The treatment involves x-ray therapy to the pituitary, adrenalectomy, or both in combination. From the point of view of pregnancy, adrenalectomy—a procedure favored by many—is of the greater importance. The resultant addisonian state is readily controlled and the patient may subsequently conceive. The outcome of pregnancy will depend to a degree on whether the patient is the victim of vascular or renal changes prior to adrenalectomy. If arteriosclerosis and nephrosclerosis are absent, the outlook is favorable and a number of patients have negotiated a pregnancy successfully after adrenalectomy for adrenal hyperplasia, benign tumor, and indeed a malignant tumor of the adrenal cortex thought to have been cured.

Primary hyperaldosteronism has been encountered in pregnancy, and with removal of the offending adenoma the gestation has continued to successful outcome. The same criteria of hypertension, meta-bolic alkalosis, hyperkalemia, and potassium loss is applicable in the diagnosis of the condition in pregnancy. However, pregnancy can mimic secondary aldosteronism. (See Normal Changes in Chapter 11 and Endocrinology of Human Pregnancy in Chapter 4.)

Although rare, both primary aldosteronism and pheochromocytoma should be on the list in the differential diagnosis of hypertension in pregnancy. Otherwise the diagnosis of these conditions is all too often postponed until several pregnancy failures have occurred or catastrophic cardiovascular or renal complications have developed.

Hyperfunction of the adrenal cortex of the newborn, the so-called **adrenogenital syndrome**, is manifested by pseudohermaphrodism and virilism in the female, and by precocious sexual development (macrogenitosomia praecox) in the male. The adult form of the adrenogenital syndrome is very rare. In the female the syndrome is evident immediately at birth, whereas in the male the disease is often not identified before he is three or four years old. The condition is characterized by a rapid somatic growth, accelerated epiphyseal maturation, and premature appearance of pubic, axillary, and facial hair. The 17-ketosteroids, which are ordinarily absent from the urine of the newborn infant of both sexes, can be recovered in amounts of 2 or 3 mg. per day soon after birth in infants with the adrenogenital syndrome and in increasing quantities as the child becomes older. In these infants, especially the males, an upset in electrolyte balance may develop, with symptoms resembling an addisonian crisis. This condition can occur soon after birth, and failure to provide adrenal replacement therapy and restore electrolyte losses may result in death. Faulty aldosterone production may be involved.

The pathophysiology of the adrenogenital syndrome is the result of failure of the adrenal cortex to produce cortisol, owing to a lack of the complete complement of enzymes responsible for its synthesis. Certain of these intermediate steroidal metabolites are converted to substances with androgenic activity.

Characteristically, the resultant female pseudohermaphrodite reveals a large clitoris, with the urogenital sinus opening onto the perineum through a small aperture near the urethra. Behind the perineum the vagina is usually normal, and the upper portion of the reproductive tract is not defective (Fig. 10). At some time in early childhood a surgical resection of the clitoris may be needed, and, by incising the perineum, a vagina is constructed.

Brilliant therapeutic results have been achieved by the administration of cortisone, with a regression of the virilizing manifestation, and through adrenal suppression stunting is avoided. Survival is assured by prevention of an addisonian crisis by cortisone and aldosterone administration. Feminization occurs and a few patients have had successful pregnancies. Two such patients have been cared for by the writer; one delivered a normal term infant without incident, and the other entered premature labor at the 26th week. Interestingly, in the latter patient, on the basis that the placenta might be secreting adrenocortical substances, before it was known otherwise,

an attempt to decrease the cortisone therapy resulted in a prompt rise in urinary 17-ketosteroids. The uterus also became hyperirritable, and, despite an increase in the dosage of cortisone, the patient delivered shortly thereafter. It is now clear that substitution therapy is required in prepregnancy dosages and perhaps even in greater amounts.

As an autosomal recessive disorder, the adrenogenital syndrome raises the question of further pregnancies. Although it is a question for individual decision, the answer is obviously influenced by the fact that endocrine therapy is now available.

Before the introduction of adrenal replacement therapy, clinicians were aware that pregnancy was a particularly hazardous time for patients with **adrenal hypofunction** (Addison's disease). Because states of adrenal insufficiency are characterized by inability of the organism to adjust to

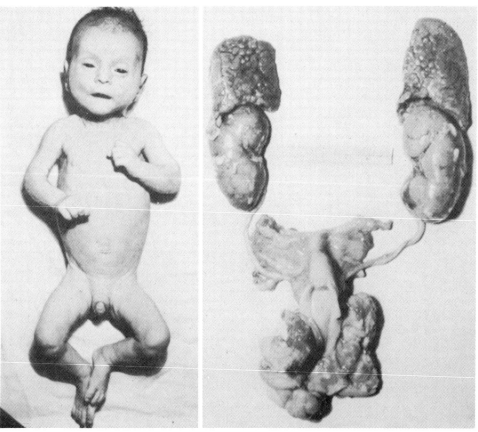

Figure 10. Adrenogenital syndrome (pseudohermaphroditism) in a neonate. The autopsy specimen shows normal-appearing uterus, upper vagina, and ovaries, and large clitoris. The fetal adrenals are not unusual in size when compared with those in the normal newborn. Note the large cervix and small uterine corpus, a normal finding at birth.

changes in the internal or external environment, one might suspect that a patient with Addison's disease would encounter difficulty in childbearing. Actually, these patients seem to improve in the latter two trimesters, or at least they may require less substitutional therapy. The favorable effect may be the result of hyperplasia of the residual adrenal cortical tissue. It is assumed that the fetus plays no part in the patient's improvement, for in cases of bilateral adrenalectomy, or in cases in which autopsy later showed the adrenals to be completely destroyed, cortisone and deoxycorticosterone were needed in amounts comparable to those required in the nonpregnant state. The same is true for patients following hypophysectomy in pregnancy.

The fact that these patients do sometimes improve during pregnancy, and immediately revert to their prepregnancy status after delivery, emphasizes the need for the careful adjustment and regulation of replacement therapy, particularly in the first trimester, when there may be nausea and vomiting, and during labor, delivery, and the early puerperium. Perhaps it is well, in the pregnant patient with Addison's disease, not to restrict salt as rigidly as is sometimes done in the normal pregnant patient. In pregnancy the average patient with Addison's disease may require approximately 10 to 25 mg. of cortisone daily. During labor these patients must be given additional cortisone up to 100 to 200 mg. daily. It must be realized that these patients are prone to infection and react poorly to trauma and blood loss. The patient in whom adrenalectomy has been performed for malignant hypertension is not a suitable candidate for pregnancy, especially if there is renal involvement.

The disease of the adrenal medulla that is particularly pertinent to pregnancy is the condition of **pheochromocytoma.** Frightening attacks of paroxysmal hypertension associated with palpitation, throbbing headache, blanching, pallor of the face and extremities, followed by flushing, tachycardia, and sweating, are the most characteristic symptoms. The signs and symptoms of a secretory medullary tumor of the adrenal may be mistaken for an indication of pre-eclamptic toxemia. The differential diagnosis of labile hypertension in pregnancy, therefore, must include pheochromocytoma as a possible cause.

The diagnosis is suspected from the patient's symptoms and the behavior of her blood pressure. Although it is sometimes possible to palpate the tumor, an attempt to do so is not without danger, for massage of the tumor may precipitate an attack of paroxysmal hypertension.

The definitive test for diagnosis is a marked elevation of urinary catecholamines and their metabolites, especially vanillylmandelic acid. Blood glucose and free fatty acids may be elevated but must be interpreted in accordance with the normal changes in pregnancy. X-ray localization of the tumor is possible in the majority of cases. Pharmacologic testing is not without its dangers and is less popular than heretofore and also is not required. The Regitine test has been used in the differential diagnosis of hypertension in pregnancy, when a fall in blood pressure would not be anticipated in essential hypertension and pregnancy toxemia.

If the patient is nearing term when the condition is suspected, continuation of the pregnancy may be indicated. A short-acting drug—phentolamine—and a longer-acting agent—phenoxybenzamine hydrochloride (Dibenzyline)—are capable of reducing the blood pressure and controlling hypertensive attacks and associated symptoms. Blocking agents to the synthesis of the catecholamines must be assessed, especially with respect to pregnancy. During labor phentolamine is best administered by slow intravenous drip, with 25 mg. added to 1000 ml. of glucose solution. The rate of administration and the amount given are titrated against blood pressure response. The objective is to maintain the systolic blood pressure near 140 mm. Hg. In the belief that fluctuations in blood pressure may be harmful to the fetus, cesarean section has been advocated as a method of delivery. There is no reason to believe, however, that labor and pelvic delivery will have any greater effect on the blood pressure than would abdominal delivery.

However, the maternal mortality with this condition is high, being reported as 40 per cent. Thus, when the condition is recognized prior to the last trimester, the wisdom of continuation of the pregnancy must be questioned. If the patient's symptoms are brought under control after one or two weeks of therapy, an alternative method of management is to remove the tumor and allow the pregnancy to continue. The possible adverse effects on the fetus from the maternal reaction to surgery deserve consideration, more particularly a hypotensive episode.

DISORDERS OF THE PARATHYROID GLANDS

Abnormal parathyroid states are rarely seen as complications of pregnancy, but pregnancy appears to furnish an impetus to increased glandular activity. The fact that hyperparathyroidism may follow pregnancy suggests that the function of this gland may be altered during gestation.

Hyperparathyroidism

Hyperparathyroidism is a disease predominantly of females, with the majority of cases occurring in the third and fourth decades of life. The probable increase in parathyroid activity during pregnancy has been suggested as a reason for the greater frequency of this condition in females. The disease develops as the result of an adenoma or hyperplasia of one or more of the parathyroid glands, producing increased bone resorption, a condition termed osteitis fibrosa cystica generalisata (von Recklinghausen's disease).

Hyperparathyroidism is characterized by large losses of urinary phosphorus with a compensatory mobilization of calcium from the bone in order to maintain ionic equilibrium of the blood. The significant laboratory findings are a hypercalcemia, calcinuria, and a low serum phosphorus. Because of marked bone resorption with osteoclastic activity, the serum alkaline phosphatase values are elevated. The bones by x-ray and pathologic examination show decalcification and areas of cyst formation. The resultant calcinuria often leads to renal changes, more particularly nephrolithiasis.

In advising about pregnancy in a patient who has been successfully treated by surgical extirpation of the offending parathyroid tissue, the decision will depend on the degree of recovery of renal function following the correction of the upset in calcium metabolism.

As to treatment when the diagnosis is made during pregnancy, the adenoma has been removed and the pregnancy has continued to term. Tetany during the neonatal period has been observed in infants of mothers with parathyroidism; it corrects itself spontaneously or through the addition of calcium and vitamin D. The explanation that the fetal parathyroid is suppressed by a rise in fetal serum calcium levels through the markedly elevated maternal serum calcium or by hyperfunction by the maternal parathyroid presupposes that parathyroid hormone crosses the placenta from maternal to the fetal circulation. At any rate, at birth there is an abrupt fall in serum calcium of the newborn with resultant tetany.

A condition referred to as neonatal familial primary hyperparathyroidism has been described. The parathyroid is hyperplastic. Bone changes have been encountered and death may occur if the disease is unrecognized and treated by subtotal parathyroidectomy.

Hypoparathyroidism

Hypoparathyroidism is usually secondary to a thyroidectomy in which the parathyroid glands were unintentionally removed or inadvertently damaged, resulting in an upset in calcium and phosphorus metabolism. Failure to maintain a normal urinary excretion of phosphorus with resultant high serum levels produces a compensatory fall in ionizable calcium in the serum. These changes lead to muscular hyperirritability and, in the extreme, to tetany. In the untreated mother with hypoparathyroidism there is a tendency toward exaggeration of symptoms, since the fetus satisfies its calcium needs even though the level in the maternal serum is low.

The treatment of hypoparathyroidism in pregnancy is little different from that in the nonpregnant patient. In fact, the patient's clinical course changes little in the event of pregnancy.

BIBLIOGRAPHY

Abelove, W. A., Rupp, J. J., and Paschkis, K. E.: Acromegaly and pregnancy. J. Clin. Endocr., 14:32, 1954.

Antoniades, H. N., Bougas, J. A., Camerini-Davalos, R., and Pyle, H. M.: Insulin regulating mechanisms and diabetes mellitus. Diabetes, 13:230, 1964.

Astwood, E. B.: Use of antithyroid drugs during pregnancy. J. Clin. Endocr., 11:1045, 1951.

Bank, H., Beer, R., Lunenfeld, B., Rabau, E., and Rumney, G.: Recurrence of adrenal carcinoma during pregnancy with delivery of a normal child. J. Clin. Endocr., 25:359, 1965.

Beetham, W. P.: Diabetic retinopathy in pregnancy. Trans. Amer. Ophthal. Soc., 48:205, 1951.

Bercovici, B., and Ehrenfeld, E. N.: Non-puerperal galactorrhea. J. Obstet. Gynaec. Brit. Comm., 70: 295, 1963.

Blair, R. G.: Phaeochromocytoma and pregnancy. J. Obstet. Gynaec. Brit. Comm., 70:110, 1963.

Bleicher, S. J., O'Sullivan, J. B., and Freinkel, N.: Carbohydrate metabolism in pregnancy; V. The interrelations of glucose, insulin and free fatty acids in late pregnancy and postpartum. New Eng. J. Med., 271:866, 1964.

Blotner, H., and Kunkel, P.: Diabetes insipidus and pregnancy; report of 2 cases. New Eng. J. Med., 227:287, 1942.

Bongiovanni, A. M., and Root, A. W.: The adrenogenital syndrome. New Eng. J. Med., 268:1283, 1391, 1963.

Burt, R. L., and Leake, N. H.: Oral glucose tolerance test during pregnancy and the early puerperium. Obstet. Gynec., 33:48, 1969.

Carrington, E. R., and Messick, R. R.: Diabetogenic effects of pregnancy. Amer. J. Obstet. Gynec., 85: 669, 1963.

Chandler, R. W., Blizzard, R. M., Hung, W., and Kyle, M.: Incidence of thyrocytotoxic factor and other antithyroid antibodies in the mothers of cretins. New Eng. J. Med., 267:376, 1962.

Charles, D., Harkness, R. A., Kenny, F. M., Menini, E., Ismail, A. A. A., Durkin, J. W., and Loraine, J. A.: Steroid excretion patterns in an adrenalectomized woman during three successive pregnancies. Amer. J. Obstet. Gynec., 106:66, 1970.

Childs, B., Grumbach, M. M., and Van Wyk, J. J.: Virilizing adrenal hyperplasia; genetic and hormonal study. J. Clin. Invest., 35:213, 1956.

Conn, J. W., and Fajans, S. S.: The prediabetic state; a concept of dynamic resistance to a genetic diabetogenic influence. Amer. J. Med., 31:839, 1961.

Cope, O., and Raker, J. W.: Cushing's disease; surgical experience in the care of 46 cases. New Eng. J. Med., 253:119, 1955.

Crooke, A. C.: Change in basophil cells of pituitary gland common to conditions which exhibit the syndrome attributed to basophil adenoma. J. Path. Bact., 41:339, 1935.

Cushing, H.: The basophil adenomas of the pituitary body and their clinical manifestations (pituitary basophilism). Bull. Johns Hopkins Hosp., 50:137, 1932.

Cushing, H.: "Dyspituitarism"; 20 years later with special consideration of the pituitary adenomas. A.M.A. Arch. Intern. Med., 51:487, 1933.

Driscoll, S. G.: The pathology of pregnancy complicated by diabetes mellitus. Med. Clin. N. Amer., 49:1053, 1965.

Echt, C. R., and Doss, J. F.: Myxedema in pregnancy. Report of 3 cases. Obstet. Gynec., 22:615, 1963.

Escamilla, R. F., and Lisser, H.: Simmonds' disease; clinical study with review of literature; differentiation from anorexia nervosa by statistical analysis of 595 cases, 101 which were proved pathologically. J. Clin. Endocr., 2:65, 1942.

Faber, H. K.: The adrenogenital syndrome, salt-losing type; case reports of two males with prolonged observation since birth. Pediatrics, 20:488, 1957.

Forbes, A. P., and Albright, F.: Comparison of 17-ketosteroid excretion in Cushing's syndrome associated with adrenal tumor and with adrenal hyperplasia. J. Clin. Endocr., 11:926, 1951.

Forbes, A. P., Henneman, P. H., Griswold, G. C., and Albright, F.: Syndrome characterized by galactor-rhea, amenorrhea and low urinary FSH. J. Clin. Endocr., 14:265, 1954.

Freedberg, I. M., Hamolsky, M. W., and Freedberg, A. S.: The thyroid gland in pregnancy. New Eng. J. Med., 256:505, 551, 1957.

Gemmell, A. A.: Phaeochromocytoma and the obstetrician. J. Obstet. Gynaec. Brit. Emp., 62:195, 1955.

Gillespie, L., White, P., and Driscoll, S.: The interrelationship of microvascular disease in diabetes and pregnancy. Diabetes, 12:364, 1963.

Gordon, R. D., Fishman, L. M., and Liddle, G. W.: Plasma renin activity and aldosterone secretion in a pregnant woman with primary aldosteronism. J. Clin. Endocr., 27:385, 1967.

Graham, W. P., III., Gordan, G. S., Loken, H. F., Blum, A., and Halden, A.: Effect of pregnancy and of the menstrual cycle on hypoparathyroidism. J. Clin. Endocr., 24:512, 1964.

Greenblatt, R. B., Carmona, N., and Hagler, W. S.: Chiari-Frommel syndrome. Obstet. Gynec., 7:165, 1956.

Greep, R. O.: Architecture of the final common pathway to the adenohypophysis. Fertil. Steril., 14:153, 1963.

Hendee, A. E., Martin, R. D., and Waters, W. C., III: Hypertension in pregnancy: Toxemia or pheochromocytoma? Amer. J. Obstet. Gynec., 105:64, 1969.

Henderson, W. R.: Sexual dysfunction in adenomas of the pituitary body. Endocrinology, 15:111, 1931.

Herbst, A. L., and Selenkow, H. A.: Combined antithyroid-thyroid therapy of hyperthyroidism in pregnancy. Obstet. Gynec., 21:5, 1963.

Herbst, A. L., and Selenkow, H. A.: Hyperthyroidism during pregnancy. New Eng. J. Med., 273:627, 1965.

Hillman, D. A., Scriver, C. R., Pedvis, S., and Shragovitch, I.: Neonatal familial primary hyperparathyroidism. New Eng. J. Med., 270:483, 1964.

Hills, A. G., Venning, E. H., Dohan, F. C., Webster, G. D., Jr., and Richardson, E. M.: Pregnancy and adrenocortical function; endocrine studies of pregnancy occurring in two adrenal-deficient women. J. Clin. Invest., 33:1466, 1954.

Hubbell, J. P., Jr., Muirhead, D. M., and Drorbaugh, J. E.: The newborn infant of the diabetic mother. Med. Clin. N. Amer., 49:1035, 1965.

Israel, S. L., and Conston, A. S.: Unrecognized pituitary necrosis (Sheehan's syndrome); a cause of sudden death. J.A.M.A., 148:189, 1952.

Jailer, J. W., Longson, D., and Christy, N. P.: Cushing's syndrome—an adrenal or pituitary disease? J. Clin. Endocr., 16:1276, 1956.

Josimovich, J. B., and Atwood, B. L.: Human placental lactogen (HPL), a trophoblastic hormone synergizing with chorionic gonadotropin and potentiating the anabolic effects of pituitary growth hormone. Amer. J. Obstet. Gynec., 88:867, 1964.

Kreines, K., Perin, E., and Salzer, R.: Pregnancy in Cushing's syndrome. J. Clin. Endocr., 24:75, 1964.

Little, B., Smith, O. W., Jessiman, A. G., Selenkow, H. A., Van't Hoff, W., Eglin, J. M., and Moore, F. D.: Hypophysectomy during pregnancy in a patient with cancer of the breast; case report with hormone studies. J. Clin. Endocr., 18:425, 1958.

Ludwig, G. D.: Hyperparathyroidism in relation to pregnancy. New Eng. J. Med., 267:637, 1962.

Malins, J. M., and FitzGerald, M. G.: Childbearing prior to recognition of diabetes; recollected birth weights and stillbirth rate in babies born to parents who developed diabetes. Diabetes, 14:175, 1965.

Maloney, J. M.: Pheochromocytoma in pregnancy;

cesarean section and adrenalectomy. New Eng. J. Med., 253:242, 1955.

McKenzie, J. M.: Review: pathogenesis of Graves' disease: role of the long-acting thyroid stimulator. J. Clin. Endocr., 25:424, 1965.

Melicow, M. M., and Cahill, G. F.: Role of adrenal cortex in somatosexual disturbances in infants and children; a clinico-pathologic analysis. J. Clin. Endocr., 10:24, 1950.

Mori, N., and Miyakawa, I.: Congenital adrenogenital syndrome and successful pregnancy. Report of a case. Obstet. Gynec., 35:394, 1970.

Ocampo, P. T., Coseriu, V. G., and Quilligan, E. J.: Comparison of standard oral glucose-tolerance test in normal pregnancy. Obstet. Gynec., 24:580, 1964.

O'Sullivan, J. B.: Gestational diabetes. New Eng. J. Med., 264:1082, 1961.

O'Sullivan, J. B., Gellis, S. S., Dandrow, R. V., and Tenney, B. O.: The potential diabetic and her treatment in pregnancy. Obstet. Gynec., 27:683, 1966.

de Paiva, L. M., Lobo, J. I., and da Silva, A. M.: Menarche and pregnancy after removal of an adrenocortical adenoma. J. Clin. Endocr., 11:330, 1951.

Pederson, L. M., Tygstrup, I., and Pederson, J.: Congenital malformations in newborn infants of diabetic women. Correlation with maternal diabetic vascular complications. Lancet, 1:1124, 1964.

Plotz, C. M., Knowlton, A. I., and Ragan, C.: The natural history of Cushing's syndrome. Amer. J. Med., 13:597, 1952.

Rankin, J. S., Goldfarb, A. F., and Rakoff, A. E.: Galactorrhea-amenorrhea syndromes: Postpartum galactorrhea-amenorrhea in the absence of intracranial neoplasm. Obstet. Gynec., 33:1, 1969.

Schneider, G. T., Weed, J. C., and Bowers, C. Y.: Pregnancy and delivery after bilateral adrenalectomy for Cushing's syndrome. Obstet. Gynec., 10:437, 1957.

Sheehan, H. L.: Simmonds's disease due to postpartum necrosis of anterior pituitary. Quart. J. Med., 8:277, 1939.

Sheehan, H. L.: The frequency of post-partum hypopituitarism. J. Obstet. Gynaec. Brit. Comm., 72:103, 1965.

Sheehan, H. L., and Murdoch, R.: Post-partum necrosis of anterior pituitary; pathological and clinical aspects. J. Obstet. Gynaec. Brit. Emp., 45:456, 1938.

Silverstone, F. A., Solomons, E., and Rubricus, J.: The rapid intravenous glucose tolerance test in obstetrical patients with a family history of diabetes. Diabetes, 12:356, 1963.

Simmonds, M.: Über embolische Prozesse in der Hypophysis. Virchow Arch. Path. Anat., 217:226, 1914.

Spain, A. W., and Geoghegan, F.: Diabetes insipidus in association with postpartum pituitary necrosis (report of two cases). J. Obstet. Gynaec. Brit. Emp., 53:223, 1946.

Spellacy, W. N., and Goetz, F. C.: Insulin antibodies in pregnancy. Lancet, 2:222, 1963.

Spellacy, W. N., Goetz, F. C., Greenberg, B. Z., and Ells, J.: Plasma insulin in normal midpregnancy. Amer. J. Obstet. Gynec., 92:11, 1965.

Steinberg, A. G.: Heredity and diabetes. Eugen. Quart., 2:26, 1955.

Veith, F. J., Brooks, J. R., Grigsby, W. P., and Selenkow, H. A.: The nodular thyroid gland and cancer; a practical approach to the problem. New Eng. J. Med., 270:431, 1964.

White, P.: Pregnancy complicating diabetes. In Joslin, E. P., Root, H. F., White, P., and Marble, A., eds.: The Treatment of Diabetes Mellitus, ed. 10. Lea and Febiger, Philadelphia, 1959, p. 704.

Wilkerson, H. L. C., and O'Sullivan, J. B.: A study of glucose tolerance and screening criteria in 732 unselected pregnancies. Diabetes, 12:313, 1963.

Wilkins, L.: The Diagnosis and Treatment of Endocrine Disorders in Childhood and Adolescence, ed. 3. Charles C Thomas, Springfield, Ill., 1965.

Wilkins, L., Lewis, R., Klein, R., Gardner, L., Crigler, J., Rosenberg, E., and Migeon, C.: Treatment of congenital adrenal hyperplasia with cortisone. J. Clin. Endocr., 11:1, 1951.

Wilson, R. B., and Keating, F. R.: Pregnancy following treatment of congenital adrenal hyperplasia with cortisone. Amer. J. Obstet. Gynec., 76:388, 1958.

DISORDERS OF THE HEMATOPOIETIC SYSTEM

The commonest diseases of the hematopoietic system encountered during pregnancy are those of the erythron (mature and immature red cells). Less rarely seen are those involving the leukocyte, the reticuloendothelial tissue, and the clotting mechanism.

DISORDERS OF THE ERYTHRON

In a high proportion of abnormalities of the red cell, the anemias and the disease entity can be characterized and classified on morphologic grounds. However, a wide variety of causes can result in the same morphologic picture. For example, in a normocytic anemia the red cells are normal in size and hemoglobin content but deficient in number. Such an anemia may occur as the result of acute blood loss or a hemolytic episode, as through failure of bone marrow function (aplastic anemia) from a host of causes. Also, in the case of blood loss unless the blood volume is restored to normal the resultant normocytic anemia in the absence of iron therapy may change to a microcytic hypochromic anemia. For at least these reasons the anemias have been classified on etiologic grounds in order to correlate more closely the factors responsible for the disease, the morphologic findings, and the therapy. An etiologic classification of anemias (Moore modified) is presented and will be employed in the discussion.

I. Anemia due to blood loss, acute or chronic, internal or external
II. Anemia due to impaired production of red cells
  A. Nutritional deficiencies
    1. Iron
    2. Megaloblastic anemia of pregnancy
  B. Aplastic anemias
III. Anemia due to excessive destruction of red cells
  A. Abnormalities of the red cell
    1. Thalassemia
    2. Hemoglobinopathies
      a. Sickle cell disease
      b. Sickle cell—hemoglobin C disease
  B. Causes other than red cell abnormalities
    1. Coombs-positive acquired hemolytic anemia
    2. Hereditary spherocytosis
    3. Thrombocytopenic purpura
    4. Thrombotic thrombocytopenic purpura

The incidence of anemia in pregnancy varies from area to area and depends largely on the economic and nutritional status of the population and the ethnic group served. The reported incidence depends to some extent on definitions of anemia in local usage.

Anemia is present when the hemoglobin concentration is below 10 to 10.5 grams per 100 ml. and the hematocrit is below 34 per cent. Equally good reasons have been presented for defining anemia as characterized by a hemoglobin concentration below 12 grams per 100 ml. and a hematocrit below 36 per cent.

Iron-Deficiency Anemia

Iron-deficiency anemia is substantially more prevalent in females than in males, reflecting a loss in body iron with each normal menses of 20 to 30 mg. or, with frequent pregnancies, with the repetitive fetal demands for iron, and, on occasion, excessive blood loss associated with a complication of pregnancy or delivery.

To recapitulate, during pregnancy the increased maternal red cell mass and the fetus each require 400 mg. of iron, for a total of 800 mg., taxing the maternal iron stores, which are normally 1000 mg. Provided the blood loss at delivery is not excessive, the mother usually recovers most of the

iron assigned to meet the demands of the increase in red cell mass, and so this represents only a temporary withdrawal from her iron stores. Iron absorption may be increased from the usual 0.5 to 1.5 mg. or more daily, although in some patients the rate of iron absorption is unchanged, thus increasing the hazard of an iron-deficiency anemia. The bone marrow is more cellular in the latter part of normal pregnancy and during the first few days post partum suggesting it is responding to the erythropoietic demands.

Through serial determinations of the plasma volume, the total hemoglobin, and the calculated red cell mass, it has been demonstrated that an iron-deficiency anemia in pregnancy becomes progressively worse as the pregnancy advances. Further, when the peripheral blood findings reveal an iron-deficiency anemia, the iron stores must be at least moderately depleted and this fact has been substantiated by a limited number of estimations of hemosiderin content of aspirated bone marrow. More important clinically is the fact that an iron-deficiency anemia of early pregnancy means that if supplementary iron is not administered the iron stores will be nearly exhausted by the increased fetal demands for iron in the last trimester. Recent evidence suggests that the fetus will fill its iron stores at the expense of the mother, who may be severely iron-deficient.

Except for fatigue, which is a common complaint of normal pregnancy, the anemia patient may be free of symptoms until the hemoglobin falls below 8 or 9 grams per 100 ml. In fact, in the pregnant patient who has a longstanding iron-deficiency anemia, dyspnea or other expected symptoms may not be apparent when the hemoglobin is 5 grams or less. Usually, however, when the anemia reaches this severity, besides pallor there is palpitation and a sensation of numbness and tingling of the extremities.

The diagnosis of iron-deficiency anemia depends on familiar hematologic tests of hemoglobin and hematocrit readings, peripheral blood smears, and erythrocyte indices. Serum iron values normally are lower in pregnancy. (See Normal Changes in Chapter 11). It must be realized that an iron-deficiency anemia may be masked by a megaloblastic anemia, and after the latter is corrected an iron-deficiency anemia may be revealed by a low serum iron and a reduction in the iron-staining granules in the reticuloendothelial cells.

The treatment of an iron deficiency depends to a degree on the stage of pregnancy at which the anemia is discovered. Iron given orally will correct the deficiency in nearly all patients. The exceptions include the few patients who fail to respond to iron in this form, in which event iron must be given parenterally. Before the oral use of iron is abandoned, if time permits, ascorbic acid and hydrochloric acid, because of their capacity to maintain iron in a reduced state, $(Fe)++$, should be added to the treatment to enhance iron absorption. In patients who are near term (34 weeks or beyond), where there is insufficient time to correct the anemia, recourse to transfusions may be indicated.

After a week of iron therapy, the hemoglobin values begin to rise, in some instances as much as 1 gram a week with a reticulocytosis; assuming an initial hemoglobin of 8 grams, to correct the anemia means the formation of approximately 300 grams of new hemoglobin. Since 3.5 mg. of iron is needed to form 1 gram of hemoglobin and assuming that the patient is some eight weeks from term, this means that about 150 mg. of iron must be absorbed weekly. Apparently the body will absorb 20 to 60 mg. daily in a severe iron-deficiency anemia. On the basis that some 10 per cent of iron ingested is absorbed, 200 to 400 mg. must be administered daily. Although the blood values may be restored within a matter of weeks, several months of iron therapy are required after delivery before the iron stores are reconstituted. Recourse to parenteral therapy may be necessary, because some 5 per cent of pregnant patients fail to respond to oral iron therapy. Whether or not these patients have depressed bone marrow function from chronic infection (e.g.,, asymptomatic bacteriuria) is perhaps worthy of consideration.

Megaloblastic Anemia of Pregnancy

A macrocytic anemia, at one time referred to as a pernicious-like anemia of pregnancy but now called a megaloblastic anemia of pregnancy, appears to be a separate entity, for it begins in pregnancy, undergoes remission with delivery, and tends to recur in subsequent pregnancies.

Pregnancy places a markedly increased demand on folate requirements, perhaps in some instances as much as ten-fold. Blood folate levels normally may rise above those of the nonpregnant in the first and second trimester and fall in the last trimester to somewhere near initial values. They are reduced below normal nonpregnant values in macrocytic anemia.

It has been demonstrated that a macrocytic anemia will develop some 20 weeks after the subject has been on a folate-deficient diet. In pregnancy this may occur in half the period of time, as observed in two patients by the writer. The point is, given the circumstance that may lead to a folate deficiency, a macrocytic anemia may develop rapidly in pregnancy.

A macrocytic anemia most commonly may result from an inadequate folate intake from diets poor in vegetables and from overcooking of vegetables. This type of anemia may be encountered in prolonged hyperemesis gravidarum. The anemia may develop in a malabsorption syndrome from whatever cause. The action of antimetabolites such as methotrexate and aminopterin and possibly Dilantin may give rise to a folate deficiency.

Macrocytic anemia is commonly associated with hemoglobinopathies, in which the folate demands are further increased by the accelerated erythropoiesis. Thus, in areas where food is in scant supply and hemoglobinopathies are frequent, macrocytic anemia is common, and in some areas of the world 20 per cent of the maternal deaths are associated with this form of anemia.

Although regarded as infrequent in this country, when a careful search is made macrocytic anemia is more common than is ofttimes appreciated. Reports of the incidence have ranged from 1 in 40 to 1 in 200 or more pregnancies.

The signs and symptoms are similar to those of other severe anemias, namely, dyspnea, tachycardia, and, in this instance, weakness, but rarely pallor. Fever is sometimes present, and the gastrointestinal complaints are often as marked as those complicating an addisonian pernicious anemia. However, the glossitis is less severe and neurologic changes are absent. The onset of the anemia is generally insidious, with the initial signs and symptoms appearing in the last trimester. But as indicated above, rapidly developing severe cases of macrocytic anemia have been encountered.

The diagnosis of megaloblastic anemia of pregnancy is based on serum and red cell folate activity, neutrophil hypersegmentation, formiminoglutamic acid excretion (FIGLU), and status of bone marrow erythropoiesis. The hematocrit is often less than 25 per cent. Serum iron values are high (100 to 300 mcg. per 100 ml.), but, again, because iron deficiency and megaloblastic anemia may coexist, the latter is not necessarily excluded by the finding of a low serum iron. The blood smear reveals the red cell pattern of a macrocytic anemia, and sometimes the characteristic megaloblast is seen. However, when the megaloblast is detected in the blood or bone marrow, it is still necessary to exclude addisonian pernicious anemia. Serum levels of vitamin B_{12} will differentiate between a macrocytic anemia due to folic acid deficiency and an addisonian pernicious anemia, the serum levels of vitamin B_{12} in the latter being less than 100 mcg. per 100 ml. of blood. All too frequently it is not until the patient has failed to respond to iron therapy that further search reveals the true nature of the underlying hematopoietic disorder.

Since it was demonstrated that tropical macrocytic anemia, seen in both pregnant and nonpregnant persons, could be reproduced in the rhesus monkey by feeding a diet similar to that of patients suffering from this form of anemia, the question was raised whether tropical macrocytic anemia and pernicious anemia of pregnancy might be somehow related. Indeed, it was proposed that the macrocytic anemia in pregnancy was the result of a dietary deficiency and not a conditioned food deficiency as is addisonian pernicious anemia. Further evidence to support this concept was furnished by the difference in hematopoietic response to refined and crude liver extract in the experimental animal and pregnant patients with tropical macrocytic anemia, in contrast to patients with addisonian anemia. Whereas crude liver extract caused a sustained remission in both tropical macrocytic and addisonian anemia, refined liver extract, highly effective in addisonian anemia, failed to elicit a hematopoietic response in tropical macrocytic anemia. The antianemia deficiency of refined liver extract was designated the Wills factor, which subsequent studies have shown is probably identical with pteroylglutamic or folic acid.

Unlike addisonian pernicious anemia, in which the response to vitamin B_{12} (extrinsic factor) is completely effective, in macrocytic anemia of pregnancy normal hematopoiesis is rarely stimulated by vitamin B_{12}, even in large doses. By contrast, there is a uniformly favorable response to folic acid unless there is a coexisting vitamin C deficiency.

Some instances have been reported in which the disorder remained refractory with continued treatment and improvement failed to occur until after delivery. With the identification and purification of substances that are specific for the treatment of the various forms of macrocytic anemia, such cases should no longer be encountered. The specific treatment is folic acid and the dosage is in excess of daily needs from 5.0 to 15.0 mg. per day. A dramatic hematopoietic response follows, with a precipitous drop in serum iron and a reticulocytosis of 10 to 20 per cent (a five- to ten-fold increase) in two or three days. When vomiting is a symptom, parenteral administration of folic acid is required.

It may be concluded that this form of anemia, although not far removed from nutritional macrocytic anemia, sprue, and tropical macrocytic anemia, deserves to be retained as a separate entity, that is, megaloblastic or macrocytic anemia of pregnancy. This is buttressed by the fact that there is spontaneous remission with delivery regardless of therapy. The anemia differs from addisonian anemia by the presence of gastric hydrochloric acid, by the absence of combined systemic disease, by the failure to respond in any appreciable degree to vitamin B_{12}, and by the fact that the serum levels of this vitamin are normal.

Pregnancy usually terminates successfully in these patients if they receive the proper hematologic and obstetric care. There is some controversy as to whether or not the newborn will be afflicted with a macrocytic anemia. It may occur apparently, but rarely, for the placenta appears to have the ability to transport to the fetus folate in amounts to satisfy its needs in the face of a marked maternal deficiency. Finally, despite many excellent studies in recent years, a controversy continues as to whether folate deficiency may be a causative factor in abortion, abruptio placentae, hypertensive pregnancy, and malformations. Most recent evidence fails to substantiate earlier claims and no correlation can be clearly established between folate deficiency and the above-listed pregnancy complications.

Aplastic Anemia

Aplastic anemia in pregnancy has a poor record. Although pregnancy has been negotiated successfully, marked improvement has been noted following therapeutic abortion. Hence, the interruption of pregnancy is strongly advised unless the patient is near term when the diagnosis is initially established.

ANEMIAS DUE TO EXCESSIVE DESTRUCTION OF RED CELLS

Faulty erythropoiesis may result from a genetic disturbance in hemoglobin synthesis. It has long been known that there are two forms of hemoglobin, fetal (Hgb F) and adult (Hgb A). Since Pauling and his collaborators demonstrated by electrophoresis that the erythrocyte of sickle cell anemia contains a hemoglobin peculiar to this disease (Hgb S), many different forms of hemoglobin have subsequently been identified, some with clinical significance, but all being important as they relate to biochemical genetics and molecular disease. These different hemoglobins have anthropologic connotations as well, serving as a means of tracing the origin of various racial groups. In addition to Hgb S, those which are clinically important are Hgb C, to a lesser degree Hgb D and Hgb E, and possibly Hgb G and Hgb H.

It is now appreciated also that the adult hemoglobin molecule is composed of two components, Hgb A$_1$ and Hgb A$_2$. Replacement or substitution of one or both of these components is responsible for certain of the hemolytic anemias. When through inheritance from one parent an abnormal form replaces a portion of the normal hemoglobin molecule, the syndrome is regarded as a trait. In this heterozygotic state the hemoglobin molecule contains more than 50 per cent of the normal adult form, and the patient may not exhibit an anemia or associated symptoms. In the homozygotic state, in which an abnormal hemoglobin is inherited from each parent, the individual

will acquire an anemia or the disease with its clinical manifestations. For example, in the case of sickle cell anemia, or sickle cell disease as it is sometimes called, the adult hemoglobin of the red cell may be completely replaced by Hgb S. Also, there are mixed forms of hereditary anemias, such as sickle cell–hemoglobin C disease. Finally, in a hereditary hemolytic disease, such as thalassemia, the erythrocytes may contain fetal hemoglobin in varying amounts.

Thalassemia (Mediterranean Anemia, Cooley's Anemia)

This disease is genetically determined and, as indicated by one of its names, was formerly thought to be found only in people of Mediterranean heritage. Actually it is encountered in people from the Mediterranean area eastward, including India and other Eastern countries. The incidence of the anemia will vary with the ethnic group studied.

The disease is characterized by increased hemolysis of the red cell believed to be due to a disturbance in hemoglobin synthesis and red cell formation. The cells are chiefly microcytic and hypochromic, but target cells and "potato chip" cells may be found. There may be anisocytosis and reticulocytosis, and nucleated red cells are seen in peripheral blood. Hemoglobin concentrations below 9 grams per 100 ml. and hematocrits of 20 per cent or less are frequently observed. There is a diminished survival time of the erythrocytes. As expected, the bone marrow is overly active in its efforts to combat the anemia.

This disease is often included in anemias associated with abnormal hemoglobins. This is based on the findings of unusually large amounts of fetal hemoglobin and A$_2$ hemoglobin in some patients with pure thalassemia. However, the abnormality consists in these *normal* hemoglobins being present in abnormal quantities and beyond the early months of life. In some cases the fetal hemoglobin may represent nearly the total amount of hemoglobin.

Extensive studies have indicated that the pattern of inheritance in this disease is through a single abnormal genetic factor in patients with thalassemia minor and that thalassemia major is characterized by two abnormal alleles. More recent studies that have clarified the geographic distribution of this disease have led to the suggestion that forms intermediate in hematologic and clinical manifestations between the major and the minor exist and that they are associated with several genetic factors rather than with a single pair of alleles. Thalassemia may be inherited along with other genetic conditions, resulting in a variety of disorders in combination, such as sickle cell–thalassemia disease.

Clinically, patients with thalassemia major (the homozygous state) are usually recognized early in life. The disease is frequently fatal in childhood and unless vigorously treated few patients survive to enter the reproductive years. Patients with thalassemia minor (the heterozygous state) are commonly free of symptoms. Pregnancy does impose a hazard for patients with the minor form, for hemolysis and anemia may occur for the first time and may recur intermittently throughout pregnancy.

The signs and symptoms are chiefly those of chronic severe anemia and associated cardiorespiratory changes. Physical examination of patients with thalassemia major reveals splenomegaly. X-ray examination of the skull characteristically reveals widening of the medullary portions of bone containing active marrow and thinning of the cortical bone.

Examination of the peripheral blood shows predominantly hypochromicity in microcytic cells of unusual shapes. The cells may be so poorly and irregularly filled with hemoglobin that only a thin rim of hemoglobin can be seen. Although morphologic similarities exist between the blood smears in thalassemia and those in iron-deficiency anemia, the disorders can be distinguished by using other laboratory aids. In thalassemia the serum may contain excessive amounts of bilirubin, and iron is always normal or increased. The peripheral blood may contain up to 10 per cent reticulocytes.

Treatment during pregnancy consists entirely of replacement of blood by transfusion, employing packed cells in some instances. No other form of therapy has been found effective. Since multiple transfusions can lead to hemosiderosis and its possible complications, they should be reserved for use during particular crises or when the hemoglobin falls to 8 grams or below. Removal of the spleen has been followed by improvement, and this procedure should be performed at a technically appropriate time.

Sickle Cell Anemia and Sickle Cell–Hemoglobin C Disease

In its homozygous form (Hgb S–Hgb S) it is referred to as sickle cell anemia, or sickle cell disease, and in the heterozygous form (Hgb S–Hgb A) it is known as the sickle cell trait. In addition, cognizance must be given to sickle cell–hemoglobin C disease (Hgb S–Hgb C), which often first comes to light under the stress of pregnancy. The precise type of sicklemia is established by identification of the various hemoglobins contained in the hemoglobin molecule by electrophoretic studies.

Although Hgb S has been considered to be genetically confined to the Negro, the S gene may well have originated in the Middle East, being carried by migration to many areas of the world. Hgb C gene appears to have its highest incidence in parts of West Africa. Patients with the heterozygous Hgb C trait (i.e., Hgb C, A_1 or A_2) rarely have symptoms. By contrast, in patients with homozygous Hgb C disease, in which the erythrocytes contain increased amounts of Hgb F and no Hgb A_1, the symptoms may resemble those of mild sickle cell anemia. A more serious disorder occurs when the individual inherits both Hgb C and Hgb S. Indeed, earlier experiences suggested that the maternal and fetal risks exceeded those recorded in patients with sickle cell disease.

A history of episodes of malaise and abdominal and bone pain, combined with the clinical findings of fever, tachycardia, pallor, and jaundice (hemolytic crisis), and sometimes leg ulcers, should arouse the suspicion of sickle cell disease. The finding of classic sickle cells in preparations of peripheral blood confirms the diagnosis. Sickling of the erythrocytes is seen whenever there is a lowering of the oxygen tension, as in the capillaries, and is thought to result from a fundamental rearrangement in the components of the hemoglobin molecule. Besides causing a hemolytic crisis, such sickling is seemingly related to pulmonary, cerebral, and splenic infarction, which are further complications of this disease. Bone changes, as seen on x-ray examination, are many and varied. There are areas of sclerosis within the long bones, the result of infarction.

Patients with sickle cell disease and sickle cell–hemoglobin C disease are particularly susceptible to infection, and are thought to have an increased incidence of pregnancy toxemia. Blood transfusions are required to combat the anemia, and even a mild infection should be treated vigorously with antibiotics and chemotherapeutic agents.

An anemia may develop rapidly with destruction of red cells and their sequestration in the liver and spleen. An associated megaloblastic anemia and the scourge of malaria adds to the maternal and fetal risk, particularly in the areas of the world where sickle cell disease is prevalent. When the hemoglobin drops by more than 2 grams per 100 ml. in 24 hours or to below 6 grams per 100 ml., exchange transfusion with normal blood has been advocated. Folic acid and antimalarial therapy is administered on indication.

Barring any unforeseen obstetric complication, the spontaneous onset of labor is awaited and pelvic delivery effected. However, the labor and delivery must be relatively normal; otherwise, cesarean section should be considered. Also, the choice of anesthesia is important, the conduction type being preferred, with avoidance of maternal hypoxia at all costs.

The perinatal mortality is influenced in no small measure by the care of the patient during pregnancy. Prematurity is a threat but the incidence of malformations is not increased in patients with sickle cell and sickle cell–Hgb C disease.

Interruption of pregnancy for sickle cell disease is only rarely indicated, but occasionally other serious medical disorders complicate the condition, making the continuation of pregnancy a decided hazard. In some patients the control of childbearing is advisable, particularly in those with sickle cell–hemoglobin C disease, which emphasizes the desirability of identifying the abnormal variety present in the hemoglobin molecule of the patient in question.

Coombs-Positive Acquired Hemolytic Anemias

These disorders are characterized by shortened life span of the patient's own or normal transfused red cells. These patients have long been known to have hemolysins in their sera, and the antiglobulin test of Coombs further demonstrated that the red cells are coated with a protein substance with many characteristics of an antibody. These hemolytic disorders may be primary (idiopathic) or they may be associated with diseases such as chronic lymphatic leukemia, lymphoma, and lupus erythematosus. The clinical course is varied and unpredictable but the condition is frequently made worse by surgery, trauma, severe infections, and pregnancy. The diagnosis is made principally on the basis of the Coombs antiglobulin test, although a variety of immunologic techniques may be required in the elucidation of the problem.

Treatment depends mainly on corticosteroid therapy or ACTH. Splenectomy is advisable in patients who fail to respond to endocrine therapy, and apparently this can safely be performed during pregnancy. Transfusions are avoided whenever possible because donor cells may be rapidly hemolyzed and the hazards of further sensitizing the patient appear to be great. When performed, transfusions should be carefully controlled; any evidence of hemolysis indicates incompatibility and the transfusion should be stopped. On the possibility that the anemia is the result of an autoimmune disease, the newborn conceivably might be temporarily afflicted.

Congenital Hemolytic Anemia

This condition, also called hereditary spherocytosis, has been encountered in pregnancy. Examination of the blood reveals evidence of hemolysis and the microcytic cells are extremely susceptible to hypotonic solutions. A hemolytic crisis requires vigorous treatment with blood transfusions. Splenectomy leads to improvement in a high proportion of cases. The results are so striking that splenectomy, if it is technically feasible, should be performed during pregnancy.

Nonspherocytic congenital hemolytic anemias are mentioned because they may be induced by drugs, such as primaquine, to which the patient is sensitive. A well known biochemical defect in these disorders is a deficiency of glucose 6-phosphate dehydrogenase which results in a shortened life span of the red cells. Other enzyme deficiencies are less well characterized.

OTHER BLOOD DYSCRASIAS

Thrombotic Thrombocytopenic Purpura (Purpura Hemorrhagica, Moschcowitz's Disease)

This condition is characterized by purpuric lesions associated with thrombocytopenia, hemolytic anemia, and severe and seemingly unrelated symptoms of central nervous system involvement. The anemia is normochromic and normocytic. Although a few nonpregnant women with this disease have survived, when this complication is encountered during pregnancy rarely if ever does the patient survive. In the differential diagnosis it is well to recall that a similar clinical picture may be seen in severe pregnancy toxemia. Indeed, it can well mimic pregnancy toxemia with the correct diagnosis being made only at autopsy.

Whatever success is achieved in the management of this profound disorder depends on early diagnosis and intensive therapy employing fresh whole blood exchange transfusions and high doses of ACTH and cortisone. Splenectomy has also been reported to produce a remission. Thus, in the early months of pregnancy splenectomy may be done following exchange transfusions. When the condition is discovered in the later months of pregnancy, when the enlarged uterus interferes with performing splenectomy, the patient should be prepared with transfusions, a cesarean section performed, and then the spleen is removed at the same time. It is the writer's personal view that the patient's chance of survival is dependent on termination of pregnancy.

Thrombocytopenic Purpura

This blood dyscrasia occurs somewhat more frequently in females than in males. Until recent times, the maternal mortality has been reportedly high (10 to 15 per cent), and the fetal mortality, 25 per cent or more. The infants may be temporarily affected by the purpura, accounting in no small measure for the high neonatal death rate. With present-day therapy, the maternal and fetal outlook is much improved. The fact that the fetus may have a transient thrombocytopenia would support the idea of an autoimmune mechanism in the etiology.

The disease in the pregnant patient, as in the nonpregnant, is characterized by spontaneous remissions and exacerbations. The diagnosis is suggested by the appearance of ecchymoses of the skin and mucous membranes, and it is established by the detection of a reduction in blood platelets, a positive tourniquet test, a prolonged bleeding time, and evidence of poor clot retraction. Unusual uterine bleeding at the time of delivery is not a feature of the disease, however, even when the platelet count is low (50,000 or less). In fact, patients with a count of less than 5000 have been delivered successfully. The treatment of thrombocytopenic purpura is the same in the pregnant state as in the nonpregnant, including ample rest, diet, iron, whole blood and platelet transfusions, and splenectomy if it seems indicated. A favorable response, however, does not always follow splenectomy in pregnancy.

Improvement of the disease in pregnancy has followed therapy with ACTH and cortisone. Although the disease will probably not respond dramatically to ACTH or cortisone therapy in each instance during pregnancy, this does not preclude the possibility that the infant will receive some benefit even though the disease fails to improve in the mother.

DISORDERS OF THE CLOTTING MECHANISMS

Bleeding disorders of the hemopoietic system must be considered in the etiology of abnormal uterine bleeding in the nonpregnant patient, but what is most pertinent here is that patients with such disorders may menstruate normally but incur serious postpartum bleeding. Moreover, these patients may bleed in the absence of trauma, presumably from the placental site which in essence is an open wound with a large surface area. Although some patients may be aware that they have a disturbance in the clotting mechanism, the deficiency may announce itself in the third stage of labor.

A systematic exposition in the field of blood coagulation is complicated from the start by continued controversies about the mechanisms involved, particularly the intermediate stages prior to the actual formation of the insoluble fibrin clot. The clotting mechanism as such is not explored here; rather, the discussion is confined to the disorders of special concern to reproduction.

Hemophilia A and Hemophilia B (Classic Hemophilia and Christmas Disease)

In this genetic clotting disorder, the biochemical congenital defect is the inability to synthesize either antihemophilia factor (AHF, hemophilia A) or plasma thromboplastic component (PTC, hemophilia B). These two factors, together with platelets and calcium, are required for blood thromboplastin formation; in short, they form part of the early pathway in the intrinsic system of prothrombin activation. They are not required in the formation of tissue thromboplastin, which accounts for normal prothrombin time usually observed in either type of hemophilia.

The development of more precise means for measuring AHF and PTC has allowed more refined studies to be done in persons with the disease and in those designated as carriers. These studies have shown that hemophilia carriers may have reduced levels of AHF and PTC and, further, that they may rarely have disorders of the clotting mechanism. These findings have been interpreted to mean that the inheritance of hemophilia may be by a mechanism that is only partially recessive.

Individuals who have a family history of the disorder and are contemplating marriage and childbearing are rightly concerned about the expected incidence of clotting difficulties in their children. The following conclusions appear to be justified: Not all hemophilic patients are severely afflicted. Hemophilia A and hemophilia B of comparable reduction in the levels of AHF or PTC will have equally severe clinical manifestations. Perhaps more than a quarter of all hemophiliacs have only mild complaints; the remainder have moderate to severe disease. The severity of hemophilia in a given family tends to be the same from generation to generation. Current concepts indicate that although a hemophiliac with levels of AHF and PTC only 5 per cent of normal may not have spontaneous bleeding, levels over 30 to 40 per cent of normal are required for adequate hemostasis during surgery or in the event of trauma. The

diagnosis of hemophilia is based on the family history and the patient's history of a bleeding tendency. The diagnosis is confirmed by examinations for plasma levels of AHF and PTC.

Pseudohemophilia (von Willebrand's Disease, Vascular Hemophilia)

This is a disease transmitted as an autosomal dominant. The basic biochemical defect in the clotting mechanism in this disorder is an inability to synthesize AHF but the specific mechanism leading to the shortage of AHF is different from that in hemophilia A. This conclusion is reached from the evidence that the infusion of plasma from a patient with hemophilia A into a patient with pseudohemophilia leads to the production of AHF in the pseudohemophilic recipient, whereas the reverse procedure has no effect in the patient with hemophilia A. In this connection, an important observation is that the amount of traumatic bleeding in pseudohemophilia is better related to plasma levels of AHF than it is to alterations in the bleeding time.

Patients with pseudohemophilia present themselves because of epistaxis, menorrhagia, easy bruising, or bruises that seem to arise spontaneously. The bleeding tendency may have variations in severity, for patients with a history of bleeding may go through surgery without incident while others may bleed excessively from minor cuts or abrasions.

The diagnosis of pseudohemophilia is made on the basis of the patient's history and the family history, together with estimates of plasma levels of AHF, or on platelet adhesiveness (PAT). Since levels of AHF may be reduced in both hemophilia A and pseudohemophilia, it may be necessary to measure the response to infusion of hemophilia A plasma or normal serum to distinguish the two conditions. The measurement of platelet adhesiveness has been found useful to make this differentiation even more reliable.

Although excessive uterine bleeding at delivery is reportedly uncommon, the writer can attest to the experience with severe postpartum bleeding in a patient that responded dramatically to the administration of factor VIII. The condition is now manageable and pregnancy need not be contraindicated.

DISORDERS OF THE LEUKOCYTES AND RETICULOENDOTHELIAL TISSUES

The Leukemias

The courses of both acute and chronic leukemias during pregnancy are characterized by exacerbations and remissions. The therapeutic measures used are the same as in nonpregnant patients, with the exception of irradiation therapy which should either be avoided or carefully controlled. There is no conclusive evidence that the use of antimetabolites or steroids has any adverse effect on the fetus if given after the first trimester. Interruption of pregnancy is of little therapeutic benefit.

The immediate prognosis for the fetus of a mother with acute leukemia is poor because of the mother's general debility, and fetal death and premature delivery are very common. By contrast, the immediate outlook for the fetus of a mother with chronic leukemia is somewhat better. Leukemia is not observed in the newborn of leukemic mothers in spite of a variety of factors that might be presumed to permit the gestational passage of the disease. For example, there is a long exposure period and it might be thought that the fetus with its incomplete immunologic mechanism would be readily inoculated by malignant cells. It has further been shown that both normal and leukemic leukocytes pass from mother to fetus. Hence, on the basis of the concordance rate of leukemia among twins it has recently been proposed that the time of origin of childhood leukemia may be the prenatal period.

Hodgkin's Disease

This is the most frequent primary lymph gland disorder encountered during pregnancy. Lymphoma and lymphosarcoma are rare, and because in pregnancy they present the same problems as Hodgkin's disease, only the latter will be considered here.

The etiology of Hodgkin's disease remains completely unknown, although it is suggested that the cause may be viral, or alternatively that the disease may have an immunologic basis. Extension of the idea that Hodgkin's disease may be viral in origin leads to the question of transmission of the disease to the fetus during pregnancy. As in the leukemias, children of mothers with active Hodgkin's disease do not appear to have an increased incidence of the disorder.

The majority of opinion holds the view that pregnancy has little effect on the course of Hodgkin's disease. This is hardly sufficient, and each patient must be individualized. In fact, for some patients, whose disease seems less stable, pregnancy may have an adverse effect. In evaluating the effect of pregnancy on the disease attention must be given to the extent of the disease and how it is to be treated. The disease should be staged in accordance with its extent and location. The answer to the variability of the apparent reaction to Hodgkin's disease may reside in repeated lymph node biopsies for the purpose of determining whether the disease may change from a paragranulomatous to a granulomatous form with its altered prognosis. When the disease is below the diaphragm as well, the question of continuation of pregnancy must be weighed against the form of therapy proposed, namely, x-ray, chemotherapy, or both in combination. Other factors influence the decision regarding therapeutic abortion—the patient's age and parity and the desires of the patient and family.

Transfusion is often required in the management of anemia. Ordinarily an uncomplicated pelvic delivery can be anticipated, although obstructive pelvic lymph node masses may make cesarean section necessary. Because extensive node involvement in the neck and mediastinum may complicate respiration, special care in the choice and administration of anesthetic is essential; tracheal intubation may be required or indeed tracheostomy to overcome upper respiratory obstruction.

Polycythemia Vera

This chronic red cell disease of unknown etiology affects men more than women and the usual age of onset is middle or later life. A familial incidence of the disease has been reported. The disease is characterized by abnormally increased activity of all the cellular elements of the bone marrow, although the red blood cell series is most extensively involved. The most common complication of untreated polycythemia vera is intravascular thrombosis, and this, together with the other clinical manifestations, including headache, paresthesias, ruddy complexion, and skin and mucous membrane hemorrhages, can reasonably be attributed to three factors characteristic of this disease. They are (1) increased blood viscosity as a result of an abnormally high number of erythrocytes per cubic millimeter (2) increased total blood volume, and (3) thrombocytosis.

Pregnancy is rarely encountered in patients with this condition. From the isolated case reports it would appear that a patient with adequate medical management can have a successful pregnancy. The tendency for thrombosis and hemorrhage to occur in the uteroplacental vasculature in this syndrome appears to modify the prognosis for the fetus and favors early delivery, at about the 35th to 37th week of pregnancy.

The management of pregnant patients with polycythemia vera appears to be the same as in the nonpregnant with the exception that irradiation therapy must be omitted.

BIBLIOGRAPHY

Aisenberg, A. C.: Hodgkin's disease; prognosis, treatment, and etiologic and immunologic considerations. New Eng. J. Med., 270:508, 565, 617, 1964.

Aisenberg, A. C.: Primary management of Hodgkin's disease. New Eng. J. Med., 278:93, 1968.

Apthorp, G. H., Measday, B., and Lehmann, H.: Pregnancy in sickle-cell anemia. Lancet, 1:1344, 1963.

Brody, J. I., Goldsmith, M. H., Park, S. K., and Soltys, H. D.: Symptomatic crises of sickle cell anemia treated by limited exchange transfusion. Ann. Intern. Med., 72:327, 1970.

Brown, D. E., and Ober, W. B.: Sickle-cell thalassemia (microdrepanocytic disease) in pregnancy. Amer. J. Obstet. Gynec., 75:773, 1958.

Burt, R. L., and Prichard, R. W.: Acquired hemolytic anemia in pregnancy. Obstet. Gynec., 10:444, 1957.

Castle, W. B.: Erythropoiesis; normal and abnormal. Bull. N. Y. Acad. Med., 30:827, 1954.

Centrone, A. L., Freda, R. N., and McGowan, L.: Polycythemia rubra vera in pregnancy. Obstet. Gynec., 30:657, 1967.

Chanarin, I., Rothman, D., Perry, J., and Stratfull, D.: Normal dietary folate, iron, and protein intake, with particular reference to pregnancy. Brit. Med. J., 2:394, 1968.

Chanarin, I., Rothman, D., Ward, A., and Perry, J.: Folate status and requirement in pregnancy. Brit. Med. J., 2:390, 1968.

Chernoff, A. I.: Human hemoglobins in health and disease. New Eng. J. Med., 253:322, 365, 416, 1955.

Chernoff, A. I.: Distribution of the thalassemia gene; historical review. Blood, 14:899, 1959.

Coopland, A. T., Firesen, W. J., and Galbraith, P. A.: Acute leukemia in pregnancy. Amer. J. Obstet. Gynec., 105:1288, 1969.

Curtis, E. M.: Pregnancy in sickle cell anemia, sickle cell-hemoglobin C disease, and variants thereof. Amer. J. Obstet. Gynec., 77:1312, 1959.

Desai, R. G., and Creger, W. P.: Maternal-fetal passage of leukocytes and platelets in man. Blood, 21:665, 1963.

Diamandopoulos, G. T., and Hertig, A. T.: Transmission of leukemia and allied diseases from mother to fetus. Obstet. Gynec., 21:150, 1963.

Evans, I. L.: Aplastic anaemia in pregnancy remitting after abortion. Brit. Med. J., 3:166, 1968.

Gabuzda, T. G., Nathan, D. G., and Gardner, F. H.: Thalassemia trait. Genetic combinations of increased fetal and A$_2$ hemoglobins. New Eng. J. Med., 270:1212, 1964.

Gaston, L. W.: The blood-clotting factors. New Eng. J. Med., 270:236, 1964.

Giles, C., and Shuttleworth, E. M.: Megaloblastic anaemia of pregnancy and the puerperium. Lancet, 2:7061, 1958.

Hendrickse, J. P. de V., and Watson-Williams, E. J.: The influence of hemoglobinopathies on reproduction. Amer. J. Obstet. Gynec., 94:739, 1966.

Herbert, V.: Experimental nutritional folate deficiency in man. Trans. Ass. Amer. Physicians, 75:307, 1962.

Herbert, V.: Megaloblastic anemia. New Eng. J. Med., 268:201, 1963.

Jonxis, J. H. P.: Hemoglobinopathies. Ann. Rev. Med., 14:297, 1963.

Kitay, D. Z., and Perrin, E. V.: Homozygous hemoglobin C disease and pregnancy. Obstet. Gynec., 32:657, 1968.

Lampkin, B. C., Shore, N. A., and Chadwick, D.: Megaloblastic anemia of infancy secondary to maternal pernicious anemia. New Eng. J. Med., 274:1168, 1966.

Lowenstein, L., and Bramlage, C. A.: Bone marrow in pregnancy and puerperium. Blood, 12:261, 1957.

Lowenstein, L., Pick, C., and Philpott, N.: Megaloblastic anemia of pregnancy and the puerperium. Amer. J. Obstet. Gynec., 70:1309, 1955.

MacMahon, B., and Levy, M. A.: Prenatal origin of childhood leukemia; evidence from twins. New Eng. J. Med., 270:1082, 1964.

May, C. D., Sundberg, R. D., Schoor, I., Lowe, C. U., and Salmon, R. J.: Experimental nutritional megaloblastic anemia; relation to ascorbic acid and pteroylglutamic acid. Amer. J. Dis. Child., 82:282, 1951.

Moore, C. V.: The anemias. In Beeson, P. B., and McDermott, W., eds.: Textbook of Medicine, ed. 13. Philadelphia, W. B. Saunders Co., 1971.

O'Leary, J. A., and Marchetti, A. A.: Thrombotic thrombocytopenic purpura in pregnancy. Amer. J. Obstet Gynec., 83:214, 1962.

Pauling, L.: Abnormality of hemoglobin molecules in hereditary hemolytic anemias. Harvey Lect., 49:216, 1954.

Peterson, O. H., Jr., and Larson, P.: Thrombocytopenic purpura in pregnancy. Obstet. Gynec., 4:454, 1954.

Pritchard, J. A., Whalley, P. J., and Scott, D. E.: The influence of maternal folate and iron deficiencies on intrauterine life. Amer. J. Obstet. Gynec., 104:388, 1969.

Quick, A. J.: Menstruation in hereditary bleeding disorders. Obstet. Gynec., 28:37, 1966.

Ricks, P., Jr.: Exchange transfusion in sickle cell

anemia and pregnancy. Obstet. Gynec., 25:117, 1965.

Rigby, P. G., Hanson, T. A., and Smith, R. S.: Passage of leukemic cells across the placenta. New Eng. J. Med., 271:124, 1964.

Robson, H. U., and Davidson, I. S. P.: Purpura in pregnancy, with special reference to idiopathic thrombocytopenic purpura. Lancet, 2:164, 1950.

Rothberg, H., Conrad, M. E., and Cowley, R. G.: Acute granulocytic leukemia in pregnancy; report of four cases with apparent acceleration by prednisone in one. Amer. J. Med. Sci., 237:194, 1959.

Ruch, W. A., and Klein, R. L.: Polycythemia vera and pregnancy; report of a case. Obstet. Gynec., 23:107, 1964.

Scott, D. E., Whalley, P. J., and Pritchard, J. A.: Maternal folate deficiency and pregnancy wastage; II. Fetal malformation. Obstet. Gynec., 36:26, 1970.

Solomon, W., Turner, D. S., Block, C., and Posner, A. C.: Thrombotic thrombocytopenic purpura in pregnancy. J.A.M.A., 184:587, 1963.

Strauss, H. S., and Bloom, G. E.: Von Willebrand's disease. Use of a platelet-adhesiveness test in diagnosis and family investigation. New Eng. J. Med., 273:171, 1965.

Strauss, H. S., and Diamond, L. L.: Elevation of factor VIII (antihemophilic factor) during pregnancy

in normal persons and in a patient with von Willebrand's disease. New Eng. J. Med., 269:1251, 1963.

Streiff, R. R., and Little, A. B.: Folic acid deficiency in pregnancy. New Eng. J. Med., 276:776, 1967.

Wendt, W. P., and LaFond, D. J.: Pseudohemophilia (von Willebrand's disease) in obstetrics and gynecology. Amer. J. Obstet. Gynec., 83:207, 1962.

Whalley, P. J., Pritchard, J. A., and Richards, J. R., Jr.: Sickle cell trait and pregnancy. J.A.M.A., 186:1132, 1963.

Whalley, P. J., Scott, D. E., and Pritchard, J. A.: Maternal folate deficiency and pregnancy wastage; I. Placental abruption. Amer. J. Obstet. Gynec., 105:670, 1969.

Whalley, P. J., Scott, D. E., and Pritchard, J. A.: Maternal folate deficiency and pregnancy wastage; III. Pregnancy-induced hypertension. Obstet. Gynec., 36:29, 1970.

Wills, L.: Treatment of "pernicious anaemia of pregnancy" and "tropical anaemia." Brit. Med. J., 1:1059, 1931.

Wills, L., Clutterbuck, P. W., and Evans, B. D. F.: New factor in production and cure of macrocytic anaemias and its relation to other haemopoietic principles curative in pernicious anaemia. Biochem. J., 31:2136, 1937.

DISORDERS OF THE URINARY SYSTEM

INFECTIONS

Incidence

Infections of the urinary tract are more prevalent during pregnancy, primarily because of the physiologic changes at this time in the renal pelvis and the ureter, including ureteral dilatation, kinking, and displacement. These changes are exaggerated by the pressure created by rotation and enlargement of the uterus. All of these factors predispose to urinary stasis, the precursor of infection. As in the nonpregnant state, calculi, aberrant blood vessels, and congenital anomalies of the urinary tract play their usual important etiologic roles.

Pathology

Controversy continues with respect to both the extent of the inflammatory process and the origin of acute infections of the urinary tract. The term pyelitis, still commonly used to describe these infections, is undoubtedly a misnomer, for the infection involves the renal parenchyma. Pyelonephritis, acute or chronic, seems a more suitable designation.

Acute pyelonephritis is a diffuse inflammatory process of the interstitial connective tissue of the kidney, with the nephron being involved only when the infection is extensive. Leukocytes and bacteria may be identified in the intertubular connective tissue, in the lymphatics surrounding the glomeruli, and within the tuft itself. On occasion the tubules may contain purulent material, and in rare instances multiple abscesses are scattered throughout the cortex and the medulla. Blood vessels may become damaged in areas where the inflammation is most marked, and deposition of fibrin may be seen within the walls and the lumen of the involved arterioles. In **chronic pyelonephritis,** in addition to the inflammatory changes described, the renal cortex is narrowed from scar tissue formation. Other connective tissue changes consist of fibrosis of Bowman's capsule and an increased thickness of the renal capsule. In the involved scarred areas, arteriolitis similar to the obliterative lesions seen in malignant nephrosclerosis have been described.

In most instances of acute pyelonephritis, the kidney heals without significant scarring or dysfunction. However, should there be recurrent attacks of infection, the disease may enter a chronic phase, producing permanent and progressive renal damage, and culminating in death from resultant hypertensive disease or renal failure. The inflammatory process is rarely blood stream in origin, but rather is ascending from the lower urinary tract.

In more than 75 per cent of the cases the offending organisms in acute pyelonephritis in pregnancy are the coliform group, with the staphylococcal and the streptococcal forms following in that order. It has been nearly four decades since it was reported that bacteriuria without symptoms occurs in otherwise normal pregnant women, with a frequency as high as 15 per cent. The majority of infected patients entering pregnancy would become febrile and develop symptoms consistent with pyelonephritis. More recently, these observations have been substantiated, with asymptomatic bacteriuria being reported in 6 to 8 per cent of all pregnant patients; furthermore, the incidence is established in the first trimester, an important observation in relation to preventive treatment. (See Conduct of Pregnancy, Chapter 23.)

Signs and Symptoms

The severity of the signs and symptoms is dependent to a degree on the extent of the inflammatory process and the type of organism involved. The systemic reaction is usually more profound when *Escherichia coli* is the organism responsible for the infection. In the milder cases the symptoms are often restricted to urinary frequency and urgency, with or without dysuria; the febrile response is minimal, and the kidney is not tender. In the more severe infections, chills, fever, and moderately severe backache are the characteristic symptoms. There is exquisite tenderness in the region of the involved kidney posteriorly, and the organ itself is tender and may be enlarged and palpable on deep inspiration. If there is ureteral obstruction and the intrapelvic pressure is significantly elevated, there may be a temporary decrease in renal function. This is manifested by a modest rise in nonprotein nitrogen. When the toxicity is severe or prolonged, a normocytic anemia may appear, and on occasion there is a precipitous fall in hemoglobin values.

Diagnosis

Diagnosis of urinary tract infection is based on the above clinical findings and is confirmed by the detection of leukocytes in the urine and the identification of bacteria in urine cultures. In the differential diagnosis of pyelonephritis, the condition most frequently considered is appendicitis. During pregnancy the differentiation between these two diseases may offer some difficulty and is at times uncertain. The growing uterus may so displace the cecum and appendix that the referred signs of appendicitis are localized well above the iliac crest, not too far removed from the lower pole of the right kidney. Moreover, a urinary tract infection is not excluded by a negative urinary sediment or culture. Occasionally ureteral blockage from kinking may cause complete urinary stasis, so that pus cells are temporarily absent from the bladder urine. Whenever the diagnosis of appendicitis remains in question, laparotomy is indicated; otherwise an occasional patient with acute appendicitis will fail to receive the benefit of surgery. Also, it must be appreciated that chronic pyelonephritis with marked renal dysfunction may occur in patients whose urine is consistently sterile. (See Hypertensive Pregnancy, Chapter 17.)

Management

The treatment of urinary tract infection begins with prevention, by treating asymptomatic bacteriuria as identified by a free midstream catch specimen of urine. (See Conduct of Pregnancy, Chapter 23.) There is general agreement that the incidence of acute pyelonephritis in the course of pregnancy can thus be reduced substantially.

Whether treating patients with asymptomatic bacteriuria will influence the prematurity rate is not so clearly established. In some series pregnancy did not appear to be affected by the presence of asymptomatic bacteriuria, and the premature rate was not especially different in the treated and the untreated groups. There are other variables in these patients that might influence prematurity, namely, impaired renal function and pregnancy toxemia. As a principle, however, labor may develop with any febrile episode regardless of cause, and hence prophylactic antibacterial therapy is warranted in a patient with asymptomatic bacteriuria to prevent an acute pyelonephritis.

The management of patients with acute

pyelonephritis of pregnancy depends to a degree on the severity of the signs and symptoms. In the more severe forms of acute pyelonephritis, when the patient is vomiting and toxic, she should be hospitalized promptly. On admission, urine is obtained for culture and examination of the urinary sediment, and blood is drawn for a blood culture, a nonprotein nitrogen determination, and studies of the peripheral blood.

The acute urinary infection is treated by forcing fluids, parenterally if vomiting occurs, to a minimum of 3500 ml. daily, with careful charting of the patient's intake and output, and by one or more broad-spectrum antibiotics. Since it is difficult to defer antibacterial therapy until the offending organism has been identified, the agent employed should at least be effective against *Escherichia coli*, which is the common offender. If the organism proves to be other than *E. coli*, the antibiotic therapy is adjusted accordingly, the selection being influenced to a degree by the findings on sensitivity tests. Usually within 48 to 72 hours the acute symptoms subside. When there is kinking of the ureter with blockage, however, the patient may fail to improve. Although it is rarely needed, ureteral catheterization is followed by dramatic improvement. In the extreme, nephrostomy may be necessary to save the kidney. Lack of favorable response and the element of chronicity are more commonly associated with enterococci, *Proteus*, and species of *Pseudomonas*, all of which are more resistant to antibacterial therapy.

Any patient with acute pyelonephritis eventually should have the benefit of at least one intravenous pyelogram to uncover or exclude any pathologic condition of the urinary tract. This examination is best performed three or four months after delivery, by which time the urinary tract will have regained its prepregnancy status.

The problems that relate to the chronicity of pyelonephritis and its effect on subsequent pregnancies and the eventual health of the mother are of the utmost importance. The question is posed, who is to be responsible for the care of patients who have experienced pyelonephritis in pregnancy or who have an asymptomatic bacteriuria? Will it be the internist, the urologist, or the obstetrician? A second question is whether such patients can be permanently cured or whether they are always subject to recurrent urinary tract infection, even though they may be unaware of its presence. Answers to these questions have a relationship to future childbearing and possible longstanding effects on the cardiovascular and renal systems. Approximately 15 to 20 per cent of cases of severe hypertension are due to chronic pyelonephritis, which in many instances began in pregnancy. All too often these patients are the victims of inadequate follow-up after an acute pyelonephritis of pregnancy. It is an example of what constitutes continuity of patient care—or lack of it—in an age of super- or subspecialization.

Although pyelonephritis is not the cause of pregnancy toxemia, as stated above it is a cause of hypertension in pregnant women. Equally significant, in women showing severe renal damage after their childbearing years no correlation can be established between the severity of the acute pyelonephritis at the time of pregnancy and the extent of subsequent renal damage. Thus, even the milder forms of acute pyelonephritis of pregnancy, if not successfully treated, seem capable of producing permanent renal damage and associated vascular disease.

The responsibilities of the obstetrician toward the problems associated with pyelonephritis in pregnancy are clear and definite. First, patients who have experienced an acute pyelonephritis should have a careful urologic and medical workup some three to four months post partum. Roughly one third of these patients will reveal a degree of abnormality of the urinary tract, renal calculi, or some other disorder. Second, the patient should not be permitted to attempt another pregnancy until she has a free interval from her urinary tract infection. Third, the patient should have periodic urologic examinations annually or biannually after her childbearing is completed.

Only by this all-out effort will cardiovascular disease and renal failure from this insidious condition be eliminated.

TUBERCULOSIS OF THE KIDNEY

Tuberculous lesions of the urinary tract may remain dormant for many months or even for years. The criterion of a bacillus-host response, which is useful in caring for patients with pulmonary tuberculosis, seems to be of little value in persons with renal tuberculosis. By its very nature the infection represents an extension of the tuberculosis, for it originates as either a hematogenous dissemination or a spread from a genital lesion.

Ideally, before pregnancy is attempted by a patient with arrested pulmonary tuberculosis, intravenous pyelography, urine culture, and guinea-pig inoculation should be performed to permit evaluation of the condition of the urinary system. During pregnancy, silent tuberculous lesions of the kidney may be reactivated, and any urinary infection that shows chronicity and fails to respond to antibiotics must be viewed with suspicion. The possibility of a tuberculous infection should be considered when a patient exhibits pyuria and the urine culture is negative.

In the pregnant patient with renal tuberculosis, when there is marked destruction of one kidney and the infection in the opposite kidney is minimal or absent, nephrectomy is the treatment of choice. However, the risk of nephrectomy is significantly increased during pregnancy. The circulatory readjustments imposed on the remaining kidney can lead to transient renal insufficiency. Furthermore, the risk of chronic infection with progressive loss of function in the remaining kidney after nephrectomy apparently is greater in the pregnant than in the nonpregnant patient, owing to the normal dilatation of the ureter with subsequent urinary stasis. Therefore, when it is decided to perform nephrectomy in the pregnant patient for renal tuberculosis or other causes, such as miliary abscesses associated with pyelonephritis, in the earlier months it is safer for the patient if the pregnancy is terminated prior to the nephrectomy. When the patient is near term, nephrectomy may be delayed until after delivery. Although pregnancy is not contraindicated following nephrectomy for unilateral renal tuberculous infection, it should be postponed for two or three years. Before conception is attempted, normal renal function must be demonstrated in the remaining kidney and the urine must be sterile.

CALCULI

The greatest significance of renal calculi in pregnancy, whether they are located in the calyces, kidney pelvis, ureter, or bladder, is the possibility that they are associated with chronic infection and renal damage. Their etiology is likewise important: namely, do they represent a single finding or a systemic disease? During the first half of gestation the resulting signs and symptoms are essentially similar to those in the nonpregnant, and include pain, hematuria, and sometimes fever. Following physiologic dilatation of the ureters, however, pain and associated hematuria is much less frequent than in the nonpregnant state. Because pain is often absent during pregnancy, the incidence of calculi may be higher than is generally appreciated. That a stone may be present without symptoms reemphasizes the importance of a complete urologic work-up post partum in patients who have had urinary tract infection during pregnancy.

The treatment of calculous disease varies, depending on the stage of pregnancy and whether or not the urine is infected. If the calculus is detected in the first half of pregnancy, the preferred treatment is surgical removal, preceded by vigorous antibiotic therapy if the urine is infected. In the latter part of pregnancy, the presence of the enlarged uterus adds to the technical difficulty of removal. With normal renal function and with little or no evidence of an infected urine, surgery to remove the stone is best postponed until after delivery. If the urinary infection is severe and fails to respond to antibiotics, renal function may become permanently impaired unless nephrostomy is performed to relieve the infection, with removal of the stone several weeks after delivery. Pregnancy following recovery from urinary calculi offers no unusual problem provided there is no residual renal damage or infection at the time of conception.

SOLITARY KIDNEY

Nephrectomy performed for the treatment of unilateral renal tuberculosis, pyelonephritis with abscess, hydronephrosis, tumor, or congenital anomalies accounts for the majority of cases of solitary kidney seen in pregnancy. The remainder of such patients are those who have a marked unilateral renal hypoplasia or congenital absence of the kidney. These latter anomalies are sometimes discovered incidental to studies of the urinary tract in toxemia or renal infection complicating pregnancy.

In offering an opinion as to the advisability of pregnancy or the continuation of an existing one in a patient with a single kidney, it is necessary to know the indication for, and the time elapsed since, the nephrectomy. When the kidney was removed for tuberculosis, pyelonephritis with miliary abscesses, or infection superimposed on congenital malformations, some time should elapse after the operation before the patient attempts a pregnancy. During the interim, periodic investigations should be made to determine the possible presence of residual infection anywhere in the urinary tract. In the event that infection can be excluded and all renal function tests are normal, pregnancy may be undertaken. There seems to be little difference in prognosis whether the right or the left kidney remains, as long as function is normal and infection is absent. It is most important, however, that the single kidney be in the normal location, for it seems that, even though an ectopic kidney functions normally, it is more vulnerable to infection. If infection of a solitary kidney is detected during the course of pregnancy, unless it responds promptly to aggressive treatment, the pregnancy should be terminated in order to preserve renal function. Frequent prenatal visits and, in the latter weeks of pregnancy, periodic nonprotein nitrogen determinations are in order to identify at the earliest moment failing renal function.

ANOMALIES OF THE URINARY TRACT

In the investigation of urinary tract infection complicating pregnancy, it is not unusual for pyelography to reveal duplication of the ureters and renal pelves, or segmented ureters, horseshoe or fused kidneys, or polycystic or ectopic kidneys. Moreover, when congenital anomalies of the reproductive tract are uncovered, a complete urologic examination should be done, for genitourinary anomalies coexist with sufficient frequency to warrant such an investigation. Unless chronic infection has resulted in renal damage and altered renal function, these types of anomalous changes are unaffected by pregnancy. On the other hand, certain congenital ano-malies, such as horseshoe kidney and polycystic disease of the kidney, are often associated with infection, diminished renal function, or both, and are a serious handicap to the pregnant woman. Patients with these conditions must be carefully evaluated, and, even though prenatal care is optimal, renal insufficiency may develop.

Polycystic disease, with its genetic aspects, has particular relevance during pregnancy. Symptoms may appear initially during this period and the diagnosis may be first established. The adult form is apparently inherited as an autosomal dominant and the infantile form as an autosomal recessive. The variants of this disease are several, with the degree of corticomedullary involvement differing appreciably. Hence, generalizations as to interaction of this disease and pregnancy are perhaps unwarranted.

However, pyelonephritis is a constant threat in these patients with secondary hypertension. Also, cerebral aneurysms are sometimes associated, adding the risk of cerebral hemorrhage in the event of pregnancy. It is evident these patients require careful study and individual evaluation both medically and genetically.

Patients with one normally located kidney and a single ectopic kidney do well during pregnancy; too few are seen with double ectopic kidneys for any conclusions to be drawn. Whether the anomaly is unilateral or bilateral, an ectopic kidney could obstruct the birth canal, making cesarean section necessary for delivery.

GROSS HEMATURIA

Spontaneous and gross unprovoked hematuria is occasionally seen in pregnancy, and when it occurs the bleeding may be sufficient to cause an appreciable fall in the hematocrit values. Distention of the renal pelvis by blood clot causes pain as well as tenderness to palpation. The hematuria is attributed to rupture of the small veins about the kidney pyramids or the renal pelvis. However, the bleeding may well be the result of any of a number of causes, including tuberculosis, pyelonephritis, and tumor. Personal experience with several patients with spontaneous hematuria in pregnancy indicates that a short observation period is justified before an investigation is made into the actual cause of the bleeding. The patient should be studied urologically when symptoms have subsided, the urine is free from gross blood, and the blood nonprotein nitrogen is known to be normal. These studies may be more informative post partum. In the absence of any demonstrable pathologic cause, the hematuria must be considered idiopathic in type, with recurrence unlikely in the current or a subsequent pregnancy.

UROLOGIC EXAMINATION IN PREGNANCY

The ordinary urologic methods are subject to some revision and modification of interpretation in pregnancy. Intravenous pyelography has several advantages over retrograde pyelography as a diagnostic procedure during pregnancy. Local trauma to the urethra, bladder, and ureters is avoided, as is overdistention of the ureters. The rapidity of the dye excretion also furnishes a rough index of the renal function. In the presence of a large uterus, it is most essential that gas shadows be minimal, and the bowel should be carefully prepared before pyelography. Concentration of the dye is best attained when fluids have been restricted for several hours before the procedure. Delayed function of one kidney, even though temporary, also limits the value of the examination, for the unaffected kidney may excrete most of the dye.

Normally the excretion of dye is somewhat delayed during pregnancy. In the nonpregnant woman, the renal pelvis and ureter are well outlined 15 minutes after injection of the dye, whereas during pregnancy the best x-ray film is obtained between 15 and 30 minutes after injection. To reduce to a minimum the amount of radiation received, a single film taken at 20 to 30 minutes may suffice. Urinary stasis with increased amounts of urine in the kidney pelves and ureters may cause dilution of the dye, but usually it is sufficiently concentrated to be opaque to x-rays. Because the ureters are generally dilated and displaced, interpretation of the significance of the pyelogram must be modified in accordance with the normal changes that occur as pregnancy advances. When used as a follow-up examination the procedure is more informative if performed three or four months post partum. The normal pregnancy changes in the urinary tract will have disappeared by that time, and any abnormalities detected will have pathologic significance.

Retrograde pyelography is less frequently performed during pregnancy, but in certain conditions the procedure must be used. When there is doubt as to the type of lesion, or the function of one kidney, or when only one kidney appears on the intravenous film, retrograde examination is indicated. Retrograde pyelography also effectively outlines the ureters, which is occasionally impossible with intravenous pyelography. Even in expert hands, however, retrograde pyelography is somewhat more difficult to perform during pregnancy. Early in gestation distortion of the trigone impedes the ready passage of catheters into the ureters. As pregnancy advances, the orifices of the trigone are further displaced as a result of the rotation of the uterus. Distending the bladder may partially correct the position of the orifices so that catheterization can be more easily accomplished.

BIBLIOGRAPHY

Anderson, G. W., Rice, G. G., and Harris, B. A., Jr.: Pregnancy and labor complicated by pelvic ectopic kidney anomalies; review of literature. Obstet. Gynec. Survey, 4:737, 1949.

Angell, M. E., Relman, A. S., and Robbins, S. L.: "Active" chronic pyelonephritis without evidence of bacterial infection. New Eng. J. Med., 278:1303, 1968.

Crabtree, E. G.: Urological Diseases of Pregnancy. Williams and Wilkins, Baltimore, 1942.

Crabtree, E. G., and Prather, G. C.: Clinical aspects of pyelonephritis in pregnancy. New Eng. J. Med., 202:357, 1930.

Crabtree, E. G., and Reid, D. E.: Pregnancy pyelonephritis in relation to renal damage and hypertension. Amer. J. Obstet. Gynec., 40:17, 1940.

Cystic diseases of the kidney (editorial). New Eng. J. Med., 274:1029, 1966.

Dixon, H. G., and Brant, H. A.: The significance of bacteriuria in pregnancy. Lancet, 1:19, 1967.

Fairweather, D. V. I.: Polycystic disease of the kidneys complicating pregnancy. J. Obstet. Gynaec. Brit. Comm., 71:277, 1964.

Hipple, R. F., and Schulman, H.: Bacteriuria in pregnancy. Obstet. Gynec. 26:396, 1965.

Hutch, J. A., Ayres, R. D., and Noll, L. E.: Vesicoureteral reflux as cause of pyelonephritis of pregnancy. Amer. J. Obstet. Gynec., 87:478, 1963.

Kass, E. H.: Bacteriuria and pyelonephritis of pregnancy. Arch. Intern. Med. 105:194, 1960.

Kincaid-Smith, P., and Bullen, M.: Bacteriuria in pregnancy. Lancet, 1:395, 1965.

Little, P. J.: Prevention of pyelonephritis of pregnancy. Lancet, 1:567, 1965.

Low, J. A., Johnston, E. E., McBride, R. L., and Tuffness, P. G.: The significance of asymptomatic bacteriuria in the normal obstetric patient. Amer. J. Obstet. Gynec., 90:897, 1964.

Roberts, A. P., and Beard, R. W.: Some factors affecting bacterial invasion of bladder during pregnancy. Lancet, 1:1133, 1965.

Schaefer, G., and Markham, S.: Full-term delivery following nephrectomy. Amer. J. Obstet. Gynec., 100:1078, 1968.

Schaefer, G., Douglas, R. G., and Dreishpoon, I. H.: Extrapulmonary tuberculosis and pregnancy. Amer. J. Obstet. Gynec., 67:605, 1954.

Schultze-Seeman, F.: Renal tuberculosis and pregnancy (translated from Deutsche Med. Wschr., 82:1003, 1957). German Med. Monthly, 2:280, 1957.

Weiss, S., and Parker, F. Jr.: Pyelonephritis; its relation to vascular lesions and to arterial hypertension. Medicine, 18:221, 1939.

DISORDERS OF THE GASTROINTESTINAL SYSTEM AND ASSOCIATED ORGANS

HIATUS HERNIA

Hiatus hernia, with or without gastric ulceration, can be first diagnosed during pregnancy. Presumably the upward displacement of the stomach by the enlarging uterus initiates or aggravates the signs and symptoms of the disorder. Episodes of gastric discomfort that continue into the middle and last trimester, combined with local tenderness below the xiphoid process, should arouse suspicion of a hiatus hernia. Additional information aiding diagnosis is gained by the observation that postural change may relieve or accentuate the symptoms of nausea and heartburn. Having eaten some hours previously, the patient often wakens from a sound sleep with violent heartburn, which is partially relieved by sitting upright, but returns on resumption of the completely supine position. Elevation of the head of the bed by suitable blocks will often afford the patient comfort and uninterrupted sleep.

When the hernia is large and an appreciable portion of the stomach is involved, ulcerations of the gastric mucosa may occur, leading to hematemesis and melena. Roentgenography after a swallow of barium is usually sufficient to confirm the diagnosis. The treatment of associated ulcers during pregnancy is conservative; when the lesions are small the symptoms are mild and subside after delivery. Even when the hernia is large and ulcerations are present, surgery is best postponed until after delivery. Vigorous supportive therapy, including multiple transfusions, have been required to carry the patient through pregnancy.

GASTRODUODENAL ULCER

This condition is regarded as a rarity in pregnancy; at least, the symptoms are rare, possibly because of the relative hypoacidity that exists during this period. Nevertheless, during pregnancy a surprising number of deaths occur from perforation, usually of the duodenum. Probably because of its apparent infrequency in pregnancy, failure to consider the diagnosis and the masking of abdominal signs by the enlarged uterus undoubtedly contribute to this high mortality. The methods for establishing the diagnosis of gastroduodenal ulcer are the same in the pregnant as in the nonpregnant state, and include gastric analysis, a barium meal, and occasionally endoscopic examination. The latter procedure is more difficult to perform in pregnancy because the stomach may be rotated and positioned transversely. There is no reason to believe that the clinical course is altered during pregnancy, and bleeding and perforation can occur. Thus, the medical and surgical management of the ulcer is the same as in the nonpregnant state.

ULCERATIVE COLITIS

Ulcerative colitis, a serious disease, is characterized by chronicity, with spontaneous remissions and relapses. The cause of the disease is unknown, and much controversy exists regarding those factors which may accelerate or aggravate its course. Among others, these include emotional situations and the personal problems of the patient.

The disease may have its onset at any age,

but the majority of the cases in the female are noted before or during the childbearing period. Severe ulcerative colitis, when it begins early in life, may be accompanied by a delay in the development of secondary sex characteristics and amenorrhea. In most adult females who have ulcerative colitis, however, the menses are usually normal and fertility is not impaired. Patients with this disorder often seek advice as to their fitness for marriage and childbearing.

The symptoms of ulcerative colitis include abdominal cramps, and frequent liquid, bloody, or mucoid stools, often accompanied by rectal tenesmus. Fever and tachycardia usually accompany the acute phase, whereas low-grade fever alone may be present during a relapse. Once the disease is suspected, the diagnosis is confirmed by sigmoidoscopic examination. Direct visualization reveals edema, ulceration, and exudate of the mucosa of the lower colon. Early in the course of the disorder, however, the mucosa may be so edematous that the characteristic ulcerations are difficult to see. The severity and extent of the disorder are not always disclosed by a barium enema. In the early stages, x-ray findings can be minimal, although the symptoms may be intense. Constriction of the lumen of the colon as revealed by roentgenography following barium enema is a late manifestation. The patients with ulcerative colitis most frequently seen in pregnancy are those whose disease has been present for some months or many years. In some instances, the patient has had extensive intestinal surgery, including partial or total colectomy and permanent ileostomy.

Opinions as to the advisability of undertaking or continuing pregnancy in the presence of this disease are often expressed with an air of finality. Some maintain that these patients tolerate pregnancy poorly, and therapeutic interruption should be performed at the earliest moment. Others are equally adamant to the effect that ulcerative colitis, being essentially a psychosomatic disease, can be so effectively controlled by psychotherapy that pregnancy can be undertaken, or, if the patient is pregnant, that there is no reason for the pregnancy to be terminated. Both of these views appear extreme and difficult to accept without qualification.

The notion that pregnancy, by virtue of an intense desire by the patient to have a child, is of therapeutic value in patients with active ulcerative colitis is a dangerous assumption. It is true that some patients appear to improve temporarily while pregnant, but relapses are common after delivery. The eventual outcome may find the disease accentuated, and any transient improvement could be attributed to an endocrine rather than a psychologic effect. The logical corollary of this psychologic approach would be to expect exacerbation of the disease if the patient emotionally "rejected" the pregnancy. However, there is no evidence to support this contention either. Psychotherapy, regardless of its form, is considered only supportive, and cannot be regarded as exclusive curative therapy.

The extent of the pathologic process and the degree of activity or quiescence of the disease must be taken into account in evaluating the question of the advisability of childbearing. The occurrence of pregnancy during either the acute phase or an exacerbation of chronic ulcerative colitis is a serious matter, and therapeutic abortion (in the early months) may be advisable. Evacuation of the uterus pelvically is preferable to an abdominal procedure, for laparotomy may aggravate the colitis. However, should the acute symptoms first appear near the time of fetal viability, continuation of the pregnancy with intensive supportive therapy, including cortisone, seems reasonable.

Whether patients with the chronic form of ulcerative colitis should attempt pregnancy depends on an appraisal of the extent of the process and any tendency for the disease to exacerbate. Despite the possibility that with cortisone therapy these patients can approach pregnancy with a greater assurance of success, if a patient with the chronic form has a history of relapses, indicative of an unstable disease, the treatment suggested for the acute form must be strongly considered.

Patients with the chronic form of the disease who are permitted to continue their pregnancy require, in addition to adrenal therapy and other medical measures, reassurance and encouragement from the physician, with considerable time being devoted to a discussion of personal problems. Labor with pelvic delivery should be anticipated, even in patients who have had extensive intestinal surgery. In the event of unproductive labor, the patient can be delivered by cesarean section, preferably the extra-peritoneal type in order to spare any insult to the bowel.

The colitis may remain quiescent throughout gestation, only to flare up after delivery. In fact, the disease may announce itself initially in the early puerperium. Ulcerative colitis therefore should always be considered among the possible causes of diarrhea or unexplained fever developing during the puerperium. These symptoms following delivery are usually attributed to parametritis, with or without pelvic abscess formation. If pelvic examination fails to disclose these conditions and the lower bowel symptoms continue, the diagnosis of ulcerative colitis should be considered. In the hope of averting exacerbation of the disease in the early weeks of the puerperium, cortisone therapy is unquestionably indicated, or, if the patient has been receiving adrenal therapy throughout pregnancy, the amounts administered should be increased and continued for two to four weeks after delivery, with gradual reduction of the dosage after this period.

In résumé, it is evident that, before the patient with ulcerative colitis attempts conception, several factors should be weighed if serious complications and sequelae are to be avoided. It behooves the physician to make a careful assessment of the patient's medical and social status. The chronicity of the disease and the effectiveness of its control are the two paramount factors determining any decision. In the presence of a tranquil emotional environment and with the disease apparently well controlled, the patient may undertake pregnancy with a favorable prognosis. When these conditions do not exist, pregnancy should be avoided, and, if conception does occur, termination of the pregnancy must be considered. A subsequent pregnancy should not be undertaken until the disease has become stabilized and the patient is well enough to cope with any emotional problem that might arise in the course of pregnancy. Even then, the outstanding feature of this disorder is the unpredictability of its course, and the physician must always be on the alert for evidence of an exacerbation.

REGIONAL ILEITIS

What has been said of ulcerative colitis as it relates to pregnancy seems to apply as well to patients with regional ileitis (Crohn's disease). With the patients grouped according to the time when the ileitis was diagnosed, that is, before, during, or after pregnancy, an attempt has been made to assess the response to pregnancy in each of the different categories. In the supposedly more favorable group, comprised of patients whose disease was present prior to pregnancy but quiescent following surgery, approximately two thirds negotiated pregnancy successfully. The remaining third of this group showed exacerbation of the disease, occurring in more than half of the instances during the puerperium. Malabsorption may reveal itself in several ways, including hypoproteinemia, anemia, and disturbance in the clotting mechanism through lack of vitamin K.

LIVER DISEASES

Until rather recent times, isolated instances of jaundice appearing in pregnancy have been diagnosed as catarrhal jaundice when the attacks were mild, and as acute yellow atrophy when they were severe. The prognosis of the latter has always been considered especially grave during pregnancy.

Characterized by degrees of hepatic necrosis, acute yellow atrophy in pregnancy was regarded as idiopathic in type, except in cases of known drug intoxication, in which a diagnosis of toxic hepatitis was made. In hepatitis of unknown etiology, endemic forms were recognized, and for a great number of years the question as to whether the condition was an infectious and contagious entity was repeatedly raised. It is now appreciated that what was designated as acute yellow atrophy in pregnancy is, in fact, viral hepatitis. Unfortunately the nomenclature remains complicated, as indicated by terms such as "true yellow atrophy" being applied to viral hepatitis and "obstetric acute yellow atrophy" being used to describe cases of a fatty metamorphosis of the liver.

Viral hepatitis accounts for nearly half of the cases of jaundice in pregnancy and has increasing implications and ramifications with regard to obstetrics. With the drug problem, the disease will be encountered with increased frequency in pregnancy. The procedure often being an emergency, the risk of transfusion will be increased in pregnancy. Time may not permit the processing of the donor blood to exclude the danger of serum hepatitis. Also, evidence is gaining that a relationship may exist between Down's syndrome and viral hepatitis in pregnancy. The recent identification of the Australian hepatitis associated antigen (HAA) has added to our knowledge about the epidemiology of hepatitis and its treatment, more specifically the effectiveness of gamma globulin. Apparently the latter neutralizes the virus of infectious hepatitis but may not be especially effective against serum hepatitis. Also, the hepatitis-associated antigen is consistently present in association with MS-2 strain of serum hepatitis and not present in the MS-1 strain of infectious hepatitis.

Hepatitis of viral etiology varies greatly in severity, but the evidence indicates that the condition is of much more serious prognostic import in the pregnant than in the nonpregnant patients. The mortality rate during pregnancy may be 5 to 10 per cent, compared with less than 1 per cent in the nonpregnant state. This increased mortality has been attributed to the added drain on the maternal nutritional stores imposed by pregnancy. In fact the nutritional state of the mother has been proposed as the crucial determinant both in the outcome of the disease and in the incidence of sequelae.

In the mild cases, the symptoms are confined to lassitude and anorexia, with slight bilirubinemia and no appreciable evidence of liver dysfunction. The majority of patients, however, present signs of urticaria, fever, jaundice, and leukopenia. The patient may complain of right upper quadrant abdominal pain, the liver is tender, and the spleen may be palpable. Telangiectases or liver spiders may become visible on the skin in greater numbers than are seen in normal pregnancy. Evidence of impaired liver function is furnished by positive cephalin-cholesterol flocculation and thymol turbidity tests, increased prothrombin time, and elevated transaminase levels. In the most severe form, persistent vomiting, progressive jaundice, tachycardia, high fever, headache, and prostration are manifest. On occasion some ascites may be present. When the disease follows a rapid downhill course with extreme liver necrosis, however, deep jaundice may fail to develop. In addition to these findings, hypoglycemia and a marked decrease in blood urea nitro-

gen are often present, which are further indications of marked liver destruction. In such instances the outlook is grave. The end stages of the disease are accompanied by cerebral manifestations of lethargy or, on occasion, excitement and delirium. The clinical duration of the severe cases in pregnancy may be relatively short, with a fatal outcome in three or four days after the onset of acute symptoms.

The liver lesions in the fatal cases of viral hepatitis are essentially the same as those previously described in the literature for acute yellow atrophy. The liver is small, and the morphologic changes are restricted to the liver cells; areas of necrosis may appear anywhere within the lobule. Hemorrhages are prevalent throughout the lung, the gastrointestinal tract, the kidney, and on the serous surfaces. In the patients who survive the severe form of the disease repeated liver biopsies during the recovery period show varying degrees of parenchymal regeneration. In most cases the repair of the cells of the liver lobules is complete. Occasionally, however, the liver cells may be replaced by fibrous tissue, and when the process is extreme the patient may eventually develop symptoms and signs compatible with a cirrhosis.

The treatment of viral hepatitis in pregnancy is for the most part medical. The therapeutic termination of the pregnancy in the hope of aiding recovery in a patient with viral hepatitis is a difficult decision; most authorities, however, favor continuation of the pregnancy. The patient's general condition, the stage of pregnancy, and the state of the clotting mechanism must all be considered in calculation of the surgical risk that termination might impose. During the acute phase of hepatitis, the wiser course is to avoid any surgical trauma to an already seriously ill patient. Following the acute phase of the disease, however, one must consider the possibility of a relapse or the effect of continuation of the pregnancy in contributing to residual liver damage. It is impossible to resolve these problems categorically, but it is a personal view that recovery is more rapid if the pregnancy is terminated. The follow-up studies that are available indicate that complete recovery is usual, and the course of subsequent pregnancies is not remarkable.

The patient must be kept at near-complete bed rest to conserve energy and promote liver repair until the disease is well under control. The medical treatment includes correction and prevention of any nutritional deficits. Sedatives and inhalation anesthetics should be avoided in the conduct of labor and delivery. When the disease fails to respond and liver damage is reaching serious proportions, exchange transfusion may be lifesaving.

Stillbirths are not uncommon, and premature labor adds to the fetal hazards. Originally, the belief was expressed that the virus did not attack the fetus, for the disease was not detected in the newborn. Fatal cases of hepatitis within the first two months of life have subsequently been reported. With the difficulty inherent in establishing the time of infection, i.e., intrauterine or extrauterine, it appears safe to conclude that the fetus is spared in infectious hepatitis, but in homologous serum hepatitis the fetus may become infected and have persistent jaundice at birth.

Pregnant patients should be made aware of the infectious nature of epidemic jaundice in event of an outbreak of the disease in their community. Avoidance of exposure must be emphasized, and, in the event of contact, gamma globulin should be administered.

Recurrent jaundice of pregnancy has now been accepted as a clinical entity characterized by mild jaundice appearing usually in the last trimester; itching and pruritis are the common symptoms. Although the serum bilirubin level may be mildly elevated and bilirubin may be present in the urine, there is little measurable change in liver function. The incidence of prematurity is somewhat increased, but the outlook for the pregnancy is favorable. The treatment is supportive and largely symptomatic. In the face of no precise etiology, hormonal changes have been assigned as the cause. Patients who exhibited cholestatic jaundice in pregnancy have had a recrudescence of their symptoms, i.e., jaundice and itching, when challenged by estrogen administration in the nonpregnant state. Liver function was likewise somewhat impaired.

Fatty metamorphosis of the liver (obstetric acute yellow atrophy) as the term would indicate reveals the entire liver lobule replaced by fatty change without evidence of necrosis. The diagnosis is not entirely certain short of liver biopsy or, unfortunately all too often, autopsy. High doses of intravenous tetracycline administered to pregnant patients have resulted in liver lesions not too different from those of fatty metamorphosis.

The disease is encountered in the last trimester, and is associated with nausea and vomiting and liver dysfunction as indicated by a marked elevation of transaminase levels and hypoglycemia. Liver coma may occur. The treatment is both medical and obstetric. Opinion appears to favor the belief that recovery is enhanced if the pregnancy can be terminated. Exchange transfusion should be considered in patients desperately ill with this disease.

Cirrhosis of the liver is occasionally encountered in pregnancy despite the disturbance in estrogen metabolism that may be associated with the disease. Risk of hemorrhagic death from esophageal varices may be reduced by portacaval shunt procedures. Pregnancy has been successful following the latter, but the results have not been uniformly favorable.

PANCREATITIS

Acute pancreatitis is a disease of the late childbearing years, and presents the same clinical picture in the pregnant as in the nonpregnant patient. The main signs and symptoms include fever, and epigastric, right upper quadrant, or back pain, which is usually constant but may come in paroxysms. The abdomen is tender to palpation, but the presence of an enlarged uterus often makes abdominal palpation somewhat unrewarding. An elevated serum amylase, of 500 Somogyi units or more, is consistent with the diagnosis. The test may apparently return to near-normal levels within 24 to 48 hours from onset of symptoms. Abdominal paracentesis with amylase determination of the ascitic fluid has been recommended. Blood sugar determination may be informative, for transient diabetes may be present. Serum calcium levels may be diminished. Chlorothiazide has been implicated as a possible etiologic factor in pancreatitis in pregnancy.

The generally accepted treatment is medical. However, should the disease be encountered at the time of exploratory laparotomy, opinion differs as to whether the abdomen should be closed promptly or biliary drainage instituted. Certainly if there are stones obstructing the pancreatic duct, they are removed. Regardless of the value of corrective biliary tract surgery, which has its advocates, because of the technical difficulties imposed by the large uterus it would seem unwise in pregnancy to perform more than the simplest palliative surgery, namely, cholecystotomy.

With respect to medical management, the losses of plasma, fluid, and electrolytes into the peritoneal and retroperitoneal spaces may be prodigious, and failure to replace these losses may lead to hypotension and early death. Fluids, electrolytes, blood, and plasma, together with antibiotics, have reduced the mortality from this serious condition.

Pregnancy has been encountered in patients with chronic recurrent pancreatitis, some of whom have had previous surgery on the extrabiliary system and procedures to improve pancreatic secretion into the duodenum. Malabsorption and diabetes may be present. These patients must be carefully evaluated and certainly careful medical management will be required if pregnancy is to be successful. The risk of recurrence and all this implies can make pregnancy a hazardous adventure.

CHOLELITHIASIS AND CHOLECYSTITIS

Pregnancy has been considered an etiologic factor in the formation of gallstones and in gallbladder disease, but attacks of cholelithiasis and cholecystitis are not especially frequent during this period. In chronic cases cholecystitis usually remains quiescent throughout pregnancy, but there is a tendency for exacerbation to occur in the early puerperium. In both the initial and recurrent attacks, fever, local or referred pain, tenderness, and spasm over the gallbladder region, with an associated leukocytosis, are the chief signs and symptoms. Food idiosyncrasies and previous episodes of indigestion prior to pregnancy are important facts to elicit in the history. Attacks usually subside during pregnancy, and thus conservative medical therapy is advisable. Three or four months after delivery the biliary tract should be carefully studied. A more accurate diagnosis and an evaluation of the extent of the disease can be made more easily at this time than is possible during pregnancy, when some degree of biliary stasis exists normally. Empyema of the gallbladder with impending rupture or common duct obstruction, however, will demand surgical intervention, regardless of the technical difficulties that may be imposed by an enlarged uterus. Biliary peritonitis with recovery has been reported in pregnancy, indicating that perforation can occur at this time.

SURGICAL ABDOMEN

A word is in order here concerning the diagnosis and general philosophy of management of the surgical abdomen in pregnancy. Surgical conditions frequently go undiagnosed, for all too often gastrointestinal symptoms are attributed to the nausea and vomiting of pregnancy, or abdominal discomfort to the vague "aches and pains" of pregnancy. This is more likely to happen in and about labor and the early puerperium. Moreover, physical examination is obviously hampered by the presence of the enlarged uterus. As usual, a careful history and physical examination can at least arouse the suspicion that the abdominal symptoms have an organic basis. Any procedure required for making a diagnosis should be performed, despite pregnancy. For example, when bowel obstruction is suspected, a scout x-ray film of the abdomen is not contraindicated. Also, there is at times a reluctance to operate and a tendency to avoid surgery when the patient is found to be pregnant. The question is frequently raised regarding the effect of the needed anesthesia on the fetus, and of exposure and manipulation of the uterus on the pregnancy. This conservative attitude is laudable, *but the decision to operate or not operate should be based on the same criteria as in the nonpregnant.* There is no evidence that harm will come to the fetus from the operation per se.

Appendicitis

Appendicitis is the most common acute surgical condition encountered in pregnancy, with an incidence rate comparable to that in the nonpregnant, but with the hazards involved decidedly increased. A number of reasons account for this, some of which have been discussed above. To repeat, for reemphasis, there is often a delay in arriving at a diagnosis because of failure of the patient or her physician to appreciate fully that nausea and vomiting and vague abdominal discomfort are not necessarily related to pregnancy and must not be disregarded. In the patient at term, abdominal distress is often attributed to the onset of labor, with the enlarged uterus interfering and concealing from the examiner the abdominal signs characteristic of appendicitis. Thus, the condition is often first recognized when the presenting signs indicate appendiceal rupture and spreading peritonitis. An additional hazard is encountered at the time of labor and delivery in the event that an appendiceal abscess has already formed. The uterus and right adnexa are often involved in the process of localization or walling off of the abscess. Commonly the uterus forms a portion of the wall of the abscess, and with delivery, as the uterus diminishes in size, the abscess ruptures, with subsequent secondary peritonitis.

It is evident that the diagnosis of appendicitis is dependent upon careful attention to the patient's history, regardless of how unimpressive the abdominal complaints may be. In the differential diagnosis, in addition to the items in the history, the height of the fever, the degree of leukocytosis, and the abdominal and vaginal findings are of special significance.

On physical examination spasm and rebound tenderness are usually elicited above the right iliac crest and toward the umbilicus. The presence of physical signs in this particular area of the abdomen is the result of the upward displacement of the cecum and appendix by the enlarged uterus. If the appendix is located retrocecally, the tenderness and spasm are commonly, but not necessarily, located more in the flank. Pressure exerted by the examining hand along the left side of the uterus may arouse discomfort in the right lower quadrant of the abdomen. This finding indicates peritoneal irritation, possibly by an inflamed appendix. Although this is a helpful sign when present, it is a rather inconstant finding in cases of acute appendicitis. In view of the upward displacement of the cecum, rectal and vaginal examinations in pregnancy find their chief value in eliminating adnexal disease as the cause of the illness. The laboratory procedures include a meticulous examination of the urinary sediment and a white blood cell count, the latter being interpreted in the light of the normal leukocyte response to pregnancy. When leukocytosis is present, an increase in the proportion of polymorphonuclear cells will favor infection rather than changes due to normal pregnancy or labor. Of the many conditions that might be included in the differential diagnosis, the more common are urinary tract disease, pathologic lesions of the adnexa, including torsion of the ovary or tube, and uterine fibroids with degeneration. A urinary tract infection is not necessarily excluded by a lack of positive findings in examination of the urinary sediment, if there is kinking of the ureter with complete urinary stasis. Occasionally the diagnosis of appendicitis cannot be confirmed short of an exploratory laparotomy.

Appendicitis treated early in the disease rarely interferes with the pregnancy. However, should diagnosis or surgical intervention be delayed and the appendix perforate with subsequent peritonitis or abscess formation, labor often ensues, regardless of the stage of pregnancy.

The treatment of appendicitis is surgical unless there is generalized peritonitis, when it becomes medical, at least until signs of localization appear. As in the nonpregnant, however, surgery in the early hours of a peritonitis, when it is still more or less localized, is indicated to avoid further peritoneal extension. Vigorous chemotherapy is needed in all cases of localized or generalized peritonitis, and, should an appendiceal or pelvic abscess develop, abdominal or cul-de-sac drainage may be required. After the patient recovers with medical treatment, the question arises as to the necessity of removing the residual appendiceal stump. Most authorities believe that surgery is indicated in order to forestall a subsequent attack of appendicitis. If such a policy is to be pursued, the patient is usually operated on six to eight weeks after recovery from the peritonitis, because any adhesions encountered are more easily lysed at that time than at a later date. Unless the patient is near term, pregnancy should not contraindicate removal of the appendiceal stump. The appendix has been known to rupture on two separate occasions during pregnancy.

Concern is often expressed regarding the effect of labor on a newly created abdominal wound. Regardless of the type of incision used, if the wound is clean and healing well, it will withstand labor. Stay sutures may give added assurance. An important point, therefore, in the technique of appendectomy is to use the type of incision that will give the best exposure in the presence of a near-term pregnancy with minimal disturbance to the uterus. If an appendiceal abscess is encountered at operation, drainage should always be through a lateral stab wound away from the uterus, for to drain toward the uterus invites premature labor and infection of the abdominal wound.

Incidental Appendectomy at Cesarean Section

There is a periodic resurgence of interest in performing an incidental appendectomy at the time of cesarean section. To justify the procedure three questions must be answered satisfactorily: (1) Is one reducing peritonitis and death from appendicitis by performing an incidental appendectomy? (2) Is it good practice to perform an incidental appendectomy at the time of other abdominal procedures? (3) Does cesarean section present a set of conditions differing from, for example, a complete abdominal hysterectomy in the nonpregnant patient? Regardless of how meticulous one may be in controlling spillage from the uterus at the time of cesarean section, some blood enters the abdominal cavity, providing a ready medium for bacterial growth. It would be presumptuous to assume that no organism escapes into the abdomen at incidental appendectomy. Also, the cecum seems more vulnerable to local thrombosis and subsequent perforation in pregnancy, so the less handling of this area the better. Some distention is common following cesarean section, and it is reassuring that it is not due to possible complications of the removal of the appendix. Even those who consider it a proper procedure perform it only in some cases. What then are the acceptable cases, and what are the criteria for selection?

Volvulus

Although infrequent, volvulus is by far the most hazardous of the abdominal conditions that may require surgical attention in pregnancy. Moreover, pregnancy may create the conditions conducive to volvulus formation, particularly in those cases in which complete torsion of the small bowel

occurs. For the latter type of volvulus to develop, the mesentery must be either extremely short or abnormally long, or have a congenitally small base. Under these circumstances the uterus, as it enlarges during pregnancy, may displace the bowel sufficiently so that the small intestine begins to rotate, usually clockwise. An extensive volvulus may suddenly develop within a period of minutes or a few hours. It can begin at the ligament of Treitz and include all of the small bowel and a portion of the ascending colon up to the region of the hepatic flexure. The writer has seen two such cases, both of them fatal and both in patients at term. The symptoms were sudden in onset in each case, and an outstanding initial complaint was midline back pain located in the region where the diaphragm would attach posteriorly. Shock developed rapidly, and at times the blood pressure was unobtainable. The abdomen quickly became tender and rigid and in each instance the fetal heart tones promptly disappeared. Premature separation of the placenta or rupture of a viscus or ovarian cyst appeared to be the most likely diagnosis. In the hope that spontaneous labor would ensue, and in face of the need for treatment of severe shock, surgical intervention was postponed. During the delay, necrosis of the entire small bowel and ascending colon developed in both of these patients.

Even when complete volvulus develops, early diagnosis and prompt treatment may save the patient's life. As soon as the diagnosis is suspected, immediate laparotomy should be performed to relieve the torsion, with simultaneous treatment of the shock.

In the partial forms of volvulus, the onset of symptoms is more gradual, and surgical treatment for the release of the intestinal obstruction may not be required immediately. In the uncertain interim, intestinal intubation and drainage should be promptly instituted to relieve the obstructive symptoms. If the signs of obstruction persist, after adequate study and proper preparation of the patient the volvulus is corrected surgically.

BIBLIOGRAPHY

Adams, R. H., and Combes, B.: Viral hepatitis during pregnancy. J.A.M.A., 192:95, 1965.
Bartlett, M. K.: Pancreatitis. New Eng. J. Med., 271:90, 1964.

Berger, R. L., Liversage, R. M., Jr., Chalmers, T. C., Graham, J. H., McGoldrick, D. M., and Stohlman, F., Jr.: Exchange transfusion in the treatment of fulminating hepatitis. New Eng. J. Med., 274:497, 1966.

Biliary peritonitis in pregnancy. Medical Memoranda. Brit. Med. J., 2:744, 1965.

Cockayne, E. A.: Catarrhal jaundice, sporadic and epidemic and its relation to acute yellow atrophy of the liver. Quart. J. Med., 6:1, 1912.

Crohn, B. B., Yarnis, H., Crohn, E. B., Walter, R. I., and Gabrilove, L. J.: Ulcerative colitis and pregnancy. Gastroenterology, 30:391, 1956.

Crohn, B. B., Yarnis, H., and Korelitz, B. I.: Regional ileitis complicating pregnancy. Gastroenterology, 31:615, 1956.

Gorbach, A. C., and Reid, D. E.: Hiatus hernia in pregnancy. New Eng. J. Med., 255:517, 1956.

Hendry, W. F., and Mackey, W. A.: Portal hypertension and pregnancy. Brit. J. Surg., 56:909, 1969.

Ioniotes, G., Clark, P. J., and Cavanagh, D.: Gastric ulcer perforation during pregnancy. Amer. J. Obstet. Gynec., 106:619, 1970.

Hsia, D. Y.-Y., Taylor, R. G., and Gellis, S. S.: Long-term follow-up study on infectious hepatitis during pregnancy. J. Pediat., 41:13, 1952.

Iber, F. L.: Jaundice in pregnancy—a review. Amer. J. Obstet. Gynec., 91:721, 1965.

Jones, R. L., and Soltau, D. H. K.: Pregnancy in association with Crohn's disease. J. Obstet. Gynaec. Brit. Emp., 65:811, 1958.

Koff, R. S., and Isselbacher, K. J.: Changing concepts in the epidemiology of viral hepatitis. New Eng. J. Med., 278:1371, 1968.

Krawitt, E. L.: Ulcerative colitis and pregnancy. Obstet. Gynec., 14:354, 1959.

Kreek, M. J., Weser, E., Sleisenger, M. H., and Jeffries, G. H.: Idiopathic cholestasis of pregnancy. The response to challenge with the synthetic estrogen, ethinyl estradiol. New Eng. J. Med., 277:1391, 1967.

Krugman, S., and Giles, J. P.: Viral hepatitis; new light on an old disease. J.A.M.A., 212:1019, 1970.

Livingston, S. H., Gold, E. M., and Narciso, F.: Acute hemorrhagic pancreatitis in pregnancy. Obstet. Gynec., 26:237, 1965.

Macdougall, I.: Ulcerative colitis and pregnancy. Lancet, 2:641, 1956.

Malkasian, G. D., Jr., Welch, J. S., and Hallenbeck, G. A.: Volvulus associated with pregnancy. A review and a report of 3 cases. Amer. J. Obstet. Gynec., 78:112, 1959.

Minkowitz, S., Soloway, H. B., Hall, J. E., and Yermakov, V.: Fatal hemorrhagic pancreatitis following chlorothiazide administration in pregnancy. Obstet. Gynec., 24:337, 1964.

Moore, H. C.: Recurrent jaundice of pregnancy. A type of intrahepatic cholestasis. Lancet, 2:57, 1963.

Nelson, P. K., and Loughead, J. R.: Pregnancy following portacaval shunt. Report of 2 cases. Obstet. Gynec., 22:725, 1963.

Ober, W. B., and Lecompte, P. M.: Acute fatty metamorphosis of the liver associated with pregnancy. A distinctive lesion. Amer. J. Med., 19:743, 1955.

Peretz, A., Paldi, E., Brandstaedter, S., and Barzilai, D.: Infectious hepatitis in pregnancy. Obstet. Gynec., 14:435, 1959.

Schultz, J. C., Adamson, J. S., Jr., Workman, W. W., and Norman, T. D.: Fatal liver disease after intravenous administration of tetracycline in high dosage. New Eng. J. Med., 269:999, 1963.

Sheehan, H. L.: Pathology of acute yellow atrophy and delayed chloroform poisoning. J. Obstet. Gynaec. Brit. Emp., 47:49, 1940.

Sheehan, H. L.: Jaundice in pregnancy. Amer. J. Obstet. Gynec., 81:427, 1961.

Snyder, W. H., Jr., and Chaffin, L.: Emergency conditions in obstetrics and general surgery. Obstet. Gynec., 13:683, 1959.

Stander, H. J., and Cadden, J. F.: Acute yellow atrophy of liver in pregnancy. Amer. J. Obstet. Gynec., 28:61, 1934.

Stokes, J., Wolman, I. J., Blanchard, M. C., and Farquhar, J. D.: Viral hepatitis in the newborn. Amer. J. Dis. Child., 82:213, 1951.

Svanborg, A., and Ohlsson, S.: Recurrent jaundice of pregnancy. Amer. J. Med., 27:40, 1959.

Zondek, B., and Bromberg, Y. M.: Infectious hepatitis in pregnancy. J. Mount Sinai Hosp. N. Y., 14:222, 1947.

DISORDERS OF THE NEUROMUSCULAR AND SKELETAL SYSTEMS AND SKIN

MULTIPLE SCLEROSIS

Multiple sclerosis, a disorder of demyelinization, is one of the more common chronic neurologic diseases encountered as a complication of pregnancy, for most of the cases develop during the childbearing years. Although it is progressive in its course, multiple sclerosis may exhibit long periods of remission. In most cases the earliest signs and symptoms are referable to more than a single locus within the nervous system. The predominant manifestations are loss of visual acuity and

incoordination of the lower limbs, with areas of paresthesia. In some of the mild and early cases, only nystagmus and diplopia may be present. When the condition becomes severe, there is scanning speech, the extremities show marked weakness, and bladder and rectal control are often impaired. A spastic paraplegic state constitutes the ultimate disability.

In the presence of these characteristic clinical features, the diagnosis of multiple sclerosis is not difficult, but during the initial phase when the signs are often fleeting one must rely more on the laboratory findings. The examination of the cerebrospinal fluid may reveal an elevated cell count, predominantly lymphocytes, and a rise in total protein. These changes, plus an altered colloidal gold reaction and a negative Wassermann test, make the diagnosis of multiple sclerosis more tenable in doubtful cases.

Opinions differ as to the direct effect of childbearing on the course of the disease. Such a situation is understandable, for the unpredictability of relapses and remissions makes it difficult to anticipate how a patient will respond. The belief is generally held that pregnancy has little influence on the course of multiple sclerosis. There is, however, both neurologic and obstetric experience to indicate that such optimism is not entirely warranted. Although attacks frequently recur without provocation, they are reputed to be precipitated by such factors as respiratory infection, over-exertion, fatigue, surgical trauma, and inhalation anesthesia; pregnancy has also been suggested as a possible precipitant of an attack. Relapses in association with pregnancy have been reported to occur with considerable frequency, but it is perhaps significant that the majority of these, as in so many other medical conditions, occur more frequently in the early puerperium.

It seems apparent that advice given patients with multiple sclerosis as to the feasibility of a pregnancy must be highly individualized. In some two thirds of the patients with multiple sclerosis seen in the childbearing years the condition is mild. In the others, the disease has progressed to the point of severe disability, and should conception occur under these circumstances, the additional danger of pyelonephritis, the respiratory difficulties that may be encountered, and the general debility of the patient, with decreased resistance to infection, create a risk that justifies therapeutic termination of the pregnancy. In women whose disease is comparatively mild and relatively stationary, however, pregnancy is not contraindicated, and even in the event of a relapse the pregnancy will proceed to a successful conclusion.

The treatment of the pregnant patient with multiple sclerosis, like that of the nonpregnant patient, is empiric, and, up to the present, none of the measures employed have been especially beneficial.

In view of the observation that multiple sclerosis has a tendency to relapse in the puerperium, ACTH or cortisone might be helpful during this period. Labor is usually uneventful, but the danger of causing a recurrent attack of the disease by an inhalation or conduction type of anesthesia demands that local block be used whenever possible at the time of delivery.

EPILEPSY

Epilepsy is a general term used to designate a condition characterized by intermittent disturbances of the sensorium with or without convulsive seizures. Patients with epilepsy present a variety of important problems in relation to childbearing. These include, among others, the differential diagnosis of convulsive seizures during pregnancy, the possible genetic factors involved, and the effect of gestation on the course of the disorder.

Epilepsy may be classified according to its etiology, the clinical manifestations, or the site within the central nervous system from which the seizures originate.

First, on the basis of etiology, cases are classified as being of idiopathic origin, or acquired, as a result of antecedent brain disease or injury. Some authorities use the terms *genetic* and *essential* interchangeably with idiopathic, implying that a hereditary factor may be present.

Second, based on clinical manifestations, the disorder is classified as being of one of three general types: grand mal, petit mal, or psychomotor. In some instances there appears to be an overlap of the signs and symptoms of these forms. Grand mal seizures are characterized by loss of consciousness and generalized convulsions. Petit mal is marked by only minor motor and sensorial disturbances, including peculiar movements of the eyes, the head, and extremities; there may also be short periods of unconsciousness. The psychomotor type of disturbance, which may be related to petit mal, is preceded by an aura; there is sensorial confusion without loss of consciousness but with purposeless movements of the body. The state of confusion may last for hours following the attack.

Third, an attempt is made to correlate the nature of the seizure with the site of origin within the areas of the motor cortex. Such a classification is especially useful to the neurosurgeon who contemplates definitive surgical treatment of the patient.

The differential diagnosis of seizures during pregnancy includes other brain diseases, physiologic disturbances such as acidosis, hyperventilation alkalosis, and various forms of intoxication, and pregnancy toxemia. Only after these causes have been excluded can the disorder be assigned to epilepsy. The diagnosis of epilepsy and determination of its type require a careful and detailed history to detect a familial tendency for seizures or to establish the possibility of brain disease or trauma. Helpful laboratory procedures include x-ray examination of the skull, lumbar puncture, determination of serum calcium and blood glucose, and electroencephalography.

Patients with epilepsy present a problem in regard to the advisability of marriage and the wisdom of having children. Epileptics request information as to the probability of having normal children, and a woman with epilepsy may question her ability to care for children. Furthermore, these patients often ask what effect pregnancy will have on the frequency and severity of the seizures. Before such questions can be answered, one must ascertain to what extent epilepsy is an inherited disease and the frequency and circumstances under which the disease is most apt to appear in the offspring.

In a classic study of approximately 4000 epileptic patients, the incidence of convulsions in near relatives was found to be 3.2 per cent. In the group with known brain damage, which represented 23 per cent of the total number of epileptics studied, the frequency of convulsions in the near relatives was 1.8 per cent. In the larger group of patients with idiopathic epilepsy, who composed 77 per cent of the total, the incidence of seizures in near relatives was 3.6 per cent. Utilizing studies of monozygotic and dizygotic twins, it was concluded that a genetic predisposition to epilepsy exists. When idiopathic epilepsy was established in a monozygotic twin, 6.6 per cent of the near relatives were epileptic, whereas no relatives of the twins with acquired epilepsy were epileptic. More important was the finding that in the monozygotic twins without brain damage the incidence of epilepsy in the cotwin was 84 per cent, whereas if epilepsy was acquired the incidence in the cotwin was 17 per cent. In the dizygotic twins, if idiopathic epilepsy was present in one, there was an incidence in the other twin of 10 per cent; if the epilepsy was secondary to brain damage, the chance of epilepsy in the cotwin was 8 per cent. Hence heredity and brain abnormality are both important, but heredity exerts a somewhat greater influence than brain injury in the etiology and frequency of epilepsy. Such data require reassessment, recognizing the possible influence of the extrauterine experience in the production of seizures after birth.

It is obvious that cautious advice concerning marriage and childbearing must be given by the physician to patients with the disease. The low overall incidence of epilepsy, even of the idiopathic type, in near relatives in both studies cited would not preclude marriage or procreation. When one parent has the idiopathic type, the chance of epilepsy appearing in the child has been quoted as 1 in 40. When both parents have the disease the incidence of seizures in the offspring undoubtedly will be increased, but the exact frequency is unknown. When epilepsy is acquired as the result of brain injury, the incidence of epilepsy in the offspring is extremely low, and chance is stated to be approximately 1 in 100.

It has been reported that some third of the patients are temporarily made worse by pregnancy, perhaps because of the normal increase in interstitial fluid and the hyperventilation that occur. Patients with epilepsy, however, do forget to take their antiepileptic drugs, which can lead to an increase in seizures that may at first be interpreted as an exacerbation of epilepsy. Rarely does pregnancy seem to precipitate an increased number of attacks in patients whose epilepsy has been well controlled. Determination of blood levels of Dilantin undoubtedly would be worthwhile in patient management and evaluation.

The usual anticonvulsive therapy may occasionally fail, and consideration must be given to therapeutic abortion. Usually, however, the frequency and severity of seizures are not altered by pregnancy, and some patients even seem to improve. Labor and delivery proceed as in the medically uncomplicated pregnancy. In the puerperium, however, the patient may show unusual concern about her ability to care for the infant. She is afraid to hold or nurse the baby for fear that a seizure will occur coincidentally and harm will come to her offspring. Reassurance and husband participation in the care of the infant will do much to allay the patient's fears. Because of the possibility of damage to the infant, it may be thought that breast feeding is contraindicated; this, however, can be overcome if the disease is controlled. These patients lactate normally, and the epilepsy apparently is not aggravated by breast feeding.

HUNTINGTON'S CHOREA

Huntington's chorea is characterized by the development of athetoid movements and mental deterioration beginning after the third decade of life. Although the children have a 50-50 chance of being normal, with such a devastating disease marriage and, certainly, propagation would appear inadvisable.

BRAIN TUMOR, CEREBRAL ANEURYSM, AND CEREBRAL VENOUS THROMBOSIS

Brain Tumor

The symptoms of brain tumors are likely to become aggravated and the condition may come to light for the first time in the presence of pregnancy. Gliomas of the brain grow with apparent rapidity, but the natural course of this type of neoplasm is so variable that it is difficult to determine whether pregnancy actually affects the rate of its growth. Meningiomas and other brain tumors increase in size temporarily during gestation, but some of the enlargement has been attributed to engorgement of cerebral vessels rather than to any significant change in the rate of tumor growth. On following a patient with a subtemporal decompression associated with a pineal tumor through a successful and asymptomatic pregnancy, it was somewhat startling to observe a herniation of the brain substance by 1 cm. or more beyond the bony aperture, mainly

in the last trimester, and then to see the brain recede a similar distance within the skull one or two days after delivery.

Cerebral Aneurysm

Intracranial aneurysms of the cerebral vessels are thought to be especially hazardous during pregnancy. The mortality rate of this complication in pregnancy has been reported as high as 25 per cent. Rupture of the aneurysm and subsequent subarachnoid hemorrhage occurs in 90 per cent of cases without prior symptoms. Sudden of onset, the initial symptom is severe headache. The sensorium is disturbed and nuchal rigidity appears. Consciousness may or may not be lost but if coma develops the prognosis is unfavorable. Besides the history and physical and neurologic examinations, bloody spinal fluid strengthens the diagnosis. An effort should be made to determine the location and extent of the vascular lesion with the hope that it will lend itself to definitive surgical treatment. Pregnancy is no contraindication to carotid or vertebral angiography studies.

The surgical treatment is based on the same indications as in the nonpregnant, although it is kept in mind that a hypotensive episode may be of some risk to the fetus. The belief of some neurologists that recurrent hemorrhage is more likely in pregnancy, along with the fact that the mortality increases if this occurs, makes surgical intervention the more urgent. Whether the pregnancy should be permitted to continue is of secondary consideration, and cases have been encountered in which pregnancy continued to a successful conclusion following surgical management.

Because of the potential danger from the rise in blood pressure with uterine contractions, there is some difference of opinion about whether a patient with congenital cerebral aneurysm should be permitted to enter labor. Until rather recently cesarean section was believed to be the safer method of delivery. There is now tangible clinical evidence to refute such a policy and to favor pelvic delivery. Methods of pain relief and choice of anesthesia are important considerations, and the avoidance of expulsive efforts by the patient by delivery with outlet forceps is basic in her management.

Cerebral Thrombosis

Although thrombosis of the dural sinuses is rare, it would seem to occur with a greater frequency with pregnancy and delivery, especially in patients with pregnancy toxemia, sepsis, vascular disease, and organic heart disease. It should therefore be considered in the differential diagnosis of convulsions and coma in the puerperium. Increase in the procoagulant factors of blood clotting during pregnancy may contribute to such a catastrophe. The usual lesion is a thrombosis of the superior longitudinal sinus and the meningeal veins entering it. Autopsy reveals softening of the brain substance with hemorrhage and subsequent necrosis in the areas that have been affected. Thrombosis of cerebral arteries has also been encountered, as observed at autopsy.

The onset of the disease is abrupt, with symptoms usually occurring some 3 to 10 days after delivery. The outstanding clinical features are headache, convulsions, and paralysis, the latter involving the face, arm, and leg. The spinal fluid, although clear, has an elevated pressure. The prognosis is relatively good if the disease is uncomplicated, but is less favorable if it is associated with the conditions listed.

Included in therapy is the control of seizures, if they be present, and prevention of the sequelae of increased intracranial pressure. This latter aspect can be managed with the use of intravenous urea solution or by controlled removal of spinal fluid. Anticoagulants are contraindicated because of the concomitant superficial cortical hemorrhages. The risk of hemorrhage is considered to outweigh any advantages anticoagulants might offer. Although recovery may be rapid and complete, if it is slow or delayed attention should be given to restoration of motor function by physical therapy. Present evidence indicates that future pregnancies can be undertaken provided full recovery has taken place.

DISORDERS OF THE PERIPHERAL NERVES

Disturbances of the peripheral nerves seen during pregnancy may be toxic, nutritional, or traumatic in origin. Many toxic substances have been implicated as the cause of the neuropathies of pregnancy; of specific interest are those contained in abortifacients. Polyneuritis has been known to follow the ingestion of apiol which is dispensed as Ergoapiol. Nerve damage in such cases may be traced to an impurity in the apiol, triorthocresyl phosphate, rather than to any ergot action. The majority of the neuropathies have been shown to be nutritional in origin. The disorder in the form of polyneuritis is seen most frequently in patients with long-standing nausea and vomiting of pregnancy (hyperemesis gravidarum). As the neurologic disorder develops, the signs and symptoms that may appear include defective memory, drowsiness, irrationality, nystagmus, decreased or absent tendon reflexes, atrophy or weakness of the muscles of the extremities, particularly the extensors, loss of sphincter control, and sensory changes. The injury to the nervous system consists of myelin degeneration of the peripheral nerves and chromatolytic changes in the ventral horn cells. Petechial hemorrhages are commonly present in the brain, especially in the hypothalamic region, the floor of the fourth ventricle, and the medulla. The response to therapy depends on the degree of nerve damage and the extent of nutritional deficiencies. In neglected cases the prognosis must be guarded, and even though the patient is receiving optimal dietary and parenteral vitamin therapy, improvement is slow.

Traumatic nerve paralysis of the lower extremities has been reported and may occur during labor or become apparent after delivery, with damage to either the lumbosacral plexus or directly to the peripheral nerves themselves. The precipitating cause has been the subject of some controversy. In the earliest reports the paralysis was said to be restricted mainly to the peroneal nerve, with foot drop being the outstanding clinical feature. The peroneal nerve originates from fibers of the fourth and fifth lumbar segments passing over the brim of the pelvis to join with fibers from the first and second sacral segments. The belief was expressed that the fibers derived from the lumbar segments were so positioned that in unusual circumstances of labor they might be compressed by the presenting part of the fetus. If the anatomic situation is indeed such as to expose the lumbosacral cord to direct injury, then whenever the pelvis is contracted, particularly in the platypelloid type, the application of forceps blades would encroach on the limited space between the fetal head and the pelvic wall and cause nerve injury. In most cases of traumatic obstetric neuritis the delivery has been regarded as difficult.

It has also been questioned whether, because of their similar origin and close anatomic relationship, the peroneal nerve could be injured without involvement of the tibial nerve.

Further, it has been proposed that in foot drop without other neurologic signs some cause other than trauma to the lumbosacral plexus is responsible. Direct pressure on the external peroneal nerve near the head of the fibula, as a result of incorrect positioning of the legs in stirrups for delivery, must be considered as a possible explanation.

The symptoms of possible traumatic neuritis may appear early in labor, with pain along the outer thigh and leg usually being the first complaint. In the unmedicated patient the pain is described as spasmodic and severe. Paresthesias are common and may even precede any discomfort in the leg. The onset of the paralysis is quite sudden and, although the flexors of the foot are always involved with resultant foot drop, neurologic examination will reveal that other muscle groups are also weakened. The ankle and knee jerks are usually absent, and there may be a complete loss of sensation in the skin area over the involved nerves. With the passage of time, muscle atrophy ensues and may become severe.

It is apparent that injury to the peroneal nerve and lumbosacral plexus is preventable and should never be encountered in current practice. In order to eliminate the possibility of pressure on the peroneal nerve, attention should be given to detail in the placing of the patient's legs in stirrups at the time of delivery. In the delivery of a patient with a contracted pelvis, one must always be mindful of the hazard of nerve injury. It is imperative that the forceps blade, when inserted into the vagina, be placed in the hollow of the sacrum, wherein lies the greatest amount of available space. The blades in turn are carefully positioned, being kept in close apposition to the head of the fetus to avoid soft tissue injury.

Before hospital discharge, it is wise to examine neurologically the lower extremities of any patient who has had a difficult labor and delivery. Such an examination may detect nerve injury at an early date and thereby prevent any unfortunate sequelae. Treatment of the injured extremity is largely confined to rest, together with a splint or cast to prevent a foot drop and deformity. The prognosis must be guarded for the patient who has experienced evident trauma to the nerve trunk and peripheral nerves; although she will usually improve, recovery is slow and occasionally there is some permanent paralysis.

MYASTHENIA GRAVIS

Myasthenia gravis, a disorder resulting from faulty transmission of nerve impulse at the neuromuscular junction, is characterized by weakness of the oculomotor, facial, laryngeal, pharyngeal, and respiratory muscles. Because the disease is subject to remissions and relapses, it is difficult to evaluate either the temporary or permanent effects of pregnancy on its course. There may be a reduction in requirements for neostigmine, indicating an improvement. In rare instances, however, the need for this drug is increased enormously during pregnancy, and may remain elevated over the prepregnancy levels after delivery.

In the majority of patients with myasthenia gravis gestation may be allowed to continue. When the disease is so severe as to require mechanical devices to maintain respiration, therapeutic termination of pregnancy would appear prudent, especially if the patient is seen in the early months. Regardless of the usual transient improvement that pregnancy may cause, it is obvious that patients with myasthenia gravis need special surveillance throughout the prenatal period and extreme care at the time of delivery.

The management of patients with myasthenia gravis is dependent on anticholinesterase compounds such as pyridostigmine and neostigmine. Great care should be taken to avoid overtreating in attempts to achieve complete control of symptoms because overdosage may lead to a dangerous state of weakness similar to that seen in untreated myasthenia. Correction of overdosage requires atropine and management of respiratory difficulties. Potassium chloride may improve the patient's strength. If an overdosage of drugs is suspected as the cause of the myasthenia, a diagnostic trial of edrophonium may be tried. If the weakness is due to a myasthenic crisis the patient will improve, but if the weakness is due to drugs the symptoms will worsen. The short action time of this compound allows the patient to be manageable during the test. These patients are unusually sensitive to quaternary ammonium compounds, so muscle relaxants should be avoided at delivery.

The contractility of the uterine musculature is apparently not impaired in myasthia gravis, and normal labor may be expected. The general fatigue of labor may exaggerate the symptoms of myasthenia gravis, however, so that additional dosages of neostigmine are required. Neostigmine has limitations in that the respiratory secretions may become so excessive from the effects of the drug that respiratory exchange may be markedly impaired. Under these circumstances, one must turn to a mechanical respirator to maintain respiratory function. Otherwise the patient could literally drown in the pulmonary secretions produced by the excessive doses of neostigmine required to control the muscular weakness. Consideration must be given especially to the choice of anesthetic at the time of delivery, and careful nursing attention provided during the period of postdelivery recovery. Most of these patients return to their prepregnancy neostigmine requirements soon after delivery.

Of significance is the observation that the newborn may reveal signs and symptoms of myasthenia gravis, which, if untreated with neostigmine, may lead to death from respiratory failure. Within three or four weeks after birth, the signs and symptoms in the infant disappear, and treatment may then be discontinued. This suggests that myasthenia may be an autoimmune disease.

OTOSCLEROSIS

Otosclerosis is a conductive type of deafness that is more frequent in women and is prone to appear initially in the age of childbearing. The disease is characterized by a deposition of calcium in the middle ear, which interferes with movement of the ossicles and results in progressive deafness. The condition appears to be aggravated by pregnancy. In most cases, however, therapeutic termination of pregnancy is not indicated, and only when it can be established beyond a reasonable doubt that the loss of hearing is unusually rapid is such a procedure justified. In multiparous patients whose previous pregnancies have resulted in a progressive loss of hearing, one must give consideration to the patient's desires.

NEUROMUSCULAR DISEASES

Muscular dystrophies are hereditary diseases characterized by progressive atrophy and wasting of muscles. The muscle is replaced with fat and connective tissue and at no time is there evidence of any muscular regeneration. The various types of the disorder have been given a variety of names, depending in part on the anatomic structures involved.

The chief obstetric interest in many of the diseases of the neuromuscular system concerns their genetic aspects. Progressive muscular dystrophy appears in three forms. One type, characterized by muscular wasting, is seen in children before the age of six. The fact that the disease is observed almost exclusively in the male suggests a sex-linked recessive inheritance. Another type, which affects both sexes in approximately equal numbers, usually occurs during adolescence, although it may not appear until after middle age. In this form the muscles of the face and pectoral girdle are involved, and the disorder is descriptively designated facioscapulohumeral dystrophy. It has an autosomal dominant pattern of inheritance.

There is an even more rare form of the disease called congenital muscular dystrophy, which resembles primary muscular atrophy and infantile spinal muscular atrophy (Werdnig-Hoffmann disease). The latter is known to recur, not necessarily as an inherited trait but perhaps as the result of a mutant. Death occurs, usually in the early years, from general wasting. The question of therapeutic abortion is difficult to decide because the birth of normal children has been known to follow that of afflicted infants.

The diagnosis of progressive muscular dystrophy is generally based on the physical examination and increased urinary creatine excretion, which is believed to reflect a decreased total body muscle mass and a decreased conversion of creatine to creatinine. Serum creatinine kinase determinations are useful in detecting female carriers of the genes for progressive muscular dystrophy. In patients with this disease the enzymatic activity may exceed the normal 3.5 units and may rise as high as 1000. In female carriers, the serum level may also be elevated. Muscle biopsy and myometric examinations are included in the diagnostic procedures.

Various forms of treatment for these rare disorders have been suggested, but none have been regularly successful in altering the course of the diseases. Recent case reports indicate that patients with these disorders may have remarkably uncomplicated pregnancies, considering the nature of their underlying disorders.

Myotonia dystrophica is a familial disease characterized by tonic spasm of the muscles, with muscular wasting occurring as a late effect. It, too, is believed to be inherited as an autosomal dominant. Peroneal muscular atrophy is a familial disease occurring mostly in males, and therefore reputed to be sex-linked inherited. In contrast to the above-named muscular disorders, incapacitation is usually not severe. The course of amyotrophic lateral sclerosis, with its poor prognosis, is not affected by pregnancy. Difficulty with deglutition and respiration must be expected. Because of the short survival time, the patient's desires as to the continuation of the pregnancy again deserve consideration.

Familial periodic paralysis is an odd disease, characterized by episodes of complete paralysis of the voluntary muscles. The patient feels and behaves quite normally during the intervening periods. Associated with these aberrations of muscular function is a precipitous drop in the serum potassium. Attacks may be prevented by proper doses of potassium chloride.

Muscle cramp is a very common complaint in pregnancy and is characterized by sustained involuntary and painful contractions. The spasms usually occur in one muscle group and the most common site during pregnancy is the calf muscles. The spasms commonly occur at night. Factors implicated have been a decrease in the plasma concentration of calcium, sodium deprivation or loss, and peripheral vascular insufficiency. In the great majority of instances the cramps occur in normal, healthy persons and the cause is completely unknown. The cramp may be relieved by thiamine chloride, 30 mg. daily, and by passive stretching of the affected muscles. The frequency of attacks can be reduced by massaging the affected group of muscles or taking a warm bath at bedtime.

DISORDERS OF THE SKELETON

The diseases of the skeleton that are of particular significance during childbearing are those conditions which, as a consequence of improper development and growth of bone from either congenital, nutritional, or metabolic causes, result in marked deformities.

Osteomalacia is a disorder of the bones occurring in the adult, as contrasted with rickets in infancy and childhood, both characterized by a defect in calcification of the newly formed bone matrix (osteoid) and accompanied by a decrease in the serum concentration of both calcium and phosphorus. The disease is produced either through insufficient calcium absorption or, in the case of renal acidosis, by excessive urinary calcium loss. The severity of renal disturbance in renal acidosis precludes pregnancy or opposes its continuation. Thus, as osteomalacia relates to pregnancy and the newborn, the concern is with failure of calcium absorption, due either directly to the lack of dietary calcium and vitamin D, or secondarily to steatorrhea in which vitamin D, being fat-soluble, is not absorbed but is lost in the feces. Such loss occurs in cases of idiopathic nontropical sprue and all conditions that come under the diagnostic umbrella of the malabsorption syndrome.

The dietary lack of calcium and vitamin D accounts for the severe form of osteomalacia reported from China and seen sporadically elsewhere in the world. In previous decades, at least in the northern areas of China, 1 to 3 per cent of all childbearing women had some degree of osteomalacia. Balanced studies have shown an increase in fecal calcium with vitamin D-deficient diets in patients with established osteomalacia.

Osteomalacia may involve all the bones of the body, and, in consequence of the upright position and weight-bearing, results in severe pelvic deformity. With bone softening, the areas about the sacral promontory and the acetabula are unable to withstand the concentration of forces created by weight-bearing, and they encroach into the excavation of the pelvis. There is forward displacement of the upper portion of the sacrum, with a convergence of the side walls of the forepelvis. As a result of these changes the pelvic inlet assumes a triangular outline, while the pubic arch becomes markedly contracted, imparting a funnel shape to the pelvis.

Osteomalacia often becomes aggravated during pregnancy, with further distortion of the skeleton. Although this distortion may be attributed to the attempt of the maternal organism to fulfill fetal requirements from her own deficient calcium stores, the major factor undoubtedly is the added stress attendant on the increase in body weight. Owing to the collapse of the skeleton, the space between the symphysis and the xiphoid process is so reduced that delivery even by abdominal hysterotomy has on occasion presented a problem.

The diagnosis of osteomalacia is made on the basis of history, evidence of demineralization with bony deformity (verified by x-ray examination), the possible presence of tetany, and a decrease in blood concentration of calcium and phosphorus associated with high serum alkaline phosphatase levels. Even the pregnant patient with osteomalacia responds readily to calcium and vitamin D therapy. The treatment should therefore include a balanced diet, with 3 to 5 grams of calcium lactate as a supplement and at least 100,000 units of vitamin D daily. When the condition results from a gastrointestinal disorder, the treatment must take into account the presence of other nutritional changes, including malabsorption of vitamin K. During pregnancy, a megaloblastic anemia may develop as the result of a defect of absorption of folic acid.

Babies born to osteomalacic mothers may present clinical evidence of fetal rickets, but, interestingly, the concentration of calcium in the cord blood of these babies is reportedly normal. During the first weeks after birth, however, these babies are subject to tetany, which is readily corrected with calcium and vitamin D therapy. Even osteomalacic mothers with tetany, and their infants on breast feeding with fetal rickets and tetany, were brought into positive calcium balance by administration of vitamin D to the mother, with relief of symptoms in both.

Osteitis fibrosa disseminata (Albright's syndrome) is an idiopathic cystic disease of bone characterized by precocious sexual development. As the result of the early closure of the epiphyses, the patient is short in stature. Cystic bone lesions, which are usually unilateral, and areas of increased bone density, especially above the base of the skull, are found roentgenologically. Irregular patches of melanin pigment are often observed in the skin over the area of the involved bone. The premature development of secondary sex characteristics with early appearance of the menses in the female is a reflection of the abnormal early release of pituitary gonadotropic activity. These patients must account for some of the reported cases of pregnancy and delivery occurring during the age of childhood.

Osteogenesis imperfecta (fragilitas ossium) is a hereditary disease of varying severity due apparently to a defect in normal osteoblastic function with failure of normal amounts of bone salts to be deposited in the matrix or osteoid tissue, despite the fact that the serum calcium and phosphorus values are normal. The disease may arise during intrauterine life, predisposing the fetal bones to fracture in utero or, more particularly, at the time of delivery. Infants in whom the disease is severe often fail to survive beyond the first few years of life. Patients seen in pregnancy with this disease, therefore, may be considered as having the milder form of osteogenesis imperfecta.

The diagnosis is established on the basis of a history of multiple spontaneous fractures and on the appearance of the eyes. The scleras are extremely thin, allowing the choroid to be visible, which gives the eyes a characteristic blue color. Inasmuch as estrogens help these patients to maintain a positive calcium balance, it might be expected that the condition would temporarily improve in pregnancy. Because of the gain in body weight during pregnancy, and its effect on a weakened skeletal system, however, great care must be taken in the conduct of pregnancy, labor, and delivery to prevent the occurrence of fractures in the patient and in the infant as well, should the latter also have the disease.

Chondrodystrophy is a condition in which the epiphyseal plate fails to produce adequate amounts of columnar cartilage. A genetic factor is apparently associated with this condition, although occasional cases appear without any hereditary background. The long bones fail to grow to normal length, which leads to dwarfism with a disproportionate rate of growth between membranous and cartilaginous bone. The cranial bones of membranous origin grow at near-normal rates, while the cartilaginous bone of the base of the skull fails to keep pace. The head is large with a prominent forehead, and the facial features are flattened. The trunk is of normal length, but there is often a marked lumbar lordosis. In the case of the latter, the sacral promontory moves forward and encroaches into the plane of the superior strait, complicating labor and delivery.

DISORDERS OF THE SKIN

The frequency of skin disorders is not increased by pregnancy and the manifestations are the same as in nonpregnant women. Spiderlike hemangiomas are common in pregnancy and disappear with delivery. Hemangiomas with bleeding requiring removal have been reported. Hirsutism is increased and in some instances deserves investigation as to possible etiology, for example, adrenal dysfunction. Hyperhidrosis and any tendency to urticaria are accentuated during pregnancy.

There are several disorders that are often described as being peculiar to pregnancy; these include prurigo gestationis, herpes gestationis, and impetigo herpetiformis. However, recent studies on disorders of the skin together with a closer study of the older literature suggest that there is no incontrovertible evidence that pregnancy invokes skin diseases not seen at other times. It appears expedient to make a diagnosis on standard dermatologic principles and to provide standard management. However, so well are the above terms entrenched that they are here considered as clinical entities.

Prurigo Gestationis

This is a rather infrequent pruritic dermatitis, manifesting itself in small, discrete, intensely itchy, papular lesions, which may become blood-encrusted from scratching. The onset of the disorder is gradual, with lesions usually first noted during the third trimester. Following delivery the papules disappear, but pigmentation may occur at their former sites. There is a tendency for prurigo gestationis to recur in subsequent pregnancies.

Herpes Gestationis

Herpes gestationis is a rare cutaneous complication that is thought to occur only during pregnancy, but the lesions may be indistinguishable from those of dermatitis herpetiformis. Some authorities believe that herpes gestationis is a variant of the latter. Dermatitis herpetiformis, however, rarely occurs in women, and the degree of pigmentation and scarring is in marked contrast to that seen in herpes gestationis. Although it is difficult to treat, the mother is not subject to risk.

The typical lesions are bullae or vesicles on an erythematous base. They usually appear on the anterior surfaces of the body and rarely, if ever, affect the mucous membranes. Burning and itching are usually intense. Following delivery, regression occurs over a period of several weeks. These herpetic lesions sometimes, but not always, recur in subsequent pregnancies.

Impetigo Herpetiformis

Impetigo herpetiformis is a rare skin condition accompanied by systemic manifestations of extreme toxicity. Fever, diarrhea, vomiting, prostration, and death may occur. The prognosis is altered adversely should it occur in pregnancy. The early lesions first appear as discrete vesicopustules on the lower extremities and trunk. As the disease increases in severity the lesions coalesce to form oozing, crusted, foul-smelling areas surrounded by a minimal area of erythema. Lesions of the mucous membranes of the mouth, together with pain, often interfere with mastication. On examination, these mouth lesions appear as grayish white plaques bordered by detached necrotic mucous membrane.

With the early use of antibiotics the systemic manifestations are alleviated, and the maternal mortality of previous years has been reduced. Delivery or termination of pregnancy results in disappearance of the disease; hence, therapeutic abortion or induction of labor must be considered in these patients.

BIBLIOGRAPHY

Albright, F., Burnett, C., Parson, W., Reifenstein, E. C., Jr., and Roos, A.: Osteomalacia and late rickets. Medicine, 25:399, 1946.

Albright, F., Butler, A. M., Hampton, A. O., and Smith, P. H.: Syndrome characterized by osteitis fibrosa disseminata, areas of pigmentation and endocrine dysfunction, with precocious puberty in females; report of 5 cases. New Eng. J. Med., 216:727, 1937.

Barter, R. H., Letterman, G. S., and Schurter, M.: Hemangiomas in pregnancy. Amer. J. Obstet. Gynec., 87:625, 1963.

Biback, S. M., Franklin, A., and Sata, W. K.: Puerperal hemiplegia; case report and review of primary puerperal cerebral venous thrombosis. Amer. J. Obstet. Gynec., 83:45, 1962.

Bruhn, D. F., Lansman, H. H., Kava, H., and Elmaleh, L. R.: Progressive pseudohypertrophic muscular dystrophy complicated by pregnancy. Obstet. Gynec., 21:438, 1963.

Bryan, W. M., Jr.: Myasthenia gravis in pregnancy and in newborn infant. Obstet. Gynec., 4:339, 1954.

Burnett, C. W. F.: Relation between epilepsy and pregnancy. J. Obstet. Gynaec. Brit. Emp., 53:539, 1946.

Cannell, D. E., and Botterell, E. H.: Subarachnoid hemorrhage and pregnancy. Amer. J. Obstet. Gynec., 72:844, 1956.

Chalmers, J. A.: Traumatic neuritis of the puerperium. J. Obstet. Gynaec. Brit. Emp., 56:205, 1949.

Crawford, G. M., and Leeper, R. W.: Diseases of the skin in pregnancy. Arch. Derm. Syph., 61:753, 1950.

Cross, J. N., Castro, P. O., and Jennett, W. B.: Cerebral strokes associated with pregnancy and the puerperium. Brit. Med. J., 3:214, 1968.

Denny-Brown, D.: Multiple sclerosis—the clinical problem. Amer. J. Med., 12:501, 1952.

Discussion on neurological complications of pregnancy. Proc. Roy. Soc. Med., 32:581, 1939.

Eckerling, B., Goldman, J. A., and Gans, B.: Intracranial sinus thrombosis; a rare complication of early pregnancy. Obstet. Gynec., 21:368, 1963.

Freda, V. J., Vosburgh, G. J., and Di Liberti, C.: Osteogenesis imperfecta congenita: A presentation of 16 cases and review of the literature. Obstet. Gynec., 18:535, 1961.

Gardy, H. H.: Dystrophia myotonica in pregnancy. Obstet. Gynec., 21:441, 1963.

Goethals, P. L., Banner, E. A., and Hedgecock, L. D.: Effect of pregnancy on otosclerosis. Amer. J. Obstet. Gynec. 86:522, 1963.

Grob, D.: Metabolic diseases of muscle. Ann. Rev. Med., 14:151, 1963.

Hadley, J. A.: Herpes gestationis; report of a case. J. Obstet. Gynaec. Brit. Emp., 66:985, 1959.

Huston, J. W., Lingenfelder, J., Mulder, D. W., and Kurland, L. T.: Pregnancy complicated by amyotrophic lateral sclerosis. Amer. J. Obstet. Gynec., 72:93, 1956.

Israel, S. L.: Hirsutism as a gynecologic problem. Amer. J. Obstet. Gynec., 87:372, 1963.

Kibrick, S.: Myasthenia gravis in the newborn. Pediatrics, 14:365, 1954.

King, A. B.: Neurologic conditions occurring as complications of pregnancy. Arch. Neurol. Psychiat., 63:471, 611, 1950.

Laubstein, M. B., Kotz, H. L., and Hehre, F. W.: Obstetric and anesthetic management following spontaneous subarachnoid hemorrhage. Obstet. Gynec., 20:661, 1962.

Lavy, S. and Kahana, E.: Cerebral arterial occlusion during pregnancy and puerperium. Report of 3 cases. Obstet. Gynec., 35:916, 1970.

Lennox, W. G.: Genetics of epilepsy. Amer. J. Psychiat., 103:457, 1947.

Lennox, W. G.: Heredity of epilepsy as told by relatives and twins. J.A.M.A., 146:529; correction, 146:662, 1951.

Lorincz, A. B., and Moore, R. Y.: Puerperal cerebral venous thrombosis. Amer. J. Obstet. Gynec., 83:311, 1962.

Maxwell, J. P.: Further studies in adult rickets (osteomalacia) and foetal rickets. Proc. Roy. Soc. Med., 28:265, 1935.

Maxwell, J. P., and Miles, L. M.: Osteomalacia in China. J. Obstet. Gynaec. Brit. Emp., 32:433, 1925.

Mealey, J., Jr., and Carter, J. E.: Spinal cord tumor during pregnancy. Obstet. Gynec., 32:204, 1968.

Pedowitz, P., and Perell, A.: Aneurysms complicated by pregnancy; aneurysms of cerebral vessels. Amer. J. Obstet. Gynec., 73:736, 1957.

Plauche, W. C.: Myasthenia gravis in pregnancy. Amer. J. Obstet. Gynec., 88:404, 1964.

Pool, J. L.: Treatment of intracranial aneurysms during pregnancy. J.A.M.A., 192:209, 1965.

Raji, M., and Vasicka, A.: Pregnancy associated with infantile muscular atrophy (Werdnig-Hoffmann disease). Obstet. Gynec., 32:70, 1968.

Rand, C. W., and Andler, M.: Tumors of the brain complicating pregnancy. Arch. Neurol. Psychiat., 63:1, 1950.

Schapira, K., Poskanzer, D. C., Newell, D. J., and Miller, H.: Marriage, pregnancy and multiple sclerosis. Brain, 89:419, 1966.

Schwab, R. S.: Management of myasthenia gravis. New Eng. J. Med., 268:717, 1963.

Tillman, A. J. B.: Traumatic neuritis in the puerperium. Amer. J. Obstet. Gynec., 29:660, 1935.

Tillman, A. J. B.: Effect of pregnancy on multiple sclerosis and its management. Ass. Res. Nerv. Ment. Dis., Proc., 28:548, 1950.

Tyler, F. H., and Wintrobe, M. M.: Studies in disorders of muscle; problem of progressive muscular dystrophy. Ann. Intern. Med., 32:72, 1950.

Walton, J. N.: Muscular dystrophy; some recent advances in knowledge. Brit. Med. J., 1:1271, 1344, 1964.

Zundel, W. S., and Tyler, F. H.: Medical progress: The muscular dystrophies. New Eng. J. Med., 273:596, 1965.

INFECTIOUS DISEASES

It has been estimated from the data of the collaborative study of the National Institutes of Health that at least 5 per cent of all pregnancies in the United States are complicated by an infection other than the common cold. Infectious diseases thus constitute an important complication of pregnancy and the parturient must be advised

TABLE 2. APPROXIMATE FREQUENCY OF
VIRUS INFECTIONS IN THE MOTHER DURING
PREGNANCY AND IN THE NEWBORN INFANT[*]

Infection	Approximate Frequency	
	Mother No./1000 Pregnancies	Neonate No./1000 Live Births
Cytomegalovirus	30–50	6–15
Rubella	1–22	0.7–7
Herpesvirus hominis (simplex)	0.5–25	Uncommon[†]
Coxsackie B	90	Uncommon[†]
Mumps	1.0	Rare[†]
Varicella-zoster	0.5	Rare[†]
Rubeola	0.06	Rare[†]

[*]From Overall, J. C., and Glasgow, L. A.: J. Pediat., 77:315, 1970.

[†]There are insufficient data to permit numerical estimates.

of the necessity of avoiding exposure to communicable diseases. In addition, the control of these diseases in the obstetric unit, including the neonatal nursery, requires the strict enforcement of rigid rules. In the case of chickenpox, diphtheria, enterovirus infection, rubella, measles, mumps, pertussis, scarlet fever, and smallpox, the pregnant patient should be cared for in a unit remote from the obstetric area or, ideally, in an infectious disease hospital equipped to care for pregnant patients. If any of these diseases develops in a patient in the obstetric unit, she should be isolated and her nurses and those who have cared for the infant should not be allowed to return to duty unless it can be verified that they are immune to the particular disease or until the incubation period has expired.

It is difficult to assess the prevalence of the more important infectious diseases complicating pregnancy. Often they produce only mild and nonspecific symptoms in the adult and their frequency in the population varies with the existence of epidemics. Systematic surveys including attempts at virus isolation and repetitive antibody studies would be needed to gain a precise insight. A recent survey of the extent of virus diseases gives the figures shown in Table 2. Even more difficult to assess is the frequency with which bacterial diseases complicate pregnancy, and their effect upon fetal well-being is more indirect. While bacterial infections are undoubtedly common, the placenta is effective in preventing their passage to the embryo, and maternal bacterial diseases during

pregnancy take a course that is generally similar to those in the nonpregnant state. There is one important exception, ascending infection of the amniotic cavity, leading to chorioamnionitis.

AMNIOTIC SAC INFECTION SYNDROME – CHORIOAMNIONITIS

Inflammation of chorion and of the fetal vessels of chorion and umbilical cord occurs frequently, the amnion being passively involved since it does not possess blood vessels. When histologic examination of all placentas is undertaken it becomes apparent that the frequency of these inflammatory reactions has an inverse relationship to gestational age and birth weight (Table 3), and in the majority of middle-trimester abortions the fetus is so affected. Characteristically, the leukocytic emigration is directional; i.e., the polymorphs are seen to migrate from the intervillous space (maternal) and from the chorionic vessels (fetal) toward the amniotic cavity. This amniotropism has suggested that within the amniotic cavity resides a chemotactic stimulus that calls forth this reaction, and the most likely of such stimuli would be bacterial infection. Indeed, in severe cases, bacteria and occasionally *Candida albicans* may be identified in the purulent exudate

TABLE 3. INCIDENCE OF CHORIOAMNIONITIS
AND ITS RELATIONSHIP TO BIRTH WEIGHT
AND GESTATIONAL AGE[*]

Birth Weight and Chorioamnionitis	
Weight (Gm.)	Percentage of Chorioamnionitis
≥2500	9.9
<2500	20.0
≥1000, <2500	18.0
<1800	36.00
<1000	50.0
(Midtrimester abortions	66.0)
All live births	10.7

Gestational Age and Umbilical Vasculitis	
Weeks Gestation	Percentage of Umbilical Vasculitis
20–28	42
>28–32	26
>32–36	15
>36–40	17
>40	19
Uncertain	24
All live births	18

[*]From Driscoll, S. G.: Pediat. Clin. N. Amer., 12:493, 1965.

or on the surface of the membranes, but systematic studies have often failed to disclose infectious organisms associated with this inflammatory reaction. Hence, other hypotheses have been suggested for the genesis of chorioamnionitis — specifically, that the inflammation results from fetal hypoxia.

There are several reasons why the infectious hypothesis is favored. In the first place, there are often bacteria found and these are most commonly identical to those that are also resident in the vaginal tract. Furthermore, chorioamnionitis frequently develops after prolonged rupture of the membranes, particularly when 24 hours or more have passed before delivery. The process is also usually limited to the first of twins, again suggesting the ascending nature of infection. Moreover, when membranes are examined routinely, chorioamnionitis is often limited to the area around that portion of membrane adjacent to the cervical os. Furthermore, there are many well documented cases of fetal hypoxia in which no inflammatory process is found and, of course, significant fetal infection or at least the need for an inflammatory response by the fetus may well compromise his well-being so that he appears in distress. The reasons why an obvious infection of the fetus may not exist at birth despite the presence of extensive chorioamnionitis are not understood. It may be that the offending agents have been successfully combated by the exudate, and also that the culture methods employed for study are inadequate. In this respect attention must be drawn particularly to the Mycoplasma organisms, which are difficult to identify and, at the same time, are well known contaminants of the urogenital tract and are capable of eliciting an acute inflammatory response.

It is perhaps most logical to envisage the pathophysiologic events of the amniotic sac infection syndrome as follows, recognizing that the entire sequence is not always documented and that exceptions may occur. During normal gestation the endocervix is occluded by the contracted state of its fibromuscular tissue and the presence of a dense mucous plug. When labor ensues or when the occluded state is disrupted by premature dilatation of the cervix or significant endocervicitis, then the decidua capsularis and chorion of the forelying membranes become exposed to the vaginal flora. Frequently, the decidua capsularis at this point has undergone degenerative changes, so that it lacks adequate vascular support. Inflammation ensues at this point and, usually following rupture of the membranes, microorganisms spread into the amniotic fluid. Occasionally it has been found that amniotic sac infection takes place without membrane rupture, particularly in ascending fungus infection. It is now assumed that the bacteria or their toxins elicit the amniotropic leukocyte migration from the placental surface which, at times, is associated with a maternal febrile response and also fetal tachycardia. The outcome varies, depending upon the virulence of the organism. More often than not, the infection is limited to the cavity and the fetus may become infected only passively by swallowing or inhaling the exudate. When delivery occurs at this point, his main difficulty may result from the obstructive nature of the exudate in his pulmonary system. Infectious symptoms may ensue later in neonatal life when a true bronchopneumonia, gastroenteritis, epidermal infection, or meningitis may become a problem. Considering the frequency of the inflammatory response in the placenta, however, it is apparent that the response ends usually with delivery, postpartum endometritis being a possible maternal complication of the infection.

The frequency of the infection around midgestational deliveries, the pathologic findings, and recent demographic studies of the syndrome suggest that endocervicitis and consequent chorioamnionitis may often be the cause of premature delivery, rather than its sequel. The finding of unusual strains of Mycoplasma organisms, particularly among the conceptuses of women with recurrent midpregnancy abortions, suggests that resident Mycoplasma endocervicitis may initiate the labor. In some cases antibiotic therapy between pregnancies, of the patient *and* her husband, has resulted in favorable outcome. The disease is much more common in lower socioeconomic groups, among whose prematurely born infants infections were found in 27 per cent of perinatal autopsies. Interestingly, the fetal adrenal glands in such cases showed morphologic changes that are consistent with chronic fetal distress (increased weight and increased width of definitive cortex).

Practical considerations include choice of delivery and administration of antimicrobial therapy. Because of the significant increase of chorioamnionitis with fetal infection when the membranes have been ruptured for more than 24 hours, it is desirable to effect delivery if fetal maturity assures extrauterine survival. Much more difficult is the decision when rupture of membranes and desultory labor commence with an immature fetus. Usually it is impossible to anticipate the type of organism that might eventually cause infectious problems, and random studies of antibiotic prophylaxis have not shown increased fetal survival when such therapy was undertaken. Although many antibiotics pass the placental membrane freely, perhaps ampicillin has the greatest advantages, although it must be recognized that the only benefit may be a reduction of postpartum complications. It is imperative when chorioamnionitis is suspected that the pediatrician receive adequate warning of the possible infection and that the placenta be examined promptly. Often it will show a milky surface, obscured by the inflammatory exudate, and at times it will have a distinct fetid odor.

The amniotic sac infection syndrome does not ensue during episodes of *maternal bacteremia*. In such rare instances, usually associated with life-threatening diseases of the mother, focal placentitis with abscesses in the villous tissue ensues. Only secondarily, after destruction of fetal villous capillaries, may the fetus suffer infectious complications. The pathway is particularly well documented for *Listeria monocytogenes* infection in which case the fetus may succumb from "granulomatosis infantiseptica," an uncommonly recognized disease in this country. It is apparently a greater problem in Europe and the agricultural communities. In a similar manner *tuberculosis* and *coccidioidomycosis* may be transferred to the fetus after having caused specific villous lesions. In tuberculosis the granulomatous lesion is usually resident in the endometrium and may secondarily involve the placenta, but it appears to be an uncommon event since the infection is more often the cause of sterility. Coccidioidomycosis, on the other hand, in epidemic areas is an important complication of pregnancy. Dissemination of benign primary disease may be initiated by pregnancy and it is almost invariably fatal. Amphotericin B therapy may be beneficial even though it carries a high risk because of the nephrotoxicity of the drug.

RUBELLA (GERMAN MEASLES)

Rubella is a common communicable disease due to a single RNA virus of the paramyxovirus group. It is usually transmitted by droplet infection. The virus is pleomorphic, relatively unstable, and excreted by the nasopharynx and in stool and urine, and it is disseminated widely during irregular periods of epidemics. The last major epidemic in the United States took place in 1964 and from its occurrence it is conservatively estimated that 30,000 infants suffered rubella-caused birth defects of one kind or another. Together with cytomegalovirus infection and congenital toxoplasmosis, rubella is the most important infectious antecedent of congenital anomalies.

The disease has an incubation period of two to three weeks with the development of a maculopapular rash in approximately half of the affected adults, fever, and tenderness of the postauricular and cervical lymph nodes. Neuritis and arthritis are frequent and often severe concomitant symptoms but they are usually self-limited. During an epidemic the disease is readily suspected, but because of the frequently minor symptomatology, during nonepidemic periods the diagnosis may be difficult and must always be entertained, particularly during the winter. Various objective means of diagnosis now exist (Fig. 11) which include isolation of the virus from the nasopharynx and neutralizing, hemagglutination-inhibiting, and complement-fixing antibody studies. During the nonepidemic periods it is assumed that approximately 85 per cent of pregnant women have prior immunity; i.e., 15 per cent are susceptible. Figures collected from 30,000 women during the collaborative perinatal research study indicate that clinical rubella occurred once in 1000 pregnancies during nonepidemic periods, while the incidence rose to 22 per 1000 during the 1964 epidemic. In addition, some women experienced seroconversion during this period, indicating clinically inapparent rubella infection (Fig. 12).

The recovery of the pregnant woman is

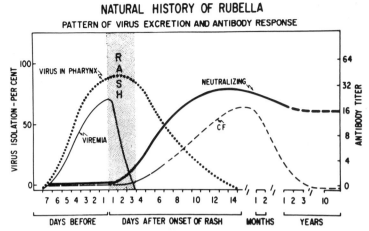

Figure 11. Pattern of virus excretion and antibody response during rubella. (From Cooper, L. Z.: Rubella: a preventable cause of birth defects. Birth Defects Original Article Series, Vol. 4. National Foundation, New York, 1968, pp. 23–35.)

prompt—barring the rare development of encephalitis—with only neuritis and arthritis lingering on at times for several weeks. The outlook for the conceptus, however, is much less favorable and depends in part on his gestational age. In general, the younger his age the more serious the sequelae. The direct relationship of fetal malformations to maternal rubella infection was recognized in 1942 by Gregg, and there is no longer any doubt that the anomalies are due to direct infection of fetus and placenta. Virus has been isolated from abortion specimens, from defective parts of the embryo, and from the placenta soon after maternal viremia, the virus being readily transmitted through the placenta in early gestation. Here it may cause a relatively mild and nonspecific villous inflammatory lesion. The virus is also found in amniotic fluid.

It is obviously of importance to know how often the fetus is infected and whether malformations are to be expected in every

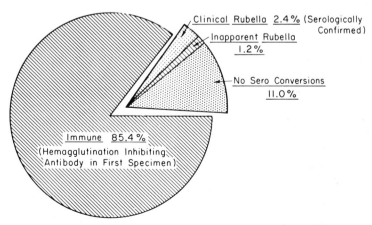

Figure 12. Breakdown of results of analysis of paired serum specimens from 500 pregnant women from 10 collaborating hospitals throughout the United States. (From Sever, J. L., In Waisman, H. A., and Kerr, G., eds.: Fetal Growth and Development. McGraw-Hill Book Co., New York, 1970.)

instance of fetal infection. Unfortunately, several facets of the complex interactions between the virus and the pregnant organism make an accurate assessment difficult. Direct isolation of virus from therapeutic abortion specimens has been the rule in almost all cases where rubella was contracted during the first three months of gestation but it is impossible to say whether lasting sequelae would necessarily have resulted in such embryos. The virus is irregularly distributed in the embryo and causes a cytotoxic effect. In part this is perhaps due to chromosomal damage; in part it may result from vasculitis in the fetus. Moreover, virus-infected cells multiply less readily and often die. As a consequence, interference with organogenesis occurs in early embryonic development while after its completion growth retardation and a variety of fetal disease states ensue that are now considered the "expanded congenital rubella syndrome." Although the virus may persist in tissues for years after its acquisition in utero, the development of specific antibodies by the fetus after the first trimester may also eradicate the infection. It has also been suggested that in later fetal life the placenta with its inflammatory response may become an effective barrier to the virus. Thus, it is difficult to anticipate precisely the fate of the fetus in any given instance. Suffice it to say, fetal infection is nearly 100 per cent during the first trimester, and because of the serious nature of most of its effects, therapeutic abortion is indicated when infection can be diagnosed this early. It was formerly suggested that malformations develop in 20 to 30 per cent of fetuses during maternal rubella. This estimate is now considered too low, particularly when minor and late-diagnosed impairment, such as hearing defects, is considered.

Among the long-term sequelae of congenital rubella, most noteworthy are congenital heart disease, deafness, cataract, and cerebral and somatic retardation (Fig. 13), but a wide variety of other congenital anomalies have been traced to the infection as well. The expanded congenital rubella syndrome consists primarily of thrombocytopenic purpura and hepatosplenomegaly but other and more variable manifestations, such as long bone lesions, pneumonitis, and encephalitis, are found. Of considerable importance is the recognition that these infants shed virus for many months

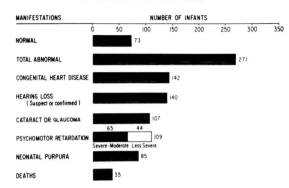

Figure 13. Clinical manifestations of congenital rubella detected during the first 18 months of life. (From Cooper, L. Z.: Rubella: a preventable cause of birth defects. Birth Defects Original Article Series, Vol. 4. National Foundation, New York, 1968, pp. 23–35.)

and thus constitute a hazard to other infants in the nursery as well as to the personnel handling the infected, and at times gravely ill, infants.

In summary, then, it emerges that a majority of fetuses show some ill effect when maternal rubella occurs during the first two trimesters. Hence, a consideration of prophylactic vaccination developed in recent years is important, recognizing that not enough experience is available at this time to answer many difficult questions concerning this disease. With this in mind the following recommendations may be advisable in the management of rubella-susceptible or infected women.

Statement on Rubella Vaccination and Control of Rubella Virus Infection in Women of Childbearing Age

(The American College of Obstetricians and Gynecologists and the National Council of Obstetrics-Gynecology)

I. In the adult female population approximately 85 to 90 per cent of individuals are thought to have a high level of naturally acquired immunity and only 10 to 15 per cent are considered to be susceptible to rubella infection.

II. The current mass vaccination program, directed at prepubertal children, seeks to eliminate or reduce wild virus rubella. However, at the present the duration of immunity acquired from vaccination remains in question. Available data indicate that antibodies persist at least for four years, the period of time the present vaccine has been available. It is possible that adult women vaccinated in childhood may be susceptible and might acquire an active rubella infection. This latter infection may express itself subclinically with only arthralgia or mild malaise and hence may go undetected. Should this occur in pregnancy, the consequences to the fetus may be comparable to a rubella infection in the absence of previous vaccination. Whether or not the vaccine per se has any teratogenic capacity is unknown, and such knowledge may not be available for a long time.

III. The following recommendations pertain to women in the childbearing age:

A. Vaccination of the pregnant woman is contraindicated under all circumstances.

B. No woman in the childbearing age should be routinely vaccinated unless it can be determined that she has a negative hemagglutin-inhibiting antibody titer (HAI) and thus is susceptible to rubella.

C. If a woman in the childbearing age has a negative HAI test, she may be vaccinated if there is reasonable assurance that she will not become pregnant for a period of at least two months.

D. All pregnant women, even those vaccinated, should be routinely tested for HAI antibodies at the first prenatal visit. If a question of rubella exposure arises in the patient with a negative test, a repeat blood specimen can be tested four weeks after the presumed exposure. A seroconversion from a negative to a positive test is indicative of a recent infection and raises the question of termination of pregnancy.*

E. Postpartum patients who had negative HAI tests prenatally can be vaccinated in the immediate puerperium if there is reasonable assurance that they will not become pregnant for at least two months.

F. All patients seen in premarital examinations who have negative HAI tests should be routinely vaccinated if there is reasonable assurance that they will not become pregnant for at least two months.

G. Patients tested in a reputable laboratory should be given a card verifying the results of the test.

H. Termination of pregnancy should be considered in a woman who initially tests negative for rubella antibody (negative HAI) and who has a seroconversion after a presumed exposure to wild type virus.

I. There is no conclusive evidence that the attenuated virus (vaccine virus) is transmitted from person to person. Hence, termination of pregnancy is not considered in women who have been exposed to recently vaccinated children or adults.

J. The administration of human immune gamma globulin to pregnant women who have been exposed or are suffering from a rubella infection is not usually recommended. There is little evidence that any significant prophylactic effect may be expected from gamma globulin in persons who are infected with a rubella virus.

CYTOMEGALOVIRUS (CMV) INFECTION

The infection with this ubiquitous virus of the herpes group is usually not recognized clinically in the adult and, except in immunologically handicapped individuals, it has no significant sequelae in adult life. Approximately 80 per cent of adults have neutralizing antibody to the virus to which they must have been exposed previously, perhaps without overt illness.

When the infection is acquired during pregnancy it may be transmitted via the placenta to the fetus and cause significant disease. In its severest form the fetal and neonatal infection has many similarities to the expanded rubella syndrome and to congenital toxoplasmosis. Thrombocytopenic purpura, hepatosplenomegaly with jaundice, and microcephaly with periventricular calcification are among the leading mani-

---

*The hemagglutination-inhibition test becomes positive within three days in about two-thirds of cases and in nearly all cases within four to seven days after onset of rash. It is a relatively reliable test and highly useful for clinical purposes.

festations. The disease is an important cause of cerebral palsy because it produces widespread cerebral degeneration.

It has recently been recognized from prospective studies that congenital infection is very much more common than is apparent from the clinically overt cases. In some of the neonates with viruria or neutralizing antibodies a variety of disease manifestations may develop in later life, but also some appear to suffer no sequelae. As with congenital rubella infection, infants with the congenital CMV infection are frequently underweight, have elevated IgM antibody levels, and excrete the virus for prolonged periods, particularly in the urine. The pathologic picture is characterized by the existence of extremely large cells with inclusion bodies in the nuclei, the so-called owl-eye cells. These may be excreted in the urine and recognized in the sediment. They were first described in the salivary glands, hence the name salivary gland virus. It is now recognized that the infection of salivary glands is but one manifestation of CMV infection, which is usually widespread throughout the body. In addition to the cerebral and hepatic involvement, frequently lung, eye, kidney, and pancreas are affected. Similar inclusion bodies have been identified in the placenta, and, rarely, fetuses of consecutive pregnancies may be infected. In such cases it is assumed that the uterus harbors a resident infection, it being well known that the virus may persist intracellularly for years despite the presence of high antibody titers. The virus has also been recovered from breast milk. Currently no specific treatment is available and there exists no vaccine.

HERPESVIRUS INFECTION

Infection of the genital tract with *Herpesvirus hominis* type 2 is a relatively frequent occurrence, and when it coincides with the advent of rupture of fetal membranes or birth it presents a major threat to the infant. In all of the approximately 150 cases of neonatal infection the acquisition of the virus can be traced to contact with vaginal or vulvar lesions of active herpes. Only on very rare occasion has transplacental infection been documented.

In the newborn the infection often takes a fulminant course ending fatally with the syndrome of "hepatoadrenal necrosis"

which may be accompanied by degenerative changes in many other systems. Probably less commonly the infection is not fatal and may then cause residual lesions such as microcephaly and microphthalmos. Recurrent vesicles have occurred in some of the infants but often the diagnosis is not suspected in the early stages.

Typical lesions of genital herpesvirus infection are illustrated in Figures 14 and 15. Commonly the symptoms include vulvar soreness, dysuria, dyspareunia, and increased vaginal discharge. The symptoms have sudden onset and usually subside within a week. The vesicles rupture early and tend to develop into shallow ulcers. On the cervix they may be mistaken for neoplastic lesions (Fig. 16). Vaginal smears and touch preparations show characteristic eosinophilic intranuclear inclusion bodies (type A), frequently also multi-nucleated giant cells and dysplastic squamous cells have been identified (Fig. 17). The disease may be regarded as a venereal disease in

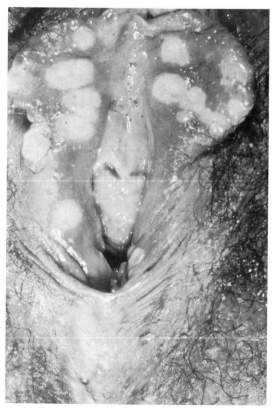

Figure 14. Extensive superficial vulvar ulcerations in primary herpes simplex infection. (From Yen, S. S. C., Reagan, J. W., and Rosenthal, M. S.: Obstet. Gynec., 25:479, 1965.)

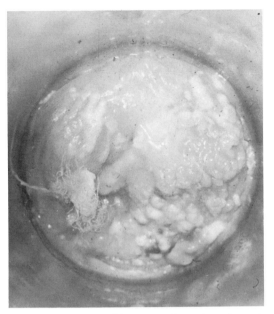

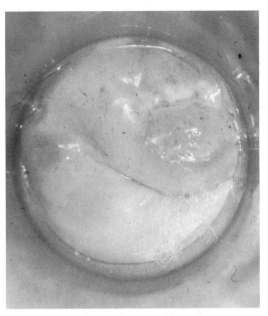

Figure 15. Cervical lesions in the patient shown in Figure 14. (From Yen, S. S. C., Reagen, J. W., and Rosenthal, M. S.: Obstet. Gynec., 25:479, 1965.)

Figure 16. Ulcerated cervical lesion in recurrent herpes simplex infection. (From Yen, S. S. C., Reagan, J. W., and Rosenthal, M. S.: Obstet. Gynec., 25:479, 1965.)

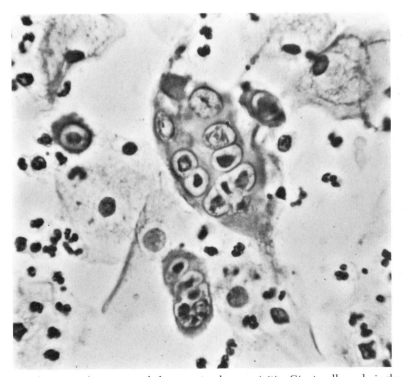

Figure 17. Cervical smear of patient with herpes simplex cervicitis. Giant cells and single-nucleated cells with typical intranuclear inclusion bodies. × 800. (From Yen, S. S. C., Reagan, J. W., and Rosenthal, M. S.: Obstet. Gynec., 25:479, 1965.)

that transmission from penile herpes lesions is well established.

Because of the serious complications in neonatal life the infant must be protected from contact with active herpetic lesions in the vulva, and elective cesarean section without labor is the preferred method of delivery. There is good evidence that in all cases of neonatal herpesvirus infection the fetal membranes had ruptured before cesarean section was undertaken. Conversely, if section was performed before labor and rupture of membranes, the infant escaped active disease.

Of the two serologically distinct types of herpesvirus only type 2 is associated with genital infections. The risk to the fetus of maternal labial infection with herpesvirus (type 1), is presumably only minimal.

ENTEROVIRUS INFECTIONS

Infection of the mother with poliovirus, Coxsackie viruses, and the numerous ECHO viruses has uncommonly recognized fetal sequelae. Although fatal infections with Coxsackie B viruses (particularly types 3 and 4) are relatively common and occur at times in epidemics in the newborn nursery, in most instances the infection is acquired in neonatal life. It then results in myocarditis and encephalitis primarily, and liver and many other organs may be involved to a lesser extent. Transplacental infection is extremely rare, if it exists. The disease is not markedly different when it occurs in pregnancy as compared to the nonpregnant state and is most common in fall and early winter. In the past, cases of transplacental poliomyelitis infection with paralysis of the fetus have been documented; however, with the advent of an effective vaccine, concern with poliomyelitis in pregnancy is restricted to patients with residual paralysis from the disease. In general, these patients do well in pregnancy. Asymmetry of the pelvis is seen in many of them but it is usually minimal and rarely causes dystocia. Except for the expulsive efforts of the second stage, labor may be expected to be normal. Although in the second stage the patient may have the desire to bear down and expel the fetus, if the abdominal muscles are paralyzed the effort is nonproductive A low forceps operation with episiotomy is usually required to accomplish delivery.

VARIOLA AND VACCINIA

Because of compulsory vaccination smallpox (variola) is an uncommon disease in the United States now. Transplacental infection of the fetus has been described and fetal variola seems to be invariably fatal.

Accumulated evidence suggests that vaccinia virus also passes the placenta and fetal vaccinia with destructive lesions in various organs, including the placenta, has been observed on several occasions. In general it is assumed that such transplacental infection occurs only when primary *vaccination* is undertaken during pregnancy, revaccination appears to be without such danger. On occasion the infection is acquired by a previously unvaccinated pregnant woman when other members of the family are vaccinated. It is therefore recommended that primary vaccination never be undertaken during pregnancy and that revaccination be done only when important epidemiologic circumstances demand the procedure.

OTHER VIRUS INFECTIONS

Several virus diseases have been reported to take a more serious course during pregnancy, occasionally leading to maternal death, fetal complications, or both. Thus, although *chickenpox* (varicella) probably does not occur more often in pregnancy, it may take a fulminant, fatal course. *Herpes zoster* is rarely recognized in the newborn and congenital anomalies have not been related to this virus infection.

Mumps does not often complicate pregnancy, but its occurrence has become of interest since it was shown that children with endocardial fibroelastosis may have positive skin tests to this antigen. Prospective studies have failed to confirm this relationship. On the other hand, growth retardation and rarely hepatomegaly and microcephaly have been observed in children whose mothers had mumps during pregnancy. Because of the general similarities of this myxovirus to the rubella virus it may be that similarities of their infectious sequelae will also become apparent when more cases are studied.

Measles is very rarely encountered during pregnancy since more than 90 per cent of the population acquire immunity in childhood. When the disease has been introduced into previously unaffected populations the mortality is appreciable and abortion common. A suggested relationship of measles virus to congenital anomalies is not clear-cut, a British study suggesting a three-fold increase over a control population. It seems thus prudent to protect a pregnant woman from contact with patients having the disease.

Influenza virus infection constitutes a significant hazard to the pregnant patient. This acute infectious disease is due to three types of myxoviruses (A, B, and C) of which types A and B with numerous antigenically different strains are responsible for the major recent epidemics. The disease may take a fulminant course in the respiratory passages with severe reduction of vital capacity through pulmonary edema, exudation, hyaline membrane formation, and erosive tracheobronchitis. During epidemics influenza may be the major cause of maternal deaths, secondary staphylococcal pneumonia being prevalent. Abortion often occurs in the course of this severe, febrile illness, but indisputable evidence of transplacental virus transmission or causation of fetal anomalies is lacking. Vaccination with specific polyvalent vaccine has proved to be highly effective in protecting pregnant patients from the serious effects of influenza infection. It has no untoward effect upon the fetus even when practiced early in pregnant patients and is therefore recommended early during epidemics.

Whether or not the *hepatitis* viruses pass the placenta is poorly understood at present. Neonatal jaundice and a variety of destructive and inflammatory lesions of the liver occur in many congenital infections (rubella, CMV infection, toxoplasmosis, Coxsackie B virus infection, and so forth). Until the hepatitis virus can be isolated, the sequelae of hepatitis during pregnancy will be difficult to assess. There is considerable hope that isolation will soon be possible.

LYMPHOGRANULOMA VENEREUM

Lymphogranuloma venereum, a virus disease acquired by sexual contact, is characterized by a marked reaction of the regional lymph nodes, often accompanied by systemic symptoms of malaise and fever. Its frequency differs greatly, depending on the populations studied, and surveys have revealed that 20 per cent or more of the individuals in some communities in the United States may give a positive complement-fixation or Frei test, 1:80 being acceptable for diagnosis.

The local involvement of the inguinal and femoral lymph nodes with suppuration is often severe and disabling. In the chronic form the rectal lymph nodes also suppurate and rectal strictures may appear. The medical treatment of the disease by tetracycline and sulfonamides is not altered by pregnancy.

As a result of the marked scarring of portions of the rectal wall, the rectovaginal septum, and the vagina, labor and delivery may be complicated by soft tissue dystocia. Although the cervix may dilate, the scar tissue surrounding the vagina and rectum, because of its rigidity, may impede progress. Equally important is the fact that forceful pelvic delivery under those circumstances may produce serious disruption of the scar tissue, with lacerations extending into the upper portion of the rectum and the posterior cul-de-sac, and death resulting from peritonitis. In some cases, therefore, abdominal hysterotomy may be the preferred method of delivery.

GRANULOMA INGUINALE

Granuloma inguinale, a disease involving the genital region, is caused by a gram-negative, nonmotile organism which typically is observed in clusters within large mononuclear cells as "Donovan bodies." The pathologic changes involve the skin and the mucous membrane of the genitalia, and, in the female, lesions of the cervix and vagina are not infrequent. The characteristic lesion is a sharp-edged, readily bleeding ulcer with a granulomatous base. Tetracycline and streptomycin are considered the treatment of choice. Marked scarring ultimately occurs, and should the cervix or the vagina be involved, soft tissue dystocia may impede descent of the fetus at the time of labor. As with lymphogranuloma venereum, abdominal hysterotomy deserves consideration, for huge exfoliative growths and scar tissue formed in and about the vagina may preclude pelvic delivery.

GONORRHEA

The incidence of infection with *Neisseria gonorrhoeae* has increased remarkably in recent years, perhaps in part because of changing behavior patterns, and in part because of increased resistance of the organism to antibiotics. An important obstacle to control of the disease is the frequently asymptomatic nature of gonorrheal infection in women, who may be totally unaware of the disease. Several recent surveys have shown approximately 5 per cent of pregnant women to have inapparent gonorrheal infection. Two recent innovations for diagnostic purposes are helpful in handling the disease. These are fluorescent antibody identification and use of a special medium (Thayer-Martin) whose antibiotic content suppresses the growth of undesirable contaminants. In a large study the diagnosis was most reliably established when cervical secretions were examined, and both methods proved equally effective, the former being more rapid. Examinations of urethral specimens were considerably less successful. After curative therapy the fluorescence method may give false-positive results for a few days because of persistence of antigens from dead bacteria. Of various schemes of treatment in current usage procaine penicillin G in a dosage of 4.8 million units (aqueous or in combination with oil) had the best results, effecting a cure rate of 89 per cent.

Although the Credé method of prophylaxis of ophthalmia neonatorum is commonly practiced and generally effective, there is no room for complacency about this disease. Neonatal eye infections are once again seen occasionally and there is also a 30 per cent puerperal morbidity associated with this infection.

SYPHILIS

Of the various chronic infectious diseases seen in pregnancy, syphilis remains one of the more important. The incidence of the disease is apparently on the increase worldwide. Prenatal examination affords a practical opportunity of making the initial discovery of the disease in the female population, and series have been reported in which only 10 per cent of the pregnant women with positive blood findings had any previous knowledge of having the disease. Recognition must be taken of the possibility of syphilis being acquired during the course of pregnancy, and in areas where the incidence of the disease is high the serologic test for syphilis should be repeated at the beginning of the last trimester of pregnancy.

When syphilis is contracted prior to or during gestation, the signs are often mild and occasionally may be completely suppressed. Symptoms of late syphilis may improve temporarily during pregnancy, especially in those patients with neurologic manifestations. Although abortion is rarely caused by syphilis, the fetus may become infected and die of a spirochetemia during any period of pregnancy, but usually after the 20th week. In one large series, nearly half of the babies of mothers who did not receive antisyphilitic treatment were stillborn, and the majority of the live-born infants had congenital syphilis. The greater frequency of fetal disease detected in later gestation is most likely due to the fact that the fetus can then muster an inflammatory response rather than to the greater placental penetrability by spirochetes, as was once believed.

In mothers with syphilis the placenta is larger, and may weigh twice as much as the normal placenta. The villi contain an increased amount of fibrous tissue with lymphocytic infiltration. The walls of the blood vessels are thickened, owing to fibrous proliferation of the intima, and the surrounding tissue may show necrosis. With the proper technique, spirochetes may be demonstrated. When syphilitic changes are seen in the placenta, the infant usually is affected with the disease, but congenital syphilis can be present in the infant without such changes being evident.

The diagnosis of syphilis during pregnancy is based on the usual findings and serologic studies. Pregnancy itself does not cause negative reactions, but incomplete or weak serologic reactions are common.

The drug of choice in the treatment of syphilis is penicillin. The infant will be free of syphilis even if treatment is instituted a few weeks preceding delivery. The serologic titer is a valuable indication of the fetal prognosis, but repeated observations are essential to detect evidence of a clinical relapse during pregnancy. Should this occur, a healthy child may be obtained if treatment is promptly reinstituted. A second course of therapy may be necessary during pregnancy in a few patients who fail to show satisfactory clinical or serologic response.

The total amount of penicillin administered is 6 million units. The incidence of Herxheimer reactions in pregnancy is great enough to warrant the giving of small doses during the first 24 hours, after which the amount of penicillin can be steadily increased. Hence, 150,000 units of penicillin can be administered during the first 24 hours. This dosage can be doubled on each of the two successive days, after which 600,000 units daily is continued. The schedule can be modified for patient convenience, sensitivity, and toxicity. Tetracycline, 0.5 gram by mouth four times daily for 10 to 12 days, may be administered in place of penicillin.

With penicillin therapy, the incidence of congenital syphilis may be reduced below 1 per cent, even though the antibiotic is administered as late as the 32nd week of pregnancy. The baby must be carefully observed and studied at birth and for the first six months of life. The serologic findings of the cord blood at delivery may be misleading, for a false positive can be the result of the presence of maternal reagin in the fetal serum. In order to exclude congenital syphilis, repeated tests should reveal a falling titer, with its eventual disappearance. The absence or presence of the disease in the offspring can be established by the end of the sixth month of life, by means of repeated serologic tests and by x-ray studies of the long bones. The long bones show an increased density and widening of the epiphyseal lines, and areas of destruction may occasionally be seen at the ends of the bones. Infants with congenital syphilis discovered at birth or recognized during the neonatal period should receive penicillin, 100,000 units per kilogram daily for a period of 7 to 10 days. The question of retreatment of the mother in a subsequent pregnancy will arise. In view of the ease and safety of administration, even patients with congenital syphilis may well be treated.

MALARIA

In certain endemic areas malaria is a more common complication of pregnancy than any other medical condition. The course of malaria is adversely affected by pregnancy, which tends to cause exacerbations in the chronic form and aggravates the severity of an acute attack. Cerebral manifestations associated with malaria are more common in the pregnant patient, and this very serious form of the disease may simulate the convulsive form of pregnancy toxemia. Indeed, pregnant patients with malaria are stated to be more prone to toxemic manifestations, and the disease predisposes the patient to albuminuria and hypertension. In the acute form, intrauterine malarial infections may develop and cause fetal death by massive parasitic infection of the placenta; the parasites can also be easily demonstrated in fetal brain tissue. Further, the fetus may die as the result of maternal toxicity or premature labor. Latent or chronic malaria, however, may have little effect on the conceptus.

Adequate treatment of malaria by Atabrine or quinine protects the baby as well as the mother. With the disappearance of the parasite from the mother's blood the chance of damage to the placenta is minimized. Moreover, effective protection is afforded to the fetus by ready passage of quinine through the placenta. In therapeutic doses, quinine does not initiate labor, but its continuous use is thought to cause congenital deafness in the newborn. Atabrine and other newer agents may be used either alone or in combination with quinine, but the latter seems to be the most effective in the pregnant patient.

TOXOPLASMOSIS

Toxoplasmosis is a ubiquitous protozoan infection which is of obstetric importance because of its tendency to affect the fetus in utero. Until the present time the diagnosis of toxoplasmosis in the adult has been uncommon, but it, together with infantile or congenital toxoplasmosis, is being recognized with increasing frequency. A high incidence of neutralizing antibodies to Toxoplasma has been found in the serum of mothers who have given birth to children with hydrocephalus, anencephaly, cerebral calcification, chorioretinitis, or convulsive seizures. The organism has been demonstrated in the placenta (Fig. 18) and may be isolated from the affected organs of the infants. It is transmitted in infected undercooked meat, and recent-

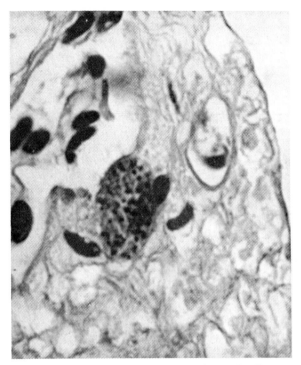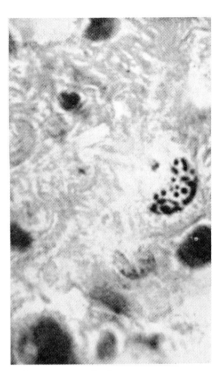

Figure 18. Toxoplasma pseudocysts in placental villi. (From Beckett, R. S., and Flynn, F. J., Jr.: New Eng. J. Med., 249:345, 1953.)

ly it has been suggested that cats serve as the most important reservoir of Toxoplasma. Approximately a third to a half of babies born to women who acquired the infection during pregnancy are found to be infected. Subsequent children are not infected.

The clinical and pathologic picture of this protozoan disease in the adult is quite different from that in the child. In the adult a peculiar type of interstitial pneumonitis and meningoencephalitis may be present but there are few, if any, symptoms. Glandular and ocular disease are relatively frequent. More important is the fact that mothers who give birth to Toxoplasma-infected babies do not themselves exhibit recognizable signs of the disease. In the child, however, granulomatous lesions of the central nervous system may result in hydrocephalus, convulsions, and spasticity. The pathologic changes in the gray matter of the cerebral cortex may vary from small foci of cellular infiltration to widespread zones of necrosis, associated at times with extensive calcification. Systemic involvement is evidenced by diarrhea, splenomegaly, hepatomegaly, jaundice, and purpura. Elevated levels of IgM antibodies are commonly found in such infants at birth.

Once the diagnosis is suspected, it may be confirmed by demonstration of the neutralizing antibodies (dye test) and complement-fixing toxoplasmic antibodies. These tests are subject to interpretation. Both of these antibodies are transmitted to the fetus quantitatively and the levels may remain near the maternal level during the first six weeks after birth, after which time there is a gradual fall. The neutralizing antibodies persist longer than the complement-fixing antibodies. In infants with congenital toxoplasmosis, antibodies persist in amounts equaling or exceeding those of the mother. In all cases the levels of neutralizing antibodies are high (dye test), but the complement-fixation test may be negative in the acute phase of the disease.

The aim of treatment is to interfere with the biosynthetic pathway to folinic acid, and sulfonamides and pyrimethamine (Daraprim) are employed. They are administered until active immunity becomes effective; however, because of the necessity of folic acid for embryonic and trophoblastic growth, treatment during pregnancy is difficult. For this reason and because the probability of fetal infection is small during the first trimester, treatment is contraindicated at that time. During the second and third trimesters therapy should include yeast and folinic acid.

HISTOPLASMOSIS

Histoplasmosis in pregnancy has been reported. It is caused by a parasitic fungus, *Histoplasma capsulatum*, which may involve the lung and, in the severe form, the reticuloendothelial system. Splenomegaly, hepatomegaly, pyrexia, leukopenia, and anemia are found in the seriously ill patient. Recovery is the rule, but the disease is not transmitted through the placenta to the fetus.

BIBLIOGRAPHY

Chorioamnionitis

Benirschke, K., and Driscoll, S. G.: The Pathology of the Human Placenta. Springer-Verlag, New York, 1967.

Driscoll, S. G.: Pathology and the developing fetus. Pediat. Clin. N. Amer., 12:493, 1965.

Gregory, J. E., and Payne, F. E.: Mycoplasma in the uterine cervix. Amer. J. Obstet. Gynec., 107:220, 1970.

Gunn, G. C., Mishell, D. R., and Morton, D. G.: Premature rupture of the fetal membranes. Amer. J. Obstet. Gynec., 106:469, 1970.

Kundsin, R. B., and Driscoll, S. G.: Mycoplasmas and human reproductive failure. Surg. Gynec. Obstet., 131:89, 1970.

Naeye, R. L., and Blanc, W. A.: Relation of poverty and race to antenatal infection. New Eng. J. Med., 283:555, 1970.

Olding, L.: Value of placentitis as a sign of intrauterine infection in human subjects. A morphological, bacteriological, clinical and statistical study. Acta Path. Microbiol. Scand. A., 78:256, 1970.

Smale, L. E., and Waechter, K. G.: Dissemination of coccidioidomycosis in pregnancy. Amer. J. Obstet. Gynec., 107:356, 1970.

Rubella

Banatvala, J. E.: Laboratory investigations in the assessment of rubella during pregnancy. Brit. Med. J., 1:561, 1968.

Cooper, L. Z.: Rubella: a preventable cause of birth defects. Birth Defects Original Article Series, Vol. 4. National Foundation, New York, 1968, pp. 23–35.

Hildebrandt, R. J., and Weber, J. M.: Immunization of young adult females with the Cendehill strain of rubella vaccine. Amer. J. Obstet. Gynec., 107:645, 1970.

Gregg, N. M.: Congenital cataract following German measles in the mother. Trans. Ophthal. Soc. Aust., 3:35, 1942.

Overall, J. C., and Glasgow, L. A.: Virus infections of the fetus and newborn infant. J. Pediat., 77:315, 1970.

Rubella Symposium. Amer. J. Dis. Child., 110:345, 1965.

Sever, J. L.: Infectious agents and fetal disease. In Waisman, H. A., and Kerr, G., eds.: Fetal Growth and Development. McGraw-Hill Book Co., New York, 1970.

Thompson, K. M., and Tobin, J. O.: Isolation of rubella virus from abortion material. Brit. Med. J., 1:264, 1970.

Cytomegalovirus Infection

Diosi, P., Babusceac, L., Nevinglovschi, O., and Kun-Stoicu, G.: Cytomegalovirus infection associated with pregnancy. Lancet, 2:1063, 1967.

Embil, J. A., Ozere, R. L., and Haldane, E. V.: Congenital cytomegalovirus infection in two siblings from consecutive pregnancies. J. Pediat., 77:417, 1970.

Hanshaw, J. B.: Cytomegaloviruses. Virology Monographs, Vol. 3. Springer-Verlag, New York, 1968, pp. 1–23.

Monif, G. R. G.: Viral Infections of the Human Fetus. Macmillan & Co., London, 1969.

Starr, J. G., Bart, R. D., and Gold, E.: Inapparent congenital cytomegalovirus infection. Clinical and epidemiologic characteristics in early pregnancy. New Eng. J. Med., 282:1075, 1970.

Herpes Virus Infection

Amstey, M. S., and Balduzzi, P. C.: Genital herpesvirus infection. Amer. J. Obstet. Gynec., 108:188, 1970.

Hass, G. M.: Hepato-adrenal necrosis with intranuclear inclusion bodies. Amer. J. Path., 11:127, 1935.

Nahmias, A. J., Dowdle, W. R., Josey, W. E., Naib, Z. M., Painter, L. M., and Luce, C.: Newborn infection with herpes virus hominis types 1 and 2. J. Pediat, 75:1194, 1969.

Witzleben, C. L., and Driscoll, S. G.: Possible transplacental transmission of herpes simplex infection. Pediatrics, 36:192, 1965.

Yen, S. S. C., Reagan, J. W., and Rosenthal, J. S.: Herpes simplex infection in female genital tract. Obstet. Gynec., 25:479, 1965.

Zavoral, J. H., Ray, W. L., Kinnard, P. G., and Nahmias, A. J.: Neonatal herpetic infection. A fatal consequence of penile herpes in a serviceman. J.A.M.A., 213:1492, 1970.

Enterovirus Infections

Barsky, P., and Beale, A. J.: The transplacental transmission of poliomyelitis. J. Pediat., 51:207, 1957.

Javett, S. N., Heymann, S., Mundel, B., Pepter, W. J., Lurie, H. I., Gear, J., Measroch, V., and Kirsch, Z. G.: A study of an outbreak associated with Coxsackie group B virus infection in a maternity home in Johannesburg. J. Pediat., 48:1, 1956.

Kibrick, S., and Benirschke, K.: Acute aseptic myocarditis and meningoencephalitis in the newborn child infected with Coxsackie virus group B, type 3. New Eng. J. Med., 255:883, 1956.

Variola and Vaccinia

Green, D. M., Reid, S. M., and Rhaney, K.: Generalized vaccinia in the human foetus. Lancet, 1:1296, 1966.

Mehta, A.: Small-pox re-vaccination during pregnancy. Bombay Hosp. J., 11:12, 1969 (Obst. Gynec. Surv., 25:1042, 1970).

Wielenga, G., Ferguson, A. H., van Tongeren, H. A. E., and van Rijssel, T. G.: Prenatal infection with vaccinia virus. Lancet, 1:258, 1961.

Other Virus Infections

Brunell, P. A.: Varicella-zoster infections in pregnancy. J.A.M.A., 199:315, 1967.

Douglas, C. P.: Lymphogranuloma venereum and granuloma inguinale of the vulva. J. Obstet. Gynaec. Brit. Comm., 69:871, 1962.

Freeman, D. W., and Barno, A.: Deaths from influenza associated with pregnancy. J.A.M.A., 78:1172, 1959.

Gorthey, R. L., and Krembs, M. A.: Vulvar condylomata acuminata complicating labor. Obstet. Gynec., 4:67, 1954.

Hulka, J. F.: Effectiveness of polyvalent influenza vaccine in pregnancy. Report of a controlled study during an outbreak of Asian influenza. Obstet. Gynec., 23:830, 1964.

Kaiser, I. H., and King, E. L.: Lymphopathia venereum complicating labor; analysis of 38 cases. Amer. J. Obstet. Gynec., 54:219, 1947.

Manson, M. M., Logan, W. P. D., and Loy, R. M.: Rubella and other virus infections during pregnancy. Report on Public Health and Medical Subjects No. 101. Ministry of Health. H.M. Stationery Office, London, 1960, pp. 1–101. (Measles)

Noren, G. R., Adams, R., and Anderson, R. C.: Positive skin reactivity to mumps virus antigen in endocardial fibroelastosis. J. Pediat., 62:604, 1963.

Pickard, R. E.: Varicella pneumonia in pregnancy. Amer. J. Obstet. Gynec., 101:504, 1968.

Gonorrhea and Syphilis

Dippel, A. L.: Relationship of congenital syphilis to abortion and miscarriage and mechanism of intrauterine protection. Amer. J. Obstet. Gynec., 47:369, 1944.

Kraus, G. W., and Yen, S. S. C.: Gonorrhea during pregnancy. Obstet. Gynec., 31:258, 1968.

Lucas, J. B., Price, E. V., Thayer, J. D., and Schroeter, A.: Diagnosis and treatment of gonorrhea in the female. New Eng. J. Med., 276:1454, 1967.

Malaria and Toxoplasmosis

Archibald, H. M.: Influence of maternal malaria on newborn infants. Brit. Med. J., 2:1512, 1958.

Beckett, R. S., and Flynn, F. J., Jr.: Toxoplasmosis; report of two new cases, with classification and with demonstration of organisms in the human placenta. New Eng. J. Med., 249:345, 1953.

Frenkel, J. K.: Toxoplasmosis. Mechanism of infection, laboratory diagnosis and management. Curr. Top. Path., 54:28, 1971.

Sabin, A. B., and Feldman, H. A.: Persistence of antibodies in congenital toxoplasmosis. Pediatrics, 4:660, 1949.

CONNECTIVE TISSUE DISORDERS

Connective tissue disorders have been attributed to hypersensitivity and autoimmune reactions. Although there may be certain morphologic similarities in certain of these diseases (collagen diseases), no correlation can be offered with respect to etiology.

RHEUMATOID ARTHRITIS

Rheumatoid arthritis tends to occur more frequently in females than in males, and the early signs and symptoms usually appear in the childbearing age. Striking remissions have been observed in the symptoms of this disease during pregnancy, but this is by no means a universal experience.

The treatment of rheumatoid arthritis during pregnancy does not necessarily differ from that during the nonpregnant state. If patients have been receiving cortisone prior to conception, the amounts required will remain the same despite increased adrenal activity. Since relapses may occur post partum, cortisone therapy should be increased for a period.

POLYARTERITIS NODOSA

The clinical features of this disease depend on how much each system of the body is affected by the diffuse arteritis. The kidney, the heart, and the gastrointestinal system are usually involved in that order of frequency, although all areas of the body are subject to morphologic change. The bizarre pattern of the disorder is the result of patchy necrotizing lesions that occur in the walls of the small and medium-sized arteries and arterioles. The vessel wall may be so weakened by these lesions that small aneurysms form and rupture. Older lesions show fibrotic repair and, in some areas, healing results in complete or partial obliteration of the lumen of the blood vessel. Hypertension follows when such anatomic changes occur in the vessels of the kidney. Once suspected, the diagnosis can be confirmed by biopsy of accessible blood vessels. It is doubtful whether pregnancy should be permitted when there is any appreciable renal damage, and therapeutic termination is indicated. In fact, the disease in the nonpregnant in its fulminating form may have a rapid downhill course.

Often confused with pregnancy toxemia, the diagnosis in pregnancy sometimes is made only at autopsy. Despite cortisone therapy, the prognosis is dismal in pregnancy.

SCLERODERMA

Scleroderma announces its presence as firm, nonpitting, painless edema of the skin. Two types of gross changes are noted in the skin and subcutaneous tissues. The first is a focal thickening which, although unsightly, is seldom serious. Only infrequently do these involved areas progress to diffuse change, which is the second type of scleroderma. Pathologically, there is swelling, proliferation, and fusion of the collagen fibrils of the corium. The lesions are peculiar in that the areas may be devoid of hair, with or without pigmentation. The second type of disease is not limited solely to the skin, but muscle and fascia and occasionally the heart, lungs, and gastrointestinal tract reveal collagen changes. The systemic signs and symptoms that often precede the skin changes are not pathognomonic, but once the characteristic thickening of the skin occurs the diagnosis is reasonably certain.

The course in pregnancy is uncertain, particularly for those with the generalized or systemic form of the disease, although the life expectancy is not affected. In the second type of the disease the increased maternal risk is definite even with expert medical management. Renal involvement may dictate the maternal and fetal outcome.

LUPUS ERYTHEMATOSUS

Lupus erythematosus occurs predominantly in females between the ages of 15 and 40. Frequently the first signs and symptoms appear after intense exposure to sunlight. Other factors, however, such as trauma, infection, pregnancy, and allergic responses, are often related to the onset of the disease.

Although variable in degree, fever and arthralgia may be present at the onset of the disease. Subsequent symptoms depend on the extent of the pathologic changes. Focal or diffuse thickening of the serous membranes may result in effusions, and clinical manifestations secondary to changes in the walls of blood vessels are noted. A diffuse lymph node involvement may accompany the disorder. A characteristic skin lesion may appear on the face, distributed over the bridge of the nose and malar regions so that it takes on a butterfly appearance. Occasionally the skin discoloration may appear before the systemic signs and symptoms but in many instances the reverse is true.

It is difficult to assess accurately the influence of pregnancy on the course of lupus erythematosus, because of its uncertain course in the nonpregnant. However, a patient with this disease should realize that it is a calculated risk to undertake pregnancy. It would appear that the disseminated form precludes acceptance of the risk that pregnancy imposes, particularly if there is significant renal damage.

Exacerbations have a much greater incidence in pregnant patients than in the nonpregnant and are especially frequent in the first trimester and immediately post partum. Prednisone therapy may influence favorably both the maternal and fetal risk. However, the presence of cardiovascular and renal involvement and the associated high fetal wastage outweigh the patient's desire to undertake or continue a pregnancy when the disease is diagnosed early in gestation.

Patients with the more chronic discoid form appear to do reasonably well during pregnancy, but a relapse is a distinct possibility. A patient with chronic discoid lupus who does not wish to accept the risk of pregnancy, therefore, deserves the benefit of a therapeutic abortion. It is perhaps well to recall that the overall fetal mortality is considerable, being 30 per cent. The discoid type has been reported in the newborn.

OTHER CONNECTIVE TISSUE DISEASES

The Marfan syndrome, a connective tissue disorder inherited as an autosomal dominant, affects principally the cardiovascular system. If pregnancy is to be undertaken it should be done at an early age for serious cardiovascular risks are involved. A recent experience attests to this in a patient with aortic dissection who fortunately survived thanks to expert cardiac surgery.

Hurler's syndrome is mentioned as another condition in which pregnancy is contraindicated for genetic reasons. Inherited as both an autosomal recessive and a sex-linked trait, the disease may not be evident at birth. Almost all body systems are involved and the intelligence may be markedly impaired.

The Ehlers-Danlos syndrome, usually inherited as an autosomal dominant, has been diagnosed with increased frequency in pregnancy. The basic defect appears to be derangement of the collagen fibers, permitting hyperextensibility of the skin. There may be generalized joint hypermobility, and dislocations have been known to occur. Bruising is common. The obstetric and gynecologic interests are many—an increased incidence of abortion and prematurity and frequent postpartum hemorrhage. Uterine prolapse, pelvic floor relaxation, and cervical incompetence can be expected. Wound healing is compromised and there has been the admonition that once a patient has been delivered by cesarean section, that method should be used in any subsequent pregnancy.

BIBLIOGRAPHY

Beighton, P.: Lethal complications of the Ehlers-Danlos syndrome. Brit. Med. J., 3:656, 1968.

Donaldson, L. B., and de Alvarez, R. R.: The Marfan syndrome and pregnancy. Amer. J. Obstet. Gynec., 92:629, 1965.

Garenstein, M., Pollak, V. E., and Kark, R. M.: Systemic lupus erythematosus and pregnancy. New Eng. J. Med., 267:165, 1962.

Jackson, R.: Discoid lupus in a newborn infant of a mother with lupus erythematosus. Pediatrics, 33:425, 1964.

Siegler, A. M., and Spain, D.: Periarteritis nodosa and pregnancy. Obstet. Gynec., 18:744, 1961.

Slate, W. G., and Graham, A. R.: Scleroderma and pregnancy, Amer. J. Obstet. Gynec., 101:335, 1968.

Stoddard, F. J., and Myers, R. E.: Connective tissue disorders in obstetrics and gynecology (Ehlers-Danlos syndrome). Amer. J. Obstet. Gynec., 102:240, 1968.

Varriale, P., Fusco, J. M., Acampora, A., and Grace, W.: Polyarteritis nodosa in pregnancy. Obstet. Gynec., 25:866, 1965.

ERRORS OF METABOLISM AND DEFICIENCY DISEASES

ERRORS OF METABOLISM

A group of disorders that arise from the incomplete fulfillment of some particular aspect of intermediary metabolism (inborn errors of metabolism) of protein, carbohydrate, fat, or pigment are of additional interest in obstetrics because of their hereditary and familial background. There is, however, limited information regarding the effect of gestation on such patients, and it is therefore assumed that they tolerate pregnancy well. It is the fetus and newborn that are of the greatest concern.

Alkaptonuria is a disease in which, in the absence of a specific enzyme, normal metabolism of phenylalanine and tyrosine fails to occur, following which homogentisic acid appears in the urine. This substance, when oxidized, turns black, and the characteristic color of the urine establishes the diagnosis. The condition apparently is inherited as an autosomal recessive trait. Albinism, characterized by the absence of pigmentation of the skin, hair, and eyes, is due to hereditary absence of the enzyme that normally acts in changing tyrosine to melanin. The disease is an autosomal recessive and varies greatly in the extent of the body surfaces involved.

The most important disease of abnormal intermediary protein metabolism is phenylketonuria. Inherited as an autosomal recessive, the diagnosis must be established at birth if mental retardation is to be prevented. (See Chapter 32, The Newborn.)

Cystinuria, inherited as a recessive trait, is characterized by the excretion in the urine of large amounts of sulfur-containing amino acids through defective renal tubular reabsorption. Cystine staghorn calculi may form, inviting infection, hydronephrosis, and disturbance in renal function. It is these latter complications that determine whether successful pregnancy can occur in the presence of this congenital disorder.

A condition distinguished by disturbance in amino acid metabolism has been described and is referred to as Fanconi's syndrome. This condition involves a marked decrease in the renal threshold for glucose, amino acid, and phosphates. The skeleton becomes demineralized, and a form of rickets develops.

Hepatolenticular degeneration (Wilson's disease) has been encountered in pregnancy and successfully managed by dimercaprol (BAL) without adverse effects on the fetus and newborn. It is inherited as a recessive autosomal trait, and the fetus is free of any biochemical evidence of the disease at birth. Besides liver cirrhosis and degeneration of the lenticular nucleus of the brain, there is marked deposition of copper in the patient's tissues with an increased urinary copper excretion associated with renal tubular dysfunction. Ceruloplasmin levels rise from their abnormal low levels as with estrogen administration and reach even higher values during pregnancy. There appears to be a slight improvement of the disease in the later stages of pregnancy and the dimercaprol needs may decrease temporarily.

Gout, with a family incidence, has been reported in pregnancy despite the fact it is rarely encountered in females and before the menopause. The outcome is influenced by the extent of renal dysfunction, but otherwise pregnancy appears not to cause an exacerbation.

The inborn errors in carbohydrate metabolism, excluding diabetes, are designated fructosuria, galactosuria, and sucrosuria. These extremely rare diseases are all hereditary and represent some particular defect in the enzyme system responsible for carbohydrate metabolism. In the first instance, fructose fails to be converted to glucose and accumulates in the blood. The kidney tubules normally fail to resorb fructose as readily as glucose, and fructose appears in large amounts in the urine. In galactosuria there appears to be a congenital defect in the enzyme responsible for the conversion of this substance to glycogen. In the condition described as sucrosuria, the defect appears to be a failure of hydrolysis of sucrose into glucose and fructose after its absorption from the gastrointestinal tract.

Glycogen disease (von Gierke's disease), inherited as an autosomal recessive, is of interest to the obstetrician because of the appearance of the disease in the newborn. The condition is characterized by deposition of enormous quantities of glycogen in many organs, particularly the liver, kidney, and heart. The disease has been observed in the newborn in succeeding pregnancies. This situation is apparently due to deficiency of the enzymes responsible for the conversion and storage of glycogen. The low blood sugar in patients with this disease is not increased following an injection of epinephrine, a further indication of a defect in glycogenolysis.

Diseases characterized by unusual deposition of lipids throughout the body have a hereditary background. These include Gaucher's disease, Niemann-Pick disease, and Tay-Sachs disease. In Gaucher's disease, an abnormal cerebroside is deposited throughout the reticuloendothelial system. Inheritance of the disease probably is by mutation. Syringomyelin is deposited in abnormal amounts in Niemann-Pick disease, and the infant of a patient with this condition frequently does not survive the first two years of life. Tay-Sachs disease results in signs similar in many respects to Niemann-Pick disease, except that the brain substance is reduced in content from the lack of normal amounts of syringomyelin. The condition is often referred to as amaurotic familial idiocy.

Other inborn errors in the metabolism of the pigments involve the porphyrins. The diagnosis of congenital porphyria is established by the appearance of burgundy red urine and discoloration of the teeth and bones. It is inherited as an autosomal dominant trait. In pregnancy the abnormal amounts of porphyrin already appearing in the urine may be increased further, and there is a tendency to exacerbations. Until more recent times the death rate precluded continuation of the pregnancy. Severe abdominal pain, vomiting, neurologic symptoms, and psychiatric reactions should arouse the suspicion of this disease. When pregnancy is involved, the type of porphyria should be carefully evaluated, and although patients have had relatively normal pregnancies, considering the genetic aspects and the unpredictability of the disease, artificial termination of the pregnancy must be given consideration.

DEFICIENCY DISEASES

In certain regions where suboptimal diets are prevalent, with the increased fetal and maternal nutritional requirements, deficiency disease may make its appearance after the onset of pregnancy. In the event that hyperemesis or other gastrointestinal upsets interfere with food intake, the signs of the deficiency disease are apt to appear earlier and be more severe. Although mixed nutritional deficiencies are often present, the signs and symptoms usually characterize the lack of a specific nutrient substance. The resultant disorders include beriberi, pellagra, scurvy, and sprue.

How deficiency disease adversely affects the course of pregnancy or the infant at birth must be stated in generalities. Undoubtedly, chronic dietary inadequacies increase maternal complications, the most common being anemia and toxemia of pregnancy. In the presence of deficient maternal nutrition, the fetus may fail to store adequate amounts of supplementary nutrients, resulting in the appearance of nutritional disease in the newborn.

Vitamin B deficiency is encountered as a polyneuritis, as a complication of severe hyperemesis gravidarum, or in the form of beriberi. Beriberi is rarely seen in pregnancy, except occasionally in those areas of the world where the disease is prevalent among the population. It has been observed in the newborn.

Although the signs are usually present only in the lower extremities in chronic and severe cases, the disease may progress to involve the upper extremities. The pathologic changes, moreover, are not confined entirely to the peripheral nerves, for the central nervous system and the autonomic system may also be affected. In rare instances swelling and chromatolysis of the sympathetic chain and, in the extreme, degeneration of the vagus nerve may occur.

The treatment of the disorder is an adequate diet supplemented with therapeutic doses of thiamine together with vitamin B complex and other vitamins.

Pellagra is a deficiency disorder resulting from insufficient ingestion of nicotinic acid (niacin), and is revealed by a typical dermatitis, glossitis, stomatitis, and diarrhea. Nervousness, insomnia, irritability, weakness, and headache are manifest. Anemia may accompany the primary disorder. Certain alterations in the skin, such as rarefaction of the corium and dilatation of the blood vessels, have been attributed to niacin deficiency. Hyperkeratosis, parakeratosis, and acanthosis may develop. The disorder is most likely to be manifest in the last trimester of pregnancy, but

should it appear in the immediate puerperium the mental symptoms may cause it to be mistaken for a postpartum psychosis. The prognosis is favorable in the mild cases when adequate therapy is instituted, but in the presence of encephalopathy the prognosis must be guarded.

Overt scurvy is rarely encountered during pregnancy, and the cases reported are those associated with severe hyperemesis gravidarum or chronic malnutrition. In these cases manifestations of an underlying capillary damage, as evidenced by hemorrhage, petechiae, ecchymoses, and hematomas, are noted. The typical gingival changes characterized by swelling and ready bleeding may be mistaken for the gingivitis of normal pregnancy. Bleeding from the mucous membranes, or other hemorrhagic manifestations, and evidence of dietary deficiency should make one suspect the true nature of the underlying disorder.

BIBLIOGRAPHY

Batt, R. E., Cirksena, W. J., and Lebherz, T. B.: Gout and salt-wasting renal disease during pregnancy. J.A.M.A., 186:835, 1963.

Bloch, B.: Porphyria variegata associated with pregnancy. J. Obstet. Gynaec. Brit. Comm., 72:391, 1965.

Dreifuss, F. E., and McKinney, W. M.: Wilson's disease; hepatolenticular degeneration and pregnancy. J.A.M.A., 195:960, 1966.

Gibson, J. R. M.: Cystinuria and bilateral renal calculi in pregnancy. Obstet. Gynec., 26:101, 1965.

Gould, S., Allison, H. M., and Bellew, L. N.: Acute porphyria complicated by pregnancy. A report of a case. Obstet. Gynec., 17:109, 1961.

Lee, F. I., and Loeffler, F. E.: Gout and pregnancy. J. Obstet. Gynaec. Brit. Comm., 69:299, 1962.

Ludwig, G. D., and Epstein, I. S.: Genetic study of two families having acute intermittent type of porphyria. Ann. Intern. Med., 55:81, 1961.

Norris, S., Eisen, A., and Bernstein, A.: Cystinuria during pregnancy. Report of a case. Obstet. Gynec., 18:187, 1961.

Petrie, S. J., and Mooney, J. P.: Porphyria with the complication of pregnancy. Case report and review of the literature. Amer. J. Obstet. Gynec., 83:264, 1962.

Van Gelder, D. W., and Darby, F. U.: Congenital and infantile beriberi. J. Pediat., 25:226, 1944.

Watov, S. E., and De Sandre, R.: Gaucher's disease and pregnancy. Report of one case involving four pregnancies. Obstet. Gynec., 23:247, 1964.

PSYCHIATRIC DISEASE

As more of the overall care of the female becomes the responsibility of the obstetrician-gynecologist, so also will he encounter emotional states with greater frequency. Certainly pregnancy will bring psychologic and emotional problems to the fore. The majority of these he may be able to resolve. But more important, he must identify the patients with psychiatric illness, especially those with a suicidal potential, for it is the physician's initial responsibility to protect such a patient from doing herself harm.

The prime concern here is to discuss briefly the psychiatric disease that may be encountered in women of the childbearing age and some of the questions that arise in their management. With psychiatry in its present state of controversy, admittedly the following remarks will not be acceptable to all and perhaps only a few will agree with them. If the nomenclature used can be categorized it is more closely allied to the British than to the Viennese school of psychiatry. It is hoped that the terms used are those that both the writer and reader understand. Furthermore, it is not the purpose here to engage in polemics concerning functional states that appear to lend themselves to subjective rather than objective interpretation.

There is no evidence to date of special psychologic problems of pregnancy causing psychiatric disturbances or diseases, although there is considerable speculation. Anxiety neurosis and hysteria are the most frequently encountered psychiatric disturbances of pregnant, as well as nonpregnant, women. Schizophrenia in the sense that this term and diagnosis are used here is an infrequent and serious illness that is seen only rarely in obstetric patients. Manic-depressive disease (or mood disturbance) offers an occasional problem in pregnancy, with its complications of low mood and suicidal threats. Delirium (or toxic psychosis) occurs occasionally with fever, with administration of drugs, or as a complication of medical disease. Finally, puerperal psychosis, as the name implies, is a complication peculiar to pregnancy; fortunately it is rare. Occasionally in patients with severe vomiting, a nutritional disturbance, Korsakoff's syndrome, may occur with the symptoms of neuritis, memory defect, and confabulation.

In addition to seeing occasional patients with the above-mentioned conditions, more often the obstetrician-gynecologist may be asked for advice in family psychiatric problems. A particular child may be slow in developing, there may be poor work in school or college, or there may be behavior problems at home or at school; or the parents may have marital problems. An understanding of psychiatric diseases gives the obstetrician-gynecologist some systematic approach to these situations. He may be able to save a marriage; or he may help a child to a sound adjustment.

The following paragraphs describe briefly the psychiatric diseases that may be seen in an obstetric-gynecologic service.

Anxiety neurosis (neurocirculatory asthenia, nervous exhaustion) is the most common of the nervous disorders. Its prevalance is possibly as high as 5 per cent of the population; women consult doctors for it twice as often as do men. The mean age of onset is about 25; onset before 20 or after 40 is unusual. The illness runs in families, and chief complaints are shortness of breath, choking, palpitation, and nervousness. There is a reduced capacity to perform muscular work or to withstand emotional strain, and there may be uneasiness in crowds. Signs include flushed face, tremor, and sighing respiration. There may be excessive increase of pulse rate and minute respiratory volume on exertion or emotional stimuli. Many women with this condition report an increase or precipitation of these symptoms during pregnancy or the puerperium. It is important not to mistake this disorder for heart disease or heart failure, thyrotoxicosis, or depressive disease. Reassurance and a few interviews are helpful in therapy. This includes how to live with one's self, with a few days away from the routine, and, if possible, a change in environment.

Hysteria (sometimes called "conversion reaction") still persists as a relatively common disorder in American women. True hysteria occurs primarily if not exclusively in women. The mean age of onset is around 19; onset before 10 or after 30 is extremely rare. There appears to be a family prevalence. Generally the patient with hysteria presents herself with abdominal pain that may be difficult to explain, or with some gynecologic problem;

the bizarre manifestations vary. In the usual case, the chief complaint is vague or multiple; it may be difficult to determine what brings the patient to the doctor.

The history usually reveals a number of previous hospitalizations and unnecessary surgical operations and procedures. Appendectomy with removal of an ovary has often been done. Too many of these patients as a consequence of multiple and unnecessary gynecologic operations are surgically sterilized at a young age. A systems review reveals many and varied symptoms, including headache, blurred vision, abdominal pain, and tales of weird reactions on eating ordinary foods. Stories of rapid loss or gain of 10 to 20 lb. of weight are common. Urinary retention occurs, "necessitating catheterization." Menstrual pains with syncope, and stories of odd menstrual cycles, such as "every two weeks," are items of history. Disinterest in sex, frigidity, and dyspareunia are characteristic. Nervousness and syncope are common complaints. Symptoms resembling those of neurologic disease, such as transient blurred vision, blindness, paralysis, seizures, or trances, are also reported by the patients. Suicide attempts in association with unhappy life events (sometimes called "reactive depression") occasionally occur.

Of special interest to gynecologists and obstetricians is the menstrual history, which includes stories of fainting, irregular periods, and severe pains in abdomen, pelvis, back, or legs. These patients report vomiting throughout pregnancy; they are apt to describe long and difficult labors and deliveries in which they "almost died." The actual number of children produced by patients with hysteria seems low; if true, this might be explained by the relative infrequency of sex activity or by the excessive amount of unnecessary gynecologic surgery, which includes the removal of comparatively normal oviducts, ovaries, and uteri. Perhaps what has been said applies to some patients with the so-called "pelvic congestion" syndrome.

When the history is taken the patients are often friendly and talkative. They show minimal ability to describe present trouble in contrast to the great detail and color with which they describe previous medical complaints and procedures. The prognosis in this illness is variable, possibly depending on its medical management.

Suggestion and reassurance constitute the recommended treatment. Avoidance of excessive disabling medical attention, especially by the surgeon or the psychiatrist, may be crucial. Mistakes can be made in management through overconcern by the physician; the other serious error is to ignore the patient's complaints when they are medical in origin. Hence, these patients tax the physician's equanimity and judgment.

Manic-depressive disease is the most important psychiatric disease that physicians will encounter. Its frequency is obscured by the variety of its presenting symptoms, such as fatigue, headache, backache, anxiety attacks, insomnia, weight loss, and inability to face further childbearing or child-rearing. A physician will see two or three cases in women to every one in men. The mean age of onset is in the forties, but some cases appear as early as infancy or as late as the eighties. There is a strong tendency to familial prevalence, suggesting that heredity may be involved. Alcoholism may be an additional complication of the disease, especially in older women.

Chief complaints may be medical, psychiatric, or both. The common medical complaints are headache, chest pain, abdominal distress, anorexia, weight loss, constipation, and urinary frequency. In women there may be amenorrhea and in men, impotence, distinct facts to keep in mind when attempting to manage this condition. These symptoms should be recognized by physicians as possible signs of manic-depressive disease.

Most patients have the depressive phase of the illness and never have the manic. However, both phases may be mixed together. The characteristic features that are unique to this disease have to do with shifts in mood and energy levels, so that usual work becomes burdensome and zest for life in general is diminished. Loss of appetite and of the enjoyment of food sometimes leads to severe weight loss. Patients may feel tired, especially in the morning, and may find it wearisome to work a full schedule, even when doing what was previously fascinating.

Mood will be described as "low," "anxious," or "worried." The patient may view her past attainments and future prospects darkly and without hope. She may feel that she is a burden to friends and family. The possibility of suicide is a grave problem. Insomnia is common, particularly with early morning waking.

Examination may reveal a fixed facial expression, stooped posture, tremor, and untidiness of dress, hair, and fingernails. The patient may be obsessed with the thought that she cannot take care of her present family, that further childbearing is impossible, and she may demand interruption of the pregnancy. Sometimes the amenorrhea of this disease will be misdiagnosed as pregnancy. This may be the background of some if not most cases of pseudocyesis. The duration of an attack of the depressive phase of this illness may range from a few weeks to a year or two; about six months is usual.

Management of the patient with depressive disease is best done by a psychiatrist or other physician experienced in the treatment of the condition. It is a personal view that the so-called "psychoanalytic techniques" are of little value. Barbital or Amytal in small doses is the drug of choice; however, the so-called "tranquilizers" or "antidepressant energizers" are perhaps more commonly used. Temporary hospital care with or without shock therapy may be necessary in some cases. Shock therapy sometimes eliminates disagreeable symptoms quickly and is not contraindicated during pregnancy. In some cases the total situation, or the type and severity of symptoms, may necessitate interruption of pregnancy.

The manic or hypomanic (mildly manic) phase of this illness leads to overactivity, overtalkativeness, irritability, and heightening of drive—to telephone, to buy many unnecessary things, or to take on new projects or crusades. Sexual urge and activity may also be heightened. Among the new projects, some patients may decide on a "new way of life" and may feel that divorce is mandatory. This accounts for some astonishing demands for divorce in couples with families who have seemed "happily married" for many years. The increase in sex urge and activity in the hypomanic state is a common cause of promiscuity in women of previously good reputation and conventional behavior. An optimistic mood and a pathologically casual disregard for consequences cause poor judgment and omission of necessary precautions. The hypomanic girl may be quite unconcerned about an illegitimate pregnancy, or the illness may swing to the depressive phase with remorse, feelings of guilt, and suicidal thoughts. The diagnosis deserves greater attention in the changing mores of the times. The writer would raise the question whether many teenagers with unplanned pregnancies are indeed victims of this psychiatric illness. In cases of this type, interruption of pregnancy with appropriate treatment in a psychiatric hospital and psychiatric follow-up is recommended. Complete recovery is the expected outcome of an attack of manic-depressive disease if properly managed and supervised. Manic-depressive disease is by far the most common serious psychiatric illness the obstetrician-gynecologist will encounter in the age spectrum from puberty to the menopause and beyond. The teenager is not immune, and the condition termed "melancholia" of the menopause is simply a depression and the word has no further meaning. To see a patient treated with various hormones for symptoms attributed to the menopause when, in fact, she has a depression, permits the obstetrician-gynecologist to conclude that in this disease treatment is often given for other illnesses before the correct diagnosis is made.

Puerperal psychosis is a special disease of the puerperium; it is possible, however, that it is a variant of manic-depressive disease. In the patients observed by the writer its onset has been in the first two or three days post partum; most have been within 48 hours of delivery. There have been no psychiatric symptoms during pregnancy, but usually there have been medical complications. These have included toxemia, hepatitis, heart failure, complicated anesthesia, or some post-partum fever.

The early symptoms are refusal of food, or becoming quiet, suspicious, and quite paranoid. There may be delusions about the baby and its care. This relative quiet or period of mutism may soon alternate with shouting, singing, pacing around the ward, and demanding to leave the hospital. Insomnia may be a problem. Such patients may be suicidal risks, but they also may do harm to their infants and children. The cause of the puerperal psychosis is unknown; no chemical or endocrinologic abnormalities have as yet been discovered.

These patients invariably require psychiatric hospital care. There is usually recovery in a few months and shock therapy aids in control of the symptoms and hastens recovery. An unpleasant by-product of this illness is the quarreling among the relatives of the patient and of her husband. The patient's relatives may insist that the husband's cruel treatment causes the trouble. The husband's relatives may express the opinion that there must have been concealed insanity in the patient before marriage. Obviously the physician must try to prevent or minimize these useless recriminations. There is no evidence that the condition will recur, and hence further pregnancies are not necessarily contraindicated.

Toxic psychosis (delirium, confusional state) occurs during pregnancy or after labor just as it does as a complication of medical or surgical disease or in association with administration of drugs or their withdrawal. It is characterized by rapid development and a short course. The patient may misinterpret noise or sights in the ward, or have hallucinations. The mood is extremely labile, and there may be fear, irritability, suspicion, anger, or euphoria. Disorientation for time, place, and person occurs at the worst of the attack. The duration is usually a few days. Treatment consists of protecting the patient and relieving her of the drug effects, infection, or the medical and environmental factors that have contributed to this state.

Korsakoff's syndrome has occurred as a result of extreme vomiting during pregnancy. It presents a combination of polyneuritis (weakness of extremities, absence of reflexes, sensory loss) and retentive memory defect. The patient is unable to recall recent events, although past memory is preserved. Confabulation (inventing stories, or bringing up telescoped old memories to fill in the gaps) is a frequent manifestation of this disorder. Treatment consists of restoration of an adequate nutritional state. Recovery may be slow in some cases.

Schizophrenia (dementia praecox) generally has its onset in young adult life. This illness is characterized by a distortion of thinking and by unusual logic. There is poor correlation between topic of conversation and emotional expression. There are unpredictable verbal associations. There may be delusions and hallucinations. Grimacing and unusual postures may be present. The illness is incapacitating and at best there is only partial recovery. A large pro-

portion of the long-term patients in psychiatric hospitals are suffering from this disorder, but in its pure form it is rarely seen in an obstetric unit. Studies including twins suggest a hereditary factor. Whether the pregnancy should continue or future pregnancies should be permitted is the question.

DISCUSSION

The above presentation has been restricted to what might be referred to as factual psychiatry, and it has avoided direct reference to the 19th century psychoanalytic, or so-called "dynamic," form of psychiatry. There are several reasons for this, but only one will be mentioned: It is suggested that psychiatric illnesses as herein defined are due to still-to-be-discovered metabolic disturbances of the brain, and are not environmental in origin. From the standpoint of the obstetrician, this preference for the factual form of psychiatry does not sacrifice the humanistic approach to patient care, but simply recognizes the limitations imposed on therapy by the present state of scientific knowledge concerning the etiology of psychiatric disease, and takes into consideration what this may mean economically to the patient and her family.

As previously indicated, the women in the childbearing age and well beyond the menopause often turn to the obstetrician-gynecologist for help and advice on general medical problems either for themselves or for members of their families. Hence, the obstetrician-gynecologist has the opportunity to observe psychiatric problems and disease, some of which he can do something about, and others in which he must act in the capacity of an advisor and referral physician to the psychiatrist. Before he can assume the responsibility for the latter, however, he must arrive at some conclusion about what he considers to be sound psychiatric care. This has many facets, including those of a socioeconomic nature, that is, the impact of prolonged ambulatory care and sometimes hospitalization.

Herein lies the controversy. Should the patient be advised to have psychotherapy of the analytic type, or should she be placed in a hospital and probably receive shock therapy if she fails to improve following a course of medical care consisting of sedation and other measures?

Undoubtedly for those physicians who are not psychiatrists their practice will be less complicated by avoiding any attempt to decide which form of psychiatric care they should recommend to their patients. In fact, certain unpleasantness may arise when one expresses a preference for one form of psychiatry over another. Perhaps this should not concern the referring physician, but it would seem to be a paradoxical attitude when in every other respect he teaches and practices that the care of the sick is based on the scientific method. This is not to deny the great need for psychiatry, although when the method is based on unproved theories without a modicum of supporting data it should be so recognized.

In addition to these definite psychiatric illnesses, there are several related clinical situations and controversies.

First, what influence has pregnancy on psychiatric disease, and is there a need for artificial or therapeutic abortion in patients so afflicted? Although the patient's symptoms and abnormal behavior may be temporarily accentuated during pregnancy, there is no convincing evidence that psychiatric disease is permanently worsened by pregnancy. However, the writer can attest from experience in the management of a few patients with manic-depressive disease that the conduct of pregnancy is indeed a most difficult task and at times an ordeal for all involved. The question is posed whether the pregnancy should be terminated, with the recognition that if the patient recovers with treatment, she can be permitted to attempt a pregnancy at some later time. If the pregnancy is allowed to continue, one must be prepared to keep the patient under constant surveillance and this may mean hospitalization.

Second, a closely related question is the matter of tubal sterilization coincident with artificial or therapeutic abortion in patients with psychiatric illness. The opinion is sometimes expressed that if the mental disease is such as to warrant termination of the pregnancy the patient should be sterilized. This sequence of management might apply to the patient with established schizophrenia but not necessarily for the patient with manic-depressive disease. On the basis of the belief that the patient with this form of illness may or will recover, the writer suggests that in the event of pregnancy therapeutic abortion may be indicated, but that in most instances sterilization should not be performed concomitantly. The patient on regaining her health should have the inherent right to decide whether she desires to have a child. In fact, the patient's total recovery may be impeded by the realization that she was sterilized at the time of the therapeutic abortion.

Third, another question difficult to answer and document is, what is the risk of suicide in patients with an unwanted pregnancy who are refused artificial termination of pregnancy? The answer to this question must take into account whether the patient has a psychiatric illness, in which case suicide is indeed a threat. Whether the risk of suicide is increased in the normal woman refused an abortion is difficult to establish.

Finally, the effect of hysterectomy on the emotional life of the patient is subject to some controversy. When there are sound indications for the operation and the patient is free of psychologic disturbance, patients remain emotionally stable following hysterectomy, especially if ovarian function is preserved. In fact, the patient who is fearful of pregnancy is relieved of anxiety and is a more effective wife and mother.

It is in patients with hysteria, anxiety states, pelvic congestion syndrome, severe premenstrual tension, and so forth, and without clear-cut gynecologic indications for the operation that adverse emotional reactions are more likely to follow hysterectomy. In short, hysterectomy is not a cure for psychologic and psychiatric conditions; in fact, it may exaggerate the patient's symptoms. However, there is the *rare* patient with essentially negative pelvic findings with seemingly uncontrolled premenstrual tension, somewhat prolonged menstrual periods, and possibly the fear of pregnancy who may benefit from hysterectomy. But one must be entirely certain that the procedure will be beneficial and will not add to perhaps an already long list of symptoms.

In addition to the complications of pregnancy that have to do with clinical psychiatry, a good deal of attention has been paid of late to the worries, problems, and anxieties of pregnant women. As could be expected, pregnant women do have some questions to ask and are curious about some problems; worries and fears do exist, some quite justifiable, about whether the baby will be normal, how the patient will get along in the hospital, and the possibility of complications of delivery and early child-rearing. Although prolonged discussion with pregnant women about fears, worries, and anxieties may allay those which are present, there is also the possibility that overstatement may arouse worse fears and create difficulties that were not present in the beginning. It is never clear what the proper emphasis should be on these matters, but perhaps it is well to recall that there is a long medical tradition against undue emphasis and exaggeration of medical details. It is possible that worries may be aroused by undue discussion and that psychologic difficulties can be artificially created.

There is no reason to believe that patients' apprehensions will lead to psychiatric disease. However, it is the responsibility of every physician to concern himself with or allay worries as they arise. It is the clinical impression that a deserved reputation for competent practice of obstetrics, an examination that permits the patient time to ask questions to which she receives reasonable and truthful answers, allowing the patient to mention things that she feels need mentioning, and giving her the feeling that what should be done will be done, and at the proper time, should provide the optimal situation for eliminating unnecessary worries and problems.

In summary, there is no reason to picture pregnancy itself as an emotional or mental disturbance or to fear that psychiatric consequences will accrue to mother or child. It appears that the psychiatric diseases in pregnant patients are much like those in other women in the same age group.

Thus, the first obligation to a psychiatrically disturbed patient is to protect her against her environment, particularly if there is any suggestion of a suicidal tendency. Her care initially depends on an immediate and accurate diagnosis of her psychiatric illness. Whatever other emotional difficulties and personal problems the patient may have can be resolved in the fullness of time.

BIBLIOGRAPHY

Arkonac, O., and Guze, S. B.: A family study of hysteria. New Eng. J. Med., 268:239, 1963.

Barker, M. G.: Psychiatric illness after hysterectomy. Brit. Med. J., 2:91, 1968.

Cohen, M. E., Badal, D. W., Kilpatrick, A., Reed, E. W., and White, P. D.: The high familial prevalence of neurocirculatory asthenia (anxiety neurosis, effort syndrome). Amer. J. Hum. Genet., 3:126, 1951.

Cohen, M. E., Robins, E., Purtell, J. J., Altmann, M. W., and Reid, D. E.: Excessive surgery in hysteria. J.A.M.A., 151:977, 1953.

Ewald, G.: Die Generationpsychosen des Weibes. In Bumke, O., ed.: Handbuch der Geisteskrankheiten, Vol. 7. Springer, Berlin, 1928.

Friederich, M. A., Romano, J., and Lund, C. J.: Psychologic aspects of obstetric-gynecologic practice. Amer. J. Obstet. Gynec., 91:1029, 1965.

Inheritance of schizophrenia. Annotations. Lancet, 1:98, 1965.

Jacobson, L., Kaij, L., and Nilsson, A.: Postpartum mental disorders in an unselected sample: Frequency of symptoms and predisposing factors. Brit. Med. J., 1:1640, 1965.

Karnosh, L. J., and Hope, J. M.: Puerperal psychoses and their sequelae. Amer. J. Psychol., 94:537, 1937.

Kimball, C. P.: A case of pseudocyesis caused by "roots." Amer. J. Obstet. Gynec., 107:801, 1970.

Kinch, R. A. H.: Sexual difficulties after 50: The gynecologist's view. Canad. Med. Ass. J., 94:211, 1966.

Kraeplin, E.: Manic Depressive Insanity and Paranoia. E. and S. Livingstone, Edinburgh, 1921.

Kraeplin, E.: Dementia Praecox and Paraphrenia. E. and S. Livingstone, Edinburgh, 1929.

Paffenbarger, R. S., and McCabe, L. J., Jr.: The effect of obstetric and perinatal events on risk of mental illness in women of childbearing age. Amer. J. Public Health, 56:400, 1966.

Paniagua, M. E., Tayback, M., Janer, J. L., and Vazquez, J. L.: Medical and psychological sequelae of surgical sterilization of women. Amer. J. Obstet. Gynec., 90:421, 1964.

Purtell, J., Robins, E., and Cohen, M. E.: Observations on the clinical aspects of hysteria; quantitative study of 50 hysteria patients and 156 control subjects. J.A.M.A., 146:902, 1951.

Schmidt, E. H., O'Neal, P., and Robins, E.: Evaluation of suicide attempts as guide to therapy; clinical follow-up study of one hundred nine patients. J.A.M.A., 155:549, 1954.

Seymour-Shove, R., Gee, D. J., and Cross, A. P.: Schizophrenia during pregnancy associated with injury to foetus in utero. Brit. Med. J., 1:686, 1968.

Sim, M.: Abortion and the psychiatrist. Brit. Med. J., 2:145, 1963.

Slater, E.: Diagnosis of "hysteria." Brit. Med. J., 1:1395, 1965.

Taylor, H. C.: Pelvic pain based on a vascular and autonomic nervous system disorder. Amer. J. Obstet. Gynec., 67:1177, 1954.

Tredgold, R. F.: Psychiatric indications for termination of pregnancy. Lancet, 2:1251, 1964.

Uhrus, K.: Some aspects of the Swedish law governing termination of pregnancy. Lancet, 2:1292, 1964.

Wallach, E. E., Garcia, C. R., and Pincus, G.: Anovulation in hospitalized mental patients. Amer. J. Obstet. Gynec., 93:72, 1965.

Watts, C. A. H.: Incidence and prognosis of endogenous depression. Brit. Med. J., 1:1392, 1956.

PART V

Neonatology

Chapter 31

Fetal Growth and Physiology

The fetus has been described anatomically in careful detail, but how and when the fetus acquires its biochemical mechanism and physiologic functions is incomplete. There is evidence to support the concept that, as the fetal organ systems assume their respective functions, these metabolic responsibilities are shifted from the placenta to the fetus. Thus, throughout pregnancy, the physiologic relationship of the feto-placental unit is undergoing constant modification.

GESTATIONAL AGE AND WEIGHT

Accurate determination and recording of the gestational age of the conceptus at the time of delivery is indispensable to studies of the fetus, to evaluation of therapeutic measures in the management of pregnancy complications, to management of the so-called "high-risk" pregnancy, and to studies of the perinatal mortality and of neonatal morbidity as it pertains to the incidence of cerebral palsy, mental retardation, and other serious conditions of the newborn and infant. Not the least of the variables that contribute to the neonatal mortality is intrauterine growth retardation with its many associated obstetric conditions. (See Chapter 20, Dysmaturity-Postmaturity, and Chapter 35, Assessment of Maternal and Fetal Care.) Moreover, the gestational age has medicolegal importance, for the law usually requires the reporting of the birth of a fetus whose gestational age is 20 or more weeks.

The World Health Organization has attempted to encourage all nations to use a uniform classification or nomenclature of what constitutes viability, prematurity, and maturity of the fetus for assessing perinatal and neonatal mortality and overall fetal wastage. As will be noted in Table 1, the classification is modified by adding the weight range for the various gestational ages. Ideally, gestational age and fetal weight both should be recorded and reported.

It is common practice for purposes of determining both obstetric and pediatric therapeutic results to subdivide group III into 1000 to 1500 grams and 1500 to 2000 grams, or 28 to 35 weeks and 35 weeks to term, respectively. This is particularly pertinent in the recognition of the dysmature syndrome, where a discrepancy exists between fetal age and weight. Also, these subdivisions are clinically useful in determining the etiology of prematurity and in its prevention and management.

FETAL DEVELOPMENT AND GROWTH

Conventionally, the development and growth of the conceptus is divided into three phases. The four weeks beyond fertilization, that is, through the two to three weeks following the first missed menstrual period, is known as the *ovular* phase. The next chronologic sequence, continuing until near the end of the second month, is called the stage of the *embryo*. During this interval, the organ systems are developed.

TABLE 1. CLASSIFICATION OF GESTATIONAL AGE AND WEIGHT

	Age	Weight
Group I	Less than 20 completed weeks	500 grams or under
Group II	20 completed weeks – less than 28 weeks	501–1000 grams
Group III	28 completed weeks and over	1001 grams plus
Group IV	Weight unknown	

Thereafter, the *fetal* phase ensues, covering the period from completion of organogenesis until the end of gestation.

The events of early intrauterine development are associated with transformation of the flat embryonic disc into a roughly cylindrical configuration in which somites are laid down at a rapid rate (Fig. 1), and by the fifth week after fertilization the full number have developed. The entire external embryonic surface is now closed and intact except for the connection which may persist between the yolk sac and the midgut (Fig. 2). Gradually the mandibular and hyoid arches become clearly differentiated over the cephalic surface of the body, while the areas destined to be occupied by the eyes and ears are identifiable (Fig. 3A). At the sixth week, the cephalad portion of the embryo is more flexed, so that the distance from the crown to the rump is not a true index of embryonic length. As a result of this flexion, the cephalic segment of the embryo comes to rest upon the protu-

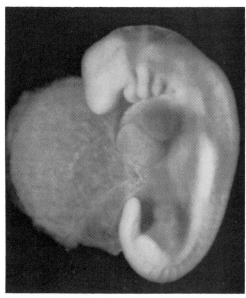

Figure 2. Human embryo at 27 days' developmental age. It measures about 5 mm. in length, and exhibits a distinct head, branchial bars, and a heart, which is already four-chambered. Along the back, the somites, which number 30 pairs at this time, are evident. The yolk sac is prominently distended and is the site of hematopoietic activity. (Courtesy of the Department of Embryology, Carnegie Institution of Washington.)

berance created by the cardiac and hepatic prominences (Fig. 3B).

The basic pattern of organogenesis is established by the eighth week, and the embryo attains fetal status, measuring approximately 1 inch in length and weighing a little more than 1 gram. At this period ossification centers appear throughout the skeleton, particularly in the skull and in the long bones. The fetal body now exhibits less flexion; its cephalic features are clearly established, and appendages and digits have become well differentiated. Growth proceeds at a rapid rate, and at the end of the first trimester the fetus weighs about 100 grams. At this time the previously undifferentiated genitalia can be grossly identified as either male or female. At the sixth lunar month the fetal body is lean and well proportioned (Fig. 4), and, inasmuch as the skin and subcutaneous tissues are thin, the superficial blood vessels over the body appear prominent. When the fetus is removed from the fluid environment of the amniotic cavity at this age, the skin covering it soon becomes wrinkled. The fetus now weighs approximately 650 grams and its crown-to-rump length averages 21 cm. The

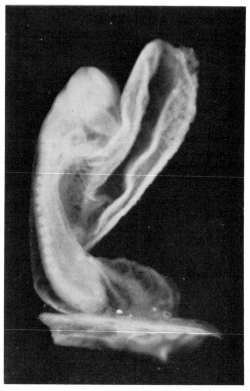

Figure 1. Early segmenting human embryo, about 20 days old. The attached yolk sac is collapsed. The row of somites is clearly seen. (Courtesy of the Department of Embryology, Carnegie Institution of Washington.)

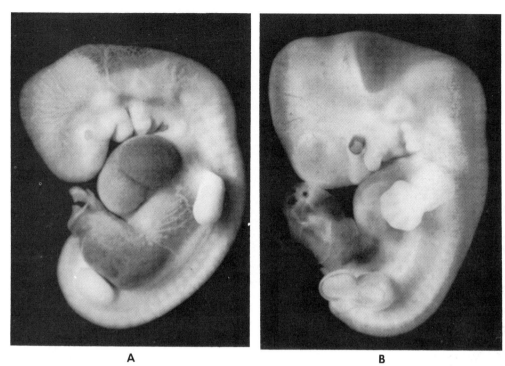

A **B**

Figure 3. Early human embryos. A, At 33 days gestational age. The rapidly growing brain causes a cephalic enlargement relatively greater than that of the rest of the body. The eye has become more conspicuous and the first branchial groove is deepening and prominent. The arm and leg buds are evident and soon will bear ridges, the precursors of digits. B, At five and one half weeks' gestational age. The liver is large and occupies most of the abdomen. The cardiac bulge is actually less prominent. The upper arm, forearm, and hand are distinguishable. However, the leg shows only a foot, with an undifferentiated segment which unites it to the body. The extreme caudal end of the embryo grows so slowly that it becomes less conspicuous and finally is incorporated into the rump. (Courtesy of the Department of Embryology, Carnegie Institution of Washington.)

fetal weight gain is rapid during the last eight weeks of pregnancy, with an increase of 200 to 250 grams each week. As the result of subcutaneous fat deposition, the skin becomes smooth and less reddened in color. The limbs become rounded and firm, and the lanugo hair covering the body begins to shed. At term, the average fetus weighs 3000 to 3500 grams (6½ to 7½ lbs.) If the infant could stand, the average height would be about 48 to 50 cm. (19 to 20 inches). The circumferences of the head, the chest, and the abdomen are about equal, ranging from 31 to 35 cm. (12.5 to 14 inches).

From the second to the third lunar month the total body length of the fetus is tripled; from the third to the fourth lunar month the length is doubled, being accompanied by a corresponding increase in body weight. Thereafter, the rate of growth declines.

A number of studies have been made to determine and define normal ovular, embryonal, and fetal growth. It was concluded from one study that the increase of the various external dimensions is always directly proportional to the increase in body length during fetal life. Consequently, the gross appearance and the length, weight, and various body diameters of the fetus may be used to estimate its age at the time of delivery. As is characteristic of biologic growth, the height and weight relationships of the fetus may deviate so as not to conform in every instance to arbitrary standards, as in the case of the dysmature syndrome. However, normal growth varies only slightly, and for clinical purposes, the age of the fetus can be determined from these accepted standards.

FETAL MENSURATION AND WEIGHT

Of the many measurements utilized in delineating normal fetal growth, the most useful indices consist of total body weight and body length, including extremities, and the circumference and the calculated diameters (Table 2) of the skull. The relationship between the length of the fetus and its age is shown in Table 3.

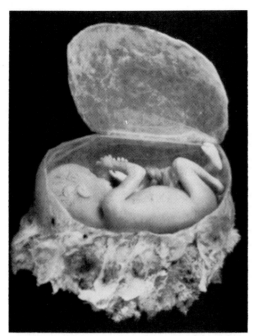

Figure 4. Human fetus of approximately six lunar months. The anterior surface of the chorioamniotic sac has been elevated to show the fetus in situ. The body is well developed. The vasculature in the corium is evident because of the thin dermis. (Courtesy of the Department of Embryology, Carnegie Institution of Washington.)

The conventional measurements of the fetus include the crown-to-rump length, or sitting height, and the crown-to-heel length, or standing height, abbreviated CR and CH, respectively. The crown-to-rump length is the distance from the vertex to the base of the spine, whereas the crown-to-heel length is the distance from the vertex to the tip of the os calcis. To standardize the measurement of the CH determination, the fetus is placed in a sitting position. With the thighs flexed and with the hip joint as the center, an arc is drawn to circumscribe the curvature of the rump. The distance to the knee from the point at which this arc intersects the femur, and that from the knee to the os calcis (Fig. 5) are added to the CR measurement to give the CH length. The relationship between the body length and the age of the fetus during the first five lunar months is such that the square root of the CH length in centimeters approximates the gestational age in months. During the last five lunar months, the CH length may be divided by five to calculate the gestational age. Conversely, during the first half of pregnancy the CH length in centimeters is equal to the gestational month squared, and in the last half of pregnancy it is equal to the number of months multiplied by 5.

At about four weeks' fertilization age the ovum is of sufficient size to permit gross examination and measurement. Ovular size, or the number of developing body somites, furnishes an index of the gestational age. The ovisac often ruptures as it is expelled from the uterus, and under these circumstances the minute embryo is usually lost and is not available for examination. Moreover, should the conceptus be abnormal, the inner cell mass may fail to develop an embryo, in which case dating the pregnancy must be accomplished by a measurement of the size of the chorion.

In patients with irregular menstrual cycles, the number of periods reported missed and the conjectured gestational age may be quite at variance with the size of the conceptus. A disparity may also exist when, in the case of an abortion, the conceptus is expelled long after it has ceased to grow in utero. Under these circumstances the menstrual history must be disregarded and pregnancy dated by ovular size.

As noted below, occasionally a discrepancy between gestational age and the weight of the fetus occurs in association with metabolic disturbances of the mother, more commonly in diabetes mellitus or in toxemia of pregnancy. In diabetes the baby's weight often exceeds values considered normal for the body length, whereas

TABLE 2.   **DIAMETERS (IN CM.) OF FETAL SKULL AT EACH LUNAR MONTH**[*]

	3 mo.	*4 mo.*	*5 mo.*	*6 mo.*	*7 mo.*	*8 mo.*	*9 mo.*	*10 mo.*
Occipitofrontal diameter	2.1	4.1	5.8	7.3	8.6	9.9	11.1	12.2
Occipitomental diameter	1.9	3.9	5.6	7.1	8.4	9.7	10.9	12.0
Suboccipitobregmatic diameter	2.0	3.7	5.2	6.4	7.6	8.7	9.7	10.6
Biparietal diameter	1.6	3.2	4.5	5.8	6.9	7.9	8.8	9.7

[*]Modified from Scammon, R. E., and Calkins, L. A.: Growth in the Fetal Period. University of Minnesota Press, Minneapolis, 1929.

**TABLE 3. LENGTH AND WEIGHT OF FETUS
IN RELATION TO AGE**

Lunar Month	Crown-Rump Length (Cm.)°	Crown-Heel Length (Cm.)†	Weight in Grams°
Second	2.3	–	1.1
Third	7.4	7.0	14.2
Fourth	11.6	15.5	108.0
Fifth	16.4	22.7	316.0
Sixth	20.8	29.2	630.0
Seventh	24.7	35.0	1,045.0
Eighth	28.3	40.4	1,680.0
Ninth	32.1	45.4	2,378.0
Tenth	36.2	50.2	3,405.0

°Streeter, G. L.: Contrib. Embryol., 11:143, 1920.
†Scammon, R. E., and Calkins, L. A.: Growth in the Fetal Period. University of Minnesota Press, Minneapolis, 1929.

in toxemia the situation is reversed. Again, the body length and measurements of the various body circumferences, rather than the body weight, serve as a more reliable index of fetal and gestational age.

The presence of ossification centers is an index of normal growth and, within limits, is useful in distinguishing the age of the fetus. The clavicle reveals a diaphyseal ossification center as early as the fifth week, while ossification centers are noted in the diaphyses of the upper and lower extremities between 6 and 12 weeks. The ossification centers of the epiphyses do not appear until late in pregnancy, near the end of the ninth lunar month.

It is readily appreciated that abdominal palpation of the pregnant patient gives only a rough estimate of fetal size. Consequently, attempts have been made to determine fetal age by x-ray visualization of the fetal skeleton, more particularly by the presence or absence of epiphyseal ossification centers. If the distal epiphyseal ossification center of the femur is visible by x-ray examination, it may be safely assumed that the fetus has reached at least 35 weeks' gestational age. By the 37th week, this ossification center is visible in 92 per cent of fetuses on roentgenography in utero. Measurement of the biparietal diameter of the vertex by ultrasound will probably replace this x-ray examination. (See Assessment of Fetus in Chapter 23.)

The growth curve of the fetus takes on increasing significance as intrauterine growth retardation comes under greater scrutiny as to its possible relationship to the

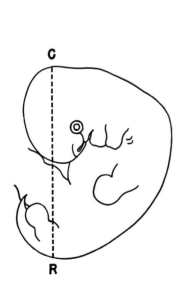

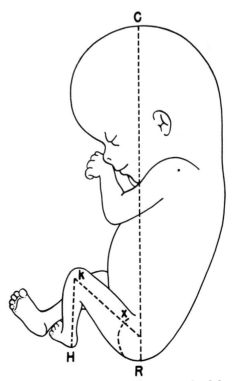

Figure 5. Diagrammatic representation of mensuration of crown-to-rump and crown-to-heel lengths. The distances x-k and k-H are added to the CR length to establish the CH length.

well-being and subsequent development of the newborn infant. What is considered the normal weight for gestational age is influenced by genetic as well as environmental factors. Thus, the actual values for the intrauterine growth curve differ from country to country and from one race to another. Regardless, the weight of the fetus triples in the last 12 weeks of pregnancy and the fetus acquires one third of its weight in the last six weeks of pregnancy. In accordance with birth weights cited below, for an infant of average weight this means a gain of slightly less than 200 grams weekly during this period.

For the United States the median weight of the newborn appears to be about 3200 to 3400 grams, with a spread of 600 grams from the average. In a given series some 10 per cent of newborns will fall in the extreme of the normal growth curve, i.e., 3800 to 4000 grams or 2600 to 2800 grams. Hence, infants born near term whose birth weight is below the lower extreme could be expected to reveal evidence of intrauterine growth retardation.

FETAL PHYSIOLOGY

Hematopoietic System

In the early days following implantation of the blastocyst the formed elements of the fetal blood originate in the blood islands of the yolk sac. Temporary centers of fetal erythropoiesis soon appear in the liver, the mesonephros, and the spleen, which in turn relinquish their hematopoietic function as the bone marrow develops. Initially, all of the blood corpuscles are nucleated, but, by the end of the 10th week, only 10 per cent of the erythrocytes contain nuclei. At term the nucleated red cells are markedly reduced in number, and a blood smear from the newborn will reveal 5 to 10 such cells for every 100 leukocytes. The leukocytes range, on the average, between 9000 and 30,000 per cu. mm., but revert to normal adult values about two weeks after birth.

The life expectancy of the fetal erythrocyte in the premature infant is about two thirds of that in the adult, which is 120 days, while that in the full-term infant is only slightly shorter than the adult figure. The osmotic fragility of the fetal red cell is not increased but the mechanical fragility is. The carbonic anhydrase content of the fetal red cell is appreciably less than that of the adult erythrocyte, but whether this decrease influences the transport of carbon dioxide is speculative.

In early fetal development the red cell counts are low, but in the premature and immature infant the erythrocyte counts are not significantly different from those in the full-term infant. The total erythrocyte count of the blood of the newborn has a higher value than the accepted standards for the adult, the initial counts ranging from 4.2 to 6 million per cu. mm. Because of the macrocytosis, hematocrit values for fetal blood range between 40 and 60 per cent. There is a transient rise in erythrocyte values immediately after birth, with a gradual fall toward adult levels after the first 24 hours.

Two concepts have been proposed to explain the erythrocytosis and macrocytosis present in the infant's blood at birth. The first of these is based on the observation that the formed elements of the peripheral blood are more mature in those species with a prolonged gestational period and less mature when pregnancy is shorter.

The second concept, and the one more generally held with respect to the human, is that the fetal blood-forming organs are stimulated to erythropoiesis by the low oxygen tension of the maternal blood in the intervillous space. The polycythemic state of the infant at birth has been compared to the hematopoietic response of individuals exposed to the low oxygen tension of high altitudes.

The fetal hemoglobin levels show a progressive increase through pregnancy, and near term the values reach 15 to 20 grams or more per 100 ml. In fact, the oxygen-carrying capacity of the fetal blood may equal that of the mother's shortly after the midpoint of pregnancy. The hemoglobin of the fetus is similar to adult hemoglobin in molecular weight but differs in chemical and physical properties. It has long been known that the hemoglobin of fetal blood (Hgb F) is highly resistant to alkaline denaturation, in comparison with the hemoglobin of adult blood (Hgb A). The fetal erythrocyte during early gestation contains only the fetal type of hemoglobin, but by midpregnancy the adult form appears in measurable amounts, on the average of 7 to 10 per cent. At term, some

55 to 85 per cent of the hemoglobin is of the fetal type (average 65 per cent), the level diminishing rapidly after birth, although the persistence of trace amounts is not abnormal. The presence of fetal hemoglobin in a concentration higher than 2 per cent after the first year of life is considered pathologic.

The fetal red cell possesses a greater attraction for oxygen than does the maternal red cell, as shown by the difference in the oxygen dissociation curves of fetal and maternal blood. When the relation between oxygen tension and percentage of saturation for adult and fetal blood is plotted, it may be seen (Fig. 6) that the curve representing fetal blood is displaced to the left. The difference in position of the two curves indicates that fetal blood acquires oxygen at a lower partial pressure than maternal blood. For example, it may be seen in Figure 6 that at an oxygen tension of 30 mm. Hg fetal blood is approximately 65 per cent saturated, whereas at the same pressure maternal blood is 50 per cent saturated. It has been suggested that the possible difference in affinity of fetal and maternal blood for oxygen may be due to altered permeability of the red cell rather than to any chemical or physical differences between adult and fetal hemoglobin. This is substantiated by the finding that the oxygen dissociation curves of adult and fetal hemoglobin in physical solution are

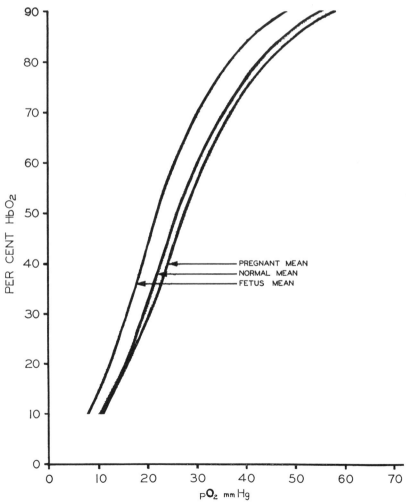

Figure 6. Superimposed oxygen dissociation curves of the nonpregnant and the pregnant woman and the human fetus. Fetal hemoglobin possesses superior ability to become both saturated and dissociated at relatively lower oxygen tension, when compared with adult hemoglobin. (From Darling, R. C., Smith, C. A., Rasmussen, E., and Cohen, F. M.: J. Clin. Invest., 20:739, 1941.)

identical. The steep slope of the lower portion of the fetal dissociation curve illustrates that the fetal blood releases an amount of oxygen per unit of tissue comparable to that in the adult but at a lower oxygen tension.

A comparison of the oxygen dissociation curves of pregnant and nonpregnant women appears relevant here. At the same pressure of oxygen, the blood oxygen saturation is slightly lower in the pregnant than in the nonpregnant female. This shift to the right in the dissociation curve of the blood of the mother may be accounted for by the slight rise in blood pH which occurs in pregnancy.

Serum iron appears in measurable amounts in the blood of the fetus by the fourth month of gestation. At birth, the serum iron values are high, averaging 150 mcg. per 100 ml., whereas the iron-binding capacity is about 225 mcg. per 100 ml. The total iron content of the fetus has been calculated to be in the neighborhood of 350 mg., of which 200 mg. is in the circulating blood as hemoglobin and the remainder is storage iron. When there has been iron-deficiency anemia in the mother, the fetal hemoglobin and serum iron values may be normal at birth, but the iron reserves may be in deficit. Some recent observations support the view that the fetus satisfies its iron needs, even if the mother is iron-deficient. (See Anemia in Chapter 30). However, iron-deficiency anemia may be encountered in the first year of life in some of these infants. A similar situation prevails in the premature infant, who is born before the full complement of storage iron is acquired. The source of iron in the newborn and early months of life is graphically displayed in Figure 7.

The major components of blood coagulation are normal in the term infant, but, despite this, hemorrhagic manifestations may occasionally be noted. Although the bleeding time of the newborn is normal, the clotting time is often delayed. Fetal blood is reputed to contain less than the normal quantity of accelerator substances, but the delay in clotting time is attributed to a prolongation of the prothrombin time. Presumably amounts of prothrombin produced or activated are inadequate because of a lack of vitamin K. Until the gastrointestinal tract of the newborn begins to absorb vitamin K, the amount contained in the infant's blood will depend upon the quantity acquired from the mother prior to

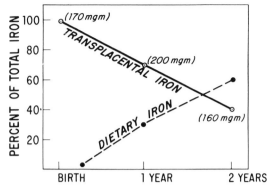

Figure 7. Persistence and utilization of maternal iron for blood formation during infancy (16 cases). Mothers given ^{55}Fe-labeled red blood cells. (From Smith, C. A., et al.: J. Clin. Invest., 34:1391, 1955.)

delivery. In most infants, the prothrombin time tends to increase during the first five days of life. The transient increase in the prothrombin time that occurs after birth may in some cases provide the background for a hemorrhagic tendency. It is common practice to administer vitamin K to the mother during labor or to the baby after delivery in order to prevent a decrease in the prothrombin time during the early neonatal period.

The blood volume tends to be relatively greater in the newborn infant than in the adult, representing some 10 to 15 per cent of the total body weight, which in an average-sized infant amounts to 300 to 370 ml. Variations in the blood volume in the newborn can reflect the amount of blood regained from the placenta at the time of birth. A considerable increment can be added to the infant's blood volume at birth by the transference of blood from the placenta, if the umbilical cord is not ligated until it has ceased to pulsate. However, it is debatable whether this addition to an already existing hypervolemia is necessary or desirable. (See Chapter 26, Conduct of Normal Labor.)

The isoagglutinins anti-A and anti-B do not appear in any quantity until weeks after birth; those present at birth are acquired from the mother and usually disappear within the first two weeks of life.

Cardiovascular System

The early circulatory system of the fetus may be considered as being made up of two components. The first of these is the portion that furnishes blood to the growing fetus itself; the second is concerned with the transport of blood within the placenta. The feto-placental component has been described previously; we are here concerned principally with the systemic circulation of the fetus.

Although the anatomic components of the fetal circulation have been known since the time of Harvey, the hemodynamics and the changes in distribution of the blood remain in some controversy. Until rather recently, most of the information had been deduced from the experimental animal, but with the introduction of angiocardiography these studies have been extended, and observations have been made in the previable human fetus.

The specific fetal characteristics of the heart and its neighboring great vessels are the patency of the foramen ovale and the function of the ductus arteriosus. The ductus arteriosus provides a connection between the pulmonary artery and the arch of the aorta at a point below the origin of the arteries that supply the cephalad portion of the body.

The umbilical vessels, while providing the anastomoses between the placental circulation and the systemic circulation of the fetus, possess certain anatomic features which may influence the direction and distribution of blood flow. The umbilical vessels contain protrusions or folds into their lumina which, in the arteries, are valve-like structures, referred to as the valves of Hoboken. These folds may assist in the closure of the umbilical vessels at the time of birth. The single umbilical vein of the cord traverses the umbilicus and divides into two branches. One of these, the hepatic branch, connects with the portal and hepatic systems; the other, the ductus venosus, anastomoses with the inferior vena cava (Fig. 8).

The direction of flow and the question of mixing of blood within the fetal heart have been the subject of longstanding interest, from which two theories have emerged. The original theory, proposed by Sabatier in 1791, states that the currents of blood from the inferior and the superior vena cava do not mix appreciably in the right atrium but retain their individuality. Supposedly this is the result of a jetlike property of the stream of blood entering from the inferior vena cava, by which it eludes being mixed with blood from other sources. A later theory (Pohlman-Kellogg)

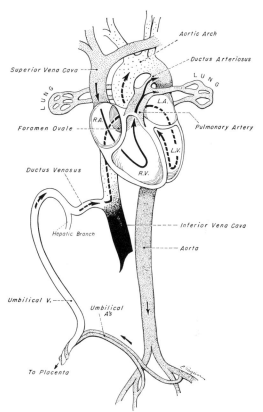

Figure 8. Routes of blood flow in the fetus. The comparative (not absolute) decrease in oxygen saturation of the blood in the various areas of the body is roughly represented by the denser stippling.

maintains that the right atrium serves as a mixing chamber for the blood of the two caval streams.

The more recent evidence has tended to support the validity of the earlier theory. The oxygen content of the blood of the carotid artery in the sheep fetus has been found to be lower than that of the blood in the umbilical vein but higher than that of the blood in the aorta and the umbilical artery. The most striking evidence that there is minimal mixing of blood in the right atrium is furnished from angiocardiographic studies. Injection of radiopaque media into the umbilical vein of human fetuses of 12 to 25 weeks' gestational age, immediately after delivery by abdominal hysterotomy, gave angiographic results supporting those based on oxygen studies in the sheep. The aorta and the subclavian and carotid arteries became well opacified, but the pulmonary artery, lung vessels, and ductus arteriosus were only faintly so (Fig. 9). It is envisioned in this study that the blood containing the contrast medium en-

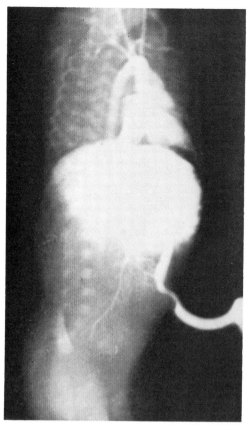

Figure 9. Angiogram of human fetus injected through the umbilical vein immediately at birth. The ductus arteriosus is visible and the vessels to the upper part of the body are prominent. (Courtesy of Dr. John Lind.)

newborn rhesus monkey of a higher oxygen content in the blood in the carotid artery than in that in the femoral artery. By such an arrangement, the brain receives blood with a comparatively high oxygen content, an important factor when oxygen transport from mother to fetus becomes compromised.

The volume of blood in the feto-placental vascular system is constantly changing throughout pregnancy. From observations in sheep (Fig. 10), in early pregnancy the greatest percentage of the blood volume is presumed to be limited to the placenta. In the second trimester, the quantities of blood in the placental and fetal beds are nearly equal. Near term, the amount of blood in the fetus is three to four times greater than that in the placenta. It is suggested from these studies that once the cotyledonary structure of the placenta is complete, which would correspond to the end of the sixth month of human gestation, the volume capacity of the placental bed remains fairly constant. Consonant with this observation, it has been shown in the subhuman primate (168 days' gestation) that the weight of the placenta changes little after the second trimester. It would appear that the later increase in blood volume of the fetal circulation is confined mostly to the enlarging vascular bed of the fetus.

In addition to meeting the metabolic demands of the fetus, the allocation of blood to various body systems in the fetus may have for its purpose the preparation of the organism for extrauterine existence. For example, it has been commonly held that the ductus arteriosus and the foramen ovale gradually close during the later weeks of pregnancy. The shunting of more and more blood through the pulmonary circulation presumably would ready the capillaries of the lung parenchyma to assume their role in pulmonary ventilation at birth. Recent cineradiographic studies have, however, cast doubt upon this concept, but until observations are made on full-term human fetuses this must remain open to question.

A decrease in the oxygen content of carotid artery blood which has been observed in the sheep near term has been related to the redistribution of the total blood volume within the fetal circulation as well as to decline in oxygen saturation of umbilical vein blood. Account must be taken of the fact that, commensurate with the growth of the fetus, the venous blood returning from the trunk and lower extremities con-

ters the right atrium and is separated into streams, perhaps by the *crista dividens*, a projection of the atrial septum. The larger stream passes through the foramen ovale and into the left atrium, for the radiopaque material rapidly appears in the arteries supplying the upper part of the body. The smaller stream remains in the right atrium to become mixed with blood entering by way of the superior vena cava. When a radiopaque medium was injected into the internal jugular vein of the human fetus, most of the material on entering the right atrium passed to the pulmonary artery, from which point the larger quantity entered the ductus arteriosus and only a minor portion entered the lungs.

In view of the disclosure that the two caval streams remain quite distinct within the fetal heart, one may conclude that the cranial portion of the fetal body is "blessed with a preferential circulation." Additional evidence that this is so is the finding in the

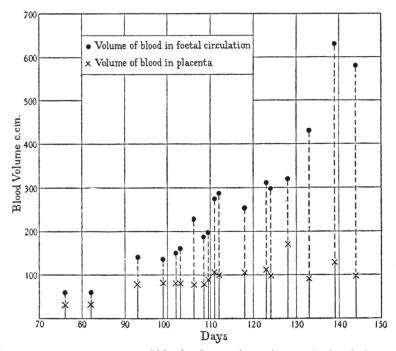

Figure 10. Diagrammatic representation of blood volume relationships in fetal and placental vascular beds throughout gestation (sheep). The capacity and blood volume of the placental bed remain relatively constant after the 110th day of gestation, while the fetal blood volume shows a progressive increase until term (Barcroft).

tributes a greater proportion of the total volume emptying into the heart from the inferior vena cava.

Other important aspects of the hemodynamics of the feto-placental circulation concern the total blood volume and the rate of and factors responsible for blood flow. While it is often stated that a leisurely rate of circulation within the placenta would be conducive to the most effective metabolic exchange between the fetal and maternal circulation, one must question whether any degree of stasis exists or is desirable. In view of the relatively constant blood volume capacity of the placenta in the last trimester and the increase in total fetal blood volume throughout pregnancy, it appears essential that the rate of flow through the placenta likewise increase if each unit of fetal blood is to participate at maximal efficiency in feto-maternal exchange. Further, a brisk flow of blood through the ductus venosus would favor maintenance of the individuality of the stream entering the right atrium from the inferior vena cava and prevent mixing. One might speculate whether, if the rate of umbilical blood flow were reduced to some critical level, mixing would occur in the right atrium, leading to aboli-

tion of the preferential circulation to the upper portion of the body and thus enhancing the chance of brain damage. It has been shown in the goat and sheep that the total amount of blood flowing through the placenta in a given period of time increases some three-fold from early to late pregnancy. From measurements of blood flow in the pregnant human uterus at term it has been determined that 400 to 500 ml. of fetal blood must circulate through the placenta per minute. This is based on the finding of almost identical values of arteriovenous oxygen difference between the uterine artery and vein and the umbilical artery and vein. The volume of fetal blood circulating through the placenta, as derived from the Fick principle, would approximate that which the mother supplies to the placenta in a given period of time, that is, 500 ml. per minute. Thus it would appear that the total blood volume of the feto-placental circulation (370 ml. per term fetus plus 125 ml. per placenta) is circulated each minute, or at a rate proportionately equal to that of the mother. This also offers some idea of the magnitude of the fetal cardiac output.

Birth is accompanied by a rapid realignment of the infant's circulation. The umbilical arteries usually cease to pulsate within a minute after birth. The umbilical vein tends to remain distended for a variable period of time, depending on the amount of blood entering from the placenta. Presumably the musculature, more especially that of the arteries, contracts because of exposure to mechanical and thermal stimuli. These vessels are reputed to contract when perfused with oxygen and relax when the carbon dioxide content of the perfusate is increased. With the onset of respiration the oxygen content of blood flowing through these vessels rises, which would tend to promote their closure. Backflow in the umbilical vein is prevented, presumably by the natural constriction of the vessel near the umbilicus and closure of a sphincter located at the umbilical end of the ductus venosus. Severance of the cord some distance from the umbilicus rarely leads to critical bleeding, and that which occurs is usually retrograde from the umbilical vein.

The onset of respiration creates a negative intrathoracic pressure which aids in opening the pulmonary capillary bed. As blood is routed through the lungs, the pressure in the right atrium falls, increasing the pressure differential between the two atria. This pressure gradient causes the closure of the foramen ovale. The additional amounts of blood returning from the pulmonary veins further increase the pressure within the left atrium, which ensures permanent closure of the foramen ovale. The fact that in the newborn lamb the carotid blood becomes 100 per cent saturated within 10 minutes after birth has led to the assumption that functionally the foramen ovale closes promptly, depending to a degree on how easily and how completely the lungs expand. The application of angiographic techniques to the human fetus, however, has given the impression that closure of the foramen ovale occurs more gradually. It is believed that the foramen ovale continues to exert more of a valvelike action, which is perhaps necessary to maintain an effective circulation during the transition to pulmonary ventilation.

In the same study, the ductus arteriosus was observed to be functionally closed soon after birth, although anatomically it may remain usable for several days. In fact, from observations on newborn lambs it was concluded that there was a reversal of blood flow from the aorta to the pulmonary circulation. The evidence was based on the auscultation of a systolic murmur in the region of the ductus arteriosus, the cineangiographic observation of the distribution of a radiopaque contrast medium injected into the arch of the aorta, and temporary occlusion of the ductus, causing a fall in pulmonary arterial pressure. The disappearance of the systolic murmur is interpreted as an indication that the ductus has closed.

The rapidity of the functional closure of the ductus is said to be related to both the expansion of the lungs and the rise in the oxygen saturation, and such closure is probably achieved through a neuromuscular mechanism. Thus, similar to that of the foramen ovale, the gradual closure of the ductus arteriosus may serve some useful function during the period when the lungs are becoming expanded. Although the ductus venosus is functionally closed through the sphincter-like action occurring in the region of the umbilicus, its complete obliteration apparently occurs at a leisurely pace, for when autopsy is performed on infants who died several weeks after birth, some patency is seen.

Two aspects of the fetal circulation are reemphasized because of their physiologic importance. First is the fact that blood with the highest oxygen saturation is shunted through the fetal heart to emerge and be distributed first to the upper part of the body. In this sense, the brain has a favored circulation, and is protected to the maximum against the threat of hypoxia. Second, the relationship between the degrees of patency of the ductus arteriosus and the foramen ovale is a matter of some physiologic significance as it pertains to the circulatory adjustments which take place with extrauterine respiration and the expansion of the lungs.

Respiratory System

Until the turn of the century, most opinion favored the belief that the fetus existed in an apneic state throughout the course of pregnancy. The thought was generally expressed that it would be undesirable for intrauterine respiration to occur, for the lungs would become filled with amniotic fluid and at birth breathing would be established with great difficulty. Then evidence began to accumulate from several sources that fetal respiratory movements may be a part of intrauterine physiology.

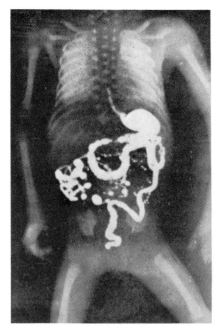 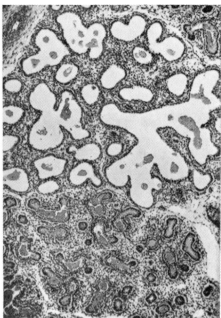

Figure 11. A, X-ray demonstration of Thorotrast in lungs and gastrointestinal tract of human fetus of 16 weeks' menstrual age. B, Microscopic section of lung tissue reveals Thorotrast in the alveolar spaces. The contrast medium was injected into the chorionic cavity 24 hours prior to abdominal hysterotomy. (From Davis, M. E., and Potter, E. L.: J.A.M.A., 131:1194, 1946.)

Evidence for the occurrence of respiratory movements by the human fetus has been furnished by the introduction of radiopaque substances such as Thorotrast into the ovisac a few days before therapeutic abortion (Fig. 11). Thorotrast was revealed in the lungs of all the fetuses during the middle trimester, although in fetuses near term this was not universally so.

Direct observation in carefully prepared animal experiments has furnished confirmatory evidence of fetal respiratory movements. The fact that respiratory excursions appear in early embryonic life and are not a completely new activity at birth has rightfully aroused curiosity as to their functional significance. The question has been proposed whether these movements are purposeful by serving to prepare the respiratory system for effective breathing at birth. More significant, however, has been the inquiry into the extent of the relationship between intrauterine respiratory behavior and the respiratory complications which are occasionally encountered at birth and in the neonatal period, that is, whether neonatal pneumonia and many cases of respiratory distress in the newborn are related to the behavior of the respiratory system during intrauterine life.

ANATOMIC DEVELOPMENT OF THE LUNG. During the first four months of fetal life the primitive lung is a series of bronchi lined with cuboidal or low columnar epithelium and surrounded by avascular connective tissue or mesenchyme (Fig. 12). This structural pattern is incompatible with extrauterine life. In the latter half of pregnancy the parenchyma of the lung becomes vascularized through an extensive network of capillaries. Although the bronchioles are numerous at first, few alveolar ducts and alveoli are discernible. With penetration of the capillaries from between the cuboidal cells lining the alveolar ducts, the alveoli begin to form. Near term the epithelial lining of the alveoli becomes sparse, and the blood and the inspired air are separated mainly by capillary endothelium. Not until a sufficient number of capillaries come in direct contact with the potential air spaces does extrauterine survival become possible, and this occurs about the 28th week, or in infants of 1000 grams (Fig. 13). The human lung at 36 weeks is sufficiently developed to be functionally mature (Fig. 14). Complete alveolar development is not acquired until near full term and under the influence of extrauterine breathing. The lung of the premature infant continues to

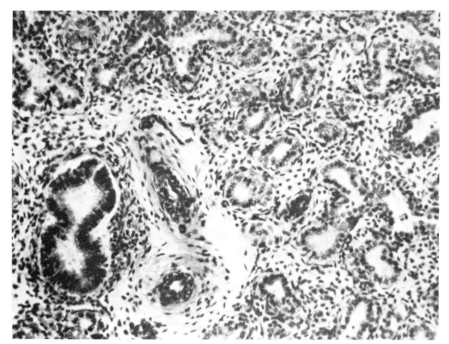

Figure 12. Microscopic section of the human lung at 16 weeks. ×150.

develop anatomically for several weeks after birth. Full alveolar growth and expansion are attained at approximately the date at which birth would have occurred at full term.

Some discussion has arisen as to the anatomic details of the capillary bed of the alveolar ducts and alveoli. The extent to which a filling of these vessels might effect alveolar expansion or the degree of resistance to the passage of blood through this capillary network could relate to respira-

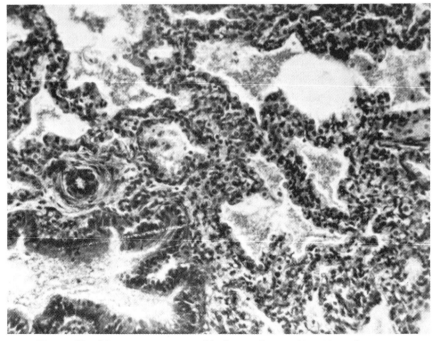

Figure 13. Microscopic section of the human lung at 26 to 28 weeks. ×150.

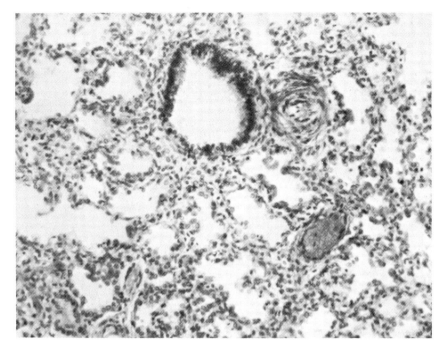

Figure 14. Microscopic section of the human lung at 36 weeks. ×150.

ory distress in the newborn. It has been suggested that a more complete filling of the capillary bed at birth is instrumental in promoting alveolar expansion. In the normal term infant there is apparently no delay in the opening of the capillaries at birth and the alveoli are expanded immediately, albeit not always completely. The amniotic fluid that is present in varying amounts in the lungs of the newborn is readily absorbed, and effective gaseous exchange across the alveolar membrane occurs almost instantaneously. In the premature infant, however, alveolar expansion at birth is less predictable. Also, a "hyaline membrane" may form over the surfaces of the alveoli and bronchioles, a special feature and additional hazard of prematurity.

Some recent observations relating to respiratory and cardiovascular adjustments at birth have bearing on the fetal distress syndrome. Cardiac catheterization revealed that in some normal infants the ductus arteriosus remained open, with a small left-to-right shunt occurring for the first 10 to 15 hours after birth. In infants in respiratory distress there was a much larger shunt, which, again, was mostly left to right. Also, it has been shown that in the premature infant there is less alveolar stability, with a greater tendency for pulmonary collapse and atelectasis.

Survival at birth is certainly dependent in large measure on the anatomic maturity of the lungs and their response to the adjustments which are required in the pulmonary and systemic circulations at birth.

THEORIES OF INTRAUTERINE RESPIRATORY MOVEMENTS. Knowledge regarding the functional development of the fetal respiratory system and the sequential appearance of the physiologic factors which influence it must necessarily be gathered largely from other than human sources. Experimentally there appears to have emerged what might be referred to as the Snyder-Rosenfeld and the Barcroft hypotheses, which attempt to explain the functional development and the physiologic meaning of the respiratory movements of the fetus. To the clinician it is of more importance to know how they may or may not relate to normal and abnormal breathing at birth or in the early days of life.

From experimental observations in the rabbit, with the fetus delivered into a saline bath and the intrauterine maternal relationship preserved, Snyder and Rosenfeld proposed the concept that fetal respirations appear early in pregnancy and, except for short episodes of apnea, continue throughout intrauterine life. Consequently, the first respiration at birth is not a new physiologic event, but is a continuation of respiratory activity established in utero. Furthermore, it was found that the behavior of the fetal respiratory system, although reacting to chemical stimuli, differed from that of the maternal organism when carbon dioxide and oxygen were administered.

It was observed that the pregnant rabbit, when it breathed a mixture containing a high concentration of carbon dioxide, reacted as anticipated and developed hyperpnea, whereas the fetus in most instances failed to respond. Under conditions of low carbon dioxide tension produced by forced respirations in the mother, fetal apnea resulted. These findings were interpreted to mean that the fetal respiratory response was under the control of pCO_2 within certain limits of concentration of the gas. The experimental observation that the fetus does not respond to carbon dioxide excess is evidence that the administration of this gas would not enhance the infant's respiration at birth. Actually such therapy could contribute to a further depression of the medullary respiratory center in babies suffering from apnea at birth.

It is further observed experimentally that when the maternal organism was placed in an anoxic atmosphere her respiratory rate increased, whereas apnea developed in the fetus. Failure of the fetus to react to hypoxia and its immediate lapse into apnea implies that the lower respiratory centers, the carotid bodies perhaps, are not functioning in intrauterine life. This is consistent with some evidence to suggest that the carotid sinus in the rabbit does not respond to asphyxia until a few days after birth. As will be seen, these experimental findings differ from those supporting the Barcroft theory, in which the conclusion is drawn that the chemoreceptors appear to respond to anoxemia, but this may be a species difference.

In résumé, this concept of Snyder and Rosenfeld maintains that fetal respirations originate in early embryonic life, but may be interrupted by states of hypercapnia or hypoxemia. These respiratory movements occur at frequent intervals, and are believed to serve a useful purpose by preparing the lung alveoli for extrauterine respiration through the tidal flow of amniotic fluid in and out of the respiratory system of the fetus. It must be realized, however, that the respiratory tract is constantly exposed to whatever particulate matter is contained within the amniotic fluid. The failure of the

respiratory system to respond in some way to an oxygen lack has caused the question to be asked whether the extramedullary respiratory centers or chemoreceptors are completely developed physiologically at birth.

Sir Joseph Barcroft, using the sheep fetus in his extensive researches on prenatal life, evolved a theory of the physiologic evolution and control of intrauterine respiratory movement. Although agreeing that there were fetal respiratory movements, he questioned whether they were necessary for normal intrauterine pulmonary development. Under normal conditions such movements as did occur were present only during the first half of pregnancy, at least in sheep. In the event of respiratory excursions in the last half of pregnancy, such movements were regarded as indicative of fetal hypoxia.

Barcroft's concept was based upon the observation that fetal activity exhibited four distinct patterns during intrauterine life. He chose to divide these into the phases of spasm, rhythm, segregation, and inhibition. By the 35th day of pregnancy, physical stimulation of the fetus elicited a spasmodic response; a few days later the response consisted of simultaneous rhythmic respiratory and somatic movements. At day 50 in the sheep, corresponding to the end of the first trimester in the human, physical stimulation evoked independent somatic and respiratory movements, denoting the phase of segregation. For the remainder of pregnancy the fetus remained quiescent. This state appeared to continue until birth except in the presence of chemical or physical stimuli.

It was emphasized that, rather than replacing its predecessor, each successive phase was superimposed upon it. Barcroft reached this conclusion by observing the effects of sectioning of the spinal cord and brain stem at various levels. This type of experiment led him to postulate that areas within the central nervous system were involved in the genesis of the movements described above. It was thought that the most primitive type of respiration is due to chemoreceptor activity, whereas the more rhythmic type of respiration is mediated through the central respiratory center. It was postulated that the phase of inhibition is brought about by the activity of a center located above the pons. The influence of this center is removed at the time of birth.

Thus, the gasping type of respiration of chemoreceptor origin, the life line in the hypoxic state, might be regarded as the first form of respiratory movement to appear in the life of the new individual, and the last to disappear, being reluctantly relinquished at the time of death, philosophically the alpha and omega of respiratory activity.

The response of the sheep fetus to carbon dioxide was found to differ at various periods of pregnancy. Prior to the phase of inhibition, carbon dioxide excess elicited respiratory movements, but the response tended to diminish as pregnancy advanced. This may have been due to the influence of the center above the pons responsible for the phase of inhibition rather than to any change in the threshold response of the central respiratory center of carbon dioxide.

Hypoxia produced by administration of a nitrogen mixture to the mother during the first trimester elicited from the fetus a gasping type of respiration. This same procedure in the latter half of pregnancy caused a vigorous somatic response prior to the gasping type of respiration. Clamping of the umbilical cord before day 39 elicited no fetal response, but such interference with the fetal circulation for the remainder of pregnancy resulted in fetal activity. Thus, in contrast to the rabbit, the sheep fetus appears to respond to hypoxia initially by exhibiting respiratory movements rather than by becoming apneic. This response to hypoxia suggests that in the sheep, at least, the chemoreceptors are functionally developed at an early fetal age.

In summary, the Barcroft theory is in agreement with the observation that intrauterine respiratory activity is present on occasion. This activity is not regarded as being essential in the preparation of the respiratory system for extrauterine function.

However, by the latter half of pregnancy the fetal respiratory system is sufficiently developed to respond to both chemical and sensory stimuli. Even at an earlier age the carotid and aortic bodies, or chemoreceptors, react. In fact, the respiratory system of the fetus of the sheep, and of the human, responds to those stimuli which regulate or influence respiratory activity in the maternal organism. It is concluded that physiologic control of the respiratory system of the newborn does not differ from that of the mother.

LEVELS OF FETAL BLOOD GASES AT VARIOUS PERIODS OF PREGNANCY. Determination of the concentration of respiratory gases in human fetal blood has been confined almost entirely to the last trimester. More complete observations at different periods of pregnancy are available in the experimental animal, especially the sheep and goat. In the sheep, the maximum blood oxygen saturation has been observed to occur between days 75 and 100. Toward the end of pregnancy (days 127 to 139) the oxygen saturation of umbilical vein blood was found to be around 70 per cent. Although the blood oxygen saturation may diminish significantly near term, the total amount of oxygen available for fetal metabolism may actually increase because of the marked rise in hematocrit and hemoglobin concentration and an acceleration in circulating minute volume.

If the oxygen saturation of the fetal carotid artery blood fell to 20 to 30 per cent, the central medullary center might become depressed and fail to respond. In such a situation the respiratory system would come under the control of chemoreceptors. The latter's influence is observed in the fetus born in an apneic state. The period of recovery is marked by irregular gasping respiration, which preserves life by initiating enough respiratory exchange to raise the oxygen saturation to a level sufficiently high to allow the central respiratory center to recover and respond. Together, the above observations could well offer an explanation that has been previously implied regarding the behavior of the human fetus in response to so-called fetal distress, which in essence is a hypoxic episode. With a decrease in the oxygen saturation of the blood entering the carotid artery, the theoretical respiratory center above the pons would no longer exert its inhibitory effect. The fetus would undergo somatic activity, including respiratory efforts, which, if amniotic fluid contaminated with meconium or other debris were aspirated, would be a dreaded complication if the infant was born alive. With further asphyxia, however, the medullary center would become completely depressed and activity would cease. This appears to fit more closely the situation observed clinically when the fetus becomes embarrassed from oxygen lack; that is, a short period of fetal hyperactivity is followed by quiescence as the oxygen deficit mounts.

In human pregnancy, a limited number of samples taken about the 30th week reveal that umbilical vein blood is 70 per cent saturated. Near term the values decrease and the blood is approximately 60 per cent saturated. Despite the decrease in oxygen saturation occurring near the end of pregnancy, the oxygen content of fetal blood may remain stationary or even rise slightly, because of the increase in oxygen capacity.

The reported values from analyses of the oxygen content of cord samples for normal newborns at term have varied considerably. The sample is usually taken from a segment of cord that has been doubly clamped and cut before the newborn takes its initial breath. Undoubtedly an important factor is the time after delivery at which the blood is removed from the cord segment. The greatest difficulty is encountered in obtaining adequate samples from the artery, for it tends to go into spasm and collapse.

A general range in volumes per cent of oxygen content of maternal and of cord blood has been reported as follows: maternal arterial blood, 15 to 16; umbilical vein blood, 8 to 12; maternal venous blood, 10 to 12; umbilical artery blood, 4 to 8. It is apparent, therefore, that the fetal blood in contact with the trophoblast membrane acquires a volume per cent of oxygen which is approximately equal to that taken up by adult arterial blood at the alveolar membrane. In both instances the quantity of oxygen transferred amounts to 4 to 5 volumes per cent.

The carbon dioxide content of the blood of the normal term newborn is 22 to 23 mM. per liter, a figure significantly lower than that of the mother. The difference is even more striking in the premature infant, in whom the carbon dioxide content is frequently as low as 15 to 18 mM. per liter. When the fetus experiences distress in utero, the carbon dioxide tension may exceed that in the maternal blood and rise to 60 to 70 mm. Hg in the arterial umbilical blood, but the hypercapnia soon disappears with the onset of normal breathing.

When an attempt is made to relate the concentration of the respiratory gases in cord blood to potential asphyxial damage to the infant, it must be established whether the reported analysis is of blood from the umbilical artery or vein or a pooled sample. For the values to be at all meaningful, one must have samples taken simultaneously from the umbilical artery and vein. For example, it might be concluded that hypoxemia exists if the umbilical vein blood at birth has an oxygen content of 5 to 6 volumes per cent. Despite this low figure, the arteriovenous oxygen difference may be normal, as indicated by an oxygen content of close to zero in the umbilical artery. In other words, in the human, the fetal tissues are apparently able to divest the blood almost completely of oxygen if the occasion demands. Secondly, as stated previously, to know the total amount of oxygen the fetus is receiving, in addition to the arteriovenous oxygen difference of cord blood, one must know the circulating minute volume of either cord or maternal uterine blood. Actually, analysis of the gaseous content of cord blood reveals the concentration at the moment of sampling only and gives no information as to whether the newborn is or is not in oxygen deficit. Although a high pCO_2 and a low pH and blood oxygen saturation are consistent with a state of asphyxia, this is not sufficient to establish either the degree of oxygen deficit in the newborn with apnea or the duration of the hypoxia associated with an episode of fetal distress.

ONSET OF RESPIRATION AND ITS CONTROL IN THE NEWBORN. Normal respiration in the newborn, brought about by physical and chemical stimuli, may be either completely irregular, rhythmic, or periodic in pattern. Regardless of the pattern, however, the normal respiratory rate is twice that of the adult, equaling about 40 excursions per minute. In general, the full-term infant tends to have predominantly periodic breathing alternating between periods of hyperpnea and apnea. The respiratory movements at the beginning are slow and shallow, reaching a maximum excursion and then subsiding and ceasing for a period of three or four seconds. This cyclic breathing, simulating the Cheyne-Stokes type of respiration, persists for some two or three weeks in the infant born at term and for a longer period in the premature.

Periodic breathing tends to disappear in the presence of those factors which are known to increase the minute volume of respiration. These include breathing of high oxygen mixtures which may first produce a momentary decrease in minute volume, stimulation of the respiratory center by carbon dioxide, and increased activity and restlessness on the part of the nfant. Because the minute volume increases with rhythmic breathing, the question might be posed as to what is the most efficient pattern of breathing for the newborn. t is conceivable that a rhythmic pattern ould operate at a much slower respiratory rate and result in a greater minute volume of alveolar exchange than periodic breathing. On the other hand, periodic breathing, with its crescendo pattern, might be a more effective type of respiration in promoting alveolar expansion.

With the initial breath, the resistance to expansion offered by the surface tension of the bronchioles and alveoli and the elasticity of the lung parenchyma must be overcome. It has been estimated that he total negative intrathoracic pressure developed momentarily with the first breath is some 40 cm. H_2O, or several imes that necessary for established normal respiration. However, this degree of pressure may not be sufficient for the premature or for the infant in respiratory distress. Anatomic immaturity of the lung, and bronchiolar and alveolar obstruction, besides possibly interfering with ventilatory exchange, make difficult the assessment of he amount of intrathoracic negative pressure required in these situations to surmount the forces resisting alveolar expansion. A deficiency of the normal alveolar lining layer that produces surfactant has been found in premature infants. This substance is important for alveolar stability. Its absence, due to prematurity or asphyxial damage, may be an important factor in the etiology of the respiratory distress syndrome.

At birth the normal infant is in a state of metabolic acidosis, as denoted by a plasma bicarbonate level of about 22 mM. per liter, a pCO_2 of 36 mm. Hg, and a pH of 7.34 to 7.39. The situation is even more pronounced in the case of the premature, in whom the plasma bicarbonate may range between 18 and 22 mM. per liter, with a further decrease in some instances in the blood pH. This metabolic acidosis may remain uncompensated for several days after birth, particularly in the premature. Also, the lactic and pyruvic acid levels of cord blood are significantly elevated over those of the mother, a condition that persists in the blood of the newborn for some time.

Thus it is seen that the normal newborn respires under chemical controls and an acid-base balance that differ somewhat from those in the adult. Despite these differences, the system is apparently efficient, for with normal respirations oxygen saturation may reach 90 per cent a few minutes after birth and 96 per cent within one or two hours. Although the blood oxygen saturation may be only 80 to 90 per cent during the first hour, there is no evidence to show that a delay of two or more hours in attaining normal levels of oxygen saturation is necessarily detrimental to the newborn.

In assessing the response of the respiratory apparatus, it has been shown that the newborn will respond to low concentrations of carbon dioxide but only for short periods of administration. When 0.5 to 2.0 per cent carbon dioxide is added to the inspired air of a newborn breathing normally, the respiratory rate increases promptly. If the administration of carbon dioxide is preceded by a period of breathing 15 per cent oxygen, the infant fails to hyperventilate. This is interpreted to mean that the stimulating effect of carbon dioxide is abolished whenever the medullary center is mildly hypoxic. It follows that increase of the pCO_2 above the physiologic level for the newborn (35 to 38 mm. Hg) is without apparent therapeutic value and, indeed, may contribute toward a further depression of the medullary respiratory center.

The physiologic status of the chemoreceptors at birth has been the subject of some debate. In the adult, when the oxygen tension falls below 70 mm. Hg, which means that the arterial blood is reduced from 97 to 92 per cent saturation, the chemoreceptors are stimulated to initiate respiratory impulses through the medullary center. The fact that the human infant has a much lower blood oxygen saturation at birth suggests that the initial respiration might arise from stimulation of the medullary center by the chemoreceptors.

It has been demonstrated that in the premature and full-term infant receiving 100 per cent oxygen the respiratory minute volume dropped 12 to 15 per cent. More impressive was the observation that when 15 per cent oxygen was administered to the infant a vigorous but short-lived respiratory response occurred. It was suggested that either the chemoreceptors, while responding well, became fatigued quickly or the medullary center failed to respond to stimulation when the newborn became even slightly hypoxic. It has been pointed out that these conclusions were based on observations made on infants a few days of age. Infants studied in the first 24 hours of life failed to hyperventilate when hypoxic, and the deduction was made that the chemoreceptors were not responding during this early period. Accordingly, it was proposed that the chemoreceptor mechanism is weak at birth but becomes more responsive during the first seven days. In spite of these observations, most workers hold the belief that the chemoreceptors are responsive at birth. In cases of apnea at birth, chemoreceptor-stimulating drugs, such as alphalobeline, could theoretically prove useful. In the presence of severe depression of the respiratory center, these drugs are apparently of little value and have been discarded from clinical practice.

Why the normal and the premature infant may continue to exist in a mild state of metabolic acidosis for several weeks after birth is an interesting question. Although the condition is subject to correction by the kidney, the cause must be looked for elsewhere, for organic acids are apparently readily excreted. Perhaps it is to the advantage of the newborn to delay correction of the very mild metabolic acidosis in order to ensure continued chemical stimulation of the medullary and extramedullary respiratory centers.

In summary, exactly how the newborn's respiratory pattern is regulated in the early weeks of life, and until the time when it assumes the adult prototype, is not entirely clear. It has been proposed that its breathing is similar to Cheyne-Stokes respiration, a "teeter" effect.

Gastrointestinal System

The injection of radiopaque substances into the ovisac discloses that as early as the second trimester the fetal digestive system is capable of mechanical function (see Fig. 11A). The fact that amniotic debris is found in the large as well as the small bowel is a further indication that some degree of intestinal motility exists. Meconium, which is an admixture of bile, lanugo hair, desquamated epithelial cells, vernix caseosa, and mucus, is normally contained within the bowel until after birth. Under anoxic situations, however, meconium may be extruded from the lower bowel into the ovisac. If this has occurred several days or weeks before birth, the infant's skin and nails, the umbilical cord, and the fetal membrane are bile-stained. Meconium staining is a striking feature of babies who are regarded as being born postmaturely, and presumably reflects hypoxia due to placental insufficiency. The absence of bile in the meconium is associated with atresia of the ileum or bile ducts.

Water and probably other substances are absorbed from the intestine during intrauterine life. The function of water absorption is important in maintaining an optimal amount of amniotic fluid. Little hydrochloric acid is present in the gastric contents of the fetus during intrauterine life but at birth there is a sudden increase in gastric acidity.

LIVER. The fetal liver begins to produce bile at about the 10th to 12th week of gestation. It has been calculated that from this time until term about 1 gram of bilirubin is formed by the fetus. Only a very small fraction (40 mg.) can usually be found in the meconium and amniotic fluid. The route by which bilirubin enters the amniotic fluid is not precisely known, but transudation through the umbilical vessels, skin, lungs, and upper gastrointestinal tract is probably the major route. The majority of bilirubin produced by the fetus is transported in the unconjugated state across the placenta for excretion by the maternal liver. During fetal life the liver is not able to conjugate bilirubin with glucuronic acid owing to the absence or inactivity of the hepatic enzyme glucuronyl transferase. This deficiency persists after birth for several days and is the most important cause of "physiologic jaundice," which is found in virtually all newborn infants but is particularly severe in small premature infants. Certain substances such as phenobarbital and alcohol can increase fetal hepatic glucuronyl transferase activity in animals. The applications of these observations of enzyme induction to possible future fetal therapy are obvious but as yet no practical application has been shown in the human.

The fetal liver cell is also deficient in the newly discovered transport proteins X and Y, which are responsible for the intracellular transport of bilirubin across the liver cell to the bile canaliculus for excretion. The slow development of these proteins in the liver cell may also be an important factor in the etiology of physiologic jaundice.

Significant amounts of glycogen are found in the human liver at 10 weeks of gestation. At term the human fetal liver contains a higher concentration of glycogen (8 grams per 100 grams wet tissue) than the adult; this indicates that the synthesizing enzymes of the glycogen cycle are present.

Urinary System

In most infants born prior to the 35th week of pregnancy or weighing less than 2500 grams there are a significant number of incompletely formed glomeruli in the kidneys. In the prematurely born infant, glomeruli continue to be formed after birth until such time as the kidney has gained its normal complement. The state of glomerular development disclosed at necropsy has been offered as a useful index of fetal maturity.

The fetal kidney is excreting at least by the fourth or fifth month, for urine can be recovered from the fetal bladder by this time. The bladder urine at birth is hypotonic, which is not surprising in view of the fact that most of the excretion of metabolites is performed by the placenta. As pregnancy advances, the contribution made by the fetal kidney to the amniotic fluid becomes progressively larger and apparently near term the fetus may have a daily urinary volume exceeding that of a normal adult. The importance of the kidney in the maintenance of amniotic fluid volume is perhaps best illustrated by oligohydramnios in cases of bilateral agenesis of the kidney.

The filtration rate in the newborn is lower than that in the adult. This is in keeping with the histologic observation that the glomerular loops tend to be matted together and covered with high columnar epithelium. After birth, the epithelial sacs burst and the loops expand. Although the renal tubules appear to be anatomically well developed at birth, they apparently have not acquired complete reabsorptive and excretory function, for the kidney of the newborn infant is said not to respond appreciably to antidiuretic substance.

Skeletal System

The fetal skeleton takes on form by the eighth to tenth week of intrauterine life, but only in the last trimester are appreciable amounts of calcium required. Actually, well over half of the total calcium content, amounting to 10 to 12 grams, is stored during the last eight weeks of pregnancy. Thus

the premature infant may be deficient in this mineral. By contrast, in those cases in which gestation is prolonged, the fetus may reveal increased deposition of calcium in the long bones and in the skull. It has been proposed that extreme calcification in the latter instance may interfere with proper molding of the fetal head to a degree sufficient to complicate labor and delivery. However, clinical experience does not bear out this contention. Moreover, molding is more concerned with overlapping of the cranial bones.

Even in full-term infants, the bones constituting the calvarium vary in thickness. Palpable softening of the skull bones, or craniotabes, is not confined to the premature but may occasionally be encountered in the term fetus. When the condition is encountered in labor, crepitation will be elicited on vaginal or rectal examination because of the parchment-like consistency of the bones of the vertex.

Endocrine System

Whether the fetal endocrine system acquires function, and if so at what period in intrauterine life, is the subject of continuing controversy, and the application to man of findings in lower species must be viewed with caution. For example, the fetal zone of the adrenal is peculiar to the human and certain other primates and is not found in other species or common laboratory animals.

Some functional autonomy of the various endocrine glands exists during the developmental period; this is perhaps best seen in the formation of the reproductive system in the male, where the interstitial cells of the testes take on a secretory appearance for a short period of time. Rabbit and rat fetuses, hypophysectomized by decapitation, continued to grow in utero to a size comparable to that of their control littermates. Although the various endocrine glands become well differentiated histologically, tropic stimulation seems necessary for the target gland to demonstrate the morphologic changes associated with function. (See Chapter 3).

FETAL METABOLISM

Water and Electrolytes

The percentage of water in the fetus in the early months is greater than that in the adult. Even at term the body water of the newborn constitutes 80 per cent of the total body weight. Measurements of the sodium (^{24}Na) or thiocyanate space reveal that 40 to 45 per cent of body weight consists of extracellular fluid, nearly twice the value for the adult. The 10 to 15 per cent decrease in weight of the newborn during the first week of life is largely the result of the extracellular fluid loss.

Evidence has been presented from studies in the sheep and goat that maternal serum has a higher colloid osmotic activity than has fetal serum. This begs the question of how the fetus is able to maintain a greater percentage of total body water than its mother or, more important, what prevents the fetus from becoming depleted of water and electrolytes. In the human, measurements of the osmolar activity of maternal and newborn sera indicate that there is no significant difference.

Protein

It is assumed that the fetus is able to synthesize plasma proteins by at least the 20th week, for small amounts of albumin are found in the fetal blood at that time. In-vitro studies furnish direct evidence that the fetus synthesizes all the known plasma proteins except gamma globulin by the third to the fourth month of gestation.

Although the total protein content of the blood of the term fetus is slightly lower than that of the maternal blood, the albumin fraction constitutes nearly the same percentage in each.

Despite the lower protein content of fetal blood, electrophoretic analysis reveals that both absolute and relative concentrations of gamma globulin in the fetus are higher than in normal adult or maternal sera. This finding is consistent with a high degree of passive immunity in the newborn.

The thymus plays a dominant role in the development of immunologic competence by the fetus. At about eight weeks of gestation small lymphocytes and Hassall's corpuscles begin to appear in this gland, and by 12 to 14 weeks lymphocytes and plasma cells can be found in the lymph nodes, gut, spleen, and bone marrow.

Immunoglobulin synthesis is well established by at least midpregnancy and probably begins within a month or two of life.

Normally IgG and IgM are present in detectable amounts. That the latter is of fetal origin is indicated by the evidence that IgM is not transferred transplacentally. This fact can be used in detecting and documenting intrauterine infection with cytomegalovirus, rubella, Toxoplasma, syphilis, and Listeria, in which IgM levels of cord and neonatal blood may be sharply elevated. IgA is barely perceptible in cord blood unless the fetus is challenged by a maternal infection.

Although the fetus possesses the capacity to make immunoglobulins, the immunity of the fetus and the infant at birth is dependent largely on passively acquired maternal antibodies.

In summary, it appears that immunogenesis in the fetus and newborn is a somewhat progressive phenomenon, starting in the human as early as the first trimester. The fetal immunologic response is not the same for all antigens at a given intrauterine age. The fetus may respond to one type of antigen but not to another at four months, although it responds to both at six or seven months. Further evidence is furnished by the pregnant patient with agammaglobulinemia, who may show antibodies of fetal origin in the circulation to a specific antigen administered late in pregnancy, having failed to reveal antibodies to the same antigen when it was administered in early pregnancy. Thus, it seems safe to conclude that a relative state of immunologic tolerance exists in the early embryo and that the achievement of immunologic competence is a step-by-step development that varies from species to species. The complete maturation of the immunoglobulin system is stated to be in the order of IgM, IgD, IgG, and IgA, the process differing somewhat as to time in the two sexes but being completed by 8 to 12 years of age.

AMINO ACIDS. Amino acids are transported transplacentally by an active transport process. The placenta functions to maintain a higher blood level of amino acids in the fetus than in the mother. All free amino acids are found in higher concentrations in the fetal circulation than in the maternal circulation. This mechanism is ideally suited to periods of maternal food deprivation but in certain circumstances (maternal phenylketonuria) where the mother's blood level of an amino acid may be quite high, this mechanism will magnify the level in fetal blood, often to the detriment of normal brain growth.

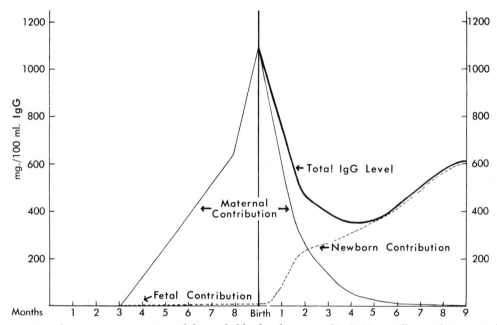

Figure 15. Schematic representation of the probable development of IgG. (From Allansmith, M., McClellan, B. H., Butterworth, M., and Maloney, J. R.: J. Pediat., 72:276, 1968.)

Fat

Acetates and free fatty acids cross the placenta rapidly, whereas cholesterol passes slowly and phospholipids do not cross. The capacity of the fetus to oxidize fatty acids is limited, but some evidence suggests that this may be an energy source available to the fetus.

Brown adipose tissue is the main site of extra heat production in the human infant. This specialized tissue produces heat by oxidizing fatty acids. White fat serves a more passive role of lipid storage in the body. Quantitative studies of the actual number of fat cells present in various areas of the body now in progress indicate that "obese" infants do have larger as well as greater numbers of fat cells than "non-obese" infants. The question of whether this number can be influenced by overfeeding in the early weeks of life is of great importance.

Carbohydrate

In-vitro studies have shown that the fetus apparently in the very early weeks of intra-uterine life acquires the enzyme system necessary for carbohydrate metabolism. The liver contains an active oxalacetic decarboxylase as early as the ninth week. The enzymes involved in the Krebs cycle are present by the eighth week, as is also the lactic dehydrogenase system. By at least the 10th week the lung, the liver, and, to a lesser degree, the kidney are all able to secrete glucose. The fetal tissues likewise take up glucose at an early age and, actually, glucose utilization is slightly higher at this period than at term, and is distinctly higher than in the middle trimester. Some tissues, however, including the heart, skeletal muscle, and cerebral cortex, are incapable of secreting glucose. It might be supposed that the liver and the lung would serve as the main source of maintaining the fetal blood glucose at physiologic levels should maternal sources fail.

The fetus is readily able to store and mobilize glycogen by the 15th week. Characteristic for the fetus is the high glycogen content of many of its tissues. Great differences have been noted, however, the liver and the heart being particularly rich in glycogen, the brain containing little.

The preservation of those tissues low in glycogen is especially dependent upon glucose derived from sources elsewhere in the body. Of particular significance to the fetus, therefore, is the ready mobilization of glycogen. In this regard, in-vitro studies of fetal tissue slices have shown that both glycogenolysis and glucose utilization occur at a more rapid rate under anaerobic than under aerobic incubation. Glucose production, on the other hand, is neither increased nor decreased by anaerobiosis.

Biologic energy is derived primarily from pyruvic acid utilization. According to in-vitro studies, pyruvic acid production is uniform throughout the intrauterine life of the fetus, indicating that anaerobic metabolism is maintained at a constant level.

Attention must be directed to the other source of energy under anaerobic conditions, namely, the production of lactic acid. The property of fetal tissues to convert glycogen to lactic acid is acquired early in development and is particularly conspicuous in heart muscle. Although glycogenolysis in the fetus is accelerated during anaerobiosis, this is not synonymous with the release of large amounts of energy, for, as stated above, the pyruvic acid production remains unchanged. In other words, although glycogen is plentiful in the fetus, its utilization is restricted except under aerobic conditions. In fact, it has been calculated that, of the total amount of energy produced from carbohydrate metabolism in the fetus, only some 13 per cent is derived from the anaerobic phase.

In summary, these in-vitro studies on human tissue furnish data indicating that from the very beginning of its embryonal development the fetus is able to carry out the anaerobic phase of carbohydrate metabolism. This continues to operate at a rather constant level of activity throughout the course of gestation.

The belief has often been expressed that a significant percentage of the fetal energy requirement is obtained from an anaerobic source. This view was based largely on the finding that the pyruvic acid and lactic acid contents of cord blood are elevated above the levels in maternal blood. Oxygen consumption of the term fetus, however, indicates that its energy requirements, under normal conditions at least, are supplied chiefly by aerobic metabolism.

Oxygen Consumption

The term fetus in utero uses oxygen in amounts comparable to its mother, but little can be said about the oxygen requirements in utero at earlier stages. In-vitro studies of the metabolism of various human fetal tissues show the oxygen consumption to be relatively constant from the beginning through the 24th week of pregnancy. Understandably, it is difficult to secure tissue suitable for this type of analysis in the period of fetal viability. Although a few observations have been made on recently dead term infants, information is lacking on the metabolism of the human fetus in the interim period of the last trimester. Expressed in microliters of oxygen per milligram of dry weight of tissue per hour, the oxygen consumption ranged between 5.4 and 1.8. The liver at the seventh week of gestation had the highest recorded oxygen consumption, but this diminished as pregnancy advanced. This was in contrast to the heart and kidney, both of which utilized oxygen in increasing amounts as pregnancy progressed. The oxygen consumption of the cerebral cortex was high throughout pregnancy, being 4.7 to 5.8 microliters. Although the oxygen consumption of the fetal lung also remained relatively stationary throughout pregnancy, it was lower, ranging between 1.8 and 3.5 microliters.

In the course of a study of uterine blood flow at cesarean section, data were obtained which afforded an opportunity to calculate the amount of oxygen consumed by the human term fetus prior to its removal from the uterus. The total oxygen consumption is the product of the uterine blood flow and the uterine arteriovenous oxygen difference. In calculating oxygen consumption by the fetus, it was determined that the myometrium, the placenta, and the fetus itself utilized oxygen in proportion to their relative weights. Indeed, the coefficient of oxygen utilization for the fetus was found by calculation to be significantly higher than that of the uterus. The evidence indicates that the fetus in utero at full term has an oxygen consumption of 5 ml. per kilogram per minute, which is comparable to that of its mother.

It seems important to reemphasize that the individual tissues and organs of the fetus require more oxygen at the time of their maximal growth and development. This would imply that the fetal oxygen needs per unit of weight could vary for different organs as pregnancy advances. The apparent ability of the fetus to withstand hypoxia better than the adult suggests that in the face of this relatively high oxygen consumption it has metabolic ways and means to reduce energy requirements or to mobilize energy by pathways which are peculiar to it.

RESISTANCE OF THE FETUS TO OXYGEN LACK. It has been demonstrated repeatedly in the experimental animal that the fetus will survive oxygen deprivation for a much longer period than will its mother. This ability of the fetus to withstand hypoxic or anoxic conditions appears to vary inversely with the comparative maturity of the fetus at birth. It must still be elucidated, however, why the fetus is able to withstand oxygen deprivation with presumably less chance of damage to its central nervous system than the adult. The answer has broad biologic implications and is not restricted entirely to fetal growth and development. Unquestionably the survival time of the fetus is dependent upon anaerobic metabolism and the high glycogen content of the fetal tissues. Fructose, which can be metabolized anaerobically by some tissues, has been suggested as a source of energy in the face of oxygen deprivation. Although found in high concentrations in the fetal fluids and blood of lower species, fructose is present in only small amounts in the human fetus.

The question has been raised whether or not the fetal oxygen consumption diminishes when the fetal blood oxygen tension falls. If true, this could be of major benefit to the fetus. In the adult, apparently the rate of oxygen consumption remains rather constant unless the oxygen tension becomes extremely low. In the lamb, with the ewe breathing a 10 per cent oxygen mixture, the fetal oxygen consumption fell when the saturation of the fetal arterial blood dropped below 35 per cent. Otherwise, under normal conditions, the rate of oxygen consumption remained fairly stationary for fetuses of different gestational ages, and did not differ greatly from that of the human term fetus, being 4.0 ml. per kilogram per minute.

To forestall the effects of oxygen lack, the fetus may react by increasing the oxygen capacity of its blood by a rise in hematocrit and hemoglobin values. Even if this is a compensatory reaction, an increase in oxygen capacity is not synonymous with an increase in the amount of oxygen being transported to the fetus in the face of a diminishing oxygen tension. The greater resistance of the fetus to hypoxia undoubtedly resides in some characteristic modification of cellular metabolism.

CONCLUSION

There is ample evidence to attest to the fact that the physiologic adjustments of birth are of greater magnitude than those occurring at any other time in the life of the individual. As has been seen, the very nature of intrauterine existence implies the presence of an evolutionary series of physiologic mechanisms which serve both temporary and permanent functions. During growth and development, the fetus is subject to the vagaries of the intrauterine environment as well as to its intrinsic genetic endowment. Alterations in these normal determinants may arrest growth and disturb body function. Moreover, at the time of labor and delivery the fetus is occasionally confronted with conditions which adversely affect both its immediate and extrauterine physical and biochemical activities. The solutions to many of the problems of abnormal growth and the complications peculiar to the newborn depend on the disclosure of more basic facts concerning the normal physiology of the fetus.

BIBLIOGRAPHY

Adams, F. H., and Lind, J.: Physiologic studies on the cardiovascular status of normal newborn infants (with special reference to the ductus arteriosus). Pediatrics, 19:431, 1957.

Adams, T. W.: Intrauterine roentgenography as an aid in determining fetal age. Obstet. Gynec., 5:43, 1955.

Allansmith, M., McClellan, B. H., Butterworth, M., and Maloney, J. R.: The development of immunoglobulin levels in man. J. Pediat., 72:276, 1968.

Allen, D. W., Wyman, J., Jr., and Smith, C. A.: The oxygen equilibrium of fetal and adult human hemoglobin. J. Biol. Chem., 203:81, 1953.

Ardran, G. M., Dawes, G. S., Prichard, M. M. L., Reynolds, S. R. M., and Wyatt, D. G.: The effect of ventilation of the foetal lungs upon the pulmonary circulation. J. Physiol., 118:12, 1952.

Arias, I.: The pathogenesis of physiologic jaundice of the newborn—a reevaluation. In Birth Defects. Original Article Series, Vol. 6. National Foundation, New York, 1970.

Avery, M. E.: The Lung and Its Disorders, 2nd Ed. W. B. Saunders Co., Philadelphia, 1968, p. 285.

Avery, M. E., and Mead, J.: Surface properties in relation to atelectasis and hyaline membrane disease. A.M.A.J. Dis. Child., 97:517, 1959.

Barcroft, J.: Researches on Prenatal Life. Charles C Thomas, Springfield, Ill., 1948.

Barnett, H. L.: The physiologic and clinical significance of immaturity of kidney function in young infants. J. Pediat., 42:99, 1953.

Brines, J. K., Gibson, J. G., Jr., and Kunkel, P.: Blood volume in normal infants and children. J. Pediat., 18:447, 1941.

Chernoff, A. I.: The human hemoglobins in health and disease. New Eng. J. Med., 253:322, 365, 416, 1955.

Christie, A.: Prevalence and distribution of ossification centers in the newborn infant. Amer. J. Dis. Child., 77:355, 1949.

Clifford, S. H.: Postmaturity—with placental dysfunction. J. Pediat., 44:1, 1954.

Cotter, J., and Prystowsky, H.: Fetal blood studies. XX. Levels of human fetal hemoglobin during pregnancy. J. Obstet. Gynec., 23:735, 1964.

Cross, K. W.: Respiratory control in the neonatal period. Symp. Quant. Biol., 19:126, 1954.

Cross, K. W., and Malcolm, J. L.: Evidence of carotid body and sinus activity in newborn and fetal animals. J. Physiol., 118:10, 1952.

Dancis, J., Braverman, N., and Lind, J.: Plasma protein synthesis in the human fetus and placenta. J. Clin. Invest., 36:398, 1957.

Davis, M. E., and Potter, E. L.: Intrauterine respiration of the human fetus. J.A.M.A., 131:1194, 1946.

Fellers, F. X., Barnett, H. L., Hare, K., and McNamara, H.: Change in thiocyanate and sodium[24] spaces during growth. Pediatrics, 3:622, 1949.

Gitlin, D.: Protein metabolism, cell formation and immunity. Pediatrics, 34:198, 1964.

Gitlin, D., and Craig, J. M.: Nature of the hyaline membrane in asphyxia of the newborn. Pediatrics, 17:64, 1956.

Good, R. H.: Agammaglobulinemia; II. Experimental study. Amer. J. Dis. Child., 90:517, 1955.

Janeway, C., Rosen, F., Merler, E., and Alper, C.: The Gamma Globulins. Little, Brown and Co., Boston, 1966.

Kellogg, H. B.: Studies on the fetal circulation of mammals. Amer. J. Physiol., 91:637, 1930.

Lester, R., Behrman, R., and Lucey, J.: Transfer of Bilirubin-C[14] across monkey placenta. Pediatrics, 32:416, 1963.

Lind, J., and Wegelius, C.: Human fetal circulation: changes in the cardiovascular system at birth and disturbances in the postnatal closure of the foramen ovale and ductus arteriosus. Symp. Quant. Biol., 19:109, 1954.

Lubchenco, L. O., Hansman, C., Dressler, M., and Boyd, E.: Intrauterine growth as estimated from live-born birth-weight data at 24 to 42 weeks of gestation. Pediatrics, 32:793, 1963.

McCance, R. A., and Widdowson, E. M.: Normal renal function in the first two days of life. Arch. Dis. Child., 29:488, 1954.

Miller, J. F. A. P.: The thymus and the development of immunologic responsiveness: The thymus directs the maturation of immunologic capabilities by means of a humoral mechanism. Science, 44:1544, 1964.

Nyhan, W.: Amino Acid Metabolism. McGraw-Hill Book Co., New York, 1967, p. 494.

Oski, F., and Naiman, J. L.: Hematologic Problems in the Newborn. W. B. Saunders Co., Philadelphia, 1966, p. 14.

Pohlman, A. G.: Fetal circulation through the heart. Bull. Johns Hopkins Hosp., 18:409, 1907.

Potter, E. L.: State of the lungs at birth. J.A.M.A., 159:1341, 1955.

Potter, E. L., and Thierstein, S. T.: Glomerular development in the kidney as an index of fetal maturity. J. Pediat., 22:695, 1943.

Romney, S. L., Reid, D. E., Metcalfe, J., and Burwell, C. S.: Oxygen utilization by the human fetus in utero. Amer. J. Obstet. Gynec., 70:791, 1955.

Rosenfeld, M., and Snyder, F. F.: Stages of development of respiratory regulation and the changes occurring at birth. Amer. J. Physiol., 121:242, 1938.

Rudolph, A. M., Drorbaugh, J. E., Auld, P. A. M., Rudolph, A. J., Nadas, A. S., Smith, C. A., and Hubbell, J. P.: Studies on the circulation in the neonatal period; the circulation in the respiratory distress syndrome. Pediatrics, 27:551, 1961.

Silverman, W.: Problems of nutrition in the perinatal period. In Report of the 60th Ross Conference on Pediatric Research, Columbus, 1969, p. 53.

Silverstein, A. M.: Ontogeny of the immune response — the development of immunologic responses by the fetus. Science, 144:1423, 1964.

Smith, R. T., Eitzman, D. V., Catlin, M. E., Wirtz, E. O., and Miller, B. E.: The development of the immune response. Characterization of the response of the human infant and adult to immunization with Salmonella vaccines. Pediatrics, 33:163, 1964.

Stenger, V., Eitzman, D., Andersen, T., Cotter, J., and Prystowsky, H.: A study of the oxygenation of the fetus and newborn and its relation to that of the mother. Amer. J. Obstet. Gynec., 93:376, 1965.

Whitehead, W. H.: A working model of the crossing caval blood streams in the fetal right atrium. Anat. Rec., 82:277, 1942.

Wintrobe, M. M., and Shumacker, H. B., Jr.: Erythrocyte studies in the mammalian fetus and newborn. Amer. J. Anat., 58:313, 1936.

Chapter 32

Erythroblastosis Fetalis

In the three decades since discovery of the Rh blood groups there has been enormous expansion of our knowledge of the normal substances in human blood that can be polymorphic. Whereas prior to 1940 there were only three known blood group systems—ABO, MN, and P—we now know of at least 15 genetically independent systems of red cell antigens, listed in the first column of Table 1. The main body of this chapter deals exclusively with the red cell antigens, and mostly with Rh. The leukocyte antigens, listed in column 2 of Table 1, are of minor clinical importance except for transplantation. However, the antigens of the NA and NB systems have been known to cause neutropenia in the newborn. The polymorphisms of the serum and intracellular proteins have no known clinical importance, but, along with all the other polymorphisms, they are enormously important in anthropology, genetics, and legal medicine. For example, one can nearly always distinguish dizygous twins if the full battery of useful tests is done. For practical purposes, two unrelated people could always be distinguished, and so could babies interchanged in the nursery. False accusation of paternity can nearly always be disproved, and the actual demonstration of parentage is now a practical possibility from the theoretical viewpoint, though it involves a good deal of labor.

There are more than 250 known antigenic factors in the various blood group systems of

TABLE 1. USEFUL HUMAN BLOOD GROUP SYSTEMS, 1971

Surface Antigens on Red Cells	Antigens on Leukocytes	Serum Proteins	Intracellular Proteins
1. ABO	16. HL-A	24. Gm	34. Hemoglobin
2. MN	17. 5	25. Inv	35. Acid phosphatase
3. P	18. 9	26. Haptoglobin	36. G-6-PD
4. Rh	19. NA	27. Transferrin	37. 6-PGD
5. Lutheran	20. NB	28. Gc	38. Phosphoglucomutase
6. Kell	21. Zw	29. Ag	39. Adenylate kinase
7. Lewis	22. Pl	30. Lp	40. Adenosine deaminase
8. Duffy	23. Ko	31. Cholinesterase	
9. Kidd		32. C'3	
10. Diego		33. Xm	
11. Yt			
12. Xg			
13. Dombrock			
14. Stoltzfus			
15. Colton			

the erythrocytes. Most of these have, at one time or another, caused transfusion reactions or erythroblastosis fetalis. Increased knowledge about all of these blood factors and storage of frozen blood from rare donors have greatly improved our ability to deal with the rare as well as the common problems of blood transfusion. With the remarkable progress in management of Rh incompatibility in pregnancy, erythroblastosis fetalis is becoming a much less difficult problem, but it will never disappear. In view of the possibilities, every newborn must be considered a candidate for erythroblastosis fetalis. Fortunately, simple and effective procedures are available for diagnosis, and within 10 to 15 years' time death or brain damage due to erythroblastosis should become almost extinct.

Erythroblastosis fetalis is a fairly common disease. Before the days of modern prevention and treatment, about one birth in 150 resulted in erythroblastosis fetalis due to Rh incompatibility. About 20 per cent of these were stillbirths, and another 30 per cent of the infants died or suffered permanent brain damage.

ETIOLOGY

Erythroblastosis fetalis (also called hemolytic disease of the fetus and newborn) is caused by feto-maternal blood group incompatibility, with maternal immunization against fetal blood group antigen. By far the most important antigen is $D(Rh_o)$, which is responsible for almost all the cases of erythroblastotic stillbirth, and almost all the early neonatal deaths (first 24 hours) from erythroblastosis.

A small proportion (probably less than 2 per cent) of all cases of erythroblastosis are the result of incompatibility with respect to $c(hr')$, $E(rh'')$, K, $C^W(rh^W)$, $C(rh')$, k, M, S, and Jk^a (and other blood factors), in about that order of decreasing frequency. In most respects the disease is the same, regardless of which blood factor is involved.

It was assumed for some years that no more than 5 per cent of cases of erythroblastosis were caused by A and B incompatibility, but active search showed that the majority of such cases may go unrecognized because of failure to observe and

properly evaluate jaundice appearing before 36 hours of age in newborn babies, and because the Coombs test is often negative.

PATHOLOGIC PHYSIOLOGY

Much remains to be learned about the pathologic physiology of erythroblastosis fetalis. This discussion does not enumerate the various alternative theories that have been advanced but indicates the simplest explanations concordant with the known facts. Exactly how primary immunization of the "negative" woman occurs in pregnancy is not known. It is, however, believed that small amounts of blood pass from the fetus to the mother in many pregnancies (perhaps 50 per cent), although the amount is usually too small to cause sensitization. (Cohen et al., 1964). Larger amounts are believed to gain access to the maternal circulation at the time of delivery, and it is quite clear that the usual time of sensitization is post partum, rather than during pregnancy. Delivery by cesarean section is more dangerous in this respect than easy pelvic delivery according to Potter (Report of the Seventh M and R Pediatric Research Conference, 1954). Massive hemorrhage from fetus to mother is known to occur (Chown, 1955). It is probable that 10 to 15 per cent of D-negative women become sensitized, although there are no exact figures for women who have completed their families.

The amount of fetal blood that reaches the maternal circulation just after delivery of the fetus depends to some extent on whether the fetal blood has been allowed to drain from the placenta immediately after the cord is cut. If the placental end of the umbilical cord is left unclamped, the fetal blood rapidly drains out of the placenta as the uterus contracts. If it is not allowed to escape in this way, feto-placental blood vessels may be ruptured and fetal blood may gain access to the maternal circulation.

Rh antibodies pass from mother to fetus with ease, except that the so-called "saline agglutinins" (IgM) apparently do not. If the baby is D-positive, anti-D that has reached its circulation attaches itself to antigen on the red cell surface. Red cells are destroyed at a greater than normal rate, resulting in a shorter than normal average life span of fetal red cells. The rapidity of red cell destruction varies widely in different cases and depends, presumably, on the amount of antibody in the baby's circulation and perhaps the "type" of antibody (albumin-active, blocking, and so forth) on the one hand, and the vulnerability of the fetal red cells on the other. The vulnerability of red cells presumably depends on the amount of available antibody that can or will be taken up by them, on the resistance or lack of resistance of the cells to whatever causes their actual destruction, and possibly on variability of the destruction mechanism in different babies (Pickles, 1949). It is well known that there are wide differences in twins with respect to vulnerability. Another factor of importance is the presence or absence in the fetus of other sites of antigen. The group A fetus has large amounts of A in tissues other than red cells, serving without doubt to protect the red cells from the full effect of passively transferred anti-A. The absence of D antigen in tissues other than red cells is presumably of paramount importance in determining, in most cases caused by D incompatibility, a much more severe hemolytic process than is ordinarily seen in A or B incompatibility.

In response to the more or less abnormal blood destruction, the fetus usually makes new red cells more rapidly, expanding its hematopoietic system in many cases to extreme degrees, particularly in the liver. In most cases, an equilibrium compatible with otherwise essentially normal intrauterine existence, growth, and development is established, often at a hemoglobin level lower, but not much lower, than normal. By-products of red cell destruction appear to be disposed of satisfactorily in utero, in almost all cases, and the circulation through the placenta is very important in removing excessive amounts of bilirubin.

Some 20 per cent of those fetuses whose disease is caused by D incompatibility fail to make a satisfactory intrauterine adjustment, and die in utero unless delivered early or given intrauterine transfusions. Presumably anemia kills these babies, and probably congestive heart failure dominates the picture at the end in most of them, the massive pitting edema so frequently seen in stillborn babies being explained on this basis (Mollison and Cutbush, 1949).

A small percentage of erythroblastotic babies (almost exclusively cases caused by D incompatibility) are very sick at birth, with marked pallor, marked enlargement of spleen and liver, and frequently some obvious edema. These very sick babies are often limp and quite unresponsive, and frequently have grunting respirations. They almost invariably have an abnormally high venous pressure (normal is 4 to 7 cm. of blood measured vertically at the umbilicus with the baby recumbent; see Postnatal Management), as well as other signs of congestive heart failure, such as enlarged heart and pulmonary rales. Loud cardiac mumurs are frequently heard. If they are breathing regularly at birth, these babies usually respond dramatically to proper treatment and go on to complete recovery. Erythroblastotic babies who at birth have massive edema almost invariably fail to breathe regularly, and usually die, but some can be salvaged by a team effort that combines immediate and essentially simultaneous intubation, thoracentesis and abdominal paracentesis to remove excessive fluid, exchange transfusion, and considerable general support (warmth, oxygen, and so forth).

Aside from this small group of very sick babies, the only real postnatal problems in clinical management are anemia and jaundice. Anemia is actually a minor problem compared with the problem of jaundice. Most erythroblastotic babies who are born alive appear perfectly normal on casual inspection, and even detailed physical examination frequently reveals no abnormalities, although the spleen and liver can be palpated with ease in more than half the patients. Detectable jaundice is almost never present at the time of birth, owing in part to the fact that the serum bilirubin is usually not very high at that time. Some other mechanism, however, keeps the baby from being jaundiced at birth with a bilirubin level at which an older baby or adult would definitely be jaundiced. The umbilical cord is commonly slightly yellow, even when the amniotic fluid looks normal. The golden yellow vernix that is occasionally seen at birth in babies with erythroblastosis must not be mistaken for true jaundice of the skin, since, when it is wiped off, the skin is found to be free of jaundice. The important point to remember is that jaundice is *not to be expected* at the time of birth; therefore, its absence does not constitute a favorable prognostic sign.

Jaundice, although absent at birth, is by far the most important sign of erythroblastosis. Not all erythroblastotic babies become jaundiced but, almost without exception, if they ever do, the jaundice is apparent in the first 24 hours of life. The corollary is also true, that nearly all babies who show any jaundice in the first 24 hours of life have erythroblastosis fetalis, whether or not the mother is Rh-negative. Actually jaundice occurs in about 90 per cent of erythroblastotic babies and it is thus much more common than anemia, hepatospleno-megaly, or (especially) erythroblastemia. It is practically certain that bilirubin ("free"—not bound by albumin) is the actual cause of the brain damage (kernicterus) that occurs in about 15 per cent of cases of erythroblastosis without proper treatment. The degrees of hyperbili-rubinemia seen in erythroblastotic babies during the second, third, and fourth days of life are commonly much higher than are seen in any other clinical situation.

One of the factors that make for excessive bilirubinemia in erythroblastosis is common to most newborn babies. This is a functional inability to dispose of bilirubin during the first 36 to 48 hours of life (or the first three or four days in premature babies). The evidence indicates that new-born erythroblastotic babies differ in no way from normal babies in this functional disability, which has been shown to consist of failure to convert bilirubin to the soluble excretable bilirubin diglucu-ronide commonly known as "direct bili-rubin" (Billing and Lathe, 1956). This failure results from a deficiency in the enzyme glucuronyl transferase (Schmid et al., 1957), which may be inhibited in the newborn by hormones of maternal origin (Lathe and Walker, 1958). A second factor that causes hyperbilirubinemia is the rapid rate of blood destruction in erythro-blastosis. Whether the rate of destruction after birth differs from that in utero is not clear, but there is no evidence that it does. (Increasing anemia after birth may result solely from less rapid production of blood, the decrease in production being initiated at birth by the change from partial to complete oxygen saturation of the hemo-globin.) A third factor important in determining the degree of bilirubinemia is the number of red cells present in the baby. It is obvious that if other conditions are the same, the higher the red blood cell count the more bilirubin will be released in a given period of time. The rate of new red cell production may be a very important element in this connection. Reticulocyte counts as high as 70 per cent have been seen at birth, indicating extremely rapid production. These three factors, and possibly others, determine the rapidity with which bilirubin accumulates during the first few days of life in erythroblastotic babies. Before the days of exchange trans-fusions, the bilirubin frequently reached 30 mg. per 100 ml. or higher, and levels of 50 mg. per 100 ml. were not rare.

The bilirubin found in the serum of the erythroblastotic baby is usually, during the first two or three days at least, almost entirely "indirect" bilirubin. This constitutes another major difference between erythro-blastosis and many other conditions in which marked jaundice is seen. For example, in infants with complete atresia of the bile ducts, not only are bilirubin levels above 20 mg. per 100 ml. rare, but no more than half of this total is indirect bilirubin. In erythroblastosis, when the bilirubin rises above 20 mg. per 100 ml. during the first two days, signs of biliary obstruction may appear, with a rise in the direct bilirubin. This sometimes clears in a few days, but may last for many weeks, in which event the intense jaundice and pale stools may lead to the mistaken diagnosis of atresia of the bile ducts. In many of these babies surgical exploration of the bile ducts has been done; this is dangerous, and fruitless, too, since the condition clears up completely, with no permanent sequelae that have been detected.

Erythroblastemia, the sign from which the disease takes its name, has been much overrated. It is quite possible that the presence in the circulating blood of numerous nucleated red cells is an indication in some cases of acute anoxia occurring during or before labor. In response to such a situation, the erythroblastotic baby, whose liver, spleen, and other tissues are crowded with growing red cells, has enormous numbers of nucleated cells available, and 200,000 to 300,000 per cu. mm. may be found in the circulating blood.

KERNICTERUS

The most important complication of erythroblastosis fetalis is brain damage, manifested by nuclear jaundice and signs of cerebral injury. This is an acute affair, never present at birth and never observed in stillborn babies. It is rare in infants whose serum bilirubin does not exceed 20 mg. per 100 ml. In erythroblastosis, the rapid development of hyperbilirubinemia occurs in the first 24 to 96 hours of life, and if kernicterus develops, it is usually during this same period. Kernicterus has developed in half the cases in which serum bilirubin exceeded 30 mg. per 100 ml. The more rapid the development of hyperbilirubinemia, the more quickly the overt signs of brain damage appear. This may be during the latter part of the first day in exceptional cases, but most commonly the first signs are observed late in the second day of life or in the third.

Kernicterus is not limited to babies with erythroblastosis, but may occur in other jaundiced newborns, particularly prematures. Data accumulated in England indicate that kernicterus does not occur in "normal" prematures unless the indirect serum bilirubin is 18 mg. per 100 ml. or higher. A rare hereditary type of jaundice, caused by deficiency of glucuronyl transferase, was described by Crigler and Najjar (1952). Five of the six infants seen at their hospital developed kernicterus; all had serum bilirubin levels above 25 mg. per 100 ml. Another patient with this disorder developed kernicterus some years later (Rosenthal et al., 1956), indicating that there is no age at which high bilirubin levels are without danger. Furthermore, there is no proof that the state of maturity of the baby is, per se, an important factor in the risk of kernicterus; the increased incidence in premature erythroblastotic infants is due in part to their tendency to become more jaundiced. In erythroblastosis, rise of serum bilirubin is slowed when exchange transfusion is given. This means that kernicterus, if it occurs in such an infant, may develop at a later age than would have been the case without treatment. Worldwide experience has demonstrated that kernicterus is generally preventable with proper treatment, but single exchange transfusions often are insufficient. Two or more exchange transfusions must be given in some cases.

Forms of Bilirubin

Kernicterus is caused by unconjugated *free bilirubin* (not bound to albumin), which is very toxic, nearly insoluble in water, but lipid-soluble (Cowger et al., 1965; Diamond and Schmid, 1966; Odell, 1959).

Conjugated ("direct-reacting") *bilirubin diglucuronide* is water-soluble, excretable in bile and urine, and nontoxic. *Unconjugated bilirubin bound to albumin* ("indirect-reacting" bilirubin) also is water-soluble and nontoxic, but can give up molecules of free bilirubin. If the infant's albumin is saturated with bilirubin, or with bilirubin plus Gantrisin (or other substances such as Madribon and salicylate that are bound by the same sites on albumin molecules), such free bilirubin molecules cannot be picked up by other albumin molecules and may be picked up by lipid-rich membranes of nerve cells. If many of the infant's albumin molecules have free binding sites (normally each molecule of albumin can bind two molecules of bilirubin), free bilirubin molecules are almost sure to be picked up by them immediately, and the nerve cells are spared. The reserve binding capacity of albumin for bilirubin is thus of critical importance so far as the risk of kernicterus is concerned; its measurement and the use of this in treatment of jaundiced newborns are described in the section on Postnatal Management.

The neurologic signs that occur in babies with kernicterus are not pathognomonic of that condition. Diminution of activity, loss of interest in feedings, and vomiting are common early signs. Opisthotonos is the first definite sign in most cases. Very common in babies with kernicterus, and very uncommon otherwise, is a tendency to extension rigidity of the arms with closed fists and inward rotation of the forearms. This sign, in a very jaundiced newborn, is very nearly diagnostic. Most babies (about 70 per cent) with kernicterus die within 48 hours of the time of onset of signs of brain damage; they usually have irregular gasping respirations, bloody discharge from nose and mouth, and pulmonary rales for some hours before death. The course is extremely rapid in a small percentage of cases, the initial sign being a state of collapse and coma, with the pulmonary signs just mentioned, and death occurring within a few hours. Those babies with kernicterus who do not die during the first five or six days of life have permanent disability, largely motor, of a type called "athetoid cerebral palsy." Many have multiple cranial nerve palsies, deafness being common. Most of them have varying degrees of athetosis. Although the damage to the intellect is usually far less than the motor damage, the overall prognosis is poor. Many patients die during the first year or two; many remain hopeless cripples. Some make excellent adjustment to their motor disability, and others turn out to have no motor disability; it is these cases that keep the initial prognosis from being quite dismal.

Evidence is very strong that if no outward neurologic signs (especially opisthotonos or a tendency to opisthotonos) are observed in the first week of life the baby has not had brain damage. This is of great importance, because parents almost always know about the possibility of brain damage, and are very worried about it whether they say so or not. If the baby has been watched *closely*, and has appeared neurologically normal, the physician should confidently reassure the parents that no neurologic sequelae are to be expected. An observant nurse can be of the greatest assistance to the physician in the frequent appraisal of the infant that is essential during the first few days of life. It is our opinion that the physician has an obligation to the parents of erythroblastotic babies to do whatever is necessary to reassure himself and them that brain damage has not occurred. Otherwise, the parents are frequently doomed to years of unnecessary anxiety.

DIAGNOSIS

PHYSICAL SIGNS AT BIRTH. Many babies with erythroblastosis fetalis appear perfectly normal on physical examination at the time of birth, even though serious trouble may arise in the next few days. At the other extreme are the very sick ones, with pallor, edema, and enlargement of the abdomen, which may contain ascitic fluid, as well as great enlargement of the liver and spleen. As explained previously, these babies do not have jaundice of the skin, although the umbilical cord may be somewhat stained. Infants with such physical findings are very sick indeed and require exchange transfusion with the least

possible delay. Infants who have no obvious pallor or edema but who do have distinct enlargement of the liver and spleen fall into an intermediate group who may or may not require exchange transfusion.

LATER PHYSICAL SIGNS. Jaundice is by far the most common physical sign in erythroblastosis fetalis, occurring in at least 90 per cent of cases. The time of onset is very variable; the earlier its onset, the more urgent is the need for exchange transfusion.

LABORATORY TESTS. A positive direct Coombs test is the diagnostic criterion of greatest importance. The Coombs test is positive when the disease is caused by anti-D, anti-C, anti-C^W, anti-c, anti-E, anti-K, anti-Jk^a, and so forth. It is usually weak, and may be negative, when the disease is caused by anti-A or anti-B.

The Coombs test is so simple, reliable, inexpensive, and valuable, and erythroblastosis is so common and so important, that the direct Coombs test should be done on the blood of all newborn infants.

The hemoglobin concentration should always be determined on the cord blood sample of an infant with erythroblastosis fetalis. When the cord blood hemoglobin is low (less than 10 grams) it indicates severe illness needing prompt exchange transfusion. On the other hand, a baby whose hemoglobin is high at birth because he is making (and destroying) blood at a very high rate may have very serious difficulties because of increase of bilirubin (or late anemia). A reticulocyte count in such babies is a very good indication of the severity of the hemolytic process. A count of the nucleated red cells is hardly worth doing, but nucleated red cells are seen in some erythroblastotic babies, sometimes in very large numbers, this being the sign from which the disease originally took its name.

Serial repetition of the hemoglobin concentration during the first two or three days is neither necessary nor advisable, because the important criteria in management during these days are the serum bilirubin concentration and the reserve albumin binding capacity, which indicate the risk of brain damage and possible necessity of repeated exchange transfusions to control the bilirubin.

Diagnosis of erythroblastosis caused by anti-A or anti-B is less accurate than diagnosis of that caused by anti-D, because diagnostic criteria are less certain. If a baby is jaundiced before 24 hours, the

TABLE 2. MAJOR BLOOD GROUP
INCOMPATIBILITIES THAT MAY RESULT IN
ERYTHROBLASTOSIS FETALIS

TABLE 2. MAJOR BLOOD GROUP
INCOMPATIBILITIES THAT MAY RESULT IN
ERYTHROBLASTOSIS FETALIS

Baby	Mother
Group A or B	Group O
Group A or AB	Group B
Group B or AB	Group A

Erythroblastosis due to anti-A or anti-B in the infants of group B or group A mothers is comparatively much less frequent than in the A or B infants of O mothers, because O mothers are much more likely than A or B mothers to have IgG antibodies that can cross the placenta. Therefore, it is more important to look for other causes of early jaundice in babies born to A or B mothers.

Coombs test is weak or negative, an incompatibility in the ABO blood groups is demonstrable (Table 2), and there are no outstanding signs of other disease, the diagnosis is almost certain. If the serum bilirubin reaches 12 mg. per 100 ml. or higher during the first 36 hours of life, the diagnosis is even more secure. Diagnosis is important, because brain damage occurs in some of these babies if they are not treated properly.

PRENATAL MANAGEMENT OF ERYTHROBLASTOSIS FETALIS

Maternal Blood Tests

During her first pregnancy, every woman should have ABO and Rh grouping done on her blood, as well as a test of her serum for irregular antibodies that might have arisen from a previous transfusion or intramuscular injection of blood. These tests should be done at the time of the first prenatal visit, along with the serologic test for syphilis. If the woman is Rh-negative, the test of her serum for antibodies should be repeated at about the 28th and 35th gestation weeks. Routine prenatal testing for ABO erythroblastosis is contraindicated—it is useless and wasteful. In Table 3 is shown the checklist for prenatal management of erythroblastosis that is used at the Boston Hospital for Women, Lying-in Division.

Amniocentesis and the Analysis of Amniotic Fluid

The present acceptance of amniocentesis as a valuable aid in the management of erythroblastosis is due to the pioneering work of Bevis (1956) and Liley (1961, 1963a) and subsequent reports by many other investigators. Amniotic fluid examination is now a major tool in assessing the degree of disease in the fetuses of sensitized Rh-negative women.

Amniocentesis is indicated if there has been a previous stillbirth or seriously affected child, or if the maternal anti-Rh titer is in the range of 32 to 64 or higher by the indirect Coombs test. The limiting titer is that level below which intrauterine death is nonexistent or rare according to each

TABLE 3. ERYTHROBLASTOSIS FETALIS: PRENATAL CARE

I. Blood tests
  A. First pregnancy, first visit, all patients
    1. History of blood transfusion or blood injection
    2. ABO and Rh typing (repeat if done elsewhere)
    3. Antibody screening and identification
      a. If Rh-positive and no antibody, regular care
      b. If Rh-negative and no antibody, repeat antibody screening at 28th and 35th weeks
      c. If Rh-negative, do Rh typing and zygosity of husband
      d. If antibody present, special care
  B. Second or later pregnancy, first visit
    1. History of blood group incompatibility in a previous pregnancy, history of jaundice or anemia in a previous newborn
    2. ABO and Rh typing if not already done by you
    3. Antibody screening and identification
      a. If Rh-positive and no antibody, regular care
      b. If Rh-negative and no antibody, repeat antibody screening at 28th and 35th weeks
      c. If antibody present, special care

II. Special care for sensitized patients
  A. Repeat titer at one-month intervals until 34 weeks of gestation, then at one- to two-week intervals
  B. Amniocentesis, if indicated
  C. Intrauterine fetal transfusion, if indicated
  D. Premature delivery, if indicated

laboratory's experience. If the titer is 16 or lower, and the history is benign, amniocentesis is inadvisable because of the danger of causing a feto-maternal bleed that can stimulate a marked rise in anti-Rh titer, and because of the possibility of other less common mishaps. Complications of amniocentesis (fetal or maternal hemorrhage, premature labor, infection) are quite uncommon in expert hands. Avoidance of the placenta by its localization with ultrasound diminishes further the risk of feto-maternal bleed.

The gestational age at which amniocentesis is begun depends upon history and titer. If there has been a previous stillbirth, amniotic fluid examination should be started at 22 to 23 weeks. If there has been serious erythroblastosis in a previous child, but no stillbirths, 25 weeks would be suitable. In cases in which the history is benign and an originally low titer has increased to 32 or 64, amniocentesis is initiated immediately, if the fetus is beyond 25 weeks.

Amniocenteses are repeated at intervals determined by the result of the previous amniotic tap. In general, a pigment level in the upper middle zone of Liley's three-zone chart warrants repetition in one week; in the lower middle zone, two weeks; and in the bottom zone, three to four weeks.

Analysis of amniotic fluid involves measurement of absorption of light of various wavelengths in a recording spectrophotometer if available, or by making isolated observations at intervals of 10 mμ from a wavelength of 700 to 350. The most important part of the spectrum is from 525 to 375 mμ; when the fetus has erythroblastosis, the absorption curve has a hump (Fig. 1) in this region with its peak at 450 mμ, the height of the hump (the "pigment peak" or "ΔO.D.") being directly and closely related to the severity of illness of the fetus. In normal fetuses, in those with mild erythroblastosis, and in those whose intrauterine disease is not worsening, the ΔO.D. tends to become lower with advancing maturity (Liley, 1963a).

Specimens must be protected from direct sunlight, which quickly decolorizes the important bilirubin pigments (Liley, 1961). The amniotic fluid must be centrifuged immediately at high speed for 20 minutes until clear, and the supernatant is removed and filtered and analyzed as described above. Every laboratory testing amniotic

fluid should be prepared to do a Kleihauer-Betke (1957) stain procedure on any red blood cells in the sediment. If the cells are fetal in origin, a direct Coombs test and Rh typing can establish whether the fetus is Rh-positive or Rh-negative, a most important consideration when the father is an Rh-positive heterozygote. Also, if the cells are derived from an Rh-positive affected fetus, the amniotic fluid will also contain fetal plasma, whose high bilirubin content will produce a falsely high ΔO.D. Liley (1963a) estimates that 5 per cent of maternal blood is the upper limit of contamination of amniotic fluid for a reading that is still considered reliable. If the amniotic fluid contains more than a minimal number of fetal cells, the ΔO.D. will not be valid because of the contamination with fetal bilirubin. Other sources of error are excessive amounts of meconium or maternal hemoglobin.

The information obtained from examination of amniotic fluid guides the management of the pregnancy. A ΔO.D. in the bottom zone (Fig. 2) would warrant delivery at or very close to term, since one could anticipate an Rh-negative fetus or a very mildly affected Rh-positive one. Such findings are most important when there is a heterozygous husband, and one or more previous pregnancies have resulted in stillbirth. Consistently low ΔO.D.'s would point toward an Rh-negative fetus, and early delivery would be avoided. Prior to the days of amniocentesis, some such pregnancies were terminated very early, with all the attendant risks of prematurity. A ΔO.D. in the lower middle zone is usually an indication for induction of labor at 37 to 38 weeks of gestation, while a figure in the upper middle zone would call for possibly earlier induction, depending on the level and the rapidity of the rise in ΔO.D. In all cases of induction of labor the pediatrician and the blood bank should be prepared in advance for treatment of the child.

A ΔO.D. in Liley's top zone appearing before 33 to 34 weeks of gestation is an indication for intrauterine fetal transfusion, but if the high level occurs at 34 weeks or later, prompt delivery is in order. Liley's original middle zone has been widened by 10 per cent in an upward direction, thus making this criterion for intrauterine transfusion a little more stringent (Liggins, 1966). There are many other systems of analysis and interpretation of amniotic

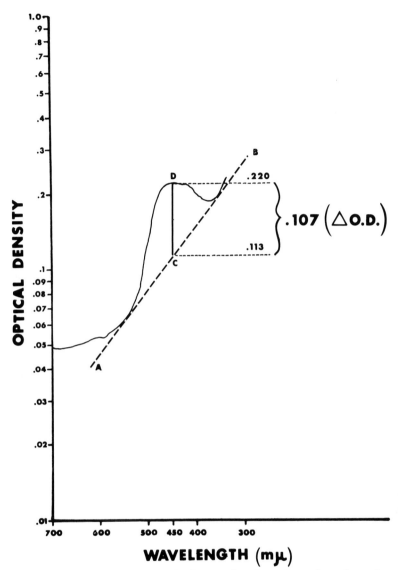

Figure 1. ΔO.D. as determined by Liley's method. Note that the ordinate has a logarithmic scale. Tangent (AB) to the spectral absorption curve of the amniotic fluid represents the expected linear curve in the absence of bilirubin pigments. Line DC represents the curve's deviation from linearity at 450 mμ caused by the bilirubin pigments in the amniotic fluid. Measurement of DC on the ordinate yields the "pigment peak" or ΔO. D.

fluid. The one outlined above, which follows Liley's system closely, is probably the one most commonly used around the world.

Intrauterine Transfusion

The recently developed technique of intrauterine fetal transfusion (Liley, 1963b) has succeeded in salvaging hundreds of fetuses that might otherwise have died in utero from severe erythroblastosis. When the amniotic fluid pigment peak (ΔO.D.) is

in the top zone (see Fig. 2), and death of the fetus seems probable, intrauterine transfusion (IU Tx) is indicated. This is particularly true if two successive amniotic taps show an increase in ΔO.D. and both are in the top zone. The criterion of at least one prior erythroblastotic stillbirth, which is sometimes used, seems unnecessary. Transfusion when the ΔO.D. is in the high middle zone is questionable unless the last level is very close to the upper zone and the upward slope is very steep. Generally it would be advisable to repeat such amniotic taps at brief intervals—one week, or even less

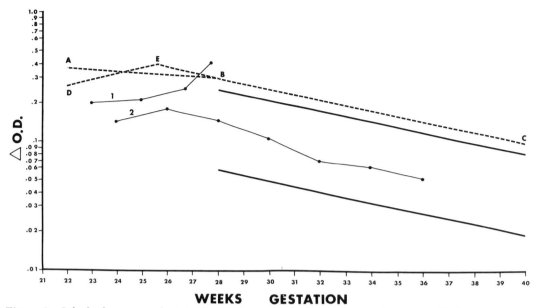

WEEKS   GESTATION

Figure 2. Liley's three-zone chart (with modifications) for interpretation of amniotic fluid ΔO.D.'s. Heavy lines represent Liley's original three zones. A ΔO.D. in the bottom zone is consistent with an unaffected or very mildly affected fetus. A ΔO.D. in the middle zone means the fetus is probably moderately affected, the degree of disease varying with the height of the ΔO.D. in the middle zone. A ΔO.D. in the top zone indicates severe erythroblastosis. Note that the original chart applies to gestational ages from 28 weeks to term.

Dashed line ABC represents Liggins' upward revision of the line between the middle and top zones (the "danger line") and its extension earlier than 28 weeks of gestation.

Dashed line DEC represents the simultaneous upward revision of the "danger line" by one of the present authors (Umansky).

Curves 1 and 2 show how two patients were followed with repeated amniotic taps. In patient 1, with ΔO.D.'s high in the middle zone, the fourth amniotic tap was done after an interval of one week. Based on the pattern of the four results, and with the fourth one in the top zone, intrauterine fetal transfusion was undertaken at 28 weeks of gestation. Patient 2 had amniocenteses at two-week intervals. All results were in the middle zone, indicating a moderately affected fetus, and labor was induced at 37 weeks of gestation.

—since borderline pigment levels sometimes turn downward and parallel the slope of the zones, and such pregnancies can be managed with early delivery.

Once the decision is made that intrauterine transfusion is indicated, there should be no delay. Prior to transfusion, an amniogram, performed by injecting about 20 ml. of Renografin* into the amniotic sac and then taking an anterior-posterior x-ray, will establish whether the fetus is grossly hydropic, with gross scalp and peripheral edema, in which case the situation would be practically hopeless, and intrauterine transfusion would not be advisable. The film may also demonstrate ascites (distended abdomen, extended legs) in the absence of gross generalized edema, a finding that points toward ascites preceding anasarca in the development of

hydrops. In such cases, intrauterine transfusion would be warranted, because an appreciable number of these fetuses have been salvaged. An additional yield of the amniogram is that it sometimes locates the placenta. If the fetus is not too sick to swallow amniotic fluid, the Renografin is concentrated in the fetal bowel after several hours, marking clearly the transfusion target, the fetal peritoneal cavity.

Most intrauterine fetal transfusions are performed according to Liley's original method, with a few minor variations. With the aid of x-rays, and fluoroscopy with an image intensifier (to keep radiation at minimum dosage), the fetal position and location are determined (biplane fluoroscopy would be ideal; Hanafee and Bashore, 1965), and if the fetal position is lateral or face up, one may proceed. If the fetus is face down, the procedure should be postponed until the position is more favorable.

---

*Renografin-60 (meglumine diatrizoate), Squibb.

A 15-gauge Tuohy needle is inserted through the mother's abdominal wall into the fetal peritoneal cavity, and its position is determined by injecting a minimal amount of Renografin or carbon dioxide (Hanafee and Bashore, 1965). If the needle is in the peritoneal cavity of the fetus, a soft plastic catheter* is inserted through the needle, with 1 or 2 feet excess of catheter coiled in the fetal peritoneal cavity (to be certain that fetal movement will not dislodge the catheter), and the needle is removed. To be absolutely certain of the location of the catheter, it should be filled with Renografin and its location verified by x-ray or fluoroscope.

Packed group O, Rh-negative blood, cross-matched against the mother's, is then pumped through the catheter into the abdominal cavity of the fetus over a period of about one hour. A dosage schedule that avoids circulatory overloading is 100 to 110 ml. at 30 gestation weeks plus or minus 10 ml. for each week later or earlier. Attempts to leave the catheter in place until the next transfusion frequently met with complications (Umansky, 1966), and so the catheter is generally withdrawn after each transfusion. About 65 per cent of the cells are absorbed into the circulation over a period of five to six days via the diaphragmatic lymphatics (Pritchard and Weisman, 1957). In the presence of ascites the absorption is less complete and slower (McKee and Stewart, 1957), but it does occur, and so the presence of ascites without anasarca should be no contraindication to treatment. Any ascitic fluid in the fetus is removed as completely as possible before the blood is infused.

Acceptable intervals for repeat transfusions are; about 10 days until the second, two and a half to three weeks until the third, and three weeks until the fourth. Rarely will more than four intrauterine transfusions be required; frequently fewer are required, depending upon the gestational age at which treatment is started. There has been almost universal lack of success when the treatment is started before 23 weeks, owing mostly to technical problems, but an appreciable number of successes when transfusion was begun at 23 to 24 weeks makes that a suitable time for a first trans-

fusion (Queenan, 1969). The later we are permitted by amniotic fluid results to start, the smaller the number of transfusions and the greater the success rate.

The transfusion procedure has serious risks and should be undertaken only by a qualified group who will be able to accumulate enough experience to develop sufficient expertise to minimize the risk and achieve a maximum of successful outcomes. The risk of fetal mortality has been variously estimated as 6.5 per cent (Lucey, 1966), to 17 per cent (Bowman and Friesen, 1964) per transfusion. Contrast material injected through the needle has been seen in the fetal spleen, bowel, bladder, kidney, pericardium, pleural cavity, and spinal canal, sometimes without any untoward effect; such unanticipated events have afforded a remarkable opportunity for the study of living fetal anatomy (Griscom et al., 1966). Additional complications include infection, rupture of membranes, bleeding, and premature delivery, frequently leading to fetal demise.

Serious infection, including gas gangrene and hepatitis (Queenan, 1969), and embolus in the mother (Barnes et al., 1965) have been reported. The overall rate of infections probably approaches 10 per cent (Queenan, 1969). Maternal bleeding has been reported to occur in 5 per cent (Queenan, 1969).

Other techniques for intrauterine fetal transfusion include: (1) hysterotomy and direct infusion of blood into the fetal peritoneal cavity (Adamsons et al., 1965); (2) hysterotomy and exchange transfusion via a fetal vessel, usually the femoral vein (Freda and Adamsons, 1964); and (3) cannulation of a fetal placental vessel, followed by exchange transfusion (Seelen et al., 1966). All of these procedures have been relatively unsuccessful because they carry a very high risk of precipitation of early premature labor, and they are not in general use.

Delivery of transfused fetuses is planned for an optimum time such that one can perform the minimum number of intrauterine transfusions required, and still avoid the hazards of extreme prematurity. A reasonable delivery time would be 36 weeks of gestation, but if fetal activity should diminish prior to that date, or if there are other signs indicating fetal distress, earlier delivery is warranted, even as early as 33 to 34 weeks. It is particularly urgent in such cases for the pediatrician and blood bank

---

*Sterile vinyl tubing, 36 inch, No. XRVX028, Becton, Dickinson & Co.

to be prepared for immediate treatment of the newborn child as required.

In addition to the usual cord hemoglobin and bilirubin tests, a Kleihauer smear should be done on all cord blood specimens to determine the percentage of fetal and adult cells in the infant's circulation. If the infant has had one or two intrauterine transfusions, there will be appreciable numbers of fetal cells in his circulation, and multiple exchange transfusions will most likely be required. After three or four intrauterine transfusions, the percentage of adult cells approaches and sometimes reaches, 100 per cent, and some of these infants can be managed without exchange transfusion. However, it is most important to follow such infants, and indeed all infants who have had intrauterine transfusions, very closely, with weekly hemoglobin and reticulocyte evaluations, because such babies frequently show a continuing drop in hemoglobin for about 8 to 10 weeks, at which time reticulocytosis generally begins. If the hemoglobin level falls below 6.5 or 7 grams before reticulocytosis begins, a booster transfusion is warranted, while in the presence of infection care must be taken not to permit the hemoglobin level to fall this low.

Data on the outcomes of intrauterine fetal transfusions have been reported by many individual centers, but there are two cooperative studies combining the results of 11 and 15 medical centers, respectively. The first study (Lucey, 1966) reported an overall salvage rate of 30.7 per cent of 238 transfused fetuses (13.6 per cent of 110 hydropic fetuses, and 45.3 per cent of 128 nonhydropic fetuses), while the second (Queenan, 1969) reported a salvage rate of 34 per cent of 607 fetuses. There is some overlap of the same patients in the two studies.

Criteria for fetal transfusion varied in the studies from ΔO.D.'s in Liley's upper middle zone to the top zone, with an occasional exception in the lower middle zone. It is apparent that the later in pregnancy fetal transfusion is initiated, the greater the salvage rate, while if at the time of the first transfusion the fetus shows signs of developing hydrops, the salvage rate is very low. There is much variation in different groups' criteria as to what constitutes fetal hydrops, but fetal scalp edema on the amniogram, or the removal of at least 25 ml. of fetal ascites at transfusion,

would be suitable criteria of hydrops, since they indicate that heart failure and accumulation of fluid have already begun.

When offering a prognosis to a prospective intrauterine fetal transfusion patient, one cannot use the total outcome results alone of any one center or of either cooperative study because of variable fetal condition in each individual case. A classification system has been recommended which groups patients by gestational age at the time of the first intrauterine transfusion, and also by whether or not the fetus was hydropic at the beginning of treatment with transfusion (Charles et al., 1967). Such a classification is valuable for prognostic purposes, and also for comparison of results of different centers.

With the accumulation of experience with intrauterine transfusions have come improvements in technique and in skill, resulting in an increase in the salvage rate up to 62 per cent in one center (Bowman et al., 1969). In centers with much experience (80 or more patients, for example), division of the data into two or more equal chronologic groups will make comparison with other centers more logical, and will yield more reasonable and reliable prognoses through use of the more recent data.

Induction of Labor

Early induction of labor has been practiced extensively, with the purpose of sparing the fetus further exposure to maternal antibodies.

Prematurity has well known hazards of its own, and prematurity carries an additional important risk in erythroblastotic babies, whose ability to conjugate bilirubin is even poorer in the first days after birth than in the mature infant. The possible benefit (decreased frequency of stillbirths) must be balanced against the known and very considerable natural variability of the disease and the risk of death from prematurity.

Beginning in 1954, at the Boston Lying-in Hospital, studies were made to evaluate the efficacy of early delivery in the prevention of stillbirth. Past experience had shown that in the group of patients with anti-Rh titer of 64 or greater and a history of erythroblastotic stillbirth, 60 per cent of the fetuses still alive in utero at 35 weeks' gestation were subsequently stillborn (Allen et al., 1954). In such a patient cesarean section is considered at 34 to 35 weeks' gestation if the baby is lively, and if the husband is believed to be homozygous for Rh. Some babies have survived, but mortality has been high. It is not certain that early delivery has reduced the mortality rate in this high-risk group. The possibility of intrauterine transfusion in these and even higher-risk babies has improved their outlook.

Since 1954 it has been routine policy to induce labor at 37 to 38 weeks' gestation when practicable, even when the maternal anti-Rh titer is low, the past history good, and the husband heterozygous. Induction, by rupture of the membranes, is done only when it is believed that labor will proceed quickly and easily. It is not done unless examination reveals that the baby is probably of the size and maturity indicated by the dates. Advantages to this procedure include better coordination of blood bank, laboratory, nursing, and medical facilities than when the time of birth is left to chance. More important is that rising titer and intrauterine death cannot occur at $39\frac{1}{2}$ weeks if the baby has been safely delivered at $37\frac{1}{2}$ weeks. It is now thoroughly established that the liberal use of exchange transfusion overcomes the increased hazard of kernicterus in immature babies. The results have been excellent. It is certain that some stillbirths have been prevented.

POSTNATAL MANAGEMENT OF ERYTHROBLASTOSIS FETALIS

EXCHANGE TRANSFUSION

Exchange transfusion, using "negative" blood, has reduced the gross case mortality in newborns to less than 5 per cent and practically eliminated kernicterus (Allen, 1965; Allen and Diamond, 1958). Almost the only babies who do not now recover completely are those who are edematous at birth and have respiratory difficulty. Exchange transfusion accomplishes two major aims that cannot be accomplished at present by other forms of treatment. The first of these is the amelioration of circulatory distress in the sickest babies. Anemia can be corrected at the same time that the blood volume is being lowered. Second is the prevention of severe hyperbilirubinemia.

The treatment of babies who seem to have congestive heart failure consists of removing, during the course of the exchange transfusion, more blood than is put in, so as to reduce the venous pressure to a normal level and keep it there. Venous pressure is measured frequently by using the plastic tubing which has been inserted into the umbilical vein as an open manometer tube, and holding a ruler vertically beside it, resting on the baby's abdomen just cephalad to the umbilicus. Normal venous pressure is usually less than 7 cm. of blood. Caution must be exercised in reducing the blood volume, since it is not difficult to overshoot the mark and produce oligemic shock, in which event the venous pressure (in the vena cava) may rise temporarily instead of continuing to fall. In these sick babies it is well also to exchange only small volumes of blood at a time (10 ml., perhaps, instead of the usual 20) to avoid as much as possible temporary circulatory overloads. The baby's heart rate should be monitored continuously during exchange transfusion.

Exchange transfusion prevents severe hyperbilirubinemia by removing the bulk of the infant's vulnerable red cells and substituting for them red cells that are compatible with the maternal antibodies. Using a volume of donor blood equal to twice the infant's blood volume results in about 85 per cent substitution. In a $7\frac{1}{2}$ lb. infant this would require about 600 ml. of blood. In actual practice, except in the case of very large babies, a single unit (500 to 600 ml.) of donor blood is used. A considerable amount of bilirubin is removed with the infant's blood, amounting to nearly a third of the total bilirubin in the body. Fresh albumin is supplied, which is able to bind bilirubin that is liberated as the result of subsequent hemolysis of newly formed red cells. Because of a number of possible factors, including some immediate hemolysis of donor red cells, less than optimal substitution of circulating red cells, and (probably most important) continued rapid production of new red cells, serum bilirubin may accumulate at a rapid rate in spite of the initial exchange transfusion. A second exchange transfusion again removes the bulk of the baby's own red cells and a substantial proportion of the bilirubin. Three, and sometimes even more, exchange transfusions have been beneficial in some cases. Bilirubin tests are done at frequent intervals, four times daily, if necessary, as a guide to prognosis and treatment. The measurement of reserve albumin binding capacity should become more and more important.

The technique of exchange transfusion is simple in principle, but there are many details of importance. The reader is referred to the description of the method used at the Boston Lying-in Hospital (Allen and Diamond, 1958). Two important improvements in technique in recent years are worthy of comment here. One is the use of plastic bags instead of glass bottles for donor blood. Since the plastic bag collapses as it empties, it can be placed with the outlet at the top (in a press, if desired; Rosenfield, 1959), so that any sedimenting red cells are allowed to collect until the end. This means that the last few syringefuls given to the baby are concentrated instead of relatively dilute blood. This is better in the average case than discarding some of the plasma in order to concentrate the donor red cells, since that reduces the total quantity of blood available for the exchange and thus reduces the efficiency of the exchange, as well as reducing considerably the amount of fresh albumin supplied to the infant. If glass blood bottles are used, the bottle may be placed on its side at the beginning of the transfusion, to allow the sedimenting cells to settle along the side of the bottle. As the transfusion nears completion, the bottle is gradually tilted to its normal position (Rosenfield, 1959). The second major improvement is the disposable exchange transfusion kit made by the Pharmaseal Corporation, which is supplied sterile, in individual packages. The umbilical vein tube has a smoothly rounded tip, which makes it very easy to introduce.

Indications for Exchange Transfusion

ANEMIA AT BIRTH. Exchange transfusion has two very different purposes. One is to prevent immediate death in erythroblastotic babies who are very anemic at birth. The other is to avoid brain damage by preventing or controlling hyperbilirubinemia when kernicterus seems to be more than a slight statistical possibility.

If the baby appears sick at birth (pallor, hepatosplenomegaly), exchange transfusion is done with the least possible delay. In the sickest infants a small exchange is often preferable to a more prolonged procedure using a larger quantity of blood.

PREVENTION OF BRAIN DAMAGE. The most common reason for doing exchange transfusion in babies with erythroblastosis fetalis is to prevent kernicterus, and with better understanding of the role of bilirubin, the criteria for exchange transfusion to prevent kernicterus will become more rational. It now appears that measurement of the reserve albumin binding capacity will provide a much more useful guide than the measurement of bilirubin alone. However, more experience with this test must be obtained before it will win widespread acceptance.

Reserve Albumin Binding Capacity

The method of measuring reserve albumin binding capacity that has been described by Porter and Waters (1966) depends on a color change in the dye hydroxy-benzine-azo-benzoic acid (HBABA) when it is bound by albumin. It is a simple and reproducible test, requiring only a small amount of serum. The method calls for the use of purified human albumin as the standard, which is a nuisance because it is expensive and difficult to procure. Johnson and Boggs (1966) demonstrated that pooled normal human serum could be used equally well as a standard, once it had been compared with purified albumin.

Porter and Waters (1966), in a limited series, found that when the reserve albumin binding capacity was at least 50 per cent of normal (based on the binding capacity of a 4 per cent solution of pure albumin) jaundiced infants escaped brain damage even when the serum indirect bilirubin concentration was as high as 30 mg. per 100 ml. Unfortunately there is no easy way of determining what the critical figure is because controlled experiments in humans cannot be so designed as to allow the development of kernicterus in an "untreated" group, and also because acidosis in the infant makes bilirubin less easily bound by albumin. Eventually, clinical experience will show what is reliable. The paper of Odell et al. (1970) should be consulted.

In the meantime, because kernicterus is preventable by exchange transfusions, and because the arbitrary figure of 20 mg. of bilirubin does still have some statistical validity, bilirubin levels should be followed closely, and repeat exchange transfusions should still be done to control high and increasing bilirubin concentrations. Initial exchange transfusions are undoubtedly still of great value in preventing kernicterus in the high-risk group of infants whose mothers have very high anti-Rh titers, who have evidence of severe hemolytic process, or whose older siblings had kernicterus. It is hoped that fewer babies will have to receive more than two exchange transfusions, and it is even more to be hoped that a method may be discovered of quickly activating the baby's own mechanisms for conjugation and excretion of bilirubin.

Criteria of No Value

1. Serial hemoglobin determinations are not only without value as indications for or against exchange transfusion, but their use is actually dangerous. Even in severe erythroblastosis, there is seldom any very great change in hemoglobin concentration attributable to the disease process in the critical first two days of life. Actually, in many infants with severe hemolytic process the hemoglobin level not only does not fall during the first two days of life, but remains high, and these infants are in special danger of developing kernicterus. To wait for falling hemoglobin as an indication for exchange transfusion in erythroblastosis is a grievous error. The initial hemoglobin test is important, of course, and it is essential to follow the hemoglobin concentration in the second, third, and fourth weeks of life in erythroblastotic babies not treated by exchange transfusion.

2. A positive Coombs test is not an indication for exchange transfusion, but is only a diagnostic test. Many infants with a positive Coombs test, although they do have erythroblastosis fetalis, do not require exchange transfusion. On the other hand, some with a negative Coombs test (as, for example, cases of erythroblastosis due to ABO incompatibility) do require transfusion to prevent kernicterus. It should be remembered, too, that the Coombs test is an essential diagnostic procedure in erythroblastosis. In a fair number of cases of Rh sensitization the infant, although genetically Rh-positive, is typed at birth as Rh-negative owing to the "blocking" of the Rh antigen sites on its red cells by maternal Rh blocking antibody. In such cases the Coombs test is positive, and it indicates the true state of affairs. This is most important in those cases of severe erythroblastosis in which there are no hematologic or physical signs of disease at birth.

Selection of Blood for Exchange Transfusion

Ideally, blood used for exchange transfusion should lack all antigens to which the mother is sensitized in order that it will survive normally in the infant's circulation and not contribute to bilirubinemia. To ensure such compatibility, donor blood must be cross-matched with the serum of the mother. This is best done before the baby is born, to avoid a last minute rush in selecting compatible blood. One of the advantages of induction of labor in these cases is that it allows time for the compatibility test to be completed before delivery. Freshness of the blood (5 days old or less) is also important, since one expects less immediate hemolysis with fresh blood and thus less contribution to bilirubinemia. Also, the fresher the blood, the higher the pH and the lower the potassium concentration. Ideally, ACD blood should not be used, because of its relatively low pH and high potassium concentration; heparinized blood should be used instead. If heparinized blood is used, a donor must be bled specially, which is easier to do if the time of the birth is planned in advance. Heparinized blood should be used within 24 hours.

In rare cases it may be impossible to have compatible blood (by the above criteria) on hand when needed. The mother's own blood is always compatible, though it is desirable to remove her plasma and substitute plasma from a normal donor of appropriate ABO group. If the mother cannot be bled, incompatible donors may have to be used. Fortunately, it is known from the work of Hubinont (1955) that kernicterus is preventable by exchange transfusion of incompatible blood, although larger quantities of blood are necessary, and more repeat transfusions may be needed. But even when the donor blood is incompatible by all criteria, one should not hesitate to use it, if no better alternative is available, when the infant is in real danger of kernicterus (Allen, 1965).

The above discussion on possible use of incompatible blood is not intended to relieve anyone of the responsibility of obtaining compatible blood if possible, or of detecting the presence of maternal antibodies potentially harmful to the fetus in the blood of all pregnant women, Rh-negative or Rh-positive. When antibodies are detected in advance of the baby's birth it is nearly always possible to obtain compatible blood in advance. Incidentally, the mother herself may need the blood more than does the baby, because it is not possible to transfuse the mother safely with incompatible blood.

Albumin in Treatment

Odell et al. (1962) have shown that albumin given before exchange transfusion (1 gram of salt-poor albumin per kilogram of body weight, as the 25 per cent solution, one hour before transfusion) results in the mobilization and removal of much more bilirubin. Porter and Waters (1966) added albumin to the blood used for exchange transfusion (12.5 grams of salt-poor albumin −50 ml. of a 25 per cent solution). The ultimate value of albumin in treatment is still to be determined. It can hardly replace exchange transfusion, but it does undoubtedly have value.

Albumin should not be given to an edematous newborn, or to one on the verge of heart failure. In fact, its use at or within a few hours of birth has questionable value.

Small Transfusions for Late Anemia

In erythroblastotic babies who have not been treated by exchange transfusion, and in a few who have been so treated, a very severe state of anemia develops during the second, third, or fourth week of life. Most of these undoubtedly are infants who have significant amounts of circulating antibody that attacks new cells as fast as they are produced and maintains the hemolytic process. Simple infusions of compatible blood to maintain the hemoglobin level above 7 grams per 100 ml. are all that is necessary. The hemoglobin concentration must be tested occasionally during this important period.

PHOTOTHERAPY OF JAUNDICE

It was first called to our attention by Cremer, Perryman, and Richards, of London, that exposure to light was to some extent effective in reducing jaundice and bilirubinemia. Experts from all over the world gathered in Chicago in 1969 to discuss phototherapy (Behrman and Hsia, 1969). It was pointed out that although the use of light does reduce the circulating bilirubin, it also may break down albumin molecules, and that there has been no proof of a diminution in brain damage from this treatment. It was also pointed out that prolonged phototherapy could have long-term side effects of an undesirable nature, and that phototherapy should not be given unless it is quite clear that the probable advantages outweigh the possible dangers. They recommend 300 to 600 mμ light, 200 to 400 foot-candles, from "daylight" fluorescent bulbs. Informed consent was considered necessary, as for a new drug. Phototherapy should not be used prophylactically for preventing hyperbilirubinemia. The eyes must be carefully protected from light as well as from possible abrasion of the cornea. More research is needed in this area.

Callahan et al. (1970) subsequently showed that light produced in-vivo conversion of bilirubin to substances that were rapidly excreted in the stool and urine of two human infants. This confirms previous in-vitro work. It seems very probable that phototherapy will eventually become one of the standard supplementary methods of dealing with the problem of neonatal jaundice of various causes, including erythroblastosis fetalis.

PHENOBARBITAL IN NEONATAL JAUNDICE

It has been demonstrated that the daily administration of 100 mg. of phenobarbital to pregnant women during the last five to six weeks of pregnancy results in lower cord blood serum bilirubin levels in the newborn, and in continued lower serum bilirubin levels during the first days of life in the treated group, as compared with a group to whom phenobarbital was not given (Bergsma and Hsia, 1970). It was also shown that the administration of phenobarbital to newborn infants in doses of approximately 8 mg. per kilogram per day results in substantially lower serum bilirubin levels and earlier clearing of bilirubin from the serum. Animal experiments seem to indicate also a greater excretion of bilirubin in the bile. The effect of phenobarbital is apparently, in part, to help activate the UDPGT (uridine disphosphoglucuronyl transferase) enzyme system in the liver, but all the effects of the drug are not known.

Were it not for the other available methods of dealing with neonatal jaundice, these findings would be even more exciting than they are. As it is, so many doubts have been expressed about the advisability of giving phenobarbital to newborn infants that this therapy seems not to be popular at the present time. It is conceivable, however, that the long-term effects of phenobarbital might be more acceptable than the long-term effects of phototherapy.

AGAR IN NEONATAL JAUNDICE

It has been suspected by a few for many years that a pool of bilirubin in the intestinal tract, from which bilirubin could be reabsorbed into the circulation, is partly responsible for neonatal jaundice. The most recent experimental work in this field, by Poland and Odell (1971), shows that feeding of agar, in the formula, to newborn infants during the first day of life resulted in a greater excretion of bilirubin, and lower serum bilirubin levels. The agar apparently protects the bilirubin from degradation by bacteria and subsequent reabsorption until it can be excreted in the stool. Such a maneuver should be helpful, when the details have been worked out, in significantly reducing the total quantity of bilirubin with which the newborn must contend, and this should help not only infants with erythroblastosis fetalis but others as well.

PREVENTION OF Rh SENSITIZATION

The great majority of cases of Rh sensitization occur as the result of pregnancy, and about 10 to 15 per cent of Rh-negative women become sensitized as a result of one or more pregnancies. It is well known that, like the kidney, the placenta is not impervious to red cells. Fetal red cells have been shown to cross the placenta during many pregnancies (Clayton et al., 1966), but generally not in sufficient number to produce a primary immune response. There is also the possibility that the pregnant woman might be less responsive to antigenic stimuli during pregnancy, which might account for the rarity of Rh sensitization during the course of a first pregnancy.

It is during the delivery process that fetomaternal bleeds large enough to produce Rh sensitization may occur. The size of such bleeds can be measured quite accurately by preparing a Kleihauer smear of the mother's blood drawn after delivery. The Kleihauer acid elution and staining technique clearly distinguishes between fetal and adult cells, and an actual count can be made of the number of fetal cells in the maternal circulation (Kleihauer et al., 1957). Adult cells show up as ghosts while fetal cells remain pink. According to Woodrow of Liverpool, a dose of less than 0.25 ml. of fetal Rh-positive cells can immunize some mothers (Woodrow et al., 1965). The greater the feto-maternal bleed, the greater the probability of maternal sensitization (Woodrow, 1970).

In 1961, Freda, Gorman, and Pollack, at Columbia University, began an investigation into the possibility of the prevention of Rh sensitization. The program was based on a principle established in 1909 by Theobald Smith that, in the presence of an excess of antibody, the corresponding antigen would not produce an immune response. They hoped that by giving recently delivered mothers an intramuscular injection of concentrated anti-D, the production of anti-D by the mother might be prevented. Following a lengthy but successful series of preliminary tests on male volunteers (Freda et al., 1964), a clinical trial in women was undertaken in 43 centers around the world. The most recent figures were reported by Dr. Gorman at the World Health Organization Conference on Rh immune globulin held in London in March, 1970. In first pregnancies, among women treated with immune globulin, 6 of 3389 women (0.2 per cent) became sensitized, while among the untreated controls 102 of 1476 (6.9 per cent) became sensitized. This was a most remarkable achievement, but the critical test was to see what happened in subsequent pregnancies. In second pregnancies, 5 of 390 treated patients (1.3 per cent) became sensitized, while among the untreated controls 23 of 155 patients (12.9 per cent) became sensitized. Although these second pregnancy numbers are relatively small, they do point toward an interesting trend: 1.3 being approximately

10 per cent of 12.9, it is apparent that, even with treatment, about 10 per cent of women who might otherwise have become sensitized, if untreated, are still producing anti-Rh. Or we might say that, in this study, Rh immune globulin decreased the frequency of sensitization by 90 per cent, an advance of most vital importance in the erythroblastosis problem. It must be emphasized again that these second pregnancy numbers are relatively small, and with time the full effect of Rh immune globulin will be determined.

It should be added that at the same time that the Columbia University group began its studies, Finn, Woodrow, and Clarke in Liverpool began a similar investigation, eventually reaching the same conclusions (Woodrow et al., 1965). Their studies were based on the observation that in the presence of ABO incompatibility between mother and child, the frequency of Rh sensitization is diminished (Levine, 1958). Reasoning that the maternal anti-A and anti-B destroyed the fetal group A or group B Rh-positive cells before a maternal response to Rh could occur, they concluded that passive immunization with anti-Rh from highly sensitized women should also destroy the Rh-positive fetal cells before they elicited a primary immune response. Rh immune globulin is produced from plasma obtained from highly sensitized men or women. The plasma is pooled and fractionated, and it is the Cohn fraction II that contains the highly concentrated IgG anti-Rh. This fraction is free of the hepatitis virus (Freda et al., 1967), a most important consideration. The antibody concentrate is distributed in 1 ml. doses containing approximately 300 mcg. of anti-D, and is to be given intramuscularly, within 72 hours after delivery, to women who meet the following criteria:

1. The mother must be Rh-negative
2. The mother must have no anti-Rh antibodies in her serum at the time of delivery (we would not regard this as a proper criterion, without qualification)
3. The baby must be Rh-positive
4. The direct Coombs test on the cord blood should be negative or, if it is positive, the cause should not be anti-D.

If all these criteria are met, a 1:1000 dilution of the immune globulin is cross-matched with the mother's cells to ensure compatibility, and 1 ml. of immune globulin is given intramuscularly within 72 hours after delivery. The 72 hour period is specified only because the clinical trial had a time limit of 72 hours and the success of Rh immune globulin has been demonstrated for that period of time. No one knows how much later than 72 hours Rh immune globulin will be fully effective, but it is suspected that administration within several days after the first 72 hours would still accomplish its purpose. Therefore, if for any reason there has been a delay of more than three days, it is probably still worthwhile to give Rh immune globulin in an attempt to prevent sensitization.

Bowman reported on 14 Rh-positive volunteers in the Winnipeg, Canada, Rh Laboratory who were given a 1 ml. dose of 300 mcg. of anti-D (World Health Organization Conference, 1970). Daily hematocrit, hemoglobin, reticulocyte, and bilirubin evaluations for 23 days showed no change, and apparently there was no harm when Rh immune globulin was given to these Rh-positive persons.

Cord blood specimens and postpartum maternal blood specimens should be drawn whenever the woman is Rh-negative. If the mother is already sensitized, the cord blood is used for Rh typing and the direct Coombs test to establish the diagnosis of erythroblastosis, and the maternal blood is used for cross-matching if exchange transfusion should be required. If the mother is not sensitized, the specimens are used for the tests previously outlined, to determine eligibility for Rh immune globulin.

The question has frequently been asked whether Rh immune globulin should be given to Rh-negative women after abortion. It has long been recognized that abortion can cause sensitization, but there was no information about the frequency of this occurrence. Recent studies in the United States and abroad have shown that fetomaternal bleeds, sufficient to sensitize, do occur with abortion (Freda et al., 1969). Such bleeds are greater after induced abortion than after spontaneous abortion (Matthews and Matthews, 1969), and they are also greater after a gestational age of 12 weeks than before 12 weeks (Voigt and Britt, 1969).

As to the actual frequency of Rh sensitization following abortion, at the World Health Organization meeting, Gorman of Columbia University reported a frequency of 4.3 per cent, and Vujaklija of Yugoslavia reported a frequency of 3.8 per cent (World

Health Organization Conference, 1970). Since that time, Galen (1970) of New York Presbyterian Hospital reported a frequency of 3.3 per cent. It appears that Rh sensitization caused by abortion occurs a little more than half as often as it does after completed pregnancies. It is therefore concluded that in order to do a thorough job of preventing sensitization, all Rh-negative women who have abortions should be given Rh immune globulin. The only exceptions would be those cases in which the father is also Rh-negative.

Another problem is how to deal with large feto-maternal bleeds, too large for a single dose of Rh immune globulin to control. A bleed of 50 to 60 ml. may be detected by an expert technician in the cross-match. The Kleihauer smear can easily detect bleeds of any size. Closely related to this is the question whether sensitization can be prevented after erroneous transfusion of Rh-positive blood into a young Rh-negative woman. A pooling of results of trial-and-error amounts of Rh immune globulin used in large feto-maternal bleeds and in incorrect transfusions, gathered from the United States, England, France, Holland, Canada, and Finland (World Health Organization Conference, 1970), indicates that about 10 mcg. of anti-D covers 1 ml. of Rh-positive blood. Thus, if there is a feto-maternal bleed of about 80 to 90 ml. an appropriate dose of Rh immune globulin would be 3 ml. which would contain 900 mcg. of anti-D. A single-unit transfusion of Rh-positive blood would require 17 ml. of Rh immune globulin. Such quantities have already been used successfully in preventing sensitization after a full-unit transfusion, and further studies are in progress to help establish doses of Rh immune globulin suitable for large feto-maternal bleeds.

PROGNOSIS IN ERYTHROBLASTOSIS FETALIS

Rh-negative women who have had a baby with erythroblastosis fetalis caused by anti-D wish to know what their chances are in a subsequent pregnancy, and many will base their decisions whether or not to try again on what the physician tells them. Because of the natural variability of the disease, the physician must adopt an attitude somewhere between complete pessimism and unbridled optimism. A few statements can be made that will be of value in considering individual cases. First, the mating of a heterozygous D-positive man with a D-negative woman produces D-negative and D-positive fetuses in equal numbers, this having been ascertained by actual counts. Therefore, if the husband is heterozygous for D, the chance of having a normal D-negative child in any particular pregnancy is exactly 50 per cent. It should be assumed, of course, that subsequent D-positive babies will have erythroblastosis, even though nothing should be assumed about the severity. The second useful fact is that there is a strong tendency to repetition, in any given family, of the degree of severity of the disease. If the erythroblastosis is mild in the first instance, subsequent babies are likely not to be seriously affected. If the first is stillborn, the chances are about 80 per cent that a subsequent D-positive baby will be stillborn.

A widely held opinion is that erythroblastosis is more and more severe in successive babies in a family. This is true only to a limited extent. The average severity of the disease in subsequent affected infants is greater than in the first affected baby (which is most commonly the second D-positive baby). The average severity of disease is very little greater, however, in third and subsequent affected babies than it is in the second affected baby. This is believed to indicate that most women attain their maximal sensitization during the second affected pregnancy. Somewhat less striking than the tendency to repetition is the variability that depends partly on fetal factors. Successive stillbirths (up to five or more) may be followed by the live birth of an infant who is not severely affected, and vice versa. Stillbirths constitute only about 5 per cent of first affected pregnancies, but about 20 per cent of all affected pregnancies (Vaughan et al., 1950).

The prognosis is much better in the case of erythroblastosis caused by anti-A or anti-B, since stillbirths do not occur and babies are almost never severely ill when born. (See preceding paragraphs, however, regarding the danger of kernicterus in this group.) Furthermore, in contrast to the case in Rh incompatibility, the husband is usually heterozygous for the offending antigen.

The prognosis in cases in which the D-negative mother has been sensitized to D by transfusion is different from that in cases in which sensitization resulted from an incompatible pregnancy. The prognosis is worse in the first incompatible pregnancy, since maximal sensitization will often have been attained during or prior to that time. The first D-positive baby is affected, and is not infrequently stillborn, which is quite uncommon in women who have not previously received blood intravenously or intramuscularly. The prognosis for *subsequent pregnancies*, however, is generally better for women who were sensitized by transfusion than for women who were sensitized by pregnancy *and who have had a baby with erythroblastosis*. This depends in large part on the fact that the husbands of women sensitized by transfusion may be D-negative, and those who are D-positive are usually heterozygous for D, whereas husbands of women sensitized by pregnancy are usually homozygous for D. The frequency of D-negative children is thus much higher in women sensitized by transfusion than in those sensitized by pregnancies. The fact that successive mildly affected babies are seen not infrequently in women sensitized by transfusion suggests that some of these women are relatively poor producers of Rh antibodies and might never have become sensitized by pregnancies alone.

Finally, there is an important relation of ABO blood groups to prognosis, first demonstrated by Levine (1943), that concerns not women who have already become sensitized but couples (woman D-negative, man D-positive) who have not yet started their families. If the husband is incompatible with his wife (could not be a blood donor to her) with respect to the ABO factors, she is much less likely to become sensitized to D by pregnancies. Table 4 gives the approximate risks in various matings. The figures are based on an estimated risk of 5 per cent for this entire group. This is undoubtedly a low estimate; it is likely nearer 10 per cent.

Artificial insemination is a possible solution in cases in which high titer and previous stillbirths make the chances of a successful outcome to another pregnancy otherwise small. By proper selection of the donor one can choose exactly what blood group genes the child may receive from the donor. It is important to match the donor, the woman, and the husband in such a way that the woman is not exposed to any new blood group antigens unnecessarily. It must be shown that she is not already sensitized to other antigens that the donor may have on his red cells. It is important also to arrange that there be no more differences than necessary between the type of the donor and that of the husband. Complete typings, for MNS, Kell, Duffy, and so forth, are worthwhile, and can be done at a number of centers. There should seldom be any difficulty in finding a suitable donor.

Sterilization of the sensitized Rh-negative woman is probably not indicated simply on the basis of high titer or previous erythroblastotic stillbirths, or both. There is seldom any significant risk to the woman beyond that incurred in any other pregnancy, and the prognosis for subsequent children is never hopeless, even without treatment. There is always the hope, too, that one can ameliorate the intrauterine disease. If such a woman becomes pregnant unintentionally, she should be told that there is a definite chance of a live-born baby that can be saved by exchange transfusion, and should be given whatever other encouragement is possible.

CONCLUSION

Although there is still much to be learned about erythroblastosis fetalis and the blood groups, there are already satisfactory practical solutions to all the clinical problems except that of repeated erythroblastotic stillbirth, and that problem too may well be capable of solution. Exchange transfusion has proved itself a marvelously effective

TABLE 4.   CHANCES OF EVENTUAL SENSITIZATION TO D, BY PREGNANCY ALONE, IN THE D-NEGATIVE WIVES OF D-POSITIVE MEN

"Zygosity" for D	A-B-O Compatibility of Husband		Total (or Unknown)
	Incompatible	Compatible	
Heterozygous	1%	3%	2%
Homozygous	4–5%	11%	9%
Total (or unknown)	2–3%	7–8%	5%

treatment for erythroblastosis, especially in the prevention of kernicterus. It is possible, however, that still better methods, in all phases of diagnosis and treatment, may be developed. Success in prevention of sensitization to Rh has exceeded early expectations, and should eventually approach 100 per cent effectiveness. There is need for some simplification, if possible, in this most esoteric field.

BIBLIOGRAPHY

Adamsons, K., Jr., Freda, V. J., James, L. S., and Towell, M. E.: Prenatal treatment of erythroblastosis fetalis following hysterotomy. Pediatrics, 35:848, 1965.

Allen, F. H., Jr.: Prevention of kernicterus. Use of incompatible blood for exchange transfusion in emergencies. Jewish Memorial Hosp. Bull., 10:86, 1965.

Allen, F. H., Jr., and Diamond, L. K.: Erythroblastosis Fetalis. Little, Brown and Co., Boston, 1958.

Allen, F. H., Jr., Diamond, L. K., and Jones, A. R.: Erythroblastosis fetalis; the problems of stillbirth. New Eng. J. Med., 251:453, 1954.

Barnes, P. H., McInnis, C., Friesen, R. F., and Bowman, J. M.: Maternal mishap following fetal transfusion. Canad. Med. Ass. J., 92:1277, 1965.

Behrman, R. E., and Hsia, D. Y. Y.: Summary of a symposium on phototherapy for hyperbilirubinemia. J. Pediat., 75:718, 1969. (Contains a review of bilirubin metabolism.)

Bergsma, D., and Hsia, D. Y. Y., eds.: Bilirubin metabolism in the newborn. National Foundation Birth Defects Original Article Series, Vol. 6, No. 2. Williams and Wilkins, Baltimore, 1970. (This conference report gives a historical review and papers on bilirubin metabolism, albumin binding, use of phenobarbitol, and phototherapy—summarized in Behrman and Hsia, 1969.)

Bevis, D. C. A.: Blood pigments in hemolytic disease of the newborn. J. Obstet. Gynaec. Brit. Emp., 63: 68, 1956.

Billing, B. H., and Lathe, G. H.: Excretion of bilirubin as an ester glucuronide, giving direct van den Bergh reaction. Biochem. J., 63:6P, 1956.

Bowman, J. M., and Friesen, R. F.: Multiple intraperitoneal transfusions of the fetus in erythroblastosis fetalis. New Eng. J. Med., 271:703, 1964.

Bowman, J. M., Friesen, R. F., Bowman, W. D., McInnis, A. C., Barnes, P. H., and Grewar, D.: Fetal transfusion in severe Rh isoimmunization. J.A.M.A., 207:1101, 1969.

Callahan, E. W., Thaler, M., Karon, M., Bauer, K., and Schmid, R.: Phototherapy of severe unconjugated hyperbilirubinemia: formation and removal of labelled bilirubin derivatives. Pediatrics, 46:841, 1970.

Charles, A. G., Alpern, W. M., and Friedman, E. A.: Rhesus-disease classification. Lancet, 1:392, 1967.

Chown, B.: The fetus can bleed. Amer. J. Obstet. Gynec., 70:1298, 1955.

Clayton, E. M., Jr., Feldhaus, W., Phythyon, J. M., and Whitacre, F. E.: Transplacental passage of fetal erythrocytes during pregnancy. Obstet. Gynec., 28: 194, 1966.

Cohen, F., Zuelzer, W. W., Gustafson, D. C., and Evans, M. M.: Mechanisms of isoimmunization. I. The transplacental passage of fetal erythrocytes in homospecific pregnancies. Blood, 23:621, 1964.

Cowger, M. L., Igo, R. P., and Lobbe, R. F.: The mechanism of bilirubin toxicity studied with purified respiratory enzyme and tissue culture systems. Biochemistry, 4:2763, 1965.

Crigler, J. F., and Najjar, V. A.: Congenital familial nonhemolytic jaundice with kernicterus. Pediatrics, 10:169, 1952.

Diamond, I., and Schmid, R.: Experimental bilirubin encephalopathy. The mode of entry of bilirubin-14C into the central nervous system. J. Clin. Invest., 45:678, 1966.

Freda, V. J., and Adamsons, K., Jr.: Exchange transfusion in utero. Report of a case. Amer. J. Obstet. Gynec. 89:817, 1964.

Freda, V. J., Gorman, J. G., Galen, R. S., and Treacy, N.: The threat of Rh immunization from abortion. Lancet, 1:694, 1969.

Freda, V. J., Gorman, J. G., and Pollack, W.: Successful prevention of experimental Rh sensitization in man with an anti-Rh gamma₂-globulin antibody preparation: a preliminary report. Transfusion, 4:26, 1964.

Freda, V. J., Gorman, J. G., and Pollack, W.: Suppression of the primary Rh immune response with passive IgG immunoglobulin. New Eng. J. Med., 277: 1022, 1967.

Galen, R. S.: Does abortion raise the risk of Rh sensitization? Med. World News, July 10, 1970.

Griscom, N. T., Harris, G. B. C., Umansky, I., Easterday, C. L., and Frigoletto, F. D.: Internal radiographic anatomy of the intra-uterine fetus. In Kaufmann, H. J., ed.: Progress in Pediatric Radiology, Vol. 2, Genito-urinary Tract. Year Book, Chicago, 1970, pp. 344–371.

Hanafee, W., and Bashore, R.: Carbon dioxide and horizontal fluoroscopy in intrauterine fetal transfusions. Radiology, 85:481, 1965.

Hubinont, P. O., and Massart-Guiot, T.: Considerations sur le traitment de la maladie hémolytique du nouveau-né en particulier sur l'utilisation du sang Rh positif lors des exsanguino-transfusions. Bruxelles Med., 35:934, 994, 1955.

Johnson, L., and Boggs, T. R.: An estimate of the kernicteric potential of jaundiced sera. Program of the American Pediatric Society, 1966.

Kleihauer, E., Braun, H., and Betke, K.: Demonstration von fetalem Hämoglobin in den Erythrocyten eines Blutausstrichs. Klin. Wschr., 35:637, 1957.

Lathe, G. H., and Walker, M.: Inhibition of bilirubin conjugation in rat liver slices by human pregnancy and neonatal serum and steroids. Quart. J. Exp. Physiol., 43:257, 1958.

Levine, P.: Serological factors as possible causes in spontaneous abortions. J. Hered., 34:71, 1943.

Levine, P.: The influence of the ABO system on Rh hemolytic disease. Hum. Biol., 30:14, 1958.

Liggins, G. C.: Current indications for intrauterine transfusion. In Lucey, J. F., and Butterfield, L. J., eds.: Report of the 53rd Ross Conference on Pediatric Research: Intrauterine Transfusion and Erythroblastosis Fetalis. Ross Laboratories, Columbus, 1966.

Liley, A. W.: Liquor amnii analysis in the management of the pregnancy complicated by rhesus sensitization. Amer. J. Obstet. Gynec., 82:1359, 1961.

Liley, A. W.: Errors in assessment of hemolytic disease from amniotic fluid. Amer. J. Obstet. Gynec., 86: 485, 1963a.

Liley, A. W.: Intrauterine transfusion of foetus in haemolytic disease. Brit. Med. J., 2:1107, 1963b.

Lucey, J. F.: In Lucey, J. F., and Butterfield, L. J., eds.: Report of the 53rd Ross Conference on Pediatric Research: Intrauterine Transfusion and Erythroblastosis Fetalis. Ross Laboratories, Columbus, 1966.

Matthews, C. D., and Matthews, A. E. B.: Transplacental hemorrhage in spontaneous and induced abortion. Lancet, 1:694, 1969.

McKee, F. W., and Stewart, W. B.: Passage of radioactive erythrocytes from the peritoneal cavity of humans. J. Lab. Clin. Med., 49:756, 1957.

Mollison, P. L., and Cutbush, M.: Haemolytic disease of the newborn; criteria or severity. Brit. Med. J., 1:123, 1949.

Odell, G. B.: Dissociation of bilirubin from albumin and its clinical implications. J. Pediat., 55:286, 1959.

Odell, G. B., Cohen, S. N. and Gordes, E. H.: Administration of albumin in the management of hyperbilirubinemia by exchange transfusions. Pediatrics, 30:613, 1962.

Odell, G. B., Storey, G. N. B., and Rosenberg, L. A.: Studies in kernicterus III. The saturation of serum proteins with bilirubin during neonatal life and its relationship to brain damage at five years. J. Pediat., 76:12, 1970.

Pickles, M. M.: Haemolytic Disease of the Newborn. Blackwell Scientific Publications, Oxford, 1949.

Poland, R. L., and Odell, G. B.: Physiologic jaundice: the enterohepatic circulation of bilirubin. New Eng. J. Med., 284:1, 1971. (Contains a bibliography going back to 1859.)

Porter, E. G., and Waters, W. J.: A rapid micro method for measuring the reserve albumin binding capacity in serum from newborn infants with hyperbilirubinemia. J. Lab. Clin. Med., 67:660, 1966.

Pritchard, J. A., and Weisman, R.: The absorption of labelled erythrocytes from the peritoneal cavity of humans. J. Lab. Clin. Med., 49:756, 1957.

Queenan, J. T.: Intrauterine transfusion: a cooperative study. Amer. J. Obstet. Gynec., 104:397, 1969.

Report of the Seventh M and R Pediatric Research Conference (on Erythroblastosis Fetalis). Ross Laboratories, Columbus, 1954.

Rosenfield, R. E.: Personal communication, 1959.

Rosenthal, I. M., Zimmerman, H. J., and Hardy, N.: Congenital nonhemolytic jaundice with disease of the central nervous system. Pediatrics, 18:378, 1956.

Schmid, R., Hammaker, L., and Axelrod, J.: The enzymatic formation of bilirubin glucuronide. Arch. Biochem. 70:285, 1957.

Seelen, J., van Kessel, H., Eskes, T., van Leusden, H., Been, J., Evers, J., van Gent, I., Peeters, L., van Der Velden, W., and Zonderland, F.: A new method of exchange transfusion in utero. Amer. J. Obstet. Gynec., 95:872, 1966.

Smith, T.: Active immunity produced by so-called balanced or neutral mixtures of diphtheria toxin and antitoxin. J. Exp. Med., 11:241, 1909.

Umansky, I.: In Lucey, J. F., and Butterfield, L. J., eds.: Report of the 53rd Ross Conference on Pediatric Research: Intrauterine Transfusion and Erythroblastosis Fetalis. Ross Laboratories, Columbus, 1966.

Vaughan, V. C., III, Allen, F. H., Jr., and Diamond, L. K.: Erythroblastosis fetalis. Pediatrics, 6:173, 441, 630, 706, 1950.

Voigt, J. C., and Britt, R. P.: Foetomaternal haemorrhage in therapeutic abortion. Brit. Med. J., 4:395, 1969.

Woodrow, J. C.: Rh immunization and its prevention. Series Hematologica, 3:1, 1970.

Woodrow, J. C., Clarke, C. A., Donohoe, W. T. A., Finn, R., McConnell, R. B., Sheppard, P. M., Lehane, D., Russell, S., Kulke, W., and Durkin, C. M.: Prevention of Rh-haemolytic disease: a third report. Brit. Med. J., 1:279, 1965.

World Health Organization Conference on the Prevention of Rh Immunization, organized by the W. H. O. Reference Center for the use of anti-D immunoglobulin. Middlesex Hospital Medical School, London, March 19 and 20, 1970.

Chapter 33

Examination of the Newborn

The initial examination of the newborn should be carried out in the delivery room by a physician as soon as possible after the birth of the infant. It need not be lengthy, but it is extremely important in determining disposition of the infant and subsequent management of any actual or potential abnormalities. The examination should be done in a warm environment, with good lighting conditions, as rapidly and gently as possible.

INITIAL EVALUATION

Some method should be used to judge the general condition of the infant quickly after birth. The Apgar scoring system is now widely used in the United States and has proved of value. Five signs—heart rate, respiratory effort, muscle tone, reflex irritability, and color—are evaluated, each given a rating of 0, 1, or 2 (see Chapter 26). The score is totaled and recorded. A score of 3 or below means that the infant is in poor condition; 10 is optimal. The score taken five minutes after birth may offer some index of neurologic residual (Fig. 1). A score of less than 5 at one minute after birth is indicative of fetal depression and the need for assisted ventilation.

The Skin at Birth

The skin of the newborn infant is usually bluish pink in color. Generalized mottling and cool extremities are common.

CYANOSIS.   The hands, feet, and perioral area are often slightly cyanotic as a result of a high hemoglobin concentration and slow capillary circulation. Generalized persistent cyanosis is abnormal, indicating central nervous system, cardiovascular, or pulmonary disease. Differential cyanosis of the lower part of the body, but not the upper portion, occurs in continued patency of the ductus arteriosus. Traumatic cyanosis of the head and chest area may occur as a result of excessive pressure over the thorax during delivery or umbilical cord compression of the neck. Cyanosis may be absent if anemia is present.

PALLOR.   Pallor of the skin may be found in asphyxia pallida due to anemia, narcosis, shock due to internal bleeding, asphyxia, or massive blood loss into the maternal circulation before birth. Marked pallor is always abnormal.

JAUNDICE.   This is rarely present at birth but may appear within one hour after birth. It is usually a sign of erythroblastosis fetalis. Jaundice first appears in the nasofacial area. The skin may be discolored, a muddy

Figure 1. Neurologic abnormalities at one year of age by birth weight and Apgar score (five minutes). (Data from Drage, J. S., and Berendes, H.: Pediat. Clin. N. Amer., 13:635, 1966.)

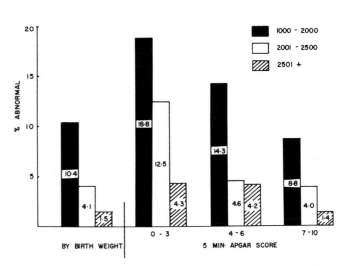

yellow, if the infant has been exposed to meconium-stained amniotic fluid. Jaundice is best judged if the skin is compressed or stretched and by the color of Wharton's jelly in the umbilical cord.

PETECHIAE. Petechiae can occur if birth has been difficult (breech or cord compression). Petechiae may also occur with intrauterine viral infections, erythroblastosis fetalis, or thrombocytopenia. The presence of ecchymoses should be noted and their location and size recorded.

EDEMA. Some edema is common in premature infants. It may also be seen in infants with erythroblastosis fetalis, infants of diabetic mothers, or those with gonadal dysgenesis.

MISCELLANEOUS. Cracked, brownish, parchment-like, peeling skin is seen in infants with the placental dysfunction syndrome. Capillary hemangiomas are commonly seen on the eyelids and forehead and neck areas.

The Attitude of Infant

The spontaneous movements of the infant should be observed. Usually the arms and legs are flexed and fists clenched. The character and symmetry of the random spontaneous movements, or their absence, should be noted. Infants dislike having their extremities extended for measurements and will cry. This crying can often be stopped by returning the infant to the fetal position. Defects of the skull, face, and extremities can also be readily observed and explained by this maneuver.

The Cry

The cry should be loud and easily provoked. If absent, or weak, central nervous system depression or asphyxia should be suspected. A weak, groaning, whining cry occurs in early respiratory distress. A high-pitched or hoarse cry may indicate local nerve injury or central nervous system disease. (See Neonatal Neurology.)

The Head

The skull may be molded, with overriding of the parietal bones. The suture lines, size, and tension of the anterior and posterior fontanelles should be determined

digitally. There is wide variation in the normal range. Soft areas (craniotabes) are occasionally found. The head circumference should be carefully measured. The presence of caput succedaneum, cephalhematomas, or forceps marks should be noted.

The Eyes

Eye movements are normally wandering and the scleras are normally blue. (See Neonatal Neurology.) The size and symmetry of the eyes should be noted and the red reflex should be checked. Subconjunctival hemorrhages are common. Mild chemical conjunctivitis may be caused by the silver nitrate instilled at birth.

The Ears

Otoscopic exam is done to prove patency of the auditory canal. Malformations of the pinnae or low-set ears suggest renal anomalies. Preauricular skin tabs and branchial cleft sinuses are relatively common.

The Nose

Infants are obligatory nose breathers. If an infant breathes through his mouth one should suspect choanal atresia and pass a nasal catheter. Mild nasal positional deformities and milia are common and will vanish quickly.

The Mouth

The palate should be inspected and palpated to detect clefts. Retention cysts of the gums and supernumerary precocious teeth may be found. The tongue appears relatively large and the frenulum is short and prominent. The throat is difficult to visualize. Excessive mucus should suggest the possibility of a tracheoesophageal fistula, and a soft plastic tube should be passed into the stomach to check the patency of the esophagus.

The Neck

The neck should be examined for masses in the sternocleidomastoid muscle (fibromas), goiter, and branchial cleft cysts. Redundant skin suggests Turner's syndrome. The clavicles should be palpated very carefully for fractures.

The Respiratory Tract

Variation of the respiratory rate between 30 and 80 per minute is common. The rate should be counted for a full minute. Breathing is predominantly diaphragmatic, and sternal retractions are common. Expiratory grunting and whining respirations usually accompany severe disturbances of respiration. Percussion is often as informative as auscultation, as it will detect pneumothorax, atelectasis, and diaphragmatic hernia. Normal breath sounds are bronchovesicular and because of the small size of the lungs these sounds are well transmitted. Rales are best heard by listening at the inspiration following a prolonged expiratory cry.

The Heart

The size of the heart is very difficult to estimate clinically. Transitory murmurs are common because of changes in neonatal circulatory shunts in this transitional period. The pulse may vary from 80 to 180 a minute between sleeping and crying. Extrasystoles are common.

The Abdomen

The abdomen should be inspected for fullness, asymmetry or localized prominences suggesting masses. A scaphoid abdomen should raise the suspicion of diaphragmatic hernia. Palpation is best carried out with the infant quiet and his hips and knees flexed. The liver is palpable 1 or 2 cm. below the costal margin on the right. The spleen is often detected if light palpation is used. In order to palpate the kidneys, slow, deep, firm, steady pressure should be used with one hand in the back. The bladder, if full, will be palpable up to the level of the umbilicus. Any firm mass detected should be investigated.

The Genitalia

The testes may be in the scrotum or palpable in the canals. The prepuce of the newborn is normally tight and adherent.

Careful inspection for hypospadias should be made. The labia minora of female infants are quite prominent and slight vaginal mucus accumulations are common.

The Anus

An imperforate anus is sometimes not obvious. If there is any doubt a soft rubber catheter should be passed into the rectum.

The Extremities

The movements of all extremities should be checked. The hips and knees should be flexed and then abducted to detect congenital dislocation of the hips.

NEONATAL NEUROLOGY

The neurologic examination in newborn infants is limited to an evaluation of primitive reflexes and motor responses because of the immaturity of the newborn's brain. Different disorders often produce similar and nonspecific abnormalities and the examination may demonstrate only the presence of dysfunction and not its cause. Knowledge of the maternal history, pregnancy, course of labor and findings at delivery, and size of the infant may give helpful clues, and diagnosis often depends on knowledge of likely etiologies and diagnostic studies.

The importance of performing a careful examination should not be minimized, because certain findings and focal abnormalities are of diagnostic significance. The following is a convenient guide for recording the findings of the examination.

General appearance and state of consciousness
Cry
Head, neck, and spine
Special senses and cranial nerves
Motor function
  posture at rest
  spontaneous movements
  muscle power
  muscle mass
  muscle tone
  reflexes
  neonatal automatisms
Sensation

GENERAL APPEARANCE AND STATE OF CONSCIOUSNESS

Morphologic abnormalities can indicate the presence of known chromosomal syndromes, i.e., Down's syndrome, holoporencephaly, and cretinism. The state of consciousness of infants varies enormously from one hour to the next, and there are many gradations between sleep and wakefulness which greatly affect the findings on neurologic examination. Thus, a particular response must be tested on different occasions before it can be concluded that it is absent or abnormal. With premature infants, particularly, it is very difficult to decide whether they are awake or asleep even under the best conditions. Depression of central nervous system activity in the newborn, whether because of maternal sedation, congenital defect, traumatic or hypoxic insult at birth, or metabolic disorder, or of other causation, clearly demands investigation.

CRY

Several types of abnormal cry may be heard. A feeble cry, or absence of cry, is most often due to general depression of central nervous system function from a wide variety of causes, including the effect of maternal anesthesia, birth injury or hypoxic insult, infection, or metabolic defect. A shrill, high-pitched cry is one of the major signs of meningeal or brain stem irritation, especially from hemorrhage or infection. It also occurs in kernicterus. A hoarse cry is likely to result from injury to the recurrent laryngeal nerve during delivery; it may be associated with respiratory distress.

HEAD, NECK, AND SPINE

The examiner looks first for obvious anomalies such as hydrocephalus or microcephaly. A small proportion of microcephalic cases may be due to premature synostosis of all of the cranial sutures, a possibility warranting the taking of x-rays of the skull.

A soft swelling over the skull in the area of one of the parietal bones or of the occipital bone is usually a cephalhematoma. After a few days a sharp edge may be felt, owing to beginning calcification, which can give an erroneous impression of a bony defect of the skull. No direct treatment is required except to rule out underlying fracture. A soft tissue swelling in another location on the skull, particularly at the midline, is more likely to be an encephalocele. Encephaloceles are by no means always associated with general cerebral defects and are compatible with normal intelligence. Similar swellings on the spine are meningomyeloceles or, less frequently, simple meningoceles. Such anomalies may require early neurosurgical attention if the sac is ruptured or extremely thin.

Opisthotonos or continuous retraction of the head in the lateral recumbent position is a sign of intracranial pressure and meningeal irritation and is seen following a variety of hypoxic or other insults to the central nervous system. One should think of kernicterus if the baby is severely jaundiced.

The size and tension of the fontanelles constitute a physical sign of paramount importance. Bulging of the fontanelles is the single most important sign of intracranial pressure, usually due either to hemorrhage or to infection. Separation and tension of the sutures of the skull are related signs. If the anterior fontanelle is normal, disproportionate size of the posterior fontanelle and separation of the sagittal suture may suggest a cystic malformation or obstruction in the vicinity of the fourth ventricle. Transillumination of the head will often document this.

Transillumination of the skull should be carried out for every baby suspected of neurologic abnormality. It should be done with a strong flashlight fitted with a scalp-tight rubber adapter, and must be done in a totally dark room after the examiner's eyes have become dark-adapted. Local malformations such as porencephaly may be seen or, more frequently, hydranencephaly (Fig. 2) with absence of the cerebral hemispheres above the basal ganglia (which may also be defective). Most such infants behave relatively or entirely normally in the newborn period. However, although hydranencephaly is rare, it can occasionally be demonstrated in an apparently normal infant if transillumination is done routinely.

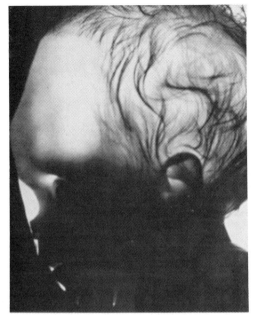

Figure 2. Abnormal total transillumination of the head in hydranencephaly. (Courtesy of Dr. Philip Dodge, Massachusetts General Hospital, Boston.)

SPECIAL SENSES

The *vision* of newborn infants is difficult to appraise and often requires repeated examination. The blink reflex should be a constant reaction to a strong flashlight, and blinking or squinting should occur even if the eyes are initially closed and the baby asleep. Newborn infants will not follow a moving light or moving object with reliability, but with persistence a following response is often obtainable by use of a large object, such as a red ring 4 inches in diameter. Pupillary constriction to light indicates that the optic nerve and parasympathetic fibers traveling with the third nerve are intact but will not rule out posterior lesions in the optic radiation and occipital cortex.

The optic fundi must be examined. Papilledema actually is not a frequent finding, as increased intracranial pressure is quickly compensated for by the open sutures and fontanelles. It must be distinguished from the anomalous but harmless persistence of myelinated nerve fibers radiating out from the optic disc. The optic discs of newborns are normally quite pale in comparison with those in adults, and a diagnosis of optic atrophy should be made very cautiously. Retinal hemorrhages are quite frequent, particularly in premature infants and those whose delivery was difficult. Numerous hemorrhages, particularly close to the optic discs, frequently accompany subdural hematomas.

Hearing can be tested by clapping the hands loudly near the baby or by using noise-making devices. A very loud sound is required, and even then response may often be absent. One may judge that an infant hears because it blinks, executes a Moro response, or otherwise startles.

CRANIAL NERVES

The position of the eyes at rest is important, as forced deviation of the eyes downward or to one side will occasionally reflect intracranial pressure or irritation. Extraocular paralyses are usually much more easily appraised in terms of eye movements induced by movement of the head up or down or to the right or left. External rectus paralysis is immediately obvious on vestibular stimulation by rotation (Fig. 3). Usually the eyes deviate ahead in the direction toward which the examiner moves the baby, with the rapid component of nystagmus backward toward the midline. The directions are reversed when rotation is stopped. Failure to obtain even deviation of the eyes usually indicates damage to the vestibular nerve or its connections. Deviation without nystagmus reflects depression of cerebral hemisphere function. It is not specific, and may be due to a wide variety of causes.

The "setting-sun" sign of the eyes (Fig. 4) is of the greatest importance. It may be a spontaneous phenomenon or may occur in response to moving the head up and down. In either event it consists in deviation of the eyes downward, usually in the midline, so that each iris appears to "set" beneath the lower lid, and white sclera is exposed between the iris and the upper lid. It usually is caused by intracranial pressure, or by irritation of the brain stem, as in kernicterus. It should not be overemphasized if it is of mild degree and is an isolated finding.

The size of the pupils is also of great importance, since dilatation of one or both pupils and failure to react to light are usually due to midbrain or third nerve injury. Unequal pupils with normal reaction to light may be without significance

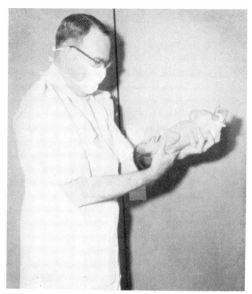

Figure 3. Position in which baby may be held for testing of eye movements by vestibular stimulation through rotation. The infant will almost always obligingly open the eyes if he is not sound asleep. It is frequently easier to keep the child quiet but alert and the eyes open in this upside-down posture than in the upright position. The latter further does not put the horizontal semicircular canals in the horizontal plane unless the baby is held above the examiner and the head inclined forward about 30 degrees. In either position the eyes deviate ahead in the direction of rotation and backward after stopping, with rapid component of nystagmus toward the midline. (From Paine, R. S.: Pediat. Clin. N. Amer., 8:577, 1961.)

(congenital anisocoria), but one should look carefully for other abnormality. There is often ptosis, slight enophthalmos, and anhidrosis, pointing to sympathetic paralysis. This may accompany a brachial palsy but more often is the result of a stretch injury of the sympathetic fibers in the neck during delivery. The condition may disappear, or may be permanent.

Unilateral ptosis may be one feature of third nerve paralysis. Less often it is part of the Marcus Gunn phenomenon, a harmless congenital anomaly in which the ptotic upper lid elevates in rhythm with sucking movements of the jaw. Bilateral ptosis should suggest myasthenia gravis or myotonic dystrophy, particularly if there is general weakness of sucking and spontaneous body activities. A transient myasthenic state occurs in infants of mothers suffering from myasthenia gravis. Recognition and prompt treatment of such babies is lifesaving, and the mortality rate is high if the condition is overlooked. Congenital myasthenia gravis, although rarely diagnosed in the neonatal period, may also occur in infants of normal mothers and under these circumstances is persistent and requires treatment indefinitely.

Facial paralysis may not be obvious except when the baby cries, but nonmovement of the paralyzed side is then obvious (Fig. 5B). There may be isolated weakness of the depressor muscles of the corner of the mouth, possibly a muscular anomaly, and a condition which must be distinguished from facial paralysis. Facial palsy in newborns is most often due to pressure of forceps on the pes anserinus or to pressure against the promontory of the mother's sacrum. The necessity of further diagnostic investigation depends on associated findings.

The ninth and tenth nerves are appraised in terms of swallowing, the gag reflex,

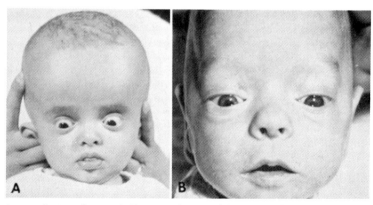

Figure 4. "Setting-sun" sign of eyes. A, Extreme degree of "setting-sun" sign of the eyes. It is due to hydrocephalus in this case but may also be encountered in the presence of intracranial pressure, of whatever cause, or of brain stem abnormality. (From Paine, R. S.: Pediat. Clin. N. Amer., 8:577, 1961.) B, Slighter degree of "setting-sun" sign in a normal premature infant.

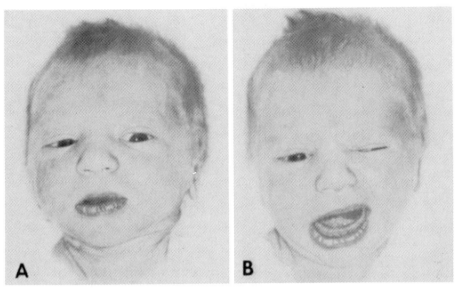

Figure 5. Right facial paralysis. A, There is only minimal asymmetry in the resting state. B, Nonmovement on the paralyzed side on crying makes the paralysis obvious. (From Paine, R. S.: Pediat. Clin. N. Amer., 7:471, 1960.)

movement of the palate, and the like. Deficiencies in this respect are, in general, most often due to universal depression of the central nervous system and less frequently to myasthenia gravis, but, aside from myasthenia gravis, the principal cause for difficulty with secretions which requires early attention is non-neurologic, namely, tracheoesophageal fistula and atresia. Hoarseness of cry due to recurrent laryngeal paralysis has already been mentioned. Torticollis is rarely primarily neurogenic; more often in the newborn it is associated with injury to the sternocleidomastoid muscle.

Twelfth nerve function can be evaluated by inspection or by observation of the elevation of the tongue produced by pinching the baby's nostrils. Fasciculations of the tongue are a more important sign but must be distinguished from synchronous tremor in crying. Fasciculations at this age are practically always due to infantile spinal progressive muscular atrophy (Werdnig-Hoffmann disease).

MOTOR FUNCTION

Posture at Rest

Opisthotonos has already been mentioned as one abnormal posture. Another is the flaccid, inactive "pithed-frog" posture (Fig. 6). This can result from very severe

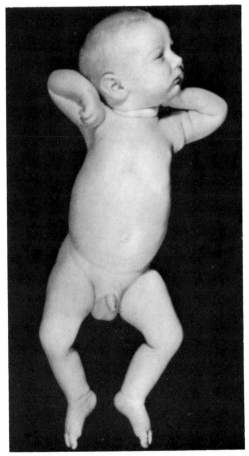

Figure 6. "Pithed-frog" posture of baby with spinal cord injury at the level of C7. Note abnormal posture of the arms due to the unopposed action of muscles innervated by C5 and C6. (From Paine, R. S.: Pediat. Clin. N. Amer., 8:577, 1961.)

general depression of the nervous system, injury to the spinal cord, and Werdnig-Hoffmann disease. In the latter condition the mother may report diminished fetal activity during late pregnancy. Muscle bulk may be diminished and deep tendon reflexes depressed or absent. The respirations are abdominal, with paradoxical retraction of the chest on inspiration because of intercostal weakness with preserved diaphragmatic function. Fasciculation of the tongue is pathognomonic if it accompanies the other features. Otherwise, the condition must be distinguished from the more benign forms of muscular hypotonia and from congenital muscular dystrophy.

Spinal cord injuries present a superficially similar picture, although the unopposed pull of the deltoids and biceps usually results in a characteristic arm posture if the lesion is low cervical in location (Fig. 6). High cervical injuries are usually immediately fatal. The diagnosis is of course further illuminated by the exaggerated automatic withdrawal following pinprick, often with extension of the opposite leg, without any evidence of perception of pain by the facial expression or cry. The abnormal posture of brachial plexus injury is depicted in Figure 7. The upper roots or trunks are usually involved, with retained finger movements (Erb type), but less commonly the lower roots are affected (Klumpke). If the roots are avulsed close to the cord, diaphragmatic paralysis, an unfavorable prognostic sign, may complicate the Erb type just as a Horner syndrome may be found in the Klumpke type. Otherwise, most of the infants with the Erb type of paralysis recover to a considerable extent.

Spontaneous Movements

Spontaneous movements should be appraised for quantity and quality, and particularly for symmetry. Brachial palsy has already been mentioned as a cause of diminished movement of one arm, but injury to the clavicle, humerus, or shoulder joint is a more common cause. Congenital hemiparesis due to such anomalies as porencephaly is very seldom evident in the newborn period, being recognized rather by disuse of one hand when cortical function emerges. Acute hemiplegia may occur in the newborn, however,

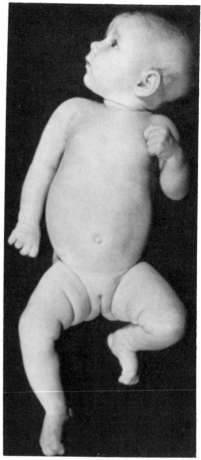

Figure 7. Right upper (Erb type) brachial palsy showing characteristic posture. (From Paine, R. S.: Pediat. Clin. N. Amer., 8:577, 1961.)

usually as a result of intracranial vascular accident. The major, and frequently the only, diagnostic sign under these circumstances is a relative lack of spontaneous movement on the affected side. Observation for some minutes and usually on more than one occasion is required to establish this. A general paucity of movement is likely to be due to Werdnig-Hoffmann spinal muscular atrophy, or may be the consequence of a spinal cord lesion.

A considerable amount of "jittery" jerky movement of the limbs may be normal, particularly in response to stimuli. More marked exaggeration may be due to an irritative insult to the central nervous system or withdrawal phenomena if the mother is addicted to narcotics. More pronounced hyperkinesis may proceed to the point of myoclonus of a more automatic and stereotyped sort. This is most often the consequence of hypoxia at birth and is often followed by various types of cerebral palsy. Similar myoclonic movements, as well as clonic convulsions, can be based on congenital errors of metabolism, of which maple syrup urine disease is the commonest, although there are several other types.

Neonatal convulsions are a neurologic problem requiring both diagnostic and therapeutic action. They are most often the result of hypoxic or traumatic insult to the brain or of meningitis. If there is nothing in the history to suggest any of these and if investigations for them prove negative, one should think more in terms of biochemical anomalies than of idiopathic epilepsy or congenital cerebral defect, as the latter only infrequently cause convulsions before a month or two of age and sometimes only after years. Tetany is by far the commonest basis of neonatal fits and can be documented by the finding of a low calcium and high phosphorus concentration in the blood. There may be two types, one beginning in the first 48 hours of life, in which birth insult is an important contributory factor, and the other beginning only after four or five days, in which intake of cow's milk, as opposed to breast milk, is implicated. Hypoglycemia may begin in the newborn period, and the blood sugar level should be checked, with the awareness that it may normally be low at this age. The urine should be checked for galactose, although glucose levels in galactosemia are seldom low enough to cause neonatal convulsions. The urine should be examined for unusual odor and for amino acids, although the interpretation of neonatal "aminoaciduria" is full of pitfalls. An excessive demand for pyridoxine is a congenital metabolic error, frequently familial, which should be considered in case of neonatal convulsions not otherwise explained. This condition is distinct from pyridoxine deficiency, which may result from inadequate dietary intake.

Convulsions in the newborn tend to be clonic rather than tonic in character and are often confined to one particular region of the body, although they quite characteristically move from one part to another in no systematic fashion. At this age, localized convulsions are very often not evidence of localized cerebral pathology. They tend to recur repeatedly over a period of hours or days and may be associated with cyanosis and the possibility of further hypoxic cerebral damage. For this reason continuous medication is usually wise. Phenobarbital in doses up to 30 mg. per day (8 mg. at a single dose) may be effective but should be used cautiously if there is any depression of respiration. Dilantin may also be useful, chiefly in conjunction with phenobarbital. It tends to produce marked drowsiness in many newborns and is best given in smaller doses than would be calculated by the usual rules (not more than 20 mg. per 24 hours).

Muscle Power, Mass, and Tone

Muscle power, mass, and tone are appraised by observation of spontaneous movement and by palpation as already discussed. The muscle tone of the neonate is appraised in several ways: the tonus at rest by palpation; the range of motion by passive manipulation; and the resistance to motion, by the amount of flapping of hand or foot produced on sudden mobilization of the limb proximally, and the "rebound" when the forearm, for example, is passively extended at the elbow and suddenly released. In full-term infants a flexor tone of the limbs normally predominates and there is limitation of extension of the knee although the ankle is hyperextensible (Fig. 8A). Premature babies lack the predominant flexor tone of full-term infants, and the limbs are often in extension, frequently showing athetotic movements as well. The range of variation of tone is considerable, and unless the infant is almost rigid or almost flaccid not too much emphasis should be placed on lesser deviations. Asymmetry, of course, is of far greater importance and points (as does asymmetry of spontaneous movement or automatisms) to a unilateral brain lesion which should be investigated.

Reflexes

Reflexes can be tested much as with older infants. The knee jerk is normally quite active, and spread to the adductor muscles, including those of the opposite side, is normal until the third or fourth month. The ankle jerk is usually unobtainable because of flexor tone in the legs unless the baby is placed in the prone position and the back of the ankle is tapped. The biceps

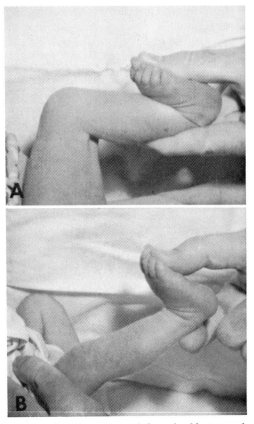

Figure 8. Hyperextensibility of ankle in newborn. A, Marked but normal hyperextensibility in full-term infant. B, More limited range of extensibility in ankle of premature.

jerk is easy enough to obtain if the infant is sufficiently quiet at the time, but the triceps jerk is suppressed by flexor tone (although it clearly exists since it can be obtained in the presence of upper brachial palsy). Up to 10 or 12 beats of ankle clonus are normally obtained in many infants, and ankle clonus is thus without much significance unless it is sustained or asymmetric.

Neonatal Automatisms

It has already been shown that it is difficult to apply to newborns the standard techniques of neurologic examination of adults. The newborns, on the other hand, present a considerable variety of postural and other automatic responses which may be exploited for examination. Absence of one or more of the more important of these usually points to a general depression of central nervous system activity.

With the infant in the supine position, the sucking response should always be obtainable by placing one's finger in the baby's mouth, preferably with the examiner wearing a finger cot or glove. A rooting response of following with the tongue, mouth, or head is obtained by touching the corners of the mouth (Fig. 9A) or the upper or lower lip in the midline (Fig. 9B). The rooting response is more variable and may

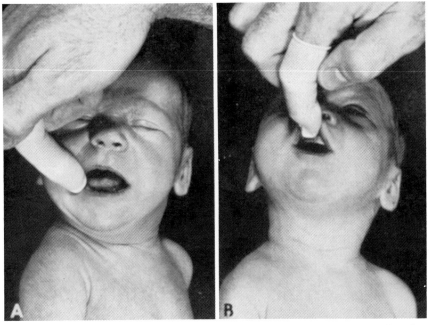

Figure 9. Rooting response in which tongue, mouth, or head follows the finger applied at the corner of the mouth (A) or middle of the upper or lower lip (B). (From Paine, R. S.: Pediat. Clin. N. Amer., 7:471, 1960.)

be absent if the baby has recently been fed. It can be reinforced in doubtful cases by testing the sucking response first.

A normal full-term infant will attempt to grasp an extended finger with his own fingers or toes. The examiner should place his finger at the base of the baby's phalanges and, if necessary, reinforce the response by gentle palmar or plantar pressure. When one pulls the baby up to a sitting position from supine, holding onto the hands firmly, a normal newborn will "assist" with the shoulder muscles and show some measure of head control when the sitting position is reached, although the head will initially flop forward and then be elevated.

The *Moro response* is the most important neonatal automatism. It can be elicited in a wide variety of ways, including slapping on the bed, making a sudden loud noise, jerking the baby by the feet, extending and pulling on the arms and then suddenly letting go, or, most reliably, letting the supported head (Fig. 10A) drop back about 30 degrees (Fig. 10B). Normally the arms first rapidly flex (although this is usually imperceptible), then extend with spreading of the fingers and a clasping movement of the arms. The femora may also flex on the pelvis. Absence of this response is definite indication of depressed nervous system activity. An asymmetric response may be due to bone injury, brachial palsy, or hemiparesis.

The behavior of the infant in the prone position is another test of vigor. Normal, healthy, full-term infants will turn the head to one side, usually bring the arm forward on that side, and make creeping movements with the legs. Asymmetry of the response on repeated examination is abnormal (it is always asymmetric at a single trial), as is failure to obtain any activity if the failure is confirmed by repeated observation. The trunk incurvation reflex is demonstrated by running the finger down the paravertebral area (Fig. 11), by pinching the skin above the pelvic brim, or by making a series of sharp touches with the fingernail running down the back of the side of the spine. The infant swings the pelvis toward the stimulated side and bends the spinal column away from it, so as to make it concave toward the stimulated side. This is a spinal reflex and is missing when there is a lesion of the spinal cord. It may also be lacking in generally depressed central nervous system activity, but such depression must be extreme.

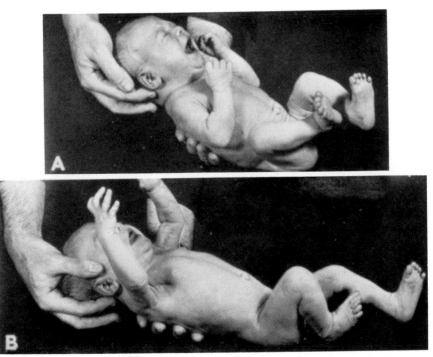

Figure 10. Method of eliciting the Moro response by dropping the head backward (see text). (From Paine, R. S.: Pediat. Clin. N. Amer., 7:471, 1960.)

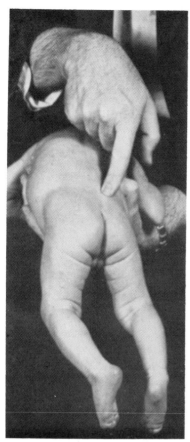

Figure 11. Trunk incurvation response in which pelvis swings to right when examiner's finger is run down paravertebral area. (From Paine, R. S.: Pediat. Clin. N. Amer., 7:471, 1960.)

In vertical suspension there are a number of automatisms which can be tested. Bringing the dorsum of a foot up against the under side of a table edge produces the placing response, in which the stimulated foot is firmly placed on the top of the table (Fig. 12A). Asymmetry in this response is one of the more sensitive signs of hemiparesis. If the observations are continued from this point, the positive supporting reaction will appear in which the foot settles firmly against the table top and there is stiffening of the leg (but not the hyperextension and locking of the knee which is seen in the positive supporting reaction of older infants). Automatic stepping may also be seen (Fig. 12B). Finally, in the most mature and vigorous full-term infants, there may be a straightening reaction of the trunk (*redressement du tronc*), but this is most easily demonstrated by holding the baby against one's chest with one hand (Fig.

13A), and manipulating the feet with the other hand. If the reaction is present, the baby will straighten up from the waist, hold the head erect, and look straight ahead (Fig. 13B). A positive reaction to all of these tests requires an alert and reasonably vigorous full-term infant. Such reactions are missing in the smaller prematures and in babies of heavily anesthetized mothers, as well as in infants whose nervous activity is depressed for any reason. Asymmetry of the responses is also important, as mentioned, but not too much emphasis should be placed on failure to obtain a single one of the more advanced automatisms.

SENSATION

Sensory function is examined by touching various parts of the body with the finger, with a piece of cotton, or with a pin, and looking for indirect evidence of perception which may include movement of the affected part or change in facial expression. Very gentle pinprick may produce an extensor response of the stimulated limb rather than withdrawal. Testing with a pin evaluates two functions, sensation and motor power. The infant with a spinal cord injury or other lesion gives no evidence of appreciation of pain in the facial expression and does not cry, but the stimulated part is jerkily and automatically withdrawn. Contrariwise, the infant with congenital muscular dystrophy or spinal muscular atrophy shows marked distress and will usually begin to cry feebly but may be too weak to withdraw. An abnormal exaggerated stereotyped crossed extension response may be seen in the presence of lesions of the spinal cord and this, as well as a mass reflex, may be obtainable from a very wide sensory area.

AUTONOMIC FUNCTION

The anal sphincter is visibly patulous and hypotonic to digital examination in babies with myelomeningocele or other spinal lesions. The reflex to pinprick of the perianal skin may also be absent. Sweating and blanching or flushing of the skin may be disturbed below a transverse spinal lesion, being either exaggerated or diminished. The triple response to scratch may be abnormal below lesions in the thoracic

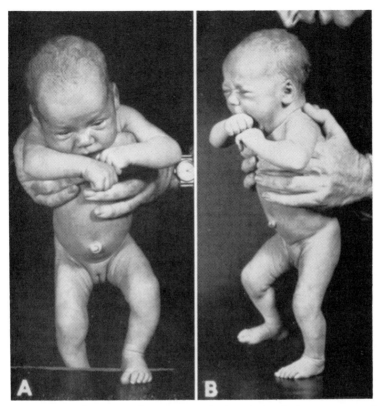

Figure 12. Automatisms tested in vertical suspension. A, Automatic placing response when dorsum of left foot is brought up under edge of table. B, Automatic stepping. This response depends more on proprioceptive stimuli from the ankle and other joints than on cutaneous contact against the surface since premature infants walk on their toes. It does not depend on position in space, and normal full-term infants will "walk" up a wall or even on the ceiling. (From Paine, R. S.: Pediat. Clin. N. Amer., 7:471, 1960.)

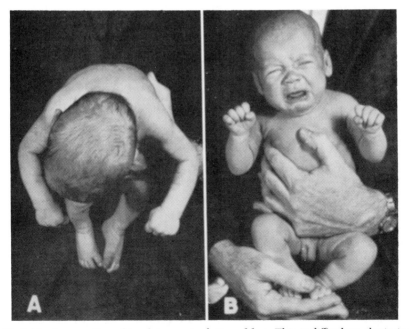

Figure 13. Straightening reaction of trunk to manipulation of feet. This is difficult to obtain in the immediate neonatal period even in vigorous normal babies. (From Paine, R. S.: Pediat. Clin. N. Amer., 7:471, 1960.)

segment of the cord, although this is an axon reflex. This is therefore one way of localizing a spinal lesion if sensory examination is unsatisfactory.

SPECIAL EXAMINATIONS AND PROCEDURES

Spinal Puncture

Spinal puncture is a source of useful information in the majority of infants with signs referable to the central nervous system. The spinal fluid should be examined for blood or infection in babies who are generally depressed, in those with signs of central nervous system irritation such as convulsions, and in babies with localizing cranial nerve signs. Because of the decompressing effect of open fontanelle and sutures, lumbar puncture is almost always innocuous even if intracranial pressure is increased.

Lumbar puncture is technically more difficult in newborns than at any other age. The smallest possible needle, No. 22 or 23, should be used, as it is very easy to push the dura loose from its attachment, making a clean puncture difficult if not impossible. If no fluid can be obtained, the tap should be repeated an interspace higher, although the spinal cord may come down to the level of L2 in newborns so that taps cannot safely be performed as high as in older infants. Cisternal puncture may be successful in obtaining fluid if lumbar puncture fails or if one cannot obtain fluid after previous successful lumbar taps. The distance between the dura and medulla is short, however, and cisternal puncture should not be done by the inexperienced operator.

Ventricular puncture may be safer than cisternal and is indicated if there is evidence of intracranial pressure coupled with inability to obtain fluid from the lumbar space, as either hemorrhage or more commonly ependymitis may become walled off. Ventricular puncture is ideally carried out by a neurosurgeon but is a proper procedure for any physician in an emergency, or if indicated when neurosurgical help is unavailable. The principal acute indication is a moribund baby with a bulging fontanelle, dilated fixed pupils, or cranial nerve paralyses. One introduces the needle through the coronal suture about 1/4 inch lateral to the corner of the fontanelle and either passes perpendicular to a plane tangent to the skull or aims for the bridge of the nose in the hope of hitting the anterior horn of the lateral ventricle. If no fluid is obtained in one pass in either direction on each side to a maximum of 1 1/4 inch (withdrawing the stylet every 1/4 inch before penetrating deeper), one can conclude that the ventricles are not greatly dilated and the procedure should usually be abandoned. The size of the lateral ventricles varies considerably, and successful puncture may be almost impossible in some instances. If blood is encountered, there may be striking improvement after removal of 10 to 15 ml.; removal of larger amounts is usually inadvisable at a single puncture. There is some difference of opinion as to whether repeated puncture should be carried out if the head enlarges and the fontanelle bulges after the first tap.

Subdural taps are performed in the same manner as ventricular puncture, except that one proceeds only to a depth of about 1/4 inch. The subdural space should be explored by removal of the stylet of the needle at this depth whenever ventricular puncture is contemplated. Subdural hemorrhage, however, is rare in the newborn, and it is reprehensible to perform subdural tap routinely in every infant with convulsions or other neonatal neurologic abnormality, particularly if there is no suggestion of increased intracranial pressure and no lateralizing signs. If a subdural hemorrhage is encountered, one should perform subdural tap every few days for 10 to 14 days. If blood or high-protein fluid continues to be obtained, craniotomy with removal of the surrounding membrane will usually be required.

Electroencephalography

Electroencephalograms are of limited value because of difficulty in interpretation at this age, but generalized slowing or spike-wave complexes occur in a number of congenital metabolic defects and in pyridoxine dependency. Changes in these in pyridoxine dependency permit evaluation of the effect of intravenously administered pyridoxine. It should be mentioned that considerable asymmetry is normal in sleep tracings in newborns.

Roentgenography

X-rays of the skull are of limited value in the newborn, as the size of the fontanelles and the possible separation of the sutures are more reliable indications of intracranial pressure. Intracranial calcification is infrequent, and x-rays are useful principally for the demonstration of fractures, although neurosurgical treatment is seldom necessary unless the fracture is depressed or extensive.

Pneumoencephalography is hazardous in the newborn because of the danger of subdural effusion in young infants following this procedure. Direct ventriculography by a neurosurgeon is preferable if contrast x-ray studies are necessary, although the types of anomalies sought are rarely treatable, and the procedure is thus more a matter of gaining information which only infrequently is the basis of any change of plans in the immediate future.

Evaluation of Positive Findings

The positive findings of the neonatal neurologic examination may well be listed in some systematic way such as that outlined at the beginning of this section. Bizarre and seemingly discrepant combinations of signs are often found, and efforts to define exquisitely localized vascular or space-occupying lesions such as can be predicted with adults are usually unsuccessful in newborns. This is only partly because of the limitations of the examination; more conspicuously it is because the type of disturbance of central nervous system function at this age is usually more extensive in nature. In any event, false-negative and sometimes false-positive signs are fairly frequent. One's general clinical impression should be thoughtfully considered even if it appears to contradict the sum of the individual signs. A high degree of suspicion needs to be maintained for hidden infection or hemorrhage. Physical signs in newborn infants change rapidly from day to day, so that reexamination at frequent intervals is necessary to adequately follow a case, and in any event should be performed before too much is made of single deviations from the expected findings.

BIBLIOGRAPHY

Apgar, V., and James, L. S.: Further observations on the newborn scoring system. Amer. J. Dis. Child., 104:419, 1962.

Craig, W. S.: Convulsive movements occurring in the first 10 days of life. Arch. Dis. Child., 35:337, 1960.

Drage, J. S., and Berendes, H.: Apgar scores and outcome of the newborn. Pediat. Clin. N. Amer., 13:635, 1966.

Greer, M., and Schotland, M.: Myasthenia gravis in the newborn. Pediatrics, 26:101, 1960.

Hunt, A. D.: Abnormally high pyridoxine requirement; summary of evidence suggesting relation between this finding and clinical pyridoxine "deficiency." Amer. J. Clin. Nutr., 5:561, 1957.

Levin, P. M.: Congenital myasthenia in siblings. Arch. Neurol. Psychiat., 62:745, 1949.

Menkes, J. H., Hurst, P. L., and Craig, J. M.: A new syndrome; progressive familial infantile cerebral dysfunction associated with an unusual urinary substance. Pediatrics, 14:462, 1954.

Moore, H.: Advantages of pyridostigmine bromide (Mestinon) and edrophonium chloride (Tensilon) in treatment of transitory myasthenia gravis in the neonatal period. New Eng. J. Med., 253:1075, 1955.

Paine, R. S.: Facial paralysis in children. Pediatrics, 19:303, 1957.

Paine, R. S.: Evaluation of familial biochemically determined mental retardation in children, with special reference to aminoaciduria. New Eng. J. Med., 262:658, 1960.

Paine, R. S.: Neurologic conditions in the neonatal period; diagnosis and management. Pediat. Clin. N. Amer., 8:577, 1961.

Pendleton, M. E., and Paine, R. S.: A visual, photographic and electro-oculographic study of eye movements in the newborn. Neurology, 11:450, 1961.

Saville, P. D., and Kretchmer, N.: Neonatal tetany; report of 125 cases and review of the literature. Biol. Neonat., 2:1, 1960.

Schneck, H.: Narcotic withdrawal symptoms in newborn infants resulting from maternal addiction. J. Pediat., 52:584, 1958.

Walker, R. P.: Congenital myasthenia gravis. Amer. J. Dis. Child., 86:198, 1953.

Chapter 34

Conditions and Diseases of the Newborn

The "high-risk" mother gives birth to the "high-risk" infant. The leading cause of problems in such infants is asphyxia, which accounts for the majority of perinatal deaths. The obstetric complications most frequently associated with fetal asphyxia are placenta praevia, premature separation of the placenta, prolapse of the umbilical cord, prolonged gestation, and maternal disease (toxemia or diabetes). Clinically it is estimated that 5 to 10 per cent of all births are accompanied by signs suggestive of fetal distress during labor. Much of the past and present confusion in this field has been caused by the fact that clinical methods of identifying fetal distress have been crude. The recently developed precise and continuous methods of detecting fetal distress, such as fetal electrocardiograph monitoring, amniotic fluid pressure recording, fetal scalp blood sampling, and amnioscopy, all show promise of giving us much better assessments of the degree and duration of the asphyxial insult.

HYPOXIA

Hypoxia is a major cause of fetal and neonatal morbidity and mortality. Recent evidence indicates that all infants are subjected to mild and varying degrees of oxygen deprivation and carbon dioxide retention during the course of labor and delivery. The umbilical cord values for pH, pCO_2, and buffer base correlate well with the five minute Apgar score and clinical condition of the infant. The mean pH of vigorous infants (Apgar score 8 to 10) was $7.26 \pm .08$, whereas depressed infants (Apgar score 0 to 4) were significantly more acidotic, with a mean arterial pH of 7.04 ± 0.14. It has long been thought, but has been very difficult to prove, that the responsiveness of the infant at birth correlates with subsequent neuro-logic development. Recent long-term studies have shown a three- to four-fold increase in neurologic abnormalities at the ages of two to four years among children who had low Apgar scores at birth.

A number of complications of pregnancy which are recognized as potential causes of intrauterine hypoxia in the premature, full-term, or postmature infant deserve recapitulation: (1) reduction of fetal oxygen through impaired maternal circulation such as might occur in hemorrhagic shock or faulty anesthesia; (2) reduction of oxygen in the fetal circulation due to faulty placenta function as in abruptio placentae, placenta praevia, or gross infarction and degeneration of the placenta; (3) reduction of fetal oxygen resulting from abnormalities of circulation through the umbilical cord, as from prolapse, true knots or stretching, or cord compression; (4) reduction of fetal oxygen due to fetal anemia as in erythroblastosis fetalis, rupture of fetal vessels in vasa praevia or in the course of amniocentesis, and vascular anastomoses in monochorial placentas in twins.

In hypoxic distress, the fetus becomes hypotonic, the anal sphincter relaxes, and meconium is passed into the amniotic fluid. The respiratory movements of the fetus are exaggerated, and amniotic fluid, with whatever debris may be present, is drawn deep into the alveolar ducts and the potential alveolar air spaces.

Regardless of the etiology, the sequence of events in fetal asphyxia follows a common course in which there is retention of carbon dioxide, accumulation of lactic acid due to anaerobic metabolism, and rapid depletion of fetal carbohydrate stores in the liver and myocardium. There is an intense pulmonary and peripheral vasoconstriction. Total asphyxia causes a reduction in the energy available to maintain the normal ionic concentration gradients across cell

848

membranes. Signs of extensive cell damage occur, with mitochondrial swelling and lysosomal destruction.

Fetal hypotension and shock cause a reduction in cerebral blood flow, and eventually increased intracranial pressure and cerebral edema. If there are repeated episodes of partial asphyxia in utero, it is impossible to predict the amount of damage that has occurred. The frequent occurrence of intracranial bleeding in areas of the brain due to capillary damage or defects in clotting which accompany asphyxia also contributes to our inability to quantitate the effects of various asphyxial insults.

RESPIRATORY DISTRESS SYNDROME (HYALINE MEMBRANE DISEASE)

The commonest cause of death in both premature and full-term infants is respiratory difficulty. The term most widely used to describe this is the respiratory distress syndrome. The postmortem findings in this syndrome are usually atelectasis and a homogeneous pink material lining the alveolar ducts (hyaline membrane). This syndrome accounts for approximately 50 per cent of all premature infant deaths. It has a mortality of about 25 per cent. The etiology of the condition is not known but certain facts have emerged which are now accepted.

Etiology

Normally pulmonary surfactant, a complex phospholipid, does not appear in the lungs until about the 20th to 24th week of gestation. Hence, premature infants in whom the respiratory distress syndrome develops have lungs with abnormally high surface tension. The amount of surface-active phospholipid is markedly lower than normal in the lungs of infants dying with hyaline membrane disease. The lack of surfactant causes the lungs to be unstable and to collapse easily, resulting in atelectasis. The important autopsy finding is the presence of eosinophilic hyaline material lining respiratory bronchioles, alveolar ducts, and alveoli. This material has been demonstrated to be of endogenous origin, consisting for the most part of fibrin.

Asphyxia, regardless of the cause, further damages pulmonary surfactant when it occurs in combination with an immature lung. In response to acidosis and hypoxia, the pulmonary arterioles of the fetus constrict, so that pulmonary blood flow is drastically reduced. This results in alveolar hypoperfusion, which damages the alveolar surface surfactant, resulting in alveolar hypoventilation.

Gluck has shown that the phospholipid content of human amniotic fluid reflects the state of development of the fetal lung. The lecithin-sphingomyelin ratio can be used to predict whether the lung is mature or susceptible to the development of hyaline membrane disease. This may prove to be a valuable test in selecting infants whose lungs are mature for elective delivery at about the 34th to 35th week of gestational age.

Clinical Course

This syndrome usually begins with rapid, shallow respirations of 60 or more per minute within the first few hours or shortly after birth. Intercostal retractions, flaring alae nasi and expiratory grunting are prominent features. On auscultation air exchange is diminished and on deep inspiration fine rales may be heard. Roentgenographically the lungs have a reticulogranular appearance which is characteristic but not pathognomonic (Fig. 1). The infant may die within a few hours or the disease may worsen over a three day period. Death is rare after the fourth to sixth day except in infants in whom the natural course of the disease may have been altered by the use of assisted ventilation.

During the course of the disease the infants often have hypotension, hypoglycemia, a decreased arterial pO_2, hypercarbia, a base deficit, and hypothermia. They also exhibit oliguria, ileus, hypotonia, and, terminally, intracranial bleeding.

Treatment

The prevention of prematurity is the single most important factor in reducing death from this cause. The conduct of labor and delivery is directed toward both the prevention of fetal distress and its early recognition and treatment.

In the newborn infant the avoidance of hypothermia, coupled with early resuscitation attempts to treat hypoxia and acidosis, is desirable therapy and may be effective

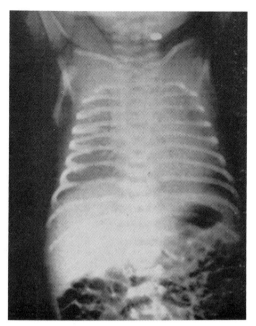

Figure 1. Roentgenogram of infant at two hours of age, showing hyaline membrane disease. (From Peterson, H. G., and Pendleton, M. E.: Amer. J. Roentgen., 74:800, 1955.)

in avoiding or at least modifying respiratory distress.

The essential element in treatment consists of the administration of oxygen in sufficient amounts to maintain arterial pO_2 values between 50 mm. Hg and 100 mm. Hg. This presents many problems as one is caught between the risks of hypoxia to the brain and the well recognized dangers of hyperoxia (arterial pO_2 above 100 mm. Hg) such as retrolental fibroplasia and pulmonary oxygen toxicity. Careful and repeated arterial gas studies are needed in the overall management. There is general agreement that the metabolic acidosis should be treated, and usually sodium bicarbonate is used for this purpose.

If these measures appear to be insufficient, then some form of assisted ventilation is indicated. This form of therapy may increase survival rates by a small amount, but it is successful only in the hands of an expert team. Recent studies suggest that mild continuous positive pressure is effective in increasing survival.

Prognosis

This condition carries a mortality rate of about 25 per cent. Controlled alternate case

studies have been very few to date so that no dogmatic statements can be made about therapy and outcome. There are no important pulmonary residua.

The survivors do have an increased incidence of neurologic residua but their etiology is difficult to determine as these infants have encountered a large number of potential biochemical insults, both in utero and following birth, such as hypoxia, acidosis, hypotension, intracranial bleeding, hypoglycemia, and hyperbilirubinemia.

MECONIUM ASPIRATION

During prolonged labors or difficult deliveries when the fetal oxygen supply is threatened, infants may attempt to breathe in utero. This condition is most apt to occur in term infants or postmature or dysmature infants. It is second in frequency to hyaline membrane disease as a cause of neonatal pulmonary problems. The possibility of this condition should be considered whenever the amniotic fluid is meconium-stained or whenever the infant shows signs of meconium staining. These infants are usually in distress from birth. The initial resuscitation procedure should include laryngoscopy and an attempt to aspirate as much of the meconium from the trachea as possible. If aspiration of acidic gastric contents has occurred, cortisone should be administered. In many infants the picture of asphyxia pallida is present, with pallor, hypotonia, apnea, hypotension, and shock. The respiratory distress that develops is clinically indistinguishable from hyaline membrane disease. The x-ray findings (Fig. 2) are different. The lungs show coarse, irregular increases in density, representing irregularities of aeration with emphysematous and atelectatic areas. A frequent and serious complication is the development of pneumothorax and mediastinal emphysema. Because of the preceding asphyxia, intracranial hemorrhage and hemorrhage in other organs often occur. These infants respond very poorly to positive-pressure artificial ventilation.

The treatment of the respiratory distress is similar to that already described, but, in addition, a constant watch must be maintained for the development of pressure pneumothorax, in which event emergency treatment may be lifesaving.

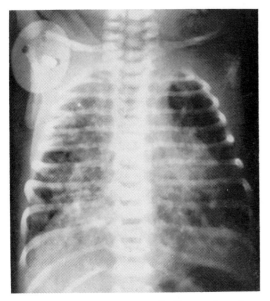

Figure 2. Roentgenogram of infant at three hours of age, showing intrauterine aspiration. The name tag is visualized. (From Peterson, H. G., and Pendleton, M. E.: Amer. J. Roentgen., 74:800, 1955.)

infants, and often are associated with prolonged rupture of the membranes or prolonged labor. It should be stressed that infection of the amniotic cavity may take place without rupture of the membranes, and, in fact, the membranes may rupture prematurely because of the existing infection, rather than the relationship being reversed. Bacterial infection progresses from the cervical area to the membranes, and to the placental and cord surfaces, with exudation into the amniotic fluid and with aspiration of infected fluid into the lungs and stomach of the fetus.

Since it is almost impossible to differentiate this variety of respiratory distress from the other types, either clinically or by x-ray, other evidence should be sought. The history is important, particularly if the mother was febrile or had prolonged rupture of the membranes or prolonged labor. In questionable cases, bacteria may be identified from smears of material aspirated from the stomach.

NONSPECIFIC ASPIRATION

There is an important group of both premature and term infants in whom distress develops, with clinical and x-ray signs similar to those in meconium aspiration, but there is no history of meconium having been passed and no meconium is found in the lungs at autopsy. The possibility of an infectious origin has also been excluded. The etiology in this group is not known, but in study of a series of stillborn and live-born infants with massive aspiration it has been suggested that toxemia and maternal diabetes might be the cause of fetal aspiration. Aspiration of gastric juice of low pH may be a factor. Rarely, live-born infants with massive aspiration but no history of any obstetric mishap may be found.

CONGENITAL PNEUMONIA

The clinical and x-ray findings in congenital pneumonia (fetal pneumonia or intrauterine pneumonia) of bacterial origin are indistinguishable from those seen in the meconium aspiration syndrome. The routes and types of fetal and newborn infection have been clarified. (See Infectious Diseases in Chapter 30.) Such infections occur more frequently in premature than in full-term

POSTNATAL ASPIRATION

A frequent and preventable cause of death occurring later in the neonatal period in otherwise normal full-term and premature infants is the regurgitation and aspiration of stomach contents. A tragic outcome can be prevented only by constant observation and immediate treatment by postural drainage and suction. The aspiration episode may be considered serious enough to warrant prophylactic treatment to prevent secondary infection in the lungs. The risk of aspiration is one reason why the propping of formula bottles is unacceptable.

INJURY AT BIRTH

Intracranial hemorrhage as the result of birth trauma has practically disappeared in modern obstetric services. If more than a rare instance occurs, it is an indication that methods of obstetric management should be critically reviewed.

The role of asphyxia in the production of intracranial injury is less well recognized. Hypoxia produces a profound disturbance of the fetus, affecting not only the central nervous system but every organ and tissue of the body. As previously stated, the changes resulting from anoxemia progress in an orderly fashion through various stages. The first stage is one of congestion with intense engorgement of the veins and capillaries. The second stage is one of congestion plus edema, the edema presumably being caused by transudation of fluid through the capillaries. In the third stage, in addition to congestion and edema, petechial hemorrhages appear, resulting from either diapedesis of red cells into the perivascular spaces or actual rupture of the capillaries. The fourth stage is characterized by all of the above findings, plus gross bleeding caused by continued capillary oozing or rupture of small veins. As is true in the event of trauma, the chances of serious injury resulting from asphyxia are increased by prematurity.

Usually the primary predisposing factor in the occurrence of intracranial injury is intrauterine asphyxia rather than trauma, but rarely there may be elements of both. The hemorrhages associated with intrauterine asphyxia are found in the ventricles, subarachnoid areas, and cerebral tissue. Trauma may result in rupture of the larger veins, particularly the vein of Galen, and tears of the falx and the tentorium; tears extending into the main sinuses of the dura may also be encountered. This type of hemorrhage involves the subdural space and is exacerbated by the presence of asphyxia.

The clinical picture in intracranial injury depends on the etiology of the hemorrhage and its anatomic location. A slowly accumulating hemorrhage in the subdural or subarachnoid space, or edema and petechial hemorrhages in the brain tissue, will produce the symptoms of cerebral irritation with convulsions that may not appear for a considerable time after birth. If these changes do not involve the region of the medulla, cyanosis may not develop. A hemorrhage in the region of the medulla or edema and petechial hemorrhages involving this area may produce immediate symptoms, and resuscitation of the infant at birth may be difficult, if not impossible.

When the injury extends above the tentorium, the fontanelle may become full and tense, but when it is below the tentorium, in the medulla, the anterior fontanelle may be normal. The findings of lumbar puncture are frequently of diagnostic value. A gross intracranial hemorrhage is revealed by a grossly bloody lumbar fluid with xanthochromic supernatant fluid. A milder degree of subarachnoid hemorrhage is indicated by blood-tinged fluid usually containing crenated red blood cells. Cerebral edema is accompanied by a marked increase in pressure of the cerebrospinal fluid, which is clear and free of red blood cells.

In treating the various types of intracranial hemorrhage, effort is made to drain all blood from the subarachnoid and ventricular spaces by repeated lumbar punctures until crystal-clear fluid is obtained. Lumbar drainage is also performed frequently enough to keep the intracranial pressure under control. Abnormal intracranial pressure is evidenced by tension of the anterior fontanelle and separation of the sutures, as well as by abnormal rate of increase in circumference of the head and by clinical symptoms.

When it is impossible to withdraw sufficient fluid from the lumbar space to relieve the intracranial pressure, or when lumbar puncture results in a "dry tap," the presence of either a block or hemorrhage in the subdural space should be suspected. A cisternal tap is then attempted; if this succeeds in relieving intracranial pressure, this route is used until tap by the lumbar approach is successful.

If the cisternal tap fails to relieve the pressure, it must then be determined whether the pressure is due to blocked drainage from the ventricles or to hemorrhage confined to the subdural space. When hemorrhage is confined to the subdural space, subdural taps may produce old blood, usually under increased pressure and free from spinal fluid. Under these circumstances the evidence points to a true subdural hematoma that is treated by frequent tapping, followed by surgical exploration to remove as much of the clot as possible, as well as the membrane which may have formed under these conditions. Unless the membrane is removed, chronic pachymeningitis hemorrhagica interna or hydrocephalus may result.

If the subdural tap fails to reveal the presence of abnormal fluid, the intracranial pressure must be controlled by direct ventricular puncture until drainage can be accomplished by the cisternal or lumbar route. Ventricular tap is always performed with reluctance, for fear of rupturing surface blood vessels and adding to the cerebral, subarachnoid, or subdural bleeding, and because the pathway of the needle may serve as a route by which the ventricular fluid, under pressure, may pass directly into the cerebral subarachnoid space and into the artificially opened subdural space.

Once the subdural space becomes filled with blood or blood and spinal fluid, if this fluid cannot be successfully drained off by repeated subdural taps, the formation of a membrane may result. Unless all signs of increased intracranial pressure disappear and the fluid clears and disappears from the subdural space, burr holes should be made in the infant's skull to prove the presence or absence of a membrane. If a membrane is present, a flap should be turned down and a liberal section of the membrane removed surgically.

Mention must be made of a particular variety of intracranial hemorrhage – intraventricular hemorrhage – to which the small premature infant is most vulnerable. Nothing in the history of the mother's pregnancy or in the infant's early history causes one to suspect this disaster. The infant's course may be uneventful or there may be mild or severe respiratory distress, without any neurologic signs, until the third or fourth day, when without warning he is stricken with this new development. Shock develops suddenly, with apneic episodes and other neurologic signs such as convulsions and shrill cry. A sharp fall in the hematocrit at this time is diagnostic. The fontanelle may become tense, but frequently the effects of the hemorrhage are so catastrophic that death occurs immediately. The only treatment available is supportive, and, if the infant lives long enough, effort should be made to relieve the intraventricular tension by puncture. The outlook for recovery from intracranial bleeding is very poor. The survivors also have a high incidence of neurologic damage but occasionally the residua are minimal.

INFECTION

The pediatric aspects of infectious diseases are considered here. (See also Infectious Diseases in Chapter 30.) A review of certain aspects of immunology as it pertains to the maternal-fetal relationship helps in the understanding of many diseases as they are encountered in the newborn infant. Many antibodies present in the mother's blood – to streptococcus, staphylococcus, and the organisms causing diphtheria, influenza, herpes simplex, vaccinia, mumps, rubella, measles, poliomyelitis, and homologous serum hepatitis – pass through the placenta and afford the infant some degree of passive immunity for four to six months. Some antibodies, such as those to the organisms causing chickenpox, smallpox, and herpes zoster, do not appear to cross the placenta as readily.

To possess antibodies, the mother must have had the specific disease either in an obvious form or, as is frequently the case, in a subclinical and unrecognized form. If a woman acquires a viral infection during pregnancy her fetus can become infected through placental transfer. If she acquires a bacterial or protozoal infection and the offending organism is present in the blood stream, as in a bacteremia or septicemia, the placenta may become the site of localized infection and of abscess formation, with breakdown of the placental barrier and invasion of the fetus.

The full-term or premature infant can form antibodies from birth, and this ability improves with age, reaching an efficient level at about two months. To a varying degree the presence of passive antibodies inhibits this production of active, permanent immunity. For both these reasons the active immunization program in infants is not started before the age of two or three months.

Viral Infections

A number of viral infections may cross the placenta and affect the fetus. Some of these may, if they occur in the first trimester of pregnancy, produce severe fetal anomalies and abortions. In Table 1 these infections are summarized and the possible fetal, neonatal, and long-term effects of such infections are listed.

The diagnosis of most of these infections is usually based on a history of exposure of the mother to the infection and often development in her of the clinical picture of the infection. Many of these, such as rubella, measles, mumps, poliomyelitis, influenza, and smallpox, are now fully preventable by adequate childhood immunization. They are thus of diminishing

TABLE 1. HUMAN VIRAL INFECTIONS AFFECTING THE FETUS OR NEWBORN

Virus	Effect
Rubella	Congenital heart anomalies; microcephaly; mental retardation; deafness, hepatosplenomegaly; cataracts; jaundice; hepatitis; encephalitis; prolonged infectiousness; growth retardation, prenatal and postnatal
Cytomegalovirus	Microcephaly; chorioretinitis; deafness; mental retardation; hepatosplenomegaly; pneumonitis; rash; persistent viruria
Toxoplasmosis (Protozoa)	Microcephaly; chorioretinitis; jaundice; hepatosplenomegaly; mental retardation; pneumonitis; rash; low birth weight
Herpes simplex	Encephalitis; death; jaundice; liver damage
Mumps	? Malformations
Rubeola	Increased rate of abortion and stillbirth
Chickenpox	Chickenpox; abortion and stillbirth
Smallpox	Abortion; stillbirth; smallpox
Vaccinia	Abortion; generalized vaccinia
Influenza	Abortion
Poliomyelitis	Paralysis
Hepatitis	Hepatitis
Coxsackie B	Hepatitis; myocarditis

clinical importance in the United States as the efficiency of programs of immunization increases. Unfortunately, no immunization is as yet available for such viruses as Coxsackie B, hepatitis, and herpes simplex. The best prevention for these remains avoidance of contact with infected persons, or, in the case of maternal genital herpes infection, delivery by cesarean section and avoidance of contact with the mother.

If one suspects an infant of having acquired an intrauterine infection, cultures of nose and throat, blood, cerebrospinal fluid, and stool should be taken at birth.

A cord blood sample should also be taken for IgM determination, as in nearly all of these intrauterine infections the IgM level will be found to be elevated above 15 mcg.

There is no effective treatment for any of these at the moment. I.D.U. (5-iodo-2-deoxyuridine) is being tried for the treatment of herpes encephalitis but clinical experience is too limited for any statement to be made about its effectiveness.

CYTOMEGALIC INCLUSION DISEASE. Cytomegalic inclusion disease is an example of an infection which may be tolerated by the mother's tissues without symptoms yet be devastating to unprotected embryonic and fetal tissue, the earlier the infection the more catastrophic being the injury. The symptoms in the newborn include jaundice, severe anemia, petechiae, thrombopenia, hepatosplenomegaly, and calcification in the ventricular walls of the brain. Infants surviving have exhibited microcephalus, hydrocephalus, cerebral palsy, mental retardation, and seizures. The diagnosis is made by culturing the virus from urine, saliva, or tissues during the first weeks of life.

In a serologic investigation of pregnant women in Boston and Philadelphia, 30 to 60 per cent had detectable antibodies and 3 to 5 per cent developed significant increases during pregnancy. It is obvious from these studies that congenital infection with cytomegalovirus is often not fatal and frequently may be subclinical. As with rubella, the infection persists in the infant for months. No effective therapy is available.

RUBELLA. The problem of rubella is largely obstetric. However, if the pregnancy continues to term the newborn may be acutely ill with anemia, thrombocytopenia, myocarditis, hepatitis, pneumonia, and encephalitis. Affected infants are often of low birth weight. Infection and viruria persist for several months after birth and such infants are contagious and must be isolated from pregnant or nonimmune women. Serum IgM levels are often but not always elevated in these infants.

COXSACKIE B VIRUS INFECTION. Coxsackie B viruses were originally found to be the cause of neonatal deaths in nursery epidemics in South Africa in 1956. Since then cases have been reported from all over the world. The mother usually has a history of an acute respiratory infection several days to a week before delivery, and investigation reveals that several members of the family have had influenza-like symptoms. The affected infants may develop a croupy cough and inspiratory crow within a few hours after birth. Fever, anorexia, lethargy, jaundice, and cyanosis may then appear. Signs of heart failure may occur, with enlargement of the liver and heart. Electrocardiography may give evidence of myocardial damage. Some infants may have convulsions from meningoencephalitis, or pneumonitis may develop. Severe bleeding may occur in the skin and in other organs.

To prevent nursery epidemics, all suspected infants should be isolated. This is particularly indicated if the mother or others in her family have had or are having an influenza-like infection, especially if pleurodynia is present.

HERPES SIMPLEX. Herpes simplex is now recognized as a serious disease of newborn infants. This disease is widespread in the adult population, and is considered more annoying than dangerous. However, if a pregnant woman acquires the disease, the fetus may be infected via the placenta, or, especially if genital lesions are present, the infant may be infected during labor and vaginal delivery. The infected baby may show vesicular lesions, lethargy, cyanosis, meningoencephalitis with convulsions and opisthotonos, and chorioretinitis; if the infant survives there may be severe neurologic defects. This condition in infants is highly fatal.

HEPATITIS. Any mother who is jaundiced during pregnancy should have a serum test for Australian antigen. If this is positive her infant should be considered potentially infected. The infected fetus may be jaundiced at birth or may later show symptoms indistinguishable from those of congenital atresia of the bile ducts, infectious hepatitis of other etiology, or obstructive jaundice associated with erythroblastosis. A high incidence of cirrhosis also occurs in survivors.

MEASLES (RUBEOLA). Measles may be transmitted from mother to fetus. If the mother is exposed late in pregnancy, the disease may develop simultaneously in the mother and the newborn infant, or the infant may be born with the rash fully developed. Passive immunity derived from the mother is lost in about six months.

SMALLPOX (VARIOLA) AND CHICKENPOX (VARICELLA). These diseases may be acquired in utero, the stage of the disease at birth depending on the time of infection.

Passive immunity in the infant, derived from the mother, lasts two or three months.

INCLUSION BLENNORRHEA. Inclusion blennorrhea is caused by contact during delivery with vaginal secretions containing the responsible virus, which belongs to the psittacosis-lymphogranuloma group. The mother may have a silent infection, as proved by recovery of the virus and by demonstration of inclusion bodies in the epithelial cells of the cervix. The incubation period is 5 to 12 days; onset is abrupt, and usually only one eye is involved, most frequently the lower lid. The acute stage lasts 10 to 14 days.

Protozoan Infections

SYPHILIS. Although it is now of rare occurrence, syphilis must never be forgotten as a possible cause of fetal infection. Syphilis rarely affects the fetus before the fifth month, and if adequate maternal treatment with penicillin is instituted before this time, the fetus is seldom infected.

MALARIA. Malaria of the fetus, in areas where the disease is prevalent, is not uncommon. It has been postulated that fetal death can result from anoxia caused by the lack of normal oxygen-bearing maternal red blood cells or from the absorption of toxic substances; the frequent premature labor may be the result of high fever in the mother. Malarial parasites have been found in cerebral vessels and abnormal pigment has been found in the fetal spleen and liver.

TOXOPLASMOSIS. Toxoplasmosis occurs in cats, dogs, sheep, rabbits, guinea pigs, and other animals; in the acutely infected animal the organisms may be present in the saliva and muscle. Enlargement of lymph nodes, in which the Toxoplasma organism may be identified and isolated, may develop in the affected human. One of the main problems in toxoplasmosis is that the infected mother, with active organisms in her blood infecting the fetus, may give no recognizable clinical sign of the disease. Only when the disease in the mother is in the active phase can the fetus be infected; of greatest importance to all concerned is the fact that *rarely will a mother produce a subsequent child with this disease.* The infant may be stillborn or may at birth exhibit various stages of the disease, depending largely on the time of acute intrauterine infection. Typically the tetrad pathognomonic of toxoplasmosis comprises:

chorioretinitis, cerebral calcification, hydrocephalus or microcephaly, and psychomotor disturbances. The calcification and chorioretinitis may not be discernible early in the newborn period. Unless the disease began early in intrauterine life, hydrocephalus or microcephaly may be lacking. In the acute phase of the disease the infant may show a rash, jaundice, meningoencephalitis with convulsions, hypertonicity, and hepatosplenomegaly.

A positive diagnosis can be made by laboratory tests. Samples of 5 or 10 ml. of blood should be drawn from both mother and baby and placed in test tubes without anticoagulants or preservatives and sent as the local or state health officer directs. Two types of tests for antibody will be performed. Both mother and child must have an antibody detectable by the "dye test." Since this antibody is stable, to rule out the infant's having acquired it by passive transfer, a second, more labile complement-fixing antibody is tested. If the mother has high antibody by both tests and if the newborn has "dye" antibody but no complement-fixing antibody, the test is positive for a current active infection with Toxoplasma in the baby.

Bacterial Infection

The ascending route of bacterial infection of the fetus has been considered in the discussion of congenital pneumonia. Such infection enters the fetus via the respiratory or digestive tract, the skin, or the eyes; only secondarily does the fetus suffer a generalized infection. The organisms commonly encountered are *Escherichia coli* and staphylococci, but hemolytic streptococcus, influenza B, pneumococcus, and meningococcus infections are not rare.

As the search for causes of infection in the newborn intensifies, other organisms are being added to the list, such as *Listeria monocytogenes.* Infection may occur transplacentally, or by the ascending route if the mother has active infection in her genital tract. Clinical symptoms which may be present at birth include septicemic fever, jaundice, skin hemorrhage, sclerema, hepatomegaly, and meningitis. Infection may also occur during passage through the birth canal, in which event the onset of the disease may be delayed two weeks. Blood and spinal fluid cultures reveal the organism. Early cases are usually fatal; in late cases recovery has followed massive antibiotic therapy.

INFECTIONS ACQUIRED AFTER BIRTH

Since the infant can acquire an infection by only three routes—air, contact, and ingestion—the problem of prevention consists of blocking these avenues of entry. Dust control is of value in reducing the number of organisms in the air, but air sterilization by glycol vapors or ultraviolet irradiation has been ineffective. The proper use of face masks for short periods of time helps to control droplet infection, but the vulnerable infants, especially the premature, should be kept continuously in an air-conditioned incubator of the Isolette type.

The control of contact infections requires strict adherence to the details of technique. Hand cleanliness is of utmost importance, and the use of antiseptic detergent solutions containing hexachlorophene has aided greatly in this respect. The detection and control of enteric infections in the mothers and nursery personnel are of great importance. Stool cultures should be done routinely on admission of all obstetric patients with intestinal symptoms. They should also be made routinely at initial employment, and when indicated, on all food handlers and nursery and pediatric personnel. All persons with actual diarrhea should be suspended from duty with pay until results of bacteriologic and clinical studies are negative.

The newborn infant can become infected through the ingestion of infected formula or fluid. This route of infection is the easiest to control, and such infection should never occur if the terminal sterilization technique is used. An approved method of terminal sterilization should be required in every nursery caring for infants.

The role of Shigella, paratyphoid, and Salmonella organisms in the outbreak of enteric disease in nurseries is well known. Certain strains of *Escherichia coli* (serogroup 0111, *B. neapolitanum*) have been recognized as responsible for diarrheal disease in the newborn. Whenever an infant is infected with one of these enteric organisms it is evidence that there has been a serious break in technique and fecal-oral contamination has taken place.

Escherichia Coli Infections

E. coli has become the commonest cause of death and of serious infections in the nursery. It can cause sepsis, diarrhea, meningitis, pneumonia, and urinary tract infections. There are at least ten serologic types of enteropathogenic *E. coli*. The ones most commonly found in infections are 0111:B4, 055:B5, 026:B6, and 0127:B8. There is some suspicion that the incidence of gram-negative infections is increasing in nurseries that use routine hexachlorophene bathing of infants to prevent staphylococcal skin infections.

Systemic infections with *E. coli* can be treated with kanamycin, 15 mg. per kilogram per 24 hours. Ampicillin, 50 to 100 mg. per kilogram per 24 hours, is also effective and may be used in combination with kanamycin. In diarrhea, oral neomycin, 50 mg. per kilogram per 24 hours, is effective.

Staphylococcal Infections

In the period 1950 to 1960 nursery epidemics of staphylococcal infection were not uncommon. In the period 1960 to 1970 there was a definite decline in epidemics. The reason for this change is not entirely clear. It is attributed by some to the use of hexachlorophene baths and hand washing, and by others to a natural cyclic change in virulence of the organism.

The staphylococcal infection in newborn infants usually begins with a simple skin infection (small pustules). This can then progress to cellulitis, furuncles, osteomyelitis, sepsis, pneumonia, and meningitis. Epidemics are usually due to certain strains (phage type 80-81). For severe infections oxacillin or methicillin is used in doses of 25 to 50 mg. per kilogram every 12 hours.

Regardless of the reasons for the decrease in nursery infections, all are agreed that the single most effective preventive measure is careful hand washing before handling each infant in the nursery.

All persons with skin infections must be excluded from the nursery and any infected mothers should be isolated and treated while their infants remain in the hospital. Avoidance of overcrowding in the nursery is very important, since the infants themselves appear to be the chief reservoir of infection. If epidemics occur, closing of the nursery and admission of all new babies to a newly established nursery is the most effective step. When this fails, the prophylactic administration to all infants of full therapeutic doses of an antibiotic effective against the responsible strain of staphylococcus is recommended.

CONGENITAL MALFORMATIONS

Infants who pass excessive amounts of mucus from the moment of birth, especially if the mother's pregnancy featured polyhydramnios, must be suspected of having a *tracheoesophageal fistula*. The condition should be strongly suspected at delivery if fluid continues to exude from the nasopharynx despite repeated aspiration or when the newborn is suspended head downward. The diagnosis can be confirmed if the passing of a catheter reveals a blind esophageal pouch. Early diagnosis and surgery have converted this once fatal anomaly into one with a favorable prognosis in full-term infants.

Obstruction of the second portion of the duodenum is intrinsic or secondary to malrotation of the cecum. The diagnosis is suspected when polyhydramnios has been present and the newborn vomits persistently from birth. A flat x-ray plate of the abdomen without a contrast meal will show the large, dilated stomach and first portion of the duodenum. Again, immediate surgery offers a good prognosis.

In slightly more than one half of the infants with prolonged *obstructive jaundice*, the cause is *congenital atresia of the bile duct*. In about one fourth of the cases it is the result of inspissated bile secondary to erythroblastosis. In the remaining one fourth it is the result of inspissated bile of unknown etiology and probably includes cases of viral or infectious hepatitis. The establishment of an accurate diagnosis is important in these patients, for in those infants in whom it is the result of inspissated bile, expectant and supportive medical treatment is accompanied by spontaneous recovery in all cases secondary to erythroblastosis and in 80 per cent of those of unknown etiology. On the other hand, congenital atresia of the bile ducts can be corrected surgically in only a small percentage of cases (10 per cent), and the operative cure rate among these is also very low.

Infants who have a condition from which they will recover spontaneously must not be exposed to the possibility of operative death caused by surgical exploration. For this reason many physicians advise a two month waiting period for all infants with jaundice before surgical exploration is attempted. Complete atresia can be diagnosed most accurately by a ^{131}I-labeled rose bengal excretion study. If the excretion in 12 to 24 hours of labeled rose bengal is less than 5 per cent, a diagnosis can be made with great accuracy. Surgical exploration should be done without further delay.

ABNORMAL BLEEDING

HEMORRHAGIC DISEASE OF THE NEW-BORN. This was once a common diagnosis, but it is now realized that this is not a true disease but a syndrome that can be the result of many causes. As the etiologic factors, such as erythroblastosis (hemolytic disease), infection, hypoxia, trauma, or accident, are recognized, the bleeding is ascribed to its proper cause and the condition is no longer referred to as "hemorrhagic disease." A small number of cases remain in which, in the light of our present knowledge, careful search fails to reveal a reasonable or positive etiology; to these cases the classification of "idiopathic hemorrhagic disease" must be applied.

CONGENITAL AFIBRINOGENEMIA. Congenital afibrinogenemia is an example of a condition once included in the "hemorrhagic disease" diagnosis in which careful laboratory investigation has revealed a specific coagulation defect. The absence of fibrinogen is assumed to be a congenital deficiency. The condition is fortunately rare. The major symptom is severe intractable bleeding that may be from the cord, in the lungs, in the intestinal tract, or into the intracranial cavity. The infant may survive the newborn period, but the defect persists and bleeding episodes recur. The blood of these infants will not clot until fibrinogen is added. Bleeding time is normal. Prothrombin content is normal. Prothrombin time cannot be determined, not because of any prothrombin defect, but because the test requires fibrinogen for its completion. Treatment is by trans-fusion with whole blood, serum, plasma, or purified fibrinogen (25 mg. per pound).

CONGENITAL DEFICIENCY OF FACTOR VII (STABLE FACTOR, PROCONVERTIN). This deficiency is the cause in certain cases of abnormal bleeding in the newborn. This condition may be a true congenital defect, the family history may be positive, and consanguinity has been reported as a factor.

In factor VII deficiency bleeding and clotting time are normal but the prothrombin time is prolonged. This prolongation can be corrected by the addition of serum (containing factor VII) or whole blood transfusion. Vitamin K is of no value.

PROTHROMBIN-COMPLEX DEFICIENCY SYNDROMES. Prothrombin-complex deficiency syndromes are still surrounded with some confusion. The *prothrombin* level is low at birth, and falls significantly for three days; it rises to a new level, well below the adult value, by one week, and reaches the adult level at one year. Vitamin K given to the mother before delivery or to the infant at birth or to both, has no effect on the prothrombin content curve.

Proconvertin (SPCA, stable factor, factor VII) is present at low levels at birth; its value follows that of prothrombin.

Proaccelerin (labile factor, Ac-globulin, factor V) is present at birth and early infancy in large amounts, from 100 to 300 per cent of the normal value for adults.

Some of the confusion in this field is due to the misinterpretation of the one-stage *prothrombin time* determination by the method of Quick. This test, instead of being an actual measurement of prothrombin, is more concerned with the ability to convert prothrombin into thrombin, and its results can be altered by all three of the above factors involved in thrombin formation. It is primarily an index of the accessory conversion factors and not of prothrombin. It is unreliable in assaying the specific deficiencies of clotting factors in the infant's blood.

The prothrombin time (Quick) is normal in all infants at birth, increases for several days, and returns to normal by about one week. The normal value at birth, despite the low levels of prothrombin and stable factor, is believed to be due to the excessive amount of labile factor present at birth. With further lowering of the amount of prothrombin and stable factor, the prothrombin time increases. Vitamin K has no effect on the amount of prothrombin, but it does increase the stable factor to about adult values.

The dilemma appears when one attempts to apply the above facts to the diagnosis and prevention or treatment of bleeding in the neonate.

The prothrombin and stable factor (factor VII) values are low in all normal infants, sometimes reaching extremely low levels without hemorrhage. Levels of 1 and 5 per cent of normal for prothrombin have been observed without hemorrhage. Many one and two day old babies have been found to have prothrombin and factor VII levels under the 20 per cent of normal that is usually considered the "safe" level, yet there was no clinical evidence of hemorrhage. It is suggested that nature may have provided factor V in great excess as a physiologic defense mechanism.

Careful hematologic investigation is revealing new specific factors in the prothrombin complex that may be deficient. A decrease of plasma thromboplastin component (PTC) in the serum of normal infants has been reported. Extremely low levels, as low as 1 and 3 per cent of normal, were found in bleeding infants. Although levels of other factors were also extremely low, deficiency of the PTC was thought to be the most important. The Stuart-Prower factor is reported to be decreased in the newborn. This factor may also be important in the clotting defect of the full-term newborn.

In summary, in all infants with bleeding every effort should be made to determine its cause. Enough has been said to demonstrate that determination of prothrombin time alone is not sufficient; it must be combined with assay methods that will reveal the amounts of prothrombin and factor VII, and other defects in the prothrombin complex. There is occasionally real danger in assuming the diagnosis to be "hemorrhagic disease" on the basis of a prolonged prothrombin time and limiting treatment to vitamin K. A case has been reported in which such an assumption was made in a true congenital deficiency of factor VII; in this condition vitamin K is of no value, and normal serum, plasma, or whole blood is required. The delay in instituting proper treatment may well have been a factor in this infant's subsequent death from intracranial hemorrhage.

FETAL MALNUTRITION (DYSMATURITY, INTRAUTERINE GROWTH RETARDATION, SMALL FOR DATES, SMALL FOR GESTATIONAL AGE)

One third of "premature infants" ($5\frac{1}{2}$ lb., 2500 grams birth weight) are actually small

Figure 3. Classification of newborns by birth weight and gestational age and by neonatal mortality risk. (From Battaglia, F. C., and Lubchenco, L. O.: J. Pediat., 71:159, 1967.)

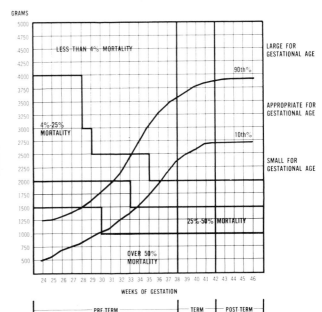

or undergrown for their gestational age. This has become apparent only in the last few years since good intrauterine fetal growth charts have become available. There are several such charts available (e.g., that of Lubchenco), and while small differences do occur from one population group to another there is remarkably good agreement among these studies on the 10th percentile distribution of birth weights at varying gestational ages. The use of both estimated gestational age and birth weight in the characterization of newborn infants has helped in their care in several ways. One can demonstrate that the following situations occur more commonly in infants below the 10th percentile.

1. Hypoglycemia (a blood sugar of less than 20 mg. per 100 ml. in a premature infant or 30 mg. per 100 ml. in a mature infant).

2. Congenital anomalies, such as Down's syndrome or D and E trisomy.

3. Low levels of blood clotting factors.

4. Asphyxia and brain damage.

5. Lower levels of average serum bilirubin.

6. Congenital viral infections such as rubella or cytomegalic inclusion disease.

7. A lower incidence of respiratory distress than in infants of the same birth weight.

Infants so afflicted may present a striking clinical picture. Described in 1954 by Clifford, the following classification of the syndrome was suggested:

STAGE I. The general appearance of the infant suggests failure of the placenta to provide for normal growth and development, and the infant's condition may suggest some malnutrition and loss of weight. The skin is unstained and generally is like parchment, and cracked and peeling. When gestation has been prolonged, the infant may appear much older than the usual newborn infant, and be open eyed and alert.

STAGE II. The infant exhibits the characteristics noted for stage I and, in addition, sufficient quantities of meconium have been liberated in utero to stain the skin, umbilical cord, nails, amniotic fluid, and placental membranes. The infant may give evidence of having aspirated meconium.

STAGE III. The infant is assumed to have passed through stages I and II in utero. At birth, all of the preceding findings are present, but to a more marked degree,

and the desquamating skin is stained a golden yellow.

The placental dysfunction syndrome may also be found in infants delivered at term. These infants present the findings outlined above, and may weigh only 3 or 4 lb. They have been called "small for dates" or dysmature infants or have been said to have fetal malnutrition. The syndrome may be associated with pregnancies that have gone beyond the expected date of confinement. (See Chapter 20, Dysmaturity-Postmaturity.)

The pathologic findings are those usually associated with intrauterine hypoxia. The most frequent findings are in the lungs, where evidence of aspiration of amniotic fluid, meconium, squamous cells, and amorphous debris is an almost universal finding. The atelectatic areas are usually of patchy distribution, and the bronchi are frequently filled with epithelial cells. Hyaline membranes are rarely encountered, and only as incidental findings of secondary importance to the aspirated material. Areas of emphysema involving the lungs and mediastinum are frequently seen.

The infants showing the features of stage I practically all recovered, but some showed findings associated with intrauterine hypoxia, intracranial injuries, convulsions, and hypertonicity. The clinical course was the same as in infants with intrauterine asphyxia and meconium aspiration with severe respiratory distress. Both the immediate and remote prognosis must be even more guarded in stage II and III infants.

INFANT OF MOTHER WITH TUBERCULOSIS

Since the introduction of isoniazid the treatment of the infant of a tuberculous mother has changed. If the mother has miliary disease in late pregnancy, the infant is at risk of congenital tuberculosis. The tuberculin test of such an infant will not become positive for three to five weeks after birth. This infant should be temporarily separated from the mother for a few weeks and treated with isoniazid, 5 to 10 mg. per kilogram per day, for at least a year. If the infant has manifest disease then streptomycin (40 mg. per kilogram on alternate days) should be used.

If the mother is thought to have active tuberculosis or suspicious recently healed tuberculosis, the infant should receive either BCG vaccination or prophylactic isoniazid therapy for one year; both of these methods have been shown to be effective in controlled studies. These methods should completely replace recommendations for long-term isolation. The psychologic problems created by separation should now no longer occur.

BIBLIOGRAPHY

Battaglia, F. C.: Recent advances in medicine for newborn infants. J. Pediat., 71:748, 1967.

Battaglia, F. C., and Lubchenco, L. O.: A practical classification of newborn infants by weight and gestational age. J. Pediat., 71:159, 1967.

Beckett, R. S., and Flynn, F. J., Jr.: Toxoplasmosis; report of two new cases with classification and with demonstration of organisms in the human placenta. New Eng. J. Med., 249:345, 1953.

Behrman, R., Fisher, D., Paton, J., and Keller, J.: In utero disease and the newborn infant. Advances Pediat., 17:13, 1970.

Benirschke, K.: Routes and types of infection in the fetus and the newborn. A.M.A.J. Dis. Child., 99:714, 1960.

Benirschke, K., and Clifford, S. H.: Intrauterine bacterial infection of the newborn infant. J. Pediat., 54:11, 1959.

Chu, J., et al.: The pulmonary hypoperfusion syndrome. Pediatrics, 35:733, 1965.

Clifford, S. H.: Postmaturity—with placental dysfunction. J. Pediat., 44:1, 1954.

Drage, J. S., and Berendes, H.: Apgar scores and outcome of the newborn. Pediat. Clin. N. Amer., 13:635, 1966.

Ferebee, S. H.: An epidemiologic model of tuberculosis. N.T.A. Bull., 53:51, 1967.

Fresh, J. W., Ferguson, J. H., Stamey, C., Morgan, F. M., and Lewis, J. H.: Blood prothrombin, proconvertin and proaccelerin in normal infancy; questionable relationships to vitamin K. Pediatrics, 19:241, 1957.

Gluck, L., and Kulovich, M.: Intrauterine assessment of pulmonary maturity by the phospholipids in amniotic fluid. Amer. J. Obstet. Gynec., 109:440, 1970.

Grossman, B. J., and Carter, R. E.: Congenital afibrinogenemia. J. Pediat., 50:708, 1957.

Hellbrugge, T. F.: Congenital abnormalities due to infectious hepatitis in pregnancy. Ann. Pediat., 179:226, 1952.

Hsia, D. Y. Y., Patterson, P., Allen, F. H., Jr., Diamond, L. K., and Gellis, S. S.: Prolonged obstructive jaundice in infancy; general survey of 156 cases. Pediatrics, 10:243, 1952.

James, L. S.: Scientific basis for current perinatal care. Arch. Dis. Child., 42:457, 1967.

Kibrick, S., and Benirschke, K.: Severe generalized disease (encephalohepatomyocarditis) occurring in the newborn period and due to infection with Coxsackie virus, Group B. Pediatrics, 22:857, 1958.

MacArthur, P.: Congenital vaccinia and vaccinia gravidarum. Lancet, 2:1104, 1952.

Nahmias, A., Alford, C., and Karones, S.: Infection of the newborn with herpesvirus hominis. Advances Pediat., 17:185, 1970.

Palmer, C. E., Shaw, L., and Comstock, G.: Community trials of BCG vaccination. Amer. Rev. Tuberc., 77:877, 1958.

Peterson, H. G., and Pendleton, M. E.: Contrasting roentgenographic pulmonary patterns of the hyaline membrane and fetal aspiration syndromes. Amer. J. Roentgen., 74:800, 1955.

Rabiner, S. F., Winick, M., and Smith, C. H.: Congenital deficiency of factor VII associated with hemorrhagic disease of the newborn. Pediatrics, 25:101, 1960.

Sabin, A. B., Eichenwald, H., Feldman, H. A., and Jacobs, L.: Present status of clinical toxoplasmosis in man. J.A.M.A., 150:1063, 1952.

Schaffer, A. J.: Diseases of the Newborn, 2nd ed. W. B. Saunders Co., Philadelphia, 1965.

Sever, J.: Infectious agents and fetal disease. In Waisman, H., and Kerr, G., eds.: Fetal Growth and Human Development. McGraw-Hill Book Co., New York, 1970, p. 316.

Sjostedt, S., Engleson, G., and Rooth, G.: Dysmaturity. Arch. Dis. Child., 33:123, 1958.

Stiehm, E., Ammann, A., and Cherry, J.: Elevated cord macroglobulins in the diagnosis of intrauterine infections. New Eng. J. Med., 275:971, 1966.

Stokes, J., Jr., Walman, I. J., Blanchard, M. C., and Farquhar, J. D.: Viral hepatitis in the newborn. A.M.A. J. Dis. Child., 82:213, 1951.

Usher, R.: The metabolic changes in respiratory distress syndrome. In Wolstenholme, G. W., ed.: Ciba Foundation Symposium on Somatic Stability in the Newly Born. Little, Brown and Co., Boston, 1961, p. 92.

Zuelzer, W. W., and Stulberg, C. S.: Herpes simplex virus as cause of fulminating visceral disease and hepatitis in infancy; report of eight cases and isolation of virus in one case. A.M.A. J. Dis. Child., 83:421, 1952.

PART VI

Public Health and Social Aspects of Human Reproduction

Chapter 35

Assessment of Maternal and Infant Care

The quality of maternal and infant care as reflected in maternal and infant death rates may also serve as an index of the socio-economic status of a particular society, nation, or ethnic group. Wherever these death rates are comparatively low, one can assume that the medical care system is superior and the economic standards are high.

To compare or assess factors that may influence the maternal mortality and the fetal and newborn death rates, uniform definitions are required and must be universally applied. Unfortunately, the definitions and their application vary to a degree from country to country and state to state. However, the World Health Organization (WHO) has attempted, with substantial success, to encourage uniform reporting in this area of vital statistics.

The determination of the maternal mortality begins with what constitutes a maternal death. With the recognition that it is subject to modification, the definition of a maternal death is given as "a woman dying of any cause whatsoever while pregnant or within ninety days of termination of the pregnancy, irrespective of duration of the pregnancy at the time of termination or the method by which it was terminated." Maternal deaths are placed into one of six categories, with subgroups based on the nature of the disorder and the stage of pregnancy when death occurred. Included are: (1) sepsis of pregnancy, childbirth, and the puerperium; (2) toxemias of pregnancy and the puerperium; (3) hemorrhage of pregnancy and childbirth; (4) abortion without mention of sepsis or toxemia; (5) abortion with sepsis; and (6) other complications of pregnancy, childbirth, and the puerperium.

It has also been recommended that maternal deaths be classified according to direct, indirect, or nonrelated obstetric causes. Death from a *direct* obstetric cause is defined as a death resulting from complications of pregnancy itself, from intervention which is elected or required, or from the chain of events initiated by the complication or the intervention. Death from an *indirect* obstetric cause is a death resulting from disease present before or developing during pregnancy (not a direct effect of the pregnancy), aggravated perhaps by the physiologic effects of the pregnancy, and the actual cause of death. Maternal death from a *nonrelated* cause is one occurring during pregnancy or within 90 days of its termination from causes unrelated to pregnancy, its complications, or management.

Despite the attention given to devising methods of review and assessing penalties for failure to report deaths, the recorded maternal mortality rate in the United States (and undoubtedly elsewhere) is only an approximation, as has been repeatedly shown by maternal mortality committee reports. For some four decades or more, maternal death studies have been conducted in some states and cities in the United States and in other countries by specially constituted maternal welfare committees. The membership of these committees is composed of representatives from various fields of medicine, particularly from pediatrics, internal medicine, public health, anesthesiology, and the preclinical sciences, as well as obstetrics and gynecology. From these studies, it is abundantly clear that the vital statistics of this country and the various states fail to contain all of the deaths associated with childbirth, perhaps in part because of the differences in the definition and interpretation of what constitutes a maternal death.

The efforts of these maternal mortality committees are important, not only because they uncover unreported maternal deaths and collect more accurate statistics, but also because they serve as an educational media for improving hospital and medical standards within the particular locale. To this end the clinical events surrounding each maternal death are carefully reviewed. Some committees collect the data by questionnaire but the most reliable data are obtained by a direct investigation of the case by a member of the committee. On review the case is assessed as to non-preventability or preventability. Because of lack of data on the hospital record, some few cases (about 10 per cent) cannot be so considered. Although the ratio of non-preventable to preventable deaths has differed rather markedly from committee to committee, depending presumably on the method by which cases are reviewed, the quality of medical care, and the patient clientele served, the majority of preventable deaths are the responsibility of the physician. In some instances inadequacy of hospital facilities and ancillary services plays a contributing role. The remaining preventable cases are assigned to patient responsibility; that is, the patient fails to seek medical care or follow medical advice or régime.

Many countries subdivide maternal deaths into obstetric and nonobstetric causes and include only the former in computing the maternal mortality. For example, death from heart disease or from a surgical condition during pregnancy is regarded as a nonobstetric death. From experiences of surveys of the different states, some 30 per cent of the maternal deaths in this country are reported as death due to non-obstetric causes and are so classified. However, the presence of pregnancy may mask the medical or surgical condition, influence the clinical course, and alter the outcome ultimately. Also, parturients or recently delivered patients who are transferred to die on surgical and medical services are ofttimes inadvertently not reported as maternal deaths. Too frequently only the immediate cause of death is listed on the death certificate, as, for example, acute renal failure, when the cause of the latter began with severe abruptio placentae and hemorrhagic shock. Unless one includes in the maternal mortality all patients who die during pregnancy or 90 days thereafter, regardless of cause, the maternal mortality will be arbitrarily derived and is hardly comparable from nation to nation or from one area of a country to another.

In this time of change and challenge it is perhaps well to recall that the available statistics on maternal mortality in this country and in England circa 1850 revealed that one death occurred in each of 150 to 200 deliveries or some 50 or more deaths per 10,000 births. This rate has been reduced by 10- to 20-fold, and ranges now from 2 to 5 per 10,000 pregnancies. Of the three major causes of death, infection has diminished greatly with the advent of antibiotics and avoidance of traumatic delivery. Through prevention, pregnancy toxemia has decreased. The same can be said of obstetric hemorrhage because of more careful patient management and facilities for immediate blood replacement.

The assessment of fetal and newborn results also requires and must begin with certain definitions. What constitutes a live birth and fetal death differs from country to country and continues to be discussed and modified. But again, the WHO definitions have gained rather wide acceptance. Accordingly, a *live birth* is the complete expulsion from its mother of a product of conception that breathes or shows any sign of life, beating of the heart or umbilical vessels, or definite movement of voluntary muscles, irrespective of the duration of pregnancy. A *fetal death* is death prior to complete expulsion from the mother, irrespective of the pregnancy, with no signs of life as defined above. The latter presupposes that life was established clinically by the physician or subjectively by the mother. Also, these definitions may include a portion of births in the middle trimester of pregnancy, when survival is highly unlikely.

The number of weeks of gestation has been recommended as the basis for determining the fetal and newborn death rate. In accordance with the WHO recommendation these rates in many countries, including the United States, are based on the 20th week to term, or the 40th week. However, the 28th week onward is the more conventional period used and reported by many nations, states, and hospitals. This is an important distinction, often ignored, for the incidence of infants born alive between the 20th and 28th week differs widely, from 5 to 6 to 20 or more per 1000 live births, being higher among the socioeconomically underprivileged peoples. Also, in accordance with the socio-economic environment the prematurity rate may reach an incidence of 15 to 18 per cent in contrast to the more acceptable incidence of 5 to 8 per cent. For these reasons it is readily understandable why the fetal and newborn death rates may differ widely from country to country and within the country or in the urban and rural areas when compared with a suburban population.

The methods of reporting births differ also, and this may influence the vital statistics. In some countries the informant may be the father who notifies the local authorities of the child's birth. In the United States the physician and hospital administrator both have the responsibility for reporting the birth. Undoubtedly, the fetus of borderline gestational age of 20 weeks may not always be reported, being considered legally nonviable. In some of the less developed countries births go unregistered and here the perinatal and infant mortality must be appraised in terms of trends rather than in absolute values.

The perinatal mortality comprises the stillbirth and neonatal deaths in the first four weeks of life from pregnancies of 20 weeks or more in duration. This rate is expressed in terms of 1000 live births. In general, the stillbirth and neonatal death rates are nearly equal. That is to say, knowing the neonatal death rate, one could assume that the perinatal rate would be approximately double. Also, fetal length and weight have been used in determining the perinatal mortality. For example, a fetus weighing 500 grams could approximate a gestational age of 20 to 28 weeks. (See Chapter 31, Fetal Growth and Physiology.)

The perinatal mortality can vary greatly in a heterogeneous population for reasons already stated. In the United States it ranges from 25 per 1000 to 50 to 60 per 1000 live births, with the national average currently being about 36 to 40 per 1000 live births. The neonatal mortality also has a wide spread but the average currently for the United States is 22 per 1000 or possibly lower (Table 1). This difference is explained by the prematurity rate and particularly the number of infants born alive between the 20th and 28th week, when the neonatal mortality is about 90 per cent. From the 28th week the neonatal mortality would be 16 per 1000, a rate that compares favorably with other countries that so report their results or that have a population with uniformly high economic standards. A summation of the perinatal and neonatal mortality rates based on the 20th and 28th week in one institution is listed in Table 2 and serves to illustrate how the infant mortality is influenced by the period in pregnancy that is used in computing the neonatal mortality. In this instance, the various mortalities were slightly lower on the house or nonprivate service than on the private patient service.

The infant mortality, namely, the mortality in the first year of life, has fallen sharply in most countries, so that the differences in the birth and death rates cause the population growth to soar. A decrease in deaths occurring after the neonatal period or first four weeks of life is largely responsible for the reduction in infant mortality. In fact, a large proportion of the deaths in the first year take place in the first week and indeed the first 24 hours of life. Also, in the United States at least, except for a modest reduction in the death rate of the mature newborn (36 weeks to term and 2000 to 3500 grams), the neonatal death rate, which accounts for more than two thirds of the infant mortality, has not decreased appreciably in the past two decades. In more recent years state and hospital committees have been established to review perinatal deaths to

TABLE 1. VITAL STATISTICS OF THE UNITED STATES

	Total Number of Events	Rates per 1000 Population				
	1968°	1968°	1965	1960	1950	1940
Births	3,470,000	17.4	19.4	23.7	24.1	19.4
Deaths	1,923,000	9.6	9.4	9.5	9.6	10.8
Marriages	2,059,000	10.3	9.3	8.5	11.1	12.1
Infant deaths	75,300	21.7	24.7	26.0	29.2	47.0

°Provisional

TABLE 2.   PERINATAL AND NEONATAL MORTALITY
(Boston Hospital for Women)

	1970	1969	1968	1967	1966
Total births	7116	7132	6644	6116	5655
Live-born	7021	7038	6542	6025	5584
Perinatal deaths[1]	169	177	200	186	153
Perinatal deaths[1] per 1000 births	23.3	24.8	30	30	27
Stillborn[2]	95	94	102	91	71
Neonatal deaths[3]	74	83	98	95	82
Neonatal deaths[4]	52	55	69	61	52
Neonatal deaths[3] per 1000 live births	10.5	11.8	15	15.7	14.5
Neonatal deaths[4] per 1000 live births	7.4	7.8	10.4	10.1	9.3

[1]Stillborn and live-born deaths from 20 weeks' gestation through 28 postnatal days.
[2]Stillborns of 20 weeks' gestation to term.
[3]20 weeks' gestation through 28 postnatal days.
[4]28 weeks' gestation through 28 postnatal days.

determine whether they are preventable or nonpreventable. Such a committee, too, can establish and maintain professional and hospital standards and serve as an educational instrument.

Whether this country ranks 13th in infant mortality among selected countries, or fourth or fifth when the infant mortality is computed from the 28th week, the unassailable fact remains that the rates differ substantially in various portions of the country, as indicated in Table 3. These wide ranges in the prematurity rate and the perinatal mortality reflect not only the posture of medical care and its utilization but socioeconomic inequities and these, too, are unacceptable.

It is apparent that any improvement in the neonatal mortality must reside in the prevention of prematurity, and, as will be noted, this applies also to the neonatal morbidity and how it may relate to the incidence of central nervous system damage. Thus, neonatal mortality must

TABLE 3.   INFANT MORTALITY RATE IN THE UNITED STATES BY PLACE OF OCCURRENCE (1968)*

Area	Infant Mortality Rate
New England	20.1
Middle Atlantic	21.2
East North Central	21.3
West North Central	19.1
South Atlantic	24.3
East South Central	26.0
West South Central	22.5
Mountain	20.6
Pacific	18.9
Puerto Rico	27.3

*From Wegman, M. E.: Pediatrics, 44:1031, 1969.

be assessed in the light of the incidence of prematurity in the various weight and gestational age groups, and the incidence may vary tremendously for reasons cited.

The neonatal morbidity is of even greater concern, for survival of the fetus and the newborn is not the ultimate in human reproduction. Rather, it is proposed that the initial right of the individual is to be born without handicap and that this is a prerequisite to the exercise of the privilege and also the responsibility of perfect freedom—which should be the hallmark of a democratic society.

The principle that prevention is preferable to curative measures has no greater application than in the events surrounding pregnancy and parturition. The incidence of cerebral palsy in its several forms may vary between 7 and 20 per 1000 births, the rate influenced largely by the numbers of prematures, in whom the incidence may reach 40 per 1000. It is accepted that 3 to 4 per cent of infants born in the United States never achieve the intelligence of a 12 year old child. Again, there are a host of variables—genetic or hereditary factors and socioeconomic environment as it bears on the incidence of prematurity, and nutrition as it may affect the mother and thus, indirectly, fetal growth and development and brain maturation in the early years of life. In a heterogeneous population it may be safe to conclude that 70 per cent or more of the cases of central nervous system deficiency are the result of the intrauterine environment and the experience of birth, while the remainder are due to cultural-familial or genetic factors. For purposes of making a prediction, there is some evidence to show that for every neonatal death of a fetus born after the 28th week of pregnancy there is a surviving infant who is neurologically compromised. In other words, the neonatal mortality computed from the 28th week onward may offer an index of the incidence of residual damage in the newborn and an overall view of the obstetric results and quality of patient care.

In recent years the term "high risk" has been applied to pregnancies of those parturients (20 to 25 per cent of the total number of maternity patients) who, either on the basis of past reproductive failure or from the signs and symptoms of the current pregnancy, are likely to develop or already have complications that may cause a disturbance in the intrauterine environment and pose a threat to life of the conceptus, or result in damage, particularly to the central nervous system, in an infant born alive.

The major obstetric conditions that contribute to neonatal morbidity have been discussed previously, and we will simply list them here: (1) hypertension in all its forms; (2) late pregnancy bleeding; (3) premature rupture of the fetal membranes with hazard of intrauterine infection; (4) abnormal presentation of the fetus; and (5) fetal malnutrition, often referred to as the dysmature or intrauterine growth retardation syndrome. Although pregnancy at high risk may develop during labor, it should be emphasized that trauma at delivery and prolonged labor with its possible adverse effects on the fetus have no place in current obstetric practice and if they occur must be construed as faulty patient management.

Also, evidence can be presented that permits the statement that the lowest incidence of mental retardation and cerebral palsy is encountered in infants of parturients between the ages of 18 and 30 years who deliver no more than four offspring, properly spaced. There might be a further decrease in the incidence of central nervous system deficiency if the number of offspring were two rather than four. It follows that family planning and population control are basic in the fight against mental retardation, cerebral palsy and genetic diseases.

Moreover, if this planet is to continue to be inhabited by man for however long, it will depend on the quality of human life rather than the quantity. With one-half of humankind either undernourished or mal-nourished, this suggests that man's survival will be determined in large measure by population size. If poverty with all its social evils is to be eliminated it is imperative that populations be stabilized and indeed reduced.

The notable and unprecedented advance in the biologic sciences has created the paradox that man's very existence may be threatened as the result of uncontrolled population as the birth rate exceeds by far the death rate.

The gravity of the situation was recorded in the United Nations report on the Future Growth of World Population over a decade ago, which stated, ". . . it took 2,000,000 years for the world population to reach 2500 million, it will take 30 years to add another 2000 million." The statement goes on to imply that the population will increase to the point at which something will happen to prevent its further growth. The question is posed, what will that something be? The disparity between the objectives of the defense technologist and scientist and those of the medical scientist leaves humanity the choice between death control and birth control. Where it is now possible that a single individual can release unlimited nuclear powers of destruction, mankind is presented the alternatives of living amicably together or facing total annihilation.

What the optimum population should be for any nation has received the attention of economists, social scientists, general theorists, and, to a degree, the medical profession. It is projected that the population of the United States will increase from 200 million to 300 million by the turn of the century. Stabilization of the population for this country requires that the annual birth rate be reduced from some 18 per 1000 to 12 per 1000. Whatever else, in the final analysis it is physicians who must accept, however reluctantly, the responsibility for population stabilization.

Despite the current methods of birth control, the birth rate in the United States exceeds by 50 to 60 per cent that required to stabilize the population. It is difficult to establish the unplanned pregnancy rate. Certainly it must be high, as measured by out-of-wedlock pregnancies.

This is not a new subject, for certainly the Greeks were concerned with population size when they asked what men should live for. When defining the form of society required for the citizen to realize the best of his nature and innate potential, Plato, in his *Republic*, also written in a period of war and revolution, was cognizant of the necessity of "keeping the number of the citizens as constant as possible, having regard to losses caused by war, epidemics, and so on." Rewards and privileges were used to enhance motivation to control population size. Also, it was recognized that each of the social classes, as defined, must participate proportionately in limiting the population; otherwise, there could be a dysgenic effect.

In the modern context, it has been suggested that motivation be replaced by the term "general will" as a means of negating the unrestricted freedom to procreate. It has further been suggested that the older idea of rewards as a deterrent to excessive reproduction be grafted onto social security, together with a bonus system, and thus provide parents with the incentive not to exceed what is for them the largest number of children, presumably two and not more than three. It is also proposed that the right to parenthood is a privilege and should be exercised only by individuals capable of meeting the responsibilities of parenthood. However unrealistic this appears at the moment, especially in a democratic society where decrees are unacceptable, any policy governing population size must consider these principles. Unquestionably it will not succeed until there is sufficient motivation through education and equality of opportunity to permit the right of every citizen to enjoy a useful and rewarding life.

The methods to control fertility are discussed only briefly, for the literature is now voluminous and readily accessible. However, all physicians need to understand the pros and cons of the current methods in order to advise patients. For ideally each female in need of fertility control should receive what is the most appropriate method for her.

Rhythm or periodic abstinence avoids intercourse during the menstrual cycle when ovulation is most likely to occur, i.e., some 14 days prior to the next menses. In a 28-day cycle it is at the midpoint, and in a 35-day cycle ovulation occurs some 21 days after the last period. Abstinence must be practiced at least from the 13th to the 17th day of a 28-day cycle or perhaps from the 12th to the 20th day, leaving approximately a week following a four or five day menses and a week prior to the expected menses when intercourse can occur with low risk of pregnancy. In those in whom the periods are irregular, the timing of ovulation is more difficult and uncertain. Charting of the daily temperature is a refinement to determine the precise time of ovulation or its absence.

The method of withdrawal prior to ejaculation is an ancient method of fertility control. Besides failure to withdraw, there is the risk that spermatozoa may be deposited in the vagina prior to male orgasm; the same disadvantage applies to the condom when it is used only before ejaculation. Douching, too, has an unacceptably high failure rate. The use of foam is a further disappointment.

The condom, a latex sheath for the male, when utilized prior to vaginal penetration, has a rather low failure rate. The method is not completely acceptable, for it may be uncomfortable to the female and regarded as not entirely physiologic by both partners.

The latex diaphragm is highly reliable if properly used. To insure a low failure rate comparable to the endocrine suppression of ovulation, the diaphragm must be of the correct size and carefully inserted to cover the cervix. Proper positioning may be difficult to attain in women in whom the uterus is retroverted and the cervix points ventrally in the mid-axis of the pelvis or above. This can be readily overcome by the use of an inserter devised to deposit the diaphragm over the cervix. Careful instruction as to its use is essential, including a demonstration by the patient herself that she is able to insert the diaphragm correctly. The diaphragm is used in conjunction with a contraceptive jelly with a low lactic acid content. A small amount of jelly is placed within the inner surface of the diaphragm, thus to contact the external cervical os. The diaphragm may remain in place for some 24 hours, giving protection during this period. This detail as to its use is given, for the failure rate is extremely low when used accordingly and inserted precoitally. The complications are nil, but obviously the method requires a high degree of patient motivation.

The more popular methods, primarily because they afford constant protection and hence are regarded as more physiologically and psychologically normal, include the endocrine control of ovulation through the medium of the "birth control pill" and a foreign body placed in the uterine cavity, the so-called intrauterine device that supposedly discourages implantation of the fertilized ovum. The oral contraceptives are highly effective. With suppression of ovulation the anticipated changes occur in the endometrium and throughout the reproductive tract, including the ovary. The side effects are definite with all the various agents, from breakthrough bleeding, accumulation of extracellular fluid consistent with pseudopregnancy, and general lassitude to outright depression. Thromboembolism and vascular problems have been recorded. Patients may develop an increase in blood pressure when on the pill, especially those with a family history of hypertension. The blood pressure usually recedes to normal following cessation of the medication. Other medical conditions preclude this method of fertility control. Failure to conceive following discontinuation of the medication is recognized, but perhaps this occurs in individuals destined to have infertility problems. Despite these limitations, it can be rightfully debated that lack of fertility control would have resulted in a complication rate and life-threatening situation in the event of pregnancy that far outweigh those associated with fertility control by suppression of ovulation.

The intrauterine device takes several forms. The failure rate is definite and the complications substantial and at times rather serious. However, the method appears to be entirely satisfactory for 75 to 80 per cent of those patients utilizing this method. The need to remove the device is mainly for hypermenorrhea and sometimes pelvic pain. Uterine perforation is the most serious complication and occurs all too often and without apparent cause. Whether the device invites pelvic infection or the latter is simply superimposed is a subject of controversy.

Abortion is a method of population control, generally practiced in Japan and other countries. It is a method that is being considered in many countries and societies and undoubtedly the debate will continue with increasing vigor. All too often statements and conclusions are made without regard to the logistics involved and who is to be medically responsible. That is to say, if the birth rate is to balance the death rate in this country, some one million to a million and a half abortions would have to be performed annually.

Also, the procedure is regarded as a minor affair and without complication. In fact, when the public is sufficiently informed and realizes that artificial abortion is subject to complications, even when performed under proper supervision and surgical environment, there will be a greater incentive toward conception control. This is supported by the decrease in recent years of the number of abortions performed for population control in Japan. Besides the complications that may arise at the time of pregnancy termination, albeit few, repeated abortion may give rise to a state of relative infertility through the syndrome of the incompetent cervix and even less well understood factors such as tubal dysfunction. However, until such time as a totally effective method of pregnancy control is available and despite psychologic and minimal physical risks, consideration must be given to abortion as a means of population control. Certainly it can no longer be ignored. The student is well advised to understand all the pros and cons of this subject, including what it all means in hospital and national policy in order to make a balanced judgment.

Finally, sterilization of both the female and male should have a high priority in planning of family size and population control. Sterilization at the time of delivery should be available as well as at other times. The laparoscope appears to have a place here in women who seek interval sterilization. Vasectomy in the male should also be part of a responsible program of fertility control. In both instances, all aspects of permanent sterilization should be discussed and understood by the patient. When accepted on this basis, any adverse psychologic sequelae appear to be remote in both male and female, and family unity is ofttimes enhanced.

It is clear that current methods of pregnancy control have limitations, as determined by side effects and failure rates, and no one method is applicable to all patients.

To cite an example, for a patient with heart disease, oral contraceptives (the pill) are contraindicated because of their influence on extracellular volume and other physiologic parameters. A foreign body (the loop) placed in the uterus is a decided risk to the cardiac patient because of the possibility of inviting endocarditis through the medium of an endometritis. This presents a principle of good medical practice that before contraceptive therapy is prescribed, a history and physical examination should be performed.

It is evident that present methods require that patients be individualized, a circumstance that fails to lend itself to population control of global scope. Even a definitive procedure such as abortion has little relevance except in the most industrialized societies. It is difficult to envision population stabilization at the world level until a totally simple, effective, and safe method of fertility control or medical abortifacient is available for the masses of humanity of whom, as previously stated, half are either undernourished or malnourished. As did the Greeks, one may ask what is the purpose of the journey?

Acknowledging that it is impossible to eliminate totally the medical risks of being born, what then is a reasonably attainable neonatal mortality and morbidity rate? Both mortality and morbidity should be reduced to 5 to 10 per 1000 live births and it is to be hoped that at the same time the incidence of cerebral palsy would be reduced to 0.5 per cent and that of mental retardation to one half or less of the present rate. To reach this perhaps unattainable objective calls for an enlightened and participating society and medical care of high quality available to all. Whatever may be the physician's contribution toward reducing the incidence of mental retardation and cerebral palsy, his efforts will be influenced in no small measure by the socioeconomic status of the patients served and their motivation to utilize the medical care available. As to the quality of the latter, methods of practice for both ambulatory and in-hospital care must be developed that will encourage the patient to seek prenatal and indeed preconceptional care, early and continuously. Implied also is the need that hospitalization be available, sometimes for prolonged periods, without any economic barriers. Thus, if cerebral palsy and mental retardation can be largely eliminated through prevention, is it not both economically wise and humanitarian to provide whatever is necessary in the treatment of patients with high-risk pregnancy, that is, the patients whose offspring are most likely to be affected adversely? It is evident that the eradication of cerebral palsy, mental retardation, and related neurologic defects is largely an obstetric responsibility. How then is this responsibility to be met in the face of a mounting physician shortage and increasing health needs of the community?

In the attempt to bring maternal and child care to all, with the emphasis on quality, a method must be sought whereby the most expertly trained and knowledgeable physicians can assume responsibility for a greater number of patients. At the current birth rate of this nation, if all deliveries were under the supervision of certified obstetrician-gynecologists (12,000 to 15,000) who were devoting all of their professional time to practice, the physician-patient ratio would be 1:300 at least. With this ratio, the time required for performing routine duties would leave the physician little time for patients with major problems besides those of an obstetric and gynecologic nature. Even now, because of the vastness of the need, the physician's attempts to serve are often only perfunctory. This also implies that this physician-to-patient ratio will apply to the inner city and rural areas, a highly unwarranted assumption.

The health team, composed of an obstetrician-gynecologist and two or more specially trained nurse assistants, would appear to be an integral part of any program to ameliorate the defects in maternal and child care. By whatever name, be they designated obstetric assistants, family nurse-practitioners, or nurse-midwives, the individuals who are to aid the physician must be recruited and trained in large numbers. The health team pattern of obstetric practice may partially answer the problem of making services available for *all*, regardless of the source of the funding of their medical care, while maintaining some semblance of personalized patient attention. It should also foster continuity of patient care—so difficult to attain in an era of specialization. Within this pattern the obstetrician-gynecologist is afforded the opportunity to care for and manage the abnormal and complicated cases as befits his years of training, and at the same time supervise the normal, a responsibility he should never relinquish.

To bring the patient and the obstetrician-gynecologist and his health team together requires an ambulatory health facility adjacent to the hospital. High priority must be given to the establishment of regional health facilities affiliated with those hospitals that are prepared to commit themselves to care for the maternal and child health needs of a designated region or section. Certainly, if paramedical personnel and ancillary services are to be adequately provided as well as most efficiently used and the patients more completely served, hospital services must be based on the population size and within natural geographic boundaries. If preventive medicine and quality of life is to be truly meaningful the case for this is surely as compelling as regional centers for heart disease, cancer, and stroke, in view of the fact that the unborn and newborn, the country's future, have a life expectancy of 67 to 72 years, in contrast to one of 12 years for those over age 60. If it is indeed a matter of priority, what contributes more to the common good, a heart transplant or expert care for 50 to 100 mothers with a high risk pregnancy? One would hope that the behavior of mankind will avoid the need to make this choice. But if it must be made, society should clearly understand the issue.

The present system of maintaining excess numbers of relatively small maternity services in the face of personnel shortages and irregular patient censuses may well be at the expense of maximum safeguards for the patient. (See Conduct of Labor.)

There must be an ideal size for the service, perhaps 3000 to 5000 deliveries annually, if it is to attract and utilize nursing skills most effectively, to acquire round-the-clock anesthesia coverage, to provide a standby nursing team for immediate cesarean section, and to offer other ancillary services. These services should include availability of pediatricians especially trained and interested in the problems of the fetus as well as the newborn.

In summary, hospitals, instead of operating relatively small services, should decide on the basis of regional planning how best to serve the medical needs of a geographic locale. The concept of fewer and larger services, at least in some areas of medicine, is basic to any solution for coping with the shortage of physicians and paramedical health services. Simply increasing the number of physicians will not necessarily correct deficiencies in the medical care system, especially in maternal and child health, where the community commitments are prodigious.

Finally, as emphasis is being placed on community medicine by medical educators, planners, those in government, and the consumer, one needs to ask what indeed does maternal and child care represent in the daily health needs of the community, whether it be inner city, suburbia, or the rural areas. Depending somewhat on the breadth of the definition, the estimates have varied between 40 and 60 per cent. The student — the future physician — dedicated to bringing care to our less privileged citizens must address himself to this need. Indeed, if he is interested in an area of medicine that encompasses both being a generalist and a specialist, he will find it in obstetrics and gynecology, provided he is suitably trained in all phases of general medicine to be the physician to women and the confidant and medical advisor to their families. There is no area of medicine that has a greater social responsibility both nationally and internationally nor the opportunity to contribute more to the common good.

BIBLIOGRAPHY

Chamberlain, R., and Jeffcoate, T. N. A.: The maternity services in Britain. Amer. J. Obstet. Gynec., 95:436, 1966.

Chase, H. E.: Ranking countries by infant mortality rates. Public Health Rep., 84:19, 1969.

Clifford, S. H.: High-risk pregnancy. I. Prevention of prematurity the *sine qua non* for reduction in mental retardation and other neurologic disorders. New Eng. J. Med., 271:243, 1964.

Corfman, P. A., and Segal, S. J.: Biologic effects of intrauterine devices. Amer. J. Obstet. Gynec., 100:448, 1968.

Davis, K.: Population policy: Will current programs succeed? Science, 158:730, 1967.

Diczfalusy, E.: Mode of action of contraceptive drugs. Amer. J. Obstet. Gynec., 100:136, 1968.

Franklin, A. W.: Leontine Young and "Tess of the d'Urbervilles" — some thoughts on illegitimacy. Brit. Med. J., 1:789, 1966.

Hendricks, C. H.: Delivery patterns and reproductive efficiency among groups of differing socioeconomic status and ethnic origins. Amer. J. Obstet. Gynec., 97:608, 1967.

Inman, W. H. W., and Vessey, M. P.: Investigation of deaths from pulmonary, coronary, and cerebral thrombosis and embolism in women of childbearing age. Brit. Med. J., 2:193, 1968.

Jacobson, H. N., and Reid, D. E.: High-risk pregnancy. II. A pattern of comprehensive maternal and child care. New Eng. J. Med., 271:302, 1964.

Legalized Abortion: Report by the Council of the Royal College of Obstetricians and Gynaecologists. Brit. Med. J., 1:850, 1966.

Parkes, A. S.: Change and control in human populations. Lancet, 1:341, 1963.

Reid, D. E.: Population control — medical and public policy. Harvard Medical School Alumni Journal, October, 1970.

Reid, D. E.: The right and the responsibility. Amer. J. Obstet. Gynec., 108:825, 1970.

Russell, J. K.: Not to be left to nature. Lancet, 1:1315, 1966.

Taylor, H. C., Jr., and Berelson, B.: Maternity care and family planning as a world program. Amer. J. Obstet. Gynec., 100:885, 1968.

Vaillant, H. W., Cummins, G. T. M., Richart, R. M., and Barron, B. A.: Insertion of Lippes loop by nurse-midwives and doctors. Brit. Med. J., 3:671, 1968.

Vessey, M. P., and Doll, R.: Investigation of relation between use of oral contraceptives and thrombo-embolic disease. Brit. Med. J., 2:199, 1968.

Wegman, M. E.: Annual summary of vital statistics — 1968. Pediatrics, 44:1031, 1969.

Williams, C. D., and Oxon, D. M.: Maternal and child health services in developing countries. Lancet, 1:345, 1964.

Willson, J. R., and Ledger, W. J.: Complications associated with the use of intrauterine contraceptive devices in women of middle and upper socio-economic class. Amer. J. Obstet. Gynec., 100:649, 1968.

Zatuchni, G. I.: International postpartum family planning program. Amer. J. Obstet. Gynec., 100:1028, 1968.

Index

Page numbers in *italics* indicate illustrations.